EMERGENCY
MEDICAL TECHNICIAN
EMT in Action

Barbara Aehlert, RN

Southwest EMS Education, Inc.

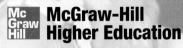 **McGraw-Hill
Higher Education**

Boston   Burr Ridge, IL   Dubuque, IA   New York   San Francisco   St. Louis
Bangkok   Bogotá   Caracas   Kuala Lumpur   Lisbon   London   Madrid   Mexico City
Milan   Montreal   New Delhi   Santiago   Seoul   Singapore   Sydney   Taipei   Toronto

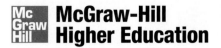

McGraw-Hill
Higher Education

EMERGENCY MEDICAL TECHNICIAN: EMT IN ACTION

Published by McGraw-Hill, a business unit of The McGraw-Hill Companies, Inc., 1221 Avenue of the Americas, New York, NY, 10020. Copyright © 2009 by The McGraw-Hill Companies, Inc. All rights reserved. No part of this publication may be reproduced or distributed in any form or by any means, or stored in a database or retrieval system, without the prior written consent of The McGraw-Hill Companies, Inc., including, but not limited to, in any network or other electronic storage or transmission, or broadcast for distance learning.

Some ancillaries, including electronic and print components, may not be available to customers outside the United States.

This book is printed on acid-free paper.

1 2 3 4 5 6 7 8 9 0 CUS/CUS 0 9 8

ISBN   978-0-07-312898-6
MHID   0-07-312898-8

Vice President/Editor in Chief: *Elizabeth Haefele*
Vice President/Director of Marketing: *John E. Biernat*
Publisher: *Linda Schreiber*
Sponsoring editor: *Claire Merrick*
Managing developmental editor: *Sarah Wood*
Freelance developmental editor: *Julie Scardiglia*
Marketing manager: *Kelly Curran*
Lead media producer: *Damian Moshak*
Media producer: *Marc Mattson*
Director, Editing/Design/Production: *Jess Ann Kosic*
Senior project manager: *Rick Hecker*
Senior production supervisor: *Janean A. Utley*
Designer: *Srdjan Savanovic*
Senior photo research coordinator: *Lori Hancock*
Media project manager: *Mark A. S. Dierker*
Cover design: *Kay Lieberherr*
Typeface: *10/12 ITC New Baskerville*
Compositor: *Aptara*
Printer: *R. R. Donnelley*
Cover credit: *Rick Brady*
Photo credits: Unless otherwise credited, all photos © The McGraw-Hill Companies, Inc./Rick Brady, photographer.

Medicine is an ever-changing science. As new research and clinical experience broaden our knowledge, changes in treatment are required. The authors and the publisher of this work have checked with sources believed to be reliable in their efforts to provide information that is complete and generally in accord with the standards accepted at the time of publication. However, in view of the possibility of human error or changes in medical sciences, neither the authors nor the publisher nor any other party who has been involved in the preparation or publication of this work warrants that the information contained herein is in every respect accurate or complete, and they are not responsible for any errors or omissions or for the results obtained from use of such information. Readers are encouraged to confirm the information contained herein with other resources.

Library of Congress Cataloging-in-Publication Data

Aehlert, Barbara.
    Emergency medical technician: EMT in action/Barbara Aehlert.
        p.   cm.
    Includes index.
    ISBN-13: 978-0-07-312898-6 (alk. paper)—ISBN-10: 0-07-312898-8 (alk. paper)
    1. Emergency medicine.   2. Emergency medical technicians.   I. Title.   II. Title: EMT in action.
    [DNLM: 1. Emergency Treatment—methods.   2. Emergency Medical
Services—methods.   3. Emergency Medical Technicians. WB 105 A246e 2009]
    RC86.7.A354   2009
    616.02'5—dc22

                                    2007037990

www.mhhe.com

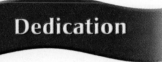 **Dedication** For my mother, Ronella Su Light

About the Author

Barbara Aehlert is President of Southwest EMS Education, Inc., in Phoenix, Arizona, and Pursley, Texas. She has been a registered nurse for more than 30 years, with clinical experience in medical/surgical and critical care nursing and, for the past 21 years, in prehospital education. Barbara is an active CPR, First Aid, ACLS, and PALS instructor. She is Director of Field Training for Southwest Ambulance in Mesa, Arizona, and an active member of the Pursley, Texas, Volunteer Fire Department.

Brief Contents

Contents

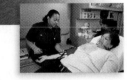

Division 2

Airway and Breathing   146

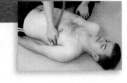

▶ **CHAPTER 7**

Airway and Breathing   147

Division 3

Scene Size-Up   183

▶ **CHAPTER 8**

Scene Size-Up   184

▶ **CHAPTER 9**

Patient Assessment   199

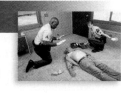

Division 4

Medical-Behavioral Emergencies and Obstetrics and Gynecology 274

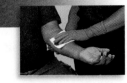

Division 8

Advanced Airway (Elective) 661

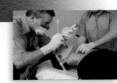

▶ CHAPTER 30
Advanced Airway Techniques 662

Appendices

Foreword

Emergency Medical Technicians (EMTs) represent the largest group of licensed prehospital care providers in this country. The emergency care system relies on the EMT to staff its ambulances, respond on fire apparatus, work in industrials settings, serve in our nation's military services, and provide care in licensed healthcare facilities.

Now, more than ever, our expectations of EMTs are high as their scope of practice broadens and they are called upon to respond to an ever-increasing number of emergencies that demand more knowledge. These emergencies include medical problems, such as heart attacks. They also include traumatic injuries from motor vehicle crashes, industrial accidents, and violent crimes. In the past few years, EMTs have also faced larger emergencies: cataclysmic hurricanes, terrorist attacks, and the fear of infectious disease outbreaks. In many of these situations, the EMT is the first medically trained person to care for critically ill or injured patients.

One of the greatest challenges for any community is having enough appropriately trained EMS providers available to respond rapidly when an emergency arises. The need to train a larger number of well-trained EMTs has never been greater. In many areas, EMTs who volunteer their time represent as many as a third or more of that community's prehospital providers. They are on call 24 hours a day, 7 days a week, to respond when their friends or neighbors are in need. These emergency healthcare professionals form the foundation for the rest of the emergency medical community. They are stationed within each community and are trained to provide rapid, timely care to sick or injured patients. Without their service, many communities would face long delays in emergency response and care.

EMTs are often the first licensed EMS personnel to arrive on the scene of an emergency, size up the situation, and provide emergency care and transportation. They practice in a wide diversity of settings—EMTs are everywhere in our community, many of them performing their EMT duties as well as their regular jobs. These providers demonstrate pride and dedication in their role on the frontline of emergency care in this country.

Barbara Aehlert wrote this text with great depth and clarity. Her easy-to-read writing style conveys a wealth of information that is essential for the student to grasp key concepts needed to become a competent EMT. Students who use this book can feel confident that they have learned accurate, up-to-date, and complete information so that they can face emergencies and provide essential emergency care in their practice setting, whatever the emergency is and wherever it occurs.

Kim McKenna, RN, EMT-P
Director of Education
St. Charles County Ambulance District
St. Peters, Missouri

Preface

This book, and the materials that accompany it, are designed to teach you how to safely and efficiently provide immediate care to an ill or injured person in accordance with the guidelines established by the U.S. Department of Transportation (DOT) Emergency Medical Technician (EMT) National Standard Curriculum. Although they may be used alone to increase your awareness of what to do in an emergency situation, these materials are best used in an EMT training program.

This book has been divided into 8 modules (divisions) that contain chapters with information relevant to each module. Each chapter begins with a list of knowledge, attitude, and skill objectives that describe what you should be able to do after completing the chapter and related exercises.

Before studying a chapter, first read the knowledge objectives. These objectives will give you an idea of the information you should obtain from reading the material in this book. Next, read the attitude objectives to learn about the behaviors that you are expected to develop as a healthcare professional. Then, read the skill objectives to discover the procedures you should be able to perform after reading about, observing, and then practicing each skill.

After reviewing the objectives, begin reading the chapter. Each chapter contains illustrations, tables, and other features to help you understand the information presented. For example, some skills discussed in this book are also demonstrated on the Delve Basic Life Support (BLS) Review DVD that is also available from McGraw-Hill. When you have finished reading the chapter, go through the objectives again to be sure that you have met them.

At the end of each module of the EMT course, time is allowed for skill practice, review, and evaluation. Video skills are provided on the Delve BLS Review DVD to help you learn and master each skill. Flashcards are also provided on the DVD. Self-test practice exam questions are provided on the McGraw-Hill Online Leaning Center (OLC) to help you prepare for the final examination.

Information that is related to your role as an EMT, but is not part of the DOT Emergency Medical Technician Curriculum, is located in Chapter 25 and in the appendices at the end of this book.

I hope you find this text helpful. If you have comments or suggestions about how I could improve this text, please visit my website, http://www.swemsed.com, and drop me a line. I would like to hear from you.

Best regards,
Barbara Aehlert, RN
Southwest EMS Education, Inc.
Phoenix, AZ/Pursley, TX

Guided Tour

Features to Help You Study and Learn

Divisions

The text is organized according to the Emergency Medical Technician National Standard Curriculum published by the U.S. Department of Transportation (DOT) and the National Highway Traffic Safety Administration (NHTSA).

Objectives Each chapter includes the knowledge, attitude, and skill objectives established by the DOT curriculum for the subject matter.

DVD Link This icon indicates the chapter skills presented on the student DVD located in the back of the text.

On the Scene These case studies represent emergency situations similar to those that EMTs may encounter in the field.

Think About It This feature presents questions related to the case study that readers should think about as they read each chapter or appendix.

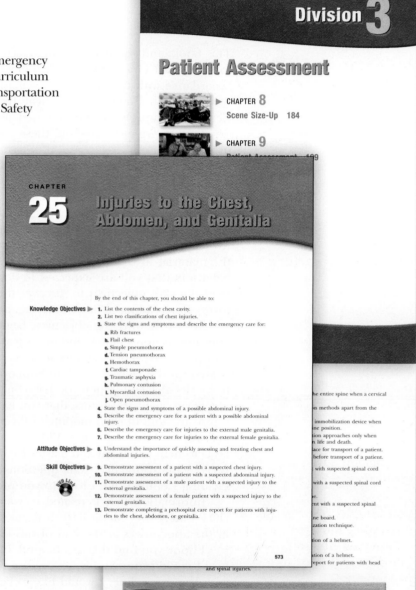

Division 3

Patient Assessment

▶ CHAPTER 8
Scene Size-Up 184

▶ CHAPTER 9
Patient Assessment 199

CHAPTER 25 Injuries to the Chest, Abdomen, and Genitalia

By the end of this chapter, you should be able to:

Knowledge Objectives ▶
1. List the contents of the chest cavity.
2. List two classifications of chest injuries.
3. State the signs and symptoms and describe the emergency care for:
   a. Rib fractures
   b. Flail chest
   c. Simple pneumothorax
   d. Tension pneumothorax
   e. Hemothorax
   f. Cardiac tamponade
   g. Traumatic asphyxia
   h. Pulmonary contusion
   i. Myocardial contusion
   j. Open pneumothorax
4. State the signs and symptoms of a possible abdominal injury.
5. Describe the emergency care for a patient with a possible abdominal injury.
6. Describe the emergency care for injuries to the external male genitalia.
7. Describe the emergency care for injuries to the external female genitalia.

Attitude Objectives ▶
8. Understand the importance of quickly assessing and treating chest and abdominal injuries.

Skill Objectives ▶
9. Demonstrate assessment of a patient with a suspected chest injury.
10. Demonstrate assessment of a patient with a suspected abdominal injury.
11. Demonstrate assessment of a male patient with a suspected injury to the external genitalia.
12. Demonstrate assessment of a female patient with a suspected injury to the external genitalia.
13. Demonstrate completing a prehospital care report for patients with injuries to the chest, abdomen, or genitalia.

573

On the Scene

You and your Emergency Medical Technician partner are dispatched to a construction site for a head injury. Upon arrival, you find a 28-year-old man lying on the floor in the construction site office. Your first impression reveals the patient is awake and aware of your approach. He appears to be breathing normally and his skin color is pink. A coworker is holding a bloodied towel to the side of the patient's head.

The patient states that while he was working, an 8-pound sledgehammer fell from about 8-10 feet above him onto his head. He then walked about 80 feet to his supervisor's office where they laid him down and controlled the bleeding from his head wound. Your partner finds an approximately 1-inch full-thickness laceration to the patient's right temporal area. The patient's initial vital signs are as follows: Pulse 110, strong and regular; respirations 16, unlabored; blood pressure 138/60. The patient denies any loss of consciousness and states that he feels dizzy and nauseated. ■

THINK ABOUT IT

As you read this chapter, think about the following questions:

• Is the patient's mechanism of injury significant?
• Should the patient receive a rapid trauma assessment or a focused physical examination?
• What emergency care should you provide for this patient?

Objective References   Each knowledge and attitude objective is referenced where it is covered in the chapter.

Key Terms   These terms are bolded within the text so that readers can review their meaning within the Glossary.

Stop and Think!   This feature contains safety tips and practical advice for the EMT.

Remember This!   This feature contains information and tips related to the EMT's role relative to other emergency care providers. This feature also provides information related to patient care.

Making a Difference   This feature contains information and tips to help the EMT provide excellent and/or specialized patient care.

You Should Know   This feature contains interesting and useful statistics and information. It also presents additional information related to the EMT's providing patient care.

- **Foodborne diseases** are spread by the improper handling of food or by poor personal hygiene. Examples include salmonella (food poisoning) and hepatitis A.
- **Sexually transmitted diseases** are spread by either blood or sexual contact. Examples include chlamydia, gonorrhea, and HIV.

You Should Know

HBV can survive up to 1 week outside the human body. HIV can survive only a short time (hours) outside the body.

Infection Control

Objective 8

An **exposure** is direct or indirect contact with infected blood, body fluids, tissues, or airborne droplets. An accidental exposure to infectious material can occur when your skin is pricked or cut, allowing the entry of germs. Germs can also enter your body through nicks or scrapes on your skin or through mucous membranes (such as your eyes, nose, and mouth). An exposure to a communicable disease does not automatically result in infection.

Remember This!

Body substance isolation precautions protect you and the patient.

Body substance isolation precautions have been developed by the **Centers for Disease Control (CDC)** to reduce the risk of exposure to infection. These standards have been adopted by the **Occupational Safety and Health Administration (OSHA),** which is a branch of the federal government responsible for safety in the workplace. **Body substance isolation (BSI) precautions** refer to self-protection against all body fluids and substances. These fluids and substances include blood, urine, semen, feces, vaginal secretions, tears, and saliva. Precautions include handwashing and using personal protective equipment. They also

Stop and Think!

When caring for patients, assume that all human blood and body fluids are infectious. For your safety, use appropriate BSI precautions during *every* patient contact.

include the proper cleaning, disinfecting, and disposing of soiled materials and equipment.

Remember This!

BSI Precautions

BSI precautions include the following:
- Handwashing
- Using personal protective equipment
- Cleaning, disinfecting, and disposing of soiled materials and equipment

Handwashing

Handwashing is the single most important method you can use to prevent the spread of communicable disease (Figure 2-13). Frequent handwashing removes germs picked up from other people or from contaminated surfaces. Wash your hands before and after contact with a patient (even if gloves were worn), after removing your gloves, and between patients.

Remember This!

Soap combined with scrubbing action is what helps dislodge and remove germs.

Proper handwashing begins with removing all jewelry from your hands and arms. Using soap and warm water, briskly rub your hands together to work up a lather. Continue washing for 10-15 seconds, washing the palm and back surface of each hand, your wrists, and exposed forearms. Scrub under and around your fingernails with a brush. With your fingers pointing

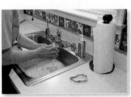

FIGURE 2-13 ▲ Handwashing is the single most important method you can use to prevent the spread of disease.

---

administration of a substance for unintended purposes, or for appropriate purposes but in improper amounts or doses, or without a prescription for the person receiving the medication. **Tolerance** occurs when an individual requires progressively larger doses of a drug to achieve the desired effect. **Addiction** is a psychological and physical dependence on a substance that has gone beyond voluntary control. **Withdrawal** is the condition produced when an individual stops using or abusing a drug to which he or she is physically or psychologically addicted. An **overdose** is an intentional or unintentional overmedication or ingestion of a toxic substance. Commonly misused and abused substances include stimulants, depressants, hallucinogens, and designer drugs.

Stimulants

Stimulants increase mental and physical activity. Examples include cocaine, amphetamines, methamphetamines, and phencyclidine (PCP). Common legal stimulants include caffeine and nicotine. Stimulants produce feelings of alertness and well-being. They may produce violent behavior. Other signs and symptoms of stimulant misuse or abuse are listed in the following *You Should Know* box. When the effects of the drug wear off, the user is often exhausted and sleeps. On awakening, the user may be confused, depressed, or suicidal.

You Should Know

Signs and Symptoms of Stimulant Misuse or Abuse
- Restlessness
- Irritability
- Combativeness
- Increased heart rate
- Increased respiratory rate
- Increased blood pressure
- Sweating
- Tremors
- Hallucinations
- Fever
- Headache
- Dizziness
- Moist or flushed skin
- Chest pain/discomfort
- Palpitations
- Nausea/vomiting
- Loss of appetite

Depressants

Depressants include alcohol, barbiturates, narcotics (opiates), and benzodiazepines. Signs and symptoms of depressant misuse or abuse are listed in the following *You Should Know* box.

You Should Know

Signs and Symptoms of Depressant Misuse or Abuse
- Drowsiness
- Slurred speech
- Decreased heart rate
- Decreased blood pressure
- Decreased respiratory rate
- Poor coordination
- Confusion

Alcohol

Alcohol slows mental and physical activity. It affects judgment, vision, reaction time, and coordination. When approaching the patient who has ingested alcohol, observe the scene for evidence of trauma. In large quantities, alcohol can cause death.

Making a Difference

Signs and symptoms of alcohol misuse or abuse can mimic those of other medical conditions such as a diabetic emergency, head injury, epilepsy, drug reaction, or central nervous system (CNS) infection. In addition, alcohol abuse can often mask potentially lethal conditions such as a head injury. Do not *assume* the patient is intoxicated. Carefully assess the patient for the presence of other injuries or illnesses. Perform a blood glucose test (if permitted by state and local protocol).

Disulfiram (Antabuse) is a medication prescribed for alcoholics to discourage them from drinking. When combined with alcohol or alcohol-containing foods, medications, or products (such as over-the-counter cough medications, mouthwash, and facial cleaning products) Antabuse produces unpleasant, and sometimes serious, reactions. Reactions last 30 minutes to 8 hours (usually 3 to 4 hours) and include nausea, vomiting, abdominal discomfort, chest discomfort, palpitations, headache,

Skill Drills These drills are step-by-step presentations of procedures and skills essential to the EMT's role.

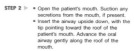

Sizing and Inserting an Oral Airway

STEP 1 ▶ Use Steps 1-4 to insert an oral airway in an unresponsive adult.
- Place the patient on his back. Position yourself at the patient's head.
- Open the patient's airway with a head tilt–chin lift maneuver. If trauma is suspected, use the jaw thrust without the head tilt maneuver to open the airway.
- Select the correct size oral airway. An oral airway is the correct size if it extends from the corner of the patient's mouth to the tip of the earlobe, or from the center of the mouth to the angle of the jaw.

STEP 2 ▶
- Open the patient's mouth. Suction any secretions from the mouth, if present.
- Insert the airway upside down, with the tip pointing toward the roof of the patient's mouth. Advance the oral airway gently along the roof of the mouth.

STEP 3 ▶ When the tip of the airway approaches the back of the throat, rotate the airway 180 degrees so that it is positioned over the tongue. Be careful not to push the tongue into the back of the throat.

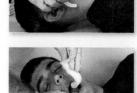
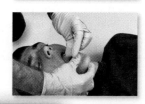

On the Scene: Wrap-Up Using the information presented in the chapter, this feature presents a wrap-up of the case study from the beginning of the chapter.

On the Scene — Wrap-Up

Any extrication is a complex event that requires great skill and a working knowledge of vehicle design and extrication operations. On the basis of the patient's condition, you decide that this patient needs to be extricated from the vehicle. You perform a 360-degree rotation around the vehicle to check for any hazards; none is found. With your PPE on, you approach the vehicle. Stabilization of the vehicle is accomplished by using cribbing. You then enter the vehicle through the back door on the driver's side. As you enter the vehicle, you notice that there is a significant amount of intrusion of the passenger side of the vehicle. This gives you an indication of the types and severity of the patient's injuries. The extrication team removes the roof of the vehicle, lifts the patient onto a long backboard, and takes the patient out of the vehicle over the trunk. The patient is placed into the back of your ambulance for transport, and you accompany the patient to the hospital. ■

Sum It Up

▶ Extrication is the process of removing machinery from around a patient to facilitate patient care and transport. The EMT on the extrication scene has an important role both as a care provider for the patient and a support member for the extrication team. Base the extrication on the patient's condition to ensure that the techniques used will provide the fastest access and best egress for the patient from the vehicle.

▶ Protective clothing that is appropriate for the situation must be worn during extrication. This includes protective boots, pants, a coat, eye protection, a helmet, and gloves. Respiratory protection may also be needed.

▶ Scene size-up is an important step in the extrication process. A proper scene size-up will reveal any hazards present and also give a good indication of the number of persons injured, the types of injury, and which patient or patients require medical attention first.

▶ Once on the scene, fire apparatus should be parked in the fend-off position, which involves parking your unit downward from the scene and in such a way that allows traveling vehicles to strike your unit and not crew members.

▶ Stabilization is the process of rendering a vehicle motionless in the position in which it is found. The purpose of stabilization is to eliminate potential movement of a vehicle (or structure) that may cause further harm to entrapped patients or rescuers.

▶ Simple extrication is the use of hand tools in order to gain access and extricate the patient from the vehicle. Complex extrication involves the use of powered hydraulic rescue tools, such as cutters, spreaders, and rams. The patient's level of entrapment will determine whether the extrication will fall into a simple or complex category.

▶ Four levels of entrapment are possible during a motor vehicle crash. The first level is no entrapment. Light entrapment means that a door or some other object will need to be opened or moved to get the patient out. Moderate entrapment is more involved, requiring removal of doors or the roof. Heavy entrapment is the highest level of entrapment and involves any situation that is above and beyond moderate entrapment.

▶ Disentanglement is the moving or removing of material that is trapping a victim.

▶ Continue your education beyond the information contained in this chapter in order to provide the best care for your patient and maintain and improve your skills as you gain more experience in Emergency Medical Services.

Sum It Up This feature is a bulleted list of the key information covered in the chapter.

Appendices

Six appendices address important and timely topics related to the EMT's role.

Glossary

The glossary provides a full definition of the key terms.

Supplements

For the Student

Workbook

Includes a full range of question types: true or false, multiple choice, sentence completion, matching, and short answer.

Pocket Guide

Contains convenient, essential information EMTs need to provide initial emergency medical care in the field.

Delve Basic Life Support Review

Available as an optional package with the text at a discounted price.

DVD

- Essential DOT EMT skills
- 150 Digital Flashcards

McGraw-Hill's Online Learning Center (OLC)—Student Site

- 200-Question Exam with Answer Key
- 150-Question Sample Final Exam with Answer Key
- 850-Question Practice Exams, organized by chapter and appendix
- McGraw-Hill's *Spanish Guide to Patient Assessment for the Emergency Medical Technician*
- Test-Taking Preparation Tips for the Emergency Medical Technician Certification Exam

For the Instructor

McGraw-Hill's Online Learning Center (OLC)—Instructor Site

- Instructor's Manual: lesson plans, end-of-chapter quizzes created exclusively for the instructor, and correlation to PowerPoint slides
- PowerPoint Slides: more than 2,300 slides
- Computerized Test Bank: more than 1,000 instructor questions created exclusively for the instructor

Acknowledgments

No book is published without the assistance of many people. Thank you to Dave Culverwell, Claire Merrick, Linda Schreiber, Rick Hecker, Lori Hancock, Srdjan Savanovic, Janean Utley, Mark Dierker, Ben Curless, Kelly Curran, and Sarah Wood of McGraw-Hill for their work in the production and design of this book and the development of the related supplements and media. A very special thanks to Julie Scardiglia and Gail Michaels, who spent hours painstakingly ensuring that the manuscripts and related files associated with each part of this project were complete.

The contributors for this book and the materials that accompany it were selected because of their experience in EMS. Whether a physician, nurse, or paramedic, they each treat their patients with compassion and respect and display professionalism every day they are on the job. Their commitment to excellence and professionalism in EMS is evident throughout this book. Thank you to Gary Smith, MD; Lynn Browne-Wagner, RN; Andrea Legamaro, RN; Terence Mason, RN; Suzy Coronel, CEP; Paul Honeywell, CEP; Captain Randy Budd, CEP; Captain Holly Button, CEP; Captain Sean Newton, CEP; Captain Jeff Pennington, CEP; Travis Kidd EMT-P; and Major Raymond Burton. Special thanks to Janet Fitts, RN, and Edith Valladares for their invaluable contributions to the *Spanish Guide to Patient Assessment for the Emergency Medical Technician,* featured on McGraw-Hill Online Learning Center (OLC).

Kim McKenna, RN, read every word in this book and the instructor's materials for accuracy. Thanks for your attention to detail and your suggestions and for making time for this project in the midst of your busy schedule. Steve Kidd and the staff of Delve Productions worked very hard to make sure that the BLS Review DVD is easy to use and useful for EMTs. Rick Brady did an outstanding job of taking the photos that appear in this book. Thanks to Carin Marter, CEP; the City of Mesa Fire Department; the City of Tempe Fire Department; and AirEvac Services (Phoenix, Arizona) for providing additional photos.

Thanks to the many EMS professionals who reviewed this text and the materials that accompany it. Each reviewer provided valuable comments and suggestions that were carefully read and discussed. Modifications have been made where needed on the basis of your comments.

Barbara Aehlert, RN
Southwest EMS Education, Inc.
Phoenix, AZ/Pursley, TX

Contributors

Lynn Browne-Wagner, RN
LBW, LLC
Phoenix, AZ

Randy Budd, RRT, CEP
City of Mesa Fire Department
Mesa, AZ

Major Raymond W. Burton (Retired)
Plymouth Academy/Plymouth County Sheriff's
  Academy
Plymouth, MA

Holly Button, CEP
City of Mesa Fire Department
Mesa, AZ

Suzy Coronel, CEP
Sportsmedicine Fairbanks
Fairbanks, AK

Janet Fitts, RN, EMT-P
Educational Consultant
Prehospital and Emergency Medical Services
Pacific, MO

Paul Honeywell, CEP
Southwest Ambulance
Mesa, AZ

Travis Kidd, EMT-P
Orange County Fire/Rescue
Orlando, FL

Andrea Legamaro, RN
Southwest EMS Education, Inc.
Dallas, TX

Terence Mason, RN
City of Mesa Fire Department
Mesa, AZ

Kim McKenna, RN, EMT-P
Director of Education
St. Charles County Ambulance District
St. Peters, MO

Sean Newton, CEP
City of Scottsdale Fire Department
Scottsdale, AZ

Jeff Pennington, CEP
City of Gilbert Fire Department
Gilbert, AZ

Gary Smith, MD
Medical Director: Apache Junction, Gilbert,
  and Mesa Fire Departments
Apache Junction, Gilbert, and Mesa, AZ

Edith Valladares
Director, Foreign Languages and Academic ESL
Central Piedmont Community College
Charlotte, NC

Reviewers

Rick Criste
Fayetteville Technical Community College
Fayetteville, NC

Bradley Dean, BBA, NREMT-P
Davidson County Emergency Services
Lexington, NC

David S. Farrow
Southwest EMS Education, Inc.
Phoenix, Arizona

Janet Fitts, RN, BSN, CEN, TNS, EMT-P
Educational Consultant
Prehospital and Emergency Medical Services
Pacific, MO

Joni J. Fowler
Alamance Community College
Burlington, NC

Lawrence A. Linder, MA. NREMTP
Hillsborough Community College
Tampa, FL

Taz Meyer, BS, EMT-P
Operations Coordinator
St. Charles County Ambulance District
St. Peters, MO

Keith Monosky, MPM, EMT-P
Assistant Professor, Department of Emergency
*   Medicine*
George Washington University
Ashburn, VA

Nikhil Natarajan, NREMT-P, CCEMT-P, I/C
SUNY Ulster
Stone Ridge, NY

Kenneth Navarro
University of Texas Southwestern Medical School
Dallas, TX

Keith A. Ozenberger, BS, LP
University of Texas Medical Branch
Galveston, TX

Anya Sanko, BS, EMT-P
Oakland Community College
Auburn Hills, MI

Brad J. Scoggins
University of Texas Medical
Galveston Branch, TX

William Seifarth
MIEMSS
Baltimore, MD

Tom Vines
Carbon Co. SAR/Mainrod
Red Lodge, MT

Division 1

Preparatory

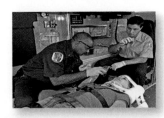
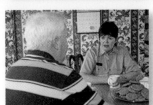
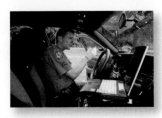
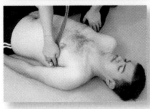

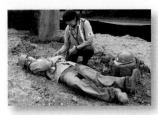
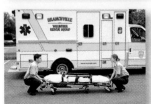

1 Introduction to Emergency Medical Care

By the end of this chapter, you should be able to:

Knowledge Objectives ▶
1. Define Emergency Medical Services (EMS) systems.
2. Differentiate the roles and responsibilities of an Emergency Medical Technician (EMT) from other prehospital care professionals.
3. Describe the roles and responsibilities related to personal safety.
4. Discuss the roles and responsibilities of the EMT toward the safety of the crew, the patient, and bystanders.
5. Define quality management and discuss the EMT's role in the process.
6. Define medical direction and discuss the EMT's role in the process.
7. State the specific statutes and regulations in your state regarding the EMS system.

Attitude Objectives ▶
8. Assess areas of personal attitude and conduct of the EMT.
9. Characterize the various methods used to access the EMS system in your community.

Skill Objectives ▶ There are no skill objectives identified for this lesson.

On the Scene

You and your Paramedic partner are called to a repair shop for an injured man. When you arrive on the scene, shop workers quickly wave you to the back of the building. A worker has been injured while repairing a gear in a lawn tractor. His hand is stuck in the engine, which still roars loudly. He is writhing in pain and soaked in sweat. Several of his fingers have been cut off. Blood is pooling on his forearm and dripping to the floor. The patient's coworkers gather around, waiting for you to take action. ■

THINK ABOUT IT

As you read this chapter, think about the following questions:

- What is your most important concern as you approach this and all emergency situations?
- What EMT skills might you need in this situation? What others may need to be provided by your Paramedic partner?
- What components of the emergency care system is this patient likely to need?

An **Emergency Medical Technician (EMT)** is a member of the Emergency Medical Services (EMS) team who responds to emergency calls, provides efficient emergency care to ill or injured patients, and transports the patient to a medical facility. EMTs are an important and essential part of the EMS system. In fact, most prehospital emergency medical care is provided by EMTs. As an EMT, you will be called to respond to many types of emergencies, such as a motor vehicle crash, life-threatening medical situation, or disaster. EMTs may be paid or volunteer fire department personnel, law enforcement officers, military personnel, members of the ski patrol, teachers, lifeguards, designated industrial/commercial medical response teams, park rangers, coaches, or athletic trainers (Figure 1-1). EMTs may work for public or private agencies. As an EMT, you will be tasked with providing medical assistance and seeking the help of other emergency caregivers as needed.

The Department of Transportation (DOT) developed the EMT Basic National Standard Curriculum to help you gain the knowledge, attitude, and skills necessary to be a competent, productive, and valuable member of the healthcare team. This curriculum was developed by representatives of federal and state agencies, professional medical organizations, and education experts. EMT training programs follow guidelines established by this curriculum.

Making a Difference

Goals of EMT Education

When you successfully complete an EMT Training Program, you will have gained the knowledge, attitude, and skills to:

- Recognize the nature and seriousness of a patient's condition or extent of injuries to determine the emergency medical care the patient requires
- Safely and efficiently provide appropriate emergency medical care based on your assessment findings of the patient's condition
- Lift, move, position, and otherwise handle the patient to minimize discomfort and prevent further injury
- Safely and effectively perform the expectations of the job description.

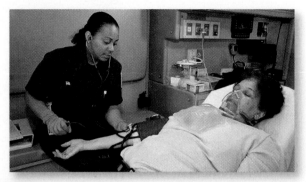

FIGURE 1-1 ▲ An Emergency Medical Technician (EMT) is a member of the Emergency Medical Services (EMS) team who provides prehospital emergency care.

Origins of Emergency Medical Services

Ancient Times to 1800s

As an EMT, you will be giving emergency care to ill or injured patients. An **emergency** is an unexpected illness or injury that requires immediate action to avoid risking the life or health of the person being treated. Emergency medical care has been given by one person to another for hundreds of years. The Egyptians splinted and dressed wounds. The ill or injured were treated at the site where the emergency happened or were carried to a designated healer or helper. The Good Samaritan stopped to provide care to a man who had been beaten and left lying on the side of the road. He wrapped bandages around the injured man's wounds and then transported him by donkey to the nearest hotel. The Romans and Greeks used chariots to remove injured soldiers from the battlefield.

EMS probably began in 1797 in the Napoleonic Wars during which a system of service was provided to the injured. Baron Dominique Jean Larrey, a French surgeon general, used light carriages to transport casualties from the field to aid stations. The medical crews operating the carriages were trained to control severe bleeding and splint fractures. The first civilian ambulance services in the United States began as hospital-based services in Cincinnati (in 1865) and New York City (in 1869).

1900 to 1960

The first civilian ambulance services in the United States began as hospital-based services in Cincinnati and New York City. The National Safety Council was established in 1913. The first known air medical transport occurred during the retreat of the Serbian army from Albania in 1915. In 1922, the American College of Surgeons established the Committee on Treatment of Fractures, which later became the Committee on Trauma.

In the mid-1940s, rural communities recognized the need for local fire protection and first aid and began volunteer services to meet the need for these services. In the 1950s, Mobile Army Surgical Hospital (MASH) units used helicopters for evacuation in the Korean War. The rapid evacuation of patients increased survival. In 1958, Dr. Peter Safar demonstrated the importance of mouth-to-mouth ventilation. Cardiopulmonary resuscitation (CPR) was shown to be useful in 1960.

1960 to 1970

In the 1960s, hospital-based mobile coronary care unit ambulances were successfully being used to treat prehospital cardiac patients in Belfast, Ireland. Meanwhile, in the United States, volunteers untrained in emergency care provided minimal stabilization at the scene of an emergency. Transport to the nearest hospital was provided by funeral homes, taxis, and automobile towing companies as an optional service.

This fragmented system of care continued in the United States throughout much of the 1960s. In 1966, the National Academy of Sciences-National Research Council (NAS/NRC) published a paper called "Accidental Death and Disability: The Neglected Disease of Modern Society" in 1966. This document is commonly called the "White Paper" or "Landmark Paper." It exposed the gaps in providing emergency care in the U.S. Some of the areas identified that needed improvement included the following:

- Improving citizen knowledge of basic first aid
- Improving ambulance design and equipment
- Improving the training of emergency responders (ambulance attendants, police, and fire personnel)
- Providing physician oversight (medical direction)
- Improving the care provided by hospital emergency departments
- Improving communications and record keeping
- Increasing local government support to provide the best possible EMS

The Highway Safety Act of 1966 charged the DOT National Highway Traffic Safety Administration (NHTSA) with the responsibility of improving EMS. This act provided funding for the development of highway safety programs to reduce the number of deaths related to highway accidents. This act also established national standards for training Emergency

You Should Know

Passage of the Highway Safety Act of 1966 was the first national commitment to reducing highway-related injuries and deaths.

Medical Technicians and the minimum equipment required on an ambulance.

The American College of Emergency Physicians (ACEP) was founded in 1968 and designated 9-1-1 as the universal emergency telephone number. In the same year, the American Trauma Society was established. In 1969, the first nationally recognized EMT-Ambulance (EMT-A) curriculum was published.

1970 to 1980

The National Registry of Emergency Medical Technicians (NREMT) was founded in 1970. The NREMT contributes to the development of professional standards. It also verifies the competency of EMS professionals by preparing and conducting examinations. Recognizing a need for an EMS training program for law enforcement personnel, NHTSA developed the Crash Injury Management for the Law Enforcement Officer training program in the early 1970s. This 40-hour course later evolved into the First Responder National Standard Curriculum in 1979.

In 1971, the television program *Emergency!* aired, featuring Paramedics Johnny Gage and Roy Desoto. This program increased the public's awareness of EMS. The Department of Labor officially recognized EMT-A as an occupational specialty in 1972. In the same year, demonstration projects were begun in some states to develop model regional EMS systems. The Emergency Medical Services System (EMSS) Act was enacted in 1973. This law mandated that there should be 15 components of EMS systems. The components identified were:

- Manpower
- Training
- Communications
- Transportation
- Facilities
- Critical care units
- Public safety agencies
- Consumer participation
- Access to care
- Patient transfer
- Coordinated patient record keeping
- Public information and education
- Review and evaluation
- Disaster plan
- Mutual aid

By this time, it was clear that patient care could be improved if the components of an EMS system worked together. The EMSS Act provided grant funding to states and communities that developed EMS systems as described in the law.

In 1975, the National Association of Emergency Medical Technicians (NAEMT) was founded. In the same year, a study in Seattle, Washington, showed that the survivability of heart attack victims was improved with early involvement of Advanced Life Support (ALS) personnel. In 1976, the American College of Surgeons Committee on Trauma published "Optimal Hospital Resources for Care of the Injured Patient." To improve hospital capabilities to care for injured patients, this document identified the need for designation of three levels of trauma centers. In 1977, national standards were developed for EMT Paramedics (EMT-P).

1980 to 1990

In 1984, the EMS for Children (EMSC) Program provided funds to improve the EMS system and better serve the needs of infants and children. In 1985, the National Research Council published "Injury in America: A Continuing Public Health Problem." This document described deficiencies in the progress of addressing the problem of accidental death and disability. In 1986, the Injury Prevention Act (followed by the Injury Control Act of 1990) established the Division of Injury Epidemiology and Control at the Centers for Disease Control (changed to the National Center for Injury Prevention and Control in 1992) to provide leadership for a variety of injury-related public health activities. In 1987, the American College of Emergency Physicians published "Guidelines for Trauma Care Systems." This document identified essential criteria for trauma systems, especially pre-hospital care components. In 1988, NHTSA began a statewide EMS system, Technical Assessment Program (TAP). This program identified 10 essential parts of an EMS system and the methods used to assess these areas. States use the standards set by NHTSA to evaluate how effective their EMS system is.

You Should Know

Components of the NHTSA Technical Assessment Program

- Regulation and policy
- Resource management
- Human resources and training
- Transportation
- Facilities
- Communications
- Public information and education
- Medical direction
- Trauma systems
- Evaluation

In 1989, *Rescue 911* aired on television. When watching this program, television viewers saw re-enactments of actual emergency calls. This was significant because previously EMS calls on TV were usually fictionalizations. Viewers saw callers dial "9-1-1" when emergency care was needed. They also saw calls to 9-1-1 being answered by trained personnel who could give lifesaving instructions over the telephone. This program increased awareness of the importance of bystander cardiopulmonary resuscitation (CPR) and resulted in increased training of the community in CPR.

1990s to Present

In 1990, the Trauma Systems Planning and Development Act created the Division of Trauma and EMS (DTEMS) within the Department of Health and Human Services. To address the needs of injured patients and match them to available resources, this law provided funding to states for the development, implementation, and evaluation of trauma systems. States were responsible for developing a system of specialized care for the triage (sorting) and transfer of trauma patients. DTEMS was disbanded in 1995. Also in 1990, the American College of Surgeons Committee on Trauma published "Resources for Optimal Care of the Injured Patient." These revised guidelines changed the focus from trauma centers to trauma systems. In 1994, the EMT-Basic National Standard Curriculum was revised.

In 1996, NHTSA published the "EMS Agenda for the Future." Because it also recommended directions for future EMS development in the United States, this paper is often called a "vision" document. This document reviewed the progress made in EMS over 30 years and proposed continued development of 14 EMS attributes. They are:

- Integration of Health Services
- EMS Research
- Legislation and Regulation
- System Finance
- Human Resources
- Medical Direction
- Education Systems
- Public Education
- Prevention
- Public Access
- Communication Systems
- Clinical Care
- Information Systems
- Evaluation

In 2000, the "EMS Education Agenda for the Future: A Systems Approach" was released. This document proposed an EMS education system made up of five integrated parts (see Table 1-1).

TABLE 1-1 EMS Education System of the Future—Components

EMS Agenda for the Future	1996 document that created the vision for EMS
EMS Education System for the Future: A Systems Approach	Outlines an EMS education system made up of five integrated parts
National EMS Core Content	Describes the domain of prehospital care
National EMS Scope of Practice Model	• Divides EMS core content into EMS levels of practice • Defines minimum skills and knowledge for each level of EMS professional
National EMS Education Standards	• Replaces National Standard Curriculum • Defines competencies, clinical behaviors, and judgments that define the performance requirements for each level of student
National EMS Education Program Accreditation	EMS education program approval based on universally accepted standards and guidelines
National EMS Certification	Standardized testing completed after graduation from an accredited EMS program that leads to state licensure

Following the events of September 11, 2001, the Department of Homeland Security was created with The Homeland Security Act of 2002. In 2003, President Bush directed the Secretary of Homeland Security to develop and administer a National Incident Management System (NIMS). The NIMS provides a consistent nationwide template to enable all government, private sector, and nongovernmental organizations to work together during domestic incidents.

In 2007, the National EMS Core Content document was released. This document defines the domain of prehospital care. "The National EMS Scope of Practice Model" is a document that was published in 2007. It divides the core content into EMS levels of practice, defining the minimum skills and knowledge for each level of EMS professional. Important dates in the history of EMS are summarized in Table 1-2.

TABLE 1-2 Important Dates in the History of EMS

Year	Event
1797	Napoleonic Wars • Beginning of system of service to the injured • Light carriages are used for transporting casualties from the field to aid stations • Medical crews operating the carriages are trained to control severe bleeding and splint fractures
1860s	• First ambulance service in United States is believed to have been in the U.S. Army in 1865 • First civilian ambulance services in United States begin as hospital-based services in Cincinnati and New York City
1915	• First known air medical transport occurs during retreat of the Serbian army from Albania
1922	• American College of Surgeons establishes Committee on Treatment of Fractures (later becomes Committee on Trauma)
Mid-1940s	Rural communities recognize need for local fire protection and first aid and begin volunteer services to meet the need for these services

Continued

TABLE 1-2 **Important Dates in the History of EMS** *Continued*

Year	Event
1950s	• MASH units use helicopters for evacuation in the Korean War; rapid evacuation of patients increases survival • American College of Surgeons develops first training program for ambulance attendants • Dr. Peter Safar demonstrates efficacy of mouth-to-mouth ventilation (1958)
1960	• CPR is shown to be useful • Ambu introduces bag-valve-mask resuscitator • Laerdal introduces Resusci-Anne
1965	PhysioControl introduces LifePak 33 heart monitor/defibrillator
1966	• Beginning of modern EMS • "Accidental Death and Disability: The Neglected Disease of Modern Society," published by National Academy of Sciences-National Research Council (NAS/NRC), identifies injury as a national healthcare problem • Highway Safety Act of 1966 charges DOT NHTSA with responsibility of improving EMS, including helping states develop EMS programs; it is the first national commitment to reducing highway-related injuries and deaths
1967	George Hurst invents Jaws of Life (Hurst Tool)
1968	• American College of Emergency Physicians (ACEP) founds and designates 9-1-1 as universal emergency telephone number • American Trauma Society is established
1969	First nationally recognized EMT-Ambulance (EMT-A) curriculum is published
1970	National Registry of Emergency Medical Technicians (NREMT) is founded
1971	*Emergency!* television program airs
1972	• Department of Labor officially recognizes EMT-A as an occupational specialty • Demonstration projects are begun in some states to develop model regional EMS systems
1973	EMSS Act provides federal guidelines and funding for development of regional EMS systems
1974	Glenn Hare patents cervical collar
1975	National Association of Emergency Medical Technicians is founded
1976	• American College of Surgeons Committee on Trauma publishes "Optimal Hospital Resources for Care of Injured Patient," which identified three levels of trauma centers • Dr. Burt Kaplan and David Clark Co. patent military antishock trousers
1977	National standards are developed for EMT-Paramedics
1981	• Omnibus Budget Reconciliation Act consolidates EMS funding into state preventive block grants; EMSS Act funding is eliminated • Rick Kendrick invents Kendrick Extrication Device
1984	EMS for Children Program provides funds to improve the EMS system and better serve the needs of infants and children
1985	National Research Council publishes "Injury in America: A Continuing Public Health Problem," which describes the lack of progress in addressing the problem of accidental death and disability

Continued

TABLE 1-2 Important Dates in the History of EMS *Continued*

Year	Event
1986	• Injury Prevention Act (followed by Injury Control Act of 1990) establishes Division of Injury Epidemiology and Control at Centers for Disease Control (changed to National Center for Injury Prevention and Control in 1992) to provide leadership for a variety of injury-related public health activities • Life Support Products develops Automatic Transport Ventilator
1988	National Highway Traffic Safety Administration establishes EMS Technical Assessment Program; 10 essential components of an EMS system are identified
1989	*Rescue 911* airs on television
1990	• Trauma Systems Planning and Development Act creates the DTEMS within the Department of Health and Human Services, provides funding to address needs of injured patients and match them to available resources, and encourages development of trauma systems • American College of Surgeons Committee on Trauma publishes "Resources for Optimal Care of the Injured Patient," which changes the focus from trauma centers to trauma systems
1993	Federal Communications Commission approves channels for exclusive emergency medical radio services use
1994	EMT-Basic National Standard Curriculum is revised
1996	NHTSA publishes "EMS Agenda for the Future," which reviews progress made in EMS over 30 years and proposes continued development of 14 EMS attributes
2000	Trauma System Planning and Development Act is reauthorized and funded
2002	Homeland Security Act of 2002 creates Department of Homeland Security
2003	Homeland Security develops and administers National Incident Management System
2005	National EMS Core Content document published defining the domain of prehospital care
2005	National EMS Scope of Practice Model is submitted to NHTSA • Divides EMS core content into EMS levels of practice • Defines minimum skills and knowledge for each level of EMS professional

Overview of the Emergency Medical Services System

Objective 1

As an EMT, you are a part of the **EMS system.** The EMS system is a network of resources that provides emergency care and transportation to victims of sudden illness or injury. An EMS system may be local, regional, state, or national. The network of resources includes emergency medical personnel, equipment, and supplies. To be efficient and effective, these resources must function in a coordinated manner.

EMS includes a wide range of emergency care including:

- Recognition of the emergency
- Accessing the EMS system
- Providing emergency care at the scene
- Providing emergency care when indicated during transport to, from, and between healthcare facilities
- Giving medical care to patients during disasters and at mass gatherings, such as a concert or sporting event

An EMS system does not exist by itself. Because EMS professionals provide care to ill or injured members of the public, EMS overlaps with other important areas such as public safety, public health, and the healthcare system. A **healthcare system** is a network of people, facilities, and equipment designed to provide for the general medical needs of the population. EMS is a part of the healthcare system.

Legislation and Regulation

Objective 7

To ensure the delivery of quality emergency medical care for adults and children, each state has laws in place that govern its EMS system. Each state must make sure that all ill or injured victims have equal access to appropriate emergency care. This includes making sure there are enough vehicles, equipment, supplies, and trained personnel on hand to meet the needs of local EMS systems. As an EMT, you must know your state and local EMS regulations and policies.

Public Access and Communications

An EMS system must have an effective communications system. The EMS system must provide a means by which a citizen can reliably access the EMS system (usually by dialing 9-1-1). To make sure appropriate personnel, vehicles, and equipment are sent to the scene of an emergency, the communication system must allow contact between different agencies, vehicles, and personnel. For example, there must be a means for:

- Citizen access to the EMS system
- Dispatch center to emergency vehicle communication
- Communication between emergency vehicles
- Communication to and between emergency personnel
- Communication to and between emergency vehicles and emergency healthcare facilities
- Communication to and between emergency personnel and medical direction
- Communication between emergency healthcare facilities
- Communication between agencies, such as between EMS and law enforcement personnel
- Methods for relaying information to the public

You Should Know

In situations involving a large number of patients, rescuers, and equipment, the **National Incident Management System (NIMS)** is often used to control, direct, and coordinate the activities of multiple agencies through **Unified Command.** Unified Command is an application of the Incident Command System that is used when multiple organizations involved in the incident coordinate an effective incident response while carrying out their own jurisdictional responsibilities at the same time.

Remember This!

The 9-1-1 network is an important part of our nation's emergency response and disaster preparedness system. Because there is no "11" on a telephone pad, 9-1-1 should always be referred to as "nine-one-one," not "nine-eleven." 9-1-1 is easily remembered, even by young children.

When an emergency occurs in the United States, the person who places a call for help expects a prompt response to the scene of the emergency. For example, law enforcement and fire department personnel are typically dispatched to the scene of a motor vehicle crash after the patient or a bystander calls 9-1-1. 9-1-1 is the official national emergency number in the United States and Canada. When the numbers 9-1-1 are dialed, the caller is quickly connected to a single location called a Public Safety Answering Point (PSAP). The PSAP dispatcher is trained to route the call to local emergency medical, fire, and law enforcement agencies. Although EMS is usually activated by dialing 9-1-1, other methods of activating an emergency response include emergency alarm boxes, citizen band radios, amateur radios, local access numbers, and wireless telephones. It is important that you know how the citizens of your community access the EMS system.

Enhanced 9-1-1, or E9-1-1, is a system that routes an emergency call to the 9-1-1 center closest to the caller and automatically displays the caller's phone number and address. Most 9-1-1 systems that exist today are E9-1-1 systems. The Federal Communications Commission (FCC) has established a program that requires wireless telephone carriers to provide E9-1-1 services. Wireless E9-1-1 provides the location of a 9-1-1 call from a wireless phone, within 50-100 meters in most cases.

You Should Know

According to the National Emergency Number Association (NENA), nearly 93% of the population of the United States was covered by some type of 9-1-1 service at the end of the 20th century. Ninety-five percent of that coverage was enhanced 9-1-1. About 96% of the geographic United States is presently covered by some type of 9-1-1.

If a 9-1-1 caller does not speak English, the 9-1-1 call taker can add an interpreter from an outside service to the line. Communications centers that answer 9-1-1 calls also have special telephones for responding to 9-1-1 calls from deaf or hearing- and speech-impaired callers.

Voice over Internet Protocol (VoIP) (also known as *Internet Voice*) is technology that allows users to make telephone calls by means of a broadband Internet connection instead of a regular telephone line.

Companies offering this service have different features. Some services only allow you to call other people using the same service. Others allow you to call anyone who has a telephone number. Some services don't work during power outages and may not offer backup power. Some services offer E9-1-1 support as an optional service. Subscribers register and pay a fee for E9-1-1. With their subscription, an emergency call is automatically routed to the PSAP that handles 9-1-1 emergencies. If the subscriber is unable to speak, the PSAP operator will know the subscriber's location and be able to dispatch the emergency. If the user declines E9-1-1 service, they do not have direct access to emergency personnel via Internet Voice.

Human Resources and Education

An EMS system must have qualified, competent, and compassionate people to provide quality EMS care. Persons working in an EMS system are expected to be trained to a minimum standard. The **National EMS Scope of Practice Model** is a document that defines four levels of EMS professionals: Emergency Medical Responders, EMTs, Advanced EMTs (AEMTs), and Paramedics. This document also defines what each level of EMS professional legally can and cannot do.

For many years, the minimum standard for education of EMS professionals was the DOT National Standard Curriculum (NSC) for each level. The **National EMS Education Standards** document is replacing the NSC. This document specifies the objectives that each level of EMS professional must meet when completing their education.

EMS education occurs in many different settings, including hospitals, community colleges, universities, technical centers, private institutions, and fire departments. To ensure quality, EMS systems should:

- Monitor educational programs regularly
- Use qualified instructors
- Use a standardized curriculum for each level of EMS professional throughout the state
- Incorporate EMS standards, using an educationally sound curriculum development process
- Use standardized testing methods

Levels of Prehospital Education

Objective 2

There are four levels of nationally recognized prehospital professionals: Emergency Medical Responder, EMT, Advanced EMT, and Paramedic (Table 1-3).

TABLE 1-3 Levels of EMS Training

Basic Life Support	Emergency Medical Responder	An EMR is the first person with medical training who arrives at the scene of an emergency. An EMR provides initial emergency care, including assessing for life-threatening conditions, opening and maintaining an airway, ventilating patients, performing CPR, controlling bleeding, caring for medical emergencies, bandaging wounds, stabilizing the spine and injured limbs, assisting with childbirth, and assisting other EMS professionals.
	Emergency Medical Technician	An EMT is more skilled than an EMR and, at the scene of an emergency, continues the care begun by EMRs. EMTs can perform all EMR skills. Additional skills include helping patients with specific prescribed medications and giving oral glucose and activated charcoal when indicated.
Advanced Life Support	Advanced Emergency Medical Technician	An AEMT is more skilled than an EMT. An AEMT can perform all EMT skills and has received additional training in patient assessment, providing IV fluids and medications, and advanced airway procedures.
	Paramedic (EMT-P)	A Paramedic has more training than an AEMT and has additional education in pathophysiology, physical examination techniques, assessing abnormal heart rhythms using a heart monitor, and invasive procedures.

Emergency Medical Responder

An **Emergency Medical Responder (EMR)** is a person who has the basic knowledge and skills necessary to provide lifesaving emergency care while waiting for the arrival of additional EMS help. EMRs were formerly called First Responders. In some states, First Responders were called Emergency Care Attendants (ECAs). Most EMRs have a minimal amount of equipment available with which to assess a patient and provide initial emergency care. An EMR is also trained to assist other EMS professionals.

Emergency Medical Technician

An EMT is a member of the EMS team who responds to emergency calls, provides efficient emergency care to ill or injured patients, and transports the patient to a medical facility. An EMT has successfully completed a minimum 110-hour training program that adheres to the National Standard Curriculum. An EMT is trained to perform a more detailed assessment and can perform more skills than an EMR. At the scene of an emergency, EMTs continue the care begun by EMRs, including stabilizing the patient and actual patient transport.

Advanced Emergency Medical Technician

An Advanced EMT (AEMT) has additional training in skills such as patient assessment, administering intravenous (IV) fluids and medications, and performing advanced airway procedures.

You Should Know

Advanced EMTs were formerly known as EMT-Intermediates.

Paramedic

A Paramedic can perform the skills of an AEMT and has had additional instruction in pathophysiology (changes in the body caused by disease), physical examination techniques, assessing abnormal heart rhythms using a heart monitor, and invasive procedures.

You Should Know

EMRs and EMTs provide basic emergency care. They are referred to as Basic Life Support, or BLS, personnel. Advanced EMTs and Paramedics provide more advanced care than EMRs and EMTs. They are often referred to as Advanced Life Support, or ALS, personnel.

You Should Know

First There, First Care

Seconds count in an emergency. A bystander who knows how to access the EMS system and give basic first aid until EMS arrives can help save a life. Realizing the importance of bystander care, the Health Resources and Services Administration (HRSA) and National NHTSA developed the *First There, First Care* program. The program encourages Americans to take five steps when they come upon an injured person:

1. Stop to help
2. Call for help
3. Assess the victim
4. Start the breathing
5. Stop the bleeding

Transportation

It has been estimated that EMS treats and transports more than 20 million patients per year in the United States. **Emergency transportation** is the process of moving a patient from the scene of an emergency to an appropriate healthcare facility. Healthcare facilities include hospitals, urgent care centers, physicians' offices, and other medical facilities. All patients who need transport must be moved safely in a properly staffed and equipped vehicle. Ground ambulances staffed by qualified emergency medical personnel are used to transport most patients (Figure 1-2). Patients with more serious injuries or illnesses may require transportation by helicopter (Figure 1-3). Boats and fixed-wing aircraft are other forms of transportation that are used in some areas.

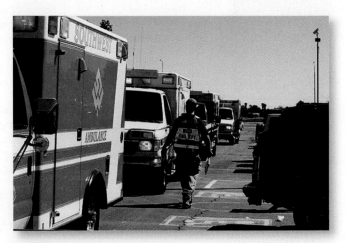

FIGURE 1-2 ▲ Most patients can be effectively transported in a ground ambulance staffed by qualified emergency medical personnel. © *The McGraw-Hill Companies, Inc./Carin Marter, photographer.*

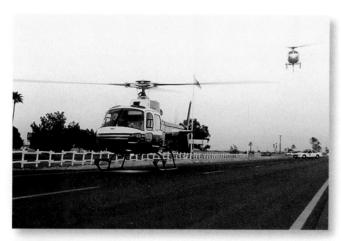

FIGURE 1-3 ▲ Patients with more serious injuries or illnesses may require rapid transportation by air medical services. © *Courtesy of Air Evac Services, Phoenix, Arizona.*

Medical Oversight

Objective 6

A physician oversees all aspects of patient care in an EMS system. In the United States, the medical care provided to patients by physicians is closely governed by laws called **medical practice acts.** These laws vary greatly from state to state and may address the ability of physicians to delegate certain skills and tasks to non-physicians, including EMTs, AEMTs, and Paramedics.

Medical oversight is the process by which a physician directs the emergency care provided by EMS personnel to an ill or injured patient. Medical oversight is also referred to as *medical control* or *medical direction.* Every EMS system *must* have medical oversight. The physician who provides medical oversight is called the **medical director.** The emergency care you give may be considered an extension of the medical director's authority; however, this may vary by state law. The medical director is responsible for making sure that the emergency care provided to ill or injured patients is medically appropriate. The two types of medical oversight are on-line and off-line.

On-Line Medical Direction

On-line medical direction, also called *direct* or *concurrent medical direction*, is direct communication with a physician by radio or telephone—or face-to-face communication at the scene—before performing a skill or administering care (Figure 1-4).

Off-Line Medical Direction

Off-line medical direction, also referred to as *indirect, prospective,* or *retrospective medical direction*, is the medical supervision of EMS personnel, using policies, treatment protocols, standing orders, education, and quality management reviews.

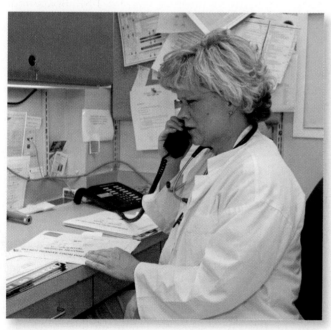
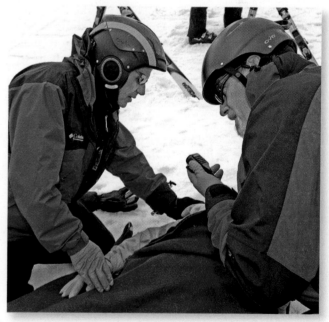

FIGURE 1-4 ▲ On-line medical direction is direct communication with a physician by radio or telephone, or by face-to-face communication at the scene.

Prospective Medical Direction

Prospective medical direction refers to activities performed by a physician medical director before an emergency call. Because it is impossible for the medical director to be physically present at every emergency, treatment protocols and standing orders are developed by the medical director, usually with the assistance of a local EMS advisory group. The development of treatment protocols and standing orders are examples of prospective medical direction.

Treatment Protocols   A **treatment protocol** is a list of steps to be followed when providing emergency care to an ill or injured patient. For example, a patient experiencing a heat-related illness may be treated by using the steps outlined in a Heat-Related Emergencies treatment protocol.

Standing Orders   **Standing orders** are written orders that allow EMS personnel to perform certain medical procedures before making direct contact with a physician. Most protocols and standing orders are consistent with state and national standards and regional guidelines.

Standing orders are used in critical situations in which a delay in treatment would most likely result in harm to the patient. They may also be used when technical or logistical problems delay establishing online communication. Direct communication with a physician should be made as soon as the patient's condition allows.

Retrospective Medical Direction

Retrospective medical direction refers to activities performed by a physician after an emergency call. The physician (or his designee) may review the documentation related to the call. This review is done as part of an ongoing quality management program to make sure that appropriate medical care was given to the patient.

Facilities

An ill or injured patient receives definitive care in the hospital. Seriously ill or injured patients must be delivered in a timely manner to the closest *appropriate* healthcare facility. Hospital care includes many specialties and patient care resources. When the patient arrives at the hospital by ambulance, healthcare professionals from the hospital's Emergency Department continue the care begun by EMTs (Figure 1-5). The patient is usually first seen by a nurse, who quickly assesses the severity of the patient's illness or injury, and then by a physician. The patient may be seen by other members of the healthcare team, depending on the patient's illness or injury and the resources of the receiving facility.

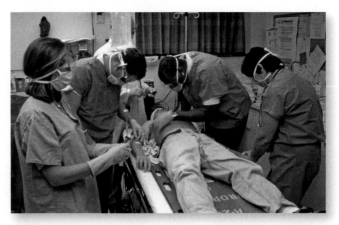

FIGURE 1-5 ▲ When the patient arrives at the hospital by ambulance, healthcare professionals from the hospital's Emergency Department continue the care begun by EMTs.

Remember This!

The healthcare facility closest to the scene of an emergency is not always the most appropriate facility.

Members of the healthcare team who are available at most hospitals include physicians and physician assistants, nurses and nurse practitioners, respiratory therapists, and laboratory and radiology technicians. Additional resources available within the hospital include surgery and intensive care, among many others.

Specialty Centers

Some hospitals provide routine and emergency care but may specialize in the care of certain conditions or emergencies. Specialty centers have resources available, such as trained personnel and equipment, to help provide the best possible care for the patient's illness or injury. A Trauma Center is one type of specialty center (Figure 1-6). In a Trauma Center, specially trained personnel and equipment are available 24 hours a day to care for patients with serious injuries. Other types of specialty centers are shown in Table 1-4.

You Should Know

In both urban and rural areas, a patient may be stabilized at a closer hospital and then transferred to a specialty center if the patient requires care beyond that available at the initial receiving facility.

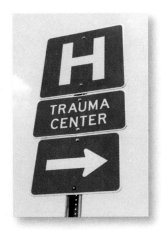
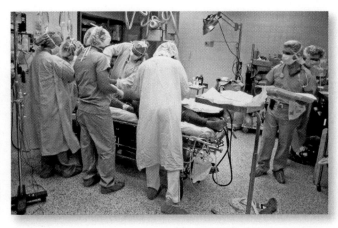

FIGURE 1-6 ▲ A Trauma Center is a specialty facility with trained personnel and equipment available 24 hours a day to care for seriously injured patients.

TABLE 1-4 Types of Specialty Centers

Burn Centers	Burn centers specialize in the care of burns ranging from relatively mild to life-threatening burn injuries. Services include helping the patient and family with the emotional stress that often comes with a burn injury and daily assistance with exercise, scar control, wound care, splinting, and activities of daily living.
Heart/Cardiovascular Centers	Heart and cardiovascular centers specialize in treating disorders of the heart and blood vessels.
Hyperbaric Centers	Hyperbaric centers specialize in hyperbaric oxygen (HBO) therapy, which uses the administration of 100% oxygen at a controlled pressure (greater than sea level) for a set amount of time. Carbon monoxide poisoning and smoke inhalation are two conditions that may be treated with HBO therapy.
Pediatric Centers	Pediatric centers have trained professionals that recognize the medical, developmental, and emotional needs of children. Children are not just small adults. Their bodies are different, and the illnesses and injuries they experience often produce signs and symptoms that differ from those of an adult.
Perinatal Centers	Perinatal centers specialize in the care of high-risk pregnancies.
Poison Centers	Poison centers specialize in providing information in the treatment of poisonings and drug interactions. Some poison centers also provide education programs for medical professionals and the public about responding to biological and chemical terrorist incidents, as well as to nonterrorist incidents, such as epidemics and hazardous material incidents.
Spinal Cord Injury Centers	Spinal cord injury centers specialize in the medical, surgical, rehabilitative, and long-term follow-up care of the patient with a spinal cord injury.
Stroke Centers	Stroke centers specialize in diagnosing and treating diseases of the blood vessels of the brain. A stroke occurs when blood vessels to a part of the brain suddenly burst or become blocked. The staff at a stroke center work very quickly to determine the cause of the stroke, where it is located, and give appropriate care.

Rehabilitation Services

Soon after their condition has been stabilized and they have been moved from the Emergency Department, some patients will require the services of healthcare professionals who specialize in rehabilitation. These healthcare professionals include rehabilitation nurses, physicians, physical therapists, occupational therapists, and social workers who work with the patient and family to return the ill or injured patient to his or her previous state of health.

Making a Difference

To be sure that your patient receives the best possible care for his illness or injury, you must be familiar with the capabilities of the healthcare facilities in your area.

Public Education and Prevention

Every EMS system should be actively involved in public education. EMTs are healthcare professionals. Healthcare professionals have a responsibility to educate the public. As an EMT, you should be actively involved in educating the public about how and when to call EMS and how to prevent illness and injuries (Figure 1-7). Public education and injury prevention programs often lead to more appropriate use of EMS resources. CPR and first aid programs can improve a citizen's ability to recognize an emergency and provide appropriate care until more advanced care arrives.

You Should Know

Examples of Injury Prevention Programs
- Bicycle safety
- Child passenger safety
- Safe boating
- Poisoning prevention
- Fire-related injury prevention
- Dog bite prevention
- Drowning prevention
- Fireworks injury prevention
- Fall injury prevention for older adults
- Playground injury prevention

Evaluation
Quality Management
Objective 5

EMS systems use quality management programs to determine the effectiveness of the service provided. **Quality management** is a system of internal and external reviews and audits of all aspects of an EMS system.

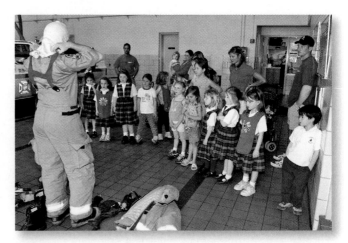

FIGURE 1-7 ▲ As an EMT, you should be actively involved in educating the public on how to access the EMS system and how to prevent injuries.

Quality management is used to identify areas of the EMS system needing improvement and to make sure that patients receive the highest quality medical care. Each state must have a program to review and improve the effectiveness of EMS services provided to adults, infants, and children.

You Should Know

The goal of an EMS quality management program is to consistently provide timely medical care that is appropriate, compassionate, cost-effective, and beneficial for the patient.

Your Role in the Quality Management Process

Quality management involves the constant monitoring of performance and is an important part of EMS. It includes:

- Obtaining information from the patient, other EMS professionals, and facility personnel about the quality and appropriateness of the medical care you provided
- Reviewing and evaluating your documentation of an emergency call (Figure 1-8)
- Evaluating your ability to properly perform skills
- Evaluating your professionalism during interactions with the patient, EMS professionals, and other healthcare personnel
- Evaluating your ability to follow policies and protocols
- Evaluating your participation in continuing education opportunities

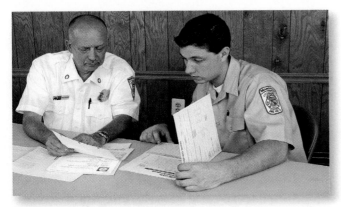

FIGURE 1-8 ▲ Quality management is an important part of EMS and involves constant monitoring of performance.

Making a Difference

Your commitment to and participation in the quality management process is important in improving the EMS system. When your medical director or another healthcare professional provides you with feedback about an area monitored by the process, be sure to maintain a positive and professional attitude. Use the information shared as an opportunity for personal and professional growth.

Phases of a Typical EMS Response

When an emergency occurs, a bystander frequently recognizes the event and activates the EMS system by calling 9-1-1 or another emergency number (Figure 1-9).

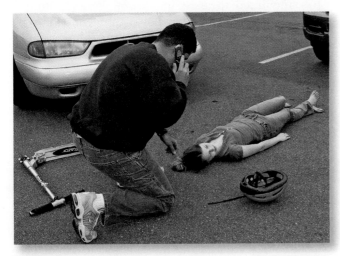

FIGURE 1-9 ▲ When an emergency occurs, a bystander frequently recognizes the event and activates the EMS system.

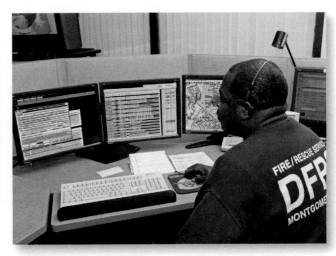

FIGURE 1-10 ▲ While in contact with the EMS dispatcher, the bystander is often provided with instructions regarding how to administer basic first aid.

The EMS dispatcher gathers information and activates an appropriate EMS response based on the information received. The bystander is often provided with instructions about how to provide basic first aid, including CPR if necessary (Figure 1-10).

On the way to the scene, EMTs prepare for the patient and situation based on the information given by the dispatcher. They consider a number of factors, including:

- The number of patients
- Possible problems in gaining access to the patient
- Scene safety
- Potential complications that could result from the patient's reported illness or injury
- The equipment and supplies that will need to be brought to the patient to begin emergency care

Upon arriving at the scene, EMTs quickly "size up" the scene to find out if it is safe to enter. A **scene size-up** is done to:

- Find out if the scene is safe
- Identify the mechanism of injury or the nature of the illness
- Identify the total number of patients
- Request additional help if necessary

The EMTs will be looking for hazards or potential hazards such as downed electrical lines, possible hazardous materials, traffic hazards, unstable vehicles, signs of violence or potential violence, and weather hazards (Figure 1-11). Scene size-up is discussed in more detail in Chapter 8.

The phases of a typical EMS response are shown in Figure 1-12 and listed in Table 1-5.

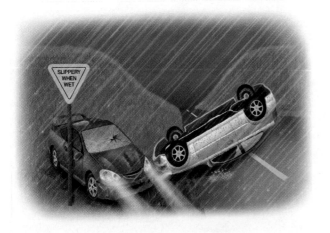

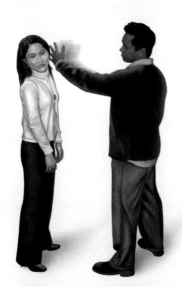

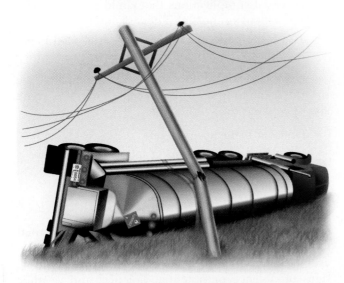

FIGURE 1-11 ▲ Arriving EMTs quickly evaluate the safety of the scene, looking for hazards or potential hazards.

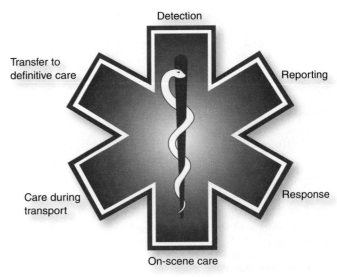

FIGURE 1-12 ▲ Phases of a typical EMS response.

TABLE 1-5   Phases of a Typical EMS Response

- Detection of the emergency
- Reporting the emergency (the call made for assistance, dispatch)
- Dispatch/response (medical resources sent to the scene)
- On-scene care
- Care during transport
- Transfer to definitive care

Stop and Think!

If the scene is not safe and you cannot make it safe, *do not enter.* If a safe scene becomes unsafe, leave. Lives have been lost when a well-meaning rescuer has attempted to assist in an emergency without enough training, assistance, or equipment. Contact the dispatcher for additional equipment/personnel if needed.

After making sure that the scene is safe, EMTs quickly perform a **patient assessment** to find out the seriousness of the patient's condition or the extent of injuries (Figure 1-13). Assessment is important to determine the emergency medical care the patient requires. EMTs provide safe and efficient emergency medical care.

You Should Know

You must know the locations of the healthcare facilities in your area and their capabilities to determine the most appropriate facility to which the patient should be transported.

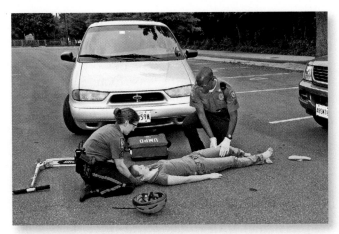

FIGURE 1-13 ▲ After making sure the scene is safe, EMTs quickly assess the patient to find out the seriousness of the patient's condition or extent of injuries.

If more highly trained medical professionals arrive at the scene, EMTs give the arriving personnel a brief description of the emergency and a summary of the care provided before transferring patient care (Figure 1-14). If the patient's condition requires further emergency care, EMTs help lift the stretcher and place the patient into an ambulance. EMTs assess the patient often and give additional emergency care as needed en route to an appropriate receiving facility, such as a hospital, for definitive care (Figure 1-15). EMT may be required to assist ALS personnel as the patient is transferred to the receiving facility.

On arrival at the receiving facility, EMTs help lift and carry the patient out of the ambulance and into the receiving facility. The EMTs give a brief description of the emergency and a summary of the care provided to a healthcare professional with the same or greater level of medical training. Patient care is

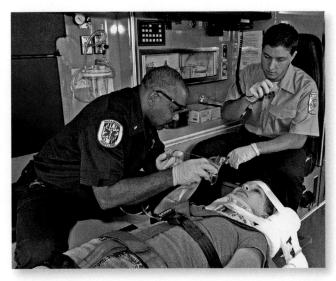

FIGURE 1-15 ▲ If the patient's condition requires further emergency care, the patient is loaded into an ambulance and transported to an appropriate receiving facility, such as a hospital.

then transferred (Figure 1-16). After documentation of the call is finished, supplies are restocked. EMTs restock and replace used linens, blankets and other supplies that were used during the emergency call. They also clean all equipment using appropriate disinfecting procedures. EMTs carefully check all equipment to make sure the vehicle is ready for the next call. They make sure that the emergency vehicle is clean, washed, and kept in neat, orderly condition. The inside of the vehicle is disinfected as needed in accordance with federal, state, or local regulations.

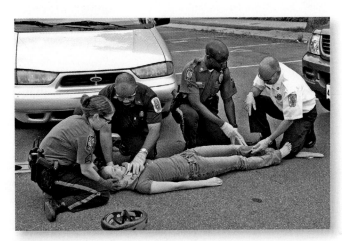

FIGURE 1-14 ▲ If more highly trained medical professionals arrive at the scene, a brief description of the emergency and a summary of the care provided are given before transferring patient care.

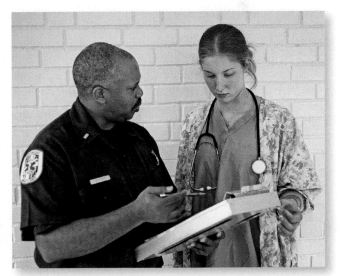

FIGURE 1-16 ▲ On arrival at the receiving facility, a brief description of the emergency and a summary of the care provided are given to a healthcare professional with the same or higher level of medical training before transferring patient care.

After the call is completed, a review may be held with the other members of the EMS crew to discuss what went well and what can go better in the future. The review also identifies opportunities for improving patient care at the scene and during transport.

Your Roles and Responsibilities as an EMT

You have many roles and responsibilities as an EMT. When you are dispatched to the scene of an emergency, you are expected to respond promptly and provide competent medical care to the ill and injured.

No matter where they work, EMTs are expected to provide the same standard of care in an emergency. **Standard of care** refers to the minimum level of care expected of similarly trained healthcare professionals. In other words, you are expected to provide the same level of care as another EMT with similar training and experience in similar circumstances.

Your Role as an EMT

Safety

Objective 3, 4

Although the patient's well-being is an important concern at the scene of an emergency, your personal safety *must* be your primary concern, followed by the safety of your crew, patients, and bystanders. When you are notified of an emergency, prepare for the patient and the situation on the basis of the information given to you. If you are responsible for driving an emergency vehicle, drive to the address or location given using the most expeditious route, depending on traffic and weather. Be sure to observe traffic laws and regulations regarding emergency vehicle operation. On arrival at the scene, park the emergency vehicle in a safe location to avoid additional injury.

Remember This!

Before approaching the patient, make sure the scene is safe for you to provide care.

When you arrive at the scene and before you begin patient care, size up the scene. You should first determine if the scene is safe. You should then identify the mechanism of the injury or the nature of the illness, identify the total number of patients, and request additional help if necessary. Before approaching the patient, put on appropriate personal protective

equipment (PPE). This helps reduce your risk of exposure to potentially infectious body fluid substances or other infectious agents (see Chapter 2). If law enforcement personnel are not present on the scene, create a safe traffic environment. This may require placing safety cones, removing debris, or redirecting traffic to protect the injured and those who are helping with their care.

Stop and Think!

Safety Priorities
1. Personal safety
2. Crew safety
3. Patient safety
4. Bystander safety

Gaining Access to the Patient

You must gain access to the patient in order to perform a **patient assessment** and provide emergency care. In some situations, you may need additional resources at the scene such as law enforcement personnel, the fire department, a utility company, or a special rescue team. In these situations, be sure to notify the dispatcher as soon as possible of the need for these resources.

If the patient has been involved in a motor vehicle crash, you must make sure the scene is safe and provide necessary care to the patient before **extrication.** You must also make sure that the patient is removed in a way that minimizes further injury. To accomplish these tasks, you will need to work closely with the rescuers responsible for extrication.

Remember This!

Patient care comes before extrication unless a delay in movement would endanger the life of the patient or rescuer.

Patient Assessment

After reaching the patient, you must perform a systematic assessment to determine what is wrong and quickly identify life-threatening conditions. Gather information about the emergency by observing the scene, speaking with the patient and bystanders, and assessing the patient. Find out who called 9-1-1.

As an EMT, you will give emergency medical care to adults, children, and infants on the basis of your findings. Depending on the patient's illness or injury, you may need to perform certain skills, including:

- Opening and maintaining an airway
- Ventilating the patient
- Providing CPR
- Operating an automated external defibrillator (AED; an AED delivers an electrical shock to the heart)
- Providing emergency medical care for victims of trauma, such as controlling bleeding, bandaging wounds, and manually stabilizing injured limbs
- Assisting in childbirth
- Assisting patients with respiratory, cardiac, diabetic, allergic, behavioral, and environmental emergencies, and suspected poisonings
- Assisting patients with prescribed medications, including sublingual nitroglycerin, epinephrine auto-injectors, and handheld aerosol inhalers
- Administering oxygen, oral glucose, and activated charcoal when indicated

Making a Difference

Once you begin emergency care, you must continue that care until:

- An individual with medical training equal to or greater than your own assumes responsibility for the patient *or*
- You are physically unable to continue providing care because of exhaustion *or*
- There is a change in the scene that weakens or endangers your physical well-being

Lifting and Moving Patients Safely

Your help may be needed to lift and move patients. For example, an unresponsive man who is found on the floor of his home will need to be lifted onto a stretcher and then into an ambulance. You must make sure that the patient and stretcher are secured in the ambulance before beginning transport. On arrival at the receiving facility, your help will be needed when removing the patient and stretcher from the ambulance and into the receiving facility. Your help may also be needed to move the patient from your stretcher to a hospital stretcher or bed.

To lift and move a patient safely, you must know about body mechanics, lifting and carrying techniques, and principles of moving patients. You must also be familiar with equipment used for lifting and moving. Lifting and moving techniques are discussed in Chapter 6.

Stop and Think!

Back injuries are common among EMS personnel. Remember: your personal safety comes first. Keep yourself (and your back) safe by learning and using proper lifting and moving techniques.

Transport/Transfer of Care

Some patients will require only Basic Life Support (BLS) care. In these situations, you will transport the patient to a healthcare facility. Other patients will require a level of care beyond that which you can give. In these situations, contact dispatch as soon as you recognize the need for advanced level care. Provide what emergency care you can and prepare the patient for transport.

You Should Know

Patients who require ALS care should be transported to the hospital without delay. When an ALS unit is called to assist a BLS unit, it is called an *ALS intercept.*

Quickly decide where you will meet the ALS unit. In some cases, the ALS unit will meet you at the scene of the emergency. However, it is sometimes necessary for you to begin transport to the receiving facility and have the ALS unit meet you at a prearranged location. This is most likely to occur when the arrival of the ALS unit to the scene is estimated to be longer than your transport time to the hospital.

Remember This!

Remember the four Cs when giving a verbal report: **C**ourteous, **C**lear, **C**omplete, and **C**oncise.

When transferring patient care to a healthcare professional with medical training equal to or greater than your own, first identify yourself as an EMT. Then give the receiving healthcare professional a brief explanation about what happened, the position in which the patient was found, your assessment findings, the emergency care you gave, and the patient's response to the treatment given.

Record Keeping/Data Collection

Documentation is an important aspect of prehospital care. Information contained in a prehospital care report (PCR) is used for many purposes (see Chapter 11). Your documentation of an EMS call must be accurate, complete, and concise. Other healthcare professionals will use the information contained in your report to note changes in the patient's condition. Changes in the patient's condition are particularly important to healthcare personnel assuming care of the patient. Your documentation should reflect what you saw and heard at the scene. It should also include the emergency care you gave and the patient's response to that care.

Some of the information contained in the PCR is used for data collection and research purposes. For example, data such as the time you were dispatched to a call, arrived on the scene, and left the scene en route to the hospital are used for quality management purposes. With this information, the quality management program can determine how long EMS units are taking to respond to calls and how much time is being spent on the scene.

Interagency Liaison

As an EMT, you will be working with persons from many other community resources. Examples of community resources include:

- Public safety agencies
- Public health departments
- Social service agencies and organizations
- Healthcare networks
- Community health educators

You will often work with public safety personnel, including police officers, firefighters, and other EMS professionals. You will be an important link in your community's healthcare system. The information you give members of these organizations about the first few minutes after the emergency will be helpful to provide continuation of patient care following the emergency response. Consider this real-life example. You are called to the home of a 93-year-old man for "difficulty breathing." When you arrive, you find the patient's home in complete disarray. He lives alone with his dog. The animal appears malnourished. The temperature outside is about 27°F and it is very cold in the patient's home. While you begin caring for the patient, your partner notices that the patient's pantry is bare. The refrigerator contains one item—a carton of milk that was outdated three weeks ago. The patient tells you he has not been feeling well for the past few days and has been too weak to go to the store for food. Because he lives on a fixed income, he does not want to turn the heat on in his home. In situations such as this, it will be important for you to relay what you saw at the scene to the healthcare professionals at the hospital who will provide further patient care. The hospital has access to many resources that can help improve the patient's situation.

Patient Advocacy

One of your responsibilities as an EMT is to serve as the patient's advocate. An advocate is a person who supports another. You must protect the patient from further injury. If the patient is unable to speak, you must be his voice and act in his best interests. You must protect the patient's rights, privacy, and dignity. For example, if it is necessary to remove the patient's clothing to assess him, you must make sure that the patient is shielded from the view of others. If bystanders ask you questions about a patient's illness or injury, you must protect the patient's privacy and not give out that information.

Your Responsibilities as an EMT

You will be expected to accept and uphold the responsibilities of an EMT according to the standards of an EMS professional. These responsibilities include preserving life, relieving suffering, promoting health, and doing no harm. You must respect and hold in confidence all information of a confidential nature that was obtained in the course of your work as an EMT, unless you are required by law to report the information.

It is not appropriate to judge a patient or vary the care you provide because of a patient's race, ethnicity, national origin, religion, gender, age, mental or physical disability, sexual orientation, or ability to pay for the care provided. The emergency medical care you provide as an EMT must be based on the patient's needs without regard to any of these factors. Every patient has the right to expect competent, considerate, respectful care from every member of the healthcare team at all times and under all circumstances (Figure 1-17).

Many patient complaints about medical care result from the patient's belief that he or she was not treated with respect. As an EMS professional, you have an obligation to do the following:

- Respect each patient as an individual
- Provide emergency medical care to every patient to the best of your ability
- Listen attentively to your patients and take their concerns and complaints seriously

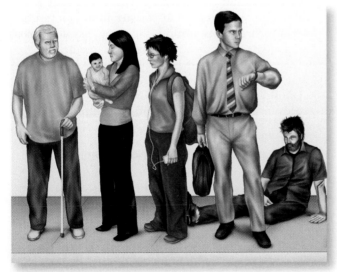

FIGURE 1-17 ▲ Healthcare personnel, including EMTs, must give all patients competent, considerate, and respectful care at all times and under all circumstances.

- Provide clear explanations
- Provide patients with emotional support to help ease fear and anxiety
- Preserve each patient's dignity during examinations

Personal Health and Safety

Your job as an EMT has physical demands that require stamina and endurance. You will have to walk, stand, and assist in lifting and carrying ill or injured patients who may weigh more than 125 pounds (250 pounds, with assistance). Climbing and balancing may be required to gain access to the patient, such as on stairs or a hillside. You may also have to help transport the patient safely. In some situations, the patient may be found in a location where patient assessment is possible only if you stoop, kneel, crouch, or crawl.

To make sure that your well-being, as well as that of the patient and your coworkers, is not at risk in these situations, you must first take care of yourself. Maintain your personal health by exercising regularly. Exercise prepares you to handle the physical demands of the job by improving muscle tone and circulation. Exercise also provides a physical release for stress. Getting enough sleep, rest, and good nutrition are important to staying healthy and doing your job well.

Making a Difference

Personal Traits of an EMS Professional
- Professional appearance, attitude, and conduct
- Professional oral and written communications
- Mastery of EMS knowledge and skills
- Confidence and leadership abilities
- Compassionate patient advocacy
- Good moral character
- Ability to use sound judgment in adapting to situations

Attitude and Communication

As an EMT, it is important that you possess and maintain a caring attitude. When you arrive at the patient's side, begin by introducing yourself: "Hello. My name is _____, and I am an Emergency Medical Technician. I am here to help you. What is your name?" An older adult should be addressed by his or her last name with Mr., Mrs., or Ms. Be considerate of your patient's personal space, physical condition, and feelings. **Personal space** refers to the invisible area immediately around each of us that we declare as our own.

TABLE 1-6 Common Zones of Personal Space in the United States

Zone	Distance	Notes
Public space	12 feet or more	Impersonal contact with others occurs in this space
Social space	4-12 feet	Much of a patient interview occurs at this distance
Personal space	1½-4 feet	Much of a physical assessment occurs at this distance
Intimate space	Touching to 1½ feet	This space is best for assessing breath and other body odors

Source: Tamparo CT, Lindh WQ, *Therapeutic Communications for Health Professionals*, 2nd ed. (Thomson Learning, 2000), pp. 31–32.

The size of your personal space can change depending on your cultural norms and who you are with, but you may feel threatened when others invade your personal space without your consent.

When talking with a patient, it is important to consider the distance between you and the patient and recognize that a "comfortable distance" differs among cultures. For example, the Japanese typically have a larger personal space than North Americans do, whereas Italians have a much smaller one. Examples of the personal space common in the United States are listed in Table 1-6.

Many of the tasks you will perform as an EMT will often occur within the boundaries of another's personal space. It is helpful to take the time to explain procedures that intrude on that personal space before beginning the procedure. If you do not, the patient may become agitated, nervous, or even aggressive because of your actions.

Composure

Many emergency calls involve minor injuries, and the medical care that is required is straightforward. However, you will come across situations involving life-threatening injuries, as well as patients and family members who are upset. As an EMT, others will look to you as the person in control of the situation. Even though you may feel anxious, you must be able to adapt to these situations, remain calm, and display confidence.

Making a Difference

Your contact with the patient, family, bystanders, and other members of the healthcare team must be respectful and professional, even in stressful or chaotic situations.

Appearance

It has been said that you never get a second chance to make a good first impression. As an EMT, you will meet individuals who are experiencing a medical emergency. In 30 seconds or less, each of them will form an opinion about you based on what they see, hear, and sense. When you approach a patient and prepare to provide needed emergency care, you are expecting the patient to place his or her trust in you. Presenting a neat, clean, and professional appearance invites trust. It also instills confidence, enhances cooperation, and brings a sense of order to an emergency.

Making a Difference

The patient, the patient's family, and bystanders often view the attention you pay to your appearance as a reflection of your care. If you are courteous and respectful and present a professional appearance, they are reassured that you will provide quality patient care. If you are ill mannered or your appearance is untidy, they may assume that the care you provide will be of poor quality.

Good personal hygiene is essential to presenting a professional appearance. It includes the following:

- Bathing daily
- Using a deodorant or antiperspirant
- Making sure your hair is clean and, if long, restrained so that is will not fall into open wounds or into your working space
- Making sure that your fingernails are clean and neatly trimmed

Good grooming includes making sure that your uniform is clean, mended, and fits well. Shoes should be clean and comfortable, provide support, and fit properly. You should wear a watch with a second hand for timing things such as a patient's heart rate, breathing rate, and labor pains. Because they may be offensive and nauseating to patients, fragrances should not be worn.

Maintaining Knowledge and Skills

Your EMT education does not end with completing the EMT course. As a healthcare professional, you must keep your knowledge and skills current through continuing education (CE) and refresher courses. CE and refresher courses are helpful because they assist you in keeping the skills and knowledge you learned during your initial training. CE and refresher courses also provide information about advances in medicine, skills, and equipment. In addition, they educate you about changes in local protocols and national guidelines that affect EMS.

CE may occur in different forms and includes skill labs, lectures and workshops, conferences and seminars, case reviews and/or quality management reviews, reading professional journals, and reviewing videotapes and/or audiotapes.

Making a Difference

Responsibilities of the Emergency Medical Technician
- Personal health and safety
- Composure and a caring attitude
- Neat, clean, and professional appearance
- Up-to-date knowledge and skills
- Current knowledge of local, state, and national issues affecting EMS

Specific Statutes and Regulations

Objective 7

Statutes are laws established by Congress and state legislatures. Every state has statutes that establish an EMS regulatory body and describe how its EMS personnel are licensed or certified. **Licensure** is the granting of a written authorization by an official or legal authority. It allows a person to perform medical acts and procedures not permitted without the authorization. **Certification** is a designation that ensures a person has met predetermined requirements to perform a particular activity.

State laws also detail the medical procedures and functions that can be legally performed by a licensed or certified healthcare professional, called the **scope of practice**. Because EMS statutes vary from state to state, ask your instructor about the laws in your area that affect you as an EMT.

EMT Certification

To be certified as an EMT, state agencies require successful completion of an EMT course that follows the DOT EMT National Standard Curriculum (or National EMS Education Standards). The NREMT provides examinations for certification and registration that may be required by your state. Recognition as a nationally registered EMT requires successful completion of a written and practical skills examination.

Certification as an EMT is good for a limited time, usually two years. Participation in CE courses or an EMT Refresher Course is required for recertification.

On the Scene   Wrap-Up

After making sure the scene is safe to enter, you quickly turn the engine off and free the patient's hand. You then lay him down in a safe area and control the bleeding. Your Paramedic partner assesses the patient and then starts an intravenous line. You check the patient's breathing rate, heart rate, and blood pressure and relay that information to your partner. After the Paramedic gives him some pain medicine, the patient's face relaxes. The patient is then transported to a trauma center, where two of his fingers are successfully reattached. He stops in to thank you two weeks later on his way home from a rehabilitation session. ∎

Sum It Up

▶ An EMT is a member of the EMS team who provides prehospital emergency care.

▶ A healthcare system is a network of people, facilities, and equipment designed to provide for the general medical needs of the population.

▶ The EMS system is part of the healthcare system. It consists of a coordinated network of resources that provides emergency care and transportation to victims of sudden illness and injury.

▶ There are four levels of nationally recognized prehospital professionals: EMR, EMT, AEMT, and Paramedic. EMRs and EMTs provide Basic Life Support. AEMTs and Paramedics provide Advanced Life Support.

▶ Every EMS system must have a medical director. A medical director is a physician who provides medical oversight and is responsible for making sure that the emergency care provided to ill or injured patients is medically appropriate.

▶ Medical oversight may be on-line or off-line. On-line medical direction is direct communication with a physician by radio or telephone, or face-to-face communication at the scene before a skill is performed or care is given. Off-line medical direction is the medical supervision of EMS personnel using policies, treatment protocols, standing orders, education, and quality management review.

▶ Quality management is a system of internal and external reviews and audits of all aspects of an EMS system. Quality management is used to identify areas of the EMS system needing improvement. This system helps to make sure that the patient receives the highest quality medical care.

▶ The phases of a typical EMS response include detection of the emergency, reporting the emergency (the call made for assistance, dispatch), dispatch/response (medical resources sent to the scene), on-scene care, care during transport, and transfer to definitive care.

▶ The roles of an EMT include personal, crew, patient, and bystander safety; gaining access to the patient; performing a patient assessment to identify life-threatening conditions; continuing care through additional EMS resources; providing initial patient care based on the assessment findings; assisting with additional emergency care; documenting the emergency per local and state requirements; and acting as a public safety liaison.

▶ The responsibilities of an EMT include personal health and safety; maintaining a caring attitude and composure; maintaining a neat, clean, and professional appearance; maintaining up-to-date knowledge and skills; and maintaining current knowledge of local, state, and national issues affecting EMS.

▶ EMTs are subject to state laws that specify the medical procedures and functions that can be performed. Recognition as a nationally registered EMT, which is known as certification, requires successful completion of a written and practical skills examination. Participating in CE courses or an EMT Refresher Course is required for recertification.

2 The Well-Being of the Emergency Medical Technician

By the end of this chapter, you should be able to:

Knowledge Objectives ▷

1. List possible emotional reactions that the Emergency Medical Technician (EMT) may experience when faced with trauma, illness, death, and dying.
2. Discuss the possible reactions that a family member may exhibit when confronted with death and dying.
3. State the steps in the EMT's approach to the family confronted with death and dying.
4. State the possible reactions that the family of the EMT may exhibit.
5. Recognize the signs and symptoms of critical incident stress.
6. State possible steps that the EMT may take to help reduce or alleviate stress.
7. Explain the need to determine scene safety.
8. Discuss the importance of body substance isolation (BSI) precautions.
9. Describe the steps the EMT should take for personal protection from airborne and bloodborne pathogens.
10. List the personal protective equipment necessary for each of the following situations: hazardous materials, rescue operations, violent scenes, crime scenes, electricity, water and ice, exposure to bloodborne pathogens, exposure to airborne pathogens.

Attitude Objectives ▷

11. Explain the importance for serving as an advocate for the use of appropriate protective equipment.

Skill Objectives ▷

12. Given a scenario with potential infectious exposure, the EMT will use appropriate personal protective equipment. At the completion of the scenario, the EMT will properly remove and discard the protective garments.
13. Given the above scenario, the EMT will complete disinfection/cleaning and all reporting documentation.

It is 3:30 a.m. Your spouse looks frustrated as the familiar beep of your volunteer fire department pager gets progressively louder. "Not again," she groans as you grab your gear and move quickly to your truck. I have to go, you think, noting the address is that of a close friend. You radio your response status and hear other members of your department notify the dispatcher that they are en route. As you walk into the living room past his wife, you see him. Your friend is slumped forward at the kitchen table. He is not aware of your approach. You can feel your heart racing. Your hand trembles as you reach for the carotid pulse. You cannot feel a pulse and note the patient's skin is cold to your touch. His wife looks on as other members of your department help you quickly move the patient to the floor. You note that his limbs are rigid and cold. His wife tells you that she got up to see why her husband had not come to bed and found him in this position at the table. ▪

THINK ABOUT IT

As you read this chapter, think about the following questions:

- How might you respond emotionally to this call?
- How will you approach the patient's wife?
- What methods will you use to tell if you should begin resuscitation?
- What personal protective equipment will you need in this situation?

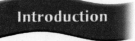

Introduction

Your Well-Being as an Emergency Medical Technician

You will encounter many stressful situations when providing emergency medical care to patients. Some of these situations will include child abuse, trauma, and death. The patients you interact with may be seriously ill or injured. They may be angry, frightened, violent, or withdrawn.

In this chapter, you will learn how to help the patient, the patient's family, your own family, and other Emergency Medical Technicians deal with stress. You will learn to recognize the signs of stress. This chapter will offer you information about how to manage stress through changes in your lifestyle and work environment. You will also learn about the professional resources that you can use to help you deal with stress. Finally, you will learn how to determine that a scene is safe, which will help you lessen your chance of being exposed to infectious disease.

Emotional Aspects of Emergency Medical Care

Stress is a chemical, physical, or emotional factor that causes bodily or mental tension. When you are dealing with an ill or injured person, the patient, the patient's family and friends, and bystanders will expect you to provide excellent medical care. They will also depend on you for emotional support. Each of us responds differently to an emergency. It is important that you learn how to anticipate and recognize the signs and symptoms of stress in yourself and others. You should also know how to manage stress when it occurs.

Stressful Situations

Objective 1

As an EMT, you will encounter stressful situations when providing emergency medical care (Figure 2-1). Examples of stressful situations are listed in Table 2-1.

The delivery of emergency medical care has an emotional impact on the patient, the patient's family,

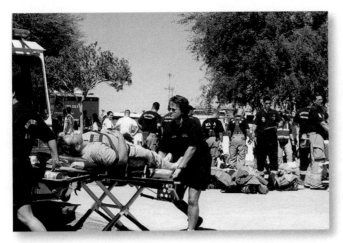

FIGURE 2-1 ▲ EMTs will respond to many different types of stressful situations. © *Courtesy of Tempe Fire Department, Tempe, Arizona.*

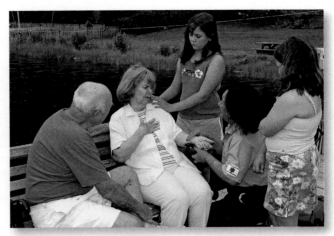

FIGURE 2-2 ▲ The delivery of emergency medical care has an emotional impact on the patient, the patient's family, bystanders, and you.

bystanders, and you. You will rarely witness the actual mishap or violent act that occurred. However, you will be repeatedly exposed to the human suffering and tragedies that result from them.

You may feel emotions such as joy, pride, and contentment when you are able to make a positive difference in a patient's life (Figure 2-2). You may experience emotions such as anger, anxiety, frustration, fear, grief, and feelings of helplessness when you are unable to relieve a patient's suffering or when a patient dies despite your best efforts to resuscitate him. You may feel sick at the sight of a severe injury. You may feel sad or anxious when dealing with a dying patient. These emotions are common and expected. You should not feel embarrassed or ashamed when these situations affect you. As you gain experience, you will learn to recognize and control these feelings while caring for patients. Despite the situation, you must act professionally. You must also be able to work quickly and confidently, think clearly, and make appropriate decisions about your patient's care.

The Stages of Grief

Grief is a normal response that helps a person cope with the loss of someone or something that had great meaning to them. Whereas grief is most often associated with death, *any* change of circumstance can cause us to go through this process (Figure 2-3). How deeply a person feels grief and for how long depends on how important the person believes the loss is. Critically ill or injured patients may experience grief. They may not recognize that they are reacting to the loss of something that was important to them. Knowing about the stages of grief will help you provide appropriate care.

TABLE 2-1 Stressful Situations and Additional Factors That May Cause Stress

Examples of Stressful Situations	Additional Factors That May Cause Stress
• Mass-casualty incidents	• Dangerous situations
• Infant and child trauma	• Challenging locations and terrain
• Death, **terminal illness**	• Weather conditions
• Amputations	• Severe time pressures
• Violence	• Media attention
• Death of a child	
• Infant, child, elder, or spousal abuse	
• Death or injury of a coworker or other public safety personnel	
• Emergency response to illness or injury of a friend or family member	

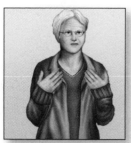 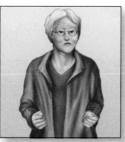 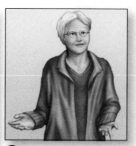 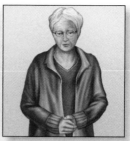 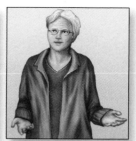

① Denial: "Not me." ② Anger: "Why me?" ③ Bargaining: "OK, but first let me…" ④ Depression: "I don't care anymore." ⑤ Acceptance: "OK, I am not afraid."

FIGURE 2-3 ▲ *Any* change of circumstance can initiate the process of grief.

You Should Know

Changes in Circumstances That Contribute to Grief

- Loss or change in status or environment (for example, retirement or relocation)
- Loss of personal possessions (such as a home destroyed by fire)
- Change in a relationship (separation, divorce, death)
- Loss of a significant other (partner, child, parent, close friend, pet)
- Loss of or change in health (including body part or function, physical or mental capacity)
- Loss of or change in security (financial, social, occupational, cultural)

Grief is a very personal and individual process. It is a natural and inevitable part of our journey through life. Elizabeth Kübler-Ross, a world-famous authority on death and dying, developed a model of the stages of grief that a person typically experiences. Although five stages of grief are presented here, a person may move back and forth between stages (see the following *You Should Know* box). An individual may also skip a stage, go through two or three stages at the same time, go through each stage more than once, or stay in one stage of the process for minutes, hours, days, or longer. Cultural differences will also affect how a person experiences grief.

You Should Know

The 5 Stages of Grief

1. Denial
2. Anger
3. Bargaining
4. Depression
5. Acceptance

Denial

"Not me."

Denial is the first phase of the grieving process. Denial is a defense mechanism. It is used to create a buffer against the shock of dying or dealing with an illness or injury. During this stage of the grief process, the person is unable or refuses to believe the reality of what has happened. The patient may try to ignore or deny the seriousness of his illness or injury. He may dismiss his symptoms with words such as "only" or "a little." During the denial stage, common reactions from the patient or family include "Not me" or "This can't be happening." During this stage, the patient or family member often does not grasp the information you provide about the illness or injury.

When dealing with a patient in this stage of the grief process, try to find a family member or close friend who can give you more information about the patient's illness or injury. The information you receive can help you make appropriate decisions regarding the patient's care.

Anger

"Why me?"

Anger is the second stage of the grief process. The ill or injured person's anger comes from several sources. It can be related to her discomfort, a limitation of activity, or an inability to control the situation. Family, friends, and medical professionals are common targets for blame. The person often experiences guilt and blames herself for either taking or failing to take specific actions ("If only I had…").

In the anger stage, common reactions from the person (or his or her family) include "Why is this happening to me?" The person's anger may be marked by the following:

- Abusive language
- Criticism of anyone who offers help

- Resentment (particularly of those who are healthy)
- Irritability
- Becoming demanding or impatient
- Physical agitation

Stop and Think!

When dealing with an angry person, remember that your safety is your priority. If the scene is not safe and you cannot make it safe, *do not enter.*

When dealing with an angry person, do not take anger or insults personally. Also, do not become defensive. Be tolerant and empathetic, and use good listening and communication skills. Speak to the person in a calm, controlled tone. It is not necessary to agree with the person, but do not challenge how he is feeling. Briefly and honestly explain what he can expect from you as well as what you expect from him.

Bargaining

"OK, but first let me . . ."

Bargaining is the third stage of the grief process. During this stage, the person is willing to do anything to change what is happening to her. The person may bargain with herself, her family, God, or medical professionals. Bargaining reflects the person's need for time to accept the situation. Bargaining is marked by statements such as the following:

- "I promise I'll be a better person if . . ."
- "If I could live to . . ."
- "OK, but first let me . . ."

Depression

"I don't care anymore."

Depression is the fourth stage of the grief process. Depression is a normal response to the loss of a significant other or the loss of some bodily function. Depression may also result from feeling a loss of control over one's destiny.

A depressed person:

- Is sad and usually silent
- Appears withdrawn and indifferent
- May take a long time to perform routine activities
- May have difficulty concentrating and following instructions
- May reject your attempts to help

- May accept your help and then fail to react to your interventions
- Shows a lack of interest

Depression is marked by statements such as, "I don't care anymore." You may feel confused, annoyed, defensive, frustrated, or even angry because of the patient's behavior. It is important to recognize these feelings. However, do not communicate them while caring for your patient. Be supportive and nonjudgmental. Provide whatever care is needed.

Acceptance

"OK, I am not afraid."

The fifth stage of the grief process is acceptance. The person has come to terms with his loss or change in circumstances and is learning to live with it. In the case of the dying patient, he realizes his fate and understands that death is certain. Acceptance does not mean that the patient is happy about dying. Instead, the patient believes that he has done all that is possible in preparing to die. For example, the patient has said what needed to be said and has completed any unfinished business. Acceptance is marked by statements such as "I am ready for whatever comes," "I know I can't change this," and "OK, I am not afraid." Friends or family members may need more support during this stage than the patient.

The Patient's Response to Illness and Injury

What a patient considers an emergency may not appear to be an emergency to a person with medical training. Some medical personnel become irritated or annoyed when they feel they have been summoned to assist a person who does not appear particularly ill or who has a minor complaint. Keep in mind that pain is what the *patient* says it is and an emergency is what the *patient* perceives it to be. As an Emergency Medical Services (EMS) professional, it is important that you accept every call for assistance without prejudice. Provide the best emergency care you can for every patient—without questioning the validity of the complaint.

Because patients react differently to an illness or injury, you must be prepared for a variety of emotions and behaviors (Figure 2-4). Depending on the nature of the illness or the severity of the injury, your patient may experience a number of emotions. Your patient's response to these emotions may be seen as distrust, resentment, despair, anger, or regression. **Regression** is a return to an earlier or former developmental state. For example, an adult patient's behavior may

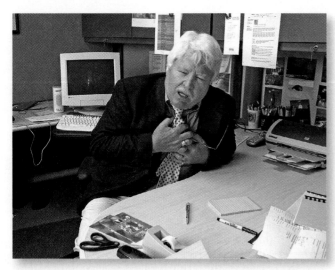

FIGURE 2-4 ▲ As an EMT, you must be prepared for a variety of emotions and behaviors from your patients.

appear childlike. This reaction is common and natural because an ill or injured patient, like a child, depends on others for his or her survival.

It is important to understand these emotions in order to be tolerant of them. For example, a busy executive experiences a heart attack. He may feel helpless because he finds himself dependent on medical professionals, whose experience and skills he cannot easily evaluate. He may be angry because his life has been disrupted. He may experience fear and anxiety because his independence is threatened. He may also wonder what the next few minutes, hours, days,

and months will bring. His concerns might include the following:

- "Why is this happening to me?"
- "Am I going to be disabled?"
- "How will I provide for my family if I can't work?"
- "Am I going to die?"

Dealing with Ill and Injured Patients

Introduce Yourself

Identify yourself and establish your role by saying "My name is Janet. I am an Emergency Medical Technician trained to provide emergency care. I am here to help you."

Treat the Patient with Respect

Recognize the patient's need for privacy, preserve the patient's dignity, and treat him with respect. Most patients are uncomfortable about being examined. In our culture, clothing is ordinarily removed in front of another in situations of trust or intimacy. Be aware that your patient will be anxious about having his clothing removed and having an examination performed by a stranger. Some patients will view these actions as an invasion of their privacy. Help ease your patient's fears by explaining what you are about to do and why it must be done (Figure 2-5). When performing a physical examination, be sure to properly drape or shield an unclothed patient from the stares of others. Conduct the examination professionally and efficiently. Talk with the patient throughout the procedure. These actions will build trust and help reduce the patient's anxiety. If your patient is a child, ask for help from a parent or family member to lessen the child's anxiety.

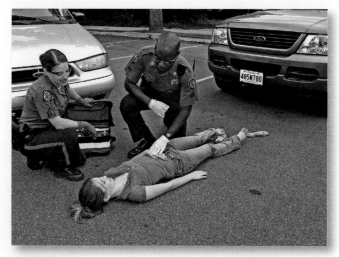

FIGURE 2-5 ▲ Explaining what you are about to do and why it must be done will help ease your patient's fears.

Do not assume that an unresponsive patient cannot hear what is being said. If your patient is unresponsive, speak in a normal tone of voice. Talk to the patient as if he were awake. Provide reassurance, offer words of comfort, and explain what you are doing. Many healthcare professionals have been embarrassed when a patient is successfully resuscitated and is able to accurately relay what was said by those caring for him.

Recognize the Patient's Need for Control

Although many patients will feel a sense of relief when you arrive, the lights, sirens, and flurry of activity involved in providing emergency care can be frightening. Even though your patient may be ill or injured, he will usually feel the need to show his independence. When possible, allow the patient to make choices, such as the hospital to which he prefers to be transported.

Listen with Empathy

Remain calm, be sympathetic, and listen with empathy. **Empathy** means to understand, be aware of, and be sensitive to the feelings, thoughts, and experiences of another. Effective listening requires concentration (Figure 2-6). Do not interrupt before your patient has finished telling you what her problem is. Do not anticipate what the patient is going to say and finish her sentences. Allow the patient time to explain what is wrong in her own words.

Do Not Give False Hope

Do not give false hope or false reassurance. You should not say, "Everything is going to be OK" when that is obviously not true. Similarly, you should not say you understand when you have not had the same experience

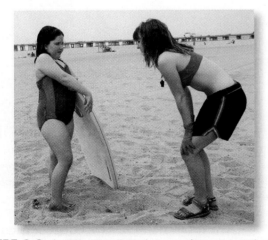

FIGURE 2-6 ▲ Effective listening requires concentration.

Cultural Considerations

Effective communication with persons of different cultures requires sensitivity and awareness. It is important to refrain from using offensive language and to avoid speaking in ways that are disrespectful to your patient's cultural beliefs. For example, you should be aware of the amount of personal space that is considered acceptable, the degree of eye contact considered acceptable, and acceptable touching.

- When speaking with most patients, 18 inches or more between people is usually considered a comfortable distance. Hispanics, Asians, and people from the Middle East generally stand closer together when talking.

- Many American Indians and patients of Mexican descent avoid direct eye contact to show respect. Sustained direct eye contact is considered rude or disrespectful. Mexican-Americans have a high respect for authority and the elderly. They should be addressed formally (by title). The Vietnamese avoid eye contact when speaking with someone they consider an authority figure or someone who is older. European-Americans use firm eye contact and look for the impact of what is being said.

- Hispanics typically find a touch on the arm, shoulder, or back comforting. Asian and Arab patients generally find touch acceptable only between members of the same gender, except within the family. Because Asians consider the area of the body below the waist private, it is almost never exposed. In addition, Asian-Americans prefer to be addressed by position and role, such as "mother" or "teacher." An individual's name is considered private and is used only by family and close friends.

- Mexican-American women may be reluctant to undress, even in the presence of a healthcare professional of the same gender.

- Pacific-Islander (native Hawaiians and Samoans) and Asian-Americans are often reluctant to ask questions or express emotion to others. They may be overly agreeable in their communications. Arab-Americans may be reluctant to reveal information about themselves to strangers. Hispanic-Americans are often vocal about illness or pain.

as your patient. Instead, reassure the patient by saying "We will do everything we can to help."

Use a Reassuring Touch

If appropriate, use a reassuring touch. Touch is a sensitive means of communication. It can be used to express feelings that cannot be expressed well with words. It is important to assess your level of comfort and that of your patient regarding the use of touch. Some healthcare professionals are uncomfortable touching patients to display concern, caring, and reassurance. Most patients will accept a reassuring touch and will respond positively to it. Others are uncomfortable when touched in this way and may misunderstand your intentions. Be sensitive to the patient's acceptance of touch. Learn to recognize when the use of compassionate touch is appropriate.

Responses of Family, Friends, or Bystanders to Injury or Illness

Family members, friends, or bystanders at the scene of an ill or injured patient may have many of the same responses as the patient. Depending on the nature of the illness or the severity of the patient's injury, family members, friends, and bystanders may be anxious, angry, sad, demanding, or impatient. A bystander's anger often results from feelings of guilt. At the scene, the family, friends, or bystanders may pressure you to move the patient to the hospital before you have completed your assessment and provided initial emergency care.

Dealing with the patient's family, friends, or bystanders requires many of the same approaches you use in dealing with patients:

- Identify yourself and take control of the situation. Use a gentle but firm tone of voice and briefly explain what you are doing to help the patient.
- Allow them to have and express their emotions, but do not let them distract you from treating the patient's illness or injury. Accept their concerns and recognize that their behavior stems from grief.
- Comfort them by being sympathetic, listening empathetically, and reassuring them that everything that can be done to help will be done.
- Do not give false hope or reassurance.
- Keep emotionally distraught individuals away from the patient. If possible, assign another EMT to care for them and their grief. You can reduce interference by well-meaning family, friends, and bystanders by assigning them a simple task to keep them occupied. Feeling useful frequently helps to lessen a person's anxiety.

Death and Dying

Dealing with death and dying patients is part of the work of an EMS professional. It is important to understand that dying is a process. Death is an event. A person's attitude about dying and death is influenced by his or her culture, experiences, religion, and age. Your reaction to a situation involving the death of a patient will also depend on the circumstances surrounding the event. It is important to look at your own fears, attitudes, and beliefs about death and dying so you will be prepared when faced with the situation. Doing so can help you understand the needs of the dying patient and his family.

You will encounter situations in which you must determine whether a patient is dead or requires emergency medical care. Dying is a process that may take minutes, hours, days, weeks, or months. As a patient dies, changes occur in the patient's level of responsiveness, breathing, and circulation.

Death occurs when the patient's organs stop functioning. When the patient's heart stops (cardiac arrest), brain death will occur within 4-6 minutes unless circulation is rapidly restored. For this reason, cardiopulmonary resuscitation (CPR) is most effective when started immediately after a cardiac arrest occurs. When you arrive at the scene of a cardiac arrest, CPR should be started immediately if the person is unresponsive, breathless, and without a pulse (heartbeat). CPR should not be started if a valid Do Not Resuscitate (DNR) order is present or in cases of obvious death.

You Should Know

In some Latin-American and Asian-Pacific cultures, a patient may not be told he has a terminal illness. It is believed to upset the patient's inner harmony and that it may hasten the progression of disease or death.

Advance Directives and Do Not Resuscitate Orders

Some patients, such as those who have been diagnosed with a terminal illness, may not want aggressive efforts aimed at reviving them when they are dying. These patients may have an advance directive or a DNR order. An **advance directive** is a legal document that details a person's healthcare wishes when he becomes unable to make decisions for himself. A **Do Not Resuscitate order** is an order written by a physician. It instructs medical professionals not to provide medical care to a patient who has experienced a cardiac arrest.

If you arrive on the scene of a cardiac arrest, begin CPR if:

- A DNR order is not present
- There are no signs of obvious death
- A DNR order is present but the DNR documentation is unclear
- A DNR order is present but you are not sure the order is valid

If you arrive on the scene of a cardiac arrest and a DNR order is present:

- Make sure the form clearly identifies the person to whom the DNR applies.
- Make sure the patient is the person referred to in the DNR document.
- Make sure the document is of the correct type approved by your state and local authorities.

If the patient requires resuscitation, Advanced Life Support (ALS) should be called to the scene. If a DNR exists but you are unsure about the validity of the order, begin CPR immediately. It is possible to stop CPR more easily than it is to begin resuscitation measures when it is too late. If you determine the DNR order is valid, follow the instructions outlined in the document. This may include stopping resuscitation if it has already been started. If required by your local protocol, call Advanced Life Support personnel to the scene to confirm that the patient is dead and/or contact medical direction.

Signs of Obvious Death

In some situations, it will be clear that a person has been dead for some time. An obvious sign of death includes decapitation (beheading). Other signs include putrefaction, dependent lividity, and rigor mortis.

Remember This!

Be sure to let the police know about your observations.

If a person shows signs of obvious death, do not disturb the body or scene. The police or medical examiner will need to authorize removal of the body. It will important for you to observe and document the following:

- The position of the patient/victim
- The patient's injuries
- The conditions at the scene
- Statements of persons at the scene
- Statements of the patient/victim before death

Putrefaction

Putrefaction is the decomposition of organic matter, such as body tissues.

Dependent Lividity

Dependent lividity refers to the settling of blood in dependent areas of the body. Dependent areas are those areas on which the body has been resting. Dependent lividity is considered an obvious sign of death only when there are widespread areas of discolored skin (reddish-purple skin) in dependent areas of an unresponsive, breathless, and pulseless person. In some EMS systems, both lividity and rigor mortis must be present to be considered signs of obvious death. Lividity is harder to detect on a person with dark skin pigmentation. In addition, lividity may be absent if there was major blood loss before death.

Rigor Mortis

Rigor mortis is the stiffening of body muscles that occurs after death. This stiffening occurs because of chemical changes in muscle tissue. After death, the muscles of the body will normally be relaxed for about three hours. They stiffen between 3 hours and 36 hours and then become relaxed again. The condition of the body, the environmental temperature, and the amount of work the muscles performed just before death affect how quickly rigor mortis occurs. The onset of rigor mortis is usually delayed in a cold environment and sped up in a hot one. A high level of muscle activity increases acid production. The presence of acid speeds up the onset of rigor mortis.

Rigor mortis begins in the muscles of the face. It then spreads downward to other parts of the body. Rigor may be more difficult to detect with obese individuals. The state of rigor usually lasts about 24-36 hours or until muscle decay occurs.

You Should Know

Signs of Obvious Death

- Decapitation or other obvious mortal injury
- Putrefaction (decomposition)
- Extreme dependent lividity
- Rigor mortis

Helping the Dying Patient

As an EMT, you may arrive to find that a patient has died or is dying. A dying patient may ask to talk with his family. If the family is not at the scene, it is appropriate to offer to pass on important messages. Write down the information. Be sure to follow through with the patient's request.

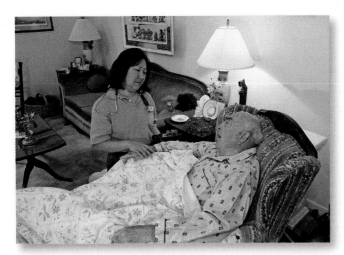

FIGURE 2-7 ▲ The dying patient may want to express his feelings and concerns to you.

A dying patient may want to express his feelings and concerns to you (Figure 2-7). Just being there and listening is often all that the patient wants from you. Remember to preserve the patient's dignity and treat him with respect.

Making a Difference

Dealing with the Dying Patient and Family Members

- The patient needs include dignity, respect, sharing, communication, privacy, and control.
- Allow family members to express their feelings.
- Listen empathetically.
- Do not falsely reassure.
- Use a gentle tone of voice.
- Let the patient know that everything that can be done to help will be done.
- Use a reassuring touch, if appropriate.
- Comfort the family.

Helping the Dying Patient's Family

When conveying news about a patient's death, speak slowly and in a quiet, calm voice. You might begin by saying, "This is hard to tell you, but . . ." Tactfully explain that the patient is dead. Use the words "death," "dying," or "dead" instead of phrases such as "passed on," "no longer with us," or "has gone to a better place." An empathic response such as, "You have my (our) sincere sympathy" may be used to express your feelings.

The patient's family will go through the grief process. If the patient had a prolonged illness, family members may have had an opportunity to share important messages. They may also have been able to resolve conflict before the patient died. When a person dies suddenly, family members and friends may experience intense grief and guilt. This may be particularly true if messages were left unsaid or harsh words were spoken before death.

The reactions of family members to a loved one's death may include anger, rage, withdrawal, disbelief, extreme agitation, guilt, or sorrow. In some cases, there may be no visible response or the response may seem inappropriate. Be sensitive to the needs of those who have suffered a loss by acknowledging their grief. They have a right to these feelings.

After a death, members of the family and close friends will often try to make sense of what happened to their loved one. Many will want to learn the details surrounding the death. They may want to talk to those who were present at the time of death. They may also want to view the body. At a possible crime scene, do not disturb the body or the scene.

Some EMS agencies have arrangements with counselors, who can be called to the scene to provide grief support for the family (Figure 2-8). Remain with the family until law enforcement personnel or the medical examiner assumes responsibility for the body. In addition, if available in your area, stay with the family until grief support personnel are on the scene to assist them. If counselors or grief support personnel are not available, give the family information packets or crisis intervention contact information so that they can seek help from mental health professionals.

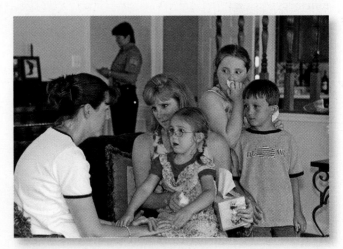

FIGURE 2-8 ▲ Many EMS agencies have arrangements with counselors who can provide grief support for the family on the scene.

Taking caring of ill or injured people is emotionally demanding. Make sure to assess your own physical and emotional response to the situation when the call is over. It may be helpful for you to talk with other EMS professionals afterward. You may find it helpful to discuss your feelings if the call involved death or dying.

Stress and Stress Management

As an EMS professional, you will experience personal stress and will encounter patients and bystanders in severe stress. A **stressor** is any event or condition that has the potential to cause bodily or mental tension. Common stressors associated with working in EMS are shown in Table 2-2.

When you encounter a stressor, your brain tells the rest of your body how to adjust to it. The part of your body that is first aware of the stressor, such as your eyes or nose, sends a message along your nerves to your brain. Your brain receives the message and tells specific body organs to release chemicals. These chemicals activate the body's fight-or-flight response (Figure 2-9). The fight-or-flight response prepares the body to protect itself.

When the stressor is removed, the body should return to its normal state. If the stress does not stop, the brain keeps the body in a state of high alert and the body becomes exhausted. Over time, this state takes its toll on the body. Stress-induced illnesses result.

Recognizing Warning Signs of Stress

Stress can affect your emotional well-being and the way in which you interact with your patients and family. Signs of stress may be physical, behavioral, mental, or emotional (Table 2-3). Become aware of your stressors and your responses to them. Recognizing the warning signs and sources of stress will help you develop a plan about what to do to avoid its occurrence or decrease its impact.

TABLE 2-2 Common Stressors Associated with Working in EMS

Environmental Stressors	Psychosocial Stressors	Personal Stressors
• Lights, siren, alarm noise • Long hours and shifts • Absence of challenge between calls • Weather conditions and temperature extremes • Confined work spaces • Emergency driving and rapid scene response • Demanding physical labor • Multiple role responsibilities • Dangerous situations	• Family relationships • Conflicts with supervisors or coworkers • Agitated, combative, or abusive patients • Dealing with critically ill and injured or dying patients • Patients under the influence of drugs or alcohol • Incompatibility with partner(s) • Getting used to new shift/assignment	• Life-and-death decision making • Personal expectations • Feelings of guilt and anxiety • Dealing with death and dying

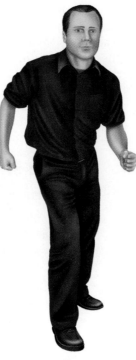

Pupils widen (dilate).

Heart rate increases.

Skeletal muscle strength increases.

Mental alertness increases.

Breathing passages dilate.

The force with which the heart contracts increases.

FIGURE 2-9 ▲ The fight-or-flight response prepares the body to protect itself.

TABLE 2-3 Signs of Stress

Physical Signs	Behavioral Signs	Mental Signs	Emotional Signs
• Increased heart rate • Pounding/racing heart	• Crying spells • Hyperactivity or under-activity	• Inability to make decisions • Forgetfulness	• Irritability • Angry outbursts
• Elevated blood pressure • Sweaty palms • Tightness of the chest, neck, jaw, and back muscles	• Changes in eating habits • Increased substance use or abuse, including smoking, alcohol consumption, medications, and illegal substances	• Reduced creativity • Lack of concentration • Diminished productivity	• Hostility • Depression • Jealousy • Restlessness • Withdrawal
• Headache • Diarrhea, constipation • Trembling, twitching • Stuttering and other speech difficulties	• Excessive humor or silence • Violence, aggressive behavior (such as driving aggressively)	• Lack of attention to detail • Disorganized thoughts • Lack of control or a need for too much control	• Anxiousness • Diminished initiative • Feelings of unreality or over-alertness • Reduction of personal involvement with others
• Nausea, vomiting • Sleep disturbances • Fatigue • Dryness of the mouth or throat • Susceptibility to minor illness	• Withdrawal • Hostility • Being prone to accidents • Impatience	• Inability to concentrate	• Tendency to cry • Being critical of others • Nightmares • Impatience • Reduced self-esteem

Managing Stress

Lifestyle Changes

Cumulative stress is common in EMS. It results from repeated exposure to smaller stressors that build up over time. Causes of cumulative stress may include not getting enough sleep for several days in a row, job-related problems, or family and relationship issues.

Objective 6

There are several things you can do to manage stress in a healthy way. These steps include developing good dietary habits, exercising, and practicing relaxation techniques.

Developing Good Dietary Habits

An excess of substances such as caffeine, sugar, fatty foods, and alcohol can exaggerate your body's response to stress. These substances can also influence your behavior. Good dietary habits include reducing or avoiding the intake of sugar, caffeine, alcohol, and foods that are high in fat.

Exercising

Regular exercise is important to keeping physically and mentally fit. It helps you meet the physical requirements of your responsibilities. Sustained aerobic activity causes the body to release endorphins. These natural chemicals can relieve stress and bring about a sense of well-being. Exercise also allows you to "burn off" pent-up emotions.

Practicing Relaxation Techniques

Meditation, deep-breathing exercises, yoga, reading, listening to music, and visual imagery can be used to help reduce stress.

Creating Balance

To effectively manage the stress associated with caring for ill or injured people, you must learn to balance work, family and friends, fitness, and recreation (Figure 2-10). Consider the following suggestions to help maintain balance in your life:

- Develop a recreational outlet or hobby.
- Get away when you can to "recharge" your emotional reserves.
- Learn to say no when you need time for yourself.
- Make sure to get adequate sleep. Be as consistent with your sleep schedule as possible.
- Develop mutually supportive friendships and relationships.

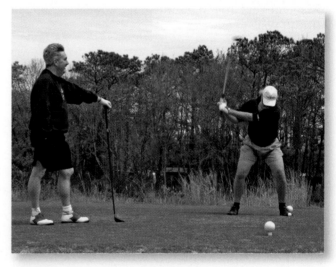

FIGURE 2-10 ▲ Learning to create balance in your life will allow you to effectively manage the stress associated with EMS work.

Family and Friends

Objective 4

Your role as an EMS professional can take a toll on those close to you. Family and friends may not understand the stressors that are a part of EMS work. After a particularly difficult call, you may arrive home too emotionally drained to take part in family activities. Family and friends may not understand the closeness and trust that develops among EMS professionals. Those who are close to you may become frustrated when you do the following:

- Eat, breathe, and sleep EMS
- Work long hours
- Sleep away from home
- Are on call when you are at home
- Agree to work yet another shift
- Miss important family events because of your shift schedule

The spouses of many EMS professionals frequently feel that they are of secondary importance, that "the job comes first."

EMS professionals may find it hard to discuss feelings about their work with others, especially loved ones. Some EMTs want to protect their loved ones from the horrors of the job. They may also need to protect confidential information. In addition, EMS professionals may be unwilling to expose themselves as being vulnerable. Family and friends become frustrated because they sense something is wrong and want to share your pain, but you refuse to do so. They may feel ignored and fear separation when you withdraw from them. These feelings often worsen if you prefer to talk with your coworkers about your feelings or spend your free time with your coworkers instead of with your family.

You Should Know

Responses to Stress by the Family and Friends of EMS Workers

- Lack of understanding of prehospital care
- Fear of separation or being ignored
- Frustration caused by the "on-call" nature of the job and the inability to plan activities
- Frustration caused by wanting to share

Although you should do your best to leave your work at work, doing so is not always realistic. Your family and friends are a base of support for you. They can help you cope with the stressors associated with

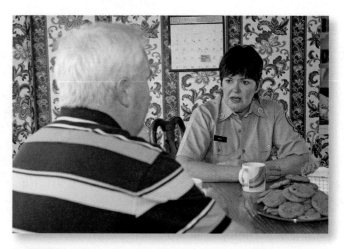

FIGURE 2-11 ▲ Your family and friends are a base of support and can help you cope with the stressors associated with caring for ill or injured people.

EMS work (Figure 2-11). *Do not assume they will not understand.* They can appreciate your feelings about a good or difficult call without knowing the details. Consider the following examples:

- "I had a tough call today. A 2-year-old drowned in a backyard pool."
- "You won't believe what happened today! I performed abdominal thrusts on a person who was choking. The patient coughed up a piece of chicken and is going to be fine."

Make it a point to talk about your day with your loved ones. Actively listen to what they have to say when they tell you about theirs. Plan time for your family and friends. Say no to work when a request would require you to alter those family plans.

Work Environment Changes

To help balance work and family, request work shifts that allow you more time for relaxation with family and friends. If you recognize the warning signs of stress, consider asking for a temporary rotation to a less stressful assignment.

Professional Help

When you need help coping with stress, seek assistance from a mental health professional, social worker, or member of the clergy. Many organizations have employee assistance programs. These programs offer confidential counseling to prehospital professionals. These resources can help you understand and effectively deal with stress.

Critical Incident Stress Management

A **critical incident** is a situation that causes a health-care provider to experience unusually strong emotions. This type of incident may interfere with the provider's mental ability to cope and function either immediately or later. Critical incident stress is a normal stress response to abnormal circumstances. Critical incident stress can affect all levels of EMS personnel. It can also affect bystanders, law enforcement officers, dispatchers, nurses, physicians, and other healthcare workers.

Objective 5

One symptom of critical incident stress is exhaustion, which often results from disturbing elements, such as the sounds, smells, or sights that occurred at the incident. When a person is awake, he may have flashbacks of the disturbing elements. Nightmares may occur during sleep. Other signs and symptoms include anxiety, depression, irritability, an inability to concentrate, indecisiveness, and either hyperactivity or under-activity.

Critical Incident Stress Management (CISM) is a program developed to assist emergency workers in coping with stressful situations. Its goal is to speed up the normal recovery process after a critical incident is experienced. CISM uses the expertise of specially trained teams of peer counselors and mental health professionals. A comprehensive CISM program includes the following:

- Pre-incident stress education
- On-scene peer support
- One-on-one support
- Disaster support services
- Defusings
- Critical Incident Stress Debriefing (CISD)
- Follow-up services
- Spouse and family support
- Community outreach programs
- Wellness programs

CISM is often necessary when any of the following occur:

- Line-of-duty death or serious injury
- Mass-casualty incident
- The suicide of a coworker
- Serious injury or the death of a child
- Events with excessive media interest or criticism
- When the victims are known to you

- Any event that has an unusual impact on personnel
- Any disaster

Techniques used by the CISM team include debriefings and defusings.

Critical Incident Stress Debriefing

A **Critical Incident Stress Debriefing** (CISD) is a formal group meeting led by a mental health professional and peer counselors. The three goals of CISD are the following:

1. To reduce the impact of a critical incident
2. To speed up the normal recovery process after experiencing a critical incident
3. To prevent the development of post-traumatic stress disorder

The benefits of CISD include:

- Allowing emergency workers to share thoughts, feelings, and emotions
- Providing emotional reassurance
- Educating emergency workers about stress reduction and coping techniques

A CISD should be held within 24-72 hours of a critical incident. Usually, all emergency workers involved in the incident participate in a CISD. Sessions are nonthreatening and confidential.

Defusing

A **defusing** is a shorter, less formal version of a debriefing. It is held for rescuers immediately or within a few hours after a critical incident. The goal of a defusing is to stabilize emergency workers so that they can return to service. The defusing process concentrates on the most seriously affected workers. If workers are at the end of their shift, the defusing helps them to return home without excessive stress. The benefits of defusing include:

- Allowing emergency workers to share thoughts, feelings, and emotions
- Providing emotional reassurance
- Educating emergency workers about stress reduction and immediate management techniques

Defusings are usually led by peer counselors, but they may be led by a mental health professional. A defusing may eliminate the need for a formal debriefing. It may also enhance the effectiveness of a debriefing, if one becomes necessary.

You Should Know

Critical Incident Stress Management

CISM was introduced to EMS in 1983. Since then, it has become widely used in EMS, fire departments, police departments, and other agencies. The effectiveness of CISM has been questioned in recent journal articles. The results of some studies raise doubts about the effectiveness of CISM. Check with your instructor about local practices following exposure to a critical incident.

Scene Safety

Objective 7

An EMT is responsible for ensuring his or her own safety as well as the safety of the crew, patient, and bystanders. Part of this responsibility includes being aware of the risks associated with emergency medical care.

Disease Transmission

As an EMT, you will provide emergency care to persons who are ill or injured. When providing care, one of the most serious risks to which you will be exposed is infection. An **infection** results when the body is invaded by **pathogens** (germs capable of producing disease), such as bacteria and viruses. A **communicable** (contagious) **disease** is an infection that can be spread from one person to another. The germs multiply and cause tissue damage, which may result in illness and disease. Signs of illness or disease may or may not be obvious.

You Should Know

Factors That Increase Susceptibility to Infection

- Age (the very young and the elderly)
- Poor nutrition
- Excessive stress or fatigue
- Chronic illness
- Poor hygiene
- Alcoholism
- Body damage resulting from trauma
- Crowded or unsanitary living conditions
- The use of drugs that decrease the body's ability to fight infection

Methods of Disease Transmission

Communicable diseases can be spread in different ways. Contact with drainage from an open sore is an example of *direct* contact. Germs can also be spread through *indirect* contact with contaminated materials or objects, such as needles, toys, drinking glasses, eating utensils, and bandages. Using gloves can help prevent the spread of disease from direct and indirect contact. Germs can also be transmitted in droplets suspended in the air through coughing, talking, and sneezing. Using a mask can help prevent the spread of infection from droplets. Using a mask that shields the eyes offers even better protection.

Classification of Communicable Diseases

Communicable diseases may be classified as airborne, bloodborne, foodborne, or sexually transmitted (Figure 2-12):

- **Airborne diseases** are spread by droplets produced by coughing or sneezing. Examples include tuberculosis, measles, meningitis, rubella, smallpox, and chickenpox (varicella).
- **Bloodborne diseases** are spread by contact with the blood or body fluids of an infected person. Examples include hepatitis B virus (HBV), hepatitis C, human immunodeficiency virus (HIV), and syphilis.

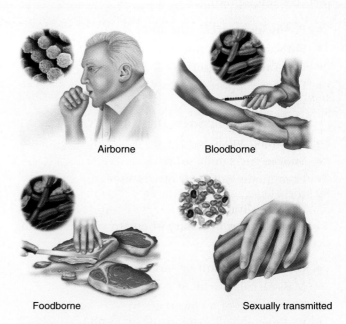

Airborne   Bloodborne

Foodborne   Sexually transmitted

FIGURE 2-12 ▲ Communicable diseases may be classified as airborne, bloodborne, foodborne, or sexually transmitted.

- **Foodborne diseases** are spread by the improper handling of food or by poor personal hygiene. Examples include salmonella (food poisoning) and hepatitis A.
- **Sexually transmitted diseases** are spread by either blood or sexual contact. Examples include chlamydia, gonorrhea, and HIV.

You Should Know

HBV can survive up to 1 week outside the human body. HIV can survive only a short time (hours) outside the body.

Infection Control

Objective 8

An **exposure** is direct or indirect contact with infected blood, body fluids, tissues, or airborne droplets. An accidental exposure to infectious material can occur when your skin is pricked or cut, allowing the entry of germs. Germs can also enter your body through nicks or scrapes on your skin or through mucous membranes (such as your eyes, nose, and mouth). An exposure to a communicable disease does not automatically result in infection.

Remember This!

Body substance isolation precautions protect you and the patient.

Body substance isolation precautions have been developed by the **Centers for Disease Control (CDC)** to reduce the risk of exposure to infection. These standards have been adopted by the **Occupational Safety and Health Administration (OSHA),** which is a branch of the federal government responsible for safety in the workplace. **Body substance isolation (BSI) precautions** refer to self-protection against all body fluids and substances. These fluids and substances include blood, urine, semen, feces, vaginal secretions, tears, and saliva. Precautions include handwashing and using personal protective equipment. They also

Stop and Think!

When caring for patients, assume that all human blood and body fluids are infectious. For your safety, use appropriate BSI precautions during *every* patient contact.

include the proper cleaning, disinfecting, and disposing of soiled materials and equipment.

Remember This!

BSI Precautions

BSI precautions include the following:
- Handwashing
- Using personal protective equipment
- Cleaning, disinfecting, and disposing of soiled materials and equipment

Handwashing

Handwashing is the single most important method you can use to prevent the spread of communicable disease (Figure 2-13). Frequent handwashing removes germs picked up from other people or from contaminated surfaces. Wash your hands before and after contact with a patient (even if gloves were worn), after removing your gloves, and between patients.

Remember This!

Soap combined with scrubbing action is what helps dislodge and remove germs.

Proper handwashing begins with removing all jewelry from your hands and arms. Using soap and warm water, briskly rub your hands together to work up a lather. Continue washing for 10-15 seconds, washing the palm and back surface of each hand, your wrists, and exposed forearms. Scrub under and around your fingernails with a brush. With your fingers pointing

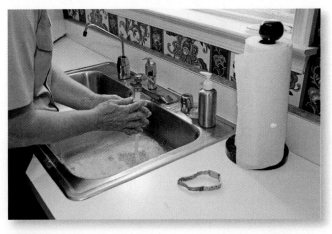

FIGURE 2-13 ▲ Handwashing is the single most important method you can use to prevent the spread of disease.

downward, rinse your wrists, hands, and fingers with running water. Use a paper towel to dry them. Also use a paper towel to turn off the faucet. Avoid touching any part of the sink once your hands are clean.

A waterless hand-cleansing solution can be used initially on the scene if you do not have access to soap and running water. Follow with a complete handwashing using soap and water as soon as possible after completing patient care.

Personal Protective Equipment

Objective 9

Personal protective equipment (PPE) and BSI precautions are a part of scene safety. PPE includes eye protection, protective gloves, gowns, and masks. These items provide a barrier between you and infectious material. The infectious condition of a patient is usually unknown. Therefore, you *must* wear PPE when an exposure to blood or other potentially infectious material may be likely, especially since this type of exposure can occur when it is not expected. Make it a habit to put on appropriate PPE before providing any patient care.

Eye Protection   Eye protection should be worn when body fluids may be splashed into your face or eyes. This splashing can occur during childbirth, when suctioning an airway, or with a coughing or spitting patient. Available eyewear includes goggles and face shields (Figure 2-14). If you wear prescription eyeglasses, removable side shields should be applied to them or form-fitting goggles should be placed over them. To prevent the transfer of germs, remove protective eyewear without touching your face.

Gloves   You should put on disposable gloves before physical contact with *every* patient. When providing patient care, use gloves made of vinyl, latex, or another

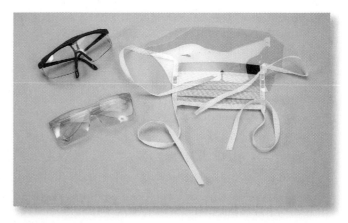

FIGURE 2-14 ▲ Goggles and face shields are types of protective eyewear.

type of synthetic material. If you have a latex allergy, wear gloves made of a non-latex material such as nitrile. If you have a cut on your hand or wrist, apply a bandage to the cut before putting on gloves. Check the condition of the gloves before putting them on. Do not use them if they have small holes or tears in them.

Remember This!

Never reuse disposable gloves.

Change your gloves between contacts with different patients. If a glove tears while providing patient care, remove it as soon as you can and replace it with a new one. Throw away contaminated gloves and other PPE in clearly labeled biohazard bags or containers.

When removing gloves, keep in mind that the outer surface of the gloves are considered contaminated. Do not let the outside surface of the gloves come in contact with your skin. Be careful not to let the gloves snap when taking them off. If the gloves snap, germs may become airborne and contact your eyes, mouth, or skin or that of a coworker or patient. The proper technique for removing gloves is shown in Skill Drill 2-1.

Removing Gloves

STEP 1 ▶
- Using your index finger and thumb on one hand, pull the bottom (cuff) of the glove away from your other hand.
- Peel the glove off your hand, being careful not to touch the skin of your wrist or hand with the outside surface of the glove. As you begin to remove the glove, it will turn inside out. This action helps prevent exposure to blood or other possibly infectious fluids on the gloves.

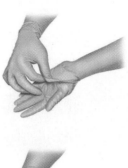

STEP 2 ▶ Place your fingers inside the bottom (cuff) of the other glove. Pull the glove off by turning it inside out.

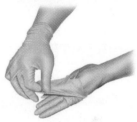

STEP 3 ▶ Dispose of the gloves in an appropriate container. Wash your hands thoroughly.

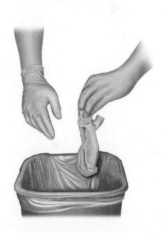

Gowns Disposable, fluid-resistant gowns should be used in situations in which large splashes of blood or body fluids might occur. Examples of such situations include childbirth, vomiting, and massive bleeding. After patient care activities are complete, properly dispose of the gown. If a gown is not available and you were exposed to the patient's body fluids when providing care, change your clothes and take a hot shower as soon as possible after contact with the patient. Wash your clothes in hot soapy water for at least 25 minutes. Launder your clothes at work, if possible. If you have to take them home, wash them in a separate load.

Masks Wear a surgical-type face mask to protect against the possible splatter of blood or other body fluids. Also wear a face mask in situations in which an airborne disease is suspected (Figure 2-15). The mask should be changed if it becomes moist. If you know or suspect that your patient has tuberculosis, wear an N-95 or High-Efficiency Particulate Air (HEPA) mask (Figure 2-16). During ambulance transport of a patient with known or suspected tuberculosis, follow these safety measures:

- Wear a HEPA mask.
- Keep the windows of the vehicle open, if possible.
- Set the vehicle's ventilation system to a non-recycling mode.

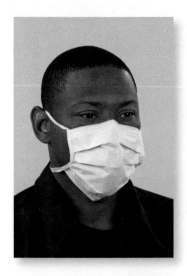

FIGURE 2-15 ◄ A surgical-type mask should cover your mouth, nose, and chin. To keep the mask from slipping, pinch the metal band at the top of the mask. This causes the mask to conform to the shape of your nose.

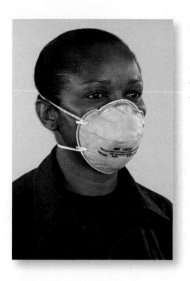

FIGURE 2-16 ◄ Wear a High-Efficiency Particulate Air (HEPA) mask if you know or suspect that your patient has tuberculosis.

Remember This!

Personal Protective Equipment

PPE includes the following:

- Eye protection
- Gloves
- Gowns
- Masks

Refer to Table 2-4 for guidelines on using PPE.

Objective 10

Immunizations

An infection can cause serious medical problems. Immunizations help your body fight infection. It is important to keep your immunizations current:

- Tetanus prevention (booster every 10 years)
- Hepatitis B vaccine
- Influenza vaccine (yearly)

- Measles, mumps, and rubella (MMR) vaccine (if needed)

Tetanus Tetanus (lockjaw) is a serious disease caused by a germ that enters the body through a cut or wound. Tetanus causes serious, painful spasms of all muscles. It can lead to "locking" of the jaw so the patient cannot open his or her mouth or swallow. The tetanus vaccine can prevent tetanus. This vaccine is usually given beginning at the age of 2 months. After receiving three doses of the vaccine (usually during childhood), a booster shot is needed every 10 years.

You Should Know

The Centers for Disease Control recommends a diphtheria vaccination every 10 years for healthcare professionals—given with the tetanus vaccine.

Hepatitis B Hepatitis B is a serious disease caused by HBV. This virus is spread through contact with the blood and body fluids of an infected person. A person can be infected in several ways, including:

TABLE 2-4 **Guidelines for Using Personal Protective Equipment**

Personal Protective Equipment	Guidelines for Use
Gloves	Any situation in which the potential for contacting blood or other body fluids exists
Gloves and chin-length plastic face shield (or mask and protective eyewear)	Any situation in which the splashing or spattering of blood or other body fluids is likely (such as suctioning, or a coughing or spitting patient)
Gloves, chin-length plastic face shield (or mask and protective eyewear), and gown	Any situation in which the splashing or spattering of blood or other body fluids is likely and clothing is likely to be soiled (such as childbirth and arterial bleeding)

- Having unprotected sex with an infected person
- Sharing needles
- Being stuck with a used needle while treating an infected patient
- Having blood splashed into your eyes, mouth, or onto a skin wound
- During birth, when the virus passes from an infected mother to her baby

HBV can cause a loss of appetite, diarrhea and vomiting, tiredness, jaundice (yellow skin or eyes), stomach pain, and pain in muscles and joints. HBV can also cause long-term illness that leads to liver damage (cirrhosis), liver cancer, and death.

The hepatitis B vaccine can prevent hepatitis B. Everyone 18 years of age and younger and adults over 18 who are at risk should receive the hepatitis B vaccine. Adults at risk for HBV infection include:

- Healthcare workers and public safety workers who might be exposed to infected blood or body fluids
- People who have more than one sex partner in 6 months
- Men who have sex with other men
- People who have sexual contact with infected individuals
- People who inject illegal drugs
- People who have household contact with individuals who have chronic HBV infection
- Hemodialysis patients

You Should Know

Hepatitis B

According to the Centers for Disease Control:
- About 1.25 million people in the United States have chronic hepatitis B infection.
- About one-third of people who are infected with hepatitis B in the United States do not know how they got it.

Each year it is estimated that:
- 80,000 people, mostly young adults, are infected with HBV.
- More than 11,000 people have to stay in the hospital because of hepatitis B.
- 4,000–5,000 people die from chronic hepatitis B.

Influenza   Influenza ("flu") is caused by a virus that spreads from infected persons to the nose or throat of others. Influenza can cause fever, sore throat, chills, cough, headache, and muscle aches. Most people are ill for only a few days. However, some people get much sicker and may need to be hospitalized. According to the CDC, influenza causes an average of 36,000 deaths each year in the United States, mostly among the elderly. All healthcare workers who breathe the same air as a person at high risk for complications of influenza and do not have a contraindication to the flu vaccine should receive an influenza vaccination every year. The flu season usually peaks from January through March. Therefore, the best time to get the flu vaccine is in October or November.

Measles, Mumps, and Rubella   Measles, mumps, and rubella are serious diseases that are spread from person to person through the air. The measles virus causes rash, cough, runny nose, eye irritation, and fever. The mumps virus causes fever, headache, and swollen glands. Rubella (German measles) is caused by the rubella virus. It causes a rash and mild fever. If a woman gets rubella while she is pregnant, she could have a miscarriage or her baby could be born with serious birth defects (see Table 2-5).

The MMR vaccine can prevent these diseases. Generally, anyone 18 years of age or older who was born after 1956 should get at least one dose of the MMR vaccine unless they can show that they have had either the vaccine or the diseases. Persons born before 1957 are generally considered immune to measles.

You Should Know

In the United States, about 100 people die each year from chickenpox.

Chickenpox (Varicella)   Chickenpox (varicella) is a common childhood disease that is usually mild. However, this disease can be serious, especially in young infants and adults. Chickenpox is caused by a virus that is spread from person to person through the air or by contact with fluid from chickenpox blisters. The virus causes a rash, itching, fever, and tiredness.

Most people who get the varicella vaccine will not get chickenpox. However, if someone who has been vaccinated does get chickenpox, it is usually very mild. All healthcare workers should be immune to varicella, as a result of either having had chickenpox or receiving two doses of the varicella vaccine.

Tuberculosis   Tuberculosis (TB) is a disease caused by bacteria that usually attack the lungs. It is spread through the air when a person with TB coughs or sneezes. You may become infected with TB if you breathe in these bacteria. To determine if you have been exposed to TB, you should have a tuberculin skin test at least yearly.

TABLE 2-5 The Signs, Symptoms, and Complications of Some Airborne Diseases

Disease	Signs and Symptoms	Complications
Measles	Rash Cough Runny nose Eye irritation Fever	Ear infection Pneumonia Seizures Brain damage Death
Mumps	Fever Headache Swollen glands	Deafness Meningitis (infection of the brain and spinal cord covering) Painful swelling of the testicles or ovaries Death (rare)
Rubella (German measles)	Rash Mild fever	Possible serious birth defects
Chickenpox (Varicella)	Rash Itching Fever Tiredness	Severe skin infection Scars Pneumonia Brain damage Death

Documenting and Managing an Exposure

If you are exposed to blood or body fluids, immediately wash the affected area with soap and water. If the eyes are exposed, flush them with water. Notify your designated infection control officer, medical director, or other designated individual as soon as possible. Get a medical evaluation and proper immunizations if necessary. Make sure to document the following:

- The date and time of the exposure
- The circumstances surrounding the exposure
- The type, source, and amount of body fluid to which you were exposed
- The actions you took to reduce the chances of infection

Know your local protocols about when and how soon to have a medical follow-up after an exposure incident. As a rule, exposure follow-up should be done immediately after the exposure. If the patient has HIV or hepatitis B, preventive care is most effective when given quickly.

Stop and Think!

Do not reuse disposable equipment.

Cleaning Equipment

Germs can be killed or inactivated by cleaning, disinfecting, or sterilizing. Different chemicals or combinations of chemicals kill or inactivate different germs. When providing patient care, use disposable equipment whenever possible. Reusable equipment used in the care of a patient with intact skin usually requires only cleaning or disinfecting.

When dealing with contaminated materials, place them in appropriately labeled leak-proof containers or bags. Double bag disposable items if the patient is known to have a communicable disease.

Cleaning Cleaning is the process of washing a contaminated object with soap and water. An item must be cleaned before it is disinfected or sterilized. To clean equipment, begin by rinsing the item with cold water to remove obvious body fluid or tissue. Then wash the item with hot, soapy water. If the item has grooves or narrow spaces, use a stiff-bristled brush to clean it. Rinse it well with moderately hot water and then dry it. The item is now considered clean.

Remember This!

Physically removing germs by scrubbing is as important as the effect of the agent you use for cleaning or disinfecting.

Disinfecting Disinfecting is cleaning with chemical solutions such as alcohol or chlorine. These agents destroy some types of germs that may be left after washing. Depending on the type and degree of contamination, items such as stethoscopes, blood pressure cuffs, backboards, and splints usually need only cleaning followed by disinfection. Isopropyl (rubbing) alcohol is often used to disinfect surfaces. However, rubbing alcohol may discolor, swell, harden, and crack rubber and certain plastics after prolonged and repeated use. When chlorine bleach is used as a disinfectant, it must be diluted. A solution of 1 part bleach and 10 parts water or 1 part bleach and 100 parts water may be used. The solution used will depend on the amount of material (such as blood, mucus, or urine) present on the surface to be cleaned and disinfected. These disinfectants are not tuberculocidal. If a patient known to have TB is transported, equipment and surfaces should be cleaned with a disinfectant solution that is tuberculocidal (the label will state that).

Many commercially available disinfectants are available. Follow the manufacturer's instructions to disinfect equipment.

Sterilizing Sterilizing is a process that uses boiling water, radiation, gas, chemicals, or superheated steam to destroy all of the germs on an object. Reusable equipment that is inserted into a patient's body should always be sterilized.

Stop and Think!

Chemical solutions can be harmful. Always protect yourself by wearing gloves and goggles.

Hazardous Materials Scenes

You may be required to respond to situations involving hazardous materials. The National Fire Protection Association (NFPA) defines a **hazardous material** as "a substance (solid, liquid, or gas) that, when released, is capable of creating harm to people, the environment, and property." A hazardous materials scene may involve liquids, solids, or gases that are toxic. To prevent further injury, you must be able to recognize that a hazardous materials situation exists.

Use binoculars to identify possible hazards before approaching the scene. Look for signs or placards that provide information about the contents. A placard is a four-sided, diamond-shaped sign. It is displayed on trucks, railroad cars, and large containers that carry hazardous materials (Figure 2-17). The placard will contain a four-digit identification number to guide you to reference information found in the *Emergency Response Guidebook*, which is

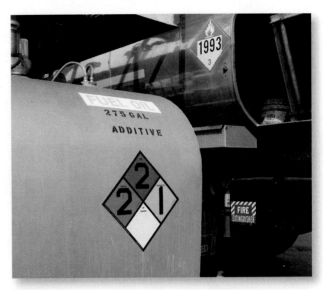

FIGURE 2-17 ▲ A placard is a diamond-shaped sign that is displayed on trucks, railroad cars, and large containers carrying hazardous materials.

published by the United States Department of Transportation (Figure 2-18). The *Guidebook* provides information to help identify the type of hazardous material involved. In addition, it outlines basic initial actions to take at the scene. The placard will also contain a class or division number that indicates whether the material is flammable, radioactive, explosive, or poisonous.

Stop and Think!

Learn how to contact your local hazardous materials team.

If you are the first person on the scene of an incident involving a hazardous material, *do not enter the scene.* Contact law enforcement and your local hazardous materials response team immediately. Stay upwind

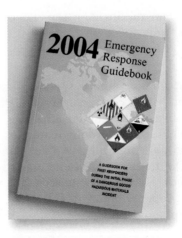

FIGURE 2-18 ◄ The four-digit identification number on a hazardous materials placard can be used to find information about the material in the *Emergency Response Guidebook*.

care only after the scene is safe and the patient is decontaminated.

Motor Vehicle Crashes and Rescue Scenes

Stop and Think!

Remember: Your personal safety is your number one priority. Think before entering a scene.

The scene of a motor vehicle crash may involve potential threats to your safety. It may also threaten the safety of your crew, the patient, and bystanders. Study the scene before entering and determine if it is safe to approach the patient. Determine the number and type of vehicles and the extent of damage. Also note the approximate number of persons injured and look for hazards (see the following *You Should Know* box). Assess the need for additional resources, such as a hazardous materials team or extrication equipment.

You Should Know

Potential Hazards at a Motor Vehicle Crash Scene

- Traffic
- Blood
- Gasoline spills
- Hazardous materials
- Sharp edges and fragments
- Exposed or downed electrical wires
- Fire or potential for fire
- Explosive materials
- Unstable vehicle or structure
- Environmental conditions (such as heavy rain, heavy snow fall, and flashfloods)

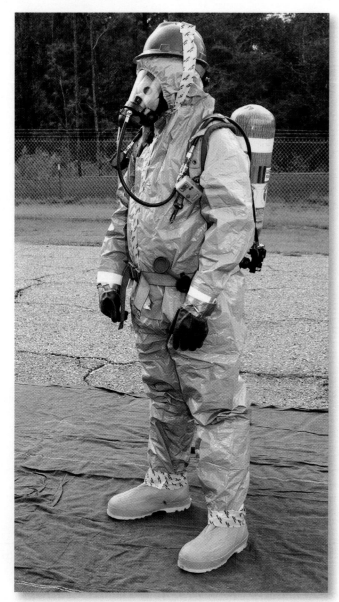

FIGURE 2-19 ▲ Protective clothing for a hazardous materials scene generally includes a hazardous material suit and a Self-Contained Breathing Apparatus (SCBA).

and on higher ground than the incident site. Keep unnecessary people away from the area.

Objective 10

Hazardous materials incidents require specialized protective equipment that is not commonly available to EMTs. In general, protective clothing for a hazardous materials scene includes a hazardous materials suit and a Self-Contained Breathing Apparatus (SCBA) (Figure 2-19.) Do not enter the scene unless you are trained to handle hazardous materials, are fully protected with the proper equipment, and know how to use that equipment. Provide emergency

Traffic

Traffic is a common danger at a crash scene. If you arrive at a crash scene in a vehicle, be very careful when preparing to exit, especially if your door will open into traffic. Put on appropriate reflective gear, if available. Make sure that the vehicle is in park or that the brake is set. Check your rearview mirror for traffic and open the door slowly. Request the help of law enforcement personnel to investigate and assist with traffic control. If the fire department responds to the scene, their large trucks are often positioned in a specific way. This positioning is done to shield the collision site and to provide protection while you care for the patient.

Power Lines

Look for downed or exposed power lines, which are a potential source of electrocution. You *must* assume that any downed wire is dangerous. Contact the power company and fire department immediately. Do not attempt to move the downed wire and make sure not to touch any metal object or water in contact with it. Wait for the power company to shut off the power to the downed line before approaching the patient. If a downed wire is in contact with the vehicle, tell those inside the vehicle to remain inside until additional help arrives. Who makes the call to the utility company varies in EMS systems. In some systems, the call is made by dispatch. In others, it is made by the senior fire officer, first engine on the scene, or the EMS unit. Follow your local protocol regarding utility company contact.

Fire Hazards

Look for fire or potential fire hazards, such as leaking fuel. Do not approach a burning vehicle unless you are trained to handle such situations and are fully protected with proper equipment.

Objective 10

Entrapped Victims

Look for entrapped victims. Request special rescue teams when an extensive or complex rescue is needed. Protective clothing for a rescue scene typically includes turnout gear, puncture-proof gloves, a helmet, eye protection (safety glasses or goggles), and boots with steel toes (Figure 2-20). In cold weather, consider wearing long underwear, a warm head covering, and gloves. In wet weather, you may want to wear waterproof boots and slip-resistant gloves.

Violent Scenes

Remember This!

Violence may occur even when police are present on the scene.

Scenes involving armed or potentially hostile persons are among the most dangerous for emergency care providers and law enforcement personnel. EMS personnel may be mistaken for law enforcement officials because of their uniform or badge. The scene should *always* be secured by law enforcement before you

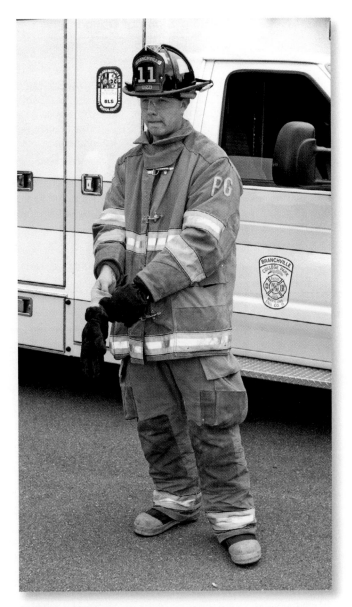

FIGURE 2-20 ▲ Protective clothing for a rescue scene typically includes turnout gear, puncture-proof gloves, a helmet, eye protection such as safety glasses or goggles, and boots with steel toes.

provide patient care. However, a scene that has been declared safe does not mean that it will *continue* to be safe. Reassess scene safety often. Notify law enforcement personnel on the scene if a condition concerning scene safety comes to your attention. Table 2-6 lists some of the warning signs of danger.

Objective 10

Some EMS professionals wear body armor (bulletproof vests). Body armor does not cover the entire body. The areas of the body that are not covered are still vulnerable to injury. Body armor protects covered areas from most handgun bullets and most knives. It

TABLE 2-6　Warning Signs of Danger

Residences	Street Scenes	Highway Encounters
• Unusual silence or a darkened residence • Past history of problems or violence • Known drug or gang area • Loud noises or items breaking • Seeing or hearing acts of violence • The presence of alcohol or other drug use • Evidence of dangerous animals (pets, non-pets, infestations)	• Crowds (large groups of people may quickly become large and unpredictable) • Voices becoming louder • Pushing, shoving • Hostility toward others at the scene (perpetrator, police, victim) • A rapid increase in crowd size • Inability of law enforcement to control crowds	• Disabled vehicles; calls for "man slumped over wheel"; motor vehicle crashes • Suspicious movements within a vehicle • Grabbing or hiding items • Arguing or fighting between passengers • Lack of activity where activity is likely • Signs of alcohol or drug use • Open or unlatched trunks (may hide people)

does not offer protection from high-velocity (rifle) bullets, from thin or dual-edged weapons (such as an ice pick), or when it is not worn. Body armor provides reduced protection when wet.

Stop and Think!

NEVER enter a potential crime scene or a scene involving a family dispute, a fight, an attempted suicide, drugs, alcohol, or weapons until law enforcement personnel have secured the scene and declared it safe for you to enter and provide patient care.

At a crime scene, law enforcement personnel are responsible for gathering evidence that is needed for investigation and prosecution. EMS personnel are responsible for patient care. Do not disturb the scene unless absolutely necessary for medical care. Evidence includes fingerprints, footprints, blood and body fluid, hair, and carpet and clothing fibers. Avoid disturbing evidence by:

- Being observant
- Touching only what is required for patient care
  —If it is necessary to touch something, remember what you touched and tell the police.
- Wearing gloves
  —Wearing gloves helps provide infection control and prevents leaving your fingerprints at the scene. However, it will not prevent you from smudging other fingerprints.
- Taking the same path in and out of the scene

- Avoiding stepping on bloodstains or splatter
- Disturbing the victim and the victim's clothing as little as possible
- Avoiding cuts to the victim's clothing that may have been caused by a knife, bullet, or other penetrating weapon
- Saving the victim's clothing and personal items in a paper bag

Stop and Think!

Scene Safety in Violent Scenes
- Communicate with dispatch and law enforcement.
- Know an alternate way out of the scene.
- Have a prearranged panic code with dispatch and your partner(s).

On the Scene　Wrap-Up

Your neighbor has no pulse. His jaw and limbs are rigid and cold, and you decide not to resuscitate him. Paramedics arrive moments later and confirm that he is dead. You sit down next to his wife and quietly tell her that her husband is dead. She screams and pushes you away angrily, asking why you didn't do anything to save him. Moments later she moans and says that she shouldn't have gone to bed, that she knew he'd been feeling ill all day.

You go back to the station after the call and tearfully explain to the crew about your lifelong friendship with the patient. Later that week a debriefing is held. Because of your ongoing dreams about the event, you visit a counselor to help you cope with the strong emotions you are feeling. ■

Sum It Up

- As an EMT, you will encounter many stressful situations. Whatever the situation, you must act professionally. It is important that you learn how to recognize the signs and symptoms of stress in yourself and others.
- Critically ill or injured patients may experience grief, which is a normal response to a loss of any kind. The five stages of grief are denial, anger, bargaining, depression, and acceptance. Remember that a person going through grief may skip a stage, go through more than one stage at the same time, or go through each stage more than once. Cultural factors will influence how a person experiences grief.
- Patients may experience any number of emotions in response to their illness or injury. As an EMT, you must be respectful of each patient. Listen with empathy to the patient's concerns but do not give the patient false hope or false reassurance. In dealing with the patient's family or friends or with bystanders, you may need to use many of the same approaches you use in dealing with patients.
- Some patients may not want aggressive efforts aimed at reviving them when they are dying. These patients may have an advance directive or a DNR order. An advance directive is a legal document that details a person's healthcare wishes when she becomes unable to make decisions for herself. A DNR order is written by a physician. It instructs medical professionals not to provide medical care to a patient who has experienced a cardiac arrest.
- The signs of obvious death include decapitation (beheading), putrefaction (decomposition), dependent lividity, and rigor mortis. If a person shows signs of obvious death, do not disturb the body or scene. The police or medical examiner will need to authorize removing the body. You should document the victim's position and his or her injuries. You should also document the conditions at the scene as well as statements of persons at the scene.
- As an EMS professional, you will experience personal stress and will encounter patients and bystanders in severe stress. A stressor is any event or condition that has the potential to cause bodily or mental tension. In order to be an effective EMT, you must learn to recognize the physical, behavioral, mental, or emotional signs of stress.
- You should manage stress through lifestyle changes. These changes include developing good dietary habits, exercising, and practicing relaxation techniques. You should also seek to create balance in your life, including time with family and friends.
- Professional help may be needed to help you cope with stress. Many organizations have employee assistance programs that offer confidential counseling to prehospital professionals.
- CISM is a program that assists emergency workers in coping with stressful situations. The results of some studies raise doubts about the effectiveness of CISM.
- An EMT is responsible for ensuring the safety of the crew, the patient, and bystanders. However, an EMT's first priority is ensuring his or her own safety at all scenes. This responsibility includes protecting one's self against disease transmission, which includes using personal protective equipment and having the proper vaccinations. It also involves safety at hazardous materials scenes, motor vehicle crashes and rescue scenes, and violent scenes.

By the end of this chapter, you should be able to:

Knowledge Objectives ▶

1. Define the EMT scope of practice.
2. Discuss the importance of Do Not Resuscitate (DNR) orders, advance directives, and local or state provisions regarding EMS application.
3. Define consent and discuss the methods of obtaining consent.
4. Differentiate between expressed and implied consent.
5. Explain the role of consent with regard to minors in providing care.
6. Discuss the implications for the EMT in patient refusal of transport.
7. Discuss the issues of abandonment, negligence, and battery and their implications for the EMT.
8. State the conditions necessary for the EMT to have a duty to act.
9. Explain the importance, necessity, and legality of patient confidentiality.
10. Discuss the considerations of the EMT in issues of organ retrieval.
11. Differentiate the actions that an EMT should take to assist in the preservation of a crime scene.
12. State the conditions that require an EMT to notify local law enforcement officials.

Attitude Objectives ▶

13. Explain the role of EMS and the EMT regarding patients with DNR orders.
14. Explain the rationale for the needs, benefits, and usage of advance directives.
15. Explain the rationale for the concept of varying degrees of DNR.

Skill Objectives ▶

There are no skill objectives identified for this lesson.

"The scene is safe. Proceed in," the dispatcher calls over the radio. A hunter has evidently shot himself while cleaning his gun. Your patient, an adult male, is sitting in a chair in the living room. He is awake, alert, and oriented, but he looks very pale. He is holding his upper leg, where you can see a small hole in his jeans. You carefully avoid touching the small handgun that is sitting on the table near the patient. The upholstery on the chair under him is soaked with blood. You introduce yourself and prepare to care for the patient, but he says, "No, man—don't touch me. I'm okay." You recognize that he is a reporter for the local news station. You carefully explain the danger of developing shock and dying if he refuses care. He insists that no care be given, so you contact your medical director for advice. ■

THINK ABOUT IT

As you read this chapter, think about the following questions:

- Can the patient refuse to allow you to care for him?
- What can you be accused of if you try to care for him without his consent?
- Is it okay to talk about his case to other coworkers because he is a reporter?
- Could you be accused of negligence in this situation?

Introduction

The Importance of Legal and Ethical Care

As an EMS professional, you will face many situations involving medical, legal, and ethical questions. Consider the following examples.

- You have completed your EMT training and are heading home after a busy day at work. While driving through town, you come upon an automobile crash that apparently happened moments ago. You can see a middle-aged man slumped over the steering wheel. Should you stop and provide emergency care to this person—even though you are off duty?

- You are on shift as an EMT and receive a call from an attorney. The attorney is representing a patient who was involved in a fall while at work. You provided emergency care for the patient about 2 months ago. Should you release patient information to the attorney on the telephone?

- You are on shift as an EMT and are called to a local park where a 7-year-old child fell off a piece of playground equipment. Her arm appears to be broken. The next-door neighbor, an adult, is present on the scene. The child's parents cannot be reached. Can you provide emergency care for this child?

You will face situations like these and other legal and ethical questions every day. You must know how to make correct decisions when these questions arise.

The first and most basic principle for any health-care professional is to *do no harm*. As an EMT, you have certain legal and ethical duties to your patients, the medical director, and the public. Your patients, the medical director, and the public also have certain expectations of you. If you act in good faith and to an appropriate standard of care, you should be able to satisfy these duties and obligations. In this chapter, we will explore common legal definitions and the expectations of your career and practice as an EMT.

Scope of Practice

Legal Duties

As an EMT, you have a legal duty to your patients, medical director, and the public. You must provide for the well-being of your patients by providing necessary medical care outlined in the **scope of practice.** The scope of practice includes the emergency care and skills an EMT is legally allowed and expected to perform when necessary. These duties are set by state laws and regulations. They are also based on generally accepted standards. States often use the U.S. Department of Transportation (DOT) Emergency Medical Technician Curriculum to define the EMT's scope of practice. Some states have adopted the National EMS Scope of Practice Model to define the scope of practice in their state. Some states modify an EMS professional's scope of practice to fit the needs or desires of the state. As a result, what is accepted EMS practice in one state may not be so in another. A medical director and/or your local, regional, or state EMS community may modify an EMT's scope of practice by using **standing orders** and **protocols.** Standing orders are written instructions that authorize EMS personnel to perform certain medical interventions before establishing direct communication with a physician. Protocols are written instructions to provide emergency care for specific health-related conditions.

You Should Know

Make sure to check your state rules and regulations to find out the specific skills you are allowed by law to perform.

Regardless of your primary occupation, as an EMT you are expected to provide the same **standard of care** in an emergency as another EMT with similar training and experience in similar circumstances. Standard of care means the minimum level of care expected of similarly trained healthcare professionals, based on education, experience, laws, and protocols. As an EMT, the laws of the state in which you practice define your scope of practice. Common skills that are within the EMT's scope of practice include:

- Patient assessment
- Inserting oral and nasal airways
- Upper airway suctioning
- Bag-valve-mask ventilation
- Supplemental oxygen therapy
- Cardiopulmonary resuscitation (CPR)

- Automated external defibrillation
- Rapid extrication
- Pulse oximetry
- Using an automatic transport ventilator
- Obtaining manual and automatic blood pressure readings
- Mechanical patient restraint
- Assisting in lifting and moving patients
- Applying the pneumatic antishock garment for fracture stabilization
- Splinting (cervical collar, spinal stabilization, extremity splinting, traction splinting)
- Assisting patients in taking their own prescribed medications
- Giving specific over-the-counter medications with appropriate medical oversight
- External hemorrhage control
- Bandaging wounds
- Using a tourniquet
- Assisting in childbirth

Your legal right to function as an EMT depends on **medical oversight.** This means that, for you to practice as an EMT, a physician must oversee your training and practice. A physician acting as medical oversight may allow you to carry out certain medical treatments in specific situations. Alternately, the physician may not allow you to provide emergency care without first making telephone or radio contact with a person of higher medical authority than you (such as a Paramedic, nurse, or physician). When you practice under medical oversight, you are, in effect, practicing under the physician's license.

Making a Difference

Legal Duties of the Emergency Medical Technician

- Provide for the well-being of the patient by giving emergency medical care as outlined in the scope of practice
- Provide the same standard of care as another EMT with similar training and experience in similar circumstances
- Before providing emergency care, make telephone or radio contact with your medical oversight authority (if required to do so)
- Follow standing orders and protocols approved by medical oversight or the local EMS system
- Follow instructions received from medical oversight

Ethical Responsibilities

Ethics are principles of right and wrong, good and bad. Ethics affect our actions and lead to consequences. Ethics are what a person *ought* to do. As a healthcare professional, you have an ethical responsibility to make the physical and emotional needs of your patient a priority. While in contact with a patient, your patient must be your primary concern. Your patient may be a person from a different ethnic or social background or a criminal. None of these circumstances can be allowed to interfere with the care you give.

Remember This!

Value judgments about a patient's character have no place at any level of medical care.

You must treat all patients with respect. Give each patient the best care you are capable of giving. To do this, you have an ethical responsibility to practice and master your skills. This includes taking advantage of continuing education and refresher programs. After a call, review how you did and look for areas in which you can improve. For example, look for ways to improve response times, patient outcomes, and communication skills.

You must be honest and accurate in your written and verbal communications. You must also respect your patient's right to privacy. Much of the information you will get from your patients is considered **protected health information (PHI).** Federal laws exist that forbid sharing patient information that you receive in the course of your work as an EMT without the patient's consent. These laws are discussed in more detail later in this chapter.

You Should Know

Ethical Responsibilities of the Emergency Medical Technician

- Responding with respect to the physical and emotional needs of every patient
- Maintaining mastery of skills
- Participating in continuing education and refresher programs
- Critically reviewing your performance and seeking improvement
- Reporting (written and verbal) honestly and accurately
- Respecting confidentiality
- Working cooperatively and with respect for other emergency care professionals

As a healthcare professional, you also have a responsibility to work cooperatively with other emergency care professionals. This includes other EMS professionals, law enforcement personnel, fire department and ambulance personnel, and members of the hospital staff. Make sure that your communications and actions with others are professional and respectful.

Making a Difference

Treat any patient with the same care and respect you would want a member of your family to receive.

Competence

Before a patient can accept or refuse the care you wish to provide, you must determine if the patient is capable (competent) of making the decision. **Competence** is the patient's ability to understand the questions you ask him. It also means the patient can understand the result of the decisions he makes about his care. A patient is considered **incompetent** if he does not have the ability to understand the questions you ask. He is also considered incompetent if he does not understand the possible outcome of the decisions he makes about his care.

You Should Know

Because state laws vary, check with your instructor to find out the requirements for legal competence in your state.

How do you determine if a patient is competent? Well-known EMS attorneys have suggested a three-part test for determining a patient's competence:

1. *Legal competence.* Determine if the patient is legally competent. In most states, this means that your patient is at least 18 years of age, is a minor who is married or pregnant, is economically independent, or is a member of the armed forces.
2. *Mental competence.* Determine if the patient is alert and oriented by asking specific questions. Assess the patient's orientation to the following:
   - Person—The patient can tell you his name
   - Place—The patient can tell you where he is
   - Time—The patient can tell you the day, date, or time
   - Event—The patient can tell you what happened

Find out if the patient has a mental condition such as Alzheimer's disease, mental retardation, or dementia that could affect his or her ability to make an informed decision.

3. *Medical/situational competence.* Some illnesses or injuries can temporarily affect a patient's ability to make an informed decision about his or her care. For example, head trauma, low blood sugar (hypoglycemia), shock, or low blood oxygen (hypoxia) can affect a patient's ability to think clearly.

In some situations, it may be difficult or impossible to determine if your patient is competent. An adult is generally considered incompetent if he or she:

- Has an altered mental status
- Is under the influence of drugs or alcohol
- Has a serious illness or injury that affects his or her ability to make an informed decision about his or her care
- Has been declared legally incompetent related to a known mental disorder

A patient who has an altered level of consciousness is often referred to as *altered*. An altered patient may be "under the influence of drugs," which include legal or prescription drugs. Medical conditions such as diabetes or epilepsy can also alter a patient's mental status. Serious injuries, such as head injuries or injuries that can lead to shock, can cause a change in the patient's mental status or level of responsiveness.

It is generally believed that any amount of alcohol or drugs can affect a patient's judgment. In most cases, a patient who is under the influence of drugs or alcohol is considered incompetent. However, determining competence can be tricky. Is a person who has had one drink or two beers intoxicated or incompetent? The person may not meet the legal definition of intoxicated by blood alcohol content. Your own state laws and medical oversight authority can help you determine the definitions of intoxicated and altered.

Some patients may be judged by the courts to be mentally incompetent. Someone who is truly mentally incompetent or legally mentally incompetent will rarely be alone. A guardian who is able to allow or refuse care for the patient will usually be present.

Consent

Objective 3

When your patient allows you to provide emergency care, he is giving you permission, or **consent.** You must have consent before assessing or treating a patient. Any competent patient has the right to decide about his care. The patient's consent is based on the information you give the patient about his condition. It is also based on the treatment you will provide and the patient's understanding of that information.

Expressed Consent

Objective 4

Consent may be expressed or implied. You must obtain expressed consent from *every* mentally competent adult before you provide any medical care. Expressed consent is given by a patient who is of legal age and competent to give consent. **Expressed consent** is a type of consent in which a patient gives specific permission for care and transport to be provided. Expressed consent may be given verbally, in writing, or nonverbally. Examples of nonverbal expressed consent include allowing care to be given or a gesture such as a nod or walking to the ambulance.

Expressed consent must be **informed consent.** This means that you must give the patient enough information to make an informed decision; otherwise the patient's expressed consent may be not considered valid. You must tell the patient what you are going to do, how you will do it, the possible risks, and the possible outcome of what is to be done. To obtain expressed consent:

- Identify yourself and your level of medical training
- Explain all treatments and procedures to the patient
- Identify the benefits of each treatment or procedure
- Identify the risks of each treatment or procedure

You must give the patient explanations using words and phrases that the patient can understand. Do not use confusing medical terms. If the patient speaks a language different from your own, you must make every attempt to find someone who can translate for you. Remember: In order for expressed consent to be valid, the patient must understand what you are saying. You must also understand what the patient is saying to you.

Remember This!

A competent adult can withdraw consent at any time during care and transport.

A competent adult may agree to some medical treatments but not to others. For example, a patient with a cut on his leg may allow you to look at his injury and bandage it but refuse transport for further care. If this situation should occur, follow your local protocol. Your local protocol may require you to contact medical direction and/or call Advanced Life Support (ALS) personnel to the scene to assess the patient and the situation.

Implied Consent

Implied consent is consent assumed from a patient requiring emergency care who is mentally, physically, or emotionally unable to provide expressed consent. Implied consent is sometimes called the *doctrine of implied consent*. Implied consent is based on the assumption that the patient would consent to lifesaving treatment if he were able to do so. It is effective only until the patient no longer requires emergency care or regains competence to make decisions. For example, an unresponsive diabetic patient with low blood sugar may be treated under implied consent. It is assumed that a patient with low blood sugar would want someone to give him sugar if he was unable to do this for himself. Implied consent does not allow you to treat a competent adult for a condition that is not life threatening.

Special Situations

Objective 5

Children and mentally incompetent adults must have a parent or guardian give consent for treatment. Each state has its own laws about when a minor child becomes of legal age to consent to his or her own treatment. A minor refers to a child under the age of 18. State laws also address emancipated minors. An emancipated minor is a person who is less than the legal age of consent but who, because of special circumstances, is given the rights of adults. Mental incompetence is also determined by state laws and sometimes involves court hearings and judgments. You must be familiar with your own state laws.

In some situations, a parent may grant permission to another person or agency to allow medical care for his or her child in an emergency. For example, many parents sign a form allowing their child's school, coach, or daycare provider to authorize care in an emergency. A life-threatening emergency may exist for a child or a mentally incompetent adult when no parent or guardian is present. In these cases, you may treat the patient under implied consent.

Remember This!

Even if there is written parental consent to treat a child, make every attempt to contact the child's parents as soon as possible.

Refusals

Objective 6

All competent adults have the right to refuse emergency care. If your patient is a child or mentally incompetent adult, only a parent or legal guardian can refuse care on behalf of the patient. If a patient refuses treatment or transport, you must inform him of the following:

- The nature of his illness or injury
- The treatment that needs to be performed
- The benefits of that treatment
- The risks of not providing that treatment
- Any alternatives to treatment
- The dangers of refusing treatment and transport

You must make sure that the patient fully understands your explanation and the consequences of refusing treatment or transport. Remember to use words and phrases the patient can understand. Call ALS personnel to the scene as soon as possible to evaluate the patient. While waiting for their arrival, make multiple attempts to try to convince the patient to accept care. The patient's refusal may stem from a lack of understanding because of the effects of his illness or injury, pain, or drugs or alcohol. If you have doubts about the competence of your patient, contact medical direction unless the situation is life threatening and you have begun treatment under implied consent.

Remember This!

As an EMT, you cannot make a decision on your own not to treat or transport a patient. You must consult with medical direction or leave this decision to ALS personnel on the scene.

Some refusals of care carry a higher risk of legal liability than others. A patient may stumble, fall to the grass, and then refuse care because he is certain he is not injured. Considering the nature of the fall, the surface the patient fell on, and the lack of signs of trauma, you may agree that the patient is competent and uninjured. In situations like this, know your EMS system's policy regarding a patient's refusal of care. You may be required to contact medical direction and/or call ALS personnel to the scene to assess the patient.

A patient involved in a high-speed motor vehicle crash may also claim he has no injuries. As a trained EMT, you know that even though there are no visible injuries or signs of trauma, there may be hidden internal injuries that require transport and a physician's evaluation. If this patient chooses to refuse emergency care, it would be considered a high-risk refusal because it is likely that the patient has experienced an injury.

You Should Know

Examples of High-Risk Refusals

Some examples of high-risk refusals involve the following:

- Abdominal pain
- Chest pain
- Electrical shock
- Foreign body ingestion
- Poisoning
- Pregnancy-related complaints
- Water-related incidents
- Falls >20 feet
- Head injury
- Vehicle rollovers
- High-speed auto crashes
- Auto-pedestrian or auto-bicycle injury with major impact (>5 mph)
- Pedestrian thrown or run over
- Motorcycle crash >20 mph or with the separation of the rider from the bike
- Pediatric patient with a vague medical complaint

Most EMS systems require an EMT to contact his or her medical oversight authority for high-risk refusals. Some systems require this contact for *any* situation in which a patient refuses treatment or transport. When contacting your medical direction authority, make sure that you clearly describe the events, your assessment, and the information you have given to the patient. This will help medical direction determine if the patient has enough information to make an informed refusal. If so, medical direction may allow the patient to refuse care. On the basis of the information you relay, if medical direction feels the patient can refuse care but does not yet have enough information to make an informed refusal, he or she can give you information to share with the patient.

In some cases, such as those involving drugs or alcohol, medical direction may instruct you to treat and transport the patient against his wishes. In these situations, ask law enforcement personnel to help you. In some cases, law enforcement will need to ride with the patient in the ambulance. It's important that you clearly explain to law enforcement what medical direction is requesting. This will help them decide whether or not to place the patient in custody.

Remember This!

If the patient refuses to allow his vital signs to be taken or will not answer your questions, make sure to document it in your report.

If you are unable to persuade the patient, parent, or guardian to receive care, you must carefully document the patient's refusal of care. Your documentation should include the patient's name, age, chief complaint, medical history, and two complete sets of vital signs. You should also document details about the patient's mental status. These details include appropriate behavior, cooperation, and the patient's ability to follow instructions or commands. Document your physical examination findings and the patient's reason for refusing treatment and/or transport. The patient's signature should be obtained on a refusal form that notes the advice the patient was given, the patient's understanding of the risks of his refusal, and the patient's understanding of the possible outcome if the advice given is not followed.

The patient's signature should be witnessed by a law enforcement officer, family member, or friend. If the patient refuses to sign the form, document this and attempt to get a law enforcement officer, if possible, to sign as a witness.

Advance Directives and Do Not Resuscitate Orders

Objective 2

An advance directive is legal document that details a person's healthcare wishes when he becomes unable to make decisions for himself. Any competent patient can refuse resuscitation. What about a patient who is unresponsive? Should all unresponsive patients be treated under implied consent regardless of the circumstances?

You Should Know

Some patients who have a DNR do not have a terminal illness.

Some patients who have been diagnosed with a terminal illness may not want further medical care, even if it could prolong their life. The patient may argue that instead of prolonging his life, you are, in fact, prolonging his death. Continued pain and suffering, a loss of dignity, and artificial life support are some of the reasons a competent patient may not want treatment or resuscitation. Whatever the reason, if it is properly documented and the documentation is available to you, you must honor the patient's request. These legal documents are called advance directives or DNR orders. A DNR order is a type of advance directive that is used when patients wish to outline their care for when they are terminally ill. Patients often fill out advance directive forms or ask their physicians to write DNR orders. In some cases, the patient's next of kin or legal guardian will begin this process for an unresponsive or mentally incompetent patient. When this occurs, it is generally based on what the patient would want if he was able to do this for himself.

All fifty states have laws or protocols to address advance directives and DNR orders. A situation may occur in which you have doubts about the legality of the order or it does not fit within the protocols of your agency. In this case, it is best to err on the side of caution and begin resuscitation. If the patient or family members on the scene request resuscitation efforts despite the presence of an advance directive, you should immediately begin resuscitation.

If you arrive on the scene to find that a patient is not breathing, has no pulse, and an advance directive is present:

- Make sure the form clearly identifies the person to whom the DNR applies.
- Make sure the patient is the person referred to in the document.
- Make sure the document you are viewing is the correct type approved by your state and local authorities.

If you determine that the document is valid, follow the instructions outlined in the document.

You Should Know

You must know your local protocol regarding advance directives before you are faced with a situation involving them. Your local protocol may require contacting medical direction and/or calling ALS personnel to the scene (if available in your area) to confirm that the patient is dead.

Different types of DNR orders exist. In some states, a DNR order may specify that the patient does not want CPR or a shock to the heart if his heart stops beating. However, the patient may want (and expect) oxygen to be given. The patient may also want medications (given by ALS personnel). Alternately, a DNR order may specifically state that the patient does not want any resuscitative measures, including CPR, heart shocks, and medications.

Some states recognize only a specific form of advance directive for EMS personnel, regardless of similar forms issued by private physicians or hospitals. Figure 3-1 is an example of the Prehospital Medical Care Directive form currently used in Arizona. This form is considered valid if it is printed on an orange background and includes specific wording on the form. Arizona EMS personnel are not required to accept or interpret medical care directives that do not meet these specific requirements. A person who has a valid Prehospital Medical Care Directive may wear an identifying bracelet on either the wrist or the ankle. In Arizona, the bracelet must be on an orange background and state three specific pieces of information: (1) Do Not Resuscitate, (2) the patient's name, and (3) the patient's physician. You must be familiar with the laws of your own state and the protocols of your agency and medical direction authority.

What should you do if you are called to a scene where a patient is seriously ill or injured and has a valid DNR order, but is not in full cardiac or respiratory arrest? Because some EMS personnel interpret the existence of a DNR order as "do not treat," confusion may exist in situations like this. As previously stated, you must be familiar with your state laws and the protocols of your agency and medical direction authority. Unless specified otherwise by your state laws or protocols, if the patient's heartbeat and breathing are adequate, treat within your scope of practice and transport as appropriate. If the patient has a valid DNR order and is not in full respiratory or cardiac arrest, but his heartbeat or breathing is inadequate, provide treatment within the scope of your practice and transport as appropriate. Providing **comfort care** means giving care to ease the symptoms of an illness or injury. Comfort care is also called palliative care or supportive care. Unless specified otherwise by your state laws or protocols, comfort care includes emotional support, suctioning the airway, giving oxygen, controlling bleeding, splinting, and positioning the patient for comfort.

Remember This!

Although a patient may have an advance directive, you must obtain consent for medical treatment from the patient as long as he is able to make decisions about his healthcare.

PREHOSPITAL MEDICAL CARE DIRECTIVE

IN THE EVENT OF CARDIAC OR RESPIRATORY ARREST, I REFUSE ANY RESUSCITATION MEASURES INCLUDING CARDIAC COMPRESSION, ENDOTRACHEAL INTUBATION AND OTHER ADVANCED AIRWAY MANAGEMENT, ARTIFICIAL VENTILATION, DEFIBRILLATION, ADMINISTRATION OF ADVANCED CARDIAC LIFE SUPPORT DRUGS AND RELATED EMERGENCY MEDICAL PROCEDURES.

Patient: _____   Date: _____
          (Signature or mark)

Attach recent photograph here or provide all of the following information below:

Date of Birth _____

Sex _____ Race _____

Eye Color _____

Hair Color _____   (Attach photo here)

Hospice Program (if any) _____

Name and telephone number of patient's physician _____

_____

I have explained this form and its consequences to the signer and obtained assurance that the signer understands that death may result from any refused care listed above.

_____   Date: _____
          (Licensed health care provider)

I was present when this was signed (or marked). The patient then appeared to be of sound mind and free from duress.

_____   Date: _____
          (Witness)

FIGURE 3-1 ▲ Sample Prehospital Medical Directive form.

Assault and Battery

Objective 7

When you hear the words "assault and battery," you may be thinking of some form of physical aggression or attack by one person on another. In medicine, assault and battery is not necessarily defined as attacking or physically striking a patient. Touching a competent adult patient without his or her consent can be considered assault or battery.

There is no universal definition of assault and battery. Each state has its own laws and definitions. In most states, **assault** is considered threatening, attempting, or causing a fear of offensive physical contact with a patient or another person. **Battery** is the unlawful touching of another person without consent. Check your local protocols and definitions concerning these terms. To protect yourself from possible legal action, clearly explain your intentions to your patient and obtain his or her consent before beginning patient care.

Abandonment

Objective 7

Abandonment is terminating patient care without making sure that care will continue at the same level or higher. You can be charged with abandonment if you turn the patient over to another healthcare professional with less medical training than you. You can also be charged with abandonment if you stop patient care when the patient still needs and desires additional care.

Stop and Think!

If a scene is unsafe, it is not abandonment if you leave the scene for your safety with the intention of returning as soon as the scene is made safe. Your safety comes first.

Remember This!

Once you have begun patient care, you must continue to provide care until it is no longer needed or patient care is transferred to another healthcare professional whose medical qualifications are equal to or greater than yours.

Negligence

Objective 7

Negligence is a deviation from the accepted standard of care resulting in further injury to the patient. When a healthcare professional is negligent, he or she fails to act as a reasonable, careful, similarly trained person would act under similar circumstances. Negligence is the cause of most lawsuits

filed against EMS personnel. Four elements must be present to prove negligence: (1) there was a duty to act, (2) the healthcare professional breached that duty, (3) injury and/or damages (physical or psychological) were inflicted, and (4) the actions or inactions of the healthcare professional caused the injury and/or damage (proximate cause). A successful negligence lawsuit can result in loss of the healthcare professional's certification or licensure and financial penalties.

You Should Know

Components of Negligence

- You had a duty to act
- You breached that duty
- Injury and/or damages were inflicted
- Your actions or lack of actions caused the injury and/or damage

Duty to Act

Objective 8

The first element that must be proved in a negligence lawsuit is a **duty to act.** The duty to act may be either a formal, contractual duty or an implied duty. A formal duty occurs when an EMS service has a written contract to provide services. For example, an EMS service may have a formal contract with a community that requires a response to 9-1-1 calls. An ambulance service may have a formal contract with a long-term care facility. Written contracts usually contain clauses that state when service to a patient must be provided or may be refused.

An implied duty occurs, for example, when a patient calls 9-1-1 and the dispatcher confirms that an EMT will be sent. If you are the EMT sent to the scene, you have an implied legal obligation (duty) to care for the patient. When you begin patient care, you have established an implied contract with the patient.

A legal duty to act may not exist. In some states, an off-duty EMT has no legal duty to act if he or she observes or comes upon an emergency. In other states, an off-duty healthcare professional is required to stop and provide care. In some states, any citizen must stop. Check your state laws and EMS agency's policies and procedures regarding your obligation to provide care if you are off duty. Although a legal duty to act may not exist, a moral or ethical duty to act may exist. You must decide if you are morally or ethically bound to provide care in emergency situations.

Whether you provide care to a patient on or off duty, the care you provide must be the same as another reasonable, prudent (sensible), similarly trained person would provide under similar circumstances.

Breach of Duty

The second element that must be proved in a negligence lawsuit is that a **breach of duty** occurred. A breach of duty occurs when the standard of care that applies in a given situation is violated. A healthcare professional can only perform skills and provide treatment within his scope of practice. Performing skills or treatments outside your scope of practice can lead to a breach of duty.

A breach of duty may be proved if you failed to act or you acted inappropriately. If you are dispatched to a scene to assist a patient and choose not to respond to the call, you are failing to act. If you respond to the call and act outside your scope of practice or do not complete an assessment or perform all treatments indicated, you are failing to act appropriately.

Remember This!

Whatever the situation, you must act as a similarly trained EMT would in a similar situation.

Damages

The third element that must be proved in a negligence case is injury or damage done to the patient. Damages occur if the patient is injured, either physically or psychologically, by your breach of duty.

Proximate Cause

Proximate cause is established when:

- Your action or inaction was either the cause of or contributed to the patient's injury
- You could reasonably foresee that your action or inaction would result in the damage

Attorneys usually use statements (testimony) from expert witnesses to prove that an EMT either failed to act or acted inappropriately and that these actions or inactions were the cause of the patient's injury. Expert witnesses can include other EMTs, Paramedics, nurses, and doctors.

You can protect yourself against negligence claims by:

- Maintaining a professional attitude and conduct
- Providing care and treatment within your scope of practice
- Maintaining mastery of your skills
- Participating in continuing education and refresher programs
- Following instructions provided by your medical oversight authority
- Following your standing orders or protocols
- Providing your patients with a consistently high standard of care
- Making sure your documentation is thorough and accurate

Confidentiality

Objective 9

Health Insurance Portability and Accountability Act

The **Health Insurance Portability and Accountability Act (HIPAA)** went into effect in 2003. This law was passed by Congress in 1996 to ensure the confidentiality of a patient's health information. HIPAA does the following:

- Provides patients with control over their health information
- Sets boundaries on the use and release of medical records
- Ensures the security of personal health information
- Establishes accountability for the use and release of medical records

Individuals who disobey HIPAA privacy rules face criminal and civil penalties. Some important points about HIPAA include the following:

- Patients have the right to review and copy their medical records. Patients can also request amendments and corrections to these records.
- Healthcare providers (and insurance plans) must tell patients with whom they are sharing their information and how it is being used.

The effects of HIPAA are widespread in medicine. As an EMT, you must protect and keep confidential any health-related information about your patients. You must keep confidential any medical history given to you in a patient interview. You must also keep private any findings you may discover during your patient assessment and any care that you provide.

Protected Health Information

PHI is information that:

- Relates to a person's physical or mental health, treatment, or payment
- Identifies the person or gives a reason to believe that the individual can be identified
- Is transmitted or maintained in *any* format, including oral statements, electronic information, written material, and photographic material

You may use and disclose the patient's PHI for three purposes without any written consent, authorization, or other approvals from the patient. These purposes are treatment, payment, and healthcare operations. Before the patient's PHI is used or disclosed for any reason other than treatment, payment, or healthcare operations, a signed authorization form must usually be obtained from the patient or his authorized representative.

In some situations, you can disclose specific PHI without the patient's authorization. These situations require an opportunity for the patient to verbally agree or object to the disclosure of information. These situations include:

- Disclosures to the patient's next-of-kin or to another person (designated by the patient) involved in the patient's healthcare
- Notification of a family member (or the patient's personal representative) of the patient's location, general condition, or death
- Disaster situations

Persons involved in the patient's care and other contact persons might include blood relatives, spouses, roommates, boyfriends and girlfriends, domestic partners, neighbors, and colleagues. In these situations, disclose only the minimum information necessary. The information you share should be directly related to the person's involvement with the patient's healthcare.

If the patient is injured or in cases of an emergency, you may use your professional judgment to decide if sharing PHI is in the patient's best interest. For example, you may tell your patient's relatives or others involved in the patient's care that he may have experienced a heart attack. You may also provide updates on the patient's condition. In these situations, reveal only the PHI that is directly relevant to the person's involvement with the patient's healthcare.

The patient's consent, authorization, or the opportunity to agree or object to the release of PHI is not required is some situations. Examples of these situations include the following:

- When you are required by law to provide this information
- For public health activities such as injury/disease control and prevention
- When the patient is a victim of abuse, neglect, or domestic violence
- For judicial and administrative proceedings
- For specific law enforcement purposes
- To avoid a serious threat to health or safety

You may accidentally reveal PHI when you are caring for a patient. Accidental disclosures usually occur during a radio or face-to-face conversation between healthcare professionals. You may freely discuss all aspects of your patient's medical condition, the treatment you gave, and any of the patient's health information you have with others involved in the patient's medical care. However, when discussing patient information with another healthcare professional, take a moment to look around you. Be sensitive to your level of voice. Make sure that persons who do not need to know this information are not able to hear what is said.

An accidental disclosure may also occur when information about a patient is left out in the open for others to access or see. For example, a prehospital care report may be left on a desk or may be visible on a computer screen when you leave to respond to another call. You must maintain the confidence and security of all material you create or use that contains patient care information. Prehospital care reports should not be left in open bins, on desktops, or on other surfaces. Store them in safe and secure areas. When using a computer, be aware of those who may be able to view the monitor screen. Take simple steps to shield the screen from unauthorized persons.

Special Situations

Medical Identification Devices

You may respond to a call and find the patient wearing medical identification. This identification device may be in the form of a bracelet, a necklace, or an identification card. Medical identification is used to alert healthcare personnel to a patient's particular medical condition. For example, the patient may have diabetes, epilepsy, a heart condition, or a specific allergy. You must consider this information while performing your assessment and patient interview.

Remember This!

Even if a patient is wearing a medical identification device, you must always perform a thorough patient assessment. The reason you were called may be completely different from the condition described by the medical identification device the patient is wearing or carrying.

Crime Scenes
Objective 11

During your career as an EMT, you may be dispatched to a crime scene. A crime scene is the responsibility of law enforcement personnel. As an EMT, your responsibilities are to ensure your own safety and then provide care for the patient. Your dispatcher should notify you of the potential crime scene at the time you are sent to the call. You may be required to stage (remain at a safe distance) and wait for an "all clear" from law enforcement personnel before entering the scene and providing patient care. Even after law enforcement personnel have declared the scene is safe to enter, you must always assess the scene yourself and ensure your safety. After you are certain the scene is safe, your first priority will be patient care.

Making a Difference

It is important to understand your obligations in providing patient care and balancing your other responsibilities on the scene. For example, a law enforcement officer may need to delay your treatment of patients until a crime scene has been secured.

Crime scenes demand certain actions and responsibilities from medical personnel. For example, you should protect potential evidence by leaving intact any holes in clothing from bullets or stab wounds. Do not disturb any item at the scene unless emergency care requires it. You should always be alert and observe and document anything unusual on a call. These actions are especially important at a crime scene. You may be called to testify in court about what you observed at the scene.

Consider talking with law enforcement personnel on the scene to discuss various crime scene issues:

- Possible victim and suspect statements
- Evidence you observed
- Collecting shoe prints from EMTs for comparison
- The names of all personnel on the scene, including EMTs and fire personnel

Special Reporting Requirements
Objective 12

State or local laws and regulations or agency protocols require you to report certain situations or conditions that you know or suspect have occurred. For example, you are required to report known or suspected abuse of a child or an elderly person and, in some locations, a spouse. You must also report injuries that may have occurred while committing a crime, such as gunshot and knife wounds. EMS agencies require you to report exposure to an infectious disease. Because state and local reporting requirements vary, you must learn the requirements for your area and act accordingly.

You Should Know

Generally, you will report special situations such as those mentioned here to law enforcement or the Emergency Department staff.

Organ Donation
Objective 10

An organ donor is a person who has signed a legal document to donate his organs in the event of his death. This document may be an organ donor card that the patient carries in his wallet. Alternately, the patient may have indicated his intent to be a donor on his driver's license. Family members may also tell you that the patient is an organ donor. A patient who is a potential organ donor should not be treated differently from any other patient who requires your care. Your responsibilities include:

- Providing any necessary emergency care
- Notifying EMS or hospital personnel that the patient is a potential organ donor when you transfer patient care

Documentation

Every organization that employs healthcare professionals has documentation requirements. As an EMT, you will be required to complete a prehospital care report (PCR). Most EMS agencies will have a documentation form that you must complete for each patient you encounter. It is important to document information in an organized, systematic manner.

The Uses of a Prehospital Care Report

A PCR has many uses. The medical uses of a PCR include helping to ensure continued patient care. The PCR may be the only source of information that hospital personnel can refer to later. This report may include important information about the scene, the patient's condition on arrival at the scene, the emergency medical care provided or attempted, and any changes in the patient's condition.

The PCR is a legal document and is considered an official record of the care provided by EMS personnel. The PCR may be used in legal proceedings. In general, the person who completed the form must go to court with the form. In many cases, the PCR may be your only reference source about a patient encounter.

The PCR may be used for billing purposes and to collect agency or service statistics. It may also be used for educational purposes to show proper documentation and how to handle unusual or uncommon calls. Data obtained from the PCR may be collected and used for research purposes. For example, the PCR may be used to determine how often specific patient care procedures are performed. It may also be used to determine continuing education needs.

The PCR is often used in quality management programs. The PCR is reviewed to assess proper documentation of information, compliance with local rules and regulations, and appropriateness of medical care.

You Should Know

The Uses of a Prehospital Care Report
- Medical use (to ensure continued patient care)
- Legal record
- Administrative use (billing as well as agency/ service statistics)
- Education
- Research (data collection)
- Quality management

On the Scene Wrap-Up

As Paramedics arrive on the scene, the patient vomits and then says, "I don't feel so good; maybe I should go to the hospital." You quickly cut away his jeans, being careful to avoid the area the bullet penetrated. As you are controlling the bleeding, he admits that his girlfriend shot him during an argument.

A few hours later, a reporter from the local news station calls to check on the patient and find out what happened. You politely tell the reporter that you are not able to share any information about the patient care because of privacy laws. The reporter is not happy with your answer and says she will call the hospital and try to get the information she wants. ■

Sum It Up

▶ The scope of practice includes the emergency care and skills an EMT is legally allowed and expected to perform. These duties are set by state laws and regulations. As an EMT, your ethical responsibilities include treating all patients with respect and giving each patient the best care you are capable of giving. You must also determine if the patient is competent (that is, if he can understand the questions you ask and the consequences of the decisions he makes about his care).

▶ A competent patient must give you his consent (permission) before you can provide emergency care. Expressed consent is one in which a patient gives specific permission for care and transport to be provided. Expressed consent may be given verbally, in writing, or nonverbally. Implied consent is consent assumed from a patient requiring emergency care who is mentally, physically, or emotionally unable to provide expressed consent.

▶ Mentally competent adults have the right to refuse care and transport. As an EMT, you must make sure that the patient fully understands your explanation and the consequences of refusing treatment or transport. In high-risk situations in which the patient's injuries may not be obvious, you must contact medical direction or call ALS personnel to the scene to assess the patient.

▶ An advance directive is a form filled out by the patient. It outlines the patient's wishes for their care if they are not able to express their wishes. A Do Not Resuscitate order is written by a physician and details the patient's wishes for care when he or she is terminally ill.

▶ Assault is considered threatening to, attempting to, or causing a fear of offensive physical contact with a patient or other person. Battery is the unlawful touching of another person without consent. Because each state has its own definitions of assault and battery, you should check your local protocols concerning these terms.

▶ Abandonment is terminating patient care without making sure that care will continue at the same level or higher. You can also be charged with abandonment if you stop patient care when the patient still needs and desires additional care.

▶ When a healthcare professional is negligent, he or she fails to act as a reasonable, careful, similarly trained person would act under similar circumstances. Negligence includes the following four elements: (1) the duty to act, (2) a breach of that duty, (3) injury or damages (physical or psychological) that result, and (4) proximate cause (the actions or inactions of the healthcare professional that caused the injury or damages).

▶ A medical identification device is used to alert healthcare personnel to a patient's particular medical condition. This identification device may be in the form of a bracelet, a necklace, or an identification card.

▶ If you are sent to a crime scene, you must wait for law enforcement personnel to declare that the scene is safe to enter. After you are certain the scene is safe and you ensure your safety, your first priority will be patient care. You should be alert and document anything unusual on the call.

▶ An organ donor is a person who has a signed legal document to donate his organs in the event of his death. The patient may have an organ donor card or may have indicated his intent to be a donor on his driver's license.

4 The Human Body

By the end of this chapter, you should be able to:

Knowledge Objectives ▶

1. Identify the following topographic terms: medial, lateral, proximal, distal, superior, inferior, anterior, posterior, midline, right and left, midclavicular, bilateral, and midaxillary.
2. Describe the anatomy and function of the following major body systems: respiratory, circulatory, musculoskeletal, nervous, and endocrine.

Attitude Objectives ▶

There are no attitude objectives identified for this lesson.

Skill Objectives ▶

There are no skill objectives identified for this lesson.

On the Scene

You and your partner respond to a report of a motor vehicle crash at a local intersection. Upon your arrival, you find the driver of the vehicle slumped forward against the steering wheel of her late-model SUV. She looks to be about 30 years old. The vehicle's airbag deployed. It is now deflated. The patient has an open airway and is breathing at about 30 times per minute. Her carotid pulse is about 120 beats per minute. You do not see any open wounds or obvious injuries. ■

THINK ABOUT IT

As you read this chapter, think about the following questions:

- What body systems may have been injured or damaged?
- How can your knowledge of the human body help you treat the patient?
- What are the possible problems that you may encounter if a vital organ system has been injured or damaged?

Understanding the Structure and Function of the Body

Anatomy is the study of the structure of an organism, such as the human body. **Physiology** is the study of the normal functions of an organism, such as the human body. As an Emergency Medical Technician (EMT), you must be familiar with the structure and function of the human body so that you can better assess an injured or ill patient. For example, if a patient was stabbed in the right upper area of the **abdomen** and you had an understanding of anatomy and physiology, you would then know the organs possibly affected. You would understand their function in the body and could anticipate possible complications. The knife blade may have injured the liver, gallbladder, intestines, blood vessels, diaphragm, lungs, and kidneys, depending on the length of the blade and the direction of the stab (for example, whether it was upward, straight, or downward). Your understanding of the human body is essential in order to give proper emergency care.

Body Systems

The human body is made up of billions of **cells**, the basic building blocks of the body. Cells are the basic units of all living tissue. Cells that cluster together to perform a specialized function are called **tissues**. For example, nervous tissue is specialized to receive and conduct electrical signals over long distances in the body. Muscle tissue is composed of similar cells that can contract, usually in response to an electrical signal from a nerve. An **organ** is made up of at least two different types of tissue that work together to perform a particular function. Examples of organs include the brain, stomach, and liver. **Vital organs** are organs such as the brain, heart, and lungs that are essential for life. An **organ system** (also called a body system) is made up of tissues and organs that work together to provide a common function. The human body consists of ten major organ systems:

- Circulatory
- Digestive
- Endocrine
- Integumentary
- Muscular
- Nervous
- Reproductive
- Respiratory
- Skeletal
- Urinary

Homeostasis

Organ systems rely on each other to maintain a constant internal environment (**homeostasis**) and perform the required functions of the entire body. Homeostasis is also called a *steady state*. The human body has various "check and balance" systems to maintain homeostasis. For example, the body's organ systems require a relatively constant temperature to function properly. If the body's temperature is too low, the muscles shiver to produce heat. If the body's temperature is too high, blood vessels near the skin's surface dilate (expand). This dilation brings more blood to the body surface and allows heat to be passed off into the environment. Sweating is another means of cooling the body through evaporation.

You Should Know

The balanced state that the body requires to function properly is very sensitive to changes caused by illness or injury.

When an organ system does not function properly because of illness or injury, other body functions are affected. For example, the circulatory and respiratory systems need the kidneys to perform their function in order for the body to maintain its balanced environment. If the kidneys fail to produce urine, the circulatory system will retain too much fluid within the bloodstream. This will cause a backup of fluid into the lungs and affect the patient's breathing, disrupting the body's internal balance.

Remember This!

Remember that, as an EMT, you are a healthcare professional. Healthcare professionals use medical terms to communicate information about a patient's illness or injury. To correctly relay what you are seeing and what the patient is saying in your written and verbal reports, you must know medical terms and their meanings.

Body Positions and Directional Terms

Objective 1

Medical terms are used to convey to others the location of a patient's injury or symptoms so that further care can be given. Directions refer to the body when it is in the **anatomical position.** In the anatomical position, a person is standing, arms to the sides with the palms turned forward, feet close together and pointed forward, the head pointed forward, and the eyes open (Figure 4-1). Definitions and examples of common directional terms are listed below.

- **Superior/Inferior. Superior** means above or in a higher position than another portion of the body. The head is the most superior part of the body. The neck is superior to the chest because it is closer to the head. **Inferior** means in a position lower than another. The soles of the feet are the most inferior part of the body. The knees are inferior to the pelvis because they are closer to the feet.

- **Anterior/Posterior. Anterior,** or ventral, represents the front portion of the body or body part. The heart is anterior to the spine. **Posterior,** or dorsal, is the back side of the body or body part. The spine is posterior to the heart.

- **Proximal/Distal.** These terms are most often used when referring to an extremity (arm or leg). **Proximal** means closer to the midline or

center area of the body. When this term is used to reference an extremity, it means nearer to the point of attachment to the body. The knees are proximal to the toes. **Distal** means farther from the midline or center area of the body. With reference to an extremity, it means farthest from the point of attachment to the body. The elbow is distal to the shoulder.

- **Midline.** The **midline** is an imaginary line down the center of the body that divides the body into right and left sides. Using the midline as a reference point will assist in describing whether an injury is **lateral** (toward the side) or **medial** (toward the midline). The **sternum** (breastbone) is medial to the left nipple. The **axilla** (armpit) is lateral to the sternum. The word **bilateral** means pertaining to both sides. **Contralateral** means on the opposite side. **Ipsilateral** means on the same side.

- **Midaxillary line.** The midaxillary line refers to an imaginary vertical line drawn from the middle of the patient's armpits (axillae), parallel to the midline. It divides the body into anterior and posterior sections.

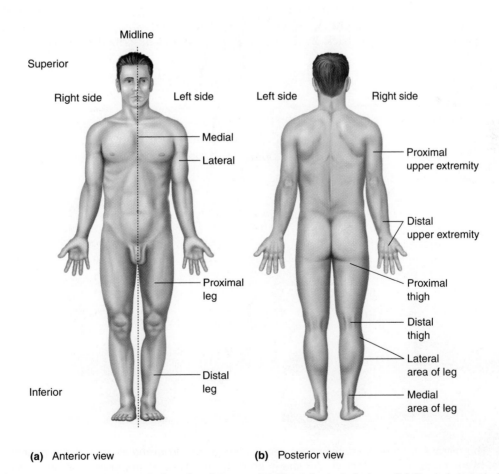

(a) Anterior view   (b) Posterior view

FIGURE 4-1 ▲ Anatomical position and directional terms. **(a)** Front (anterior) view. **(b)** Back (posterior) view.

- **Midclavicular line.** The midclavicular line refers to an imaginary vertical line drawn through the middle portion of the collarbone (clavicle) and nipple, parallel to the midline (Figure 4-2).

Remember This!

- When you look at a patient in the anatomical position, describe the patient's injuries from the patient's perspective. In other words, right and left always refers to the *patient's* right and left.
- If you forget the proper medical term for something, use a plain, understandable description instead. For example, if you forget that the back is posterior, then refer to the "back of the patient." Do not make up or guess at terms—it could be embarrassing. It could also lead to misinterpretation by others.

Ill and injured patients are found in many positions. When a person is standing upright, he is said to be **erect**. A person lying flat on his back (face up) is said to be in a **supine** position. A person lying face down and flat is in a **prone** position. If a person is found on his side, he is in a **lateral recumbent position**. If he is found on his left side, he is in a left lateral recumbent position. If he is on his right side, he is in a right lateral recumbent position.

Remember This!

It is important to properly use body position and directional terms so that you can describe the position in which the patient is found and transported.

As an EMT, you may choose to place a patient in a specific position based on the patient's condition. For example, in the **Trendelenburg position**, the patient is lying on his back with the head of the bed lowered and his feet raised in a straight incline. **Fowler's position** is lying on the back with the upper body elevated at a 45- to 60-degree angle. A patient who is short of breath is often placed in this position. These positions are illustrated and described in more detail in Chapter 6.

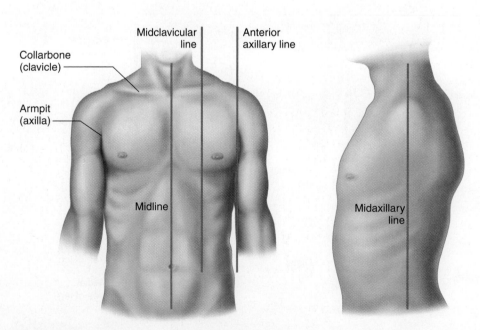

Collarbone (clavicle)

Armpit (axilla)

Midclavicular line

Anterior axillary line

Midline

Midaxillary line

FIGURE 4-2 ▲ The midaxillary line is an imaginary vertical line drawn from the middle of the patient's armpits (axillae), parallel to the midline. The midclavicular line is an imaginary vertical line drawn through the middle portion of the collarbone (clavicle) and nipple, parallel to the midline.

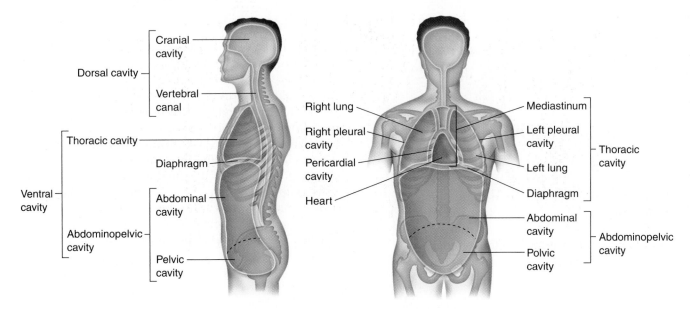

FIGURE 4-3 ▲ Body cavities.

Body Cavities

A **body cavity** is a hollow space in the body that contains internal organs (Figure 4-3). The **cranial cavity** is located in the head. It contains the brain and is protected by the skull. The **spinal cavity** extends from the bottom of the skull to the lower back. It contains the spinal cord and is protected by the vertebral (spinal) column. The brain and spinal cord make up the **central nervous system**. This system allows the body to carry electrical signals from the body's organ systems to the brain and spinal cord as well as to the various organ systems of the body.

The **thoracic (chest) cavity** is located below the neck and above the diaphragm and is protected by the rib cage. The thoracic cavity contains the heart, major blood vessels, and the lungs. The heart is surrounded by another cavity, the **pericardial cavity.** The lungs are surrounded by the **pleural cavities.** The right lung is located in the right pleural cavity; the left lung is located in the left pleural cavity.

The abdominal and pelvic cavities are often called the abdominopelvic cavity. The **abdominal cavity** is located below the diaphragm and above the pelvis. The abdominal cavity contains the stomach, intestines, liver, gallbladder, pancreas, and spleen. Although not separated by any kind of wall, the area below the abdominal cavity is called the **pelvic cavity.** The pelvic cavity contains the urinary bladder, part of the large intestine, and the reproductive organs.

To make things easier when identifying the abdominal organs and the location of pain or injury, the abdominal cavity is divided into four quadrants

(Figure 4-4). These quadrants are created by drawing two imaginary lines that intersect with the midline through the navel (umbilicus). The right upper quadrant (RUQ) contains the liver, the gallbladder, portions of the stomach, the right kidney, and the major blood vessels. The left upper quadrant (LUQ) contains the stomach, spleen, pancreas, and left kidney. The right lower quadrant (RLQ) contains the appendix. The left lower quadrant (LLQ), along with the other three quadrants, contains the intestines. In females, the right and left lower quadrants contain the ovaries and fallopian tubes. The uterus is in the

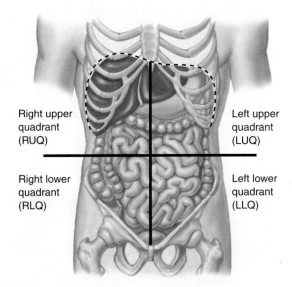

Right upper quadrant (RUQ)

Left upper quadrant (LUQ)

Right lower quadrant (RLQ)

Left lower quadrant (LLQ)

FIGURE 4-4 ▲ The abdominal area is divided into four quadrants.

midline above (superior to) the pelvis and just behind (posterior to) the bladder. Knowing the organs found within each of the four quadrants will help you describe the location of an injury or the symptoms of a sick or injured patient.

The Musculoskeletal System

Objective 2

The musculoskeletal system gives the human body its shape and ability to move and protects the major organs of the body. It consists of the skeletal system (bones) and the muscular system (muscles).

The Skeletal System

The skeletal system consists of 206 bones of varying types. Bones store minerals for the body, such as calcium and phosphorus. Many bones have a hollow cavity that contains a substance called bone marrow. Bone marrow produces the body's blood cells—the red blood cells, white blood cells, and platelets.

The skeletal system is divided into two groups of bones. The **axial skeleton** is the part of the skeleton that includes the skull, spinal column, sternum, and ribs (Figures 4-5 and 4-6). The **appendicular skeleton** is made up of the upper and lower extremities (arms and legs), the shoulder girdles, and the pelvic girdle. The **shoulder girdle** is the bony arch formed

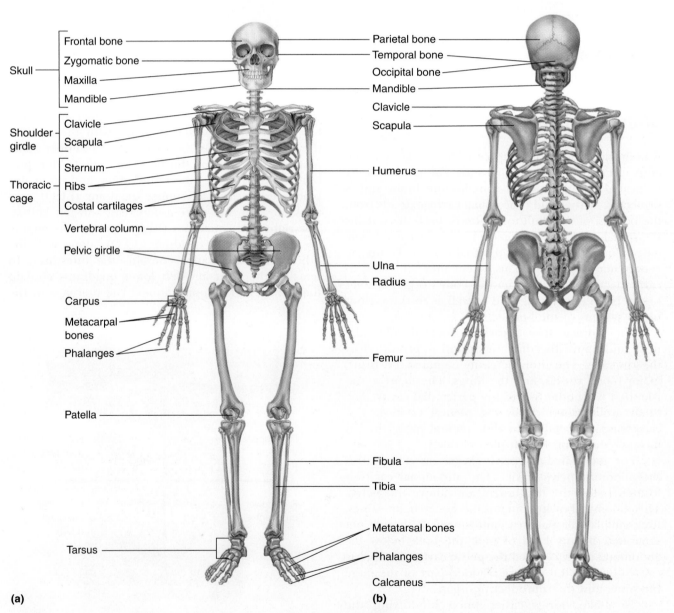

FIGURE 4-5 ▲ The adult skeleton. **(a)** Anterior view. **(b)** Posterior view. The appendicular skeleton is colored blue and the rest is axial skeleton.

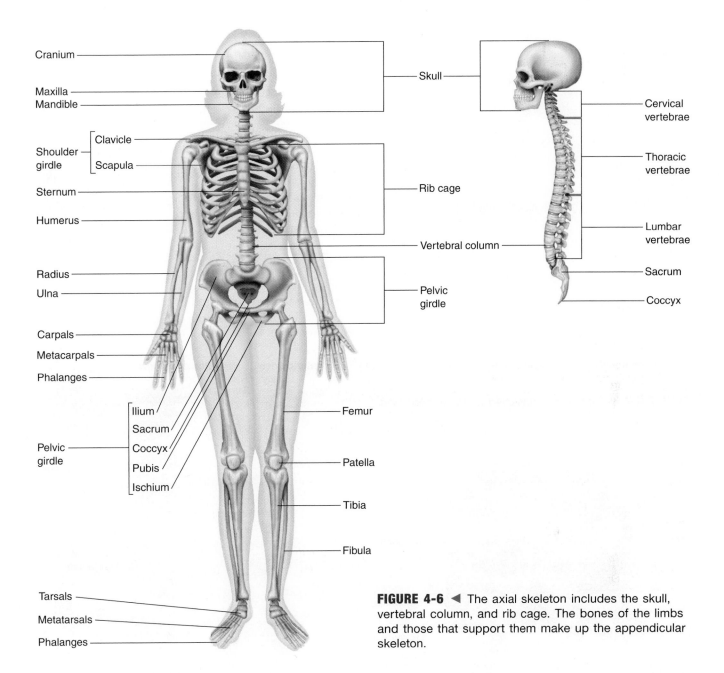

Cranium

Maxilla
Mandible

Shoulder girdle
— Clavicle
— Scapula

Sternum

Humerus

Radius

Ulna

Carpals

Metacarpals

Phalanges

Ilium
Sacrum
Pelvic girdle
Coccyx
Pubis
Ischium

Tarsals

Metatarsals

Phalanges

Skull

Rib cage

Vertebral column

Pelvic girdle

Femur

Patella

Tibia

Fibula

Cervical vertebrae

Thoracic vertebrae

Lumbar vertebrae

Sacrum

Coccyx

FIGURE 4-6 ◄ The axial skeleton includes the skull, vertebral column, and rib cage. The bones of the limbs and those that support them make up the appendicular skeleton.

by the collarbones (clavicles) and shoulder blades (scapulae). The **pelvic girdle** is made up of bones that enclose and protect the organs of the pelvic cavity. It provides a point of attachment for the lower extremities and the major muscles of the trunk. It also supports the weight of the upper body.

Bones are classified by their shape and size—long, short, flat, and irregular (Figure 4-7). Long bones are the relatively cylindrical bones of the upper and lower extremities, such as the humerus of the upper arm. Short bones can be found in the carpal bones of the hand and the tarsal bones of the feet. The shoulder blade (scapula) is an example of a flat bone. The vertebrae are examples of irregular bones.

The Skull

The **skull** is the bony skeleton of the head that protects the brain from injury and gives the head its shape. It is made up of two main groups of bones, the bones of the cranium and the bones of the face (Figure 4-8). The **cranium** contains eight bones that house and protect the brain:

- Frontal (forehead) bone
- Two parietal (top sides of cranium) bones
- Two temporal (lower sides of cranium) bones
- Occipital (back of skull) bone
- Sphenoid (central part of floor of cranium) bone
- Ethmoid (floor of cranium, nasal septum) bone

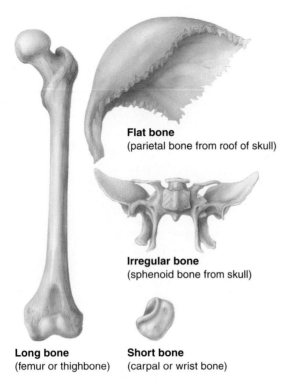

Flat bone
(parietal bone from roof of skull)

Irregular bone
(sphenoid bone from skull)

Long bone
(femur or thighbone)

Short bone
(carpal or wrist bone)

FIGURE 4-7 ▲ Bones are classified by their shape and size.

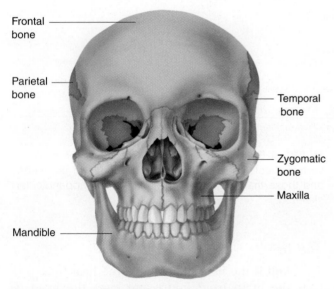

Frontal bone

Parietal bone

Temporal bone

Zygomatic bone

Maxilla

Mandible

FIGURE 4-8 ▲ The anterior view of the skull.

The skull is supported by the neck, which receives its strength from the vertebrae. Attached to the skull are many facial bones. Muscles attached to these bones allow eye movements and facial expressions. These muscles also allow the tongue to be held in position so that the airway remains open. Without these important mouth muscles, a person would not be able to swallow food or fluids without gagging and choking. The face contains 14 bones:

- Orbits (eye sockets)
- Nasal bones (upper bridge of nose)
- Maxilla (upper jaw)
- Mandible (lower jaw)
- Zygomatic bones (cheek bones)

The mandible is the largest and strongest bone of the face. It is the only movable bone of the face. The ear contains six bones, which are located in the middle ear and are called the auditory ossicles. The tongue is anchored to the hyoid bone. The hyoid bone is only bone in the body that does not connect to another bone.

The Spine

The spine (vertebral column) is made up of 32-33 vertebrae that are arranged in regions (Figure 4-9 and Table 4-1). The vertebrae of each region have a

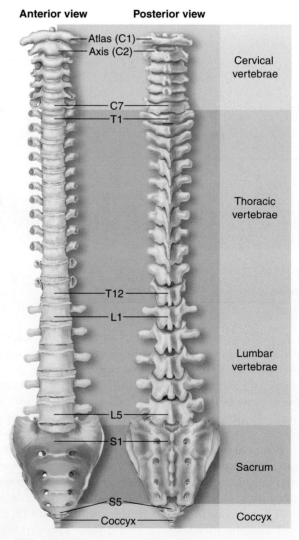

Anterior view   Posterior view

Atlas (C1)
Axis (C2)

Cervical vertebrae

C7
T1

Thoracic vertebrae

T12
L1

Lumbar vertebrae

L5
S1

Sacrum

S5
Coccyx

Coccyx

FIGURE 4-9 ▲ The vertebral column, anterior and posterior views.

TABLE 4-1   Regions of the Spinal Column

Region	Number of Vertebrae
Cervical spine (neck)	7
Thoracic spine (chest, upper back)	12
Lumbar spine (lower back)	5
Sacrum	5 (fused)
Coccyx	3 to 4 (fused)

distinctive shape. The vertebral column is made up of 7 cervical (neck) vertebrae, 12 thoracic vertebrae, 5 lumbar vertebrae, 5 fused vertebrae that form the sacrum, and 3-4 fused vertebrae that form the coccyx (tailbone). The vertebral column provides rigidity to the body while allowing movement. It also encloses and protects the spinal cord. It extends from the base of the skull to the coccyx.

The 7 cervical vertebrae of the neck hold up the head and allow it to rotate left and right as well as move backward, forward, and side to side. At the scene of an emergency, rescuers often refer to the cervical spine as the *c-spine*. The first cervical vertebra, the atlas, supports the skull. The second cervical vertebra is called the axis. The 12 thoracic vertebrae form the upper back and posterior portion of the thorax. Below the thoracic vertebrae are five lumbar vertebrae. The lumbar vertebrae are the largest and strongest of the vertebrae because they carry the bulk of the body's weight. Below the lumbar vertebrae are five fused vertebrae that form the sacrum (the back wall of the pelvis) and eventually attach to three to four fused vertebrae that form the coccyx. The fused sacral vertebrae are connected to the pelvis, which attaches the lower appendicular skeleton to the axial skeleton.

You Should Know

The adult spinal cord is about 16-18 inches in length and about three fourths of an inch in diameter in the midthorax. The length of the spinal cord is shorter than the length of the bony vertebral column. It extends down to only about the second lumbar vertebra. In the cervical and thoracic areas of the vertebral column, the spinal cord lies very close to the walls of the vertebrae. The spinal cord is at risk of injury in these areas.

Between each vertebra is a disc. Each disc is a tiny pad that is made up mainly of water (Figure 4-10). These discs help protect the spinal nerves. The discs between the vertebrae are soft and rubbery, cushioning each of the vertebrae and acting as shock absorbers. The spinal nerves exit the spinal cord at openings between the vertebrae. They send signals to the body's muscles and organs (Figure 4-11).

The Chest

The chest (thorax) is made up of the 12 thoracic vertebrae, 12 pairs of ribs, and the breastbone (sternum). (Figure 4-12.) These structures form the thoracic cage, serving to protect the organs within the thoracic cavity, such as the heart, lungs, and major blood vessels. The sternum is attached to the ribs and collarbones (clavicles). All of the ribs are attached posteriorly to the thoracic vertebrae by ligaments. Pairs 1 through 10 are attached to the front of the sternum. Pairs 1 through 7 are attached to the front of the sternum by cartilage and are called **true ribs.** Rib pairs 8 through 10 are attached to the cartilage of the seventh ribs. These ribs are called **false ribs.** Pairs 11 and 12 are not attached to the front of the sternum; these ribs are called **floating ribs.**

The sternum (breastbone) consists of three sections. The **manubrium** is the uppermost (superior) portion; it connects with the clavicle and first rib. The body is the middle portion. The **xiphoid process** is a piece of cartilage that makes up the inferior portion. This landmark is important when determining the proper hand position for chest compressions in cardiopulmonary resuscitation (CPR). The superior portion of the sternum is attached to the clavicles, which join the axial skeleton to the appendicular skeleton.

The Upper Extremities

The upper extremities are made up of the bones of the shoulder girdle, the arms, the forearms, and the hands (Figure 4-13). The **humerus** is the upper arm bone where the biceps and triceps muscles are attached, allowing the shoulder to rotate, flex, and extend. The humerus is the largest bone of the upper extremity and is the second longest bone in the body. The clavicles (collarbones) and the scapulae (shoulder blades) form the capsule into which the proximal portion of the humerus inserts to form the shoulder joint. The forearm contains two bones, the **radius** (lateral, thumb side), and **ulna** (medial side). The ulna is the longer of the two bones. The **olecranon** (elbow) is the joint where the humerus connects with the radius and the ulna. The forearm is connected to the **carpals** (wrist) and then to the **metacarpals** (hand), and the **phalanges** (fingers). There are multiple bones and joints within the wrist and hand, allowing humans to have a greater deal of flexibility, movement, and use.

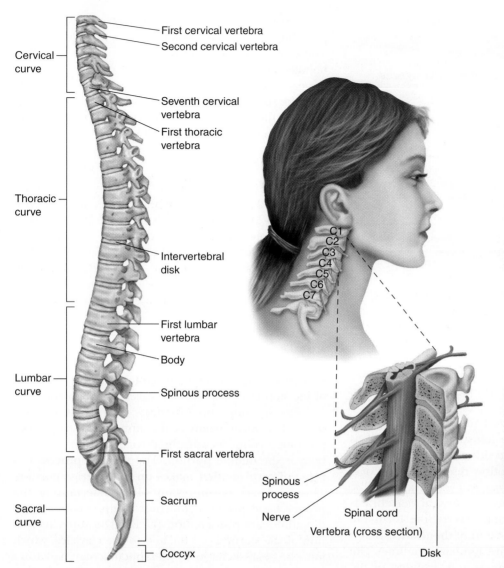

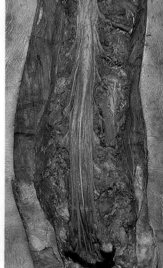

FIGURE 4-10 ▲ The vertebral column.

Cervical curve

First cervical vertebra
Second cervical vertebra

Seventh cervical vertebra
First thoracic vertebra

Thoracic curve

Intervertebral disk

First lumbar vertebra
Body

Lumbar curve

Spinous process

First sacral vertebra

Sacral curve

Sacrum

Coccyx

C1
C2
C3
C4
C5
C6
C7

Spinous process
Nerve
Spinal cord
Vertebra (cross section)
Disk

FIGURE 4-11 ▲ A dissected spinal cord and roots of the spinal nerves.
© The McGraw-Hill Companies, Inc./Karl Rubin, photographer.

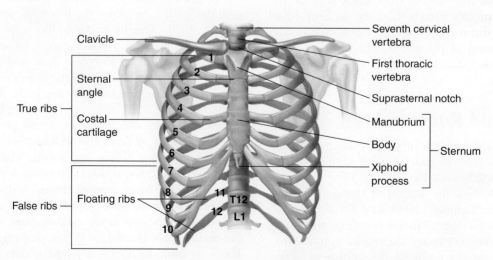

Clavicle

Seventh cervical vertebra
First thoracic vertebra
Suprasternal notch

Sternal angle

True ribs

Costal cartilage

Manubrium
Body
Sternum

Xiphoid process

1
2
3
4
5
6
7
8
9
10
11
12

T12
L1

False ribs

Floating ribs

FIGURE 4-12 ▲ The thoracic cage (anterior view). The thoracic cage includes 12 pairs of ribs and the 12 thoracic vertebrae with which they join. The thoracic cage also includes the breastbone (sternum).

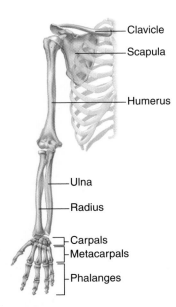

FIGURE 4-13 ▲ The shoulder girdle consists of two pairs of bones that attach the upper limb to the body. Each pair is composed of a scapula (shoulder blade) and a clavicle (collarbone).

The Lower Extremities

The lower extremities are made up of the bones of the pelvis, upper legs, lower legs, and feet (Figure 4-14). In general, the bones of the lower extremities are thicker, heavier, and longer than the upper extremity bones. The bones of the lower extremities support the body and are essential for standing, walking, and running. The **pelvis** is a bony ring formed by three separate bones that fuse to become one by adulthood. The lower extremities are attached to the pelvis at the hip joint. The hip joint is formed by the socket of the **acetabulum** (hip bone) and the head of the **femur** (thigh bone). The femur is the longest, heaviest, and strongest bone of the body. The **greater trochanter** is the large, bony prominence on the lateral shaft of the femur to which the buttock muscles are attached. The head of the femur is the upper end of the bone and is shaped like a ball.

The knee is the largest joint in the body. It is a hinge joint that allows the distal leg to move in flexion and extension. The knee is protected anteriorly by the **patella** (kneecap). It attaches the femur to the two lower leg bones, the **tibia** (shinbone) and **fibula.** The tibia is the larger of the two bones of the lower leg. The lower leg attaches to the foot by the ankle, which is similar to the wrist of the upper extremities. Like the hand, the foot contains several smaller bones and joints, allowing free movement of the foot at the ankle. The **tarsal** bones make up the back part of the foot and heel. The **metatarsal** bones make up the main part of the foot. The toes (**phalanges**) are the foot's equivalent to the fingers.

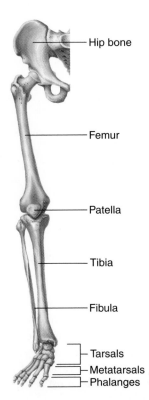

FIGURE 4-14 ▲ Lower extremity bones.

The Muscular System

The muscular system provides several functions for the body:

- Gives the body shape
- Protects internal organs
- Provides for movement of the body
- Maintains posture
- Helps stabilize joints
- Produces body heat

Muscles allow you to smile, open your mouth, breathe, speak, blink, walk, talk, and move food through your digestive system. The heart is a muscle that pumps blood through the body.

Muscles are classified according to their structure and function: skeletal (voluntary) muscle, smooth (involuntary) muscle, and cardiac muscle.

Skeletal Muscles

Skeletal muscles move the skeleton, produce the heat that helps maintain a constant body temperature, and maintain posture. Skeletal muscles are *voluntary* because you can determine how they move. Most skeletal muscles are attached to bones by means of tendons. **Tendons** are strong cords of connective tissue that firmly attach the end of a muscle to a bone. The tendons of many muscles cross over joints, which helps to stabilize

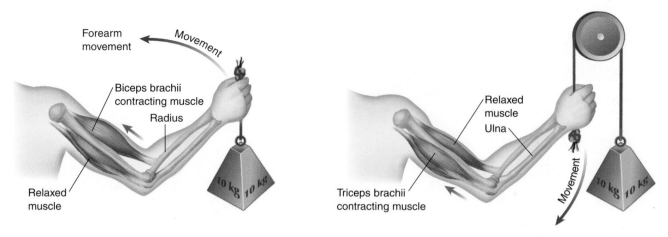

FIGURE 4-15 ▲ When the forearm bends or straightens at the elbow, the bones and muscles function as a lever.

the joint. Skeletal muscles produce rapid, forceful contractions but do not contract unless they are stimulated by a nerve. When a skeletal muscle contracts it shortens, pulling on the structure next to it to cause movement. Although the contractions produced are forceful, skeletal muscle tires easily and must rest after short periods of activity. Regular exercise maintains or increases the size and strength of skeletal muscles. When contraction occurs, the bones work together with muscles to produce body movement. For example, when the forearm bends or straightens at the elbow, the bones and muscles function as a lever (Figure 4-15).

Even when you are not moving, your muscles are in a state of partial contraction. This state is referred to as **muscle tone.** Because of electrical signals sent from nerve cells, some muscle fibers are continuously contracted at any given time. This state of constant tension keeps your head in an upright position, your back straight, and the muscles of your body prepared for action.

Smooth Muscle

Smooth (involuntary) **muscle** is found within the walls of tubular structures of the gastrointestinal tract and urinary systems, blood vessels, the eye, and the bronchi of the respiratory system. Smooth muscle is *involuntary* because you cannot control its movement. Smooth muscle contractions are strong and slow. They respond to stimuli such as stretching, heat, and cold. In the iris of the eye, smooth muscle regulates pupil size. The contraction of the smooth muscle that surrounds the intestines causes food and feces to move along the digestive tract. In blood vessels, smooth muscle helps maintain blood pressure. In the bronchi, the constriction of smooth muscle may result in breathing problems.

A person has no voluntary control over smooth muscle. The contraction and relaxation of smooth muscle is controlled by the body's needs. For example, when a person eats, he does not think about the digestive process. The food is broken down in the stomach and moved forward to the intestinal tract. Nutrients are absorbed and waste is excreted. This process occurs involuntarily (without thought) and with each meal eaten.

Cardiac Muscle

Cardiac muscle, found in the walls of the heart, produces the heart's contractions and pumps blood. Cardiac muscle is found *only* in the heart and has its own supply of blood through the coronary arteries. It can tolerate an interruption of its blood supply for only very short periods. Normal cardiac muscle contractions are strong and rhythmic.

Like smooth muscle, cardiac muscle is involuntary. The heart has the ability to change its rate, rhythm, and strength of contraction according to the needs of the other muscles and organ systems within the body. The heart is the body's hardest working muscle. It beats about 100,000 times every day, without rest, year after year, to move blood through the body.

A comparison of the different muscle types is found in Table 4-2.

Infants and Children

The skull of an infant and child is thin and flexible. When an infant or child suffers trauma to the head, force is more likely to be transferred to the brain instead of fracturing the skull. In infants and young children, the ligaments of the neck are underdeveloped and the muscles of the neck are relatively weak. The head is also larger and heavier relative to the rest of the body. In addition, young children have less muscle mass and more fat and cartilage than older children.

TABLE 4-2 Comparison of Muscle Types

	Location	Function	Type of Control
Skeletal	Attached to bone	• Move the skeleton • Produce heat that helps maintain a constant body temperature • Maintain posture	Voluntary
Smooth	Walls of the esophagus, stomach, intestines, bronchi, uterus, blood vessels, glands	• Move food through the digestive tract • Adjust the size of blood vessels to control blood flow	Involuntary
Cardiac	Walls of the heart	• Contract and relax the heart • Move blood through the body	Involuntary

Injuries to the spinal cord and spinal column are uncommon in infants and young children. When they do occur, children younger than eight years of age tend to sustain injury to the uppermost area of the cervical spine.

The Respiratory System

Objective 2

The body's cells need a continuous supply of oxygen to sustain life. Working with the circulatory system, the respiratory system supplies oxygen from the air we breathe to the body's cells. It also transports carbon dioxide (a waste product of the body's cells) to the lungs. Carbon dioxide is removed from the body in the air that we exhale.

The respiratory system is divided into the upper and lower airways (Figure 4-16). The upper airway is made up of structures outside the chest cavity. These structures include the nose, the **pharynx** (throat), and the **larynx** (voice box). The lower airway consists of parts found almost entirely within the chest cavity, such as the **trachea** (windpipe) and the lungs.

Air enters the body through the nose or the mouth (Figure 4-17). The nostrils are also called the **external nares.** The nostrils open into the nasal cavity. Air is warmed, moistened, and filtered as it moves over the damp, sticky lining (mucous membrane) of the nose. The nasal septum [a wall (partition) that separates two cavities] divides the nasal cavity into right and left portions. The floor of the nasal cavity is bony and is called

the **hard palate**. The **soft palate** is fleshy and extends behind the hard palate. It marks the boundary between the nasopharynx and the rest of the pharynx.

Four nasal **sinuses** (spaces or cavities inside some cranial bones) drain into the nose. Sinuses produce mucus and trap bacteria; they can become infected when bacteria become entrapped in the sinus tissues. Because they are filled with air, sinuses lighten the weight of the bones that make up the skull. They provide additional surface area to nasal passages for warming and humidifying air. Each side of the nose has several **turbinates** (shelf-like projections that protrude into the nasal cavity). As air moves within the

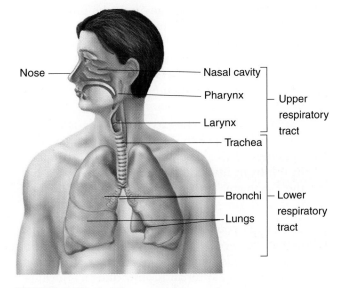

FIGURE 4-16 ▲ The respiratory system.

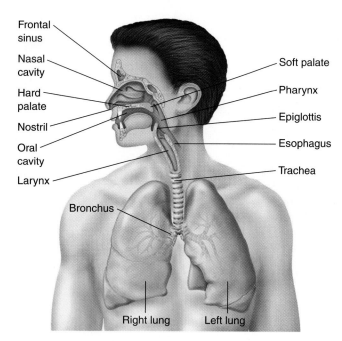

FIGURE 4-17 ▲ Structures of the respiratory system.

turbinates, it is warmed, humidified, and filtered. The turbinates protect structures of the lower airway from foreign body contamination.

Air then travels down the throat through the larynx and the trachea. The pharynx is a muscular tube that is about 5 inches long. It is used by both the respiratory and the digestive systems. It serves as a passageway for food, liquids, and air. The pharynx is made up of three parts.

- **Nasopharynx**. The nasopharynx is located directly behind the nasal cavity. It serves as a passageway for air only. The tissues of the nasopharynx are extremely delicate and bleed easily.

- **Oropharynx**. The oropharynx is the middle part of the throat. It opens into the mouth and serves as a passageway for both food and air. It is separated from the nasopharynx by the soft palate. The **uvula** is the small piece of tissue that looks like a mini punching bag and hangs down in the back of the throat.

- **Laryngopharynx**. The laryngopharynx is the lowermost part of the throat. It surrounds the openings of the esophagus and larynx. It opens in the front into the larynx and in the back into the esophagus. It serves as a passageway for both food and air.

The larynx connects the pharynx with the trachea. It functions in voice production; the length and tension of the vocal cords determine voice pitch. The larynx provides a passageway for air to enter and exit the lungs. It is made up of nine cartilages connected to each other by muscles and ligaments. The **thyroid cartilage** (Adam's apple) is the largest cartilage of the larynx and is shaped like a shield. It can be felt on the front surface of the neck. The hyoid bone is a U-shaped bone that sits above the larynx. It helps move the larynx upward during swallowing. The epiglottis is the uppermost cartilage and is shaped like a leaf. It is attached along the interior anterior border of the thyroid cartilage in a hinge-like fashion. You cannot swallow and breathe at the same time because the **epiglottis,** a special flap of cartilage, covers the trachea when you are eating or drinking so that food or liquids do not enter the lungs (Figure 4-18). The **cricoid cartilage** is the lowermost cartilage of the larynx. It is the only complete ring of cartilage in the larynx. The cricoid cartilage forms the base of the larynx on which the other cartilages rest. The vocal cords stretch across the inside of the larynx. The space between the vocal cords is called the **glottis.**

You Should Know

Cricoid pressure (also called the Sellick maneuver) is a technique used in unresponsive patients. When pressure is applied to the cricoid cartilage, the trachea is pushed backward and the esophagus is compressed (closed) against the cervical vertebrae. This compression helps decrease the amount of air entering the stomach during artificial ventilation.

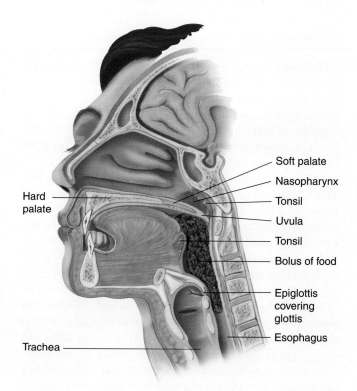

FIGURE 4-18 ▲ The structures involved in swallowing.

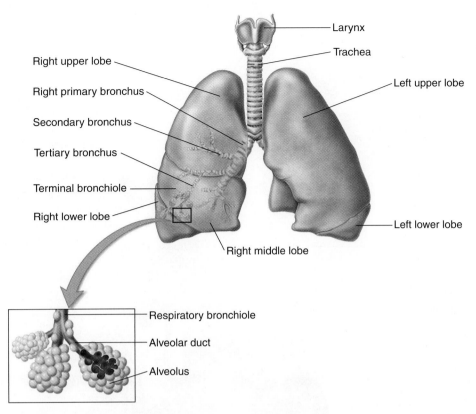

Larynx
Trachea
Right upper lobe
Right primary bronchus
Secondary bronchus
Tertiary bronchus
Terminal bronchiole
Right lower lobe
Left upper lobe
Left lower lobe
Right middle lobe

Respiratory bronchiole
Alveolar duct
Alveolus

FIGURE 4-19 ▲ The bronchial tree consists of the passageways that connect the trachea and the alveoli.

The trachea is located in the front of the neck. It is kept permanently open by C-shaped cartilages. The **esophagus,** which is part of the digestive system, is a muscular tube located behind the trachea. It serves as a passageway for food. The open part of each C-shaped cartilage faces the esophagus. This allows the esophagus to expand slightly into the trachea during swallowing.

The trachea continues into the chest, where it branches into large airway tubes called the right mainstem bronchus and left mainstem bronchus (Figure 4-19). The right mainstem bronchus is shorter, wider, and straighter than the left. Each **bronchus** is joined to a lung, so one tube leads to the right lung and the other leads to the left lung. The inside walls of the bronchi are covered with mucus, which traps dirt and germs that get into the lungs. Small, hair-like structures (cilia) work like brooms to get rid of the debris caught in the mucus. The mainstem bronchi branch into smaller and smaller tubes called **bronchioles**. Bronchioles end in microscopic tubes called alveolar ducts. Each alveolar duct ends in several alveolar sacs. At the end of each alveolar duct, the collections of air sacs (**alveoli**) looks like a cluster of grapes.

You Should Know

The bronchi and bronchioles serve as passageways for air to enter and exit the alveoli. The point at which the trachea divides into two primary bronchi forms an internal ridge called the **carina.** The mucous membrane of the carina is one of the most sensitive areas of the respiratory system and is associated with the cough reflex.

Alveoli are the sites where gases—oxygen and carbon dioxide—are exchanged between the air and blood. There are about 300 million alveoli in the human body. The wall of an alveolus consists of a single layer of cells. A thin film of **surfactant** coats each alveolus and prevents the alveoli from collapsing. Each alveolus is surrounded by a network of pulmonary capillaries (Figure 4-20). Oxygen-rich air enters the alveoli each time you breathe in. Oxygen-poor blood in the capillaries passes into the alveoli. Oxygen enters the capillaries from the alveoli as carbon dioxide enters the alveoli from the capillaries.

The **lungs** are spongy, air-filled organs. They are bound from above (superiorly) by the clavicles

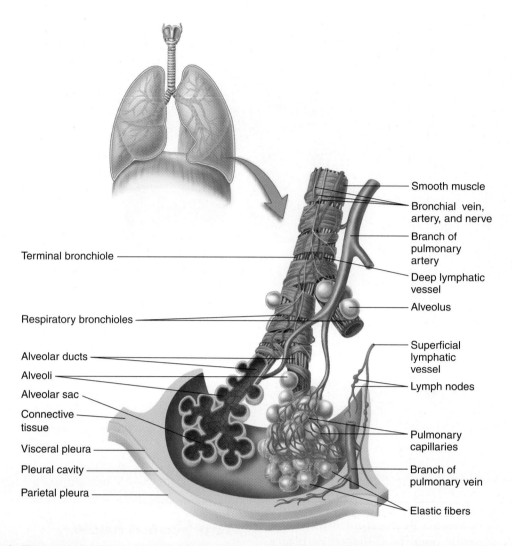

Terminal bronchiole

Respiratory bronchioles

Alveolar ducts

Alveoli

Alveolar sac

Connective tissue

Visceral pleura

Pleural cavity

Parietal pleura

Smooth muscle

Bronchial vein, artery, and nerve

Branch of pulmonary artery

Deep lymphatic vessel

Alveolus

Superficial lymphatic vessel

Lymph nodes

Pulmonary capillaries

Branch of pulmonary vein

Elastic fibers

FIGURE 4-20 ▲ The mainstem bronchi branch into smaller and smaller tubes called bronchioles. At the ends of the bronchioles are tiny sacs that look like clusters of grapes. These tiny sacs are called the alveoli. Alveoli are the sites of gas exchange between the air and blood.

and from below (inferiorly) by the diaphragm (Figure 4-21). The lungs bring air into contact with the blood so oxygen and carbon dioxide can be exchanged in the alveoli. The apex of the lung is the uppermost portion of the lung; it reaches above the first rib. The base of the lung is the portion of the lung resting on the diaphragm. The **mediastinum** is part of the space in the middle of the chest, between the lungs. The mediastinum extends from the sternum (breastbone) to the spine. It contains all of the organs of the thorax—the heart, major blood vessels, the esophagus, the trachea, and nerves—except the lungs.

The lungs are divided into lobes. The right lung has three lobes. It is shorter than the left lung because the diaphragm is higher on the right to make room for the liver that lies below it. The left lung has two lobes. Because two thirds of the heart lies to the left

of the midline of the body, the left lung contains a notch to make room for the heart.

The lungs "float" within separate pleural cavities. They are separated from the chest wall by a space containing pleural fluid. The **pleurae** are the serous (oily) double-walled membranes that enclose each lung (Figure 4-22). The **parietal pleura** is the outer lining and lines the wall of the chest cavity (the rib cage, diaphragm, and mediastinum). The **visceral pleura** is the inner layer and covers the surface of the lungs. The **pleural space** is a space between the visceral and parietal pleura filled with a small amount of oily fluid. Pleural fluid allows the lungs to glide easily against each other as the lungs fill and empty during breathing. Certain illnesses or injuries can cause air, blood, or both to fill the pleural space. This can cause a collapse of the lung on the affected side.

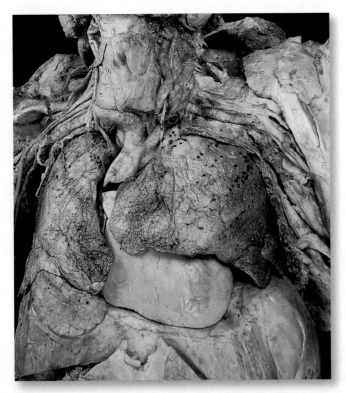

FIGURE 4-21 ▲ Anterior view of the chest. © *The McGraw-Hill Companies, Inc./Karl Rubin, photographer.*

The Mechanics of Breathing

Breathing (also called *pulmonary ventilation*) is the mechanical process of moving air into and out of the lungs. **Inspiration** (inhalation) is the process of breathing in and moving air into the lungs. **Expiration** (exhalation) is the process of breathing out and moving air out of the lungs. **Respiration** is the exchange of gases between a living organism and its environ-ment. Oxygen is the component of air that is an essential "fuel" needed by all body cells for survival. Most cells begin to die if their oxygen supply is interrupted for even a few minutes.

The rate and depth of breathing is controlled by the brain. The brain is sensitive to the level of carbon dioxide in the bloodstream. Carbon dioxide is a waste product produced by the body's cells. When the level of carbon dioxide in the blood is increased, a person breathes faster and deeper to get rid of the carbon dioxide and bring in more oxygen, which is necessary for cell function.

Every three to five seconds, nerve impulses stimulate the breathing process. When the brain senses a rise in the carbon dioxide level in the bloodstream, it sends a signal to the diaphragm and **intercostal** muscles (muscles between the ribs), causing them to contract. The **diaphragm** is the dome-shaped muscle below the lungs. It is the main muscle of respiration and separates the chest cavity from the abdominal cavity. The external intercostal muscles are located between the ribs. The internal intercostal muscles and abdominal muscles may be used during forceful expiration.

You Should Know

In most people, a rise in the level of carbon dioxide in the bloodstream is the stimulus that triggers the respiratory center in the brain. However, chronic respiratory diseases may alter the normal respiratory drive over time. Instead of an increase in carbon dioxide levels stimulating breathing, low levels of oxygen in the blood become the breathing stimulus. This kind of breathing stimulus is called **hypoxic drive.**

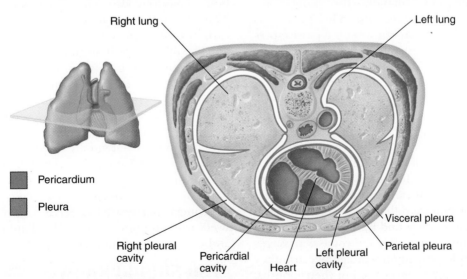

FIGURE 4-22 ▲ Each lung is surrounded by a pleural cavity. The parietal pleura lines each pleural cavity and the visceral pleura covers the surface of the lungs. The potential spaces between the pleural membranes (the left and right pleural cavities) are shown here as actual spaces.

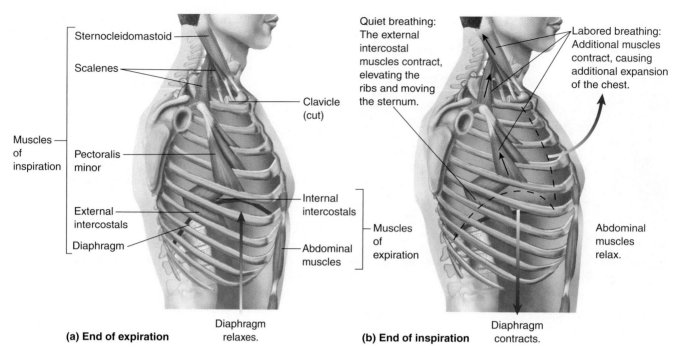

Muscles of inspiration
- Sternocleidomastoid
- Scalenes
- Clavicle (cut)
- Pectoralis minor
- External intercostals
- Diaphragm

Internal intercostals

Muscles of expiration
- Abdominal muscles

(a) End of expiration

Diaphragm relaxes.

Quiet breathing: The external intercostal muscles contract, elevating the ribs and moving the sternum.

Labored breathing: Additional muscles contract, causing additional expansion of the chest.

Abdominal muscles relax.

(b) End of inspiration

Diaphragm contracts.

FIGURE 4-23 ▲ **(a)** Muscles of respiration at the end of expiration. **(b)** Muscles of respiration at the end of inspiration. During inhalation, the diaphragm and external intercostal muscles between the ribs contract causing the volume of the chest cavity to increase. During a normal exhalation these muscles relax and the chest volume returns to normal.

The mechanics of breathing can be compared with a bellows: When it is opened, air enters; as it closes, air is forced out. When the diaphragm and external intercostal muscles contract, the chest cavity enlarges and fills with air. This process is called inspiration. Inspiration is considered an active process because it requires muscle contraction. When the diaphragm and external intercostal muscles relax, the chest cavity becomes smaller, the lungs are compressed, and air is forced out. This process is called expiration. Expiration is normally a passive process because the lungs recoil as a result of their elasticity (Figure 4-23). Methods used to assess adequate and inadequate breathing are discussed in Chapters 5, 7, and 9.

Infants and Children

The respiratory anatomy of infants and young children differs from that of older children and adults. In general, all structures are smaller. Because they are smaller, they are more easily blocked than in adults. The nasal passages are soft and narrow and have little supporting cartilage. It is important to keep the nasal passages clear in infants under six months of age because they breathe mostly through their noses, not their mouths. If the nasal passages are blocked as a result of tissue swelling or a buildup of mucus, difficulty in breathing and problems with feeding can result.

The tongue takes up proportionally more space in the mouth of a child than in an adult. The tracheal rings are softer and more flexible in infants and children. This puts the airway at risk of compression if the neck is not positioned properly.

The chest wall of an infant and young child is softer and more elastic than that of an older child and adult. This is because it is made of more cartilage than bone. Children also have fewer and smaller alveoli. Thus, the potential area for exchanging oxygen and carbon dioxide is less. Because the chest wall is soft and flexible, rib and sternum fractures are less common in children than in adults. However, the force of the injury is more easily transmitted to the delicate tissues of the underlying lung. This results in bruising of the lung and bleeding in the alveoli, which reduces the number of alveoli available for gas exchange. This type of injury is potentially life-threatening.

Infants and young children depend more heavily on the diaphragm for breathing than adults. Air can build up in the stomach during rescue breathing or improperly performed CPR. As a result, the stomach swells with air, movement of the diaphragm is limited, and effective breathing is reduced.

You Should Know

The main cause of cardiac arrest in infants and children is an uncorrected respiratory problem.

The Circulatory System

The circulatory system is made up of the cardiovascular and lymphatic systems. The **cardiovascular system** is made up of three main parts: a pump (the heart), fluid (blood), and a container (the blood vessels). The **lymphatic system** consists of lymph, lymph nodes, lymph vessels, tonsils, the spleen, and the thymus gland. The spleen and liver are also associated with the circulatory system because they form and store blood.

The functions of the circulatory system are the following:

- Deliver oxygen-rich blood and nutrients to body tissues
- Help maintain body temperature
- Protect the body against infection
- Remove waste and by-products of metabolism from the body tissues
- Transport hormones and other chemical messengers to targeted tissues of the body

The Heart

The **heart** is located slightly to the left of the center of the chest. It is attached to the chest through the **great vessels** (pulmonary arteries and veins, the aorta, and the superior and inferior vena cavae). With its thick walls of cardiac muscle, the heart functions to pump blood through the vessels of the body (Figure 4-24).

The heart has four hollow chambers. The two upper chambers are the right and left **atria.** The job of the atria is to receive blood from the body and lungs. The two lower chambers of the heart are the right and left **ventricles.** The ventricles are larger and have thicker walls than the atria because their job is to pump blood to the lungs and body.

The right atrium receives blood that is low in oxygen from the body by means of veins. Blood flows from the right atrium through a one-way valve, the tricuspid valve. The tricuspid valve forces the blood to always move in the correct direction, into the right ventricle. When the right ventricle contracts, blood is pumped through another one-way valve, the pulmonic valve, into the pulmonary arteries. Blood flows from the pulmonary arteries to the lungs, where it receives a fresh supply of oxygen. From the lungs, the oxygen-rich blood flows along the pulmonary veins to the left upper chamber of the heart, the left atrium. The left atrium pumps the blood through the mitral (bicuspid) valve to the left ventricle. The left ventricle is about three times thicker than the right ventricle because it has to produce enough pressure to push

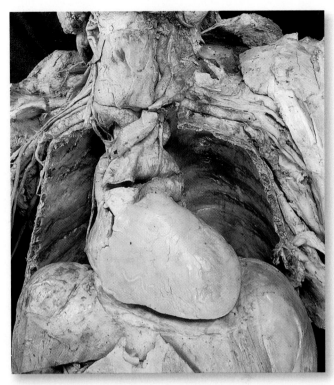

FIGURE 4-24 ▲ Anterior view of the human heart in the chest with the lungs removed. © The McGraw-Hill Companies, Inc./Karl Rubin, photographer.

the blood out of the heart, through the aortic valve, and into the aorta, the body's largest artery (Figure 4-25). The aorta and its branches distribute the oxygen-rich blood throughout the body.

The normal heartbeat begins as an electrical signal in a small area of specialized tissue in the upper right atrium of the heart. The impulse spreads through a system of pathways called the conduction system. A disruption of these pathways can cause the heart to malfunction. For example, a heart attack disrupts the flow of oxygen and nutrients to the heart's cells. This disruption can cause the heart to beat too quickly or too slowly. It can also affect the heart's ability to contract and pump blood to the rest of the body.

Blood

Blood is a type of transport system. It is the means by which oxygen, food, hormones, minerals, and other essential substances are carried to all parts of the body. An adult has about 5-6 liters of blood flowing through his or her circulatory system. Blood carries carbon dioxide and other waste material from the body's cells to the lungs, kidneys, or skin for removal. To help maintain body temperature, blood vessels narrow (constrict) and widen (dilate) as needed to keep or lose heat at the skin's surface. The blood and lymphatic system work together to protect the body against infection.

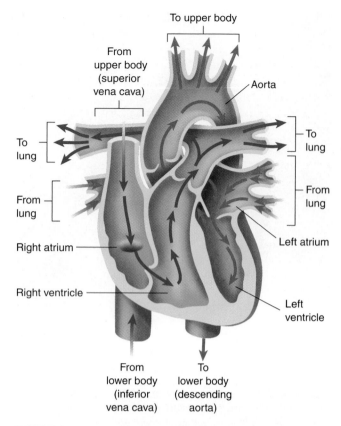

FIGURE 4-25 ▲ Blood flow through the heart and lungs.

the lungs and transports it to the body's cells. Hemoglobin is red and therefore gives blood its red color.

After delivering oxygen to the cells, red blood cells gather up carbon dioxide and transport it to the lungs, where it is removed from the body when we exhale. White blood cells (**leukocytes**) attack and destroy germs that enter the body. **Platelets** (thrombocytes) are irregularly shaped blood cells that have a sticky surface. When a blood vessel is damaged and starts to bleed, platelets gather at the site of injury. The platelets begin sticking to the opening of the damaged vessel and seal it, stopping the flow of blood.

Blood Vessels

Blood vessels that carry blood away from the heart to the rest of the body are called **arteries** (Figure 4-27). Remember: **A**rteries = **A**way. Blood is forced into the arteries when the heart contracts. Arteries have thick walls because they transport blood under high pressure. Arteries normally carry oxygen-rich blood. However, the pulmonary artery and its two branches, the left and right pulmonary arteries, carry oxygen-poor blood.

Arterioles are the smallest branches of arteries. They connect arteries to capillaries. **Capillaries** are the smallest and most numerous blood vessels. They are very thin (thinner than a human hair) and connect arterioles and venules. The exchange of oxygen, nutrients, and waste products between blood and body cells occurs through the walls of capillaries. **Venules** are the smallest branches of veins. They connect capillaries and veins. **Veins** are vessels that return blood to the heart. Veins normally carry oxygen-poor blood. However, the pulmonary vein and its two branches (the left and right pulmonary veins) carry oxygen-rich blood. (There are four pulmonary veins, two from each lung). The walls of veins are thinner than arteries. Because the pressure in the veins is low, veins contain one-way valves that help keep the blood flowing toward the heart (Figure 4-28).

Blood is made up of liquid and formed elements (Figure 4-26). The liquid portion of the blood is called **plasma**. Plasma carries blood cells, vitamins, proteins, glucose, and many other substances throughout the body. The formed elements of the blood include red blood cells, white blood cells, and platelets. Red blood cells (**erythrocytes**) contain hemoglobin. Each red blood cell has about 250 million hemoglobin molecules. Hemoglobin is an iron-containing protein that chemically bonds with oxygen. Thus, hemoglobin is the part of the red blood cell that picks up oxygen in

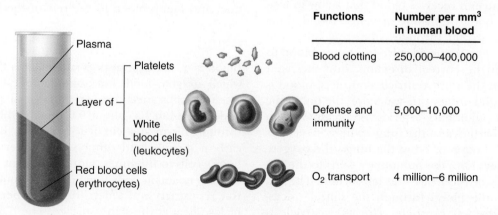

	Functions	Number per mm³ in human blood
Platelets	Blood clotting	250,000–400,000
White blood cells (leukocytes)	Defense and immunity	5,000–10,000
Red blood cells (erythrocytes)	O₂ transport	4 million–6 million

FIGURE 4-26 ▲ Blood is made up of liquid (plasma) and formed elements (red blood cells, white blood cells, and platelets).

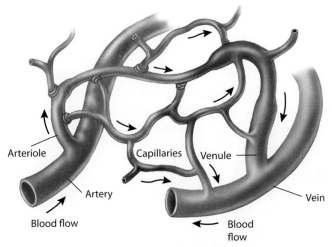

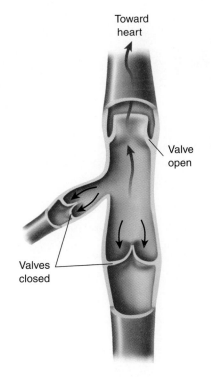

FIGURE 4-27 ▲ Blood flow from the heart through the body moves through the following vessels: Arteries → arterioles → capillaries → venules → veins.

FIGURE 4-28 ▶ Veins contain one-way valves that help keep blood flowing toward the heart.

Major Arteries

Blood flows from the **aorta**, the largest artery in the body, to all parts of the body. The aorta lies in front of the spine in the thoracic and abdominal cavities (Figure 4-29). Because the heart must have a constant blood supply, it supplies itself with oxygenated blood first through the coronary arteries. The coronary arteries are the first blood vessels that branch off the aorta. When the heart relaxes, the coronary arteries fill with blood in between beats and supply the heart muscle with the oxygen it needs.

Branches of the aorta form the carotid and subclavian arteries. The left and right carotid arteries are the major arteries of the neck, supplying the head and neck with blood. A carotid pulse can be felt on either side of the neck. The subclavian arteries run under the clavicles and supply blood to the upper extremities. The subclavian arteries branch into the axillary and brachial arteries in the upper arm. A brachial pulse can be felt on the inside of the arm between the elbow and the shoulder. This artery is used when determining a blood pressure (BP) with a BP cuff and stethoscope. The brachial arteries branch into the radial and ulnar arteries. These arteries supply the forearm with blood. The radial artery is the major artery of the lower arm. A radial pulse can be felt on the side of the wrist below the thumb.

The femoral arteries are the major arteries of the thigh, supplying the lower extremities with blood. A femoral pulse can be felt in the groin area (the crease between the abdomen and the thigh). Behind the knees, the femoral arteries become the popliteal arteries. The popliteal arteries supply blood to the lower legs. Slightly below the knee, the popliteal arteries become the tibial arteries. The posterior tibial pulse is located just behind the ankle bone. At the ankle, one of the tibial arteries becomes the dorsalis pedis artery, which supplies blood to the foot. A dorsalis pedis pulse (often called a *pedal pulse*) can be felt on the top of the foot.

Major Veins

The two largest veins in the human body are the inferior vena cava and the superior vena cava. These two veins empty oxygen-poor blood into the heart's right atrium. The superior vena cava returns blood from the head and upper extremities to the heart. The inferior vena cava returns blood from the trunk and lower extremities to the heart.

You Should Know

Coronary Artery Bypass Graft

A coronary artery bypass graft (CABG) is a surgical procedure that may be performed to fix a blocked coronary artery. The bypass graft is usually part of a healthy blood vessel that is taken from the patient's leg, chest, or arm. The blood vessel is sewn from one healthy area of the heart to another. This newly placed vessel creates a detour around the blocked area. The vessel most often used for the graft is the saphenous vein in the leg. This vessel is used because it is long, reaching from the ankle to the thigh, and is about the same diameter as a coronary artery.

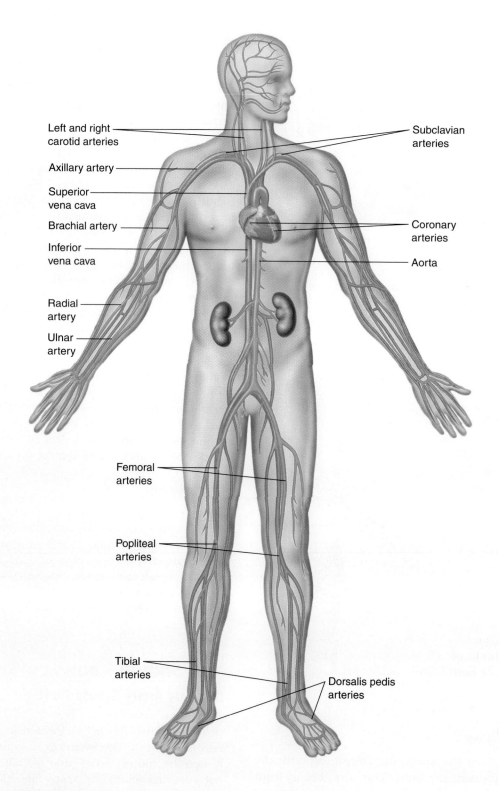

Left and right carotid arteries

Subclavian arteries

Axillary artery

Superior vena cava

Brachial artery

Coronary arteries

Inferior vena cava

Aorta

Radial artery

Ulnar artery

Femoral arteries

Popliteal arteries

Tibial arteries

Dorsalis pedis arteries

FIGURE 4-29 ▲ Major arteries and veins.

The Physiology of Circulation

Pulse

When the left ventricle contracts, a wave of blood is sent through the arteries, causing the arteries to expand and recoil. A **pulse** is the regular expansion and recoil of an artery caused by the movement of blood from the heart as it contracts. A pulse can be felt anywhere an artery passes near the skin surface and over a bone. Central pulses are located close to the heart, such as the carotid and femoral pulses. Peripheral pulses are located farther from the heart, such as the radial, brachial, posterior tibial, and dorsalis pedis pulses.

Blood Pressure

Blood pressure is the force exerted by the blood on the inner walls of the heart and arteries. The **systolic blood pressure** is the pressure in an artery when the heart is pumping blood (systole). The **diastolic blood pressure** is the pressure in an artery when the heart is at rest (diastole). A blood pressure measurement is made up of both the systolic and the diastolic pressures. It is measured in millimeters of mercury (mm Hg). Blood pressure is written as a fraction (for example, 115/78), with the systolic number first. In an adult, a normal systolic blood pressure ranges from 100 to 119 mm Hg. A normal diastolic blood pressure ranges from 60 to 79 mm Hg. Blood pressure is dependent on the contraction of the heart, blood volume, and the condition of the blood vessels. A slow or fast heart rate, a loss of blood, or changes in the elasticity of the blood vessels may lead to changes in the blood pressure. Methods used to measure blood pressure are discussed in Chapter 5.

Perfusion

Perfusion is the flow of blood through an organ or a part of the body. **Shock** (hypoperfusion) is the inadequate flow of blood through an organ or a part of the body.

The Nervous System

Objective 2

The nervous system is a collection of specialized cells that conduct information to and from the brain. The functions of the nervous system are to:

- Control the voluntary (conscious) and involuntary (unconscious) activities of the body
- Provide for higher mental function (such as thought and emotion)

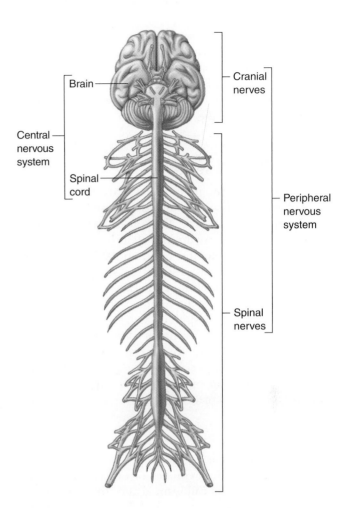

FIGURE 4-30 ▲ The central nervous system (CNS) consists of the brain and spinal cord. The peripheral nervous system (PNS) consists of cranial nerves, which arise from the brain and spinal nerves, which arise from the spinal cord. The nerves actually extend throughout the body.

The nervous system has two divisions: the central nervous system (CNS) and the peripheral nervous system (PNS). (Figure 4-30.)

The Central Nervous System

The **central nervous system (CNS)** consists of the brain and the spinal cord. The brain is made up of many nerve cells (**neurons**) that are involved in higher mental function. These higher functions include the ability to think, to perform unconscious motor functions such as breathing and the control of blood vessel diameter, and to experience and express emotion.

The brain is located in the **cranium**, where it is protected. The spinal cord is protected in the spinal canal where it travels through the **foramen magnum**, which is the opening in the base of the skull, and down the vertebral column. The central nervous system is also protected by the **meninges**, a covering over the brain and spinal cord, and **cerebrospinal fluid (CSF),** a clear liquid that is circulated continuously. CSF acts as a shock absorber for the central nervous system. It also provides a means for the exchange of nutrients and wastes between the blood, the brain, and the spinal cord.

You Should Know

Meninges (literally, membranes), are three layers of connective tissue coverings that surround the brain and spinal cord. The pia mater (literally, "gentle mother") forms the delicate inner layer that clings gently to the brain and spinal cord. It contains many blood vessels that supply the nervous tissue. The arachnoid (literally, "resembling a spider's web") layer is the middle layer with delicate fibers resembling a spider's web; it contains few blood vessels. The dura mater (literally, "hard" or "tough mother") is the tough, outermost layer that sticks to the inner surface of the skull. **Meningitis** is an inflammation of the tissue coverings of the brain and spinal cord.

The **cerebrum** is the largest part of the human brain (Figure 4-31). It consists of two cerebral hemispheres. The **corpus callosum,** a very thick bundle of nerve fibers, joins the two hemispheres. Although no area of the brain functions alone, each cerebral hemisphere is divided into four lobes named for the bones that lie over them:

- *Frontal.* The frontal lobes control goal-oriented behavior, personality, short-term memory, elaboration of thought, inhibition of emotions, and programming and integrating motor activity, including speech.
- *Parietal.* The parietal lobes receive and process information about touch, taste, pressure, pain, heat, and cold.

- *Occipital.* The occipital lobes receive and interpret visual information.
- *Temporal.* The temporal lobes receive auditory signals and interpret language. They are also involved in personality, behavior, emotion, long-term memory, taste, smell, and have some influence on balance.

You Should Know

Think of the CNS as a computer system. The right and left hemispheres of the brain are two computers in the network. The corpus callosum is the cable that connects (networks) the two computers.

The **cerebellum** is the second largest part of the human brain. It is responsible for the precise control of muscle movements as well as maintaining posture and balance. The **diencephalon** is the part of the brain between the cerebrum and the brainstem. It contains the thalamus and hypothalamus. The **thalamus** functions as a relay station for impulses going to and from the cerebrum. The **hypothalamus** plays an important role in the control of thirst, hunger, and body temperature. It also serves as a link between the nervous and endocrine systems.

The **brainstem** is made up of the midbrain, the pons, and the medulla oblongata. The midbrain connects the pons and cerebellum with the cerebrum. It acts as a relay for auditory and visual signals. The pons, which means "bridge," connects parts of the brain with one another by means of tracts. It influences respiration. The medulla oblongata is the lowest part of the brainstem. It joins the brainstem to the spinal cord. The medulla contains nerves that pass from the spinal cord to the brain and nerves that pass from the brain to the spinal cord. The medulla is involved in controlling blood vessel diameter, respiration, and centers that control reflexes such as coughing, swallowing, sneezing, and vomiting.

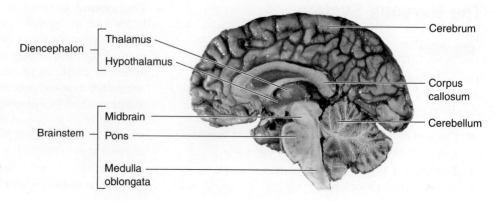

FIGURE 4-31 ▶ The areas of the brain. © *Branislav Vidic.*

TABLE 4-3 Effects of Stimulation of the Autonomic Nervous System

Effects of Sympathetic Stimulation	Effects of Parasympathetic Stimulation
"Fight or Flight"	"Rest and Digest"
• Heart rate increases	• Heart rate decreases
• Heart's force of contraction increases	• Heart's force of contraction decreases
• Pupils widen	• Pupils narrow
• Digestion decreases	• Digestion increases
• Mouth and nose secretions decrease	• Mouth and nose secretions increase
• Bronchial muscles relax	• Bronchial muscles constrict
• Urine secretion decreases	• Urine secretion increases

The **spinal cord** is continuous with the medulla and is the center for many reflex activities of the body. It relays electrical signals to and from the brain and peripheral nerves.

The Peripheral Nervous System

The **peripheral nervous system (PNS)** is made up of nerves that connect the brain and spinal cord to the rest of the body. Twelve pairs of **cranial nerves** are linked directly to the brain. Even though the cranial nerves exit from the brain, they are still considered a part of the peripheral nervous system. The cranial nerves are involved in special senses such as vision, hearing, smell, and taste. They are also involved in eye, face, and tongue movements. Cranial nerves relay signals to and from the brain.

Spinal nerves are any of 31 pairs of nerves that relay impulses to and from the spinal cord. There are three types of spinal nerves: sensory, motor, and mixed nerves. Sensory nerve cells receive information from the body. They send electrical signals *to* the brain and spinal cord, allowing the body to respond to sensory input. The brain and spinal cord's response is sent along motor nerve cells. Motor nerves send electrical signals *from* the brain and spinal cord. For example, when a person touches hot water, the sensory nerve signal travels up to the brain and then back down via motor nerve cells to the muscles of the involved extremity, causing movement away from the hot water.

The PNS has two divisions. The **somatic** (voluntary) **division** has receptors and nerves concerned with the external environment. It influences the activity of the musculoskeletal system. The **autonomic** (involuntary) **division** has receptors and nerves concerned with the internal environment. It controls the involuntary system of glands and smooth muscle and functions to maintain a steady state in the body.

The autonomic division is further divided into the sympathetic division and parasympathetic division. The **sympathetic division** mobilizes energy, particularly in stressful situations. This is called the "fight-or-flight" response. Its effects are widespread throughout the body. The **parasympathetic division** conserves and restores energy; its effects are localized in the body (Table 4-3).

The Integumentary System

The **integumentary system** is made up of the skin, hair, nails, sweat glands, and oil (sebaceous) glands (Figure 4-32). The skin protects the body from the environment, bacteria, and other organisms, as well as keeps the fluids inside the body. Blood vessels and the sweat glands in the skin help control and maintain body temperature. The skin acts as a sense organ, detecting sensations such as heat, cold, touch, pressure, and pain. The skin relays this information to the brain and spinal cord.

The skin has multiple layers, including the epidermis, dermis, and subcutaneous tissue, which lie over muscle and bone. Each layer contains different structures. The **epidermis** is the outer portion of the skin. It does not contain blood vessels and is thickest on the palms of the hands and the soles of the feet. The **dermis** is the thick layer of skin below the epidermis. The dermis contains hair follicles, sweat and oil glands, small nerve endings, and blood vessels. The **subcutaneous layer** is thick and lies below the dermis. It contains fat and insulates the body from changes in temperature. This layer is loosely attached to the muscles and bones of the musculoskeletal system.

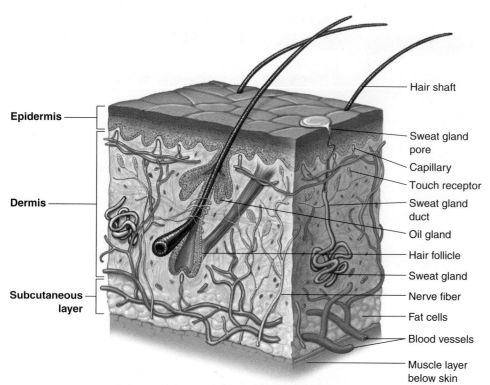

FIGURE 4-32 ◄ Human skin consists of the epidermis and dermis. The subcutaneous layer is beneath the dermis. Associated structures include hair follicles, sweat glands, and sebaceous (oil) glands.

Labels on figure:
- Hair shaft
- Epidermis
- Sweat gland pore
- Capillary
- Touch receptor
- Sweat gland duct
- Dermis
- Oil gland
- Hair follicle
- Sweat gland
- Nerve fiber
- Subcutaneous layer
- Fat cells
- Blood vessels
- Muscle layer below skin

You Should Know

The skin is the largest organ system of the human body. In a 150-pound man, the skin weighs about 9 pounds and covers an area of about 18 square feet.

The Digestive System

Function

The digestive system performs the following functions:

- **Ingestion.** The digestive system brings nutrients, water, and electrolytes into the body.
- **Digestion.** It chemically breaks down food into small parts so absorption can occur.
- **Absorption.** It moves nutrients, water, and electrolytes into the circulatory system so they can be used by body cells.
- **Defecation.** It eliminates unabsorbed waste.

Components

The primary organs of the digestive system are the mouth, pharynx, esophagus, stomach, small intestine, large intestine, rectum, and anal canal (Figure 4-33). The **accessory organs of digestion** are the teeth and tongue, salivary glands, liver, gallbladder, and pancreas. **Peristalsis** is the involuntary wavelike contraction of smooth muscle that moves material through the digestive tract.

The mouth, teeth, and salivary glands begin the process of digestion. The tongue manipulates food for chewing and swallowing. Chemicals (enzymes) in the salivary glands begin the breakdown of food. The salivary glands also moisten and lubricate food so it can be swallowed. The teeth mince food into small pieces so it can be swallowed when mixed with saliva.

Swallowing moves food from the pharynx into the esophagus. The esophagus transports food from the pharynx to the stomach by peristalsis. The stomach stores food. It mixes food with gastric juices and breaks it down into chyme. The **chyme** (partially digested food) is moved into the small intestine by peristalsis.

The **small intestine** is about 20 feet (7 meters) long. It is smaller in diameter than the large intestine. It receives food from the stomach and secretions from the pancreas and liver. It completes the digestion of food that began in the mouth and stomach. Most digestion and absorption occurs here. It selectively absorbs nutrients that can be used by the body. It is composed of three sections (listed in the order in which food passes through them): **duodenum, jejunum,** and **ileum.**

The **large intestine** is about 5 feet (1.5 meters) in length. It absorbs water and electrolytes from the remaining chyme and changes it from a fluid to a semi-solid mass. It excretes waste as feces. The large intestine is subdivided into the following sections (listed in the order in which food passes through them): **cecum, ascending colon, transverse colon, descending colon, sigmoid colon, rectum,** and **anal canal.**

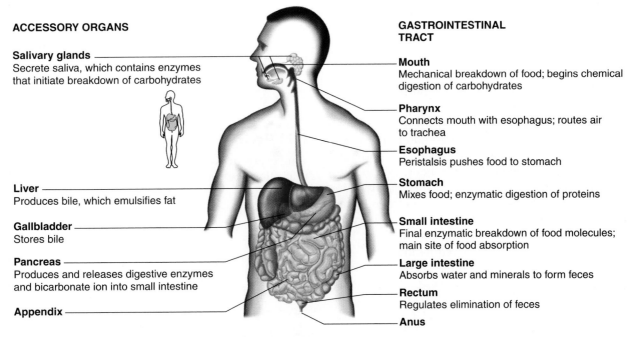

Salivary glands
Secrete saliva, which contains enzymes that initiate breakdown of carbohydrates

Liver
Produces bile, which emulsifies fat

Gallbladder
Stores bile

Pancreas
Produces and releases digestive enzymes and bicarbonate ion into small intestine

Appendix

GASTROINTESTINAL TRACT

Mouth
Mechanical breakdown of food; begins chemical digestion of carbohydrates

Pharynx
Connects mouth with esophagus; routes air to trachea

Esophagus
Peristalsis pushes food to stomach

Stomach
Mixes food; enzymatic digestion of proteins

Small intestine
Final enzymatic breakdown of food molecules; main site of food absorption

Large intestine
Absorbs water and minerals to form feces

Rectum
Regulates elimination of feces

Anus

FIGURE 4-33 ▲ Primary and accessory organs of the digestive system.

The **liver** is the largest internal organ of the body. It produces bile, which breaks up (emulsifies) fats. It stimulates the gallbladder to secrete stored bile into the small intestine. It stores minerals and fat-soluble vitamins (A, D, E, and K). It also stores blood. The **gallbladder** stores bile until it is needed by the small intestine. The **pancreas** secretes juices that contain enzymes for protein, carbohydrate, and fat digestion into the small intestine.

The Endocrine System

Objective 2

Function

The **endocrine system** is a system of glands that secrete chemicals (hormones) directly into the circulatory system (Figure 4-34). The chemicals released into the bloodstream trigger a response in specific body cells. As a result, the endocrine system influences body activities and functions. The endocrine system works closely with the nervous system to maintain homeostasis.

Components

The **thyroid gland** lies in the neck, just below the larynx. Its shape resembles that of a butterfly. The thyroid gland produces hormones that stimulate body heat production and bone growth. It also controls the body's metabolic rate. The **parathyroid glands** are located behind the thyroid gland. They secrete a hormone that

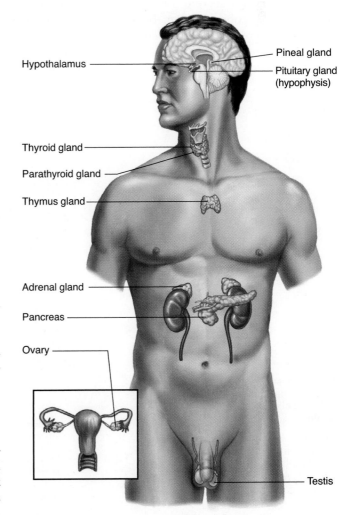

Hypothalamus

Thyroid gland

Parathyroid gland

Thymus gland

Adrenal gland

Pancreas

Ovary

Pineal gland

Pituitary gland (hypophysis)

Testis

FIGURE 4-34 ▲ The endocrine system.

maintains the calcium level in the blood. **Adrenal glands** are located on top of each kidney. The outer tissue of an adrenal gland is called the cortex. The inner tissue of an adrenal gland is called the medulla. The adrenal medulla releases epinephrine and norepinephrine. Epinephrine and norepinephrine help prepare the body for its "fight or flight" response.

The **pituitary gland** is buried deep in the cranial cavity at the base of the brain. In an adult, it is about the size and shape of a garbanzo bean. The pituitary gland is the "master gland" of the body. It regulates growth and controls other endocrine glands. The hypothalamus produces or controls hormones released by the pituitary. It controls the part of the nervous system that controls involuntary body functions, hormones, and functions such as regulating sleep and stimulating appetite. The **pineal gland** is located near the center of the brain. It is responsible for producing **melatonin**, which has a role in regulating daily rhythms, such as sleep. Levels of melatonin increase at night and are low or undetectable during the day.

The **islets of Langerhans** are located in the pancreas. Alpha cells secrete glucagon, which increases blood glucose concentration. Beta cells secrete **insulin**, which decreases blood glucose concentration.

Other glands of the endocrine system include the **thymus gland**, ovaries, and **testes**. The thymus gland plays a role in the body's immune system. The ovaries secrete estrogens, which are female sex hormones. The testes secrete testosterone and other male hormones.

The Reproductive System

Function

The **reproductive system** makes cells (sperm, eggs) that allow continuation of the human species.

Components

Male

The testes produce sperm and the hormone testosterone (Figure 4-35). Reproductive ducts allow passage of sperm. Ducts include:

- Epididymis
- Ductus (vas) deferens
- Ejaculatory duct
- Urethra

Seminal vesicles secrete fluid that nourishes and protects sperm. The **prostate gland** secretes fluid that increases sperm movement and neutralizes the acidity

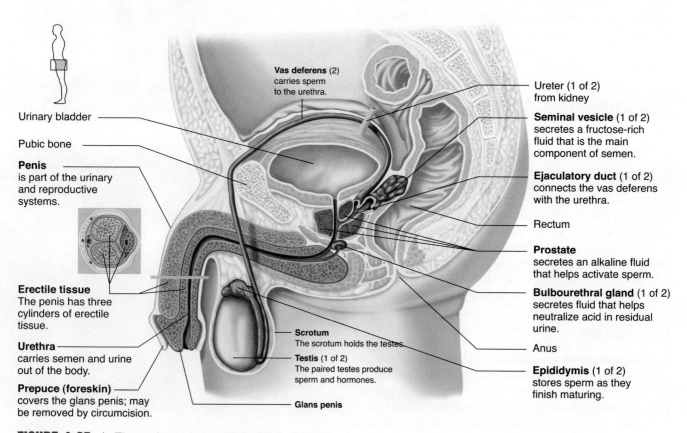

FIGURE 4-35 ▲ The male reproductive system.

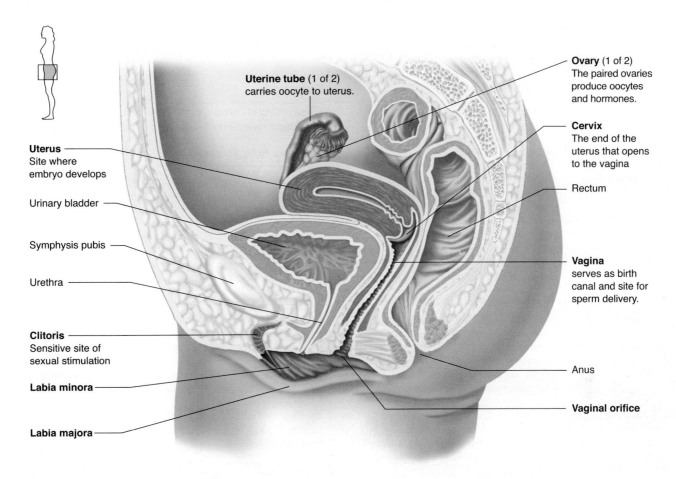

Uterine tube (1 of 2) carries oocyte to uterus.

Ovary (1 of 2)
The paired ovaries produce oocytes and hormones.

Cervix
The end of the uterus that opens to the vagina

Rectum

Uterus
Site where embryo develops

Urinary bladder

Symphysis pubis

Urethra

Vagina
serves as birth canal and site for sperm delivery.

Clitoris
Sensitive site of sexual stimulation

Labia minora

Labia majora

Anus

Vaginal orifice

FIGURE 4-36 ▲ The female reproductive system.

of the vagina during intercourse. The **penis** serves as the outlet for sperm and urine. The **scrotum** is the loose sac of skin that houses the testes.

Female

The **ovaries** are a pair of almond-shaped organs that produce eggs (ova) (Figure 4-36). They are located on either side of the uterus in the pelvic cavity. The ovaries produce the hormones estrogen and progesterone. **Fallopian tubes** (oviducts) receive the ovum and transport it to the uterus after ovulation. The **uterus** is a hollow, muscular organ in which a fertilized ovum implants and receives nourishment until birth. The **vagina** (birth canal) receives the penis during intercourse and serves as a passageway for menstrual flow and delivery of an infant. Accessory organs include the **mammary glands** (breasts), which function in milk production after delivery of an infant.

The external genitalia include the mons pubis, clitoris, urethral opening, Bartholin's gland, vagina, labia minora, labia majora, and hymen. The **perineum** is the area between the vaginal opening and anus.

The Urinary System

Function

The urinary system produces and excretes urine from the body.

Components

The **kidneys** are located at the back of the abdominal cavity on each side of the spinal column. They produce urine, maintain water balance, aid in regulation of blood pressure, and regulate levels of many chemicals in the blood. The **ureters** are tubes that drain urine from the kidneys to the urinary bladder. The **urinary bladder** serves as a temporary storage site for urine. The **urethra** is a canal that passes urine from the urinary bladder to the outside of the body (Figure 4-37). In males, the urethra transports semen from the body. The male urethra is longer than that of females.

TABLE 4-4 Organ Systems

System	Components	Function
Muscular	Skeletal muscle, smooth muscle, and cardiac muscle	Gives the body shape, protects internal organs, provides movement of parts of the skeleton
Skeletal	Ligaments, cartilage, and bones	Gives the body shape, protects vital internal organs
Respiratory	Air passages (mouth, nose, trachea, larynx, bronchi, and bronchioles) and lungs	Brings oxygen into the body, removes carbon dioxide from the body
Circulatory	Heart, blood, blood vessels, lymph, and lymph vessels	Delivers oxygen and nutrients to the tissues, removes waste products from the tissues
Nervous	Brain, spinal cord, and nerves	Controls the voluntary and involuntary activity of the body, provides for higher mental function (thought, emotion)
Integumentary	Skin, hair, fingernails, toenails, sweat glands, and sebaceous glands	Protects the body from the environment, bacteria and other organisms; helps regulate the temperature of the body; senses heat, cold, touch, pressure, and pain
Digestive	Mouth, esophagus, stomach, liver, pancreas, and intestines	Ingestion and digestion of food is absorbed into the body through the membranes of the intestines
Endocrine	Pituitary gland, thyroid gland, parathyroid glands, adrenal glands, thymus gland, ovaries, testes, pineal gland, and the islets of Langerhans in the pancreas	Interacts with the nervous system to regulate many body activities; secretes chemicals (hormones) to stimulate many body functions
Reproductive	Female: ovaries, uterus, vagina, and mammary glands Male: testes and penis	Manufactures cells (sperm, eggs) that allow continuation of the species
Urinary	Kidneys, urinary bladder, ureters, and urethra	Removes body wastes, assists in regulating blood pressure

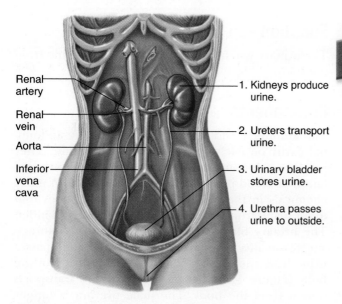

Renal artery
Renal vein
Aorta
Inferior vena cava

1. Kidneys produce urine.
2. Ureters transport urine.
3. Urinary bladder stores urine.
4. Urethra passes urine to outside.

FIGURE 4-37 ▲ The urinary system.

On the Scene **Wrap-Up**

Your knowledge of the human body helps you understand that your patient has potentially life-threatening injuries to the lungs, heart, and abdomen. You call for an ALS crew, and the Paramedics arrive within twenty minutes. By the time they arrive, your patient is complaining of difficulty breathing. You note that she is working hard to breathe. Her skin color is now pale and cool. You have trouble getting her to remain still because she is so anxious. Oxygen is given with no improvement. The patient is rapidly secured to a long spine board. Within eight minutes, the patient and the Paramedics have left the scene. The organs and organ systems that have been damaged will adversely alter the body's ability to transport oxygen and may lead to the patient's death. Early recognition of the potential for life-threatening injuries can and will make a difference for your patient. ■

Sum It Up

▶ The body's most basic building block is a cell. The human body contains billions of cells. Clusters of cells form tissues. Specialized types of tissues form organs such as the brain and the liver. An organ system (also called a body system) consists of tissues and organs that work together to provide a specialized function. The circulatory and respiratory systems are examples of organ systems (Table 4-4).

▶ Organ systems work together to maintain a state of homeostasis (balance). These systems need a constant internal environment to perform the required functions of the body.

▶ In your role as an EMT, it is important to know the terms used to describe body positions and directions. You must be able to use these terms correctly so that you can describe the position in which a patient is found and transported. You will also need to know body positions so that you can place a patient in a specific position based on the patient's condition.

▶ A body cavity is a hollow space in the body that contains internal organs. Knowing the body cavities and the organs found within each cavity will help you describe the location of the injury or symptoms of a sick or injured patient.

▶ The musculoskeletal system gives the human body its shape and ability to move and protects the major organs of the body. It consists of the skeletal system (bones) and the muscular system (muscles).

▶ The respiratory system supplies oxygen from the air we breathe to the body's cells. It also removes carbon dioxide (a waste product of the body's cells) from the lungs when we breathe out. This system is made up of an upper and a lower airway. The upper airway includes the nose, the pharynx (throat), and the larynx (voice box). The lower airway consists of structures found mostly within the chest cavity, such as the trachea (windpipe) and the lungs.

▶ The circulatory system is made up of the cardiovascular and lymphatic systems. This system has three main functions: (1) to deliver oxygen-rich blood and nutrients to body tissues, (2) to help maintain body temperature, and (3) to protect the body against infection. The cardiovascular system consists of the heart, blood, and blood vessels. The lymphatic system consists of lymph, lymph nodes, lymph vessels, tonsils, the spleen, and the thymus gland.

▶ The nervous system is a collection of specialized cells that transfer information to and from the brain. The two main functions of the nervous system are to control the voluntary (conscious) and involuntary (unconscious) activities of the body and to provide for higher mental function (such as thought and emotion). The nervous system has two divisions: (1) the CNS and (2) the PNS. The PNS has two divisions. The somatic (voluntary) division has receptors and nerves concerned with the external environment. It influences the activity of the musculoskeletal system. The autonomic (involuntary) division has receptors and nerves concerned with the internal environment. It controls the involuntary system of glands and smooth muscle and functions to maintain a steady state in the body. The autonomic division is divided into the sympathetic division and parasympathetic divisions. The sympathetic division mobilizes energy, particularly in stressful situations. This is called the fight or flight response. Its effects are widespread throughout the body. The parasympathetic division conserves and restores energy; its effects are localized in the body.

▶ The integumentary system is made up of the skin, hair, nails, sweat glands, and oil (sebaceous) glands. The skin is the largest organ of the body. It protects the body from the environment, bacteria, and other organisms and plays an important role in temperature regulation.

▶ The digestive system brings nutrients, water, and electrolytes into the body (ingestion). It chemically breaks down food into small parts so absorption can occur (digestion). It moves nutrients, water, and electrolytes into the circulatory system so they can be used by body cells (absorption). It also eliminates undigested waste (defecation). The primary organs of the digestive system are the mouth, pharynx, esophagus, stomach, small intestine, large intestine, rectum, and anal canal. The accessory organs are the teeth and tongue, salivary glands, liver, gallbladder, and pancreas.

▶ The endocrine system is a system of glands that secrete chemicals (hormones) directly into the circulatory system. It influences body activities and functions. The endocrine system works closely with the nervous system to maintain homeostasis.

▶ The reproductive system makes cells (sperm, eggs) that allow continuation of the human species. The urinary system produces and excretes urine from the body.

5 Baseline Vital Signs and SAMPLE History

By the end of this chapter, you should be able to:

Knowledge Objectives ▶

1. Identify the components of vital signs.
2. Describe the methods to obtain a breathing rate.
3. Identify the attributes that should be obtained when assessing breathing.
4. Differentiate between shallow, labored, and noisy breathing.
5. Describe the methods to obtain a pulse rate.
6. Identify the information obtained when assessing a patient's pulse.
7. Differentiate between a strong, weak, regular, and irregular pulse.
8. Describe the methods to assess the skin color, temperature, condition, and capillary refill (in infants and children).
9. Identify the normal and abnormal skin colors.
10. Differentiate between pale, blue, red, and yellow skin color.
11. Identify the normal and abnormal skin temperature.
12. Differentiate between hot, cool, and cold skin temperature.
13. Identify normal and abnormal skin conditions.
14. Identify normal and abnormal capillary refill in infants and children.
15. Describe the methods to assess the pupils.
16. Identify normal and abnormal pupil size.
17. Differentiate between dilated (big) and constricted (small) pupil size.
18. Differentiate between reactive and nonreactive pupils and equal and unequal pupils.
19. Describe the methods to assess blood pressure.
20. Define systolic pressure.
21. Define diastolic pressure.
22. Explain the difference between auscultation and palpation for obtaining a blood pressure.
23. Identify the components of the SAMPLE history.
24. Differentiate between a sign and a symptom.
25. State the importance of accurately reporting and recording the baseline vital signs.
26. Discuss the need to search for additional medical identification.

Attitude Objectives ▶

27. Explain the value of measuring the baseline vital signs.
28. Recognize and respond to the feelings patients experience during assessment.

29. Defend the need for obtaining and recording an accurate set of vital signs.
30. Explain the rationale of recording additional sets of vital signs.
31. Explain the importance of obtaining a SAMPLE history.

Skill Objectives ▶ 32. Demonstrate the skills involved in assessment of breathing.
33. Demonstrate the skills associated with obtaining a pulse.
34. Demonstrate the skills associated with assessing the skin color, temperature, condition, and capillary refill in infants and children.
35. Demonstrate the skills associated with assessing the pupils.
36. Demonstrate the skills associated with obtaining blood pressure.
37. Demonstrate the skills that should be used to obtain information from the patient, family, or bystanders at the scene.

On the Scene

You and your Emergency Medical Technician partner have been dispatched to a report of a motor vehicle crash (MVC). Upon arrival, you see two vehicles that have been involved in a head-on collision. Law enforcement personnel have secured the scene and are directing traffic. Vehicle #1 is a late model sports utility vehicle. It has extensive damage to the front of the vehicle. You note that the airbag has deployed. Vehicle #2 is an older model pickup truck. Law enforcement personnel quickly tell you that the driver of vehicle #1 is an 80-year-old woman with no complaints or injuries. They direct your attention to the driver of vehicle #2. You find the driver slumped forward against the steering wheel of his vehicle. He looks to be about 35 years of age. He is unresponsive to your questions. Inspection of the vehicle reveals a bent steering wheel and a broken windshield. Your initial assessment reveals that the patient has an open airway but that his breathing is irregular. He has a radial pulse of 40 beats per minute and a blood pressure of 180/100. ■

THINK ABOUT IT

As you read this chapter, think about the following questions:

- What is the normal range of vital signs for this patient?
- What specific vital signs may be of help in determining the type of injury that this patient has?
- How will the assessment of this patient's vital signs affect your care?
- Could your on-scene vital signs change or vary as time passes?

Introduction

As an Emergency Medical Technician (EMT), you must be able to accurately assess and record a patient's vital signs. This chapter explains the difference between signs and symptoms. It discusses the usual vital signs, including pulse, respirations, skin findings, pupils, and blood pressure. A less common but equally important vital sign, pulse oximetry, is also discussed. This chapter explains the importance of these vital signs when assessing a patient's condition. Obtaining a SAMPLE history is also discussed.

Signs and Symptoms

A **sign** is a medical or trauma condition of the patient that can be seen, heard, smelled, measured, or felt by the examiner. Examples of signs include unusual chest movement, bleeding, swelling, pale skin, and a fast pulse. A **symptom** is a condition described by the patient. Shortness of breath, nausea, abdominal pain, chills, chest pain, and dizziness are examples of symptoms.

You Should Know

Because signs can be seen, heard, smelled, measured, or felt, they are considered **objective findings.** Some of the ways signs (also called *clinical findings*) can be determined include physical or psychological examination, laboratory tests, and imaging studies (such as x-rays). Symptoms are **subjective findings** because they are dependent on (subject to) the patient's interpretation and description of his complaint.

Vital Signs

Objective 1

Vital signs are measurements of breathing, pulse, skin temperature, pupils, and blood pressure. Measuring vital signs is an important part of patient assessment. Vital signs are measured to:

- Detect changes in normal body function
- Recognize life-threatening situations
- Determine a patient's response to treatment

Objective 25

Baseline vital signs are an initial set of vital sign measurements. Later measurements are compared against baseline vital signs. When possible, take two or more sets of vital signs. Doing so will allow you to note changes (trends) in the patient's condition and response to treatment. For example, after obtaining the first set of vital signs (the baseline), you will be able to spot if the patient's heart rate is increasing, staying about the same, or decreasing when you take them a second or third time. Watching these trends in your patient's condition is very important. With this information and your patient assessment findings, you will be able to recognize life-threatening emergencies, such as shock.

To take a patient's vital signs, you will need:

- A watch with a second hand or a digital watch that shows seconds. The watch will be used to count your patient's respirations and pulse as well as to note the time of events for your documentation.
- A penlight or flashlight. This will be used to look at your patient's pupils.
- A **stethoscope**. A stethoscope is an instrument used to hear sounds within the body, such as respirations. It is also used to measure blood pressure.
- A sphygmomanometer (blood pressure cuff) to take your patient's blood pressure.
- A pen and paper to record your findings.

Making a Difference

It is not enough to be able to take a patient's vital signs—almost anyone can be taught to do that. A good EMT knows how to take a patient's vital signs correctly, knows normal values, interprets the results, relays the findings to other healthcare professionals as needed, documents the findings, and gives appropriate care based on the patient's signs and symptoms, vital signs, history, and physical examination findings.

Pulse

Arteries are large blood vessels that carry blood away from the heart to the rest of the body. Blood is forced into the arteries when the heart contracts. A pulse is the rhythmic contraction and expansion of the arteries with each beat of the heart. A pulse can be felt anywhere an artery passes near the skin surface and can be pressed against firm tissue, such as a bone.

Objective 5

A **central pulse** is a pulse found close to the trunk of the body (Figure 5-1). Examples of central pulses are the carotid pulse and femoral pulse (Table 5-1). The carotid artery is the major artery of the neck. It supplies the head with blood. Pulsations can be found on either side of the neck. To find the carotid pulse, place your index and middle fingers in the soft hollow area just to the side of the patient's windpipe. The femoral artery is located in the fold between the thigh and pelvis. In the field, a femoral pulse is not often used because the patient's clothing prevents easy

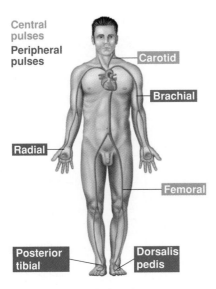

Central pulses

Peripheral pulses

Carotid

Brachial

Radial

Femoral

Posterior tibial

Dorsalis pedis

FIGURE 5-1 ▲ Location of central (carotid and femoral) and peripheral pulses (radial, brachial, posterior tibial, and dorsalis pedis).

access to the femoral artery. To adequately feel a femoral pulse, you may have to apply more pressure than is required at other sites.

A peripheral pulse is located further from the trunk of the body than a central pulse. A peripheral pulse can be felt at several locations:

- The radial pulse is located in the wrist at the base of the thumb. Check for a radial pulse first when assessing a responsive adult or a child one year of age or older.
- The brachial pulse is located on the inside of the upper arm, midway between the shoulder and the elbow. Always check for a brachial pulse in an infant.
- The posterior tibial pulse is located just behind the ankle bone.
- The dorsalis pedis pulse is located on the top surface of the foot.

TABLE 5-1 Central and Peripheral Pulses

Central Pulses	
Carotid	• Major artery of the neck • Supplies the head with blood • Pulsations can be found on either side of the neck • Check this pulse first when assessing an *unresponsive* adult or child 1 year of age or older • Avoid applying excess pressure • Never assess the carotid pulse on both sides of the neck at the same time, this can decrease blood flow to the brain and slow the patient's heart rate
Femoral	• Located in the fold between the thigh and pelvis • In the field, not often used because of the presence of patient clothing • To adequately feel, may require more pressure than at other sites
Peripheral Pulses	
Radial	• Located in the wrist at base of the thumb • Used to assess circulation in the upper extremities • Check this pulse first when assessing a *responsive* adult or a child 1 year of age or older
Brachial	• Located on the inside of the upper arm, midway between the shoulder and the elbow • Used to assess circulation in the upper extremities • Always check this pulse in an infant
Posterior Tibial	• Located just behind the ankle bone • Used to assess circulation in the lower extremities
Dorsalis Pedis	• Located on the top surface of the foot • Used to assess circulation in the lower extremities

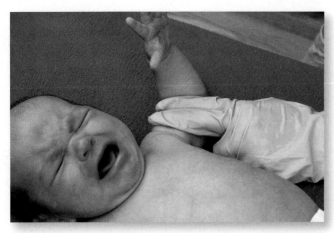

FIGURE 5-2 ▲ To feel for a pulse, use the pads of your index and middle fingers and apply gentle pressure to the artery.

TABLE 5-2 Normal Pulse Rates at Rest

Life Stage	Age	Beats per Minute
Newborn	Birth to 1 month	120 to 160
Infant	1 to 12 months	80 to 140
Toddler	1 to 3 years	80 to 130
Preschooler	4 to 5 years	80 to 120
School-age child	6 to 12 years	70 to 110
Adolescent	13 to 18 years	60 to 100
Adult	18 years and older	60 to 100

To feel for a pulse:

- Use the pads of your index and middle fingers and apply gentle pressure to the artery (Figure 5-2). The pads on the tips of the finger are used because they are the most sensitive areas. Do not use your thumb to assess a pulse—it has a pulse of its own and could be mistaken for the patient's pulse. If you use too much pressure, you will cut off blood flow through the artery and will not be able to feel a pulse.
- Count the number of beats for 30 seconds. Then multiply the number by two to determine the number of beats per minute. If the pulse is irregular, count it for one full minute. Normal pulse rates for patients at rest are shown in Table 5-2.

Objectives 6, 7

A patient's pulse rate varies with age and physical condition. When checking the pulse, note if the pulse rate feels very slow, very fast, or within the normal range for the patient's age. Also note if the rhythm of the pulse is regular or irregular. A slow heart rate may be normal in well-conditioned athletes. However, a slow heart rate may occur because of a medical or trauma-related problem. A fast heart rate occurs as a normal response to the body's demand for more oxygen.

Pulse "quality" refers to the strength of the heartbeat felt when taking a pulse. A normal pulse is easily felt and the pressure is equal for each beat. This kind of pulse is said to be a "strong" pulse. A pulse is said to be "weak" if it is hard to feel. A pulse that is weak and fast is called a "thready" pulse. Pulses are normally of equal strength on both sides of the body.

You Should Know

Possible Causes of a Slow Heart Rate
- Coughing
- Vomiting
- Straining to have a bowel movement
- Heart attack
- Head injury
- Very low body temperature (hypothermia)
- Sleep apnea
- Some medications

Possible Causes of a Rapid Heart Rate
- Fever
- Fear
- Pain
- Anxiety
- Infection
- Shock
- Exercise
- Heart failure
- Substances such as caffeine and nicotine
- Cocaine, amphetamines, "Ecstasy," cannabis
- Some medications

Respirations

Respiration is the exchange of gases between a living organism and its environment. A single respiration consists of one inhalation and one exhalation. Inspiration (inhalation) is the process of breathing in and moving air into the lungs. Expiration (exhalation) is the process of breathing out and moving air out of the

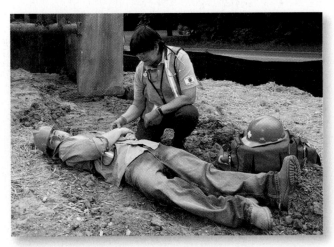

FIGURE 5-3 ▲ To count the respiratory rate, place the patient's arm across his chest or abdomen. Hold the patient's wrist as if you are assessing the radial pulse. Watch the rise and fall of the chest or abdomen. Begin counting when the chest or abdomen rises. Count each rise and fall of the chest or abdomen as one respiration.

lungs. During inhalation, the chest rises and oxygen is taken into the lungs. During exhalation, the chest falls and carbon dioxide is moved out of the lungs.

Objective 2

To count the patient's respirations:

- Place the patient's arm across his chest or abdomen. Hold the patient's wrist as if you are assessing the radial pulse. Watch the rise and fall of the chest or abdomen. Begin counting when the chest or abdomen rises. Count each rise and fall of the chest or abdomen as one respiration (Figure 5-3). Watch to see if respirations are regular and if the chest rises equally. Ask the patient not to speak during this time.

- Count respirations for 30 seconds. Multiply the number by two to determine the rate for one minute. If the patient's respirations are irregular or slow, count the rate for one full minute.

- In infants and young children, it is often easier to observe the rise and fall of the abdomen to determine the respiratory rate. Count an infant's respirations for one full minute.

The normal respiratory rates for an adult, child, and infant at rest are shown in Table 5-3. The number of respirations per minute can be influenced by many factors. For example, exercise, stress, anxiety, pain, fever, and the use of stimulants can increase the respiratory rate. The use of narcotics or sedatives decreases the respiratory rate.

Remember This!

- Do not tell the patient you are counting his respiratory rate. If he knows that it is being assessed, he may vary his breathing without realizing it.
- Make it a habit to count the patient's pulse first. When you have finished, keep your hands in place but shift your attention to the patient's chest and abdomen and count his respiratory rate.

Objectives 3, 4

Normal respirations are evenly spaced and of adequate depth. Infants and young children tend to breathe less regularly than adults do. Irregular respirations may be associated with conditions such as a diabetic emergency or head injury. A patient is said to breathe *shallowly* if it is difficult to see movement of the chest or abdomen during breathing. Only a small volume of air is exchanged during shallow breathing.

Normal breathing is relaxed and effortless. *Labored* breathing is an increase in the work (effort) of breathing. If a patient is having difficulty breathing, he is usually irritable, anxious, or restless. You may see the following signs during labored breathing (Figure 5-4):

- Gasping for air
- Excessive widening of the nostrils with respiration (nasal flaring)
- The use of neck muscles to assist with inhalation
- The use of the abdominal muscles and the muscles between the ribs (intercostal muscles) to assist with exhalation

TABLE 5-3 Normal Respiratory Rates at Rest

Life Stage	Age	Breaths per Minute
Newborn	Birth to 1 month	30 to 50
Infant	1 to 12 months	20 to 40
Toddler	1 to 3 years	20 to 30
Preschooler	4 to 5 years	20 to 30
School-age child	6 to 12 years	16 to 30
Adolescent	13 to 18 years	12 to 20
Adult	18 years and older	12 to 20

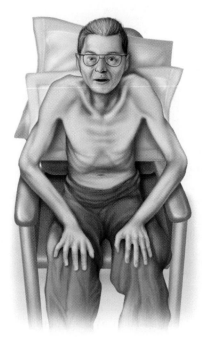

Gasping for air

Excessive widening of the nostrils with respiration (nasal flaring)

Use of muscles in the neck to assist with inhalation

Skin color changes (cyanosis around the mouth)

"Sinking in" of the soft tissues between and around the ribs or above the collarbones (retractions)

Use of the abdominal muscles and muscles between the ribs to assist with exhalation

FIGURE 5-4 ▲ Signs of respiratory distress.

- A "sinking in" of the soft tissues between and around the ribs or above the collarbones (retractions)
- Skin color changes (blue or cyanotic skin)

Normal breathing is quiet. While counting the patient's respirations, listen for any abnormal respiratory sounds. Abnormal respiratory sounds include:

- **Stridor,** which is a harsh, high-pitched sound (like the bark of a seal). Stridor is associated with severe upper airway obstruction and is most often heard during inhalation
- **Snoring,** which results from partial obstruction of the upper airway by the tongue

- **Wheezing,** which is a high-pitched whistling sound heard on inhalation or exhalation that suggests a narrowed or partially obstructed airway
- **Gurgling,** which is the sound heard as air passes through moist secretions in the airway
- **Crowing,** which is a long, high-pitched sound heard on inhalation

Skin Color, Temperature, and Condition

While assessing the patient's pulse, quickly check the patient's skin. Assessing the patient's skin condition can provide important information about the flow of blood through the body's tissues (**perfusion**). Perfusion is assessed by evaluating the following:

- Skin color
- Skin temperature
- Skin condition (moist, dry)
- Capillary refill (in infants and children younger than six years of age)

Skin Color
Objectives 8, 9, 10

Assess the patient's skin color by looking at areas of the body that are not usually exposed to the sun. For example, look at the palms of the hands, soles of the feet, oral mucosa (mucous membranes of the mouth), and conjunctiva (mucous membrane that lines the inner surface of the eyelid).

Pale (whitish color) skin occurs when the blood vessels in the skin have severely narrowed (constricted) (Figure 5-5). This condition may be seen in shock, fright, anxiety, and with other causes. **Cyanosis,** a blue-gray color of the skin or mucous membranes, suggests inadequate breathing or poor perfusion. It often appears first in the fingertips or around the

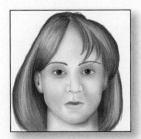 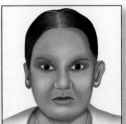 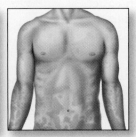 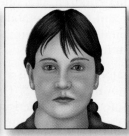 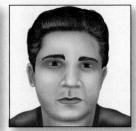

(a) Pale skin   **(b)** Cyanosis   **(c)** Mottled skin   **(d)** Flushed skin   **(e)** Jaundice

FIGURE 5-5 ▲ Assess an adult patient's skin color in the nail beds, inside the mouth, and inside the eyelids.

mouth. Nail beds are an unreliable site to assess skin color. They are easily affected by air temperature and many medical conditions.

Cyanosis may be seen in:

- Respiratory distress
- Airway obstruction
- Exposure to cold
- Blood vessel disease
- Shock
- Cardiac arrest

Mottling refers to an irregular or patchy skin discoloration that is usually a mixture of blue and white. Mottled skin is usually seen in patients in shock, with hypothermia, or in cardiac arrest. Jaundiced (yellow) skin may be seen in patients with liver or gallbladder problems. Flushed (red) skin may be caused by the following:

- Heat exposure
- Late stages of carbon monoxide poisoning
- Allergic reaction
- Alcohol abuse
- High blood pressure

Skin Temperature

Objectives 11, 12

Assess skin temperature by placing the back of your hand against the patient's face, neck, or abdomen (Figure 5-6). The back surfaces of the hands and fingers are used because the skin in these areas is thin and sensitive to temperature changes. Normal skin temperature is warm. Hot skin may be caused by fever or heat exposure. Cool skin may be caused by inadequate circulation or exposure to cold. Cold skin may be caused by extreme exposure to cold or shock. Clammy (cool and moist) skin may be caused by shock, among many other conditions. An infection, inflammation, or burn can cause localized warmth. Localized coolness may occur because of poor arterial blood flow to a limb.

Skin Condition

Objective 13

Assess the patient's skin condition (moisture). Normal skin is dry. Wet or moist skin may indicate shock, a heat-related illness, or a diabetic emergency. Warm and moist skin may be seen with anxiety, a warm environment, or exercise. Excessively dry skin may indicate dehydration. Abnormal skin findings and possible causes are shown in Table 5-4.

Capillary Refill

Objective 14

Assess **capillary refill** in infants and children younger than six years of age. To assess capillary refill, firmly press on the child's nail bed until it blanches (turns white) and then release (Figure 5-7). Observe the time it takes for the tissue to return to its original color. If the temperature of the environment is normal to warm, color should return within two seconds. Other sites may be used to assess capillary refill, including the forehead, chest, abdomen, or fleshy part of the palm. A capillary refill time of three to five seconds is said to be *delayed*. This may indicate poor perfusion or exposure to cool temperatures. A

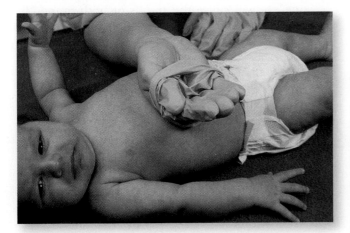

FIGURE 5-6 ▲ Assess skin temperature by placing the back of your hand against the patient's face, neck, or abdomen.

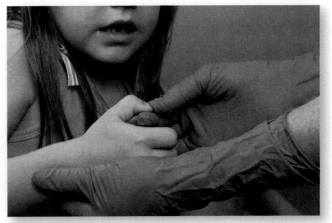

FIGURE 5-7 ▲ Assess capillary refill in infants and children less than six years of age.

TABLE 5-4 Abnormal Skin Findings and Possible Causes

Skin Finding	Possible Cause
Color	
Pale (white) skin	Shock, fright, anxiety
Cyanotic (blue) skin	Respiratory distress, airway obstruction, exposure to cold, blood vessel disease, shock
Mottled (patchy blue and white) skin	Shock, hypothermia, cardiac arrest
Jaundice (yellow)	Liver or gallbladder problems
Flushed (red) skin	Heat exposure, late stages of carbon monoxide poisoning, allergic reaction, alcohol abuse, high blood pressure
Temperature and Condition (Moisture)	
Hot and dry or moist	Heat exposure
Warm and moist	Anxiety, warm environment, exercise
Cool and dry	Inadequate peripheral circulation, exposure to cold
Cool or cold and moist	Shock
Localized warmth	Infection, inflammation, or burn
Localized coolness	Poor arterial blood flow to a limb

capillary refill time of more than five seconds is said to be *markedly delayed* and suggests shock.

Pupils
Objectives 15, 16, 17, 18

Examine the patient's pupils. The pupils are normally equal in size, round, and equally reactive to light (Figure 5-8). Briefly shine a light into the patient's eyes and assess the size, equality, and reactivity of the patient's pupils.

- *Size.* Dilated (very big) pupils in the presence of bright light may be caused by trauma, fright, poisoning, eye medications, or glaucoma. Constricted (small) pupils in a darkened area may be caused by narcotics, treatment with eye drops, or a nervous system problem.
- *Equality.* Unequal pupils, a condition called **anisocoria,** are a normal finding in 2% to 4% of the population. In most patients, unequal

pupils suggest a head injury, a stroke, the presence of an artificial eye, or cataract surgery on one eye.

- *Reactivity.* Reactivity refers to whether or not the pupils change in response to light. Normally, a light that is shined into the pupil of one eye will cause the pupils of both eyes to constrict. Nonreactive pupils do not change when exposed to light. This condition may occur because of medications or cardiac arrest. Unequally reactive pupils (one pupil reacts but the other does not) may occur because of a head injury or stroke.

Abnormal pupil findings and possible causes are shown in Table 5-5.

Blood Pressure
Objective 19

Blood pressure is the force exerted by the blood on the walls of the arteries. Blood pressure is usually

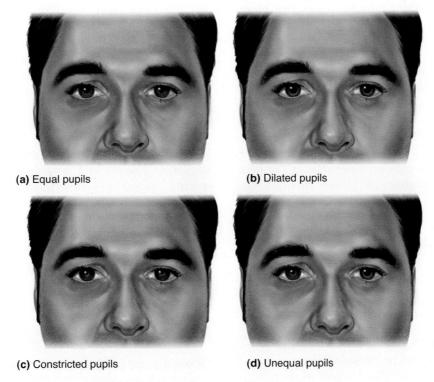

(a) Equal pupils   (b) Dilated pupils

(c) Constricted pupils   (d) Unequal pupils

FIGURE 5-8 ▲ Assess the size, equality, and reactivity of your patient's pupils.

TABLE 5-5 Abnormal Pupil Findings and Possible Causes

Pupil Finding	Possible Cause
Constricted (small)	Narcotics, treatment with eye drops, head injury, exposure to organophosphate insecticides (such as malathion), some mushrooms, nerve agents
Dilated (very wide)	Trauma, fright, poisoning, eye medications, glaucoma, use of amphetamines, caffeine, cocaine, methamphetamine
Unequally reactive (one pupil reacts but the other does not)	Normal finding in some individuals, head injury, stroke, presence of an artificial eye, cataract surgery on one eye
Nonreactive (pupils do not change when exposed to light)	Medications, cardiac arrest

assessed using a blood pressure cuff and stethoscope. This method of taking a blood pressure is called *blood pressure by auscultation* because it involves the use of a stethoscope. Electronic sphygmomanometers, which do not require the use of a stethoscope, are also available. Blood pressure is abbreviated as *BP*.

Objectives 20, 21

When a blood pressure cuff is applied to a patient's arm and inflated, blood flow in the artery under the cuff is momentarily cut off. If a stethoscope is applied over the artery, sounds can be heard that reflect the patient's blood pressure. As the cuff is slowly deflated, blood flow resumes through the partially compressed artery. The first sound heard is the systolic pressure. Systolic pressure is the pressure in an artery when the heart is pumping blood. As the pressure in the cuff continues to drop, a point is reached where sounds are no longer heard because the artery is no longer compressed. The point at which the sound disappears is the diastolic pressure. Diastolic pressure is the pressure in an artery when the heart is at rest. A blood pressure measurement is made up of both the systolic and the diastolic pressure. It is written as a fraction

(116/78), with the systolic number first. The blood pressure is recorded as an even number since most gauges have a scale marked in increments of 2 millimeters of mercury (mm Hg). If you are using a digital blood pressure device, the readings obtained may include both odd and even numbers.

A noninvasive blood pressure (NIBP) monitor does not require the use of a stethoscope to measure blood pressure. The machine's blood pressure cuff is applied to the patient's arm. As the cuff is deflated, the machine monitors the changes in pressure caused by the flow of blood through the artery.

Using a Stethoscope

A stethoscope is used to listen to body sounds. It consists of four major parts: the chest piece, tubing, binaurals, and earpieces (Figure 5-9). The earpieces should fit snugly but comfortably in the ears. For the best sound reception, the earpieces should normally point toward the EMT's face as the stethoscope is put on. The earpieces should be cleaned before and after use. The **binaurals** are the metal pieces of the stethoscope that connect the earpieces to the plastic or rubber tubing. When you are using a stethoscope, the binaurals should be angled so the earpieces remain in the ears without causing discomfort. The stethoscope's plastic or rubber tubing should be flexible and about 12 to 18 inches in length. Longer tubing decreases sound wave transmission.

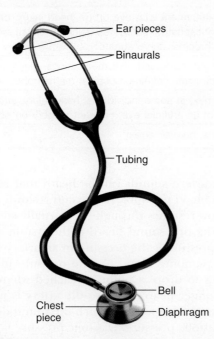

FIGURE 5-9 ▲ A stethoscope consists of four major parts: the chest piece, tubing, binaurals, and earpieces.

The chest piece of the stethoscope may consist of a diaphragm and/or bell. The diaphragm is the circular, flat part at the end of the tubing. It has a thin plastic disk on the end. The diaphragm is used to detect high-pitched sounds, such as breath sounds. The diaphragm should be firmly held against the patient's skin with the fingertips of the index and middle fingers.

Some stethoscopes are also equipped with a bell. The bell has a deep, hollow, cuplike shape. It is used to detect low-pitched sounds such as those heard during blood pressure measurement. The bell should be lightly held against the patient's skin, just enough to form a seal. When possible, the stethoscope should be placed directly on the patient's skin because clothing makes sounds harder to hear. Skill Drill 5-1 explains how to assess a patient's blood pressure by auscultation.

Remember This!

Obtain a blood pressure by auscultation before applying a NIBP monitor.

Objective 22

Sometimes the presence of noise on the scene makes it impossible to hear sounds through a stethoscope. In situations like this, assess the patient's blood pressure by palpation. Skill Drill 5-2 explains how to assess a patient's blood pressure by using this method. When a blood pressure is obtained by palpation, the diastolic pressure cannot be measured. Document the patient's blood pressure as the systolic pressure over a capital "P," such as 110/P.

Many factors can influence a patient's blood pressure. For example, anxiety, fear, fever, pain, emotional stress, and obesity increase blood pressure. Blood loss may decrease blood pressure. Table 5-6 shows normal blood pressures for patients of different ages.

When taking a blood pressure, it is important to use a blood pressure cuff of the correct size. The width of the cuff should not be more than two-thirds the length of the patient's upper arm. Blood pressure readings will be wrong if the cuff is the wrong size.

For an unstable patient, vital signs should be assessed and recorded every five minutes. At a minimum, for a stable patient, vital signs should be assessed and recorded every 15 minutes. Remember, a stable patient can become unstable very quickly. Reassess frequently!

Measuring Blood Pressure by Auscultation

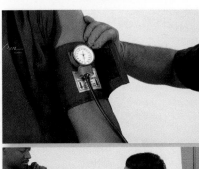

STEP 1 ▶ • Expose the patient's upper arm. Select the correct size blood pressure cuff for the patient.
• Wrap the pressure cuff evenly around the patient's upper arm at least one inch above the elbow. Place the arrow on the cuff over the patient's brachial artery.

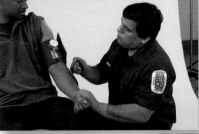

STEP 2 ▶ • Locate the patient's radial artery.
• Rapidly inflate the cuff until you can no longer feel the radial pulse. Inflate the cuff 30 mm Hg beyond the point at which you last felt the pulse.

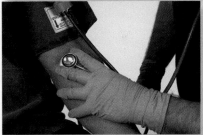

STEP 3 ▶ • Place the stethoscope in your ears.
• Place the diaphragm of the stethoscope over the brachial artery and hold it in place.

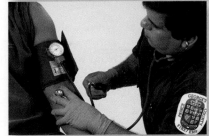

STEP 4 ▶ • While watching the gauge, deflate the cuff slowly and evenly at a rate of 2 to 3 mm Hg per second.
• Listen for sounds. The first sound is the systolic pressure and should be near the point where the radial pulse disappeared.

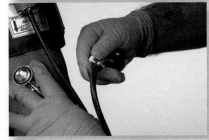

STEP 5 ▶ Continue to deflate the cuff, noting the point where the sound disappears. This is the diastolic pressure.

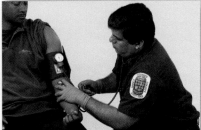

STEP 6 ▶ • Deflate the cuff completely.
• Record the blood pressure as systolic/diastolic pressure.

Measuring Blood Pressure by Palpation

STEP 1 ▶ • Expose the patient's upper arm. Select the correct size blood pressure cuff for the patient.
• Wrap the pressure cuff evenly around the patient's upper arm at least one inch above the elbow. Place the arrow on the cuff over the patient's brachial artery.

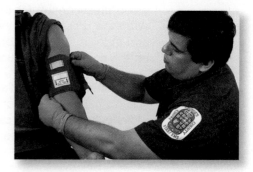

STEP 2 ▶ • Locate the patient's radial artery.
• Rapidly inflate the cuff until you can no longer feel the radial pulse. Inflate the cuff 30 mm Hg beyond the point at which you last felt the pulse.

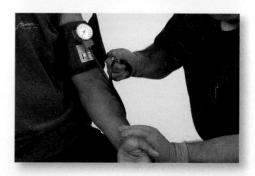

STEP 3 ▶ • While watching the gauge, deflate the cuff slowly and evenly at a rate of 2 to 3 mm Hg per second.
• Note the point on the gauge when you feel the return of the radial pulse. This is the systolic pressure and should be near the point where the radial pulse disappeared. The diastolic pressure cannot be accurately measured by palpation.

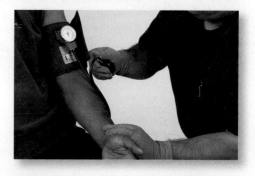

STEP 4 ▶ • Deflate the cuff completely.
• Record the blood pressure as systolic/P (for example, 148/P).

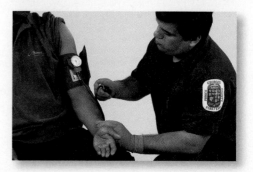

TABLE 5-6 Normal Blood Pressure at Rest

Life Stage	Age	Systolic Pressure	Diastolic Pressure
Newborn	Birth to 1 month	74 to 100	50 to 68
Infant	1 to 12 months	84 to 106	56 to 70
Toddler	1 to 3 years	98 to 106	50 to 70
Preschooler	4 to 5 years	98 to 112	64 to 70
School-age child	6 to 12 years	104 to 124	64 to 80
Adolescent	13 to 18 years	118 to 132	70 to 82
Adult	18 years and older	100 to 119	60 to 79

Remember This!

Common Errors in Blood Pressure Measurement

Errors that produce a falsely low reading:

- The patient's arm is above the level of the heart
- The cuff is too wide

Errors that produce a falsely high reading:

- The cuff is deflated too slowly
- The patient's arm is unsupported
- The cuff is too narrow
- The cuff is wrapped too loosely or unevenly

Errors that produce either falsely high or low readings:

- Retaking a blood pressure too quickly may produce a falsely high systolic or low diastolic reading. Wait 2-3 minutes before reinflating the cuff.
- Deflating the cuff too quickly may produce a falsely low systolic and high diastolic reading. Deflate the cuff at a rate of 2-3 mm Hg per second.

Remember This!

Learning to take accurate vital signs is very important. Because vital signs allow you to detect changes in your patient's condition, take them often.

Additional Vital Signs

Pulse Oximetry

Pulse oximetry is a method of measuring the amount of oxygen saturated in the blood. Pulse oximetry is commonly referred to as *pulse ox*. An oximeter is a small machine used to obtain this measurement (Figure 5-10). A small sensor is placed on an area of the patient's body in which a pulsation can be detected, such as a fingertip or ear lobe. The sensor is connected to the oximeter, which is a small computer. The sensor passes red and infrared light waves through the tissue to which it is attached.

Most of the body's oxygen is attached to hemoglobin molecules in the arterial blood. Hemoglobin absorbs red and infrared light waves differently when

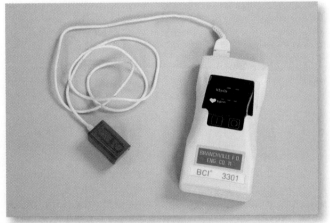

FIGURE 5-10 ▲ A pulse oximeter is used to check the amount of oxygen in the patient's blood.

it is bound with oxygen than when it is not. The oximeter calculates the amount of hemoglobin saturated with oxygen. This calculation is called the **saturation of peripheral oxygen (SpO2).** The oximeter displays this value as a percentage on its screen, as well as the patient's pulse rate.

Pulse oximetry is used to detect and provide warnings about low levels of oxygen in the blood. A reading between 96% and 100% generally indicates adequate oxygenation. A reading between 91% and 95% suggests a mild lack of oxygen in the tissues (hypoxia). A reading below 91% generally indicates severe hypoxia. Supplemental oxygen is usually given to patients whose readings are below 91%.

To use a pulse oximeter, start by making sure there is no dirt or obstruction on the oximeter's red light. If dirt is present, remove it and clean the device before putting it on the patient. Clean the tissue to which the oximeter will be attached, such as the fingertip or earlobe. If the patient's fingertip is used, remove any dark or metallic nail polish, if present. Attach the pulse oximeter to the patient (Figure 5-11). If the fingertip is used, insert the patient's finger into the oximeter. Make sure the patient's tissue is centered over the light and detector. Turn the pulse oximeter on. To make sure the pulse oximeter's measurements are accurate, check the patient's pulse to be sure that the pulse rate shown on the oximeter is consistent with what you feel (palpate) when assessing the patient (Figure 5-12).

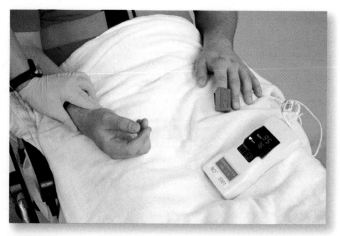

FIGURE 5-12 ▲ To make sure the pulse oximeter's measurements are accurate, check the patient's pulse to be sure that the pulse rate shown on the oximeter is consistent with what you feel when assessing the patient.

You Should Know

Indications for Pulse Oximetry

Altered mental status

Respiratory rate outside the normal range for age

Increased work of breathing

Respiratory or cardiac chief complaints

History of respiratory difficulty or respiratory disease

During delivery of supplemental oxygen

During and after endotracheal intubation

During transport of a sick or injured child

Remember This!

- A pulse oximeter measures oxygen saturation. It does not measure the effectiveness of ventilation.

- Too often, Emergency Medical Services (EMS) professionals use a pulse oximeter as their only source for determining the patient's heart rate and oxygen level. Although a pulse oximeter is a useful device, *it is not a replacement for patient assessment.*

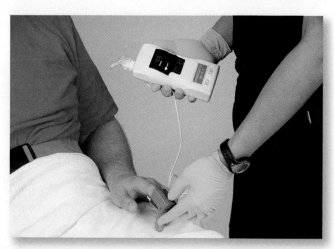

FIGURE 5-11 ▲ Clean the tissue to which the oximeter will be attached, such as the fingertip. Remove any dark or metallic nail polish, if present. Attach the pulse oximeter to the patient. Insert the patient's finger into the oximeter. Make sure the patient's tissue is centered over the light and detector. Turn the pulse oximeter on.

Pulse oximeter readings may be inaccurate in the following circumstances:

- Poor capillary blood flow
- Abnormal hemoglobin concentration
- Abnormal shape of the hemoglobin molecule

Examples of conditions that may cause these situations, resulting in misleading pulse oximetry readings, include the following:

- Cardiac arrest
- Shock
- Hypothermia
- Carbon monoxide poisoning
- Sickle cell disease
- Patient movement, shivering
- Patient use of nail polish

End-Tidal Carbon Dioxide

Some EMS agencies consider end-tidal carbon dioxide an additional vital sign. An **end-tidal carbon dioxide (ETCO$_2$) detector** measures a person's exhaled carbon dioxide (Figure 5-13). Although an ETCO$_2$ detector is most often used to confirm the position of a tube that has been placed in a patient's trachea, some detectors can be used with oxygen delivery devices, such as a nasal cannula or bag-valve-mask device.

Pain Assessment

Some regulatory agencies consider an assessment of a patient's pain an additional vital sign. EMS and other healthcare professionals often underestimate a patient's pain. Some of the reasons for this may include the following:

- Some healthcare professionals believe it is a "waste of time" to ask a patient about his pain.
- Because pain is unique to the person experiencing it, it is difficult for another person to accurately tell how severe the pain is.
- The patient may be unable to relay his needs about the pain. For example, it may be difficult

to adequately assess pain in an infant or young child. It may also be difficult to assess pain if the patient speaks a language different from your own or has an illness that prevents him from verbalizing his needs.

If the patient is able to express pain, the way in which it is expressed varies. A patient may have tremendous pain, yet show no outward signs of his discomfort. On the other hand, a patient may cry, be very loud and expressive, or revert to childhood behavior when in pain. Tools that you can use to assess a patient's pain are discussed later in this chapter.

Making a Difference

Cultural Considerations

A person's culture may influence how pain is expressed. Asians, Chinese, Filipinos, Japanese, American Indians, Russians, and East Indians often show no signs of pain. Cubans, Haitians, and Puerto Ricans tend to be very loud and outspoken about their pain. Because Mexican Americans value inner control and self-endurance, they often show no signs of pain. Most Korean men are reserved, but some Koreans may be very expressive.

SAMPLE History

Components of the SAMPLE History
Objective 23

The **patient history** is the part of the patient assessment that provides pertinent facts about the patient's current medical problem and medical history. **SAMPLE** is a memory aid used to remind you of the information you should get from the patient. SAMPLE stands for:

- **S**igns and symptoms
- **A**llergies
- **M**edications
- (Pertinent) **P**ast medical history
- **L**ast oral intake
- **E**vents leading to the injury or illness

With medical patients, take the patient's history before performing the physical exam. With trauma patients, perform the physical exam first. When possible, ask the patient questions. Try to avoid questions that the patient can answer with a "yes" or "no." Questions that can be answered with "yes" or "no" or with one- or two-word responses are called *closed questions*.

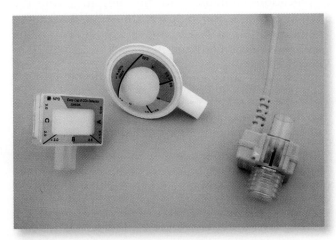

FIGURE 5-13 ▲ End-tidal carbon dioxide detector (ECTO$_2$). Left, Electronic CO$_2$ detector. Right, Colorimetric CO$_2$ detector.

This type of questioning is useful for focusing on specific points. For example, "Do you have any allergies?" "Is this the first time you have ever had chest pain?" However, closed questions do not allow an opportunity for the patient to explain what is wrong. Instead, ask questions that will give you as much information as possible. Questions that allow the patient an opportunity to express his thoughts, feelings, and ideas are called *open-ended questions*. Open-ended questions encourage the patient to describe and explain what is wrong. An example of an open-ended question is "Can you tell me why you called us today?" After asking the question, allow the patient time to answer. Do not anticipate what the patient is going to say and finish sentences for him. *Listen* closely to what the patient tells you, instead of thinking ahead to the next question you want to ask.

Objective 26

In some situations, the patient will not be able to answer your questions. For example, the patient may be unresponsive or too short of breath to provide detailed answers. If the patient is unresponsive, gather as much information as possible by looking at the scene. Also look for medical identification tags and question family members, coworkers, or others at the scene.

Signs and Symptoms

Objective 24

A sign is any medical or trauma condition displayed by the patient that can be:

- Seen, such as bleeding
- Heard, such as snoring or wheezing
- Smelled, such as an unusual breath odor
- Measured, such as a fast pulse or fever
- Felt, such as cold skin

A symptom is any condition described by the patient. Examples of symptoms include nausea, shortness of breath, headache, and pain.

You Should Know

Ask your patient about the frequency with which his symptoms occur. Use this guide to help pinpoint symptom frequency:

- Constant means about 90-100% of the time.
- Frequent means about 75% of the time.
- Intermittent means about 50% of the time.
- Occasional means about 25% of the time.

Allergies

Allergies are common and may be the reason you were called to the scene. Find out if the patient has an allergy to medications, food, environmental causes (such as pollen or bees), and products (such as latex). Ask the patient (or bystanders if the patient is unresponsive):

- Do you have any allergies to medications?
- Are you allergic to latex?
- Do you have any food allergies or allergies to insect stings, pollen, dust, or grass?

Check for a medical identification tag. The patient may be wearing a bracelet or necklace, or carrying a wallet card that identifies a serious medical condition, allergies, or medications she is taking.

Medications

Find out if the patient is currently taking any medications. You will need to ask specific questions because some patients do not consider some substances medications, such as vitamins or aspirin. Examples of questions to ask include:

- Do you take any prescription medications? Is the medication prescribed for you? What is the medication for? When did you last take it? Are you taking birth control pills? (If applicable)
- Do you take any over-the-counter medications, such as aspirin, allergy medications, cough syrup, or vitamins? Do you take any herbal medication?
- Have you recently started taking any new medications? Have you recently stopped taking any medications?
- Do you use any recreational substances (cocaine, marijuana, or alcohol)?

If the patient is taking medication, send the medication containers to the hospital with the patient. This action helps the hospital staff determine what the patient's medical condition is, if he sees a doctor regularly, and if he has been taking his medication correctly.

Pertinent Past Medical History

Ask the patient about medical conditions he may have that may help you determine what the problem is today. If the patient is unresponsive, check for a medic alert tag. Examples of questions to ask include the following:

- Are you seeing a doctor for any medical or psychological condition?
- Do you have a history of heart problems, respiratory problems, high blood pressure, diabetes, epilepsy, or other ongoing medical condition?

- Have you been in the hospital recently? Have you had any recent surgery?

Last Oral Intake

It is important to determine when the patient last ate or had anything to drink. This is especially important if the patient is a diabetic or may need immediate surgery. Determine what he last ate or drank, how much he ate or drank, and when.

Events Leading to the Injury or Illness

Ask the patient to tell you what happened. This information can provide important clues about the patient's current situation. For example, you arrive on the scene of a MVC. After making sure there are no immediate life threats, you ask the patient what happened. She tells you she is a diabetic. She remembers taking her insulin this morning. She was running late for her doctor's appointment and did not have time to eat breakfast. She thinks she may have "blacked out." The information provided by the patient tells you that although you must look for possible injuries caused by the motor vehicle crash, some of the signs you will find during your physical exam may be caused by her medical condition.

If your patient is complaining of pain or discomfort, OPQRST is a memory aid that may help identify the type and location of the patient's complaint:

- **O**nset: "How long ago did the problem or discomfort begin?" "What were you doing when the problem started?" "Did the problem begin suddenly (acutely) or slowly (gradually)?"
- **P**rovocation/Palliation: "What makes the problem better or worse?"
- **Q**uality: "What does the pain feel like (dull, burning, sharp, stabbing, shooting, throbbing, pressure, or tearing)?"
- **R**egion/Radiation: "Where is the pain?" "Is the pain in one area or does it move?" "Is the pain located in any other area?"

- **S**everity: "On a scale of 0 to 10, with 0 being no pain and 10 being the worst, what number would you give your pain or discomfort?"
- **T**ime: "How long has your discomfort been present?" "Have you ever had this discomfort before?" "When?" "How long did it last?"

Remember This!

SAMPLE History

Signs/symptoms
Allergies
Medications
(Pertinent) **P**ast medical history
Last oral intake
Events leading to the injury or illness

To assess pain in a child three years or older, use the Wong-Baker FACES Pain Rating Scale (Figure 5-14). This scale shows six cartoon faces ranging from a smiling face representing "no hurt" to a tearful, sad face representing "worst hurt." To use the scale, explain to the child that each picture is a person's face. "Face 0 is very happy because he doesn't hurt at all. Face 1

Making a Difference

Cultural Considerations

Some healthcare professionals end an interview with a child by patting him on the head. Although this gesture is meant to show friendliness, it may be viewed differently by people of other cultures. For example, this gesture is considered an insult by Southeast Asians. They believe the head is the seat of the soul and the most sacred part of the body. Intentionally touching a child's head without the consent of the parents may make the parents or relatives angry.

TRANSLATIONS OF WONG-BAKER FACES PAIN RATING SCALE*

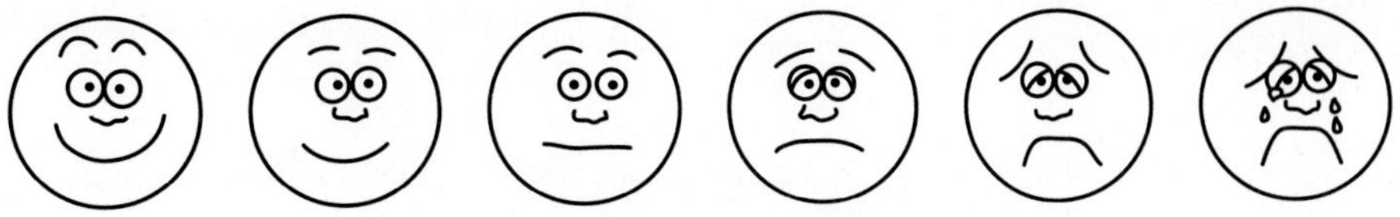

0–5 coding	0	1	2	3	4	5
0-10 coding	0	2	4	6	8	10

FIGURE 5-14 ▲ Wong-Baker FACES Pain Rating Scale.

hurts just a little bit. Face 2 hurts a little more. Face 3 hurts even more. Face 4 hurts a whole lot. Face 5 hurts as much as you can imagine, although you don't have to be crying to feel this bad." Ask the child to point to the face that best describes how he is feeling. Document the number indicated by the child. For example, "Patient rates pain 4 out of 10 on Faces Pain Scale." In real life, this is usually simplified when documenting on a prehospital care report to, "Pain 4/10 on FACES Pain Scale."

On the Scene Wrap-Up

Your knowledge of the "normal" range of vital signs helps you determine whether or not the patient has any life-threatening injuries. This patient is breathing irregularly, has a pulse of 40 beats per minute and a blood pressure of 180/100. You recognize that the patient's heart rate is too slow, his blood pressure is too high, and his respiratory pattern is not normal. All of these signs are indicators that the patient has a life-threatening injury. You begin care while your partner calls dispatch to request that an Advanced Life Support (ALS) crew meet you as you begin transport to the closest appropriate facility. The paramedic crew responds and quickly begins ALS care. The patient is rapidly transported to a trauma center. After a rapid assessment by the trauma team, the patient is wheeled to surgery to repair a bleeding vessel in his head. Two weeks later the patient stops by your station to thank you for the care you provided. Your early recognition of this patient's abnormal vital signs led to a positive outcome for this patient ■

Sum It Up

▶ Vital signs are measurements of breathing, pulse, temperature, pupils, and blood pressure. Measuring vital signs is an important part of patient assessment. Vital signs are measured to:
  • Detect changes in normal body function
  • Recognize life-threatening situations
  • Determine a patient's response to treatment

▶ Additional vital signs include pulse oximetry, $ETCO_2$, and pain assessment. Pulse oximetry is a method of measuring the amount of oxygen saturated in the blood.

▶ A sign is any medical or trauma condition displayed by the patient that can be seen, heard, smelled, measured, or felt. A symptom is any condition described by the patient.

▶ SAMPLE is an aid to remind you of the information you should get from the patient:
  • **S**igns/symptoms
  • **A**llergies
  • **M**edications
  • (Pertinent) **P**ast medical history
  • **L**ast oral intake
  • **E**vents leading to the injury or illness

▶ OPQRST is a memory aid that may help identify the type and location of a patient's complaint.
  • **O**nset
  • **P**rovocation/Palliation
  • **Q**uality
  • **R**egion/Radiation
  • **S**everity
  • **T**ime

▶ The Wong-Baker FACES Pain Rating Scale is a tool used to assess pain in children three years or older.

Lifting and Moving Patients

By the end of this chapter, you should be able to:

Knowledge Objectives ▶

1. Define body mechanics.
2. Discuss the guidelines and safety precautions that need to be followed when lifting a patient.
3. Describe the safe lifting of cots and stretchers.
4. Describe the guidelines and safety precautions for carrying patients and/or equipment.
5. Discuss one-handed carrying techniques.
6. Describe correct and safe carrying procedures on stairs.
7. State the guidelines for reaching and their application.
8. Describe correct reaching for log rolls.
9. State the guidelines for pushing and pulling.
10. Discuss the general considerations of moving patients.
11. State three situations that may require the use of an emergency move.
12. Identify the following patient carrying devices:
    - Wheeled stretcher
    - Portable stretcher
    - Stair chair
    - Scoop stretcher
    - Long spine board
    - Basket stretcher
    - Flexible stretcher

Attitude Objectives ▶ 13. Explain the rationale for properly lifting and moving patients.

Skill Objectives ▶ 14. Working with a partner, prepare each of the following devices for use, transfer a patient to the device, properly position the patient on the device, move the device to the ambulance, and load the patient into the ambulance:

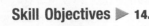

- Wheeled stretcher
- Portable stretcher
- Stair chair
- Scoop stretcher
- Long spine board
- Basket stretcher
- Flexible stretcher

15. Working with a partner, the Emergency Medical Technician will demonstrate techniques for the transfer of a patient from an ambulance stretcher to a hospital stretcher.

On the Scene

A fire at a nursing home is everyone's nightmare. And here you are, living it. Residents from the wing that is on fire are being evacuated to the recreation area until units can be brought in to evacuate them from the facility. A firefighter arrives, carrying an elderly man over his shoulders. The man is confused but pleasant and does not appear injured. Another firefighter appears in the doorway, dragging an approximately 250-pound woman with a blanket. As he turns around to go back, two of his coworkers burst through the fire doors holding a frightened man in a two-person seat carry.

You quickly begin to sort the new arrivals and assess for any injuries while trying to calm them. Your chief radios that the fire is spreading through the attic. These people will need to be moved outside within the next 10 minutes. You quickly survey your situation. There are eight residents who can walk, four on the floor, two who are unconscious in hospital beds, and three in wheelchairs. You are on the third floor. "Send me the following…," you calmly radio to your chief. ■

THINK ABOUT IT

As you read this chapter, think about the following questions:

- What additional equipment will you need to evacuate the residents?
- What type of carriers can be used to move some of these residents?
- What lift can you use to safely move the patients from the floor onto a stretcher?
- What general safety measures should be taken each time you lift one of the residents?

Introduction

Safe Moving and Lifting

Many Emergency Medical Technicians (EMTs) are injured every year because they attempt to lift or move patients improperly. In fact, surveys show that almost one in two (47%) Emergency Medical Services (EMS) personnel have sustained a back injury while performing EMS duties. Improper lifting and moving techniques can result in muscle strains and tears, ligament sprains, joint and tendon inflammation, pinched nerves, and related conditions. These conditions may develop gradually or may result from a specific event, such as a single, heavy lift. Pain, a loss of work, and disability may result. In most cases, these injuries are preventable. More EMTs leave the profession because of disability and complications resulting from a back injury than any other cause.

There is no one best way to move all patients. Many circumstances will affect the method you choose to use. The key is to take a brief moment to analyze the situation and think of all your options. Then choose the method that is safest for you, your coworkers, and the patient.

The Role of the Emergency Medical Technician

You will most often provide initial emergency care to a patient in the position in which he is found. Your responsibility is to distinguish an emergency from a non-emergency situation. Your role will also include:

- Positioning patients to prevent further injury
- Recognizing when to call for more help
- Assisting other EMS professionals in lifting and moving patients

Principles of Moving Patients

Objectives 10, 11

THE BIG DECISION... What is an emergency that requires immediately moving a patient from the area? In general, a patient should be moved *immediately* (an **emergency move**) when one of the following situations exists:

1. *Scene hazards.* The patient may need to be moved if you are unable to protect the patient from hazards in the area and there is an immediate danger to you or the patient if he is not moved. Examples of possible scene hazards include:

   - Fire or the danger of fire
   - Uncontrolled traffic
   - Explosives or the danger of an explosion
   - Electrical hazards
   - Rising flood water
   - Toxic gases
   - Radiation
   - Structural collapse or the threat of a structural collapse
   - Potentially violent scenes (such as a shooting or domestic violence)

2. *The inability to reach other patients who need lifesaving care.* For example, if there are multiple patients in a vehicle, you may need to move a patient to reach one who is more seriously injured.

3. *The inability to provide immediate, lifesaving care because of the patient's location or position.* For example, a patient in cardiac arrest who is sitting in a chair or lying on a bed must be moved to the floor in order to provide effective cardiopulmonary resuscitation (CPR).

All of these situations put you at great risk. Always consider your safety first and then make the decision whether to attempt an emergency move or wait for additional resources.

The greatest danger in moving a patient quickly is the possibility of aggravating a spinal injury. Always drag the patient in the direction of the length (the long axis) of the body. This action will provide as much protection as possible to the patient's spine. Never push, pull, or drag a patient sideways. In the rare event that you need to perform an emergency move, realize that you will be putting yourself at risk for injury as well as possibly complicating the patient's injury. Using an emergency move to remove a patient from a vehicle makes it impossible to provide the same level of spine protection that would be accomplished with spine stabilization devices. *Think before you act!* Remember that in most cases—except in those situations stated earlier—a patient is better off being treated in place until additional help arrives.

Remember This!

Bystanders are often eager to provide assistance in emergencies. Before asking a bystander to assist you, check your agency's policy regarding these situations. This is particularly important in situations in which there is a risk of injury to you, the patient, or the bystander, such as when lifting or moving a patient. If you are permitted to use bystanders to help you, make sure to provide them with specific instructions to avoid injury of all involved. You should remain in charge of the patient at all times, not allowing a bystander to direct care or make movement decisions.

If no immediate threat to life exists, when ready for transport, move the patient using a **non-urgent move.** Non-urgent moves are the types of moves you will perform most often. They will be done with the help of other EMTs. It is important to communicate with each other and the patient before, during, and after the lift. Work as a team for success.

Body Mechanics and Lifting Techniques

Objective 1

Safety Precautions and Preparation

Body mechanics refers to the way we move our bodies when lifting and moving. Body mechanics includes body alignment, balance, and coordinated body

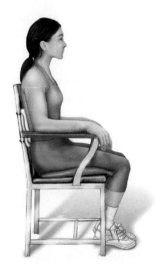

FIGURE 6-1 ▲ Good body mechanics includes good posture.

movement. Proper body alignment is synonymous with good posture and is an important part of body mechanics (Figure 6-1). Good posture means that the spine is in a neutral position when standing, sitting, or lying. This position recognizes that the spine has four natural curves. These curves are in the areas of the cervical, thoracic, lumbar, and sacral vertebrae (Figure 6-2). When you use good posture, there is minimal strain on your muscles, ligaments, bones, joints, and nerves. By maintaining proper body alignment, you reduce strain on your spine as well as on the muscles and ligaments that support it.

You also improve your balance when you use good posture. Balance can be further improved by:

- Separating your feet to a comfortable distance
- Bending your knees
- Flexing your hips to reach a squatting position

These actions broaden your base of support and help reduce your risk of injury. To protect yourself and the patient, you should prepare and plan *before* you actually move a patient. Important factors to consider include:

- The patient's weight
- The patient's condition
- The presence of hazards or potential hazards at the scene
- The terrain
- The distance the patient must be moved
- Your physical abilities and any limitations
- The availability of any equipment or personnel to assist with the move

In some cases, a patient may be in an awkward position or a tight space. The patient's position or

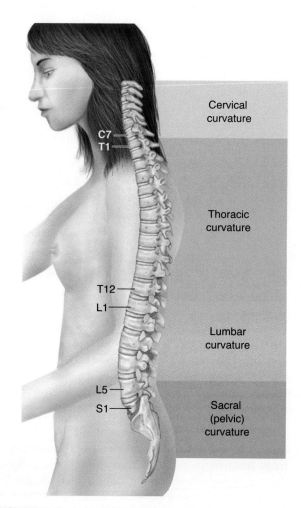

FIGURE 6-2 ▲ The adult spine has four natural curves in the areas of the cervical, thoracic, lumbar, and sacral vertebrae.

location may require you to bend or move out of balance. In these situations, it is best to call for additional help before moving the patient. In some situations, the *patient* may be able to tell you the best technique to move him. In all cases, it is very important to communicate clearly and frequently with your partner and the patient throughout the process. Work as a team and remind each other to use proper lifting techniques.

The Power Grip

When lifting, your arms and hands are strongest when positioned with your palms up. Use the **power grip** (underhand grip) when lifting an object to take full advantage of the strength of your hands, forearms, and biceps. With your palms up, grasp the object you are preparing to lift. Position your hands a comfortable distance apart, usually about 10 inches. Your palms and fingers should be in complete contact with the object, with all fingers bent at the same angles (Figure 6-3).

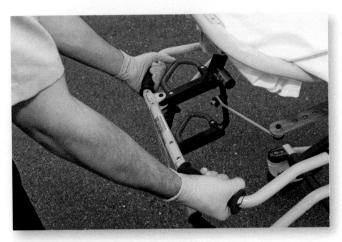

FIGURE 6-3 ▲ The power grip.

Guidelines for Safe Lifting of Cots and Stretchers

Objectives 2, 3

Safe lifting means keeping your back aligned as vertically as possible, using your leg strength, and maintaining your center of balance while lifting. Follow these important rules to prevent injury when lifting:

- Know or find out the weight to be lifted. Consider the weight of the patient, the weight of the equipment being used, and the need for additional help. Know or find out the weight limitations of the equipment being used. Know what to do with patients who exceed the weight limitations of the equipment.
- Know your physical ability and limitations.
- Plan how you will move the patient and where you will move him. It is often helpful to mentally picture the patient's final position and work backward to the patient's current position. Working in this way helps prevent arms from getting crossed and bodies from becoming twisted during the actual move. It also prevents you from being stuck in a position in which you are unable to complete the move safely.
- Make sure your path is clear of obstructions.
- Make sure that enough help is available. Use at least two people to lift. If possible, always use an even number of people to lift to maintain balance. Determine in advance who will direct the move. *One* person (usually the person at the patient's head) must assume responsibility for directing the actions of the others. "On my count, lift on three: one, two, three." "On my count, turn on three: one, two, three." Agree in advance that if anyone involved in the move says "no," the move will immediately be stopped.

The person stopping the move must state what needs to be done in order to complete the move. Sometimes, it's just stopping to turn a corner and get a better grip.

- Position your feet a comfortable distance apart (usually a shoulder's width) on a firm surface. Wear proper footwear to protect your feet and maintain a firm footing.
- Tense the muscles of your abdomen and buttocks before lifting. This tensing helps relieve the stress on your back muscles.
- Bend at your knees and hips, not your waist, and keep your back straight. All movement in the lift comes from your *legs*.
- Use your legs to lift, not your back. Your legs are much stronger than your back.
- Lift using a smooth, continuous motion. *Do not jerk or twist* when lifting. Jerking or twisting increases your risk of injury.
- Keep the patient's weight as close to you as possible. "Hug the load." Doing so moves your center of gravity closer to the patient, helps maintain balance, and reduces muscle strain.
- When possible, move forward rather than backward.
- Walk slowly, using short steps.
- Look where you are going.
- Move slowly, communicating clearly and frequently with other EMS personnel and the patient throughout the move.

Remember This!

You must think about these guidelines before *every* lift.

The **power lift** is a way to lift heavy objects, using the proper body mechanics just described. Skill Drill 6-1 shows a two-person power lift being used to lift a wheeled stretcher.

Stop and Think!

Always practice proper lifting techniques. Learning to lift by using proper body mechanics takes training and practice. When practicing, use "spotters" to alert you when you are performing a technique incorrectly. Practice and practice again until using correct lifting techniques become a habit. One bad lift can damage your back for the rest of your life!

Two-Person Power Lift

STEP 1 ▶ Position your feet a shoulder's width apart on a firm surface. Wear proper footwear to protect your feet and maintain a firm footing.

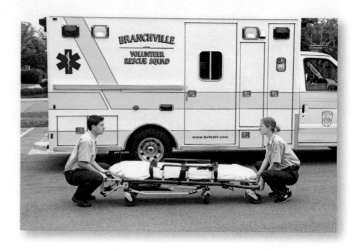

STEP 2 ▶ Use the power grip to grasp the stretcher. Tense the muscles of your abdomen and buttocks. Bend at your knees and hips, not at your waist, and keep your back straight.

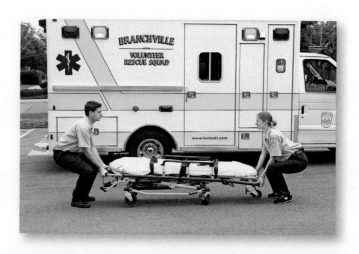

STEP 3 ▶ Communicating with each other and the patient, lift at the same time with your legs, not your back. Use a smooth, continuous motion.

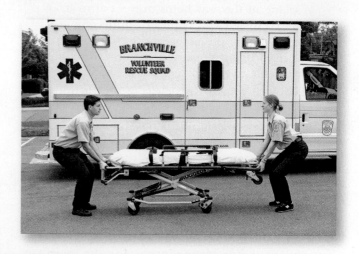

Carrying Patients and Equipment

Objectives 4, 5

To avoid injury when carrying patients and equipment, follow these important guidelines:

- Whenever possible, transport patients on devices that can be rolled.
- Know or find out the weight to be lifted.
- Know your physical abilities and limitations and that of your crew.
- Work in a coordinated manner and communicate frequently with your partner and the patient.
- Keep the weight as close to the body as possible.
- Keep your back in a locked-in position and avoid twisting.
- Flex at the hips, not at the waist, and bend at the knees.
- Do not hyperextend the back (do not lean back from the waist).
- Whenever possible, you and your partner should be of similar height and strength.
- When carrying a stretcher or backboard with only two crew members, face each other from either the sides or ends of the stretcher.

When using a one-handed carrying technique, pick up and carry with the back in a locked-in position. Avoid leaning to either side to compensate for the imbalance.

Carrying Procedure on Stairs

Objective 6

Follow these guidelines when carrying patients and equipment down stairs:

- When possible, use a commercially made stair chair instead of furniture or a stretcher when transporting patients down stairs.
- Make sure that the stairway is free of obstructions.
- Have another rescuer act as a guide or "spotter," especially if going down the stairs. This person can alert you to the number of steps, changes in footing surfaces, or any potential hazards.
- Make sure that the patient is secured to the stair chair before lifting.
- Carry patients head first up the stairs and feet first down the stairs.
- Keep your back in a locked-in position.
- Flex at the hips, not at the waist, and bend at the knees.

- Keep the weight and your arms as close to your body as possible.
- Always communicate with your partner during the move.

Guidelines for Safe Reaching

Objective 7

To avoid injury when reaching, follow these important rules:

- Keep your back straight.
- Avoid stretching or leaning back from your waist (hyperextending) when reaching overhead. Lean from your hips.
- Avoid twisting while reaching.
- Avoid reaching more than 15-20 inches in front of your body to grasp an object.
- Avoid situations in which prolonged strenuous effort (more than a minute) is needed.

Objective 8

A **log roll** is a technique used to move a patient from a facedown to a faceup position while keeping the head and neck in line with the rest of the body. This technique is also used to place a patient with a suspected spinal injury on a backboard. Correct reaching for log rolls includes the following guidelines:

- Keep your back straight while leaning over the patient.
- Lean from the hips.
- Use your shoulder muscles to help with the roll.

Guidelines for Safe Pushing and Pulling

Objective 9

To avoid injury when pushing and pulling, follow these guidelines:

- Push, rather than pull, whenever possible.
- Keep your back straight.
- Avoid twisting or jerking when pushing or pulling an object.
- Push at a level between your waist and shoulders.
- When the patient or object is below your waist, kneel to push or pull.
- When pulling, avoid reaching more than 15-20 inches in front of your body. Change your position (move back another 15-20 inches) when your hands have reached the front of your body.

- Keep the line of the pull through the center of your body by bending your knees.
- Keep the weight close to your body.
- Keep your elbows bent and your arms close to your sides.
- If possible, avoid pushing or pulling from an overhead position.

Remember This!

When you are called to the scene of an emergency, it is the patient's emergency. Treat the patient to the best of your ability until you can *safely* move him. If you are injured in the process of lifting and moving, you have done nothing but caused an additional problem.

Emergency Moves

Drags

Drags are a good way to move patients already on the ground. Dragging or pulling is more difficult than pushing. You will be surprised by how tired you become in a short time. Stabilize the patient's head and neck as much as possible before beginning the move. The clothes drag and blanket drag may be used when the patient must be moved quickly and an injury to the head or spine is suspected. Although it is not ideal material to stabilize the spine, the patient's clothing or a blanket provides material against which the patient's head and neck is cradled during the move. The patient's clothing or blanket is not used as a pillow, but rather as stabilization around the sides of the head to prevent rolling.

When dragging a patient, always pull along the length of the spine from either the patient's shoulders or the patient's feet and legs. The surface should be smooth to prevent bobbing of the patient's head over uneven terrain. *Never* pull the patient's head away from his neck and shoulders. Broaden your base of support by moving your rear leg back (if you are facing the patient) or by moving your front foot forward (if you are facing away from the patient).

Stop and Think!

Before performing an emergency move, make sure your path is clear of obstructions. Doing so will protect the patient from being dragged through broken glass, metal fragments, or other sharp objects that can cause additional injury.

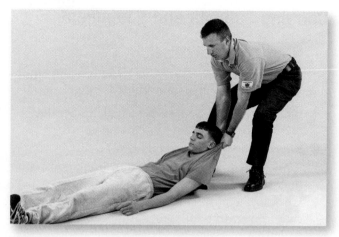

FIGURE 6-4 ▲ The clothes drag.

Clothes Drag

To perform a **clothes drag** (also called the *clothing pull* or *shirt drag*), position yourself at the patient's head (Figure 6-4). To prevent the patient's arms from being pulled upward during the move, consider securing the patient's wrists together or tucking his hands into his waistband. Gather the shoulders of the patient's shirt and pull him toward you so that a cradle is formed for the patient's head and neck. Make sure you have a firm grasp on the patient's clothing and begin pulling the patient to safety. When using this move, check often to make sure you are not choking the patient as his clothes slide up around his neck.

Blanket Drag

To perform a **blanket drag,** lay a blanket, sleeping bag, tarp, bed sheet, bedspread, or similar material lengthwise beside the patient. Make sure there is approximately two feet of the blanket above the patient's head. The uppermost section of the blanket will provide a cradle for the patient's head. It will also be used as the handle with which you will drag the patient. Kneel on the opposite side of the patient and roll him toward you (Figure 6-5a). Grasp the blanket and tuck half of the blanket under the patient. Leave the remainder of the blanket lying flat (Figure 6-5b). Quickly but gently, roll the patient onto his back. Pull the tucked portion of the blanket out from under the patient. Wrap the corners of the blanket securely around the patient (Figure 6-5c). Using the blanket "handle" that you created above the patient's head, keep the pull as straight and as in-line as possible and drag the patient to safety. Remember to use your legs, not your back, and keep your back as straight as possible (Figure 6-5d).

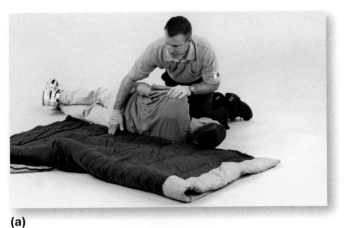
(a)

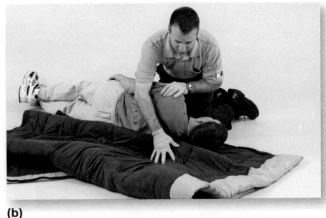
(b)

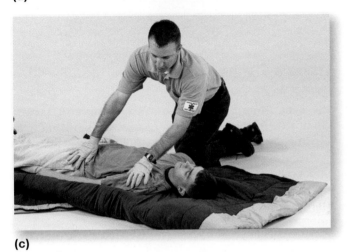
(c)

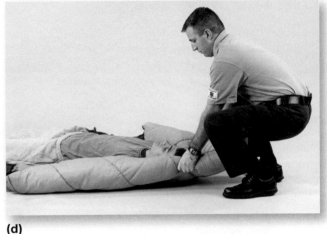
(d)

FIGURE 6-5 ▲ The blanket drag.

Shoulder Drag

A **shoulder drag** is an emergency move that is often used because it does not require any additional materials. To perform a shoulder drag, position yourself behind the patient and prop him up into a sitting position. From your position behind the patient, slide your hands under his armpits and drag him to safety (Figure 6-6).

Forearm Drag

To perform a **forearm drag** (also called the *bent-arm drag*), position yourself as you would in a shoulder drag. After sliding your hands under the patient's armpits, grasp his forearms and drag him to safety (Figure 6-7). Note that the forearm drag or shoulder drag provide *no* protection for the patient's spine.

Ankle Drag

To perform an **ankle drag**, grasp the patient's ankles or pant cuffs (Figure 6-8). This emergency move is not recommended because the patient's head is not supported and it may bounce if the patient is not pulled over a smooth surface. However, it is presented here because it is possible that you will

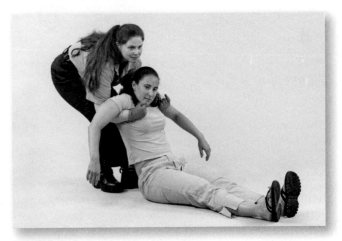

FIGURE 6-6 ▲ The shoulder drag.

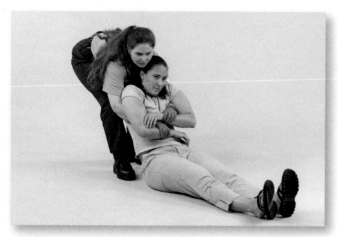

FIGURE 6-7 ▲ The forearm drag.

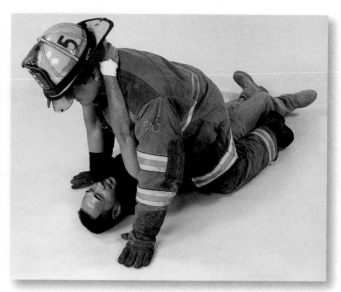

FIGURE 6-9 ▲ The firefighter's drag.

his back (Figure 6-9). Cross his wrists and secure them together with gauze, a triangular bandage, or a necktie. Straddle the patient and lift his arms over your head so that his wrists are behind your neck. As you crawl forward, be sure to raise your shoulders high enough so that the patient's head does not hit the ground.

Remember This!

Dragging Tips

- Always drag the patient along the length (long axis) of the spine.
- Never push, pull, or drag a patient sideways.
- Never pull the patient's head away from his neck and shoulders.

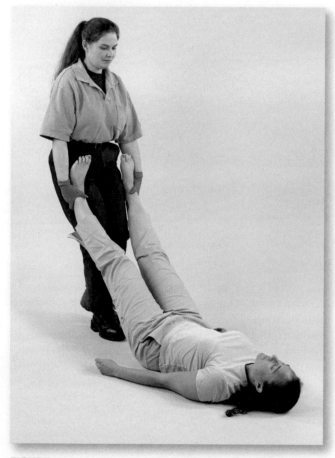

FIGURE 6-8 ▲ The ankle drag.

encounter a situation in which you have no other means to move the patient.

Firefighter's Drag

The **firefighter's drag** is particularly useful when you must crawl underneath a low structure for a short distance or move a patient from a smoke-filled area. To perform a firefighter's drag, place the patient on

Carries

Firefighter's Carry

The **firefighter's carry** can be used to quickly move a patient. The patient's abdomen bears the weight with this move. To perform the firefighter's carry, position yourself toe to toe with the patient. Crouch down, grasp the patient's wrists, and pull the patient to a sitting position (Figure 6-10a). Step on the patient's toes with the tip of your shoes. While grasping the patient's wrists, pull the patient to a standing position (Figure 6-10b). Remove your shoes from the patient's toes. Quickly place your shoulder into the patient's abdomen and pull the patient lengthwise across your shoulders (Figure 6-10c). Place one arm through the

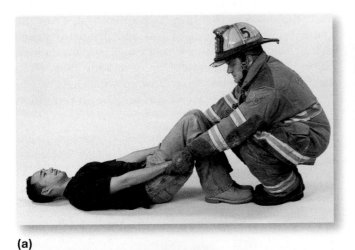

(a)

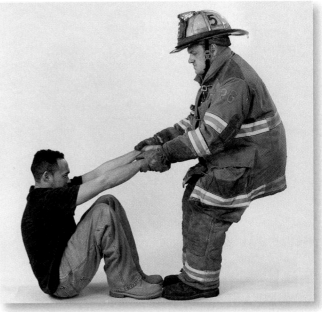

(b)

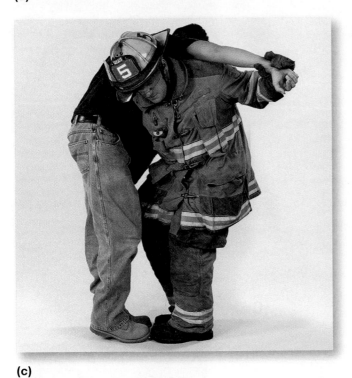

(c)

(d)

FIGURE 6-10 ▲ The firefighter's carry.

patient's legs. Use your other hand to grasp one of the patient's arms, secure the patient in position on your shoulders, and then stand up (Figure 6-10D). Remember to lift with your legs and not your back.

Cradle Carry

The **cradle carry** (also called the *one-person arm carry*) may be used if the patient is a child or a small adult. To perform a cradle carry, kneel next to the patient.

Place one hand under the patient's shoulders and the other under his knees, and then stand up, using the strength of your legs (Figure 6-11).

Pack-Strap Carry

The **pack-strap carry** requires no equipment. It is best used with a conscious patient unless someone is available to help you position the patient. To perform the pack-strap carry, kneel in front of a seated patient with

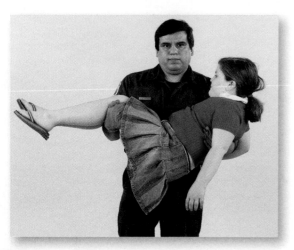

FIGURE 6-11 ▲ The cradle carry.

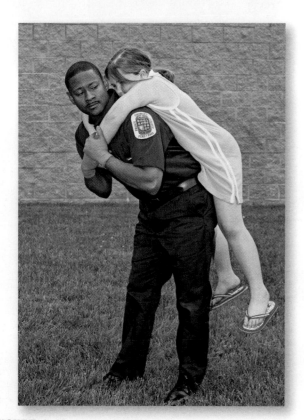

FIGURE 6-12 ▲ The pack-strap carry.

Piggyback Carry

The **piggyback carry** is used when the patient cannot walk but can use his arms to hold onto you. To perform this move, kneel in front of a seated patient with your back to him. Have the patient place his arms over your shoulders so that they cross your chest. Cross the patient's wrists in front of you and grasp his wrists. While holding his wrists, lean forward, rise up on your knees, and pull the patient up onto your back. Hold both of the patient's wrists close to your chest as you stand up (Figure 6-13a). As you prepare to reposition

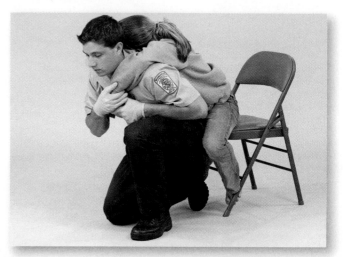

(a)

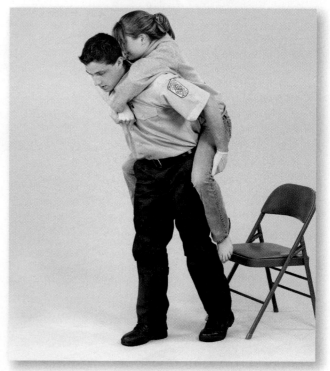

(b)

FIGURE 6-13 ▲ The piggyback carry.

your back to him. Have the patient place his arms over your shoulders so that they cross your chest. Be sure the patient's armpits are over your shoulders. Cross the patient's wrists in front of you and grasp them. While holding the patient's wrists, lean forward, rise up on your knees, and pull the patient up onto your back. Hold both of the patient's wrists close to your chest as you stand up (Figure 6-12). If the patient is small, it may be possible to grasp both of his wrists with one hand. This action leaves your other hand free to open doors and move obstructions.

your arms and hands, instruct the patient to hold onto you with his arms. Position your forearms under the patient's knees and grasp his wrists (Figure 6-13b).

Two-Person Carry

If the patient is unable to walk, two people can make a "seat" for the patient. It is best to have two rescuers of about the same height and size perform this move.

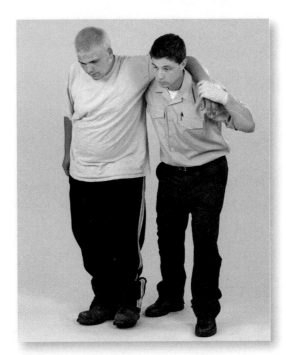

FIGURE 6-15 ▲ The human crutch move.

To perform the **two-person carry** (also called the *two-person seat carry*), place one arm under the patient's thighs and the other across the patient's back. Grasp the arms of the other rescuer and lock them in position at the elbows, forming a "seat." Both rescuers then rise slowly to a standing position (Figure 6-14).

Human Crutch Move

In some situations, the patient may be able to walk but requires assistance. You can assist him to safety by acting as a crutch. One or two rescuers may be used for this move. To perform the **human crutch move** (also called the *rescuer assist* or *walking assist*), place the patient's arm across your shoulders and hold his wrist with one hand. Place your other hand around his waist and help him to safety (Figure 6-15).

Urgent Moves (Rapid Extrication)

A patient should be moved quickly (**urgent move**) when there is an immediate threat to life, such as in the following situations:

- Altered mental status
- Inadequate breathing
- Shock (hypoperfusion)

Rapid extrication must be accomplished quickly, without compromise or injury to the spine. Skill Drill 6-2 shows the steps for rapid extrication.

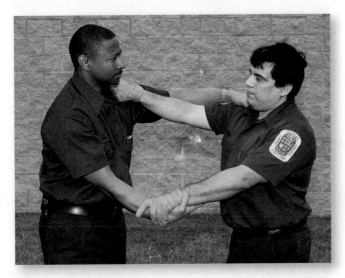

(a)

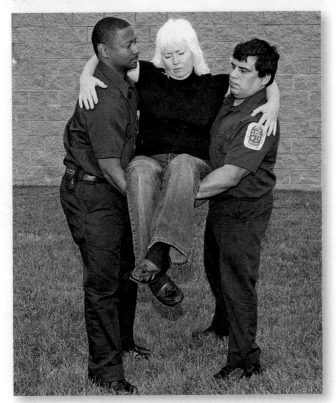

(b)

FIGURE 6-14 ▲ The two-person seat carry.

Rapid Extrication

STEP 1 ▶ One EMT positions himself behind the patient. This EMT then places his hands on either side of the patient's head, bringing the cervical spine into a neutral in-line position and providing manual stabilization. At the same time, the EMT begins assessment of the patient's airway.

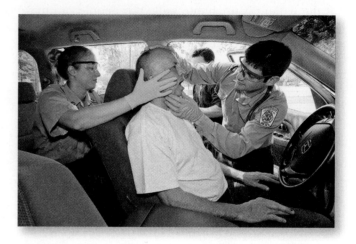

STEP 2 ▶ • A second EMT performs a primary survey and applies a cervical immobilization device.
   • At the same time, a third EMT places a long backboard near the door.

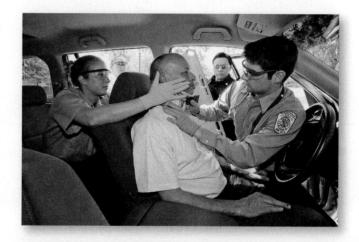

STEP 3 ▶ The second EMT supports the patient's chest and back as the third EMT moves to the passenger seat and frees the patient's legs from the pedals and floor panels.

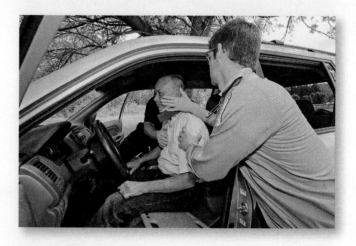

STEP 4 ▶ At the direction of the EMT at the patient's head, the patient is rotated in several short, coordinated moves until the patient's back is in the open doorway and his feet are on the passenger seat.

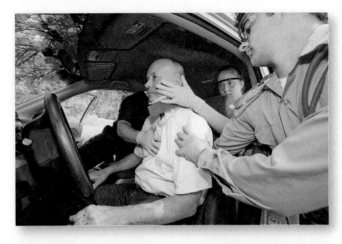

STEP 5 ▶ Because the first EMT cannot usually support the patient's head any longer, another available EMT or emergency worker supports the patient's head as the first EMT gets out of the vehicle and takes support of the head outside the vehicle. The end of the long backboard is placed on the seat next to the patient's buttocks.

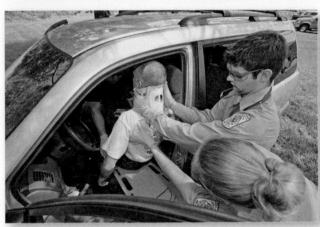

STEP 6 ▶ • Assistants support the other end of the board as the first EMT and the second EMT lower the patient onto it.
• The second and third EMTs slide the patient into proper position on the board in short, coordinated moves.

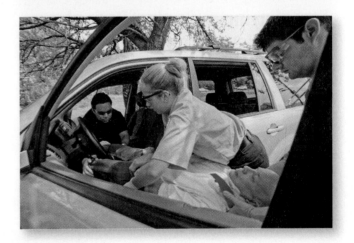

Non-Urgent Moves

If no threat to life exists, the patient should be moved when ready for transportation (non-urgent move).

Direct Ground Lift

The **direct ground lift** is used to lift and carry a patient with no suspected spinal injury from the ground to a bed or a stretcher. If the patient is going to be transferred to a stretcher, place the stretcher as close to the patient as possible. Although this lift can be performed with two rescuers, three is the safest method. A lot of communication and teamwork is necessary to lift and move patients safely. Skill Drill 6-3 shows the steps for a three-person direct ground lift.

Remember This!

Do *not* perform a direct ground lift or an extremity lift if trauma to the patient's head, neck, or back is suspected because the head is not stabilized during these moves. The extremity lift must also be avoided if an extremity is injured.

Extremity Lift

The extremity lift is used to lift a patient onto a carrying device, such as a stretcher. Two rescuers are needed to perform an extremity lift. This lift should *not* be used on a patient with a suspected head, neck, back, or extremity injury. Skill Drill 6-4 shows a two-person extremity lift.

Transferring a Supine Patient from Bed to Stretcher

There are two common methods used to transfer a supine patient from a bed to a stretcher. The first method is the direct carry. It is used when you are required to move a patient to a stretcher that cannot be placed parallel to the bed. The second, the draw sheet method, is by far the most common. This method requires the stretcher to be placed parallel to the patient's bed. In both cases, you will be assisting hospital personnel or another EMS professional. As with previous moves, teamwork and coordination are essential.

Direct Carry

The direct carry is used to move a patient with no suspected spinal injury from a bed to a stretcher. Skill Drill 6-5 illustrates a direct carry.

Draw Sheet Transfer

A **draw sheet** is a narrow sheet placed crosswise on a bed under the patient. It is used to assist in moving a patient or when changing soiled bed sheets. The draw sheet transfer requires a minimum of two people to perform; however, the use of four rescuers is preferred. To move a patient by using a draw sheet, follow the steps outlined in Skill Drill 6-6.

Patient Positioning

Although patient positioning is often overlooked, it is an essential part of your patient care. In some cases, simply changing the patient's position can improve condition. Consider the following situations:

- Your patient was golfing when he suddenly felt hot and lightheaded. He sat down in the grass to rest. As you approach, he lies down. Your patient is now unresponsive without a possible head, neck, or back injury. He is breathing and a pulse is present. This patient should be placed in the **recovery position** (Figure 6-16). To place a

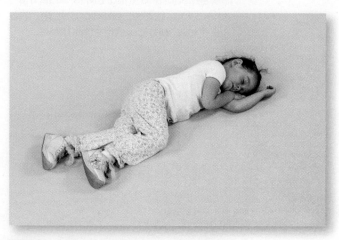

FIGURE 6-16 ▲ The recovery position.

Three-Person Direct Ground Lift

STEP 1 ▷
- Three rescuers line up on the same side of a supine patient. If three rescuers are available, position one at the patient's head, the second at the patient's waist, and the third at the patient's knees.
- To maintain balance throughout the move, all rescuers should kneel on one knee. The same knee should used by all rescuers. If possible, place the patient's arms across his chest.
- If only two rescuers are available, position one at the patient's chest and the other at the patient's thighs.

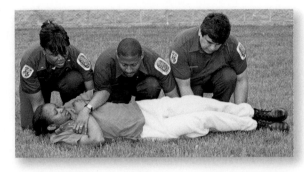

STEP 2 ▷
- The rescuer at the head places one arm under the patient's neck and shoulders, cradling the patient's head. The first rescuer's other arm is placed under the patient's lower back. The second rescuer places one arm above and one arm below the patient's waist. The third rescuer places one arm under the patient's knees and the other under the patient's ankles.
- If only two rescuers are available, the first rescuer places one arm under the patient's head and neck and cradles the patient's head. He places the other hand under the patient's shoulders. The second rescuer places his arms under the patient's lower back and buttocks.

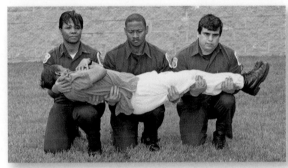

STEP 3 ▷
- On the command of the rescuer at the patient's head, everyone should lift the patient to their knees.
- Once everyone is balanced, the patient is rolled toward the rescuers' chests. This action keeps the weight of the patient close to the rescuer's body, reducing the risk of back injury to the rescuer.

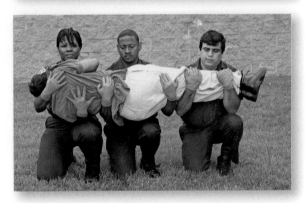

STEP 4 ▷
- On the command of the rescuer at the patient's head, all rescuers should stand and move the patient to the desired location.
- To lower the patient, simply reverse the steps.

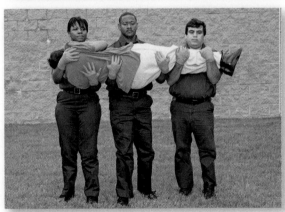

Two-Person Extremity Lift

STEP 1 ▶ One rescuer kneels at the patient's head. The second rescuer kneels between the patient's bent knees with his back to the patient.

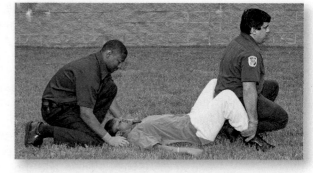

STEP 2 ▶ The rescuer at the patient's head places one hand under each of the patient's armpits and grasps the patient's wrists. The second rescuer slips his hands behind the patient's knees.

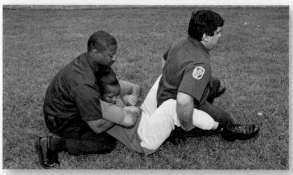

STEP 3 ▶ On a signal from the rescuer at the patient's head, both rescuers move up to a crouching position.

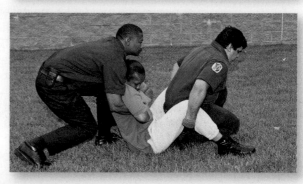

STEP 4 ▶ On a signal from the rescuer at the patient's head, both rescuers stand at the same time and move with the patient.

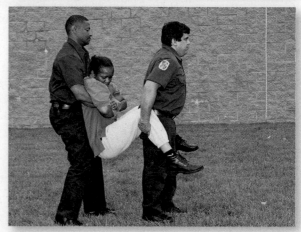

Direct Carry

STEP 1 ▶
- Place the stretcher at a 90-degree angle to the bed, with the head end of the stretcher at the foot of the bed. Prepare the stretcher by unbuckling the straps, adjusting the height of the stretcher to be even with the bed, and lowering the side rails. Set the brakes on the stretcher (if so equipped) to the "on" position.
- Both rescuers should stand between the bed and the stretcher and face the patient.

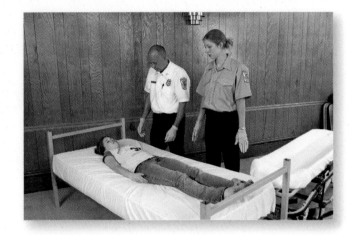

STEP 2 ▶
- The rescuer at the head slides one arm under the patient's neck, cupping the patient's far shoulder with his hand and cradling the patient's head. The rescuer then slides his other arm under the patient's lower back.
- The second rescuer slides one hand under the patient's hip and lifts slightly. She then places her other arm under the patient's hips and calves.

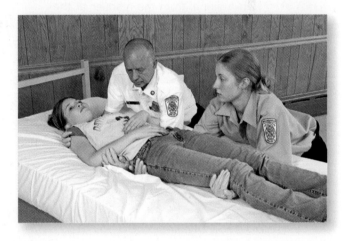

STEP 3 ▶ On a signal from the rescuer at the patient's head, both rescuers slide the patient toward them to the edge of the bed. Both rescuers should lift with their legs.

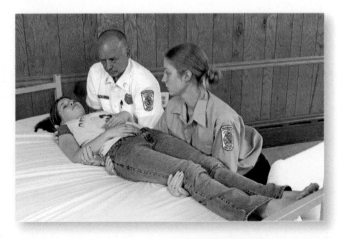

Continued on next page

Direct Carry (*continued*)

STEP 4 ▶ On a signal from the rescuer at the patient's head, the patient is lifted and curled toward the rescuers' chests. Both rescuers should be careful not to jerk or twist.

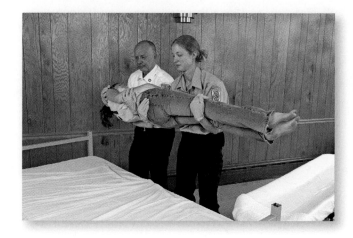

STEP 5 ▶ On a signal from the rescuer at the patient's head, both rescuers then rotate together, lining up with the stretcher, and gently place the patient onto the stretcher.

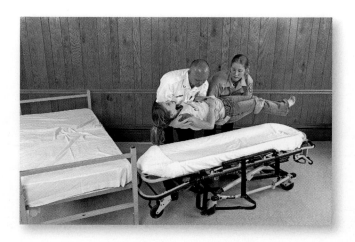

Draw Sheet Transfer

STEP 1 ▶
- Loosen the draw sheet on the bed and form a long roll to grasp.
- Prepare the stretcher by unbuckling the straps, adjusting the height of the stretcher to be even with the bed, and lowering the side rails.
- Set the brakes on the stretcher (if so equipped) to the "on" position.
- Position the stretcher next to and touching the patient's bed.

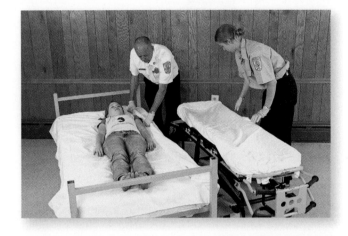

STEP 2 ▶ Both rescuers should stand on the same side of the stretcher and then reach across it to grasp the draw sheet firmly at the patient's head and hips.

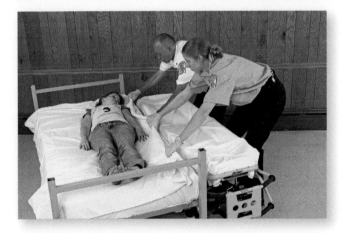

STEP 3 ▶ On a signal from the rescuer at the patient's head, gently slide the patient from the bed to the stretcher.

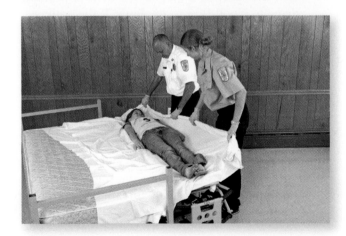

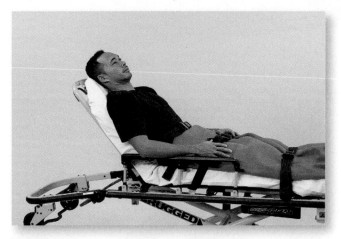

FIGURE 6-17 ▲ The Fowler's position.

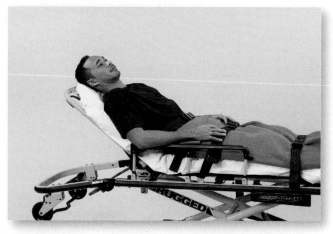

FIGURE 6-18 ▲ The semi-Fowler's position.

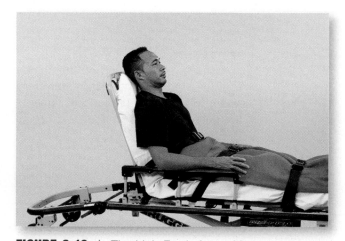

FIGURE 6-19 ▲ The high-Fowler's position.

patient in the recovery position, raise the patient's left arm above his head so that his head will rest on his arm once he is log-rolled onto his left side. Kneel on the left side of the supine patient. Grasp the patient's leg and shoulder and roll him toward you, onto his left side. This positioning allows the patient's head to rest on his raised left arm with his face in a slightly downward position. It also helps secretions drain from the patient's nose and mouth, reducing the risk of a blocked airway. Be aware that nerve and blood vessel injury can occur if the patient lies on one arm for a prolonged period. Bend both of the patient's legs to help stabilize the patient. The left side is preferred so that the patient faces the EMT during ambulance transport. Positioning the patient on the left side is also preferred when transporting a pregnant patient to promote adequate blood flow to the fetus. If the patient stops breathing or no longer has a pulse, roll him onto his back and begin CPR.

- Your patient has fallen from a ladder while trimming tree branches. You suspect a head, neck, or back injury. This patient should *not* be moved until additional personnel are on the scene to help you assess the patient and stabilize his spine before moving him to a stretcher. Be sure to have suction readily available should vomiting occur.

- Your patient was running at the track and is now experiencing difficulty breathing. This patient should be allowed to assume a position of comfort. Most often, this will be a seated position. In a Fowler's position, the patient is lying on his back with his upper body elevated at a 45- to 60-degree angle (Figure 6-17). In a **semi-Fowler's position**, the patient is sitting up with his head at a 45-degree angle and his legs out straight (Figure 6-18). In a **high-Fowler's position,**

the patient is sitting upright at a 90-degree angle (Figure 6-19).

- Your patient is experiencing a sudden onset of severe abdominal pain or non-traumatic back pain. Patients with this complaint are often most comfortable on their back or side with their knees slightly bent.

- Your patient is vomiting. She is awake and alert with a strong pulse. There is no history or evidence of trauma. This patient should be allowed to assume a position of comfort. Be prepared to manage her airway and place her in the recovery position if her level of consciousness decreases.

- Your patient is complaining of weakness. He has had flu symptoms for three days. He is confused. His skin is pale, cool, and moist, and his heart rate is fast. A patient with signs and symptoms of shock should be placed flat on his back. In the past, the shock position was

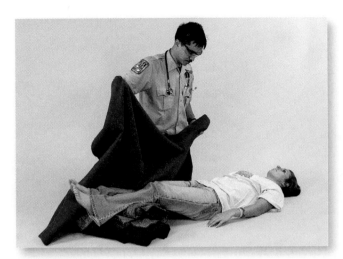

FIGURE 6-20 ▲ The shock position is no longer recommended.

recommended. In this position, the patient was placed on her back with her legs raised about 8-12 inches (Figure 6-20). This position is no longer recommended

Remember This!

- Any patient with a suspected spinal injury should be fully stabilized on a long backboard.
- Do not place a patient in the recovery position if you suspect the patient has experienced an injury to his head, neck, or spine.
- *Do not permit a patient complaining of chest pain or difficulty breathing to walk to the stretcher or ambulance.*
- If the stretcher will not fit into a particular area, it may be necessary to place the patient in a chair and then move the patient in the chair to the stretcher.

Equipment

Objective 12

You will encounter many different types of equipment that are used to assist in stabilizing and moving your patients. Most equipment works under the same basic principle with slight design and cosmetic variations. It is important to become familiar with the equipment used in your area. Following are descriptions of commonly used equipment.

Wheeled Stretcher

A wheeled stretcher is a rolling bed that is commonly found in the back of an ambulance (Figure 6-21). It is used more often than any other patient transfer device. There are many different manufacturers, but all wheeled stretchers have certain characteristics that make them compatible with the need to transfer and maneuver patients from the scene to the transport vehicle. The main bed (patient platform) is about 76 inches in length and usually about 23 inches wide. It is typically padded with a comfort mattress that will need to be covered with a sheet. It should also include a cover that will stop fluids from penetrating into the mattress. The head of the stretcher can be adjusted to several different angles. Most patients will be more comfortable with their head and body inclined at a slight angle. Cardiac and respiratory patients will generally be unable to lay flat. The platform can incline to a semi-sitting position and into a Trendelenburg position.

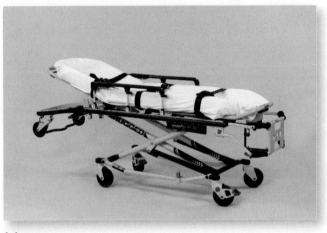

(a)

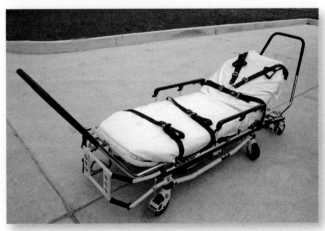

(b)

FIGURE 6-21 ▲ **(a)** A wheeled stretcher. **(b)** A bariatric stretcher.

All patient transport devices must have an effective method of securing the patient to the device. This is generally accomplished with a restraint system. Current recommendations are for restraint devices that incorporate an "over the shoulder" system. This can protect the patient during rapid deceleration. In addition, patient transport equipment must have the ability to be securely fastened to the floor to prevent movement during a "rollover" type of accident. The actual movement of the patient on the stretcher will be influenced by many factors such as the size and weight of the patient and even the terrain over which you are traveling. Many newer stretchers have large, inflatable tires that allow for movement over uneven ground.

Wheeled stretchers have handles used for lifting and rolling. If you are lifting a wheeled stretcher with someone who does not operate it often, take the control end so that you can make sure the wheels will drop properly. Be sure you know the weight limitations of the stretcher you are using. Exceeding it could cause injury to the patient, the crew, or both.

Newer types of lifting devices are available that offer some type of "power" assist to help reduce your risk of back strain or injury. A bariatric stretcher is designed to hold larger or heavier patients (Figure 6-21). It may have an ability to be moved into the transport vehicle on a ramp by using a pulley or winch system. Request additional resources if this equipment is unavailable and the patient is large. Lifting a heavy or large patient not only puts your back at risk, but there is also a greater possibility of dropping the patient.

Remember This!

Keep the stretcher in the lowest, most comfortable position during patient moves. This will keep the patient's center of gravity lower, and the stretcher will be less likely to tip over.

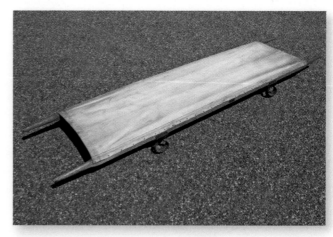

FIGURE 6-22 ▲ A portable stretcher.

Portable Stretcher

A portable stretcher usually folds or collapses when it is not in use. It is often made of heavy canvas or heavy plastic (Figure 6-22). It may be used in the following situations:

- To carry patients down stairs, downhill, or over rough terrain
- To remove patients from spaces too confined or narrow for a wheeled stretcher
- In incidents in which you need to quickly transfer a large number of people from one place to another

Scoop Stretcher

A **scoop (orthopedic) stretcher** is unique in that it is hinged and opens at the head and feet to fit around and under the patient (Figure 6-23). The scoop stretcher is also called a *split litter*. To use this device,

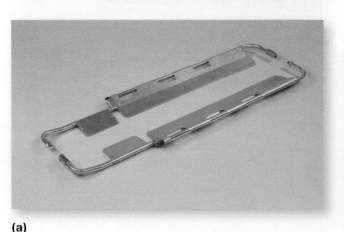

(a)

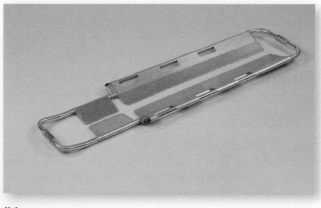

(b)

FIGURE 6-23 ▲ A scoop (orthopedic) stretcher, **(a)** sides separated; **(b)** sides together.

you must have access to both sides of the patient. The two halves of the stretcher are adjusted to the patient's length. Each piece is then slid under the patient and reconnected, effectively scooping the patient onto the device. The scoop stretcher may be used to carry a supine patient up or down stairs. However, a scoop stretcher does not adequately stabilize the spine. If a spinal injury is suspected, the patient and scoop stretcher should be secured to a long backboard for stabilization.

Basket Stretcher

A **basket stretcher** (Figure 6-24) is shaped like a long basket and can hold a scoop stretcher or a long backboard. A basket stretcher is also called a *basket litter* or *Stokes basket*. Some basket stretchers are too narrow to hold all widths of backboards. If you will be using a basket stretcher, be sure to check how wide it is to make certain your backboard will fit. There is a military version of basket stretcher that has a leg divider. This device will not accept a long backboard, no matter what the width.

The basket is made of fiberglass-plastic composites, plastic with an aluminum frame, or a steel frame with wire or plastic mesh. Some basket stretchers have holes in the bottom of the stretcher to allow for water drainage. A basket stretcher is used for moving patients over rough terrain, in water rescues, or in high-angle rescues. A basket stretcher that has a solid bottom can also be pulled over snow and ice (and other terrain), much like a sled.

Flexible Stretcher

A **flexible stretcher** can be rolled up for easy storage and carrying but forms a more rigid surface that conforms to the sides of the patient when in use. Examples of flexible stretchers include the Reeves stretcher

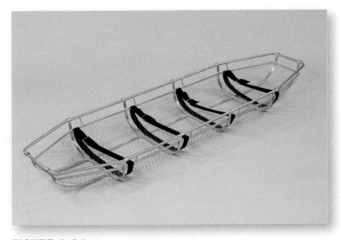

FIGURE 6-24 ▲ A basket stretcher.

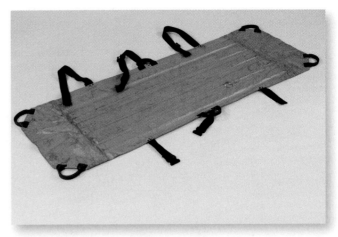

FIGURE 6-25 ▲ A flexible stretcher.

(Figure 6-25), SKED, and Navy stretcher. Flexible stretchers are made of canvas or flexible, synthetic material with carrying handles. Straps are used to secure the patient. This type of stretcher is particularly useful when space is limited to access the patient. It can be used in narrow hallways, stairs, cramped corners, high-angle rescues, and hazardous materials situations. Because the flexible stretcher conforms around the patient, it may not be possible to access all areas of the patient when giving emergency care. Flexible stretchers do not provide the kind of impact protection for the patient provided by many basket stretchers. You will need to have greater concern about spinal precautions and exercise greater care when moving your patient in a flexible stretcher. Patients carried in a flexible stretcher should be carried in a supine position to prevent accidental suffocation.

Stair Chair

A **stair chair** is a commercially made chair (Figure 6-26). At least two rescuers are required to move the patient in a stair chair. It is used to transfer patients up or down stairways, through narrow hallways and doorways, into small elevators, or in narrow aisles in aircraft or buses. It is a very helpful device when a patient does not need to lie flat. The stair chair has belts and straps with which to secure the patient. It also has handles for lifting.

Backboards

Backboards (also called *spine boards*) come in many different shapes, sizes, and colors. The **long backboard** has holes spaced along the head and foot ends as well as the sides of the board (Figure 6-27). These holes are made for handholds and inserting straps. A long backboard is relatively inexpensive, easy to store, and very versatile. The long backboard is used in the following situations:

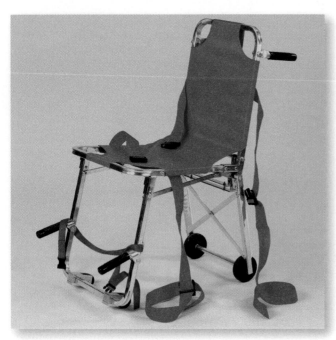

FIGURE 6-26 ▲ A stair chair.

- Securing a patient who is either lying or standing and needs to be immobilized to prevent worsening a potential spinal injury
- Lifting and moving patients
- Providing secondary support when a short backboard or scoop stretcher is used
- As a firm surface on which to perform CPR

Securing a patient properly to a long backboard is essential in order to minimize spinal movement. This is particularly important if it is necessary to tilt the backboard. Tilting the backboard may be necessary if an immobilized patient vomits and during transport of a woman in her second or third trimester of pregnancy.

Although the use of a long backboard helps to stabilize a patient's spine, it is uncomfortable for the patient. Although most prehospital patient encounters are relatively short, the patient may remain on the board for hours after his arrival in an Emergency Department. Patients can develop pressure injuries at body contact points along the board. In some cases, the backboard itself can cause pain and lead to unnecessary tests (such as x-rays) at the hospital to identify the source of the pain. The three most common areas for pressure pain are the back of the head, lower back, and sacrum. Padding at points of contact between the bones in these areas and the backboard can help reduce the patient's discomfort without compromising spinal stabilization.

Vacuum mattresses are being used with increasing frequency in the field. A vacuum mattress can provide spinal stabilization, as does a backboard, and is much more comfortable for the patient than a backboard. A vacuum mattress is particularly helpful for long transports where a hard backboard will cause the patient great discomfort and pain (and possible minor injury). Another benefit of using a vacuum mattress is that it is easier to position a patient who has been immobilized on his side when it is necessary to clear his airway. One drawback of using a vacuum mattress is that access to the posterior aspect of the patient may be difficult. A vacuum mattress is also susceptible to punctures and tears. Carrying a patient on a vacuum mattress requires the assistance of more than two people. The mattress will collapse if it is supported solely at each end, with potentially disastrous results.

The **short backboard** is used to secure the head, neck, and back of a stable patient found in a seated position (Figure 6-28). Once secured, the patient can then be transferred to a long backboard for full stabilization that includes the hips and legs. A vest-type device can be used in place of a short backboard.

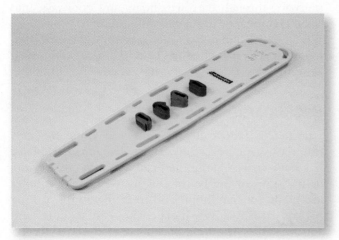

FIGURE 6-27 ▲ A long backboard.

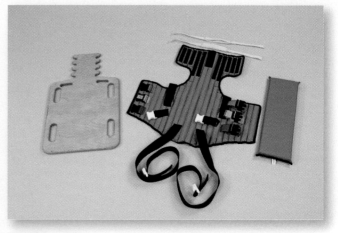

FIGURE 6-28 ▲ A short backboard and vest-type device.

On the Scene Wrap-Up

Equipment and personnel begin to arrive quickly. You direct them to take the unconscious patients, using available stretchers. Stair chairs are used to evacuate others who are too large and too weak to walk. One elderly woman is able to walk with a firefighter who uses the human crutch move to assist her. As you wait for the equipment to return, your aide reports that the fire doors are becoming very hot. You can see a wisp of smoke curling around them at the ceiling. You pick up the last tiny woman in a cradle carry and evacuate the building. Thirty minutes later, the ceiling collapses, crushing the room you and your patients were in. ■

Sum It Up

▶ As an EMT, you will most often give initial emergency care to a patient in the position in which he is found. You will need to be able to distinguish an emergency from a non-emergency situation. Your role will also include positioning patients to prevent further injury and assisting other EMS professionals in lifting and moving patients.

▶ Body mechanics refers to the way we move our bodies when lifting and moving. Body mechanics includes body alignment, balance, and coordinated body movement. Good posture is key to proper body alignment.

▶ In order to lift safely, you should use the power grip (underhand grip). To perform this grip, you should position your hands a comfortable distance apart (about 10 inches). With your palms up, grasp the object you are preparing to lift. The power grip allows you to take full advantage of the strength of your hands, forearms, and biceps.

▶ Safely lifting patients requires you to use good posture and good body mechanics. You should consider the weight of the patient and call for additional help if needed. Plan how you will move the patient and where you will move him. It is also important to remember to lift with your legs and not your back. When lifting with other EMS professionals, communication and planning are key.

▶ An emergency move is used when there is an immediate danger to you or the patient. These dangers include scene hazards, the inability to reach patients who need lifesaving care, and a patient location or position that prevents you from giving immediate and lifesaving care.

▶ Safely lifting patients requires you to use good posture and good body mechanics. You should consider the weight of the patient and call for additional help if needed.

▶ Drags are one type of emergency move. When dragging a patient, remember to stabilize the patient's head and neck as much as possible before beginning the move. Also, always remember to pull along the length of the spine. *Never* pull the patient's head away from his neck and shoulders. You should also never drag a patient sideways. Carries are the second major type of emergency move. As an EMT, you should become familiar with the different types of carries.

▶ An urgent move is used to move a patient when there is an immediate threat to life, such as in the following situations: altered mental status, inadequate breathing, or shock. Rapid extrication is an example of an urgent move. It must be accomplished quickly, without compromise or injury to the spine.

▶ Non-urgent moves are used to move, lift, or carry patients with no known or suspected injury to the head, neck, spine, or extremities. The direct ground lift and the extremity lift are the two main types of non-urgent moves.

▶ The direct carry and the draw sheet method are the two primary methods used to transfer a supine patient to a bed or stretcher. In both transfer types, you will be assisting hospital personnel or another EMS professional. Therefore, teamwork and coordination are essential.

▶ Patient positioning is an important part of the patient care you provide. In some cases, simply changing a patient's position can improve his condition. As an EMT, you should become familiar with the different types of positions and when to use them.

▶ Many different types of equipment are used to assist in stabilizing and moving patients. In your role as an emergency care provider, it is important to become familiar with the equipment used in your area. Commonly used equipment includes various types of stretchers and backboards as well as the stair chair.

Division 2

Airway

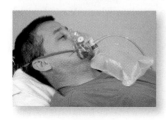

7 Airway and Breathing

By the end of this chapter, you should be able to:

Knowledge Objectives ▶

1. Name and label the major structures of the respiratory system on a diagram.
2. List the signs of adequate breathing.
3. List the signs of inadequate breathing.
4. Describe the steps in performing the head tilt–chin lift.
5. Relate mechanism of injury to opening the airway.
6. Describe the steps in performing the jaw thrust without head tilt maneuver.
7. State the importance of having a suction unit ready for immediate use when providing emergency care.
8. Describe the techniques of suctioning.
9. Describe how to artificially ventilate a patient with a pocket mask.
10. Describe the steps in artificially ventilating a patient with a bag-mask while using the jaw thrust without head tilt maneuver.
11. List the parts of a bag-mask system.
12. Describe the steps in artificially ventilating a patient with a bag-mask for one and two rescuers.
13. Describe the signs of adequate artificial ventilation using the bag-mask.
14. Describe the signs of inadequate artificial ventilation using the bag-mask.
15. Describe the steps in artificially ventilating a patient with a flow-restricted, oxygen-powered ventilation device.
16. List the steps in performing mouth-to-barrier device and mask-to-stoma artificial ventilation.
17. Describe how to measure and insert an oropharyngeal (oral) airway.
18. Describe how to measure and insert a nasopharyngeal (nasal) airway.
19. Define the components of an oxygen delivery system.
20. Identify a nonrebreather face mask and state the oxygen flow requirements needed for its use.
21. Describe the indications for using a nasal cannula versus a nonrebreather face mask.
22. Identify a nasal cannula and state the flow requirements needed for its use.

Attitude Objectives ▶

23. Explain the rationale for artificial ventilation and airway protective skills taking priority over most other basic life support skills.
24. Explain the rationale for providing adequate oxygenation through high inspired oxygen concentrations to patients who, in the past, may have received low concentrations.

On the Scene

You and your Emergency Medical Technician partner pull up to a house for "an unconscious person." As you grab your emergency kit and approach the door, a tearful woman directs you to the bathroom. She tells you, "I think he's taken a heroin overdose." A 21-year-old man is seated limply on the toilet, taking an occasional weak gasp. His skin is gray, cool, and wet. "Let's get him out of here," you tell the police officer. You struggle to drag him to the next room, aware that he is unconscious. As you lay him on his back, you perform a head tilt–chin lift. You listen carefully for airway movement from his nose or mouth. As you look at his chest, you can see that he is only taking three or four breaths each minute. You quickly assemble your bag-mask device and deliver two breaths and then slide your fingers into the groove in his neck. You can feel a strong pulse. Your partner quickly notifies dispatch to send a Paramedic unit to the scene. ▪

THINK ABOUT IT

As you read this chapter, think about the following questions:

- What findings suggest that he is not breathing adequately?
- Are there other measures that are needed to open his airway?
- How can you assist his breathing?

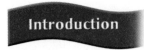
Airway Emergencies

All living cells of the body require oxygen and produce carbon dioxide. Oxygen is particularly important to cells of the nervous system because, without it, brain cells begin to die within four to six minutes. The most stressful and chaotic scene usually involves a difficult airway. A nonbreathing patient or a patient with difficulty breathing is experiencing a true emergency. To prevent death, you must be able to recognize early signs of breathing difficulty and know what to do.

The Respiratory System

The Functions of the Respiratory System

One of the major functions of the respiratory system is to deliver oxygen from the atmosphere to the bloodstream. Another major function is to remove carbon dioxide from the bloodstream that is produced by the body cells and release it to the atmosphere. As an Emergency Medical Technician (EMT), you must make sure these functions happen by maintaining an open airway and ensuring that the patient has adequate respirations. Maintaining an open airway allows a free flow of air into and out of the lungs.

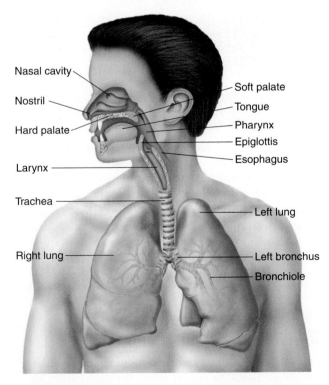

Nasal cavity

Nostril

Hard palate

Larynx

Trachea

Right lung

Soft palate

Tongue

Pharynx

Epiglottis

Esophagus

Left lung

Left bronchus

Bronchiole

FIGURE 7-1 ▲ The anatomy of the respiratory system.

When we breathe in, the air entering the body from the atmosphere is rich in oxygen and contains little carbon dioxide. Carbon dioxide is the waste product we rid the body of when breathing. The oxygen-rich air enters the alveoli in the lungs and passes through the walls of capillaries into the bloodstream. Carbon dioxide passes from the blood through the capillary walls into the alveoli. It leaves the body in the air we breathe out (Figure 7-1).

Anatomy Review
The Nose and Nasal Cavity
Objective 1

The nose warms, humidifies, and filters the air before it enters the lungs. A wall of tissue called the **septum** separates the right and left nostrils. The nose is lined with a mucous membrane that is fragile. When the nose is subjected to trauma, it is prone to bleed and become inflamed, which can cause an airway obstruction. The nose is susceptible to trauma because of its location on the face. The nasal cavity is separated from the cranium by a thin bone that can become fractured as a result of head trauma.

The Mouth and Oral Cavity

The mouth and its structures serve many functions. The most important function is its ability to move fresh air in and out of the lungs. Air enters the body through the mouth or nose and passes down the pharynx (throat), past the epiglottis, down the trachea, and into the lungs. Air entering the mouth is not filtered or warmed as efficiently as air entering the nostrils.

The upper airway is the most common place for an airway obstruction to occur. When a patient becomes unresponsive, the tongue falls back into the posterior oropharynx (the back of the mouth). This can cause a complete airway obstruction. Other common causes of upper airway obstruction are dislodged teeth or dentures, blood, body secretions, and foreign objects. You must be able to recognize signs of an airway obstruction and act quickly to remove the object in order for the patient to survive.

The epiglottis is a piece of cartilage that protects the lower airway from **aspiration.** When we swallow, the epiglottis closes off the trachea and prevents food from entering it. Choking may result if the epiglottis fails to close, allowing food or liquids to enter the airway. Placing an unresponsive, uninjured patient on his side (recovery position) while suctioning out the airway will allow material to flow from the mouth by gravity and reduce the risk of aspiration.

The Larynx and Trachea

The larynx contains the vocal cords. This area is the narrowest part of an adult's airway. The vocal cords are responsible for sound production. An airway obstruction at or below this level will affect the ability to produce sound. The space between the vocal cords is called the glottis. The largest cartilage of the larynx is the thyroid cartilage, also called the Adam's apple. The cricoid cartilage is the most inferior (lowest) of the cartilages of the larynx. The narrowest part of a child's airway is at the level of the cricoid cartilage.

The next section of the windpipe is the trachea, which extends to the level of the upper and middle portion of the breastbone (sternum). The trachea is protected and supported by C-shaped rings of cartilage. This allows for some expansion during breathing and coughing. At about the middle of the breastbone, the trachea divides into two main branches. One branch, the right mainstem bronchus, allows air in and out of the right lung. The other, the left mainstem bronchus, allows air in and out of the left lung.

The Lungs

The lungs are very elastic and are made up of many tiny air sacs (alveoli). The lungs are divided into three separate lobes on the right and two lobes on the left. Even a tiny blockage in the lower airways can completely collapse a segment of the lung, making breathing much more difficult. This situation can also occur because of a penetrating injury to the lung, such as a stabbing or gunshot wound. If an opening occurs between the outside atmosphere and the lung, the lung will collapse and require emergency treatment.

The Diaphragm

Below the lungs is the diaphragm, a major muscle used for breathing. The dome-shaped diaphragm divides the chest cavity from the abdominal cavity.

The job of the lower airway is the exchange of oxygen and carbon dioxide. Lower airway problems usually take longer to develop than upper airway problems. Although the patient must be watched closely, lower airway problems are less likely to cause sudden changes in the patient's condition while you are providing care.

The Mechanics of Breathing
The Muscles of Breathing

The diaphragm is the primary muscle of breathing. It works in concert with the external intercostal muscles, which are located between the ribs. The external intercostal muscles assist with inhalation. The internal intercostal muscles and abdominal muscles may be used during forceful **exhalation.**

As the diaphragm moves down and in, the external intercostal muscles move the ribs up and out and the chest expands, increasing the volume of the chest cavity. The pressure within the lungs decreases to allow for inspiration. After inhalation, tiny air sacs (alveoli) are inflated while oxygen and carbon dioxide cross their membranes. Oxygen enters the circulation, while carbon dioxide enters the alveoli. Carbon dioxide is exhaled into the atmosphere as the diaphragm returns to its resting state, reducing the volume of chest cavity and pushing air from the lungs.

Respiratory Physiology
Alveolar/Capillary Exchange

Alveolar/capillary exchange is the exchange of gases in the lungs. Blood pumped from the right ventricle of the heart enters the pulmonary artery and eventually enters the lungs. The blood then flows through the lung capillaries that are close to the alveoli. The blood from the right heart is low in oxygen (oxygen-poor) and high in carbon dioxide. Oxygen is continuously used by the cells of the body. Carbon dioxide is a waste product of cellular work. Air entering the alveoli from the atmosphere during inspiration is rich in oxygen (oxygen-rich) and contains little carbon dioxide. Oxygen-rich air enters the alveoli and passes through the capillary walls into the bloodstream. Carbon dioxide passes from the blood through the capillary walls into the alveoli and leaves the body in exhaled air.

Capillary/Cellular Exchange

Capillary/cellular exchange is the exchange of gases in tissues. Oxygen-rich blood moves out of the tissue capillaries and into the tissue cells. Tissue cells use oxygen. Carbon dioxide, a waste product, is produced. Carbon dioxide moves from the tissue cells into the tissue capillaries and is transported in the bloodstream to the lungs for removal from the body.

Tidal Volume and Minute Volume

Tidal volume is the amount of air moved into or out of the lungs during a normal breath. Think of tidal volume as the depth of a patient's breathing. You can indirectly assess tidal volume by watching the rise and fall of the patient's chest and abdomen. The tidal volume of a healthy adult at rest is about 500 mL.

Minute volume is the amount of air moved in and out of the lungs in one minute. Minute volume is determined by multiplying the tidal volume by the respiratory rate. A change in either the tidal volume *or* respiratory rate will affect minute volume.

Infant and Child Anatomy

The airway of infants and young children differs from that of older children and adults. The epiglottis is large and floppy. The teeth are either absent or very delicate. Infants less than 6 months of age breathe primarily through the nose, not the mouth. Their airway is much smaller, allowing a greater opportunity for obstruction. One such obstruction is their tongue, which is large in size compared to the size of their mouth.

The trachea is softer and more flexible in infants and children. The supporting cartilage of a child's trachea is less developed than an adult's, making it prone to compression with improper neck positioning. Be sure to place an infant's head in a neutral position, which may require slight elevation of the infant's shoulders. This can be done by placing padding under the shoulders to compensate for the proportionately larger head.

The narrowest part of a child's airway is at the cricoid cartilage, which is lower in the airway than it is in an adult. A small change in airway size (because of conditions such as swelling or inflammation) can result in significant breathing problems. These differences allow for easier airway obstruction in an infant or child.

The chest wall of the infant and young child is flexible because it is composed of more cartilage than bone. Because of the flexibility of the ribs, children are more resistant to rib fractures than adults. The force of the injury, however, is easily transmitted to the lungs. Chest injury may result in bruising of the lungs (pulmonary contusion) or more serious injury.

Infants and children depend more heavily on the diaphragm for breathing. Gastric distention (swelling) is common in the ventilation of infants and children. If enough air builds up in the child's stomach to push on the lungs and diaphragm, effective breathing can be compromised. When assisting the breathing of an infant or child, avoid using too much volume. Use only enough volume to cause gentle chest rise.

Remember This!

The primary cause of cardiac arrest in infants and children is an uncorrected respiratory problem.

A is for Airway

You must perform a primary survey on *every* patient. The primary survey begins after the scene or situation has been found or made safe and you have gained access to the patient. The purpose of the primary survey is to find and care for immediate life-threatening problems.

As you approach the patient, you will first form a general impression of him to determine if he appears "sick" or "not sick." You will also determine the urgency of further assessment and care. Using your senses of sight and hearing (look and listen), quickly determine if the patient is ill (a medical patient) or injured (a trauma patient). Look at the patient and determine if he has a life-threatening problem. If a life-threatening condition is found, you must treat it immediately. Examples of life-threatening conditions include:

- Unresponsiveness
- An obstructed airway
- Absent breathing (respiratory arrest)
- Severe bleeding

After forming a general impression of your patient, you must assess the patient's level of responsiveness.

Begin by speaking to him. If the patient appears to be awake, tell the patient your first name and identify yourself as an EMT. Explain that you are there to help. You may ask, "Why did you call 9-1-1 today?" If the patient appears to be asleep, gently rub his shoulder and ask, "Are you OK?" or "Can you hear me?" Do not move the patient.

A patient who is alert and talking clearly or crying without difficulty has an open airway. If the patient is unable to speak, cry, cough, or make any other sound, his airway is completely obstructed. If the patient has noisy breathing, such as snoring or gurgling, he has a partial airway obstruction.

Remember This!

When resuscitating a patient, it is important to know the definitions of an infant, a child, and an adult:

- Infant: Less than one year of age
- Child: 1 to 12 to 14 years of age
- Adult: More than 12 to 14 years of age

Opening the Airway

A patient without an open airway has no chance of survival. If the airway is not open, there is no breathing. Without breathing, the patient's heart will stop beating unless you open the airway and begin breathing for him. Therefore, one of the most important actions that you can perform is to open the airway of an unresponsive patient. An unresponsive patient loses the ability to keep his own airway open because he loses muscle tone. This loss of muscle tone causes the soft tissues of the throat

and the base of the tongue to relax. If the patient is lying on his back, the tongue falls into the back of the throat, blocking the airway (Figure 7-2). Because the tongue is attached to the lower jaw, moving the jaw forward will lift the tongue away from the back of the throat.

Stop and Think!

Because the risk of exposure to blood, vomitus, or potentially infectious material is high, you must remember to take appropriate body substance isolation precautions when managing a patient's airway.

Opening the Mouth

The crossed-finger technique may be used to open the mouth of an *unresponsive* patient (Figure 7-3). To perform this technique:

- Kneel above and behind the patient.
- Cross the thumb and forefinger of one gloved hand.
- Place the thumb on the patient's lower front teeth and your forefinger on the upper front teeth.
- Use a scissors motion or finger-snapping motion to open the mouth.

Head Tilt–Chin Lift

The **head tilt–chin lift maneuver** is the most effective method for opening the airway in a patient with no known or suspected trauma to the head or neck. It requires no equipment and is simple to perform.

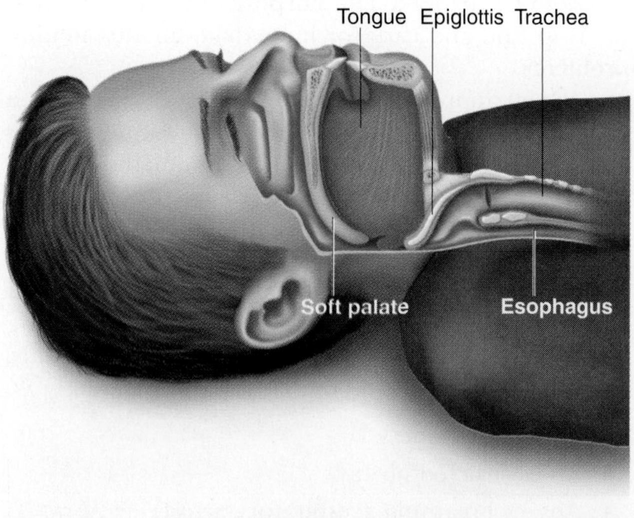

Tongue Epiglottis Trachea

Soft palate   Esophagus

FIGURE 7-2 ▲ An unresponsive patient loses the ability to keep his own airway open because he loses muscle tone. The tongue falls into the back of the throat, blocking the airway.

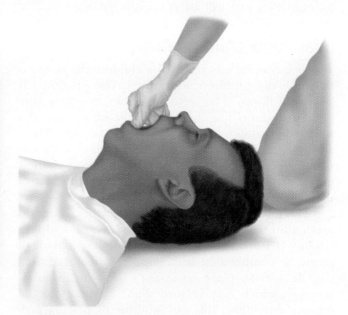

FIGURE 7-3 ▲ Opening the mouth by using the crossed-finger technique.

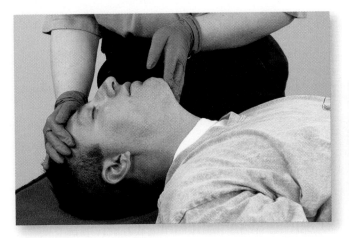

FIGURE 7-4 ▲ The head tilt–chin lift.

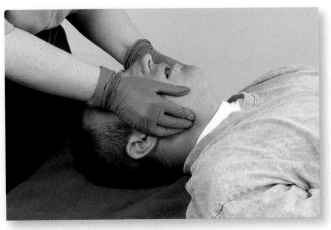

FIGURE 7-5 ▲ The jaw thrust without head tilt.

When done correctly, the base of the tongue will be displaced from blocking the back of the throat (Figure 7-4). Examples of patients who are likely to need the head tilt–chin lift maneuver include:

- An unresponsive patient with no known or suspected trauma to the head or neck
- A patient who is not breathing with no known or suspected trauma to the head or neck
- A patient who is not breathing and has no pulse (cardiac arrest) with no known or suspected trauma to the head or neck

Objective 4

Follow these steps to perform a head tilt–chin lift:

- Position the patient on his back.
- Place your hand closest to the patient's head on his forehead. Apply back pressure with your palm, gently tilting the patient's head backward.
- Place the fingers of your hand that is closest to the patient's feet under the bony part of his chin. Do not compress the soft tissues under the chin; doing so can result in an airway obstruction.
- Lift the chin forward and support the jaw.
- Make sure the patient's mouth is open. If the patient is wearing dentures and they fit well, leave them in place. If the dentures are loose or do not fit well, remove them.
- Look, listen, and feel for breathing.

Jaw Thrust Without Head Tilt

Objective 5

Use the **jaw thrust without head tilt maneuver** to open the airway of an unresponsive patient when trauma to the head or neck is suspected (Figure 7-5). The jaw thrust without head tilt maneuver is also called the *jaw thrust without head extension maneuver*. Although this method of opening the airway is effective, it is less effective than the head tilt–chin lift and is more tiring. Because this technique requires the use of both hands, a second rescuer will be needed if the patient requires ventilation. Examples of patients who are likely to need the jaw thrust without head tilt maneuver include:

- An unresponsive trauma patient
- An unresponsive patient with an unknown mechanism of injury

Objective 6

Follow these steps to perform a jaw thrust without head tilt:

- Position the patient on his back and kneel at the top of the patient's head.
- While keeping the patient's head and neck in line with the rest of his body, place your hands on each side of the patient's lower jaw. It may be helpful to rest your elbows on the surface on which the patient is lying.

You Should Know

The head tilt–chin lift and jaw thrust without head tilt maneuvers may cause some movement of the cervical spine when they are performed. Health-care professionals should use the jaw thrust without head tilt maneuver to open the airway of a trauma victim if cervical spine injury is suspected. However, "because maintaining a patent airway and providing adequate ventilation is a priority in CPR, use a head tilt–chin lift maneuver if the jaw thrust does not open the airway."

- Gently grasp the angles of the patient's lower jaw. Lift with both hands, gently moving the lower jaw forward. Make sure the patient's mouth is open. If the patient's lips close, gently pull back the lower lip with your gloved thumb.
- Look, listen, and feel for breathing.

Inspecting the Airway

After opening the airway, look in the mouth of every unresponsive patient and any responsive patient who cannot protect his airway. This can be done by opening the patient's mouth with your gloved hand. Look inside the patient's mouth for an actual or potential airway obstruction such as a foreign body, blood, vomitus, teeth, or the patient's tongue. If you see a foreign body in the patient's mouth, attempt to remove it with your gloved fingers. If there is blood, vomitus, or other fluid in the patient's airway, clear it with suctioning.

Clearing the Airway

There are three methods you can use to clear an unresponsive patient's airway: the recovery position, finger sweeps, and suctioning. The patient's situation will dictate which technique is most appropriate.

The Recovery Position

The recovery position involves positioning an uninjured patient on his side (Figure 7-6). There are several variations of the recovery position. The 2005 Resuscitation Guidelines note that no single position is perfect for all victims. In the recovery position, gravity allows fluid to flow from the mouth and helps keep the airway clear. Follow these steps to place a patient in the recovery position:

- Raise the patient's left arm above his head and then cross the patient's right leg over his left leg. (Use the opposite side if the patient has a contraindication to lying on one side.)
- While supporting the patient's face, grasp his right shoulder and roll him toward you onto his

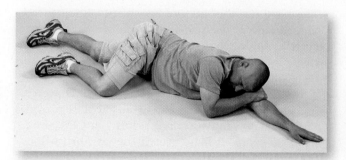

FIGURE 7-6 ▲ The recovery position.

left side. The patient's head should be in as close to a midline position as possible. The patient's head, torso, and shoulders should move at the same time without twisting.
- Place the patient's right hand under the side of his face.
- Continue to monitor the patient while he is in your care.

Remember This!

- Do *not* place a patient with a known or suspected spinal injury in the recovery position.
- There is a potential risk for nerve and vessel injury if the patient lies on one arm for a prolonged period in the recovery position. To avoid these types of injuries, it may be necessary to roll the patient to the other side.

Finger Sweeps

The removal of foreign material from the airway is critical for patient survival. You should use a finger sweep only when you can *see* solid material blocking the upper airway of an unresponsive patient. A finger sweep is *not* performed on responsive patients or on unresponsive patients who have a gag reflex.

Follow these steps to perform a finger sweep:

- If the patient is uninjured, roll him to his side.
- Wipe out liquids from the airway, using your index and middle fingers covered with a cloth.
- Remove solid objects, using your gloved index finger positioned like a hook. Use your little finger when performing a finger sweep in an infant or child.

Remember This!

A "blind" finger sweep is performed without first seeing foreign material in the airway. Blind finger sweeps should *never* be performed. Doing so may cause the object to become further lodged in the patient's throat.

Suctioning

Objectives 7, 8

Suctioning may be needed if the recovery position and performing finger sweeps are not effective in clearing the patient's airway. It may also be needed if trauma is suspected and the patient cannot be placed in the recovery position. **Suctioning** is a procedure used to vacuum vomitus, saliva, blood, food particles, and other material from the patient's airway. You should always have suction equipment available when you are managing a patient's airway or assisting a patient's breathing. Having the equipment available means having it within arm's reach. If you hear a gurgling sound as a patient breathes, he needs to be suctioned immediately.

Suction Units

Suctioning requires the use of a device that creates negative pressure. Suction units consist of tubing, a collection chamber, and a manual or electrical power source. Some suction units also have a regulator. Most suction units are inadequate for removing solid objects like teeth, foreign bodies, and food.

Mounted suction devices are mounted (built-in) on ambulance walls and are usually powered by the vehicle's battery (Figure 7-7). Mounted suction devices are also called *fixed suction units*. They provide a vacuum that is strong and adjustable. The parts of the suction unit that come in contact with body fluids are disposable. Disadvantages of mounted suction devices are that they are not portable and cannot be used with an alternative power source.

Battery-operated portable suction units are often used in Emergency Medical Services (EMS). They are lightweight and generally have good suction power (Figure 7-8). The suction unit must be checked daily to make sure it functions properly. Because most of these devices use rechargeable batteries, it is important that the suction unit be kept charged when not in use. Over time, rechargeable batteries will lose their ability to hold a charge and need to be replaced. In most battery-operated suction units, the parts that come in contact with body fluids are disposable. However, in others the parts are not disposable and must be cleaned after each use.

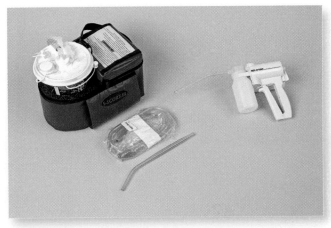

FIGURE 7-8 ▲ A battery-powered and manual (hand-powered) suction unit.

Hand-powered devices are lightweight, portable, and reliable (Figure 7-9). They are easy to use and relatively inexpensive. To create the vacuum necessary for suctioning, hand-powered units must be pumped or squeezed. This limits the length of time suctioning can be applied. The collection chamber of a hand-powered device is small. This limits the volume that can be suctioned.

Suction Catheters

Suction catheters may be rigid or soft. Rigid suction catheters are able to quickly suction large amounts of fluid (Figure 7-10). A rigid suction catheter is also called a *hard suction catheter*, a *Yankauer catheter*, a *tonsil tip catheter*, or a *tonsil sucker*. Use a rigid suction catheter to remove secretions from a patient's mouth.

Soft suction catheters are also called *flexible, whistletip,* or *French suction catheters* (Figure 7-11). These catheters are used to clear the mouth and throat and remove secretions from a tracheal tube in intubated

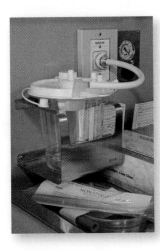

FIGURE 7-7 ◄ A mounted suction device is mounted (built-in) on the wall of an ambulance and is usually powered by the vehicle's battery.

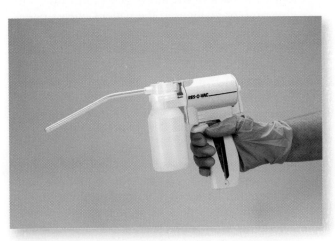

FIGURE 7-9 ▲ To create the vacuum necessary for suctioning, hand-powered units must be pumped or squeezed.

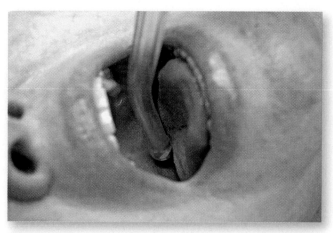

FIGURE 7-10 ▲ A rigid suction catheter can be used to remove secretions from a patient's mouth. This type of catheter should be inserted no deeper than to the base of the tongue.

patients. They are available in many sizes. The inside diameter of soft suction catheters is smaller than that of rigid catheters.

Suctioning Technique

Follow these steps to suction a patient's mouth:

- If possible, give the patient 100% oxygen for two to three minutes before suctioning.
- Turn on the suction unit and make sure it is working. If the unit is equipped with a pressure gauge, be sure it can generate a vacuum of 300 millimeters of mercury (mm Hg).
- Attach the suction catheter.
- *Without* applying suction, place the tip of the catheter in the patient's mouth. Gently advance the catheter tip along one side of the mouth. Insert the catheter tip only as far as you can see. Do not touch the back of the airway. This can cause vomiting and/or changes in the patient's heart rate.
- Apply suction while moving the tip of the catheter from side to side as you withdraw it from the patient's mouth. Because you are removing air (oxygen) from the patient when suctioning, do not suction an adult for more than 15 seconds at a time. When suctioning an infant or child, do not apply suction for more than 10 seconds at a time.
- If the patient has secretions or vomit that cannot be removed quickly and easily by suctioning, log roll him and clear the mouth manually. If the patient produces blood or secretions as rapidly as suctioning can remove, suction for 15 seconds, artificially ventilate for 2 minutes, then suction for 15 seconds, and continue in that manner. Consult medical direction when this situation occurs.

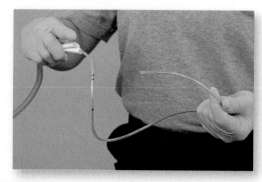

FIGURE 7-11 ▲ A soft suction catheter is used to clear the mouth and throat and remove secretions from a tracheal tube in an intubated patient.

- If necessary, rinse the catheter and tubing with water to prevent blockage of the tubing from dried or large (chunky) material.

Because suctioning can cause serious changes in your patient's heart rate, you must watch your patient closely when you perform this procedure. The patient's heart rate may slow or become irregular because of a lack of oxygen or stimulation by the catheter of the back of the tongue or throat. These changes in the heart rate can occur in any patient. However, they are particularly common in infants and children. If the patient's heart rate slows, stop suctioning and provide ventilation with oxygenation.

Keeping the Airway Open: Airway Adjuncts

Airway adjuncts are devices used to help keep a patient's airway open. When using an airway adjunct, you must first open the patient's airway by using one of the techniques already described. You should then insert the airway adjunct and maintain the proper head position while the device is in place.

Remember This!

The use of an airway adjunct does not eliminate the need for maintaining proper head positioning.

Oral Airway

An oral airway is a curved device made of rigid plastic. An oral airway is also called an *oropharyngeal airway (OPA)*. An OPA is inserted into the patient's mouth and used to keep the tongue away from the back of the throat. It may only be used in unresponsive patients without a gag reflex.

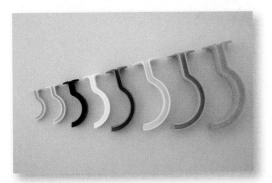

FIGURE 7-12 ▲ Oral airways are available in a variety of sizes.

Objective 17

OPAs are available in a variety of sizes (Figure 7-12). Before inserting an OPA, you must determine the correct size for your patient. To select the correct size, hold the OPA against the side of the patient's face. Select an OPA that extends from the corner of the patient's mouth to the tip of the earlobe, or from the center of the patient's mouth to the angle of the jaw. If you select an OPA of the wrong size, you can cause an airway obstruction. An OPA that is too long can press the epiglottis against the entrance of the larynx, resulting in a complete airway obstruction (Figure 7-13). An OPA that is too short may come out of the mouth or it may push the tongue into the back of the throat, causing an airway obstruction (Figure 7-14).

Skill Drill 7-1 shows the steps for sizing and inserting an oral airway.

Special Considerations

An oral airway should not be used in a patient who has a gag reflex. If you try to use an OPA in a patient with a gag reflex, he may vomit and aspirate the vomitus

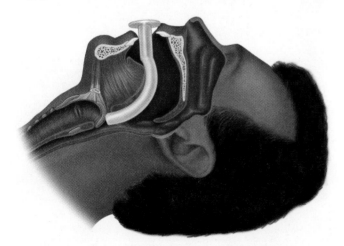

FIGURE 7-13 ▲ An oral airway that is too long can press the epiglottis against the entrance of the larynx, resulting in a complete airway obstruction.

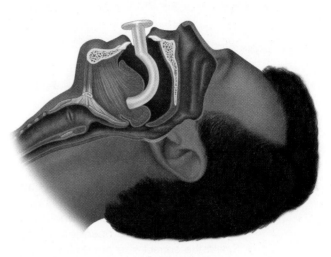

FIGURE 7-14 ▲ An oral airway that is too short may come out of the mouth or it may push the tongue into the back of the throat, causing an airway obstruction.

into his lungs. Use of an oral airway does not eliminate the need for maintaining proper head position.

Nasal Airway

Objective 18

A **nasal airway** is a soft, rubbery tube with a hole in it that is placed in the patient's nose (Figure 7-15). A nasal airway is also called a *nasopharyngeal airway* (NPA) or *trumpet airway*. The NPA allows air to flow from the hole in the NPA down into the lower airway. To select an NPA of proper size, hold the NPA against the side of the patient's face. Select an airway that extends from the tip of the patient's nose to his earlobe. When an NPA of the proper size is correctly positioned, the tip rests in the back of the throat. This positioning helps to keep the tongue from blocking the upper airway (Figure 7-16). It can be placed in either nostril to help maintain an open airway. Remember that the bevel of the NPA needs to be kept against the nasal septum.

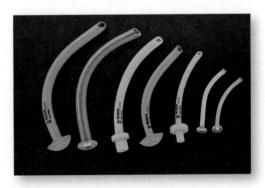

FIGURE 7-15 ▲ Nasal airways are available in different sizes.

A is for *Airway* ◀ **157**

Sizing and Inserting an Oral Airway

STEP 1 ▶ Use Steps 1-4 to insert an oral airway in an unresponsive adult.
- Place the patient on his back. Position yourself at the patient's head.
- Open the patient's airway with a head tilt–chin lift maneuver. If trauma is suspected, use the jaw thrust without the head tilt maneuver to open the airway.
- Select the correct size oral airway. An oral airway is the correct size if it extends from the corner of the patient's mouth to the tip of the earlobe, or from the center of the mouth to the angle of the jaw.

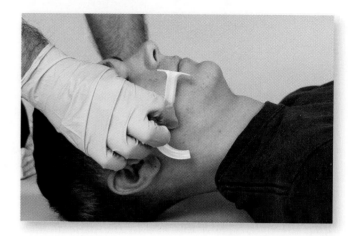

STEP 2 ▶
- Open the patient's mouth. Suction any secretions from the mouth, if present.
- Insert the airway upside down, with the tip pointing toward the roof of the patient's mouth. Advance the oral airway gently along the roof of the mouth.

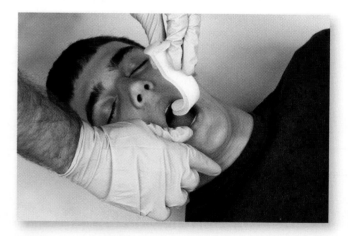

STEP 3 ▶ When the tip of the airway approaches the back of the throat, rotate the airway 180 degrees so that it is positioned over the tongue. Be careful not to push the tongue into the back of the throat.

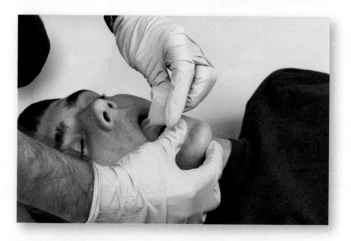

STEP 4 ▶ • When the oral airway is correctly positioned, the flange end should rest on the patient's lips or teeth. Remove the device *immediately* if the patient begins gagging as you slide it between the tongue and the back of the throat.
• Ventilate the patient.

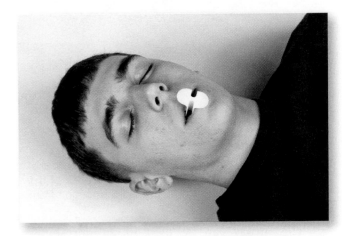

STEP 5 ▶ Use the following steps to insert an oral airway in an unresponsive infant or child:
• Place the patient on his back. Position yourself at the patient's head.
• Open the patient's airway.
• Select the correct size oral airway.
• Open the patient's mouth. Suction any secretions from the patient's mouth, if present.
• Use a tongue blade to press the tongue down.
• Insert the oral airway with the tip following the base of the tongue.
• Advance the device until the flange rests on the patient's lips or teeth.
• Remove the oral airway *immediately* if the patient begins gagging as you slide it between the tongue and the back of the throat.
• Ventilate the patient.

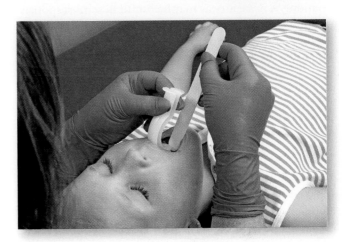

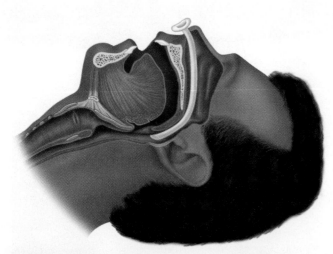

FIGURE 7-16 ▲ When a nasal airway of the proper size is correctly positioned, the tip rests in the back of the throat. This positioning helps to keep the tongue from blocking the upper airway.

This airway can be used in an unresponsive patient. A nasal airway may be useful in semi-responsive patients who have a gag reflex. Situations in which a semi-responsive patient may need this type of airway include the following:

- Intoxication
- Drug overdose
- Stroke
- After a seizure
- Low blood sugar

Skill Drill 7-2 shows the steps for sizing and inserting a nasal airway.

Special Considerations

Use of a nasal airway does not eliminate the need for maintaining proper head position. If the airway cannot be inserted into one nostril, try the other nostril. A nasal airway should be inserted gently into the nose along the "floor" of the nasal cavity. Do not try to insert the nasal airway up the nose along the "roof" of the nasal cavity.

Forceful insertion of an NPA may cause cuts or tears of the delicate mucous membranes of the nose. In some cases this can result in significant bleeding that may not be controlled by direct pressure.

If the nasal airway is too long, it may enter the esophagus. This can cause gastric distention and inadequate ventilation. A nasal airway does not prevent aspiration. This means that although a nasal airway may be properly positioned, it is still possible for blood, vomitus, or other secretions to enter the patient's lungs if they are not quickly removed with suctioning.

A nasal airway should not be used in situations involving trauma to the middle of the face or if a skull fracture is suspected (blood or clear fluid coming

from the nose or ears). Check your local protocols in these situations.

B is for *Breathing*

Is the Patient Breathing?

After making sure that the patient's airway is open, check for breathing. **Breathing** is the mechanical process of moving air into and out of the lungs. Normal breathing is quiet, painless, and occurs at a regular rate. Both sides of the chest rise and fall equally. Normal breathing does not require excessive use of the muscles between the ribs, above the collarbones, or in the abdomen during inhalation or exhalation. These muscles are called **accessory muscles** for breathing. Breathing assessment is described in more detail in Chapter 9.

Is Breathing Adequate or Inadequate?

Objective 2

If the patient is breathing, quickly determine if breathing is adequate or inadequate. To do this, you need to be able to see the rise and fall of the patient's chest and abdomen. If the patient has on many layers of clothing or bulky clothing, such as a jacket or coat, you will need to uncover him enough to watch him as he breathes.

A patient who is breathing adequately:

- Does not appear to be in distress
- Speaks in full sentences without pausing to catch his breath
- Breathes at a regular rate and within normal limits for his age
- Has an equal rise and fall of the chest with each breath
- Has an adequate depth of breathing (tidal volume)
- Has normal skin color

A patient who is having difficulty breathing is working hard (laboring) to breathe. He may be gasping for air. You may see him use the muscles in his neck to assist with inhalation. He may use his abdominal muscles and the muscles between the ribs to assist with exhalation. You may see **retractions** (a "sinking in") of the soft tissues between and around the ribs or above the collarbones.

A patient who is having difficulty breathing often naturally assumes a position to improve his breathing. For example, the patient may instinctively avoid lying down if he feels as if he is suffocating or if it is harder to breathe when he does so. If the increase in difficulty breathing occurs slowly over a period of days or weeks, the patient may increase the number of pillows he uses at night in order to breathe more easily. As

Sizing and Inserting a Nasal Airway

STEP 1 ▶ • Place the patient on his back. Position yourself at the patient's head.
• Open the patient's airway.
• Choose the proper size nasal airway. To select an airway adjunct of proper size, hold the nasal airway against the side of the patient's face. Select an airway that extends from the tip of the patient's nose to his ear lobe.

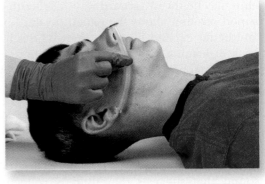

STEP 2 ▶ Lubricate the outside of the nasal airway with a water-soluble lubricant, if available.

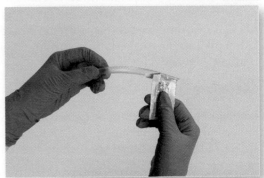

STEP 3 ▶ • Gently push the tip of the patient's nose back slightly.
• Gently insert the nasal airway with the bevel pointing toward the nasal septum. During insertion, do not direct the airway upward. Do not force the device into position. Serious bleeding that is hard to control can result.

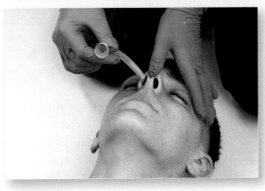

STEP 4 ▶ • Stop advancing the nasal airway when the bevel of the device is flush against the opening of the nostril.
• Assess placement by feeling for air coming from the device.

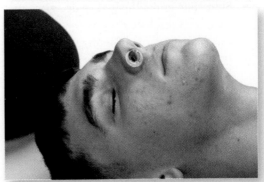

breathing becomes more difficult, a patient may prefer to sit and sleep in a chair, such as a recliner. When breathing is particularly difficult, the patient may prefer to sit up and lean forward, with the weight of his upper body supported by his hands on his thighs or knees. This is called the **tripod position.** The patient's chin may be thrust forward with his mouth open. The tripod position allows the patient to draw in more air and better expand his lungs than if he is lying on his back or leaning back in a sitting position.

Normal breathing is quiet. Noisy breathing is usually abnormal breathing and a sign that the patient is in distress. Stridor is a harsh, high pitched sound that suggests the upper airway is partially blocked. It is usually heard during inhalation. The sound of snoring suggests the upper airway is partially blocked by the tongue or soft tissue of the palate. Gurgling is a wet sound that suggests that fluid is collecting in the patient's upper airway. Wheezing is a high- or low-pitched whistling sound that is usually heard on exhalation. Wheezing suggests that the lower airways are partially blocked with fluid or mucus.

Objective 3

Inadequate breathing must be treated aggressively before it becomes absent breathing (respiratory arrest). The signs of inadequate breathing include the following:

- Anxious appearance, concentration on breathing
- Confusion, restlessness
- A breathing rate that is too fast or slow for the patient's age
- An irregular breathing pattern
- A depth of breathing that is unusually deep or shallow
- Noisy breathing (stridor, snoring, gurgling, wheezing)
- Sitting upright and leaning forward to breathe
- Being unable to speak in complete sentences
- Pain with breathing
- Skin that looks flushed, pale, gray, or blue; skin that feels cold or sweaty
- Physical signs of difficulty in breathing (such as retractions, flared nostrils, or pursed lips)

If your patient is awake but appears to have trouble breathing, ask," Can you speak?" "Are you choking?"

You Should Know

When assessing your patient, look to see if he is breathing through pursed (sometimes called puckered) lips. Pursed lip breathing may be seen in patients who have a history of long-term respiratory illnesses, such as emphysema.

You Should Know

Many factors affect a person's rate of breathing. For example, breathing slows during sleep. The rate of breathing increases with fever, pain, and emotions. Drugs may increase or decrease a person's breathing rate depending on the actions of the drug.

If he is able to speak or make noise, air is moving past his vocal cords. If he is unresponsive, open his airway. Place your ear close to the patient's mouth and nose. Look, listen, and feel for breathing:

- Look for a rise and fall of the chest
- Listen for air escaping during exhalation
- Feel for air coming from the mouth or nose

If a complete airway obstruction is present, you may initially see a rise and fall of the chest but you will not hear or feel air movement. If the patient's heart stops, you may see irregular, gasping breaths (agonal respirations) just after this occurs. Do not confuse gasping respirations with adequate breathing.

You Should Know

Breathing-related problems are the most common medical emergencies encountered in children.

Respiratory Distress, Respiratory Failure, and Respiratory Arrest

A patient who is showing signs of respiratory distress will often progress to respiratory failure if you do not work quickly to relieve his symptoms. **Respiratory distress** is increased work of breathing (respiratory effort). A patient who has signs and symptoms of inadequate breathing must be considered to be experiencing respiratory distress. In **respiratory failure,** there is inadequate blood oxygenation and/or ventilation to meet the demands of body tissues. A patient in respiratory failure looks very sick and often very tired. Signs of greatly increased work of breathing are usually present. The patient's skin may appear pale, mottled, or blue. If respiratory failure is not corrected, it will usually progress to **respiratory arrest,** which is an absence of breathing. If not corrected, respiratory arrest will, in turn, rapidly lead to cardiac arrest. **Agonal breathing** is slow and shallow breathing that is sometimes seen just before the onset of respiratory arrest. Other signs and symptoms of respiratory arrest include the following:

- Unresponsiveness
- No air movement from the mouth or nose
- No chest rise and fall
- Changes in skin color caused by a lack of oxygen

- The best way to learn how to assess a patient's normal work of breathing is to watch a person without medical problems breathing while he or she is asleep. This is a good baseline to see comfortable breathing without signs of respiratory distress. It is also a good picture to recall when you have to artificially ventilate a patient.

- Think of respiratory distress, failure, and arrest as increasing levels of severity of a respiratory problem. If you do not move quickly to resolve it, the respiratory problem will also become a cardiac problem.

How to Ventilate

If your patient's breathing is inadequate or absent, you will need to begin breathing for him immediately. When a patient is not breathing, he has only the oxygen-rich blood remaining in his lungs and bloodstream to survive on. You can assist breathing by forcing air into the patient's lungs. This action is called **positive-pressure ventilation.** Mouth-to-mask ventilation, mouth-to-barrier ventilation, mouth-to-mouth ventilation, and bag-mask ventilation are methods used to deliver positive-pressure ventilation.

Applying Cricoid Pressure

If positive-pressure ventilation is performed too rapidly or with too much volume, air can enter the stomach. The cricoid cartilage is the lowermost cartilage of the larynx. It is the only complete ring of cartilage in the larynx (Figure 7-17). When pressure is applied to the cricoid cartilage, the trachea is pushed back-

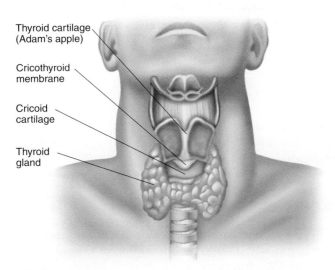

Thyroid cartilage (Adam's apple)

Cricothyroid membrane

Cricoid cartilage

Thyroid gland

FIGURE 7-17 ▲ The cricoid cartilage is the lowermost cartilage of the larynx.

ward and the esophagus is compressed (closed) against the cervical vertebrae. This compression helps decrease the amount of air entering the stomach during positive-pressure ventilation, which reduces the likelihood of vomiting and aspiration. **Cricoid pressure** (also called the *Sellick maneuver*) should be used only in unresponsive patients. It is usually applied by a third person during positive-pressure ventilation. The earlier cricoid pressure is applied, the less likely air will enter the stomach during ventilations. Be sure to release cricoid pressure if the patient begins to vomit.

Follow these steps to apply cricoid pressure (Figure 7-18):

- Using your index finger, locate the patient's Adam's apple on the front of his neck. Slowly move your finger downward until you feel a depression. Just below this depression is a firm ring of cartilage. This is the cricoid cartilage.

- Make sure the cricoid cartilage is between your thumb and index finger and apply firm pressure. Pressure is applied in a downward direction (toward the patient's back). The cricoid cartilage should remain in the midline position; it should not move to either side.

- Maintain pressure until the patient begins breathing on his own; a tube has been inserted in the patient's trachea by appropriately trained personnel; or the patient becomes responsive as evidenced by moving, coughing, or gagging.

You Should Know

- The cricoid cartilage may be difficult to find in women, obese patients, and patients with thick necks.

- Applying too much pressure on the cricoid cartilage can cause an airway obstruction.

Mouth-to-Mask Ventilation

The piece of equipment used for mouth-to-mask ventilation is the **pocket mask,** also called *pocket face mask, ventilation face mask,* or *resuscitation mask.* The mask provides a physical barrier between you and the patient's nose, mouth, and secretions. The mask used should have a one-way valve, which directs the patient's exhaled breath away from you (Figure 7-19). This helps prevent exposure to infectious disease. The mask should also have a disposable, High-Efficiency Particulate Air (HEPA) filter. A HEPA filter snaps inside the mask and is used to trap respiratory particles from patients with diseases such as tuberculosis. All masks should be transparent so that vomiting can

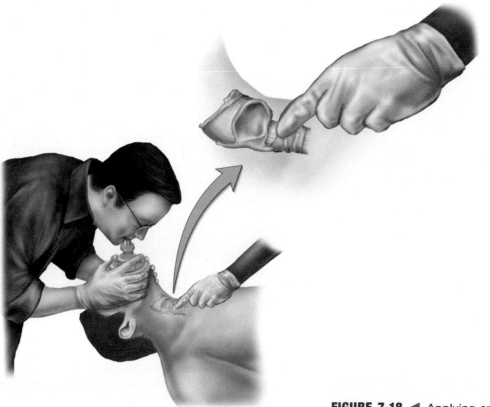

FIGURE 7-18 ◄ Applying cricoid pressure.

be seen and suctioned from the airway. Some pocket masks have an oxygen inlet on the mask that allows oxygen delivery. If oxygen is available, connect the mask to oxygen at 15 liters per minute (L/min).

Mouth-to-mask ventilation is very effective because you can use two hands to hold the mask in place on the patient's face and maintain proper head positioning at the same time. It also allows you to get a better face-to-mask seal, reducing the likelihood that air will leak from the mask. With a pocket mask you can also adjust the volume of air to meet the patient's needs.

You can do this by increasing or decreasing your own breath. When ventilating the patient through the mask, watch the rise and fall of his chest to determine if you need to adjust the volume of your breath. Rates for positive-pressure ventilation are shown in Table 7-1.

Objective 9

Skill Drill 7-3 shows the steps for mouth-to-mask ventilation.

Making a Difference

Use the following guidelines when providing mouth-to-mask ventilation:

- Position the narrow portion of the mask over the bridge of the patient's nose. The wide portion of the mask should rest in the groove between the patient's lower lip and chin.
- You are providing adequate ventilation if you see the patient's chest gently rise and fall with each breath.

Remember This!

The position of the mask is critical. If the mask is too large, turn it upside down and place the patient's nose in the chin piece of the mask.

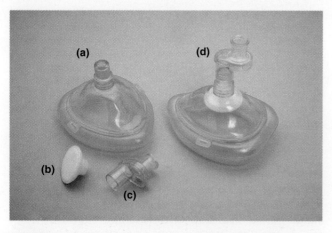

FIGURE 7-19 ▲ A pocket face mask. (a) The mask. (b) HEPA filter. (c) One-way valve. (d) Pocket face mask assembled with mask, HEPA filter, and one-way valve.

Mouth-to-Mask Ventilation

STEP 1 ▶
- Connect a one-way valve to the mask. Place the patient on his back. Open his airway with a head tilt–chin lift maneuver. If trauma is suspected, use the jaw thrust without head tilt to open the airway.
- Position yourself at the top of the patient's head. Lower the mask over the patient's nose and mouth. Create a face-to-mask seal by forming a "C" around the ventilation port with your thumb and index finger. Place the third, fourth, and fifth fingers of the same hand along the bony portion of the lower jaw. (These fingers form an "E".) Lift up slightly on the jaw with these fingers.

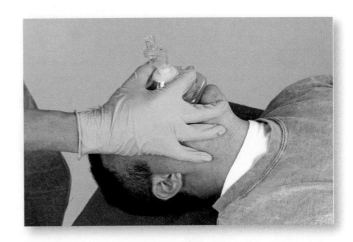

STEP 2 ▶
- Take a deep breath and place your mouth around the one-way valve. Exhale slowly with just enough volume to make the chest rise. Deliver each breath over one second. (See Table 7-1.)
- Watch for the rise and fall of the patient's chest with each ventilation. Stop ventilation when adequate chest rise is observed. Remove your mouth from the one-way valve and allow the patient to exhale between breaths.
- If air does not go in or the chest does not rise, reposition the patient's head. Reapply the mask to the patient's face and try again to ventilate. If the air still does not go in, suspect an airway obstruction.
- Ventilate once every three to five seconds for an infant or child and once every five to six seconds for an adult.

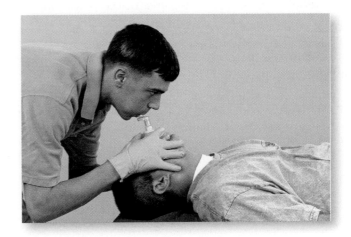

TABLE 7-1 Rates for Positive-Pressure Ventilation

Patient	Breaths/Minute	Length of Each Breath
Adult	10 to 12 (1 breath every 5 to 6 seconds)	1 second
Infant/Child	12 to 20 (1 breath every 3 to 5 seconds)	1 second
Newborn	40 to 60 (1 breath every 1 to 1.5 seconds)	1 second

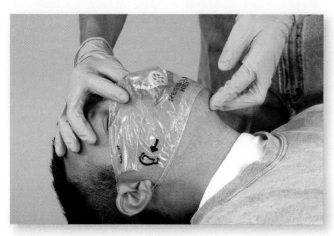

FIGURE 7-20 ▲ Mouth-to–barrier device ventilation.

Mouth-to–Barrier Device Ventilation

A **barrier device** is a thin film of plastic or silicone that is placed on the patient's face. It is used to prevent direct contact with the patient's mouth during positive ventilation (Figure 7-20). Face shields, a type of barrier device, are compact awernd portable. Some face shields are equipped with a short tube (1-2 inches) that is inserted in the patient's mouth. Use a barrier device if a pocket mask is not available.

You Should Know

Air leaks are common when a barrier device is used.

Although their features vary, most barrier devices have a one-way valve or filter in the center of the face shield. This allows the patient's exhaled air to escape between the shield and the patient's face when you lift your mouth off the shield between breaths.

Objective 16

Follow these steps for mouth-to-barrier device ventilation:

- Place the patient on his back. Open his airway with a head tilt–chin lift maneuver. If trauma is suspected, use the jaw thrust without head tilt to open the airway.
- Position yourself at the patient's head. Place the barrier device over the patient's mouth and nose. The opening at the center of the device should be placed over the patient's mouth. If a tube is present on the device, insert the tube in the patient's mouth over the tongue.
- Gently close the patient's nostrils with your thumb and index finger. Take a normal breath and place your mouth over the mouthpiece on the barrier device. Give a breath over one second, with just enough volume to make the chest gently rise.
- Watch for the rise and fall of the patient's chest with each ventilation. Stop ventilation when an adequate chest rise is observed. Too large a volume of air or a breath given too fast will cause the air to enter the stomach. Remove your mouth from the one-way valve and allow the patient to exhale between breaths. Continue ventilation at the proper rate.
- If the patient's chest does not rise, ventilation is not effective. In this case, the airway is obstructed or more volume or pressure is needed to provide effective ventilation. Readjust the position of the patient's head, make sure the mouth is open, and try again to ventilate. If the chest still does not rise, suspect an airway obstruction.

Mouth-to-Mouth Ventilation

Mouth-to-mouth ventilation is the delivery of your exhaled air to a patient while making mouth-to-mouth contact. Room air contains 21% oxygen. Your exhaled air contains 16% to 17% oxygen, which is enough oxygen to support life. Mouth-to-mouth ventilation is a quick and effective method of delivering oxygen to a nonbreathing patient. Should you choose to ventilate a patient by using the mouth-to-mouth technique, you must be aware of the risks. The most significant risk is being exposed to the patient's body fluids, including blood, vomit, and exhaled air.

The decision to perform mouth-to-mouth ventilation is not recommended but will be your personal choice. Whenever possible, you should use a barrier device or a pocket mask.

Follow these steps for mouth-to-mouth ventilation:

- Place the patient on his back. Position yourself at the patient's head. Open his airway with a head tilt–chin lift maneuver. If trauma is suspected, use the jaw thrust without head tilt to open the airway.
- If the patient is an adult or child, gently close the patient's nostrils with your thumb and index finger. Take a deep breath and place your mouth over the patient's mouth, creating an airtight seal. If the patient is an infant, place your mouth over the infant's mouth and nose.
- Give a breath over one second with enough volume to make the chest gently rise.
- Remove your mouth and release the patient's nose to allow the patient to exhale.
- Ventilation is adequate if there is adequate rise and fall of the chest and escaping air is heard or felt during exhalation. Continue ventilation at the proper rate.
- If the chest does not rise, either the airway is obstructed or more volume or pressure is needed to provide effective ventilation. Readjust the position of the patient's head, make sure the patient's mouth is open, and try again to ventilate. If the chest still does not rise, suspect an airway obstruction.

Bag-Mask Ventilation

Bag-Mask Features

Objective 11

A **bag-mask (BM) device** is a self-inflating bag with a one-way valve and an oxygen reservoir. The one-way valve on the BM prevents the patient's exhaled air from reentering the bag. The reservoir is an oxygen collector, allowing the delivery of a higher concentration of oxygen to the patient. A see-through mask with an air-filled cuff is attached to the bag (Figure 7-21). The see-through mask allows you to notice blood, vomit, or other secretions in the patient's mouth. The mask on most BMs has an inflatable cushion. A syringe is used to increase or decrease the amount of air in the cushion. Adjusting the amount of air in the cushion is important. Too much air in the cushion will not allow a tight seal between the patient's face and the mask. Inflate the cushion with

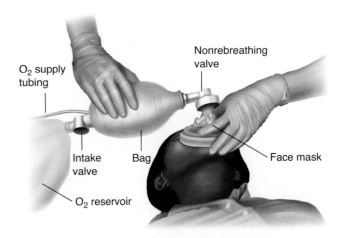

FIGURE 7-21 ▲ The components of a bag-mask (BM) device.

air so that it is flexible enough to make a tight seal over the patient's mouth and nose. This will limit the amount of room air that enters or oxygen that escapes from the mask.

You Should Know

A BM device is also called a *bag-mask device*.

It is important to select a mask of the proper size. A properly sized mask extends from the bridge of the patient's nose to the groove between his lower lip and chin. If a mask of the proper size is not used, air will leak from between the mask and the patient's face. This will result in less oxygen being delivered to the patient.

BM devices are available in adult, child, and infant sizes. Most adult BM devices can hold a volume of about 1600 mL. When connected to oxygen, the reservoir collects a volume of 100% oxygen equal to the capacity of the bag. When the bag is squeezed, oxygen is delivered to the patient. When pressure on the bag is released, it expands and refills with oxygen. Most BM devices used in the field today are disposable and come equipped with a built-in oxygen reservoir.

A BM device that is used during a cardiac arrest should not have a pop-off (pressure-release) valve or, if a pop-off valve is present, it should be one that can be manually disabled during resuscitation. To disable a pop-off valve, depress the valve with a finger during ventilation or twist the pop-off valve into the closed position. Failure to disable a pop-off valve may result in inadequate artificial ventilation.

Ventilating with a Bag-Mask

Ventilation performed with a BM device is often referred to as *bagging*. Although BM ventilation can be done using one person, it is best performed with two rescuers. It is not easy for one person to maintain the proper position of the patient's head, make sure the mask is sealed tightly on the patient's face, and compress the bag at the same time. When two people are available, one takes responsibility for compressing the bag. The other is responsible for maintaining the patient's head in the proper position and making sure the mask is sealed tightly on the patient's face.

One of the advantages of ventilating a patient with a BM device is the ability to feel the compliance of the patient's lungs. **Compliance** refers to the ability of the patient's lung tissue to distend (inflate) with ventilation. A patient who has healthy lungs requires relatively little pressure with the BM device (or other device used to deliver positive-pressure ventilation) to inflate the lungs. However, some diseases and injuries can cause changes in the patient's lung compliance. When delivering positive-pressure ventilation, it is important to notice if there is a change in the ease with which you can ventilate the patient. For example, if it was initially easy to ventilate a patient with a BM device but you now notice that it is becoming increasingly difficult to ventilate him, the patient's condition is changing. You will need to reassess him and search for the cause of this change.

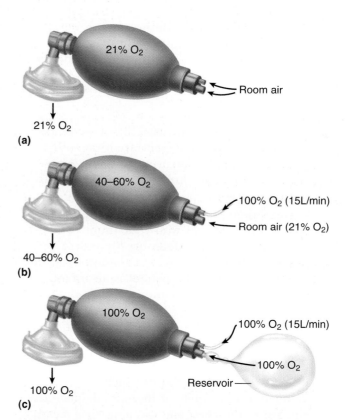

FIGURE 7-22 ▲ **(a)** A bag-mask device without supplemental oxygen will deliver 21% oxygen (room air) to the patient. **(b)** A bag-mask device used with supplemental oxygen at a flow rate of 15 L/min will deliver about 40-60% oxygen to the patient, provided there is a good face-to-mask seal. **(c)** A reservoir (an oxygen-collecting device) is attached to this bag-mask device. The reservoir collects a volume of 100% oxygen equal to the capacity of the bag. When the bag refills, 100% oxygen is drawn into the bag from the reservoir. With the oxygen flow rate set at 15 L/min, a bag-mask can deliver about 90-100% oxygen to the patient, provided there is a good face-to-mask seal.

You Should Know

Compliance refers to the distensibility (ability to inflate) of the lungs as measured by the resistance it creates to ventilation.

Although a BM device can be used to assist ventilations in a patient with inadequate breathing, it is more commonly used to ventilate a nonbreathing patient. When a BM device is not connected to supplemental oxygen, 21% oxygen (room air) is delivered to the patient (Figure 7-22a). If a BM device is connected to supplemental oxygen set at a flow rate of 15 L/min but no reservoir is used, about 40-60% oxygen can be delivered to the patient, provided there is a good face-to-mask seal (Figure 7-22b). If the BM device is connected to supplemental oxygen at a flow rate of 15 L/min and a reservoir is present on the bag, about 90-100% oxygen can be delivered to the patient, provided there is a good face-to-mask seal (Figure 7-22c).

Making a Difference

Assisting the Ventilations of a Spontaneously Breathing Patient

There are times that you will need to assist the breathing of a patient who is breathing on his own but whose breathing is too slow or shallow to be effective. For example, a patient who took a drug overdose and now is breathing shallowly at 4 times/minute needs assisted ventilation.

Assisting a patient's breathing requires patience and practice. If the patient is awake, be sure to explain what you are going to do. For instance, "Mrs. __, I'm going to use this special bag and mask to help you breathe." Connect supplemental oxygen to the BM device. Because a patient who is having difficulty breathing may feel smothered when a mask is applied, begin by holding the mask near the patient's face. While explaining what you are doing, squeeze the bag a couple of times so the patient can feel the air escape from the bag. Then apply the mask to the patient's face. Match squeezing the bag with the patient's inspiration. As the patient starts to breathe in, gently squeeze the bag. Stop squeezing as the chest starts to rise. If the patient's breathing rate is too slow, insert artificial breaths between the patient's own breaths.

Objectives 10, 12

Follow these steps if you are by yourself and are using a BM device to ventilate a patient who is not breathing:

- Connect the bag to the mask.
- Place the patient on his back. Open his airway with a head tilt–chin lift maneuver. If trauma is suspected, use the jaw thrust without head tilt to open the airway. Size and insert an oral or nasal airway.
- Position the narrow portion of the mask over the bridge of the patient's nose. Position the wide portion of the mask between the patient's lower lip and chin. Lower the mask over the patient's nose and mouth.
- Create a face-to-mask seal by forming a "C" around the ventilation port with your thumb and index finger. Place the third, fourth, and fifth fingers of the same hand along the bony portion of the lower jaw, avoiding the soft tissue area. (These fingers form an "E"). If no injury to the head or spine is suspected, lift up slightly on the jaw with these fingers, bringing the patiensst's jaw up to the mask as you tilt the patient's head backward. If injury to the head or

spine is suspected, do *not* tilt the patient's head backward. Instead, bring the patient's jaw up to the mask without moving the head or neck.

- With your other hand, squeeze the bag until you see a gentle chest rise (Figure 7-23a). Deliver each ventilation over one second. Watch for gentle rise and fall of the patient's chest with each ventilation. Stop ventilation when you see adequate chest rise. Allow the patient to exhale between breaths.
- Ventilate at an age-appropriate rate: once every three to five seconds for an infant or child and once every five to six seconds for an adult.
- If oxygen is available, connect the bag to oxygen at a flow rate of 15 L/min and attach the reservoir.

Remember This!

You can deliver a greater tidal volume with a pocket mask than with a BM device. There are two reasons for this. First, you can use both hands to hold a pocket mask securely in place and keep the patient's head in proper position at the same time. Second, you can adjust the depth of your breaths to make up for any leaks between the mask and the patient's face. This allows greater lung ventilation.

Follow these steps if two rescuers are present and are using a BM device:

- Connect the bag to the mask.
- Place the patient on his back. Open his airway with a head tilt–chin lift maneuver. If trauma is suspected, use the jaw thrust without head tilt to open the airway. Size and insert an oropharyngeal or nasopharyngeal airway.
- Position the narrow portion of the mask over the bridge of the patient's nose. Position the

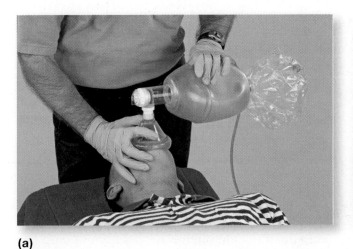

(a)

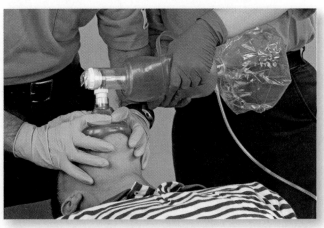

(b)

FIGURE 7-23 ▲ Bag-mask device ventilation. **(a)** One-person technique. **(b)** Two-person technique.

wide portion of the mask between the patient's lower lip and chin. Lower the mask over the patient's nose and mouth.

- Create a face-to-mask seal by forming a "C" around the ventilation port with your thumb and index finger. Place the third, fourth, and fifth fingers of the same hand along the bony portion of the lower jaw, avoiding the soft tissue area. (These fingers form an "E"). Lift up slightly on the jaw with these fingers, bringing the patient's jaw up to the mask.
- Have an assistant squeeze the bag with two hands until you see gentle chest rise (Figure 7-23b). Deliver each ventilation over one second. Watch for the rise and fall of the patient's chest with each ventilation. Stop ventilation when you see adequate chest rise. Allow the patient to exhale between breaths.
- Ventilate once every three to five seconds for an infant or child and once every five to six seconds for an adult.
- If oxygen is available, connect the bag to oxygen at a flow rate of 15 L/min and attach the reservoir.

Making a Difference

The ability to provide positive-pressure ventilation is a very important EMT skill. You must practice this skill in order to do it effectively. During your initial training program and in later continuing education classes, take advantage of all opportunities to practice this important skill.

Adequate and Inadequate Artificial Ventilation

Objective 13

Artificial ventilation (also called *rescue breathing*) is adequate when:

- The chest rises and falls with each artificial ventilation
- The rate of ventilations is sufficient. Sufficient rates are:
  - About 10-12 times per minute for adults (once every five to six seconds)
  - About 12-20 times per minute for infants and children (once every three to five seconds)
- The patient's heart rate improves
- The patient's color improves

Objective 14

Artificial ventilation is inadequate when:

- The chest does not rise and fall with each ventilation
- The ventilation rate is too slow or too fast
- The heart rate does not improve with ventilation
- The patient's color does not improve

Troubleshooting Bag-Mask Ventilation

If the chest does not rise and fall with BM ventilation, reassess the patient. Start by reassessing the patient's head position. Reposition the airway and try again to ventilate.

The tidal volume delivered to the patient depends on a tight mask seal and adequate compression of the bag. If an air leak is present because of an improper mask seal, an inadequate tidal volume will be delivered to the patient. If air is escaping from under the mask, reposition your fingers and the mask. Incomplete bag compression will also result in the delivery of an inadequate tidal volume to the patient. This can occur if the bag is large or the EMT's hands are small and only one hand is used to squeeze the bag. If the patient's chest does not rise and fall during BM ventilation, recheck the technique you are using to squeeze the bag. If the patient's chest does not rise, check for an obstruction. Lift the patient's jaw and suction the airway as needed. If the chest still does not rise, use a different method of artificial ventilation, such as a pocket mask or flow-restricted, oxygen-powered ventilation device.

Remember This!

Situations in which ventilation with a BM device is most likely to be difficult include the following:

- Patients older than 55 years of age
- Patients with facial trauma
- Large patients
- Presence of a beard
- Lack of teeth or ill-fitting dentures

If the patient has dentures and they do not fit well, remove them so that they do not block the airway.

Making a Difference

Advanced Life Support Assist

Endotracheal intubation is the placement of a plastic tube into a patient's trachea to keep the airway open. In most EMS systems, this skill is performed only by appropriately trained Advanced Life Support (ALS) personnel. However, you also have an important role during this procedure. You must be prepared to:

- Suction the patient.
- Hand the ALS provider a curved or straight laryngoscope blade.
- Ventilate the patient with a BM device before the procedure.
- Apply cricoid pressure.
- Hand the ALS provider the tracheal tube when asked.
- Keep track of time. Endotracheal intubation should take no longer than 30 seconds. Time starts with the last ventilation of the BM device before the tube is inserted and ends with the first ventilation of the BM device after the tube has beesn inserted. In other words, time is from breath to breath. When the elapsed time approaches 20 seconds, be sure to let the ALS provider know.
- Keep an eye on the patient's heart rate, and skin color during the procedure. If you have a pulse oximeter available, monitoring the patient's oxygen saturation level is also important.
- Remove the mask from the BM device and hand the bag-valve device to the ALS provider after the tracheal tube is in place, or ventilate the patient with the bag-valve device through the tracheal tube if asked to do so.
- Hand a securing device such as tape or a commercial tube holder to the ALS provider when asked to do so.
- Listen for breath sounds with a stethoscope if asked to do so. (This skill is discussed in detail in Chapter 9.)

Flow-Restricted, Oxygen-Powered Ventilation Device

A **flow-restricted, oxygen-powered ventilation device** (FROPVD, also called a *manually triggered ventilation (MTV) device*, is used to give positive-pressure ventilation with 100% oxygen (Figure 7-24). It can be attached to a face mask, tracheal tube, or tracheostomy tube.

A FROPVD consists of high-pressure tubing that connects the oxygen supply and a valve that is activated by a lever or push button. When the valve is open, oxygen flows into the patient. The major advantages of this device are that it provides high concentrations of oxygen and allows the EMT to use two hands to maintain a tight face-to-mask seal. Although the FROPVD is easy to use, it is not carried on every EMS vehicle. In addition, it cannot be used for infants and

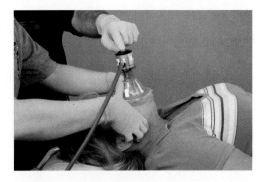

FIGURE 7-24 ▲ A flow-restricted, oxygen-powered ventilation device (FROPVD).

children. The FROPVD can cause gastric distention in patients who are not intubated. When using this device, you will be unable to feel the compliance of the patient's lungs. Because a FROPVD delivers oxygen under high pressure, pressure injury (barotrauma) to the lungs is a possible complication of this device.

Objective 15

Skill Drill 7-4 shows the steps to use a FROPVD for a nonbreathing patient.

Making a Difference

A common phrase in EMS is "BLS before ALS"— Basic Life Support before Advanced Life Support. This is particularly true when managing a patient's airway. Common problems in airway management involve the use of poor technique. Examples include improper positioning of the patient's head, failure to obtain (and maintain) a good seal with a BM device, and delivering ventilations at an improper rate (usually too fast). Another common problem is failure to reassess the patient after each intervention. Rise above these common mistakes. Aspire to provide excellent care. Practice your skills often, perform them to the best of your ability, and reassess your patient often while he is in your care.

Special Considerations

Tracheal Stomas

A **laryngectomy** is the surgical removal of the larynx. A person who has had a laryngectomy breathes through a stoma. A **stoma** is an artificial opening. A **tracheal stoma** is a permanent opening at the front of the neck that extends from the skin surface into the trachea. It opens the trachea to the atmosphere. A **tracheostomy** is the surgical formation of an opening

Flow-Restricted, Oxygen-Powered Ventilation for a Nonbreathing Patient

STEP 1 ▶ Prepare the flow-restricted, oxygen-powered ventilator. Select a mask of the correct size while another EMT ventilates the patient using another method. Connect the ventilator to the mask.

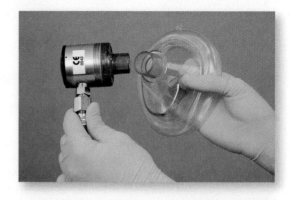

STEP 2 ▶ Position yourself at the patient's head. Position the mask on the patient's face. Seal the mask in place with one hand.

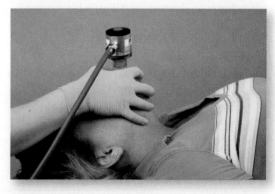

STEP 3 ▶ While holding the mask in place, open the patient's airway. If no trauma is suspected, use a head-tilt chin-lift (as shown here). If trauma is suspected, open the airway using a jaw thrust without head tilt maneuver.

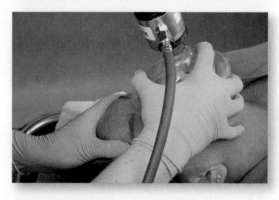

STEP 4 ▶ Trigger the valve (depress the button) on the ventilator to inflate the patient's lungs. Inflate only until you see adequate chest rise. Repeat once every five seconds. Watch for gastric distention. If seen, reposition the patient's head and recheck ventilation.

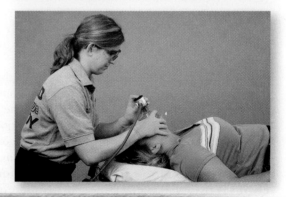

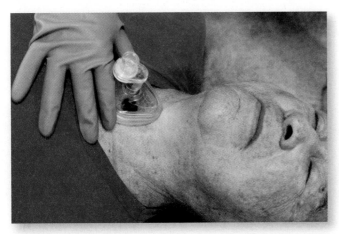

FIGURE 7-25 ▲ Pocket mask-to-stoma breathing.

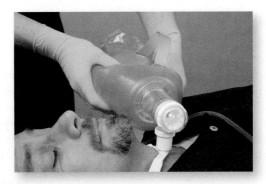

FIGURE 7-26 ▲ Ventilating through a tracheostomy tube.

into the trachea. There are many reasons why a person may have a tracheal stoma:

- A throat tumor or infection
- A severe injury to the neck or mouth
- A disease or infection that affects swallowing
- The need for long-term breathing assistance with a mechanical ventilator

Patients who have a tracheal stoma breathe through this opening in the neck because it is their airway. If artificial ventilation is required, it should be delivered through the stoma.

Objective 16

Follow these steps to perform mask-to-stoma breathing:

- If present, remove any garment (scarf, neck tie) covering the stoma.
- Place a pediatric face mask or barrier device on the patient's neck over the stoma. Make an airtight seal around the stoma (Figure 7-25).
- Slowly blow into the one-way valve on the mask until the chest rises.
- Remove your mouth from the mask to allow the patient to exhale.

Follow these steps to perform BM-to-stoma breathing:

- If present, remove any garment (scarf, necktie) covering the stoma.
- If available, connect oxygen to the BM device. If the patient has a tracheostomy tube in place, remove the mask from the device. Connect the bag-valve device to the patient's tracheostomy tube (Figure 7-26). Squeeze the bag while watching for chest rise. Allow the patient to exhale

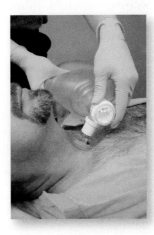

FIGURE 7-27 ◄ Bag-mask-to-stoma breathing.

passively. If you are unable to ventilate through the tracheostomy tube, suction it with a flexible suction catheter and then try to ventilate again. Seal the patient's nose and mouth and reattempt ventilation. Release the seal to allow the patient to exhale.

- If a stoma is present (but no tracheostomy tube), attach a pediatric mask to the BM device. Center the mask over the stoma and make an airtight seal around the stoma (Figure 7-27). If the chest does not rise and fall, seal the patient's mouth and nose and try again to ventilate. Release the seal to allow the patient to exhale. Suction the stoma with a soft suction catheter if foreign matter is present and try again to ventilate.

Dental Appliances

Dentures that fit well in the patient's mouth should be left in place. If they become loose or dislodged, remove them from the mouth because they can become a foreign body obstruction. Note that when you ventilate a patient with his dentures removed, it is harder to obtain a seal.

Infants and Children

Ventilating an infant or a child with a BM device requires special consideration. The flat bridge of an infant's or a child's nose makes it more difficult to obtain a good mask seal. Place the head in neutral position for an infant and slightly extended position for a child. Extending the head too far back may kink the airway, resulting in an airway obstruction. An oral airway may be needed when other procedures fail to provide a clear airway.

Use a pediatric BM device for full-term newly born infants, infants, and children. Use an adult bag for larger children and adolescents. To remember the correct timing for ventilating an infant or child, think "squeeze, release, release." As you begin compressing the bag say, "squeeze." As soon as you see the chest rise, release the bag and say, "release, release." This pattern makes sure that there is enough time for exhalation. Watch for improvement in skin color and/or heart rate.

Gastric distention is common when ventilating infants and children. To help avoid this, do not use excessive bag pressure when ventilating an infant or a child. Use only enough pressure to make the chest gently rise. When using a BM device during a cardiac arrest, make sure it does not have a pop-off valve. If a pop-off valve is present, it must be disabled (placed in closed position) for adequate ventilation.

Supplemental Oxygen

Objective 19

Oxygen is considered a medication. It is the most common medication that an EMT gives a patient. An oxygen delivery system is used to deliver oxygen from an oxygen cylinder to the patient. An oxygen delivery system consists of an oxygen cylinder, pressure regulator, flow meter, oxygen delivery tubing to carry oxygen to the patient's face, and an oxygen mask or cannula to deliver the oxygen to the patient's airway (Figure 7-28).

Oxygen Cylinders

Oxygen is stored in steel or aluminum cylinders. Oxygen cylinders (also called O₂ *tanks* or *bottles*) may be green, or they may be silver or chrome with green around the valve stem. Despite their characteristic color, it is best to identify the contents of a cylinder by checking its label or tag. Cylinders that contain gas have a pin index safety system. This system is designed to prevent accidental connection of oxygen equipment to the wrong gas, such as nitrous oxide. A yoke is used to connect a regulator to the cylinder. Each type of gas cylinder has a specific arrangement of protruding pins on the yoke hanger that must fit into matching depressions on the cylinder's valve. In this way, an oxygen cylinder will accept a regulator designed only for use with oxygen.

Letters are used to identify the size of an oxygen cylinder. "D" and "E" O2 cylinders are small, portable, and often used by EMTs. They weigh between 10 and 17 pounds when full. **Onboard oxygen** refers to the large oxygen cylinders carried on an ambulance. The amount of oxygen in various size cylinders is noted in Table 7-2.

Oxygen cylinders must be handled carefully because their contents are under pressure. It is important to take the steps necessary to make sure an oxygen tank is secure, including when moving a patient. Oxygen cylinders should be hydrostatically tested every five years to make sure they are safe to use.

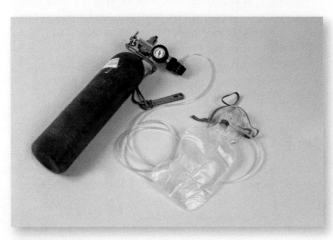

FIGURE 7-28 ▲ An oxygen delivery system.

TABLE 7-2 Oxygen Cylinders

Cylinder Type	Amount of Oxygen in Liters
Portable	
D	425
Jumbo D	640
E	680
Onboard	
M	3450
G	5300
H	6900

Using Oxygen Safely

- Never use combustible materials around oxygen equipment.
- Never place an oxygen cylinder where it may become part of an electrical circuit.
- Never use oil, grease, or other petroleum-based products on oxygen equipment.
- Never use adhesive tape or similar materials to seal connections or repair leaks.
- Never allow smoking around oxygen equipment.
- Never use oxygen around an open flame or spark.
- Never store oxygen cylinders in areas of extreme temperature.
- Never position any part of your body in front of or behind the cylinder's valve.
- Never leave an oxygen cylinder unattended.
- Never drag, roll, slide, or drop an oxygen cylinder.
- Never lift an oxygen cylinder by its cap; the sole purpose of the cap is to protect the valve.
- Never carry an oxygen cylinder by its attached regulator.
- Always store oxygen cylinders in well-ventilated areas.
- Always secure an oxygen cylinder when moving a patient.
- Always secure cylinders upright to keep them from falling or being knocked over.
- Always store full and empty cylinders separately. Use a first-in, last-out (FILO) system to prevent storing full cylinders for long periods.
- Always open the cylinder valve slowly to a full open position.
- Always use equipment (such as pressure gauges and regulators) designed for use with oxygen.

Pressure Regulators

The tank pressure of a fully pressurized cylinder is approximately 2000 pounds per square inch (psi), but tank pressure varies with the temperature. Tank pressure increases with increased temperature and decreases with decreased temperature. Because 2000 psi is too high a pressure to be delivered to a patient, a **pressure regulator** is used to release oxygen from the oxygen cylinder in a controlled manner (Figure 7-29). It reduces pressure in the oxygen cylinder to a safe range, about 40-70 psi. Regulators may decrease

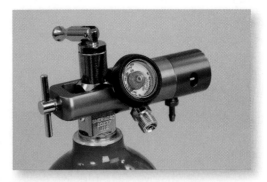

FIGURE 7-29 ▲ An oxygen pressure regulator.

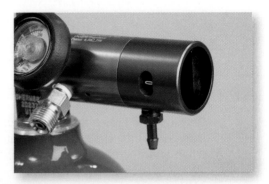

FIGURE 7-30 ▲ An oxygen flow meter.

the cylinder pressure in one or two stages. A one-stage (also called a single-stage) regulator decreases the cylinder pressure to a pre-set working pressure of about 40-70 psi. A two-stage (also called a double-stage) regulator creates two steps in the pressure drop. The pressure is first decreased as the gas leaves the cylinder and enters the regulator. It is reduced again when it meets the liter flow gauge.

A pressure regulator contains a gauge, which tells you how much oxygen is left in the cylinder. An oxygen cylinder is best refilled when the pressure gauge reads 200-300 psi. Some regulators also have a flow meter connected to it. A flow meter is a valve that controls the liters of oxygen delivered per minute (Figure 7-30). Oxygen flow is measured in liters per minute. The range of the flow meter is usually from 0 to 25 L/min. Skill Drill 7-5 shows the steps needed to set up an oxygen delivery system. Skill Drill 7-6 shows the steps to discontinue oxygen administration.

Humidifiers

Medical oxygen is very drying to airway and lung tissue. A humidifier is a bottle filled with sterile or distilled water (Figure 7-31). When the bottle is connected to oxygen, oxygen passes through the water to gather moisture. In some EMS systems, humidified oxygen is used when caring for patients with smoke inhalation, when caring for children with certain respiratory

Setting Up an Oxygen Delivery System

STEP 1 ▶ • Place the cylinder in an upright position and position yourself to the side of the cylinder. Verify the contents of the cylinder by checking the label or tag.
• After making sure that it is an oxygen cylinder, remove the protective seal covering the inlet.

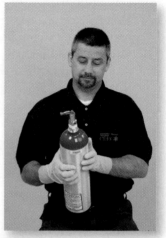

STEP 2 ▶ • Check the regulator and cylinder valve to make sure they are in good operating condition and free of dust and debris, such as oil and grease.
• Make sure that a washer or gasket is in place at the opening of the cylinder or regulator.

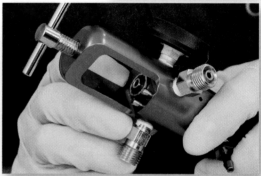

STEP 3 ▶ After making sure that the cylinder valve is aimed away from people or objects, quickly crack (open and close) the main valve on the top of the cylinder to blow out any dust and debris from its opening that might cause the valve to stick. You may need to use an oxygen wrench to open the valve. Then close the valve.

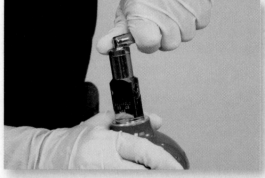

STEP 4 ▶ • Attach the pressure regulator to the cylinder. Carefully line up the pins on the regulator with the holes in the cylinder valve.
• Use an appropriate washer or gasket between the regulator and cylinder valve to ensure an airtight fit.

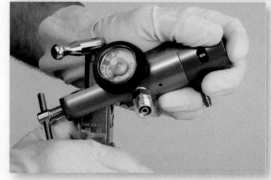

STEP 5 ▶ Hand-tighten the clamp on the regulator.

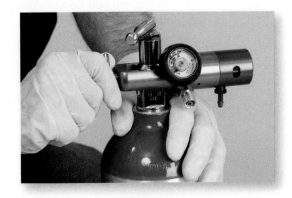

STEP 6 ▶
- Open the cylinder valve by turning it counterclockwise.
- Check the pressure in the cylinder and listen for leaks. If you hear a leak, close the valve and remove the regulator.
- Recheck the condition and position of the washer/gasket. Then repeat Steps 4, 5, and 6.

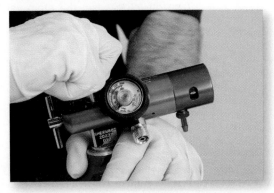

STEP 7 ▶
- Attach the oxygen delivery device to the regulator.
- Adjust the liter flow to the desired setting by turning the appropriate valve/knob on the regulator.

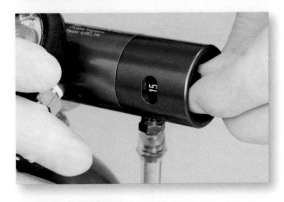

STEP 8 ▶ Apply the oxygen delivery device to the patient. Secure the oxygen cylinder.

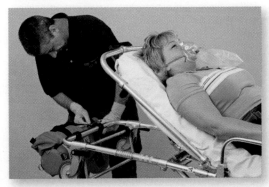

Discontinuing an Oxygen Delivery System

STEP 1 ▶ Remove the oxygen delivery device from the patient. Turn off the flow of oxygen.

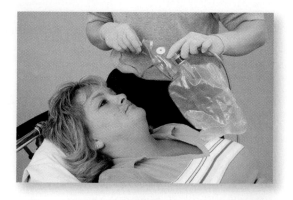

STEP 2 ▶ Turn off (clockwise) the main valve on the top of the cylinder.

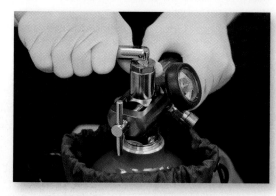

STEP 3 ▶
- Bleed oxygen out of the system by opening the flow meter valve until the flow stops.
- Close the flow meter valve.

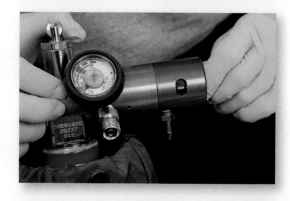

STEP 4 ▶
- Loosen the clamp and remove the regulator from the cylinder.
- Store the oxygen cylinder appropriately.

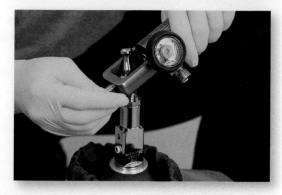

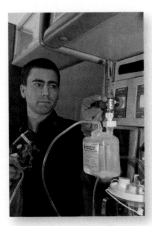

FIGURE 7-31 ◀ An oxygen humidifier.

conditions, and during long transports. In adults, oxygen does not generally need to be humidified if the flow rate is 4 L/min or less. When a humidifier is used, it should be changed after each use to prevent the growth of bacteria in the container.

Making a Difference

It is unacceptable to respond to an emergency and find out that your oxygen cylinder is empty. Make it a habit to check the pressure remaining in an oxygen cylinder at the start of every shift and after every call in which oxygen was given. Replace an oxygen cylinder when the pressure within it is low.

Oxygen Delivery Devices

Nonrebreather Mask

In most situations, a **nonrebreather (NRB) mask** is the preferred method of oxygen delivery in the field for a patient who is breathing adequately (Figure 7-32). It allows the delivery of high-concentration oxygen to a breathing patient. At 15 L/min, the oxygen concentration delivered is about 90%. A one-way valve allows exhaled air to escape the mask but prevents room air from being breathed in.

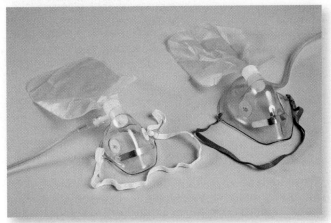

(a)

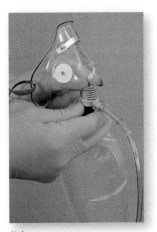

(b)

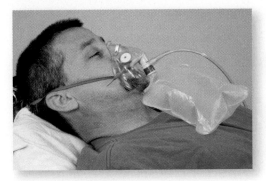

(c)

FIGURE 7-32 ◀ **(a)** A pediatric and adult nonrebreather mask (NRB). **(b)** Before placing it on the patient, attach the nonrebreather mask to an oxygen regulator. Set the flow rate so that when the patient inhales, the bag does not collapse (usually 15 L/min). Prefill the oxygen reservoir on the nonrebreather mask by placing two clean, gloved fingers inside the mask and closing off the valve. Hold the valve closed until the bag is full. **(c)** Apply the mask to the patient's face. Make sure the mask makes a good seal by forming the metal nosepiece to the patient's nose. Adjust the mask's elastic straps to secure the mask to the patient's face.

When using a NRB mask, be sure to fill the reservoir bag with oxygen *before* placing the mask on the patient. The reservoir bag of a NRB mask must never be less than two thirds full. This helps to make sure that there is enough supplemental oxygen available for each breath. Adjust the flow rate so that the bag does not completely deflate when the patient inhales (usually 15 L/min). The mask must fit snugly on the patient's face to prevent room air from mixing with the oxygen from the reservoir bag. Make sure the mask makes a good seal by forming the metal nosepiece to the patient's nose. Adjust the mask's elastic straps to secure the mask to the patient's face.

Remember This!

Using a Nonrebreather Mask

Indications:

Delivery of high concentration oxygen

Contraindications:

Nonbreathing patient

Patient who has poor respiratory effort

Nasal Cannula

Objectives 21, 22

A **nasal cannula** is a piece of plastic tubing with two soft prongs that stick out from the tubing (Figure 7-33). The prongs are inserted into the patient's nostrils and the tubing is secured to the patient's face. The use of a nasal cannula requires a breathing patient. This oxygen delivery device is often used for patients who have chest pain and are breathing adequately. It is also the preferred method of oxygen delivery in some EMS systems for patients showing signs and symptoms of a possible stroke (and who are breathing adequately).

A nasal cannula can deliver an oxygen concentration of 25-45% at 1-6 L/min. Flow rates of more than 6 L/min are irritating to the nasal passages. This method of oxygen delivery will provide little benefit to the patient who is breathing through his mouth and not his nose. A nasal cannula is also ineffective if the patient's nose is plugged with mucus or blood.

Remember This!

Using a Nasal Cannula

Indications:

Delivery of low- to medium-concentration oxygen

Contraindications:

Nonbreathing patient

Patient who is unable to breathe through his nose

Patient who has poor respiratory effort

You Should Know

To figure out the approximate percentage of oxygen a patient may receive by means of a nasal cannula, consider this. Room air is about 21% oxygen. For each L/min of oxygen flow, add 4%. For example, at 1 L/min, the approximate percentage of oxygen delivered by a nasal cannula would be 21% (room air) + 4% = 25%.

1 L/min = 25%	4 L/min = 37%
2 L/min = 29%	5 L/min = 41%
3 L/min = 33%	6 L/min = 45%

Blow-By Oxygen

Some patients will not tolerate oxygen delivered by means of a nasal cannula or face mask. If you are faced with a situation like this, consider **blow-by oxygen.** When oxygen is delivered by using this method, the device used to deliver the oxygen does not make actual contact with the patient. For example, oxygen

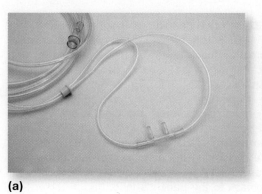

(a)

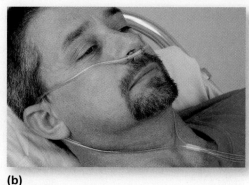

(b)

FIGURE 7-33 ◀ **(a)** A nasal cannula. **(b)** Place the prongs of the nasal cannula in the patient's nostrils. Place the tubing around the patient's ears and under the chin.

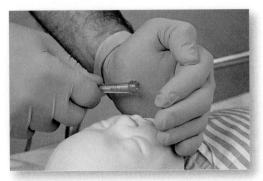

(a)

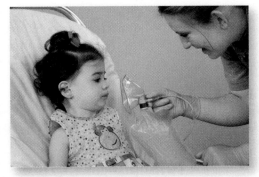

(b)

FIGURE 7-34 ◄ Giving blow-by oxygen.

tubing can be attached to a toy or inside a paper cup (Figure 7-34). Oxygen is then "blown-by" when the toy or cup is held near the patient's face. Although this method is not ideal for delivering oxygen, it is better than breathing room air.

On the Scene   Wrap-Up

You carefully slide an oral airway into the patient's mouth. Positioning your pocket mask over his nose and mouth, you deliver rescue breaths at the proper rate, pausing to let him exhale each time you see his chest rise. Your partner notes that the patient's pupils are very small. He connects a BM to oxygen and you continue to ventilate him. The Paramedics arrive and quickly start an intravenous line and give the patient a drug to reverse the effects of the narcotic. You can feel your patient's breathing rate increase between the breaths you are giving. Within minutes his eyes are open, he is breathing on his own, and he is trying to sit up. As you prepare to load the patient into the ambulance, his sister tearfully tells you she thought he had quit taking drugs and was trying to get clean. You realize that if she had waited a few more minutes to call, he would have been in cardiac arrest. ■

Sum It Up

► As an EMT, you must maintain an open airway in order to allow a free flow of air into and out of the patient's lungs. You must be familiar with the structures of the upper and lower airways. You must also understand the mechanisms of breathing.

► One of the most important actions that you can perform is to open the airway of an unresponsive patient. You must become familiar with the two main methods of opening an airway: the head tilt–chin lift and the jaw thrust without head tilt maneuver.

• The head tilt–chin lift maneuver is used to open the airway if trauma to the head or neck is not suspected.

• When trauma to the head or neck of an unresponsive patient is suspected, you should use the jaw thrust without head tilt (also called the jaw thrust without head extension maneuver) to open the patient's airway. However, use a head tilt–chin lift maneuver if the jaw thrust does not open the airway. This method of opening the airway is effective, but it is less effective than the head tilt–chin lift and is more tiring. Because this technique requires the use of both hands, a second rescuer will be needed if the patient requires ventilation.

► If a patient's airway is obstructed, you must clear it. The three primary ways of clearing the airway of an unresponsive patient are with the recovery position, finger sweeps, and suctioning.

• In some situations, the recovery position can be used to help maintain an open airway in an unresponsive patient. This position involves positioning a patient on his side. As an EMT, you must become familiar with placing a patient in this position. You must also remember not to place a patient with a known or suspected spinal injury in the recovery position.

• If you see foreign material in the patient's mouth, you must remove it immediately. If foreign material is seen in an unresponsive patient's upper airway, a finger sweep may be used to remove it. A "blind" finger sweep is never performed. Performing a blind finger sweep may cause the object to become further lodged in the patient's throat.

• You should always have suction equipment within arm's reach when you are managing a patient's airway or assisting a patient's breathing.

Suctioning is a procedure used to vacuum vomitus, saliva, blood, food particles, and other material from the patient's airway.

▶ After you have opened a patient's airway, you may need to use an airway adjunct to keep it open. After the airway adjunct is inserted, maintain the proper head position while the device is in place.

- An oral airway (also called an oropharyngeal airway or OPA) is a device that is used only in unresponsive patients without a gag reflex. An OPA is inserted into the patient's mouth and used to keep the tongue away from the back of the throat.

- A nasal airway (also called a nasopharyngeal airway or NPA) is a device that is placed in the patient's nose. An NPA keeps the patient's tongue from blocking the upper airway. It also allows air to flow from the hole in the NPA down into the patient's lower airway.

▶ After making sure that the patient's airway is open, you must check for breathing. If the patient is breathing, you must determine if the patient is breathing adequately or inadequately. You must also be able to recognize the sounds of noisy breathing, which include stridor, snoring, gurgling, and wheezing.

▶ If your patient's breathing is inadequate or absent, you will need to assist the patient by forcing air into the patient's lungs during inspiration. This action is called positive-pressure ventilation and includes the following: mouth-to-mask ventilation, mouth-to-barrier ventilation, mouth-to-mouth ventilation, and bag-mask ventilation. As an EMT, you must be familiar with performing all of these ventilation methods. You must also learn how to remove foreign body airway obstructions in patients of every age.

▶ A flow-restricted, oxygen-powered ventilation device is used to give positive-pressure ventilation with 100% oxygen. It can be attached to a face mask, tracheal tube, or tracheostomy tube.

▶ You may need to give patients supplemental oxygen. Become familiar with the features and functioning of oxygen cylinders. Remember to always keep combustible materials away from oxygen equipment and never position any part of your body over the cylinder.

▶ The two most common oxygen delivery devices are the nonrebreather mask and the nasal cannula. In most situations, the nonrebreather mask is the preferred method of oxygen delivery. It allows the delivery of high-concentration oxygen to a breathing patient. At 15 L/min, the oxygen concentration delivered is about 90%. The nasal cannula is often used for patients who have chest pain and are breathing adequately. It is also the preferred method of oxygen delivery in some EMS systems for patients showing signs and symptoms of a possible stroke (and who are breathing adequately). A nasal cannula can deliver an oxygen concentration of 25-45% at 1-6 L/min.

Division 3

Patient Assessment

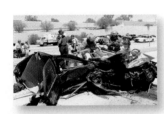
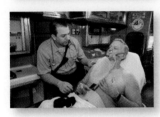
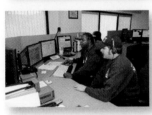
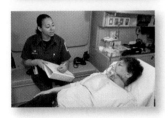

Scene Size-Up

By the end of this chapter, you should be able to:

Knowledge Objectives ▶

1. Recognize hazards and potential hazards.
2. Describe common hazards found at the scene of a trauma and a medical patient
3. Determine if the scene is safe to enter.
4. Discuss common mechanisms of injury and nature of illness.
5. Discuss the reason for identifying the total number of patients at the scene.
6. Explain the reason for identifying the need for additional help or assistance.

Attitude Objectives ▶

7. Explain the rationale for crew members to evaluate scene safety before entering.
8. Serve as a model for others by explaining how patient situations affect your evaluation of mechanism of injury or illness.

Skill Objectives ▶

9. Observe various scenarios and identify potential hazards.

You are dispatched to a private residence for a "welfare check." Law enforcement personnel are already on the scene, and they are requesting your assistance for a 56-year-old man. Although there is no additional information available at the time of dispatch, you recognize the address as a house that you and your partner have been to several times in the past. As you arrive at the scene, you note three police cruisers. Officers are standing in the entryway of the house. You and your partner note two newspapers on the driveway. As you walk up the sidewalk, an officer tells you that a friend of the patient called the police department because he was concerned about the health of the man inside but gave no other information. The officers do not have any other information except that there are no immediate safety concerns that they can find. Officers are inside the house. You take the information, relay it to your partner, and enter the house to speak with the patient. ■

THINK ABOUT IT

As you read this chapter, think about the following questions:

- What is scene size-up, and why is it important to the Emergency Medical Technician?
- What are the components of an effective scene size-up?
- Who is responsible for the scene size-up?
- Why is it important to note subtle details in every emergency scene?

The Importance of Scene Size-Up

Scene size-up is the first and most important aspect of patient assessment. Scene size-up begins as an Emergency Medical Technician (EMT) approaches the scene. During this phase, you will survey the scene to determine if any threats may cause injury to you, other rescuers, the patient, or bystanders. This evaluation also allows you to determine the nature of the call and the need for additional resources as necessary.

An Overview of Scene Size-Up

As an EMT, you will be called to provide emergency care to patients in many different settings. Your patients will include infants, children, young adults, middle-aged adults, the elderly, and patients with special healthcare needs. These patients may experience an emergency resulting from trauma or a medical condition. These emergencies may occur in a person's home, on a busy highway, in a shopping mall, or in an office. In every situation, you must quickly look at the entire scene before approaching the patient (Figure 8-1). You must size up the scene to find out if there are any threats that may cause injury to you, other rescuers, or bystanders, or that may cause additional injury to the patient.

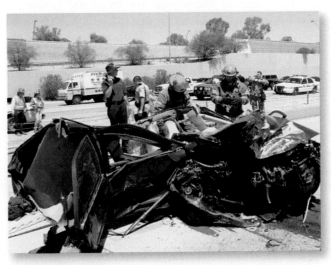

FIGURE 8-1 ▲ You must quickly survey the entire scene for safety on every emergency call. *Courtesy of City of Tempe Fire Department, Tempe, Arizona.*

Scene size-up is the first phase of patient assessment and is made up of five parts:

1. Body substance isolation precautions
2. Evaluating scene safety
3. Determining the mechanism of injury or the nature of the patient's illness
4. Determining the total number of patients
5. Determining the need for additional resources

The scene size-up begins with the information received about the emergency. The information given to the EMS dispatcher by the caller may help you determine the following:

- The location of the emergency
- If the call is a trauma emergency (such as a motor vehicle crash) or a medical emergency (such as a seizure)
- The number of vehicles involved
- The number of patients involved
- The ages and genders of all patients (if known)
- When the emergency occurred
- If the call involves fire or other potential hazards such as leaking materials, downed power lines, broken gas lines, hazardous materials, a violent patient, or dangerous pets
- If law enforcement or fire department personnel are on the scene
- If Advanced Life Support (ALS) personnel have been sent to the scene
- If special resources will be required, such as a hazardous materials team, a confined space rescue team, a water rescue team, extrication equipment, or air medical transport

En route to the scene, try to create a mental picture of the call by using the information given to you by the dispatcher. Be prepared for the unexpected. What additional help might be needed on the scene? Law enforcement personnel? The fire department? A utility company? ALS personnel? How will you gain access to the patient? What questions will you ask the patient or family?

Remember This!

The information given to you by a dispatcher is often limited to that provided by the caller. You may arrive at the scene of an emergency to find the patient with injuries or a complaint that differs from that reported by the caller to the dispatcher.

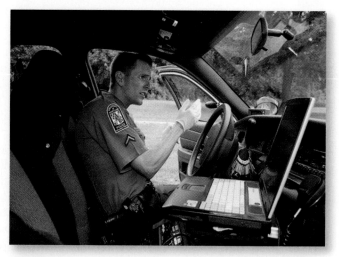

FIGURE 8-2 ▲ Put on appropriate personal protective equipment on the basis of the dispatch information received and your initial survey of the scene.

Body Substance Isolation Review

You must take appropriate body substance isolation (BSI) precautions on *every* call. Consider the need for BSI precautions before you approach the patient. Put on appropriate personal protective equipment (PPE) on the basis of the information the dispatcher gives you and your initial survey of the scene (Figure 8-2). This equipment includes gloves, eye protection, mask, and gown, if necessary. Consider the following examples of real emergency situations:

- You are called to a fitness club for a woman with a rapid heart rate. The dispatcher tells you that the woman was using the treadmill when she felt weak, became dizzy, and felt her heart race. Because gloves should be worn before physical contact with *every* patient, put on gloves while en route to the scene.
- You are called to respond to a single vehicle rollover. The bystander who called 9-1-1 said the vehicle rolled twice and is resting on its side. There is heavy damage to the vehicle. He believes there are three patients. En route to the scene, put on gloves because it is likely that blood will be present on the scene. Once on the scene, put on a chin-length face shield (or protective eyewear and mask) if you see serious bleeding that could spray or splash into your eyes, nose, or mouth. Put on a gown if there is a chance of splashing blood or other body fluids and your clothing is likely to be soiled. If you are trained in fire or rescue techniques and will be responsible for that role during the rescue, wear appropriate clothing to protect yourself from fire, glass, sharp edges and fragments, and

other debris at the scene. Protective clothing includes turnout gear, puncture-proof gloves, a helmet, eye protection (safety glasses or goggles), and boots with steel toes.

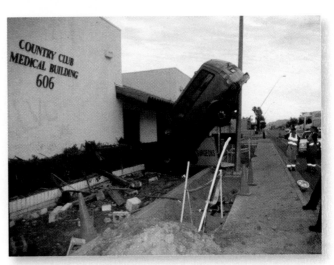

FIGURE 8-3 ▲ Study the scene before approaching the patient. Look for possible hazards. *Courtesy of City of Mesa Fire Department, Mesa, Arizona.*

Scene Safety

Objective 3

Scene safety is an assessment of the entire scene and surroundings to ensure your well-being and that of other rescuers, the patient(s), and bystanders. Remember, you are of no help to the patient if you become a patient yourself!

Personal and Other Rescuer Safety

Objectives 1, 2

Study the scene before approaching the patient (Figure 8-3). Consider the following questions at a crash or rescue scene:

- Is the area marked by safety lights or flares?
- Is traffic controlled by law enforcement personnel?
- Does the vehicle, aircraft, or machinery appear stable?
- Do you see any leaking fluids?
- Are downed power lines present?
- Do you see fire, smoke, or potential fire hazards?
- Do you see entrapped victims?

At a scene involving toxic substances, obvious hazards may be present. At other scenes, the hazards may not be as obvious. Look for clues that suggest the presence of hazardous materials:

- Placards on railroad cars, storage facilities, or vehicles
- Vapor clouds or heavy smoke
- Unusual odors
- Spilled solids or liquids
- Leaking containers, bottles, or gas cylinders
- Chemical transport tanks or containers

When you arrive at a scene, park at a safe distance that is upwind or uphill from the incident. Contact your local hazardous material response team immediately. Do not enter the area unless you are trained to handle hazardous materials and are fully protected with proper equipment. Do not walk or drive an emergency vehicle through spilled liquids. Keep unnecessary people away from the area. Provide emergency care only after the scene is safe and the patient is decontaminated.

Emergencies that occur in a confined space such as a mine, well, silo, or an unreinforced trench may be low in oxygen (Figure 8-4). Rescues in these situations require specially trained personnel and equipment. Do not enter the area unless you have all the necessary equipment and have been trained in this type of rescue.

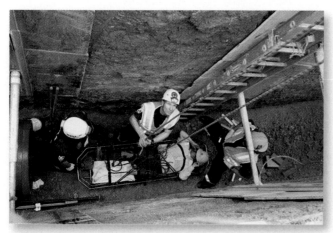

FIGURE 8-4 ▲ Confined space rescue requires specially trained personnel and equipment. *Courtesy of City of Mesa Fire Department, Mesa, Arizona.*

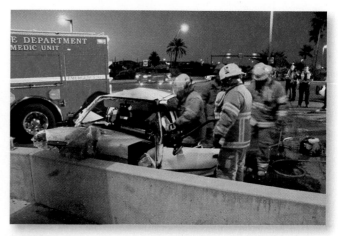

FIGURE 8-5 ▲ You are responsible for ensuring the patient's safety, including protecting the patient from glass and other debris during extrication procedures. *Courtesy of City of Tempe Fire Department, Tempe, Arizona.*

At a crime scene or hostile situation, assess the potential for violence. Clues include:

* A knowledge of prior violence at a particular location
* Evidence of alcohol or other substance use
* Weapons visible or in use
* Loud voices, fighting, or the potential for fighting

Assess the crowd and look for hostile bystanders. *Never* enter a potential crime scene or a scene involving a family dispute, fight, attempted suicide, drugs, alcohol, or weapons until law enforcement personnel have secured the scene and declared it safe for you to enter and provide patient care.

Remember This!

Notify appropriate law enforcement personnel immediately in the event that a crime scene is suspected. It is important to realize that as healthcare professionals, our primary responsibility is to the patient. At the same time, law enforcement personnel are looking to protect any evidence that may be associated with the crime scene. In these situations, it is important that EMS and law enforcement personnel work cooperatively together.

Consider the environment before approaching the patient. If a surface or slope is unstable or if water, ice, fire, or downed power lines are present, call for specially trained personnel as needed. Do not enter a body of water unless you have been trained in water rescue and the necessary safety measures are in place. Do not enter fast-moving water or venture out on ice unless you have been trained in this type of rescue. If the scene is safe

but extremes of heat or cold are a concern, move the patient to an ambulance as quickly as possible.

Patient Safety

You are responsible for ensuring the patient's safety. This responsibility includes:

* Protecting the patient from curious onlookers
* Assessing for traffic and other hazards
* Protecting the patient from glass and other debris during extrication procedures (Figure 8-5)
* Protecting the patient from environmental temperature extremes

Bystander Safety

At the scene of an emergency, bystanders may become so engrossed in the situation that they fail to watch out for themselves. Look for bystanders who may be in danger or who may endanger your safety or that of the patient. Help bystanders avoid becoming patients by preventing them from getting too close to the scene. If the scene is safe and you need assistance, ask bystanders to help you. Reassure your patient and bystanders by working confidently and efficiently.

The Mechanism of Injury or the Nature of the Illness

During the scene size-up, try to determine the nature of the patient's problem. A **trauma patient** is one who has experienced an injury from an external force. In trauma situations, look for the mechanism of injury.

A **medical patient** is one whose condition is caused by an illness. In medical situations, try to determine the nature of the patient's illness.

Making a Difference

Trauma and medical emergencies can occur at the same time. For example, a patient with low blood sugar may be involved in a motor vehicle crash or a patient may have had a seizure before falling. A patient with a history of asthma may develop difficulty breathing after an airbag deploys in a motor vehicle crash. Don't get tunnel vision!

The Mechanism of Injury

Mechanism of injury (MOI) refers to the way in which an injury occurs, as well as the forces involved in producing the injury. **Kinetic energy** is the energy of motion. The amount of kinetic energy an object has depends on the mass (weight) and speed (velocity) of the object. **Kinematics** is the science of analyzing the mechanism of injury and predicting injury patterns. The amount of injury is determined by the following three elements:

- The type of energy applied
- How quickly the energy is applied
- To what part of the body the energy is applied

Physical injury is the result of different sources of energy (Table 8-1). Injuries may be intentional or unintentional (Table 8-2). If you understand the types of forces that were involved in producing an injury, you will be able to look for specific injuries and injury patterns. On a trauma scene, you must quickly decide if the MOI is significant or not. If the patient is unresponsive, considering the mechanism of injury may be the only way you can determine what the injuries (or

Making a Difference

When providing care for a seriously injured trauma patient, make every effort to limit your time on the scene to 10 minutes or less. These patients require definitive care at the hospital. The longer it takes to deliver a seriously injured patient to the hospital, the less likely patient survival becomes.

TABLE 8-1 Sources of Energy and Mechanisms of Injury

Energy Source	Mechanism of Injury
Kinetic (mechanical) energy	Motor vehicle crashes Motorcycle crashes Firearms Falls Assaults
Thermal energy	Heat Steam Fire
Radiant energy	Rays of light (sun rays) Sound waves (explosions) Electromagnetic waves (x-ray exposure) Radioactive emissions (nuclear leak)
Chemical energy	Plant and animal toxins Chemical substances
Electrical energy	Lightning Exposure to wires, sockets, plugs

Modified from *Trauma Nursing Core Course Provider Manual,* 5th ed. (Emergency Nurses Association, 2000), p. 27.

TABLE 8-2 Examples of Unintentional and Intentional Injuries

Unintentional Injuries	Intentional Injuries
• Motor vehicle crash • Motorcycle crash • Bicycle crash • Pedestrian injuries • Fire, burn • Fall • Farm machinery (pin, crush, fall, run over, rollover) • Ejection from motor vehicle (including motorcycles, mopeds, all-terrain vehicles, or open bed of pick-up trucks) • Snowmobile injuries • Snowskiing injuries • Poisoning • Water-related incident (drowning, diving) • Choking • Explosion • Electrocution • Entrapment • Ejection from a horse	• Assault • Suicide • Homicide

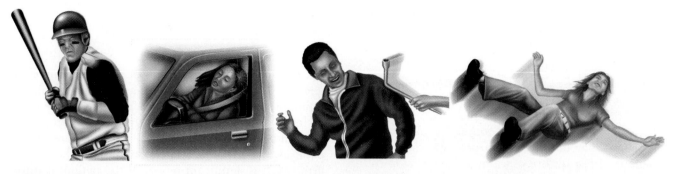

FIGURE 8-6 ▲ Blunt trauma is any mechanism of injury that occurs without actual penetration of the body. Examples of mechanisms of injury causing blunt trauma include motor vehicle crashes, falls, sports injuries, or assaults with a blunt object.

medical situation) might be. Survey the scene and talk to the patient, family, and bystanders to determine the mechanism of injury.

Objective 4

Trauma is generally divided into two categories: blunt and penetrating. **Blunt trauma** is any mechanism of injury that occurs without actual penetration of the body. Examples of mechanisms of injury causing blunt trauma include motor vehicle crashes, falls, sports injuries, or assaults with a blunt object (Figure 8-6). Blunt trauma produces injury first to the body surface and then to the body's contents. This results in compression and/or stretching of the tissue beneath the skin. The amount of injury depends on how long the compression occurred, the force of the compression, and the area compressed.

Penetrating trauma is any mechanism of injury that causes a cut or piercing of the skin. Examples of mechanisms of injury causing penetrating trauma include gunshot wounds, stab wounds, and blast injuries (Figure 8-7). Penetrating trauma usually affects organs and tissues in the direct path of the wounding object.

Making a Difference

The extent and seriousness of a patient's injuries may not be obvious. When evaluating the mechanism of injury, try to picture the organs that may have been damaged. This technique will help you predict the patient's injuries.

Motor Vehicle Crashes

A motor vehicle crash (MVC) can involve automobiles, motorcycles, all-terrain vehicles (ATVs), and tractors. Most motor vehicle crashes (75%) occur within 25 miles of home. Most crashes also occur in areas where the speed limit is 40 mph or less. In an MVC, three separate impacts occur as kinetic energy is transferred (Figure 8-8):

1. The vehicle strikes an object.
2. The occupant collides with the interior of the vehicle. Interior elements include seatbelts, airbags, and the dashboard.

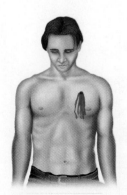
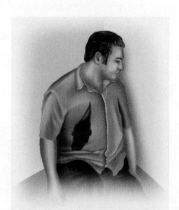
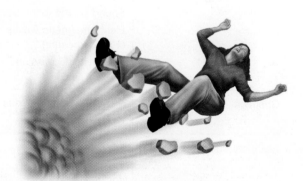

FIGURE 8-7 ▲ Penetrating trauma is any mechanism of injury that causes a cut or piercing of the skin. Examples of mechanisms of injury causing penetrating trauma include gunshot wounds, stab wounds, and blast injuries.

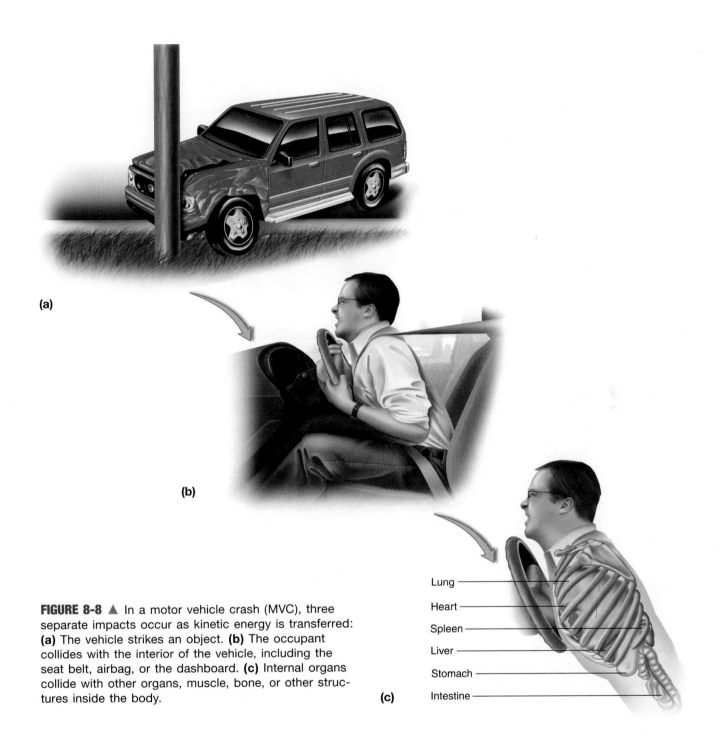

FIGURE 8-8 ▲ In a motor vehicle crash (MVC), three separate impacts occur as kinetic energy is transferred: **(a)** The vehicle strikes an object. **(b)** The occupant collides with the interior of the vehicle, including the seat belt, airbag, or the dashboard. **(c)** Internal organs collide with other organs, muscle, bone, or other structures inside the body.

Lung
Heart
Spleen
Liver
Stomach
Intestine

(a)

(b)

(c)

3. Internal organs collide with other organs, muscle, bone, or other structures inside the body. The lungs, brain, liver, and spleen are particularly vulnerable to trauma.

Note that a fourth impact may occur if loose objects in the vehicle become projectiles.

A motor vehicle crash is classified by the type of impact. The five types of impact include head on (frontal), lateral, rear end, rotational, and rollover (Figure 8-9). The injuries that result depend on the type of collision, the position of the occupant inside the vehicle, and the use or nonuse of active or passive restraint systems. Restraint systems are used to absorb the energy of the impact before the occupant hits something hard. They also limit the distance the body has to travel.

In a frontal impact, such as a head-on collision, the vehicle stops and the occupants continue to move forward by one of two pathways: down and under or up and over. In the down and under pathway, the victim's

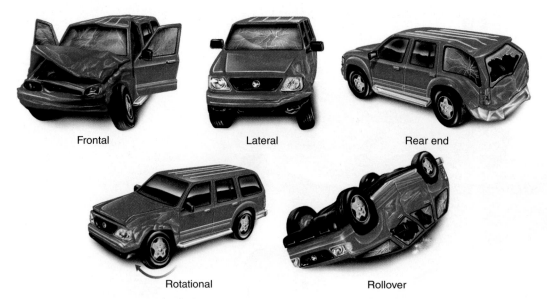

Frontal   Lateral   Rear end

Rotational   Rollover

FIGURE 8-9 ▲ A motor vehicle crash is classified by the type of impact. The five types of impact include head on (frontal), lateral, rear end, rotational, and rollover.

knees impact the vehicle's dashboard. The down and under pathway may be seen when the occupant is not wearing a lap and shoulder restraint system, or when the occupant is wearing only the shoulder harness and not a lap belt. Predictable injuries include a knee dislocation and/or patella fracture. The impact may also result in fractures of the femur or hip or a posterior dislocation of the hip socket (acetabulum). In the up and over pathway, the victim's upper body strikes the steering wheel, resulting in injuries to the head, chest, abdomen, pelvis, and/or spine. The up and over pathway may be seen when the occupant is not wearing a lap and shoulder restraint system or when the occupant is wearing only a lap restraint (not the shoulder har-

ness). Predictable injuries based on common mechanisms of injury are listed in Table 8-3.

Other Considerations

Although mechanism of injury is important, it is not the only factor to consider when assessing a trauma patient and determining whether or not he is a priority patient. For some patients, the risk of significant injury is increased because of their age or a preexisting medical condition, despite what may appear to be a "minor" mechanism of injury.

In some EMS systems, other factors for designating "priority" status are considered in addition to the

TABLE 8-3 Predictable Injuries Based on Common Mechanisms of Injury

Mechanism of Injury		Predictable Injuries
Motor vehicle crashes	Head-on collision	Below the steering wheel: • Lower extremity fractures • Dislocated knees and hips At the level of and above the steering wheel: • Trauma to the head, brain, and face • Serious chest injuries
	Lateral (side) collision	• Head and cervical spine injuries • Injuries to the chest and pelvis • Internal injuries may be present without outward signs of injury

(Continued)

Mechanism of Injury		Predictable Injuries
Motor vehicle crashes *(Continued)*	Rear-end collision	• Head, brain, and cervical spine injuries • Possible chest, abdomen, long-bone, and soft-tissue injuries
	Rotational collision	• Head and cervical spine injuries • Internal injuries that may be present without outward signs of injury
	Rollover	• Head and cervical spine injuries • Crushing injuries • Soft-tissue injuries, multiple broken bones
Motor vehicle–pedestrian crashes	Adult	• Injuries to both lower legs • Secondary injuries may occur when the body strikes the hood of the car and then the ground
	Child	• Trauma to the lower extremities from the bumper • Chest and abdominal trauma from striking the hood • Injuries to the head and face from hitting the hood or windshield
Falls	Adult	• Compression injuries of the spine • Upper- or lower-extremity trauma
	Child	• Head, face, and neck trauma (young children tend to fall head first) • Upper- or lower-extremity trauma
Bicycle crashes	Without helmet	• Injuries to head, face, and spine; broken clavicles, ribs • Extremity fractures • Abdominal injuries (from striking the handlebars)
	With helmet	• Upper- or lower-extremity trauma • Abdominal injuries (from striking the handlebars)
Motorcycle crashes	Head-on collision	• At the level of and above the handlebars: lower-extremity fractures with serious soft-tissue injuries and blood loss • Head, face, and neck trauma likely on landing
	Lateral collision	• Pelvic or lower-extremity injuries; crushing injuries
	Ejection	• The type and severity of injuries depend on how the victim lands and the nature of the object struck
	Laying down the bike	• Scrapes, burns, possible fractures of lower extremities
Penetrating traumas	Low-velocity weapons (knife, ice pick)	• Injury that is usually limited to the area penetrated • Blood loss
	Medium- and high-velocity weapons (shotgun, high-powered rifle, assault weapon)	• An injured area that is larger than the area penetrated • Fluid-filled organs (bladder, heart, great vessels, and bowel), which can burst because of the pressure waves generated • Liver, spleen, and brain, which are easily injured

TABLE 8-4   Factors to Consider when Identifying Priority Trauma Patients

Mechanism of Injury	Anatomy	Physiology	Patient Factors
• Motor vehicle crash • Motorcycle crash • Bicycle crash • All-terrain vehicle (ATV) crash • Pedestrian injuries • Fire, burn • Fall • Farm machinery (pin, crush, fall, run over, rollover) • Ejection from motor vehicle (including motorcycles, mopeds, ATVs, or open bed of pick-up trucks) • Poisoning • Water-related incident (drowning, diving) • Choking • Explosion • Electrocution • Entrapment	• Penetrating trauma • Blunt trauma • Fracture • Burn • Significant soft tissue injury • Significant deformity • Injury to eyes, hands, feet, genitalia	• Altered mental status • Slow heart rate • Fast heart rate • Nausea/vomiting • Sweating • Shortness of breath • Chest pain • Headache • Severe pain • Hypotension • Respirations <10 or >40 • Fever >101° • Abdominal pain • Inability to walk	• Age <5 or >55 • Cardiac disease • Respiratory disease • Seizure disorder • Liver disease • Insulin-dependent diabetes • Obesity • Pregnancy • Immunosuppressed patients • Patients with a bleeding disorder or patients on blood thinners • Use of alcohol or drugs • Recent surgery/illness

mechanism of injury (Table 8-4). These include anatomy, physiology, and patient factors. For instance, the patient in our previous example was involved in a motor vehicle crash (mechanism of injury). The appearance of the bent steering wheel and starred windshield leads us to suspect he experienced blunt trauma to his chest and head (anatomy). A physical exam has not yet been completed, but our initial assessment reveals the patient has an altered mental status (physiology). A SAMPLE history has not yet been obtained, so we do not yet know if there are other patient factors to consider. Some trauma experts have also noted that significant injury may also be suspected from key phrases said by patients (Table 8-5). The more of these factors that are present, the more likely the patient has experienced a serious injury.

Motor Vehicle–Pedestrian Crashes

Adult pedestrians will typically turn away if they are about to be struck by an oncoming vehicle. This action results in injuries to the side or back of the body. A child will usually face an oncoming vehicle, which results in injuries to the front of the body.

TABLE 8-5   Patient Complaints and Possible Significant Injury

Possible Significant Injury	Patient Complaint
Compromised airway	"I can't breathe." "I can't swallow." "I'm choking."
Breathing problem, lack of oxygen, cardiac tamponade	"Let me sit up."
Blood loss, lack of oxygen	"Please help me." "I'm going to die."
Blood loss	"I'm thirsty."
Spinal cord injury	"I can't move my legs."
Irritation of the abdominal lining	"My belly hurts."
Significant injury	"Please do something for my pain."

Adapted from: Rhodes M, "Trauma Resuscitation," in *The Trauma Manual*, Peitzman A, Rhodes M, Schwab CW, Yealy DM (eds.) (Philadelphia: Lippincott-Raven, 1998), p. 82.

Bicycle Crashes

Most severe and fatal bicycle injuries involve head trauma. Other injuries associated with bicycle crashes include trauma to the face, limbs, and abdomen (from striking the handlebars). The most common bicycle crashes include the following:

- Riding into a street without stopping
- Turning left or swerving into traffic that is coming from behind
- Running a stop sign
- Riding against the flow of traffic

Bicycle helmets protect against injuries to the mid and upper face. They can also reduce the risk of head injury. A helmet absorbs some of the energy and disperses the blow over a larger area for a slightly longer time. It is estimated that helmets reduce the risk of head injury by 85% and brain injury by 88%.

Among children five to nine years of age, pedestrian injuries are the most common cause of death from trauma. Children are susceptible to pedestrian injuries because of the following factors:

- They have less accurate depth perception.
- They tend to "dart" into traffic.
- They cannot accurately judge the speed of a vehicle.

Children under the age of five years are at risk of being run over in the driveway. Most pedestrian injuries occur during the day, peaking in the period after school. About 30% of pedestrian injuries occur while the child is in a marked crosswalk.

Falls

Falls are a common mechanism of injury. Factors to consider in a fall are:

- The height from which the patient fell
- The patient's weight
- The surface the patient landed on
- The part of the patient's body that struck first

Infants are more likely to fall from changing tables, countertops, and beds. Preschool children usually fall from windows. Older children fall more often from playground equipment. Adults who have jumped rather than fallen from a height tend to land on their feet and then fall onto their buttocks or outstretched hands. Of older adults who fall, 20-30% suffer moderate-to-severe injuries such as hip fractures or head trauma.

The Nature of the Illness

The **nature of the illness** (NOI) describes the medical condition that resulted in the patient's call to 9-1-1. Examples include fever, difficulty breathing, chest pain, headache, and vomiting. Try to find out the nature of the illness by talking to the patient, family, coworkers, and bystanders. If the patient is uncooperative or unresponsive, look to family members or others at the scene as a source of information. Look for clues that may help explain the patient's condition, such as pills, spilled medicine containers, or household or gardening chemicals.

While in a patient's home, look around you. Note the orderliness, cleanliness, and safety of the home (Figure 8-10). Sometimes homes are hazardous because of large collections of paper, trash, or animal waste. Look at the general appearance of the patient and other members of the family. Check if there are any medical devices that may be used by the patient, such as home oxygen equipment or a breathing machine.

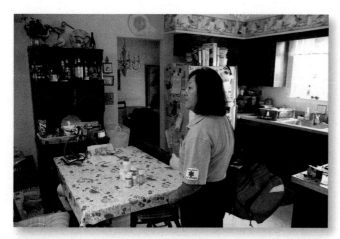

FIGURE 8-10 ▲ While in a patient's home, look around and note the orderliness, cleanliness, and safety of the home.

The Number of Patients

Objective 5

At the scene, you should take appropriate BSI precautions, evaluate scene safety, and determine the mechanism of injury or the nature of the patient's illness. After taking these steps, determine the number of patients. The need for additional resources is based on the correct count of patients at any emergency scene. The number of patients for a medical call in which the patient complains of chest pain may be easy to answer. However, a rollover accident with multiple persons involved may be more difficult to assess. Be alert for patients in addition to the first patient you observe at the scene. Look for clues that other patients may be present. Clues might include toys, diapers, bottles, school books, a purse, or a child safety seat.

It is important to quickly find out the number of patients on the scene in order to request additional resources if necessary. In most situations, one EMS professional is needed for each patient, with one additional professional designated to drive each transporting vehicle. If a patient is severely ill or injured, two or more EMS professionals may be needed to provide emergency care. If there are more patients than you can effectively handle, call for additional help.

Remember This!

Call for additional help *before* you make contact with the patient. Once you begin patient care, you will have fewer chances to make the call.

While waiting for the arrival of more resources, determine the patients that must be treated first. The process of sorting patients by the severity of their illness or injury is called **triage.** This information is covered in more detail in Chapter 29.

Additional Resources

Objective 6

Determine if more help is needed at the scene. Types of additional help that may be needed are shown in Table 8-6. Contact the dispatcher as soon you recognize the need for more resources.

TABLE 8-6   Scene Hazards and Possible Resources

Scene Hazard	Possible Resources
Traffic control, crime or violent scene	Law enforcement personnel
Complex extrication	Fire department, special rescue team
Hazardous materials	Fire department, hazardous materials team
Confined space	Fire department, special rescue team
Swift-water rescue	Fire department, special rescue team
High-angle rescue	Fire department, special rescue team
Trench rescue	Fire department, special rescue team
Downed power lines	Fire department, electric utility company
Natural gas leak	Fire department, gas utility company
Dangerous pets	Animal control
Mass-casualty incident	Law enforcement, fire department, Advanced Life Support personnel, ground ambulances, air ambulances, municipal and public school bus services (if needed), Federal Emergency Management Agency (FEMA) (if needed), National Guard (if needed)

Remember This!

Scene size-up is an ongoing process. Alter your plan of action as necessary based on the information obtained at the scene, your patient assessment findings, and available resources.

On the Scene Wrap-Up

In each of the emergencies that an EMT responds to, the safety of the crew, the patient, and bystanders rests solely with the concept that scene size-up will dictate the course of action leading to the safest outcome for all personnel on the scene. This is a call where you must pay particular attention to details about the scene, e.g., there are newspapers in the driveway; there is no technical rescue or access problem.

As you cautiously enter the house, you notice a man lying on the living room sofa. You approach him and shake him gently as you say, "I'm an EMT. Sir, are you all right?" There is no response. You place a hand on his forehead, lift his chin, and look, listen, and feel for breathing. He is breathing quietly, about 16 times per minute. When you reach to feel his radial pulse, you notice his skin is cool, dry, and pale. His heart rate is about 100 beats per minute. Your partner tells you the patient's blood pressure is 114/66. You do not find any other abnormal findings in your examination. A police officer performs a quick search of the patient's home and finds a number of prescribed medicines for a heart condition but nothing that is unusual.

You apply oxygen by nonrebreather mask at 15 L/min. You quickly check the patient's blood sugar, which is normal. You contact medical direction and are instructed to load the patient immediately and transport to the closest appropriate hospital. You leave the scene with lights and sirens on to hasten your arrival to the hospital. When transporting another patient to the same hospital later in your shift, you learn that the patient had a stroke. He was transferred to the critical care unit. ■

Sum It Up

▶ As an EMT, you must quickly look at the entire scene before approaching the patient. You must size up the scene to find out if there are any threats that may cause injury to you, other rescuers, or bystanders or that may cause additional injury to the patient.

▶ Scene size-up is the first phase of patient assessment and is made up of 5 parts:
1. BSI precautions
2. Evaluating scene safety
3. Determining the mechanism of injury (including considerations for stabilization of the spine) or the nature of the patient's illness
4. Determining the total number of patients
5. Determining the need for additional resources

▶ You must take appropriate BSI precautions on *every* call. Consider the need for BSI precautions before you approach the patient. Put on appropriate PPE on the basis of the information the dispatcher gives you and your initial survey of the scene. This equipment includes gloves, eye protection, mask, and gown, if necessary.

▶ Scene safety is an assessment of the entire scene and surroundings to ensure your well-being and that of other rescuers, the patient(s), and bystanders.

▶ During the scene size-up, try to determine the nature of the illness or mechanism of injury.

▶ A medical patient is one whose condition is caused by an illness. The nature of the illness (NOI) describes the medical condition that resulted in the patient's call to 9-1-1. Examples include fever, difficulty breathing, chest pain, headache, and vomiting. You should try to find out the nature of the illness by talking to the patient, family, coworkers, and bystanders.

▶ Mechanism of injury (MOI) refers to the way in which an injury occurs as well as the forces involved in producing the injury. Kinetic energy is the energy of motion. The amount of kinetic energy an object has depends on the mass (weight) and speed (velocity) of the object. Kinematics is the science of analyzing the mechanism of injury and predicting injury patterns. The amount of injury is determined by the following three elements: (1) the type of energy applied, (2) how quickly the energy is applied, and (3) to what part of the body the energy is applied.

▶ A trauma patient is one who has experienced an injury from an external force. Traumatic situations include motor vehicle crashes, motor vehicle–pedestrian crashes, falls, bicycle crashes, motorcycle crashes, and penetrating traumas.

▶ Blunt trauma is any mechanism of injury that occurs without actual penetration of the body. Examples of mechanisms of injury causing blunt trauma include motor vehicle crashes, falls, sports injuries, or assaults with a blunt object. Blunt trauma produces injury first to the body surface and then to the body's contents.

► Penetrating trauma is any mechanism of injury that causes a cut or piercing of the skin. Examples of mechanisms of injury causing penetrating trauma include gunshot wounds, stab wounds, and blast injuries. Penetrating trauma usually affects organs and tissues in the direct path of the wounding object.

► A motor vehicle crash is classified by the type of impact. The five types of impact include head on (frontal), lateral, rear end, rotational, and rollover.

► In a frontal impact, such as a head-on collision, the vehicle stops and the occupants continue to move forward by one of two pathways: down and under or up and over.

- In the down and under pathway, the victim's knees impact the vehicle's dashboard. The down and under pathway may be seen when the occupant is not wearing a lap and shoulder restraint system or when the occupant is wearing only the shoulder harness and not a lap belt.

- In the up and over pathway, the victim's upper body strikes the steering wheel, resulting in injuries to the head, chest, abdomen, pelvis, and/or spine. The up and over pathway may be seen when the occupant is not wearing a lap and shoulder restraint system, or when the occupant is wearing only a lap restraint (not the shoulder harness).

► Although mechanism of injury is important, it is not the only factor to consider when assessing a trauma patient and determining whether or not he is a priority patient. For some patients, the risk of significant injury is increased because of their age or a preexisting medical condition, despite what may appear to be a "minor" mechanism of injury. In some EMS systems, other factors for designating "priority" status are considered in addition to the mechanism of injury. These include anatomy, physiology, and patient factors.

► Adult pedestrians will typically turn away if they are about to be struck by an oncoming vehicle. This action results in injuries to the side or back of the body. A child will usually face an oncoming vehicle, which results in injuries to the front of the body.

► Falls are a common mechanism of injury. Factors to consider in a fall are include the height from which the patient fell, the patient's weight, the surface the patient landed on, and the part of the patient's body that struck first.

Patient Assessment

By the end of this chapter, you should be able to:

Knowledge Objectives ▶

1. Summarize the reasons for forming a general impression of the patient.
2. Discuss methods of assessing altered mental status.
3. Differentiate between assessing the altered mental status in the adult, child, and infant patient.
4. Discuss methods of assessing the airway in the adult, child, and infant patient.
5. State reasons for management of the cervical spine once the patient has been determined to be a trauma patient.
6. Describe methods used for assessing if a patient is breathing.
7. State what care should be provided to the adult, child, and infant patient with adequate breathing.
8. State what care should be provided to the adult, child, and infant patient without adequate breathing.
9. Differentiate between a patient with adequate and inadequate breathing.
10. Distinguish between methods of assessing breathing in the adult, child, and infant patient.
11. Compare the methods of providing airway care to the adult, child, and infant patient.
12. Describe the methods used to obtain a pulse.
13. Differentiate between obtaining a pulse in an adult, child, and infant patient.
14. Discuss the need for assessing the patient for external bleeding.
15. Describe normal and abnormal findings when assessing skin color.
16. Describe normal and abnormal findings when assessing skin temperature.
17. Describe normal and abnormal findings when assessing skin condition.
18. Describe normal and abnormal findings when assessing skin capillary refill in the infant or child patient.
19. Explain the reason for prioritizing a patient for care and transport.
20. Discuss the reasons for reconsideration concerning the MOI.
21. State the reasons for performing a rapid trauma assessment.
22. Recite examples and explain why patients should receive a rapid trauma assessment.
23. Describe the areas included in the rapid trauma assessment and discuss what should be evaluated.

24. Differentiate when the rapid assessment may be altered in order to provide patient care.

25. Discuss the reason for performing a focused history and physical exam.

26. Describe the unique needs for assessing an individual with a specific chief complaint with no known prior history.

27. Differentiate between the history and physical exam that is performed for responsive patients with no known prior history and the history and physical exam that is performed for responsive patients with a known prior history.

28. Describe the unique needs for assessing an individual who is unresponsive or has an altered mental status.

29. Differentiate between the assessment that is performed for a patient who is unresponsive or has an altered mental status and other medical patients requiring assessment.

30. Discuss the components of the secondary survey.

31. State the areas of the body that are evaluated during the secondary survey.

32. Explain what additional care should be provided while you are performing the secondary survey.

33. Distinguish between the secondary survey that is performed on a trauma patient and the one performed on the medical patient.

34. Discuss the reasons for repeating the primary survey as part of the ongoing assessment.

35. Describe the components of the ongoing assessment.

36. Describe trending of assessment components.

Attitude Objectives ▶ **37.** Explain the importance of forming a general impression of the patient.

38. Explain the value of performing a primary survey.

39. Recognize and respect the feelings that patients might experience during assessment.

40. Attend to the feelings that these patients might be experiencing.

41. Explain the rationale for the feelings that these patients might be experiencing.

42. Explain the value of performing an ongoing assessment.

43. Recognize and respect the feelings that patients might experience during assessment.

44. Explain the value of trending assessment components to other health professionals who assume care of the patient.

Skill Objectives ▶ **45.** Demonstrate the techniques for assessing mental status.

46. Demonstrate the techniques for assessing the airway.

47. Demonstrate the techniques for assessing if the patient is breathing.

48. Demonstrate the techniques for assessing if the patient has a pulse.

49. Demonstrate the techniques for assessing the patient for external bleeding.

50. Demonstrate the techniques for assessing the patient's skin color, temperature, condition, and capillary refill (infants and children only).

51. Demonstrate the ability to prioritize patients.

52. Demonstrate the rapid trauma assessment that should be used to assess a patient on the basis of mechanism of injury.

53. Demonstrate the patient assessment skills that should be used to assist with a patient who is responsive with no known history.

54. Demonstrate the patient assessment skills that should be used to assist with a patient who is unresponsive or has an altered metal status.

55. Demonstrate the skills involved in performing the secondary survey.

56. Demonstrate the skills involved in performing the ongoing assessment.

On the Scene

You are dispatched to a local park for a person who has an unknown problem. Upon arrival, you find a 20-year-old man lying next to his bicycle. He has a severely angulated left forearm and is bleeding from a cut on his left forehead. You notice that his lips are slightly blue and his respiratory rate is 30 breaths per minute. He is responsive and responds to your questions but cannot remember what happened. He keeps asking the same questions repeatedly. ■

THINK ABOUT IT

As you read this chapter, think about the following questions:

- What do you suspect happened?
- How does the size-up of the scene give you information about the patient's condition or possible injuries? Is that information pertinent to your initial assessment?
- What does your patient's mental status indicate?
- Should you be concerned about the patient's respiratory rate and the bluish color of his lips?

Introduction

The Importance of Patient Assessment

You will be taught many skills during your Emergency Medical Technician (EMT) course. Of all the skills you will learn, the most important skill is patient assessment. Every decision you make about the care of your patient is based on what you find during your patient assessment. In this chapter you will learn the steps needed to properly assess a patient. In Chapter 8, you learned that the scene size-up is the first phase of patient assessment. In this chapter you will learn about the primary and secondary surveys, and differences in the assessment of trauma and medical patients.

An Overview of Patient Assessment

The ability to properly assess a patient is one of the most important skills you can master. You must learn to work quickly and efficiently in all types of situations.

Some situations may include poor lighting conditions, temperature extremes, large numbers of people, and being in a moving ambulance. To work efficiently, you must approach patient assessment systematically. The emergency care you provide to your patient will be based on your assessment findings.

While assessing your patient, you will discover his signs and symptoms. You must provide emergency medical care based on those signs and symptoms. Discovering the patient's signs and symptoms requires you to use your senses of sight (look), sound (listen), touch (feel), and smell.

- *Look.* You will use your sense of sight to assess parts of the patient's body and his behavior. Does he look sick or poorly nourished? Do you see obvious problems such as a rash, external bleeding, vomiting, seizures, an arm or leg deformity, pale or flushed skin, or sweating?

- *Listen.* You will use your sense of hearing to find out why your patient called for assistance. You will also listen to find out if the patient is breathing normally, if he is having difficulty breathing, or if breathing is absent. You will use a stethoscope to listen to the patient's lung sounds. You will use a stethoscope and blood pressure cuff to take a blood pressure.

- *Feel.* You will use your sense of touch to find out important information about your patient. Using your hands or forearms, you can find out if the patient's skin is hot, warm, cool, or cold. You can also determine if a body part is hard, soft, or swollen. You will also determine if touching a part of the patient's body causes pain.
- *Smell.* Your will use your sense of smell to identify odors associated with specific problems. For example, a sweetish (fruity) breath odor can indicate a diabetic problem. The smell of alcohol may explain why a patient is slow to answer your questions.

Patient assessment consists of the following components (Figure 9-1):

- Initial assessment
  —Scene size-up (see Chapter 8)
  —Primary survey (ABCDE assessment)

PATIENT ASSESSMENT

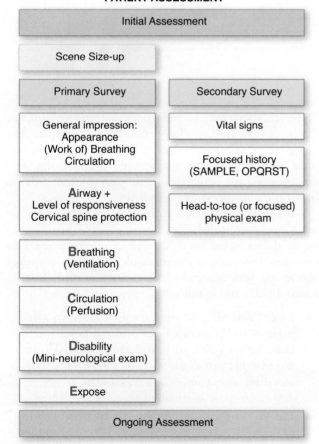

FIGURE 9-1 ▲ The initial assessment.

  —Secondary survey
  - Vital signs
  - Focused history
  - Head-to-toe physical examination
- Ongoing assessment

The primary survey is a rapid assessment to find and treat all immediate life-threatening conditions. During this phase of patient assessment, you will look for and treat life-threatening conditions as you discover them ("find and fix"; "treat as you go") and decide if the patient needs immediate transport or additional on-scene assessment and treatment. The secondary survey is a physical examination performed to discover medical conditions and/or injuries that were not identified in the primary survey. During this phase of the patient assessment, you will also obtain vital signs, reassess changes in the patient's condition, and determine the patient's chief complaint, history of present illness, and significant past medical history. The secondary survey does not begin until the primary survey has been completed and treatment of life-threatening conditions has begun.

You Should Know

An organized approach to patient assessment helps to make certain that no significant findings or problems are missed.

Performing the Primary Survey

As mentioned above, the primary survey is a rapid assessment of the patient to find and care for immediate life-threatening conditions. You must perform a primary survey on *every* patient. The primary survey begins after the scene or situation has been found safe or made safe and you have gained access to the patient. It usually requires less than 60 seconds to complete. However, it may take longer if you must provide emergency care to correct an identified problem. Remember to wear appropriate personal protective equipment (PPE) before approaching the patient.

The primary survey has several parts (Table 9-1):

- General impression
- *A*irway/level of responsiveness/cervical spine protection
- *B*reathing (ventilation)
- *C*irculation with bleeding control (perfusion)
- *D*isability (mini-neurological exam)
- *E*xpose (for examination)
- Identification of priority patients

TABLE 9-1 Components of Patient Assessment

Initial Assessment

Scene size-up	• Take body substance isolation precautions • Evaluate scene safety • Determine the mechanism of injury or the nature of the patient's illness • Determine the total number of patients • Determine the need for additional resources
Primary survey	• General impression 　—Appearance 　—(Work of) Breathing 　—Circulation • *A*irway, level of responsiveness, cervical spine protection • *B*reathing (Ventilation) • *C*irculation (Perfusion) • *D*isability (mini-neurological exam) • *E*xpose • Identify priority patients
Secondary survey	• Vital signs, pulse oximetry • Focused SAMPLE history, OPQRST • Head-to-toe or focused physical examination
Ongoing Assessment	• Repeat the primary survey • Reassess vital signs • Repeat the focused assessment regarding patient complaint or injuries • Reevaluate emergency care

General Impression

Objective 1

Whenever you meet someone for the first time, you form a first impression—sometimes without realizing it. You will do the same thing with every patient. A **general impression** (also called a *first impression*) is an "across-the-room" assessment. As you approach him, you will form a general impression without the patient's telling you what his complaint is. You can complete it in 60 seconds or less. The purpose of forming a general impression is to decide if the patient looks "sick" or "not sick." If the patient looks sick, you must act quickly. As you gain experience, you will develop an instinct for quickly recognizing when a patient is sick.

Before you speak to your patient and find out what is wrong, stop a short distance from her

Remember This!

Your patient's condition can change at any time. A patient that initially appears "not sick" may rapidly worsen and appear "sick." Reassess your patient often.

(Figure 9-2). Look and listen. What things stand out in your mind when you first see her?

- Does the patient look ill (medical patient) or injured (trauma patient)? If the patient looks ill, are there clues around you that suggest the nature of the illness? For example, the presence of an oxygen tank suggests that someone in the home has a chronic medical condition. If the patient is injured, what is the mechanism of injury (MOI)?
- How old do you think the patient is? Is the patient male or female?

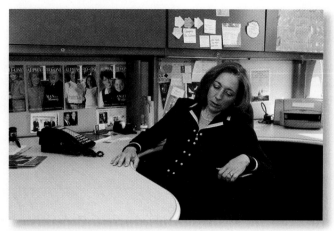

FIGURE 9-2 ▲ Form a general impression by pausing a short distance from the patient.

- Does the patient look sick? If she looks sick, she may have a life-threatening problem. Life-threatening problems must be treated immediately. Examples of life-threatening problems include unresponsiveness, a blocked airway, absent breathing (respiratory arrest), and severe bleeding. If you find a life-threatening condition, you must treat it before going on to the next step.

Making a Difference

Some say that your "intuition" helps you form a general impression of a patient. Actually, a combination of knowledge, careful observation, effective communication, and experience is what forms that "intuition."

You will base your general impression of a patient on three main areas: (1) appearance, (2) breathing, and (3) circulation. Remember: Approach a patient only after making sure that the scene is safe.

1. *Appearance.* Unless the patient is sleeping, his eyes should be open. His eyes should follow you as you move. If he looks agitated, limp, or appears to be asleep, approach him immediately and begin the primary survey.
2. *(Work of) Breathing.* With normal breathing, both sides of the chest rise and fall equally. Normal breathing is quiet, painless, and occurs at a regular rate. Approach the patient immediately and begin the primary survey if the patient:
   - Looks as if he is struggling (laboring) to breathe
   - Has noisy breathing
   - Is breathing faster or more slowly than normal
   - Looks as if his chest is not moving normally

3. *Circulation.* The patient's skin color should be normal for his ethnic group. Approach the patient immediately and begin the primary survey if the patient's skin looks flushed (red), pale (whitish color), gray, or blue (cyanotic).

Some refer to the general impression as the "big picture." If your general impression reveals an urgent problem, move quickly. Begin emergency care and arrange for immediate patient transport. If your general impression does not reveal an urgent problem, work at a reasonable pace and continue your patient assessment. Remember to explain what you are doing to the patient and family.

Remember This!

During the primary survey, find the answers to these five questions:

1. Is the patient awake and alert?
2. Is the patient's airway open?
3. Is the patient breathing?
4. Does the patient have a pulse?
5. Does the patient have severe bleeding?

Airway, Level of Responsiveness, and Cervical Spine Protection

After forming a general impression, begin the primary survey by assessing the patient's airway and level of responsiveness. Assessment of a patient's airway and level of responsiveness occur at the same time. If the patient appears to be awake, start by telling him your first name. Let him know you are an EMT. Explain that you are there to help. Next, ask your patient a question like, "Why did you call 9-1-1 today?" His answer will give you some important information.

You Should Know
Chief Complaint

In many cases, the patient's chief complaint will be the reason you were called to the scene. However, the patient's chief complaint may turn out to be different from the reason you were called. For example, a family member may call 9-1-1 and tell the dispatcher that the patient is complaining of difficulty breathing. When you arrive and speak directly to the patient, you may find that he is complaining of chest pain and has no complaint of difficulty breathing. Document the chief complaint using the patient's description of what is wrong.

First, it will tell you if his airway is open. Second, it will tell you his level of responsiveness. Third, the patient's answer should be his **chief complaint.** A chief complaint is the reason Emergency Medical Services (EMS) was called, usually in the patient's own words.

Airway

The human body must have a continuous supply of oxygen to survive. Air containing oxygen enters the body through the nose and mouth. It travels down the throat (pharynx), through the windpipe (trachea), and into the lungs. In the lungs, oxygen is transferred to the blood. The oxygen-rich blood is circulated to every cell in the body. The cells of the body cannot live long without oxygen. Therefore, a life-threatening emergency can result if the flow of air is blocked (obstructed) or if oxygen-rich blood is not circulated throughout the body.

Objective 4

A patient who is alert and talking clearly or crying without difficulty has a **patent** (open) airway. The airway is the pathway from the nose and mouth to the lungs. If the patient is unable to speak, cry, cough, or make any other sound, his airway is completely obstructed. If the patient has noisy breathing, such as snoring or gurgling, he has a partial airway obstruction.

Objective 11

If the patient is unresponsive and you do not suspect trauma, open his airway by using the head tilt–chin lift maneuver (Figure 9-3). If the patient is unresponsive

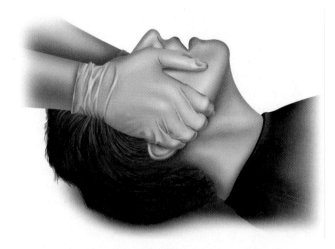

FIGURE 9-4 ▲ If you suspect trauma, use the jaw thrust without head tilt maneuver to open the airway of a patient who is unresponsive.

and you suspect trauma, open his airway by using the jaw thrust without head tilt (extension) (Figure 9-4). Both of these maneuvers lift the tongue away from the back of the throat, allowing air to enter the lungs. If you are unable to open the airway (or maintain an open airway) by using the jaw thrust without head tilt maneuver, use the head tilt–chin lift maneuver. If the patient is an unresponsive infant or child, do not hyperextend the neck when opening the airway.

Look for an actual or potential airway obstruction, such as a foreign body, blood, vomitus, teeth, or the patient's tongue. The tongue is the most common cause of a blocked airway in an unresponsive patient. If there is blood, vomitus, or other fluid in the patient's airway, clear it with suctioning.

Level of Responsiveness (Mental Status)
Objective 2

Level of responsiveness is also called *level of consciousness* or *mental status.* These terms refer to a patient's level of awareness. A patient's mental status is "graded" using a scale called the **AVPU scale** as follows.

- A = *A*lert
- V = Responds to *V*erbal stimuli
- P = Responds to *P*ainful stimuli
- U = *U*nresponsive

If the patient looks as if he is sleeping, gently rub his shoulder and ask, "Are you OK?" or "Can you hear me?" Unresponsiveness may indicate a life-threatening condition. If the patient does not answer, family or bystanders may be able to supply information. You may ask, "Can you tell me what happened?"

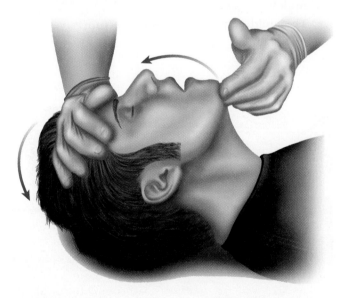

FIGURE 9-3 ▲ If you do not suspect trauma, use the head tilt–chin lift maneuver to open the airway of a patient who is unresponsive.

Determine if the patient is awake and responds appropriately to questions. Evaluate his orientation to the following:

- Person (the patient can tell you his name)
- Place (the patient can tell you where he is)
- Time (the patient can tell you the day, date, or time)
- Event (the patient can tell you what happened)

A patient who is speaking or crying is responsive (conscious), breathing, and has a pulse. A patient who is oriented to person, place, time, and event is said to be "alert and oriented × ('times') 4" or "A and O × 4." If your patient is awake but cannot answer these questions correctly, the patient is said to be confused or disoriented. For example, if your patient is awake and knows his name (alert and oriented to person) and where he is (alert and oriented to place) but does not know what day it is and cannot tell you what happened, he is said to be "alert and oriented × 2."

If the patient is not awake but responds appropriately when spoken to, he is said to "respond to verbal stimuli." For example, the patient will respond correctly to a request such as "squeeze my fingers." If the patient is not awake but responds to a painful stimulus, such as pinching the skin on the back of the hand or ear lobe, he is said to "respond to painful stimuli" (Figure 9-5). The patient is unresponsive if he does not respond to a verbal or painful stimulus. Again, it is important to note what kind of stimulus is applied and what the patient's response to it is.

As you continue your assessment, note any changes in the patient's mental status. The brain requires a constant supply of oxygen and sugar. Changes in the patient's level of responsiveness may result from a decreased supply of oxygen or sugar. These changes may also come from the use of alcohol or drugs, brain swelling caused by injury, or other causes. In a trauma patient, agitation and combativeness may be caused by a decreased supply of oxygen.

It is important to document (and report) which realms of orientation the patient is disoriented to. If Advanced Life Support (ALS) personnel arrive on the scene, be sure to tell them about any changes in the patient's mental status. Otherwise, relay this information to the staff person who takes the report from you at the hospital. In your prehospital care report, document the patient's response to a specific stimulus and any changes in mental status, for example, "The patient opened his eyes on command," "The patient moaned in response to a pinch on the wrist," or "The patient knows his name but does not know the date, where he is, or what happened."

Infants and Children

Objective 3

An alert infant or young child (younger than three years of age) smiles, orients to sound, follows objects with her eyes, and interacts with those around her (Figure 9-6). As the infant or young child's mental status decreases, the following changes may be seen (in order of decreasing mental status):

- The child may cry but can be comforted.
- The child may show inappropriate, persistent crying.
- The child may become irritable, agitated, and restless.
- The child may have no response (unresponsive).

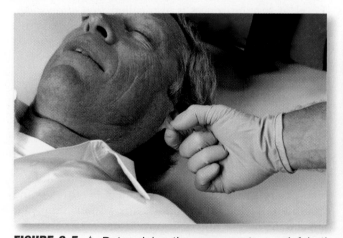
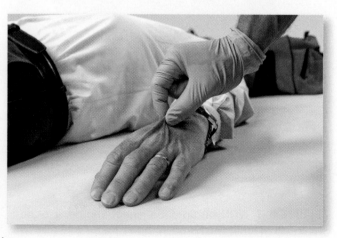

FIGURE 9-5 ▲ Determining the response to a painful stimulus.

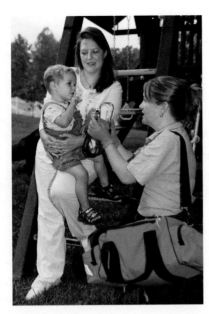

FIGURE 9-6 ▲ An alert infant or young child smiles, orients to sound, follows objects with her eyes, and interacts with those around her.

Assessing the mental status of a child older than three years of age is the same as assessing the mental status of an adult.

Making a Difference

Assessing a young child can be difficult. Toddlers distrust strangers and are likely to resist your attempts to examine them. They do not like having their clothing removed. They fear pain, separation from their caregiver, and separation from their favorite blanket or toy. When possible, assess the child in the arms or lap of his caregiver. Approach the child slowly and talk to him at eye level. Use simple words and phrases and a reassuring tone of voice. The child will understand your tone even if he does not understand your words.

Cervical Spine Protection

Objective 5

For trauma patients or unresponsive patients with an unknown nature of illness, take **spinal precautions.** Spinal precautions are used to stabilize the head, neck, and back in a neutral position. This stabilization is done to minimize movement that could cause injury to the spinal cord. The technique used to minimize movement of the head and neck is called **in-line stabilization.** The term *in-line* refers to keeping the head and neck anatomically in line with the body. In-line stabilization

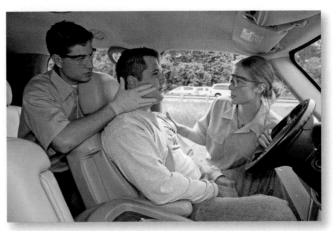

FIGURE 9-7 ▲ In-line stabilization requires keeping the head and neck anatomically in line with the body.

is first performed by using your hands. This is called manual stabilization. Manual stabilization is a temporary maneuver. The patient's head is not considered stabilized until it is secured to a long backboard.

If the patient is awake and you suspect trauma to the head, neck, or back, face the patient so that he does not have to turn his head to see you. Instruct him not to move his head or neck. Position your hands on both sides of the patient's head and spread your fingers apart (Figure 9-7). Place the patient's head in a neutral position (eyes facing forward and level) and in line with the body. If the patient complains of pain or you meet resistance when moving his head and neck to a neutral position, stop and stabilize the head and neck at the point just before resistance was met. Once begun, manual stabilization of the patient's head and neck must be continued without interruption until the patient is properly secured to a long backboard with the head and neck stabilized (Figure 9-8).

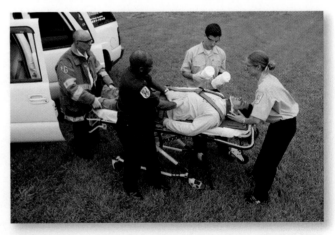

FIGURE 9-8 ▲ Manual stabilization of the patient's head and neck must be continued until the patient is properly secured to a long backboard with the head stabilized.

You Should Know

Examples of emergency care that may be needed to manage the patient's airway during the primary survey include the following:

- Spinal stabilization as needed for trauma
- Head tilt–chin lift or jaw thrust without head tilt
- Suctioning
- Repositioning
- Removal of a foreign body
- Insertion of an oral or nasal airway

Breathing

Objectives 6, 9, 10

The priorities for assessing breathing and providing necessary treatment for infants and children are the same as for adults. After you have made sure that the patient's airway is open, assess his breathing. If the patient is responsive, watch and listen to him as he breathes. Quickly determine if his breathing is adequate or inadequate (see the following *You Should Know* box). Keep in mind that normal respiratory rates for infants and children are faster than for adults.

If the patient is unresponsive, look, listen, and feel for breathing (Figure 9-9). Look for a rise and fall of the chest. Because the diaphragm is the main muscle used for breathing in infants and young children, watch the abdomen when assessing breathing. Look at the chest to assess breathing in older children and adults. Listen for air movement. Determine if breathing is absent, quiet, or noisy. Feel for air movement from the patient's nose or mouth against your chin, face, or palm. If breathing is present, quickly

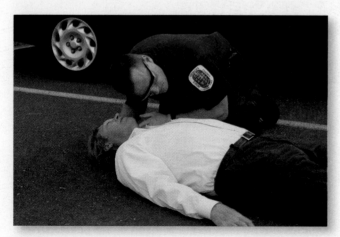

FIGURE 9-9 ▲ If the patient is unresponsive, look, listen, and feel for breathing.

determine if breathing is adequate or inadequate. Breathing that is too fast or too slow for the patient's age is a "red flag" that requires a search for the cause.

You Should Know

Characteristics of Adequate and Inadequate Breathing

Adequate Breathing

- The breathing effort (work of breathing) is quiet, relaxed, and effortless.
- The breathing rate is within normal limits for the patient's age.
- The breathing pattern is regular.
- Both sides of the chest rise and fall equally.
- The depth of breathing is adequate.
- Skin color is normal; skin is warm and dry to the touch.

Inadequate Breathing

- The patient's appearance is anxious; the patient concentrates on breathing.
- The patient is confused and restless.
- The breathing rate is too fast or slow for the patient's age.
- The breathing pattern is irregular.
- The depth of breathing is unusually deep or shallow.
- Breathing is noisy (snoring, gurgling, wheezing).
- The patient is sitting upright and leaning forward to breathe.
- The patient is unable to speak in complete sentences.
- The patient has pain with breathing.
- The patient's skin may look flushed, pale, gray, or blue, and feel cold and sweaty.
- The chest rise and fall is unequal.
- Muscles in the neck, above the collarbone, between the ribs, or below the rib cage are used to breathe.

Objective 7

If breathing is adequate and the patient is responsive, allow him to assume a comfortable position. Remember that emergency care for life-threatening conditions is given during the primary survey. For example, if your primary survey reveals that the patient needs oxygen, give oxygen by means of a nonrebreather mask or other oxygen delivery device before continuing the rest of the steps in the assessment.

If the patient is unresponsive and his breathing is adequate, maintain an open airway. Use airway adjuncts, such as an oral airway, if needed. Place the patient in the recovery position if there are no contraindications. Provide oxygen by nonrebreather mask. Watch the patient closely to make sure that adequate breathing continues.

Objective 8

If the patient is unresponsive and breathing is inadequate or if the patient is not breathing, begin positive-pressure ventilation using a pocket mask, mouth-to-barrier device, or bag-mask (BM) device. If the patient has dentures and they fit well, leave them in place to help provide a good mask seal. If the dentures are loose, remove them so that they do not fall back into the throat and obstruct the airway. Watch the patient's chest while you ventilate the patient. If your ventilations are going in, you should see the patient's chest rise gently with each breath. Continue breathing for the patient until he begins to breathe adequately on his own or another trained rescuer takes over.

Remember This!

If the patient is not breathing, his heart will stop beating unless you begin breathing for him. When giving positive-pressure ventilations, give breaths with just enough force to see the patient's chest rise gently with each breath. If you ventilate the patient too fast or use too much force, you can blow air into the patient's stomach. Too much air in the stomach can cause vomiting.

If your initial breath does not go in, gently reposition the patient's head and breathe for him again. If there is still no chest rise, begin cardiopulmonary resuscitation (CPR). Check the patient's mouth for a foreign body each time you open the airway to give rescue breaths (see Appendix A).

You Should Know

Examples of emergency care that may be needed to manage the patient's breathing during the primary survey include the following:

- Giving oxygen
- Suctioning
- Repositioning
- Removal of a foreign body
- Insertion of an oral or nasal airway
- Positive-pressure ventilation

Circulation

The assessment of circulation involves evaluating the following:

- Signs of obvious bleeding
- Central and peripheral pulses
- Skin color, temperature, and condition
- Capillary refill (in children less than six years of age)

Obvious Bleeding

Objective 14

Look from head to toes for signs of significant external bleeding. Control major bleeding, if present, by applying direct pressure over the bleeding site. Apply a pressure bandage if needed.

Stop and Think!

Dark clothing, waterproof clothing, or many layers of clothing may mask severe bleeding. Expose the injury site and look closely for bleeding in these situations.

Pulses

Objectives 12, 13

When assessing a *responsive* adult or a child one year of age or older, first check the radial pulse in the wrist. Use the carotid artery in the neck to check the pulse of an *unresponsive* adult or child older than one year of age (Figure 9-10). Feel for a brachial pulse in the upper arm of an infant (Figure 9-11). Feel for a pulse for at least 5 but no more than 10 seconds. A heart rate that is too fast or too slow for the patient's age is a "red flag" that requires a search for the cause. If there is no pulse, you must begin chest compressions.

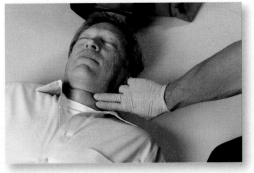

FIGURE 9-10 ▲ Use the carotid artery to check the pulse of an unresponsive adult or child older than one year of age.

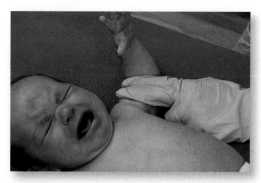

FIGURE 9-11 ▲ In infants, feel for a brachial pulse.

Making a Difference

Practice finding pulses on adults and children of various ages. Knowing how to find a normal pulse in a healthy patient will help you recognize what is abnormal.

Skin Color, Temperature, and Condition

While assessing the patient's pulse, quickly check the patient's skin. Assessing the patient's skin condition can provide important information about the flow of blood through the body's tissues (perfusion). Assess perfusion by evaluating skin color, temperature, and condition (moist, dry). In infants and children younger than six years of age, capillary refill is also used to assess perfusion.

You Should Know

Perfusion is the flow of blood through the body's tissues. Perfusion requires a functioning pump (the heart), adequate blood volume (fluid), and an intact vascular system (container).

Skin Color

Objective 15

Assess the patient's skin color in the palms of the hands, soles of the feet, inside the mouth, and inside the eyelids. In infants and children, assess the palms and soles. In Caucasians, normal skin color is pink. Abnormal skin colors include the following:

- Pale skin suggests poor perfusion (impaired blood flow) resulting from shock, fright, anxiety, blood loss or other causes.
- Cyanotic (blue) skin suggests low levels of oxygen resulting from inadequate breathing or poor perfusion.

- Mottled (patches of blue and white) skin may be seen in shock, hypothermia, or cardiac arrest.
- Jaundiced (yellow) skin suggests liver or gallbladder problems.
- Flushed (red) skin suggests heat exposure, high blood pressure, an allergic reaction, alcohol abuse, or the late stages of carbon monoxide poisoning.

Skin Temperature

Objective 16

Assess skin temperature by placing the back of your hand against the patient's face, neck, or abdomen. Normal skin temperature is warm. Hot skin may be caused by fever or heat exposure. Cool skin may be caused by inadequate circulation or exposure to cold. Cold skin may be caused by extreme exposure to cold or shock. Clammy (cool and moist) skin may be caused by shock, among many other conditions.

Skin Condition

Objective 17

Assess the patient's skin condition (moisture). Normal skin is dry. Wet or moist skin may indicate shock, a heat-related illness, or a diabetic emergency. Excessively dry skin may indicate dehydration.

Capillary Refill

Objective 18

Assess capillary refill in infants and children younger than six years of age. Firmly press the skin over the warmest point on the child's body (such as the chest or abdomen) and release. If the temperature of the environment is warm, color should return within two seconds. Other sites used to assess capillary refill include the forehead or fleshy part of the palm. Capillary refill in adults is an unreliable indicator of perfusion because it is easily affected by medications, chronic medical conditions, cold weather, and smoking.

Remember This!

Capillary Refill

1. Normal: less than two seconds
2. Delayed: refill time of three to five seconds
3. Markedly delayed: refill time of more than five seconds

Disability

Altered mental status means a change in a patient's level of awareness. Altered mental status is also called an *altered level of consciousness* (ALOC). Common causes of an altered mental status are shown in the following *You Should Know* box. A patient who has an altered mental status is at risk of an airway obstruction. As awareness decreases, muscle tone decreases. When this occurs, the tongue can fall back into the throat and cause an airway obstruction. The breathing muscles may not expand and contract as strongly as normal. This can result in inadequate breathing, low blood oxygen, and respiratory failure.

The AVPU scale is used early in the primary survey to assess responsiveness. Most EMS systems use the Glasgow Coma Scale (GCS) during the disability phase of the primary survey to obtain a more detailed assessment of the patient's neurological status. This mini-neurological examination is used to establish a baseline level of responsiveness and note any obvious problem with central nervous system (brain and spinal cord) function. Three categories are assessed with the GCS: (1) eye opening, (2) verbal response, and (3) motor response (see Table 9-2). The Glasgow Coma Scale score is the sum of the scores in three categories. The lowest possible score possible is 3. The highest possible score is 15. A patient who has a score in the range of 3 to 8 is usually said to be in a coma. When relaying GCS information to the healthcare professional assuming care of your patient, do not provide only the sum of the three categories. Instead, provide him with the sum in each category *and* the total score. For example, "Eye opening = 3, verbal response = 4, and motor response = 4. Total GCS score = 11." In this way, improvement or worsening of the patient's condition can be more closely assessed.

If the patient has an altered mental status and cannot maintain his own airway, open (or position) the airway by using a manual maneuver and insert an oral or nasal airway as needed. Suction as necessary. Give oxygen. If the patient's breathing is adequate, apply oxygen by mask at 15 L/min. If the patient's breathing is inadequate, assist his breathing with a BM or mouth-to-mask device. Position the patient. If the patient is sitting or standing, help him to a position of comfort on a firm surface. If there is no possibility of trauma to the head or spine, place him in the recovery position. Assess the patient's blood glucose level per local protocol (see Chapter 18).

Expose

When assessing a patient, you can't treat what you don't find. Expose pertinent areas of the patient's body for examination. Factors that you must consider when exposing the patient include protecting the patient's modesty, the presence of bystanders, and environment/weather conditions.

TABLE 9-2 Adult, Child, and Infant Glasgow Coma Scale

Eye Opening	Spontaneous, opens with blinking	4	Spontaneous
	Responds to verbal command, speech, or shout	3	Responds to verbal
	Responds to pain	2	Responds to pain
	No response	1	No response
Best Verbal Response	Oriented	5	Coos, babbles
	Confused, but able to answer questions	4	Irritable cry but can be comforted
	Confused; answers with inappropriate words	3	Inappropriate crying or screaming
	Incomprehensible sounds	2	Grunting or agitated, restless
	No response	1	No response
Best Motor Response	Obeys commands	6	Spontaneous
	Purposeful response to pain	5	Purposeful response to touch
	Withdraws from pain	4	Withdraws from pain
	Abnormal flexion (decorticate)	3	Abnormal flexion (decorticate)
	Abnormal extension (decerebrate)	2	Abnormal extension (decerebrate)
	No response	1	No response
	Total = E + V + M	3 to 15	

Removing the clothing of a medical patient may reveal a medical identification bracelet or necklace, implanted pacemaker or defibrillator, surgical scars, swollen tissue, or other important findings. Removing clothing of a trauma patient may reveal injured areas that would otherwise go unnoticed. Clothing that might impair patient movement, respirations, or distal circulation should be removed. Remember to keep the patient warm.

Identifying Priority Patients

Objective 19

Determine if the patient requires on-scene stabilization or immediate transport with additional emergency care en route to a hospital. Patients who require immediate transport ("load and go") include the following:

- Patients who give a poor general impression
- Unresponsive patients
- Responsive patients who cannot follow commands
- Patients who have difficulty breathing
- Patients who are in shock
- Women who are undergoing a complicated childbirth
- Patients with chest pain and a systolic blood pressure less than 100 mm Hg
- Patients with uncontrolled bleeding
- Patients with severe pain anywhere

Performing the Secondary Survey

Objectives 30, 33

A secondary survey is typically a head-to-toe examination. The reason the secondary survey is performed is to find other injuries or signs of illness that may affect the emergency care you provide. This examination is performed only after you have found and treated all life-threatening injuries or illnesses.

The secondary survey is patient, situation, and time dependent. For instance, a patient with an isolated injury, such as a painful ankle, would typically not require a head-to-toe physical examination. However, a secondary survey should be performed in the following situations:

- Trauma patients with a significant MOI
- Trauma patients with an unknown or unclear MOI
- Trauma patients with an injury to more than one area of the body
- All unresponsive patients
- All patients with an altered mental status
- Some responsive medical patients, as indicated by history and focused physical examination findings

The phrase **physical examination** implies a head-to-toe assessment of the patient's entire body. A quick secondary survey (head-to-toe assessment) of a trauma patient with a significant MOI is called a **rapid trauma assessment.** A *significant* MOI is one that is likely to produce serious injury. A quick secondary survey of a medical patient who is unresponsive or has an altered mental status is called a **rapid medical assessment.** The phrase **focused physical examination** is used to describe an assessment of specific body areas that relate to the patient's illness or injury.

The procedure for performing a secondary survey is the same for trauma and medical patients. However, the physical findings that you are looking for and discover may have a different meaning depending on whether the patient is a trauma or medical patient. For instance, a swollen ankle in a trauma patient may be a sign of a sprain or broken bone. Swollen ankles in a patient with difficulty breathing and a history of a heart condition are more likely to be a sign of heart failure.

When examining your patient, first look (inspect), listen (auscultate), and then feel (palpate) body areas to identify potential injuries. Use your stethoscope to listen to (auscultate) the movement of air into and out of the patient's lungs. Use your sense of smell to identify unusual odors during the exam, such as alcohol on the patient's breath, body, or clothing. Because it can cause pain, palpation should be performed last.

DCAP-BTLS is a helpful memory aid to remember what to look and feel for during the physical exam:

- **D**eformities
- **C**ontusions (bruises)
- **A**brasions (scrapes)
- **P**unctures/penetrations
- **B**urns
- **T**enderness
- **L**acerations (cuts)
- **S**welling

Depending upon the severity of the patient's injury or illness, a secondary survey may not be completed. This is because treatment of life-threatening conditions takes priority over performing this examination. A secondary survey is usually performed en route to the receiving facility. However, the exam should be performed on the scene if transport is delayed.

When examining your patient, ease your patient's fears by explaining what you are about to do and why it must be done. Remember to properly drape or shield an unclothed patient from the stares of others. Conduct the exam professionally and efficiently, and talk with the patient throughout the procedure. If your patient is a child, ask a parent or family member to help you. Doing so should lessen the child's anxiety.

Making a Difference

You must be able to tell the difference between a seriously ill or injured patient who needs a rapid assessment and a less seriously ill or injured patient who needs a focused exam. If a life threat is discovered during the secondary survey, stop and treat it and repeat the primary survey.

Assessment of Vital Signs

Remember to take two or more sets of vital signs. Doing so will allow you to note changes (trends) in the patient's condition and response to treatment. Reassess and record vital signs at least every 5 minutes in an unstable patient, and at least every 15 minutes in a stable patient.

Assess respirations by evaluating rate, depth/equality, and rhythm. Assess any changes in respiration, including abnormal respiratory sounds. Assess the patient's pulse. Initially, a radial pulse should be assessed in all patients one year of age or older. In patients younger than one year of age, a brachial pulse should be assessed. If a pulse is present, assess its rate and quality. The quality of a pulse includes assessment of pulse strength (absent, weak, strong/full [normal], or bounding), rhythm, and equality.

Assess the skin for color, temperature, and condition (moisture). Assess capillary refill in infants and children younger than six years of age. Assess the pupils for size, equality, and reactivity. Assess the patient's blood pressure. Blood pressure should be assessed in any patient older than three years of age. Whenever possible, blood pressure should be assessed by auscultation. If available, attach a pulse oximeter and monitor the patient's oxygen saturation.

The Patient's Medical History

The conclusion you reach about what is wrong with your patient is called a **field impression.** The emergency care you provide is based on your field impression. Arriving at a correct field impression of what is wrong with your patient can be compared with putting together the pieces of a puzzle. The patient's answers to your questions about his medical history are pieces of the puzzle. Forgetting to ask specific questions or not listening to the patient's answers to the questions you ask will result in missing pieces of the puzzle and an inaccurate field impression. Each finding you uncover during the physical exam is another piece of the puzzle. The field impression is the finished puzzle.

If the patient is responsive, obtain a SAMPLE history from the patient after sizing up the scene and performing a primary survey. If the patient is unresponsive or has an altered mental status, quickly size up the scene, perform a primary survey, and then proceed to the rapid trauma or medical assessment. Obtain a SAMPLE history from the family or bystanders.

History of the Present Illness (HPI)

Although a medical history is important to obtain for all patients, it is especially important for the medical patient. To obtain a good history, it is best to use an organized approach so that key information is not overlooked.

The **history of the present illness (HPI)** is a chronological record of the reason a patient is seeking medical assistance. It includes the patient's chief complaint and the patient's answers to questions about the circumstances that led up to the request for medical help.

Chief Complaint

The **chief complaint** is the reason why the patient called for assistance. It is best to document the chief complaint by using the patient's own words in quotes. For example, "I can't catch my breath."

Objectives 26, 27

Some patients who call for medical help will have a history of a medical condition that is related to their current complaint. For instance, a patient whose chief complaint is difficulty breathing may have a history of asthma or heart failure. However, some patients will have a chief complaint that they have never experienced before. Some patients will have more than one chief complaint. In each case, listen carefully to what the patient's concerns are and then ask questions that will help you form an accurate field impression.

When asking questions to find out the patient's medical history, use open-ended questions when possible. **Open-ended questions** require the patient to answer with more than a "yes" or "no." For example, you might ask, "What is troubling you today?" or "How can I help you?" There are times when asking questions that require a simple yes or no answer is appropriate. For instance, when asking the patient if he has a history of high blood pressure, diabetes, and other illnesses, a yes or no answer is appropriate, as it is when the patient is having difficulty communicating (because of severe pain or difficulty breathing or a language barrier). Questions that require a yes or no answer are called **direct questions.**

When you are caring for patients, a "yes" answer pertaining to an illness or injury is considered a pertinent positive or positive finding. A "no" answer is considered a pertinent negative or negative finding. For example, when you are caring for a patient who has asthma, pertinent positive findings would include shortness of breath and/or a feeling of tightness in throat or chest. Pertinent negative findings would include no history of a recent cold, bronchitis, pneumonia, or other infection. When you are caring for a female patient who is complaining of abdominal pain, pertinent positive findings include a sexually active woman whose last menstrual period was six weeks ago. Pertinent negative findings include no recent abdominal trauma or illness and no recent history of abdominal surgery or a vaginal infection.

Making a Difference

Taking a medical history is not simply a matter of asking a series of rapid-fire questions in order to complete a report. Obtaining a useful medical history is an art. It requires thoughtful questions, good listening skills, and practice.

OPQRST and SAMPLE History

It is important to obtain a SAMPLE history from all responsive patients. Using the SAMPLE history format provides an organized approach to gathering important patient information. As we discussed in Chapter 5, OPQRST is a great tool to use when you have a

TABLE 9-3 OPQRST

Letter	What It Means	Possible Questions
O	**O**nset	"How long ago did the problem or discomfort begin?" "What were you doing when it started?"
P	**P**rovocation/Palliation	"What causes the problem or discomfort?" "What makes it worse?" "What makes it better?"
Q	**Q**uality	"What does the pain feel like?" (sharp, dull, burning, stabbing, shooting, crushing, throbbing, pressure, or tearing)
R	**R**egion/Radiation	"Where is the pain?" "Is the pain in one area or does it move?" "Is the pain located in any other area?"
S	**S**everity	"On a scale of 0 to 10, with 0 being no pain and 10 being the worst, what number would you give your pain or discomfort?"
T	**T**ime	"How long has your discomfort been present?" "Is it constant or does it come and go?" "Have you ever had this problem before?" "When?" "How long did it last?"

patient who is complaining of pain or discomfort. As you learn more about specific injuries and illnesses, you will be able to modify the sample questions provided in Tables 9-3 and 9-4 to address those complaints. For example, questions that you might ask of a pregnant patient experiencing an obstetrical emergency might include:

- When is your baby due?
- Are you carrying only one baby?
- Have you been seeing a doctor regularly?
- Are you having pain or contractions? How long are your contractions?
- Have you had any vaginal bleeding or discharge?
- Do you feel the need to push?

If a patient loses consciousness, knowing what his symptoms were before he lost consciousness can help identify possible causes of his condition. If the patient is unresponsive, attempt to find out information from family members, neighbors, bystanders, or others present at the scene.

In some situations, the patient's condition will be so critical that there is no time to collect detailed information. Ask the important questions while on the scene and as you are providing care. For example, you should ask the patient about any allergies while providing care at the scene. It is important that this information be documented and relayed to the healthcare professionals who assume patient care.

Leave the less important questions to ask the patient while en route to definitive care.

Trauma Patient Considerations
Reconsidering the Mechanism of Injury
Objective 20

At a scene that involves trauma, perform a scene size-up and primary survey, and then reconsider the mechanism of injury. In Chapter 8, we defined mechanism of injury (MOI) as the way in which an injury occurs, as well as the forces involved in producing the injury.

Suppose you and your EMT partner are called to the scene of a motor vehicle crash. You arrive to find a 16-year-old male lying on the side of the road. He was the restrained driver of an older model vehicle (no airbags) that struck a bridge abutment at a high rate of speed. There is intrusion of about 12 inches to the front of the vehicle. The steering wheel is bent. The windshield is starred, but not broken. According to bystanders, the patient was initially walking around at the scene and then stumbled and lost consciousness. They estimate he was "out" for about three to five minutes. At this time, the patient is awake and can tell you his name. He is not certain of the place or time. He remembers the crash, but does not remember the loss of consciousness.

TABLE 9-4 SAMPLE History

Letter	What It Means	Possible Questions
S	**S**igns and symptoms	"Can you tell me how you are feeling right now?"
A	**A**llergies	"Do you have any allergies to medications?" "Are you allergic to latex?" "Do you have any food allergies or allergies to insect stings, pollen, dust, or grass?"
M	**M**edications	"Do you take any prescription medications?" "Is the medication prescribed for you or for someone else?" "What is the medication for?" "When did you last take it?" "Are you taking birth control pills?" (if applicable) "Do you take any over-the-counter medications, such as aspirin, allergy medications, cough syrup, or vitamins?" "Do you take any herbs?" "Have you recently started taking any new medications?" "Have you recently stopped taking any medications?" "Do you use any recreational drugs (cocaine, marijuana)?" "Have you consumed any alcohol?"
P	**P**ast medical history	"Are you seeing a doctor for any medical condition?" "Do you have a history of heart problems, breathing problems, high blood pressure, diabetes, epilepsy, or any other ongoing medical condition?" "Have you been in the hospital recently?" "Have you had any recent surgery?"
L	**L**ast oral intake	"When did you last have something to eat or drink?" "What was it?"
E	**E**vents prior	"What events led up to this illness?"

This situation involves a significant MOI. Any visible deformity of the steering wheel is an indicator of potentially serious internal injury. The patient needs a rapid trauma assessment. Some injuries may be obvious while other injuries may be hidden. As you prepare to examine the patient, you must be suspicious of potentially serious internal injuries. This is called having an **index of suspicion.** By evaluating the MOI, you can often predict the types of injuries the patient is most likely to experience.

If the MOI is significant, time is of the essence. A severely injured patient has the greatest chance for survival if he reaches definitive care within one hour of the injury. This is commonly referred to as the **golden hour.** Definitive care for a severely injured trauma patient is surgery. Since the golden hour starts at the time the patient is injured, every action you take

ticks away minutes until the patient reaches the operating room. The goal for prehospital trauma care

Remember This!

Factors to Consider in a Motor Vehicle Crash

Rate of speed

Seatbelt use

Impact site

Amount of intrusion

Airbag deployment

Vehicle size

Condition of steering wheel

Condition of windshield

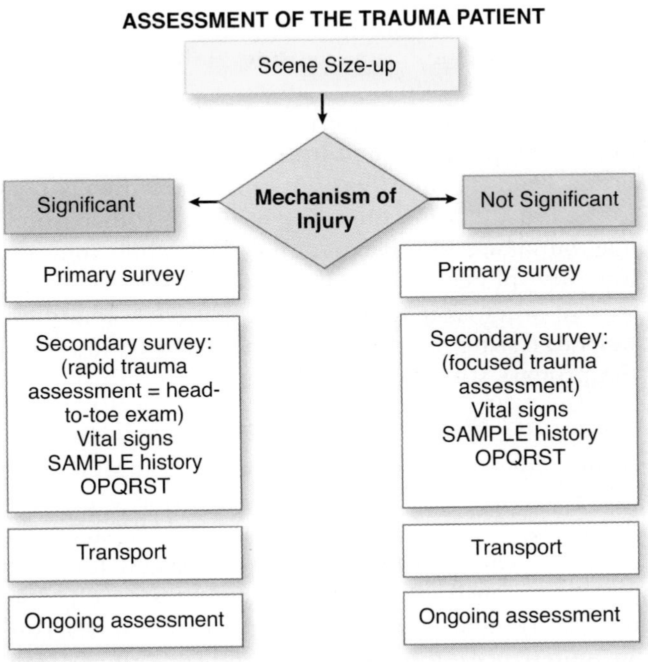

ASSESSMENT OF THE TRAUMA PATIENT

```
                    ┌──────────────┐
                    │ Scene Size-up│
                    └──────┬───────┘
                           │
                           ▼
                      ╱─────────╲
  ┌─────────────┐    ╱ Mechanism ╲    ┌───────────────┐
  │ Significant │◄──┤     of      ├──►│ Not Significant│
  └──────┬──────┘    ╲  Injury   ╱    └───────┬───────┘
         │            ╲─────────╱             │
         ▼                                    ▼
  ┌─────────────┐                    ┌───────────────┐
  │Primary survey│                   │Primary survey │
  └──────┬──────┘                    └───────┬───────┘
         ▼                                    ▼
  ┌──────────────┐                   ┌───────────────┐
  │Secondary     │                   │Secondary      │
  │survey:       │                   │survey:        │
  │(rapid trauma │                   │(focused trauma│
  │assessment =  │                   │assessment)    │
  │head-to-toe   │                   │Vital signs    │
  │exam)         │                   │SAMPLE history │
  │Vital signs   │                   │OPQRST         │
  │SAMPLE history│                   └───────┬───────┘
  │OPQRST        │                           │
  └──────┬───────┘                           ▼
         ▼                           ┌───────────────┐
  ┌─────────────┐                    │  Transport    │
  │  Transport  │                    └───────┬───────┘
  └──────┬──────┘                            ▼
         ▼                           ┌───────────────┐
  ┌──────────────┐                   │Ongoing        │
  │Ongoing       │                   │assessment     │
  │assessment    │                   └───────────────┘
  └──────────────┘
```

FIGURE 9-12 ▲ Assessment of the trauma patient flow chart.

is to limit scene time to 10 minutes. Therefore, your decision regarding the significance of the MOI must be made quickly, using your best judgment. If the MOI is significant, you need to perform a rapid trauma assessment (Figure 9-12). This means that you must move quickly and efficiently, examining the patient from head to toe for obvious and potential injuries. You will also need to determine the need for ALS personnel and immediate transport. EMTs give important emergency care during the golden hour. This care includes making sure the patient has an open airway, giving oxygen, controlling bleeding, and rapidly transporting the patient to the closest appropriate facility.

Remember This!

All healthcare professionals who are involved in trauma care know about the golden hour and the importance of time. If your trauma patient is a priority patient and your scene time is more than 10 minutes, be prepared to answer questions about your extended scene time to medical personnel at the receiving facility. Sometimes there are logical reasons for an extended scene time. For example, a patient may require special tools and trained personnel before removal from a wrecked vehicle. Or time may be spent trying to convince a patient who initially refuses care to allow treatment and transport. In these situations, it may be helpful to notify medical direction by phone or radio to give them a "heads up" about the delay.

Making a Difference

Significant Mechanisms of Injury

If the patient has any of the following injuries, transport the patient to a Trauma Center:

- Penetrating injury to the head, neck, or torso (excluding superficial wounds in which the depth of the wound can be easily determined)
- Penetrating injury to the extremities above the elbow or knee
- Flail chest
- Combination trauma with burns
- Two or more proximal long-bone fractures
- Pelvic fractures
- Open or depressed skull fracture
- Paralysis
- Amputation above the wrist or ankle
- Major burns

If you determine the MOI is not significant, you will perform a focused physical exam. This means that you will begin the secondary survey with an assessment of the injured body part. Other areas of the body would be examined as needed.

Consider transport to a Trauma Center if the MOI is from any of the following causes:

- Ejection from a vehicle (including motorcycles, mopeds, ATVs, open beds of pickup trucks)
- Dead occupant in the same passenger compartment
- Falls more than 15 feet (or three times the patient's height); falls greater than 10 feet if the patient is less than 14 years of age or older than 55
- Vehicle rollover
- High-speed auto crash with an initial speed of more than 40 miles per hour (mph)
- High-speed auto crash with intrusion and major auto deformity of more than 20 inches
- High-speed auto crash with intrusion into the passenger compartment of more than 12 inches
- Injury from an auto-pedestrian or auto-bicycle crash with significant impact (more than 5 mph)
- Pedestrian thrown or run over
- Motorcycle crash at more than 20 mph or with separation of the rider from the bike

Also consider transport to a Trauma Center for significant mechanisms of injury for infants and children:

- Falls more than 10 feet (or three times the child's height)
- Bicycle collision
- Vehicle collision at a medium speed
- Any vehicle collision in which the infant or child was unrestrained

Trauma Patient with Significant Mechanism of Injury

Objectives 21, 22

A rapid trauma assessment should be performed when:

- A significant MOI exists
- Additional injuries are suspected
- A critical injury is found during the focused physical examination
- A previously stable patient with no significant MOI becomes unstable during the focused physical examination
- After providing any emergency intervention

Assessment of a trauma patient requires a consistent, organized approach. If a patient has experienced a significant MOI, follow the primary survey with a rapid trauma assessment. Because life-threatening injuries should have been identified during the primary survey, a rapid trauma assessment is a head-to-toe exam performed to detect the presence of additional injuries. If you found life-threatening injuries in the primary survey, it is possible that you may never get to perform the rapid trauma assessment. In situations like this, ask another EMT to perform a rapid trauma assessment while you manage the life-threatening injuries already identified.

Remember This!

If the patient is unstable, a rapid trauma assessment should be done en route to the hospital.

Objectives 23, 24

Begin the rapid trauma assessment by reassessing the patient's mental status and then checking the patient's head. Then examine the neck, chest, abdomen, pelvis, lower extremities, upper extremities, and the back. Compare one side of the body to the other. For example, if an injury involves one side of the body, use the uninjured side as the normal finding for comparison.

Although the steps for performing a rapid trauma assessment are presented in this chapter in a specific order, keep in mind that some tasks are usually performed at the same time. For example, your partner may be taking the patient's vital signs while you perform the physical exam. If you find a serious injury, treat it when you find it. If the patient's condition worsens during the physical exam, go back and repeat the primary survey.

Transport of the Priority Trauma Patient

If the patient's physical exam findings and MOI (and other factors) indicate you have a priority patient, determine the timeliest method to get the patient to definitive care. To make the best decision for your patient, you will need to consider the distance to the nearest Trauma Center, availability of ground versus air ambulances, time of day (traffic conditions), and weather. Contact the receiving facility as soon as possible so its personnel can prepare for the patient's arrival. Let them know the patient's condition, the treatment you have given, and the patient's estimated time of arrival. Be sure to notify the receiving facility of significant changes in the patient's condition while he is in your care.

Trauma Patient with No Significant Mechanism of Injury

Objective 25

If a trauma patient has no significant MOI, perform a focused physical examination. A focused physical exam performed on an injured patient is also called a **focused trauma assessment.** The focused physical examination concentrates on the specific injury site (and related structures) based on what the patient states is wrong and your suspicions based on the MOI and primary survey findings. For example, if your patient presents with a possible fracture of his lower arm, you will assess the injured area. You will also assess pulses, movement, and sensation distal to the injury. A focused physical examination also identifies other injuries that could be life threatening if not cared for quickly.

Assess the injured area for DCAP-BTLS. Be sure to assess for a pulse, movement, and sensation if the injured area involves an extremity. After completion of the focused physical exam, assess vital signs and obtain a SAMPLE history. Provide emergency care on the basis of the type and severity of the injury. If the patient's injury requires further care, prepare the patient for transport to the most appropriate facility.

Medical Patient Considerations

A medical patient is a person whose complaint is related to an illness. For the medical patient, the patient's level of responsiveness is the first important factor in determining the type of physical examination you need to perform (Figure 9-13). If your primary

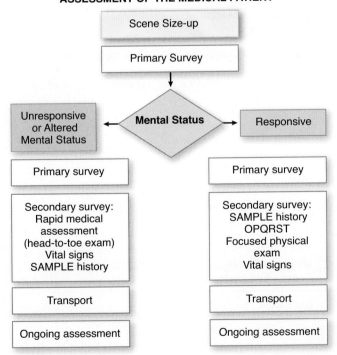

ASSESSMENT OF THE MEDICAL PATIENT

FIGURE 9-13 ▲ Assessment of the medical patient flow chart.

survey reveals that the patient is unresponsive or has an altered mental status, a rapid secondary survey (head-to-toe assessment) needs to be done to find out what is wrong. A quick secondary survey of a medical patient who is unresponsive or has an altered mental status is called a **rapid medical assessment.** A focused physical exam is usually performed for a responsive medical patient because he can usually tell you the problem that prompted a call for medical help.

The Unresponsive Medical Patient

Rapid Medical Assessment

Objectives 28, 29

After performing a scene size-up and making sure the scene is safe to enter, an unresponsive medical patient or a patient who has an altered mental status needs a primary survey and then a quick secondary survey, similar to a rapid trauma assessment. Remember to treat problems as you find them. The DCAP-BTLS memory aid used for the rapid trauma assessment is also used for the rapid medical assessment.

As you begin the rapid medical assessment, it is important not to have "tunnel vision." For instance, although you may have been called for a diabetic emergency, do not assume that this is the actual (or only) problem. If you approach the patient looking only for signs and symptoms consistent with a diabetic emergency, you may miss important indicators of other illnesses or injuries. An unresponsive patient who is known to have a history of diabetes may have fallen when he lost consciousness. In situations like this, you must consider the possibility of an injury to the head, neck, or back. Assign another rescuer to manually stabilize the head and neck in a neutral position while you examine the patient. Begin by reassessing the patient's mental status and then checking the patient's head. Then examine the neck, chest, abdomen, pelvis, lower extremities, upper extremities, and the back. Compare one side of the body to the other.

After the rapid medical assessment, assess the patient's vital signs and then proceed with getting the patient's medical history from family and friends and from clues in the area. Examples of clues include a "puffer" (inhaler), nitroglycerin tablets or other medications, and medical identification, such as a necklace or bracelet. Provide emergency care based on your physical exam findings.

Do not forget about family members at the scene. Explain to the family the emergency care provided and where the patient will be transported for further care.

Remember This!

If the patient's condition worsens during the physical exam, go back and repeat the primary survey. In situations like this, you may never complete the physical exam.

The Responsive Medical Patient

The focused exam is guided by the patient's chief complaint and presenting signs and symptoms. If your patient is responsive and ill (not injured), find out his medical history first. Finding out the patient's medical history will often help you pinpoint the patient's present problem. The information you collect will help guide where you look and what you are looking for in the focused physical exam. For example, if your patient is complaining of abdominal pain, your physical exam will be focused on that area. Performing the physical exam helps to establish if your initial assumption about what is wrong is accurate.

TABLE 9-5 Focused Medical Assessment by Chief Complaint

Chief Complaint	Body Area	Possible Medical Condition
Abdominal pain	Abdomen, pelvis	Ectopic pregnancy, heart attack, appendicitis, gall bladder disease, disease of the colon, bowel obstruction, spontaneous abortion
Altered mental status	Head, neck, chest, abdomen, back, extremities	Stroke, low blood sugar, overdose, seizure, heat-related illness, hypothermia, anaphylaxis, hypoxia, shock
Back pain	Back	Kidney stone, back strain, aortic aneurysm
Chest discomfort	Neck, chest, abdomen, extremities	Heart attack, respiratory infection, gall bladder disease, anxiety disorder
Difficulty breathing/ shortness of breath	Head, neck, chest, lower extremities	Asthma, emphysema, heart failure, heart attack, anxiety disorder, toxic exposure, pulmonary embolism, anaphylaxis
Dizziness	Head, chest	Dehydration, abnormal heart rhythm, viral infection
Fainting	Head, chest (and any body part that may have been injured if the patient fell)	Dehydration, low blood sugar, abnormal heart rhythm
Headache	Head, neck	Stroke, seizure, meningitis
Arm complaint	Head, neck, chest, upper extremities	Heart attack–related pain, insect stings, musculoskeletal problems
Leg complaint	Head, neck, chest, lower extremities	Heart failure, bite or sting, blood clot, stroke, peripheral vascular disease
Nausea/vomiting	Chest, abdomen	Heart attack, bowel obstruction, toxic exposure, anaphylaxis, viral illness, pregnancy, foodborne illness, dehydration
Neck pain or stiffness	Head, neck	Meningitis
Palpitations	Neck, chest	Abnormal heart rhythm, anxiety, subarachnoid hemorrhage
Weakness	Head, chest	Shock, abnormal heart rhythm, nervous system disorder, anemia, electrolyte imbalance

After the focused physical exam, obtain vital signs. Assess the patient's pulse, respirations, and blood pressure. Assess oxygen saturation by using a pulse oximeter. Assess the skin for color, temperature, and condition (moisture). Assess the pupils for size, equality, and reactivity. Check capillary refill in infants and children younger than six years of age.

Table 9-5 shows a few examples of the body areas that should be assessed on the basis of the patient's chief complaint. Although it may seem overwhelming right now, knowing the body areas to assess on the basis of a patient's chief complaint will become easier as you learn more about specific illnesses and injuries.

The Head-to-Toe Examination

Objectives 31, 32

Reassessment of Mental Status

As you begin the head-to-toe exam, it is very important to note any changes in a patient's mental status. Decreased blood flow to the brain can cause the patient's mental status to worsen. For example, if the patient was alert during the primary survey and now responds only to voice or pain, his mental status has worsened. On the other hand, if the patient was unresponsive during the primary survey and now responds to pain, his mental status has improved.

If the patient is alert, he can direct the physical exam with his complaints and response. A patient who is not awake may still react during the physical examination. For example, the patient may respond to your voice or may withdraw from pain. A patient displays *purposeful movement* when he attempts to remove the stimulus. *Nonpurposeful movement* is displayed when the patient moves in response but does not attempt to remove the stimulus. Be sure to document the patient's response to a specific stimulus. For example, "The patient responded to a pinch on the wrist by pulling both arms toward his chest."

Changes in a patient's level of responsiveness are important findings that must be relayed to the healthcare professionals to whom you transfer care. It is also important to document these findings in the prehospital care report.

Head and Face

The head contains many blood vessels. Wounds of the face or scalp may bleed heavily. Before examining the head of a trauma patient, have someone manually stabilize the patient's head and neck to keep them from moving—if this has not already been done. Using your gloved hands, gently feel the patient's scalp for deformities, depressions, tenderness, and swelling (Skill Drill 9-1, Step 1). Look for any open wounds or dis-

colored areas. Run your fingers through the patient's hair and examine your gloves for the presence of blood. Gently slide your gloved hands behind the patient's head and feel for tenderness, swelling, or depressions that may indicate a skull fracture. If you feel a depression or an indentation in the skull, you may hear and feel crackling. This is called **crepitation** or *crepitus*. It is caused by the grating of broken bone ends against each other. Control bleeding from a scalp wound by applying gentle, direct pressure with a dry, sterile dressing. If you suspect a skull fracture, do not apply direct pressure to the center of the wound. Doing so could force bone fragments down into the brain. Instead, apply gentle pressure around the edges of the wound and over a broad area.

Remember This!

Assume that any patient who has significant facial trauma also has a cervical spine and head injury until proven otherwise.

Assess the face for DCAP-BTLS (Skill Drill 9-1, Step 2). Swelling of the face is often first seen around the eyes and cheeks because the subcutaneous tissue is relatively loose in these areas. Look at the patient's face for **symmetry** (evenness). Assess for symmetry by comparing one side of the face with the other. Examples of uneven (**asymmetrical**) facial movements that may be seen include an eye on one side of the face that does not close completely or drooping of the lower eyelid and mouth (Figure 9-14). These are signs of a possible stroke.

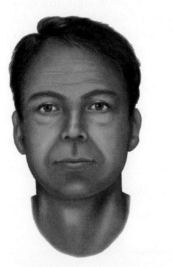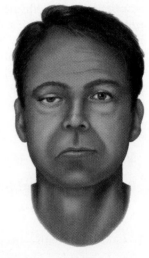

FIGURE 9-14 ▲ Examples of asymmetrical facial movements that may be seen include an eye on one side of the face that does not close completely or drooping of the lower eyelid and mouth.

Gently palpate the facial bones—eye sockets (orbits), nasal bones, cheek bones, maxilla (upper jaw bone), and mandible (lower jaw bone)—for instability or tenderness (Skill Drill 9-1, Steps 3-6). The orbits are often fractured in patients who have experienced facial trauma. Assess for crepitation. If the patient is responsive and has experienced facial trauma, ask him if he has any facial numbness. If facial numbness or weakness is present, the patient may have possible nerve damage associated with the facial injury.

Look for blood or fluid from the nose and singed nasal hairs (Skill Drill 9-1, Step 7). Singed facial hairs suggest a possible airway burn. Do not insert a nasal airway if the patient has known or suspected trauma to the midface. Look for signs of increased breathing effort, such as **nasal flaring** (widening of the nostrils). Complaints of nasal stuffiness and drainage from the nose can be caused by environmental allergies. Although swelling around the nose and eyes may be seen in a patient who has experienced trauma to the face, these findings may also be seen in a patient who has a medical condition (such as a sinus infection). A patient who has a sinus infection may complain of pain or tenderness when you feel the areas just above or below the eyes.

Look in the mouth for blood; vomitus; absent, broken, or loose teeth; an injured or swollen tongue; and foreign material (Skill Drill 9-1, Step 8). Suction as needed. Note the color of the patient's lips and the mucous membranes of the mouth. They should appear pink and moist. A bluish tinge of the lips and mucous membranes is common in dark-skinned patients. Swelling of the lips may be caused by trauma or an allergic reaction to medications, foods, or other allergens. Lips that are dry and cracked may be caused by exposure to the sun, wind, or a dry environment, or dehydration. Note the presence of any unusual odors on the patient's breath, body, or clothing (see the following *You Should Know* box and Skill Drill 9-1, Step 9). If the patient is coughing up sputum, note its color, amount, and consistency. If the patient is unresponsive, insert an oral airway to maintain an open airway. Suction the mouth to clear the airway if necessary.

You Should Know

Possible Causes of Breath Odors

- Acetone or "fruity" breath—diabetic ketoacidosis
- Musty breath—liver failure
- Ammonia—kidney failure
- Bad breath—tooth decay; poor oral hygiene; disease of the gums, tonsils, or sinuses

Eyes and Ears

Look for injury to the eyes, but do not touch the eyes to find out if an injury is present. Assess for DCAP-BTLS. Look for bluish discoloration (**ecchymosis**) around the eyes (**raccoon eyes**). This sign can occur because of direct trauma to the face. It can also be associated with a possible skull fracture. Look for the presence of blood in the anterior chamber of the eye (**hyphema**). Look for the presence of redness, contact lenses, or a foreign body. Use a penlight or flashlight to check the pupils for size, shape, equality, and reactivity (Skill Drill 9-1, Step 10). The pupils are normally equal, round, and react briskly to light. Unequal pupils in the presence of head trauma suggest swelling (**edema**) of the brain. Do a quick check of the patient's vision by asking, "How many fingers am I holding up?"

Look at the eyelids for discoloration, cuts, or swelling. Assess the whites of the eyes (sclerae) for discoloration. A yellow discoloration (jaundice) of the sclerae suggests liver disease. Red or bloodshot sclera may be caused by allergies, trauma, or an infection. The sclera is lined with a paper-thin mucous membrane called the **conjunctiva.** If the conjunctiva becomes infected (conjunctivitis), it can produce a red eye with pus, mucus, or watery discharge.

Remember This!

Use a penlight or flashlight to look in the ears, nose, and mouth and to examine the eyes.

Look for blood or fluid leaking from the ears (Skill Drill 9-1, Step 11). If fluid is seen in the ears, do not attempt to stop the flow. Cover the ear with a loose, sterile dressing. A bluish discoloration of the mastoid process (behind the ear) is called **Battle's sign** and is a sign of a possible skull fracture (Skill Drill 9-1, Step 12). Note the color of the earlobes. They may appear pale or blue in a cold environment. Excessive redness may indicate inflammation, fever, or high blood pressure in some patients.

Patients who have an infection of the external or middle ear often pull or tug at the affected ear. Middle ear infections are common, particularly in patients who have seasonal allergies. Inflammation of the outer ear can be caused by an allergic reaction to personal care products, such as hair dye and perfume.

You Should Know

Raccoon eyes and Battle's sign are signs of a possible skull fracture. These signs may not be present for several hours after the injury.

Neck

Examine the front and back of the neck. Assess for DCAP-BTLS. Look to see if the patient has a **laryngeal stoma** (surgical opening in the neck). Is the patient using the accessory muscles in the neck during breathing? Look at the jugular veins on the side of the neck (Skill Drill 9-1, Step 13). The jugular veins run from the angle of the jaw to the shoulders. The neck veins normally bulge slightly when a patient is supine. Flat neck veins in a supine patient suggest decreased blood volume. Bulging (**distention**) of the neck veins when the patient is placed in a sitting position at a 45-degree angle indicates a backup of blood from the heart because of fluid overload or an injury to the chest, lungs, or heart. Distention of the neck veins is commonly called **jugular venous distention** (JVD).

Look for open wounds and for medical identification (ID) tags (Skill Drill 9-1, Step 14). Medical alert tags may be worn on a necklace or bracelet. These ID tags contain important medical information, such as the patient's medical condition, important prescription medications, and allergies. Do not consider the information on a medical alert tag a complete listing of the patient's medication or medical history.

Gently feel the front and back of the neck to detect areas of tenderness or deformity (Skill Drill 9-1, Step 15). Feel for tenderness or crepitation of the cervical spine. Feel the position of the trachea just above the manubrium in the suprasternal notch (Skill Drill 9-1, Step 16). It should be in a midline position. In an injured patient, shifting of the trachea (**tracheal deviation**) from a midline position suggests a collapsed lung (**pneumothorax**). When a **tension pneumothorax** is present, the trachea deviates away from the injured lung (see Chapter 25). Feel for air trapped beneath the skin (**subcutaneous emphysema**). Subcutaneous emphysema is a crackling sensation under the fingers felt while palpating the chest. It feels and sounds like crisped rice cereal or bubble wrap. The presence of subcutaneous emphysema suggests a collapsed lung or ruptured bronchial tube and the leakage of air into the pleural space.

If there is an open wound of the neck, cover the wound with an airtight (**occlusive**) dressing to prevent air from entering the wound. Apply a cervical immobilization device if a spinal injury is suspected or if the patient is unresponsive and the MOI is unknown. Ask another EMT to continue to maintain in-line spinal stabilization while you continue the assessment. Remember: Once begun, manual stabilization must continue until the patient has been completely immobilized on a long backboard. If the patient has difficulty swallowing, monitor the patient's airway closely. Be prepared to suction if needed.

Chest

To examine the chest, it is usually necessary to remove the patient's clothing. Protect the patient's privacy and shield him from curious onlookers. Assess for DCAP-BTLS (Skill Drill 9-1, Step 17). Assess the patient's work of breathing. Check for the use of accessory muscles during breathing. Look for surgical scars, an equal rise and fall of the chest, bruises, open wounds, or obvious deformities. The presence of a long scar over the patient's breastbone indicates a cardiac history. Unequal chest expansion may occur when part of the lung is obstructed or collapsed because of injury (such as a flail chest, pneumothorax) or illness (such as pneumonia). When **paradoxical** chest movement is present, a part of the chest wall moves in an opposite direction during breathing. This finding is a sign of a flail segment. When the patient breathes in, the flail segment is drawn inward instead of moving outward. When the patient breathes out, the flail segment moves outward instead of moving inward with the rest of the chest. **Flail chest** occurs when two or more adjacent ribs are broken in two or more places or when the sternum is detached (see Chapter 25). The section of the chest wall between the broken ribs becomes free-floating because it is no longer in continuity with the thorax. This free-floating section of the chest wall is called the *flail segment*. The forces necessary to produce a flail chest cause bruising of the underlying lung (**pulmonary contusion**).

You Should Know

Paradoxical chest wall movement may be most easily seen in an unresponsive patient. In patients with thick or muscular chest walls, it may be hard to see paradoxical movement. In some conscious patients, spasm and splinting of the chest muscles may cause paradoxical motion to go unnoticed.

If you see an open chest wound, immediately cover it with your gloved hand and then apply an airtight dressing. Tape the dressing to the chest on three sides. Leave the fourth side open to allow air to escape but not enter the wound. If the patient appears to worsen after covering the wound with the dressing (or your hand), remove it to let air escape. Then reapply your hand or the dressing to the wound. If you see an object impaled in the chest, such as a knife, do not try to remove it. Removing it can result in bleeding and the entry of air into the chest. Leave the object where it is and stabilize it in place with bulky dressings. If a flail segment is present, the patient will usually need positive-pressure ventilation with a BM device.

Performing the Secondary Survey

STEP 1 ▶ Using your gloved hands, gently feel the patient's scalp for deformities, depressions, tenderness, and swelling. Look for any open wounds or discoloration.

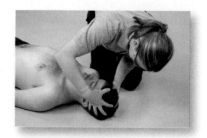

STEP 2 ▶ Assess the face for DCAP-BTLS. Look at the patient's face for symmetry (evenness).

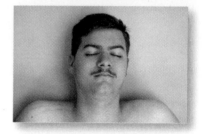

STEP 3 ▶ Gently palpate the eye sockets (orbits) for instability or tenderness.

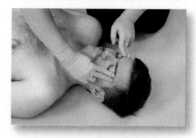

STEP 4 ▶ Gently palpate the nasal bones for instability or tenderness.

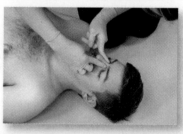

STEP 5 ▶ Gently palpate the cheek bones for instability or tenderness.

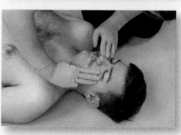

STEP 6 ▶ Gently palpate the upper jaw bone (maxilla) and lower jaw bone (mandible) for instability or tenderness.

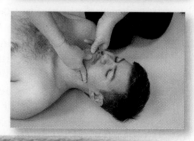

STEP 7 ▶ Look for blood or fluid from the nose and singed nasal hairs. Also look for nasal flaring (widening of the nostrils).

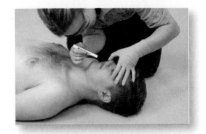

STEP 8 ▶ Look in the mouth for blood; vomitus; absent, broken, or loose teeth; an injured or swollen tongue; or foreign material. Note the color of the patient's lips and the mucous membranes of the mouth.

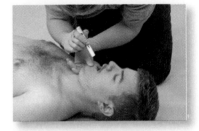

STEP 9 ▶ Note the presence of any unusual odors on the patient's breath, body, or clothing.

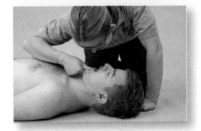

STEP 10 ▶ Assess the size and shape of the pupils and their response to light. Look at the eyelids for discoloration, cuts, or swelling. Look at the whites of the eyes for discoloration. Look at the conjunctivae for redness, pus, and foreign bodies.

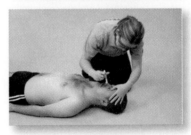

STEP 11 ▶ Look for blood or fluid leaking from the ears.

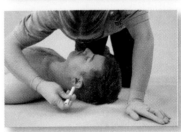

STEP 12 ▶ Look for bruising behind the ears.

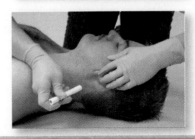

Continued on next page

Performing the Secondary Survey (*continued*)

STEP 13 ▶ Assess the neck for DCAP-BTLS, open wounds, a laryngeal stoma, use of accessory muscles, and jugular venous distention.

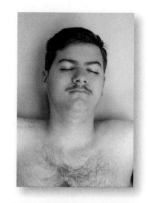

STEP 14 ▶ Medical alert tags may be worn on a necklace or bracelet. These ID tags contain important medical information, including the patient's medical condition, important prescription medications, and allergies.

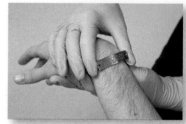

STEP 15 ▶ Gently feel the front and back of the neck to detect areas of tenderness or deformity.

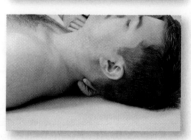

STEP 16 ▶ Feel the position of the trachea just above the manubrium in the suprasternal notch.

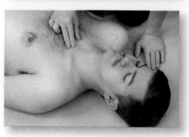

STEP 17 ▶ Assess the chest for DCAP-BTLS. Note the shape of the patient's chest. Assess the patient's work of breathing, including the use of accessory muscles during breathing. Look for surgical scars, an equal rise and fall of the chest, bruises, open wounds, obvious deformities, or signs of a rash.

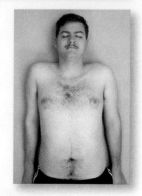

STEP 18 ▶ Listen for breath sounds. Listen at the top (apices) of the lungs in the midclavicular line on both sides of the chest. Listen at the bottom (bases) of the lungs and in the midaxillary line on both sides of the chest. Compare from side to side.

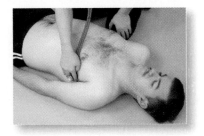

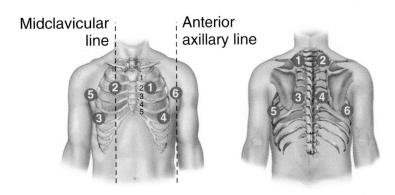

Midclavicular line   Anterior axillary line

STEP 19 ▶ Feel the collarbones, shoulders, breastbone, and ribs for tenderness and deformity. Check for subcutaneous emphysema. Gently reach under the patient to assess the back of the chest.

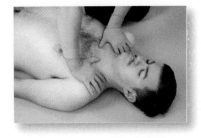

STEP 20 ▶ Using the pads of your fingers, gently feel the upper and lower areas of the abdomen for injuries or tenderness.

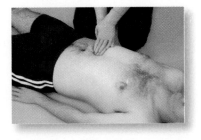

Continued on next page

Performing the Secondary Survey (*continued*)

STEP 21 ▷ Gently reach under the patient to assess the lower back.

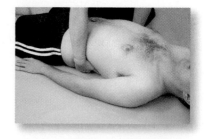

STEP 22 ▷ If the patient has not complained of pain and there are no obvious signs of pelvic injury, assess the pelvis by applying gentle downward pressure on the pubic bone. Press the iliac crests of the pelvis inward toward each other and posteriorly toward the back.

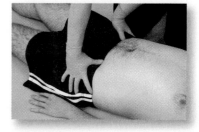

STEP 23 ▷ • Examine the upper leg.
   • Examine the lower leg.
   • Assess the dorsalis pedis pulse in each lower extremity. Remember to assess movement and sensation in each extremity.

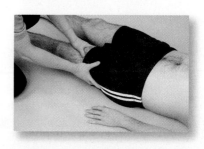

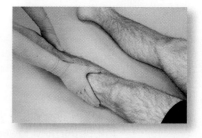

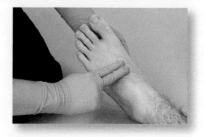

STEP 24 ▷ • Examine the upper arm.
         • Examine the lower arm.
         • Assess the radial pulse in each upper extremity.

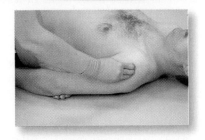

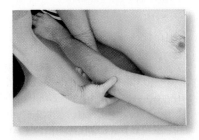

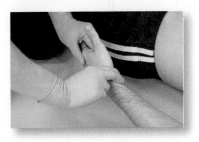

STEP 25 ▷ If the patient is awake, assess movement by asking the patient to squeeze your fingers.

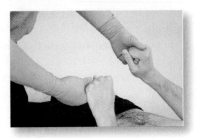

STEP 26 ▷ Logroll the patient to assess the patient's back.

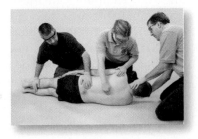

Note the shape of the patient's chest. A barrel-shaped chest suggests a history of chronic lung disease. Look at the skin for signs of a rash. The presence of a rash may indicate the patient's problem is to the result of an allergic reaction.

Use a stethoscope to listen to the movement of air into and out of the patient's lungs. Starting at the apices of the lungs (about the second intercostal space), listen for breath sounds in six places (Skill Drill 9-1, Step 18):

- At the apices, midclavicular line on each side of the chest
- At the bases on each side of the chest
- In the midaxillary line on each side of the chest

Listen to one full respiratory cycle (inhalation and exhalation) in each location, comparing from side to side. Breath sounds on the back of the chest are best assessed later in the physical exam when the rest of the back is examined. Watch and listen to see if the patient has any signs of difficulty breathing or pain with breathing.

Determine if breath sounds are present, diminished, or absent; equal or unequal; and/or clear, muffled, or noisy. Normal breath sounds are clear and equal on both sides of the chest. Diminished or absent lung sounds may be caused by spasm of the bronchioles, a foreign body, pneumonia, a completely or partially collapsed lung (pneumothorax), or blood in the pleural space (**hemothorax**). A hemothorax can produce muffled breath sounds, which appear distant.

Abnormal breath sounds may include crackles, rhonchi, and wheezes. **Crackles** (also called *rales*) indicate the presence of fluid in the alveoli or larger airways. Crackles can be heard in patients with congestive heart failure, pulmonary edema, pneumonia, or trauma. They sound like hair rolled between the thumb and forefinger close to one's ear. **Rhonchi** are sounds produced when air flows through passages narrowed by mucus or fluid. They sound like "rattling" or "rumbling" in the lungs. Rhonchi can be heard in patients with pneumonia, upper respiratory infection, and chronic obstructive pulmonary disease (COPD). **Wheezes** are musical whistling sounds caused by the movement of air through narrowed airways. There are many possible causes of wheezes, including asthma and COPD (see the following *You Should Know* box).

A patient who has experienced trauma to the head or brain may have an abnormal breathing pattern. This occurs as the brain swells and pushes on lower structures in the brain. An abnormal breathing pattern is an important assessment finding. Be sure to document this finding and relay it to the healthcare professional to whom you transfer patient care.

Gently feel the collarbones, shoulders, breastbone, and ribs for tenderness and deformity (Skill Drill 9-1, Step 19). Check for subcutaneous emphysema. Gently reach under the patient to assess the back of the chest. Examine your gloves for the presence of blood.

You Should Know

Possible Causes of Wheezing

Anaphylaxis
Asthma
Bronchiolitis
Bronchospasm
Chronic bronchitis
Congestive heart failure
Croup
Emphysema
Foreign body obstruction
Inhalation injury
Pulmonary edema
Pneumonia
Tumor

Abdomen

Remember that the abdominal cavity is divided into four imaginary quadrants (Figure 9-15). These quadrants are created by drawing two imaginary lines that intersect with the midline through the navel (umbilicus).

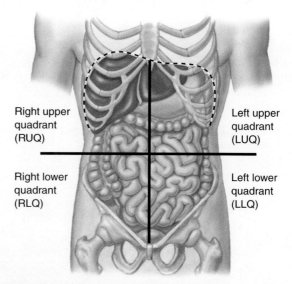

Right upper quadrant (RUQ)

Left upper quadrant (LUQ)

Right lower quadrant (RLQ)

Left lower quadrant (LLQ)

FIGURE 9-15 ▲ The abdominal cavity is divided into four imaginary quadrants created by drawing two imaginary lines that intersect with the midline through the navel (umbilicus).

The abdomen contains solid and hollow organs. Solid organs, such as the liver and spleen, bleed. When hollow organs are cut or burst, their contents spill into the abdominal cavity. This results in pain and soreness. Hollow organs include the stomach, intestines, and gallbladder.

Assess the abdomen for DCAP-BTLS. When assessing the abdomen, look for the following:

- Surgical scars
- Bruising
- Open wounds
- Obvious bleeding
- Protruding abdominal organs
- An impaling object
- Distention
- Generator for an implantable cardioverter-defibrillator
- Catheter for an insulin pump
- Signs of obvious pregnancy

Look to see if abdominal distention is present (the abdomen appears larger than normal). Abdominal distention can be caused by blood, fluid, or air. It is difficult to assess in obese patients. If exposed abdominal organs are present, do not attempt to reinsert them into the abdominal cavity. Cover them with a moist, sterile dressing. If you see an object impaled in the abdomen, leave the object in place and stabilize it in place with bulky dressings.

The abdomen is normally soft and is not painful or tender to touch. To examine the abdomen, place one hand on top of the other. Use the pads of the fingers of the lower hand and gently feel the upper and lower areas of the abdomen for injuries or tenderness (Skill Drill 9-1, Step 20). If the patient is responsive, ask him to point to the area that hurts (point tenderness). Assess the area that hurts last. Watch the patient's face while you palpate the abdomen. A grimace may indicate tenderness over a particular abdominal area. Determine if the abdomen feels soft or hard (rigid). Note the presence of any masses or pulsations. In a pregnant patient, note movement or the absence of movement in the fetus. Gently reach under the patient to assess the lower back (Skill Drill 9-1, Step 21). Examine your gloves for the presence of blood.

Patients with abdominal pain may present in different positions. The patient with inflammation of the abdominal lining (**peritonitis**) usually prefers to lie absolutely still. The patient with a bowel obstruction is often restless and often moves in an attempt to find a position of comfort. Patients may also present with their knees in a flexed position (fetal position) to decrease tension on the abdominal muscles.

Abdominal pain is not always felt directly over the affected organ. For example, gallbladder pain may radiate to the right scapula and shoulder. Pancreatic pain may radiate to the back and improve when the patient sits forward. A ruptured aortic aneurysm may present with pain radiating to the back.

Pelvis

The pelvic area contains large blood vessels. Therefore, an injury to the pelvic ring can result in life-threatening internal and external bleeding. Assess the pelvis for DCAP-BTLS. If the patient complains of pain in the pelvic area or if obvious deformity is present, do not palpate or compress the pelvis. If the patient has not complained of pain and there are no obvious signs of pelvic injury, assess the pelvis by directing gentle downward pressure on the pubic bone, using the heel of one hand. Press the iliac crests of the pelvis inward toward each other and posteriorly toward the back (Skill Drill 9-1, Step 22). Do not rock the pelvis. If applying pressure results in tenderness, instability, or crepitation, suspect a pelvic fracture. When examining the pelvic area, check to see if the patient lost control of his bowels or bladder. Examples of situations in which this may occur include seizures, stroke, or cardiac arrest.

Severe blood loss may occur from a break in the continuity of the pelvis. If tenderness, instability, or crepitation of the pelvis is present, give oxygen and secure the patient to a long backboard. The patient will need rapid transport to the closest appropriate facility.

Remember This!

If the patient complains of pain in the pelvic area or if obvious deformity is present, do not palpate or compress the pelvis.

Extremities

Assess the extremities for DCAP-BTLS. Look for open wounds, swelling, and abnormal positioning, such as an unequal length, etc. Look at the wrists and ankles for a medical ID tag. Look for swelling (edema) of the hands, feet, and ankles. Look for signs of a possible insect bite or sting, signs of possible intravenous drug abuse, or the presence of a dialysis shunt/fistula.

Assess pulses, motor function, and sensation in each extremity. Feel the dorsalis pedis pulse (on the top of the foot) in each lower extremity (See Skill Drill 9-1, Step 23). Assess the radial pulse in each upper extremity (Skill Drill 9-1, Step 24). Gently feel the upper and lower portion of each extremity for bone or joint deformities.

Assess movement and sensation in each extremity. If the patient is awake, assess movement of the lower extremities by asking if he can push both of his feet into your hands at the same time. Assess movement of the upper extremities by asking the patient to squeeze your fingers using both of his hands at the same time (Skill Drill 9-1, Step 25). Compare the strength of his grips and note if they are equal or if one side appears weaker. If the patient is awake, assess sensation by touching the hands and toes of each extremity and asking him to tell you where you are touching. If the patient is unresponsive, assess movement and sensation by applying a pinch to each foot and hand. See if the patient responds to pain with facial movements or movement of the extremity.

A fractured femur (open or closed) may result in significant blood loss. Injury to both femurs may cause life-threatening bleeding. Even if there is no break in the skin, internal bleeding may be present. Comparing one extremity to the other may reveal differences in size as blood builds up in the soft tissues. If you suspect a femur fracture, give oxygen, control significant bleeding if present, and immobilize the patient on a long backboard. Transport to the closest appropriate medical facility. If the patient has experienced multiple injuries or his vital signs are unstable, a splint should be applied during transport if time permits. If the patient's injuries are not critical and his vital signs are stable, immobilize the injured body part with an appropriate splint before transport.

Remember This!

Check PMS in each extremity. PMS = *pulse*, *movement*, and *sensation*. Compare each extremity to the opposite extremity. Assess PMS in each of your patient's extremities *before* and *after* immobilization. Be sure to document your findings.

Posterior Body

After making sure that there are enough personnel to assist you, logroll the patient to assess the patient's back (Skill Drill 9-1, Step 26). Make sure to maintain in-line spinal stabilization while rolling the patient. Assess the back for DCAP-BTLS. Look for swelling in the sacral area. In patients confined to bed, fluid collects in this area. If possible, listen to breath sounds on the posterior chest. Feel for swelling, tenderness, instability, and crepitation. If present, cover any open wounds with an airtight dressing. Control significant bleeding if present. Immobilize the patient to a long backboard.

Emergency Care During the Secondary Survey

Life-threatening conditions must be managed as soon as they are found. Less critical conditions can be managed as they are found during or after completing the secondary survey. Examples include:

- Abrasions, burns, and lacerations: Provide wound care
- Swollen, discolored, deformed extremity: Provide immobilization
- Minor bleeding: Control bleeding and provide wound care

You Should Know

Patient assessment has been described as an input/output process. The assessment findings are the input. The treatment you provide to the patient is the output.

Performing an Ongoing Assessment

Purpose of the Ongoing Assessment

You must frequently reevaluate a patient to make sure that you deliver appropriate emergency care. These reevaluations are called **ongoing assessments.** An ongoing assessment should be performed on *every* patient. The ongoing assessment allows you to:

- Reevaluate the patient's condition
- Assess the effectiveness of the emergency care provided
- Identify any missed injuries or conditions
- Observe subtle changes or trends in the patient's condition
- Alter emergency care as needed

Components of the Ongoing Assessment

Objective 35

An ongoing assessment consists of the following components:

- Repeating the primary survey
- Reassessing and documenting vital signs
- Repeating the focused assessment
- Reevaluating the emergency care provided

Repeating the Primary Survey

Objective 34

Begin the ongoing assessment by repeating the primary survey (Skill Drill 9-2, Step 1). This is done in order to identify and treat life-threatening injuries that may have been missed. Reassess the patient's level of responsiveness and note any changes in the patient's mental status. If the patient has an altered mental status, document the patient's response to a specific stimulus. Communicate any changes in mental status to the healthcare professionals to whom you transfer patient care. Document any changes in mental status in the prehospital care report (PCR).

Reassess the patient's airway. If the patient is able to talk clearly and without difficulty, assume his airway is open. If the patient is unresponsive, look in the patient's mouth for an actual or potential obstruction (such as a foreign body, blood, vomitus, or broken teeth). Check placement of any airway adjuncts that are inserted. If necessary, insert one to maintain an open airway. Document and communicate any changes or trends to those to whom you transfer patient care.

Reassess the patient's breathing rate and quality. Assess the rise and fall of the patient's chest, respiratory rate, depth/equality of breathing, and rhythm of respirations. Look for signs of increased work of breathing (respiratory effort) and signs of chest trauma. Note if the patient's respirations are absent, quiet, or noisy. Give appropriate treatment as necessary. For instance, give oxygen (if not already done) and suction the airway if needed. Document and communicate any changes or trends to those to whom you transfer patient care.

Reassess the patient's circulation. Reassess the patient's perfusion by assessing the patient's pulse rate and quality and skin temperature, color, and condition. Note any changes since you last assessed the patient's pulse. For example, if the patient's pulse was initially strong and regular and is now weak and irregular, this important finding suggests the patient's condition is worsening. On the other hand, if the patient's pulse was initially hard to feel and is now strong, this finding suggests the patient's condition is improving. If you were initially able to feel a carotid pulse but were unable to feel a radial pulse, be sure to reassess the patient's radial pulse to see if there has been a change in this finding. Look for changes in skin color. Feel for changes in skin temperature and condition (moisture). Remember to reassess capillary refill in infants and children younger than six years of age. Reassess the patient for signs of obvious external bleeding. Major bleeding should have been controlled during the primary survey. If there are any sites of minor bleeding, bleeding should be controlled and dressings applied as needed. Document

and communicate any changes or trends to those to whom you transfer patient care.

If the ongoing assessment is performed en route to the hospital and the patient's condition worsens, it may be necessary to change the patient's destination or mode of transport. For example, let's suppose you are en route to a trauma center with a patient injured in a motor vehicle crash. Your primary survey revealed a patient who was awake and alert with an open airway, adequate breathing, and strong radial and carotid pulses. You decided to perform a secondary survey en route to the hospital. Since the patient's condition appeared stable, you opted to transport to a trauma center but without the use of lights or siren. En route to the hospital, your secondary survey reveals the patient's abdomen is firm and distended. Your ongoing assessment reveals the patient is no longer awake and alert. He now responds only to a painful stimulus. His airway is open but his respiratory rate has slowed to 8 breaths per minute and his breathing is shallow. You can feel a carotid pulse but are unable to feel a radial pulse. The patient's skin is cool, pale, and moist. It is clear that the patient's condition is worsening. In situations such as this, consider your local protocols and contact medical direction as needed. You may need to alter the mode of patient transport to include lights and siren (if consistent with your protocols and medical direction).

If the ongoing assessment is performed on the scene, reconsider your transport decision (patient destination and mode of transport) on the basis of your assessment findings.

Reassessing Vital Signs

Reassess and document the patient's vital signs (Skill Drill 9-2, Step 2). Reassess each of the following:

- Respiratory rate and quality
- Pulse rate and quality
- Blood pressure
- Pupils
- Skin color, temperature, and condition (moisture)
- Capillary refill in infants and children younger than six years of age

Objective 36

Compare the vital signs taken during the ongoing assessment with the baseline vital signs taken earlier. Having two or more sets of vitals allows you to note changes (trends) in the patient's condition and response to treatment. For example, by comparing the values obtained for the patient's heart rate, you will be able to see if it is increasing, staying about the same, or decreasing. Watching these trends will enable you to recognize life-threatening emergencies, such as shock.

Ongoing Assessment

STEP 1 ▶ Repeat the primary survey.

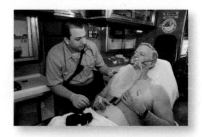

STEP 2 ▶ Reassess and document the patient's vital signs.

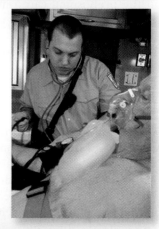

STEP 3 ▶ Repeat the focused assessment of the patient's specific complaint or injury.

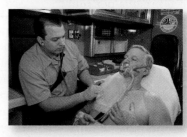

STEP 4 ▶ Reassess the treatments you have provided to be sure that they are effective.

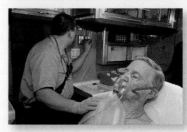

Repeating the Focused Assessment

Repeat the focused assessment of the patient's specific complaint or injury (Skill Drill 9-2, Step 3). If the patient develops a new complaint or if a previously identified symptom changes, perform a focused assessment on the area of complaint.

Reevaluating Emergency Care Interventions

Reassess the treatments you have provided to be sure that they are effective (Skill Drill 9-2, Step 4).

Remember This!

When providing patient care, always make sure that suction is within arm's reach.

Airway and Breathing

After making sure that the patient's airway is open, check to see if the method you chose to deliver oxygen during the initial assessment is still appropriate. For example, if the patient was initially breathing adequately and was placed on oxygen by nonrebreather mask but is now breathing shallowly at a rate of 6 breaths per minute, you will need to remove the nonrebreather mask and assist the patient's breathing with a BM device that is connected to supplemental oxygen. On the other hand, if you were assisting a patient's breathing with a BM device but his respiratory effort and rate are now adequate, consider switching to a nonrebreather mask to deliver oxygen. In any case, close monitoring of the patient's airway and breathing is essential.

If the patient is unresponsive and an oral or nasal airway was inserted, check to make sure that the device is properly positioned. If the patient is being ventilated with a BM device, make sure it is connected to oxygen at 15 L/min. If a reservoir bag is used, make sure that the reservoir is inflated. Reassess the effectiveness of BM ventilation by ensuring there is adequate rise and fall of the chest. Check to make sure that there is an adequate face-to-mask seal. Reassess the patient's lung compliance (resistance to ventilation). Increasing resistance suggests an airway obstruction.

If oxygen is being delivered by nonrebreather mask, make sure the mask is connected to oxygen at 15 L/min. Make sure the reservoir bag is not pinched off and remains inflated. Make sure the inhalation valve is not obstructed.

If oxygen is being delivered by nasal cannula, make sure the oxygen flow rate is set at no more than 6 L/min. Make sure the prongs are properly placed in the patient's nose. Make sure open chest wounds have been properly sealed with an airtight dressing taped on three sides. Also, make sure that there is no trapped air under the fourth side of the dressing. Loosen it if needed.

Remember This!

Regardless of the method used to deliver it, be sure to check the amount of oxygen left in the tank often.

Circulation

If the patient is injured, make sure that bleeding from previously identified wounds is controlled and there is no fresh bleeding. If time and the patient's condition permits, make sure that open wounds are properly dressed and bandaged and the patient is properly positioned.

Other Interventions

If the patient is injured and a head or spinal injury is suspected, make sure the patient's spine is adequately stabilized. Make sure the cervical collar used is of appropriate size and fits properly. Make sure that the patient remains properly secured to a long backboard.

Make sure injured extremities are effectively immobilized. Check to make sure that dressings, bandages, and splints applied to an extremity are not too tight.

Reassess the patient's response to any medications you may have given or assisted the patient in taking. For example, if you assisted the patient in taking prescribed nitroglycerin (NTG) for chest discomfort, assess the patient's response, vital signs, and degree of discomfort after taking the medication. If glucose was given to a patient experiencing a diabetic emergency, reassess the patient's mental status and vital signs. If you assisted a patient with asthma in taking a prescribed metered dose from an inhaler, reassess the patient's breath sounds, degree of breathing difficulty, and vital signs.

How often you need to do an ongoing assessment is guided by the length of time spent with the patient or the patient's condition. Repeat the ongoing assessment at least every 15 minutes for a stable patient and every 5 minutes for an unstable patient. Reassess the patient's mental status and maintain an open airway. Monitor the patient's breathing, pulse, skin color, temperature, and condition. Repeat the physical exam as needed. Continue to calm and reassure the patient.

It is important that your documentation and verbal report to other healthcare professionals accurately reflects your assessment findings and the emergency care provided. Be sure to accurately record all times associated with the care given.

On the Scene   Wrap-Up

The scene size-up provides clues that point to a bicycle crash with traumatic injuries. On the basis of your scene size-up, you should suspect head, neck, and spine trauma in addition to the visible injuries. Your general impression and primary survey will confirm these suspicions and help you to prioritize your treatment plan. You must also consider that this patient may have an altered mental status because of another problem, such as low blood sugar.

It cannot be stated too frequently that the purpose of the primary survey is to "find and fix" life-threatening injuries. This patient has signs and symptoms of potentially life-threatening problems to both the nervous system and the respiratory system. When you remove the patient's shirt, you see a wound on his chest that appears to be "bubbling." You immediately call an ALS unit for an intercept. The patient is transported rapidly to the closest trauma center. The patient survives because you recognized this deadly chest injury. ∎

Sum It Up

▶ The ability to properly assess a patient is one of the most important skills you can master. As an EMT, you must learn to work quickly and efficiently in all types of situations. To work efficiently, you must approach patient assessment systematically. The emergency care you provide to your patient will be based on your assessment findings.

▶ While assessing your patient, you will discover his signs and symptoms. You must provide emergency medical care based on those signs and symptoms. Discovering the patient's signs and symptoms requires you to use your senses of sight (look), sound (listen), touch (feel), and smell.

▶ Patient assessment consists of the following components:
  ● Initial assessment
    —Scene size-up
      ● Take BSI precautions.
      ● Evaluate scene safety.
      ● Determine the MOI or the nature of the patient's illness.
      ● Determine the total number of patients.
      ● Determine the need for additional resources.
    —Primary survey
      ● General impression
        —Appearance
        —(Work of) Breathing
        —Circulation
      ● **A**irway, level of responsiveness, cervical spine protection
      ● **B**reathing (ventilation)
      ● **C**irculation (perfusion)
      ● **D**isability (mini-neurological exam)
      ● **E**xpose
      ● Identify priority patients
    —Secondary survey
      ● Vital signs, pulse oximetry
      ● Focused SAMPLE history, OPQRST
      ● Head-to-toe or focused physical examination
  ● Ongoing assessment
    —Repeat the primary survey.
    —Reassess vital signs.
    —Repeat the focused assessment regarding patient complaint or injuries.
    —Reevaluate emergency care.

▶ The primary survey is a rapid assessment to find and treat all immediate life-threatening conditions. It begins after the scene or situation has been found safe or made safe and you have gained access to the patient. During this phase of patient assessment, you will look for and treat life-threatening conditions as you discover them ("find and fix", "treat as you go") and decide if the patient needs immediate transport or additional on-scene assessment and treatment. You must perform a primary survey on *every* patient.

▶ The secondary survey is a physical examination performed to discover medical conditions and/or injuries that were not identified in the primary survey. During this phase of the patient assessment, you will also obtain vital signs; reassess changes in the patient's condition; and determine the patient's chief complaint, history of present illness, and significant past medical history. The secondary survey does not begin until the primary survey has been completed and treatment of life-threatening conditions has begun.

▶ A general impression (also called a first impression) is an "across-the-room" assessment. As you approach him, you will form a general impression without the patient's telling you what his complaint is. You can complete it in 60 seconds or less. The purpose of forming a general impression is to decide if the patient looks "sick" or "not sick." If the patient looks sick, you must act quickly. As you gain experience, you will develop an instinct for quickly recognizing when a patient is sick. You will base your general impression of a patient on three main areas: (1) appearance, (2) breathing, and (3) circulation.

▶ After forming a general impression, begin the primary survey by assessing the patient's airway and level of responsiveness. Assessment of a patient's airway and level of responsiveness occur at the same time. Level of responsiveness is also called level of consciousness or mental status. These terms refer to a patient's level of awareness. A patient's mental status is "graded" using a scale called the **AVPU scale** as follows.

- A = *A*lert
- V = Responds to *V*erbal stimuli
- P = Responds to *P*ainful stimuli
- U = *U*nresponsive

▶ A patient who is oriented to person, place, time, and event is said to be "alert and oriented ✕ ('times') 4" or "A and O ✕ 4." Assessing the mental status of a child older than 3 years of age is the same as that of an adult.

▶ For trauma patients or unresponsive patients with an unknown nature of illness, take spinal precautions. Spinal precautions are used to stabilize the head, neck, and back in a neutral position. This stabilization is done to minimize movement that could cause injury to the spinal cord.

▶ After making sure that the patient's airway is open, assess the patient's breathing to determine if breathing is adequate or inadequate. If the patient is unresponsive and breathing is inadequate or if the patient is not breathing, begin rescue breathing by using a pocket mask, mouth-to-barrier device, or BM device.

▶ Assessment of circulation involves evaluating for signs of obvious bleeding, central and peripheral pulses; skin color, temperature, and condition; and capillary refill (in children less than 6 years of age). Look from the patient's head to toes for signs of significant external bleeding. Control major bleeding, if present.

▶ Altered mental status means a change in a patient's level of awareness. Altered mental status is also called an altered level of consciousness (ALOC). A patient who has an altered mental status is at risk of an airway obstruction. Most EMS systems use the GCS during the disability phase of the primary survey to obtain a more detailed assessment of the patient's neurological status. This mini-neurological examination is used to establish a baseline level of responsiveness and note any obvious problem with central nervous system (brain and spinal cord) function. Three categories are assessed with the GCS: (1) eye opening, (2) verbal response, and (3) motor response.

▶ Expose pertinent areas of the patient's body for examination. Factors that you must consider when exposing the patient include protecting the patient's modesty, the presence of bystanders, and environment/weather conditions.

▶ Determine if the patient requires on-scene stabilization or immediate transport ("load-and-go" situations) with additional emergency care en route to a hospital.

▶ The secondary survey is patient, situation, and time dependent. For instance, a patient with an isolated injury, such as a painful ankle, would typically not require a head-to-toe physical examination. However, a secondary survey should be performed in the following situations:

- Trauma patients with a significant MOI
- Trauma patients with an unknown or unclear MOI
- Trauma patients with an injury to more than one area of the body
- All unresponsive patients
- All patients with an altered mental status
- Some responsive medical patients, as indicated by history and focused physical examination findings

▶ A quick secondary survey (head-to-toe assessment) of a trauma patient with a significant MOI is called a rapid trauma assessment. A significant MOI is one that is likely to produce serious injury. A quick secondary survey of a medical patient who is unresponsive or has an altered mental status is called a rapid medical assessment. The phrase focused physical examination is used to describe an assessment of specific body areas that relate to the patient's illness or injury. The procedure for performing a secondary survey is the same for trauma and medical patients. However, the physical findings that you are looking for and discover may have a different meaning depending on whether the patient is a trauma or medical patient.

- When examining your patient, first look (inspect), listen (auscultate), and then feel (palpate) body areas to identify potential injuries.
- DCAP-BTLS is a helpful memory aid to remember what to look and feel for during the physical exam:
  - **D**eformities
  - **C**ontusions (bruises)
  - **A**brasions (scrapes)
  - **P**unctures/penetrations
  - **B**urns
  - **T**enderness
  - **L**acerations (cuts)
  - **S**welling
- Remember to take two or more sets of vital signs. Doing so will allow you to note changes (trends) in the patient's condition and response to treatment. Reassess and record vital signs at least every 5 minutes in an unstable patient, and at least every 15 minutes in a stable patient.
- The conclusion you reach about what is wrong with your patient is called a field impression.
- The history of the present illness is a chronological record of the reason a patient is seeking medical assistance. It includes the patient's chief complaint and the patient's answers to questions about the circumstances that led up to the request for medical help. The chief complaint is the reason the patient called for assistance.
- When asking questions to find out the patient's medical history, use open-ended questions when possible. Open-ended questions require the patient to answer with more than a "yes" or "no." Questions that require a yes or no answer are called direct questions.
- It is important to obtain a SAMPLE history from all responsive patients. Using the SAMPLE history format provides an organized approach to gathering important patient information. OPQRST is a great tool to use when you have a patient who is complaining of pain or discomfort.
- At a scene that involves trauma, perform a scene size-up and primary survey and then reconsider the mechanism of injury. Mechanism of injury (MOI) is the way in which an injury occurs, as well as the forces involved in producing the injury. By evaluating the MOI, you can often predict the types of injuries the patient is most likely to experience.
- If the MOI is significant, time is of the essence. The goal for prehospital trauma care is to limit scene time to 10 minutes. If the MOI is significant, you need to perform a rapid trauma assessment. This means that you must move quickly and efficiently, examining the patient from head-to-toe for obvious and potential injuries. You will also need to determine the need for ALS personnel and immediate transport. If you determine the MOI is not significant, you will perform a focused physical exam. This means that you will begin the secondary survey with an assessment of the injured body part. Other areas of the body would be examined as needed.
- If a patient has experienced a significant MOI, follow the primary survey with a rapid trauma assessment. Begin the rapid trauma assessment by reassessing the patient's mental status and then checking the patient's head. Then examine the neck, chest, abdomen, pelvis, lower extremities, upper extremities, and the back. Compare one side of the body to the other. For example, if an injury involves one side of the body, use the uninjured side as the normal finding for comparison.
- If a trauma patient has no significant MOI, perform a focused physical examination. The focused physical exam concentrates on the specific injury site (and related structures) based on what the patient states is wrong and your suspicions based on the MOI and initial assessment findings.
- For the medical patient, the patient's level of responsiveness is the first important factor in determining the type of physical examination you need to perform. If your primary survey reveals that the patient is unresponsive or has an altered mental status, a rapid secondary survey (head-to-toe assessment) needs to be done to find out what is wrong. A quick secondary survey of a medical patient who is unresponsive or has an altered mental status is called a rapid medical assessment. A focused physical exam is usually performed for a responsive medical patient because he can usually tell you what is wrong that prompted a call for medical help.
- An ongoing assessment consists of four main areas:
  - Repeating the primary survey
  - Reassessing vital signs
  - Repeating the focused assessment
  - Reevaluating emergency care
- An ongoing assessment should be performed on every patient. It is performed after the secondary survey, if a secondary survey is performed. In some situations, the patient's condition may prevent performance of a secondary survey. An ongoing assessment is usually performed en route to the receiving facility. However, if transport is delayed, the ongoing assessment should be performed on the scene.
- Repeat the ongoing assessment at least every 15 minutes for a stable patient and every 5 minutes for an unstable patient. Continue to calm and reassure the patient throughout the on-going assessment.

10 Communications

By the end of this chapter, you should be able to:

Knowledge Objectives ▶
1. List the proper methods of initiating and terminating a radio call.
2. State the proper sequence for delivery of patient information.
3. Explain the importance of effective communication of patient information in the verbal report.
4. Identify the essential components of the verbal report.
5. Describe the attributes for increasing effectiveness and efficiency of verbal communication.
6. State legal aspects to consider in verbal communication.
7. Discuss the communication skills that should be used to interact with the patient.
8. Discuss the communication skills that should be used to interact with the family, bystanders, and individuals from other agencies while you are providing patient care, and the difference between skills used to interact with the patient and those used to interact with others.
9. List the correct radio procedures in the following phases of a typical call:
   - To the scene
   - At the scene
   - To the facility
   - At the facility
   - To the station
   - At the station

Attitude Objectives ▶
10. Explain the rationale for providing efficient and effective radio communication and patient reports.

Skill Objectives ▶
11. Perform a simulated, organized, concise radio transmission.
12. Make an organized, concise patient report that would be given to the staff at a receiving facility.
13. Make a brief, organized report that would be given to an Advanced Life Support provider arriving at an incident scene at which the Emergency Medical Technician was already providing care.

You have been dispatched to a report of an unknown medical problem. The address is just a few blocks away from your quarters. You and your partner immediately respond from your station to the scene. Upon arrival at the scene, you find a residence on a quiet city street. A very angry elderly man meets you at the door. He grudgingly allows you into the house. Your patient is an elderly woman. You find her seated on the couch. As you begin to ask her some basic questions, she leans toward you and says, "Please get me out of here. I'm very frightened of this man. I don't know who he is." ■

THINK ABOUT IT

As you read this chapter, think about the following questions:

- What do you need to know about this scene?
- What questions will you ask?
- Is there any danger to you or your partner?
- How will you get help if it is needed?
- What is the best way to interact with the patient and family members?
- What information will need to be relayed to the hospital if you transport this patient?

Introduction

One of the most amazing abilities we possess is the capacity for communication. We can express fear, describe symptoms, ask questions, inform crewmembers, give a radio report, relay information to hospital staff, and even offer condolences when needed. This special ability is an important component of prehospital care. As an Emergency Medical Technician (EMT), you must be able to communicate effectively with crewmembers, emergency dispatchers, medical direction, and other healthcare professionals; law enforcement personnel and other public safety workers; the patient; and the patient's family. Communication with medical direction may be necessary when a patient refuses care, when you encounter difficult patient management situations, or when you need to obtain orders to give medications. As an EMT, you must learn to communicate patient information to other healthcare professionals in a concise, organized manner. You must also learn to communicate early with the receiving facility to make sure that adequate resources are mobilized to care for the patient.

Communication requires more than knowing the proper words and their meaning. Communicating in a respectful manner may mean the difference between acquiring information and missing it. This chapter focuses on the basic requirements to successfully communicate with your dispatch center, your partner, your patients, and the hospital or receiving facility staff.

Remember This!

Advanced Life Support Assist

In many instances, the EMT will be transmitting information to the receiving facility, even if he is partnered with a Paramedic.

Communications Systems

Communication is the process of sending and receiving information. This interaction may occur on a radio or cell phone with dispatch personnel, between crewmembers, with a patient's family, or with the staff of the receiving facility. Effective communication requires that we send and receive this information using an understandable and commonly recognized language. This "language" requirement is not just as simple as speaking English or Spanish. Using terminology that is too technical or too advanced may create confusion. Information that is misunderstood can lead to inappropriate treatment or care. To alleviate this potential problem, most Emergency Medical Services (EMS) systems in the United States require the use of clear text or speech to relay data from one point to another. To understand its importance, we must consider the history, terminology, and basic concepts of communication.

History

Modern EMS communication began with the use of telephones to contact local rescue squads or personnel. This usually required calling a specific local number or the local operator, who then contacted EMS personnel. In many towns across the United States, this contact may have initiated the sounding of a bell or siren located on a tower near the station that housed the ambulance. Sounding of the bell notified local volunteers to assemble for a call. You can imagine the time that may have elapsed from the original call to arrival at the scene.

Communication Centers

Communication capabilities and equipment have changed significantly in just the past two decades. Cellular phones that used to be the size of a toaster are now small enough to fit in your pocket. This has helped reduce the overall time needed to find a telephone to report a medical problem. Despite all of the advances in technology, we still rely heavily on the ability of all of the people connected with the EMS system to verbally communicate with each other.

Regulation

The **Federal Communications Commission (FCC)** is the United States government agency responsible for regulation of interstate and international communications by radio, television, wire, satellite, and cable. The FCC is charged with the development and enforcement of rules and regulations pertaining to radio transmissions. In addition, the FCC is mandated to do the following:

- Control licenses and allocate frequencies
- Establish technical standards for radio equipment
- Monitor frequencies for appropriate usage
- Spot-check for licenses and records

Remember This!

Always speak in a professional manner during radio communication. Inappropriate language or use of radio frequencies may lead to enforcement action by the FCC. Keep in mind that many people have scanners in their homes and may hear all communications shared back and forth.

Radio Frequencies and Ranges

In the United States, the FCC regulates the use of non-governmental radio frequencies. The **Interagency Radio Advisory Committee (IRAC)** is responsible for coordinating radio use by agencies of the federal government. The **Emergency Medical Radio Service (EMRS)** is a group of frequencies designated by the FCC exclusively for use by EMS providers. EMRS includes many frequencies in the **VHF** (very high frequency) and **UHF** (ultra-high frequency) bands (a band is a group of radio frequencies close together).

Very High Frequency (VHF)

VHF radio frequencies can be subdivided into low band and high band. Low-band frequencies generally have a greater range than high-band VHF frequencies.

Radio waves in the low-band frequency range bend and follow the curvature of the Earth, allowing radio transmission over long distances. These radio waves are subject to interference by atmospheric conditions, including weather disturbances, and electrical equipment. These waves do not penetrate solid structures (such as buildings) well, making VHF low band less effective for use in metropolitan areas.

Radio waves in the high-band frequency range travel in a straight line. This straight-line quality means that the radio wave is easily blocked by topography such as a hill, mountain, or large building. Although less interference occurs in this band than in VHF low band, its susceptibility to interference by solid structures may result in gaps or "holes" in radio coverage. This band is generally better for use in metropolitan areas than VHF low band.

Ultra-High Frequency (UHF)

Radio waves in the UHF frequency travel in a straight line but do have an ability to reflect or bounce around buildings. This band has a shorter range than VHF high or low bands. This type of frequency has a greater ability to enter buildings or structures through openings or mediums that are radio frequency permeable. UHF frequently requires the use of repeaters because of its short range. A **repeater** is a device that receives a transmission from a low-power portable or mobile radio on one frequency and then retransmits it at a higher power on another frequency so it can be received at a distant location.

You Should Know

"Line-of-sight" and "straight-line" radio coverage problems are generally overcome with the use of repeaters placed on high ground or on top of a large structure or tower.

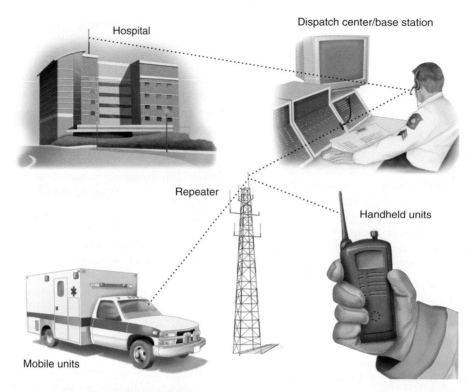

FIGURE 10-1 ▲ Example of an EMS communication system.

Hospital

Dispatch center/base station

Repeater

Handheld units

Mobile units

800-Megahertz Frequencies

The 800-megahertz (MHz) frequencies are UHF radio signals that use computer technology to make transmissions more secure than the other types of radio transmission. These frequencies allow clear communication with minimal interference. They also use a trunking system, which allows routing of a transmission to the first available frequency. Many channels are available to choose from. Although 800-MHz frequencies generally have a limited range and are very straight line, these problems are overcome by using multiple repeaters. This makes 800-MHz frequencies very effective for use in urban areas.

Remember This!

Knowing the capabilities of your equipment may mean the difference in communicating effectively with a distant site.

Equipment

Base Station

A **base station** is a **transmitter**/receiver at a stationary site such as a hospital, mountaintop, or public safety agency (Figure 10-1). At a minimum, a base station is made up of a transmitter, a receiver, a transmission

line, and an antenna. A transmitter is a device that sends out data on a given radio frequency. A radio signal generated by the base station may be sent directly to a receiving unit or to a repeater as needed.

Mobile Two-Way Radio

A **mobile two-way radio** is a vehicular-mounted communication device (Figure 10-2). It usually transmits at a lower power than base stations (typically 20B50 watts). The typical transmission range is 10B15 miles over average terrain. Transmission over flat land or water

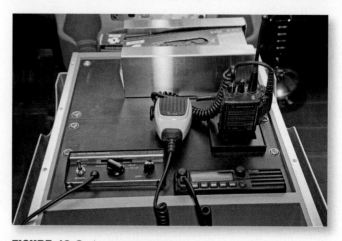

FIGURE 10-2 ▲ A mobile radio.

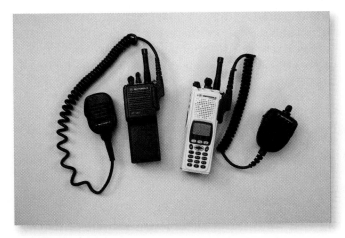

FIGURE 10-3 ▲ Portable (handheld) radios.

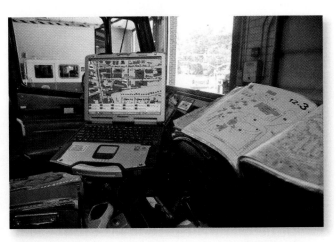

FIGURE 10-4 ▲ Mobile data computers display information pertaining to the calls for which EMS personnel are dispatched.

increases range. Urban areas, mountains, and dense foliage decrease transmission range.

Portable Radio

A **portable radio** is a handheld communication device (Figure 10-3). Typical power output is 1 to 5 watts, which limits its range. Portable radios are used for radio communication away from the emergency vehicle. They may have a single or multiple channels. A portable radio is often used in conjunction with repeaters to increase transmission range.

Repeater

A repeater is designed to receive a lower-powered transmission and then boost the signal for retransmittal. This may allow for greater geographical coverage and can assist with the transmission of portable signals to other units in the system. Repeaters can be fixed or mobile. For portable communications, repeaters may be located in the vehicle or on radio towers. Mobile communications use repeaters on radio towers. Repeater signals can be retransmitted by radio waves, microwaves, or telephone landlines.

Digital Radio Equipment

Digital pagers are used in many EMS systems. An audible signal and/or text message can be transmitted quickly by the dispatch center to alert EMS personnel to respond to a call.

Some EMS systems use **mobile data computers** (**MDCs**) (also called *mobile data terminals* or *MDTs*). A MDC is a computer that is mounted in an emergency vehicle (Figure 10-4). The computer displays information pertaining to the calls for which EMS personnel are dispatched. Examples of information displayed include text from dispatch pertaining to the call, the address of the incident, and a local map pointing

directly to the incident. The computer is used to log response times and indicate the status of the EMS crew/vehicle (in service and available for calls, on the scene, responding to a call, en route to the hospital, etc.). The computer is also used to send and receive text messages between the EMS crew and the dispatch center.

Many EMS vehicles are equipped with an **Automatic Vehicle Locator (AVL).** An AVL is a device that uses the **Global Positioning System (GPS)** to track a vehicle's location. GPS uses a system of satellites and receiving devices to compute the receiver's geographic position on the Earth. If the MDC is equipped with the necessary software, EMS vehicles equipped with an AVL appear on the local map that is displayed on the computer terminal.

Cellular Telephones

Geographical areas are divided into "cells." Each cell has a base station to transmit and receive signals. Cellular communication systems can track a mobile unit's movements from cell to cell and transfer the unit's radio activity to the appropriate cell base station.

Transmission Modes

Four transmission modes are generally used in an EMS communication system: one-way, simplex, duplex, and multiplex. A one-way transmission mode is generally used for paging systems. In one-way mode, a signal is sent to any unit monitoring the appropriate frequency, but the receiving unit has no ability to transmit a message.

A **simplex system** uses a single frequency to transmit and receive messages. As a result, only one signal may be transmitted or received at a time. Simultaneous radio transmissions will block a message from being received. An advantage of this type of system is that it allows the speaker to relay his message without interruption. However, communication using a simplex system takes away the ability for discussion regarding a patient or situation.

A **duplex system** is a mode of radio transmission that uses two frequencies to transmit and receive messages, allowing simultaneous two-way communication. An advantage of using this system for radio transmission is that either party can interrupt as necessary. Two-way communication aids discussion regarding a patient or situation. A disadvantage of this type of system is that the user at each end has a tendency to interrupt the other.

A **multiplex system** is a mode of radio transmission that permits simultaneous transmission of voice and other data, using one frequency. Advantages of using this system for radio transmission are that either party can interrupt as necessary and two-way communication aids discussion regarding a patient or situation. Disadvantages of this type of system are that voice signals can interfere with data transmission.

The Call

An EMS communications network must provide a means by which a citizen can reliably access the EMS system (usually by dialing 9-1-1). To ensure adequate EMS system response and coordination, there must also be a means for dispatch center to emergency vehicle communication, communication between emergency vehicles, communication from the emergency vehicle to the hospital, hospital-to-hospital communication, and communication between agencies, such as between EMS and law enforcement personnel.

9-1-1 is the official national emergency number in the United States and Canada. When the numbers 9-1-1 are dialed, the caller is quickly connected to a single location called a **Public Safety Answering Point (PSAP).** A PSAP is a facility equipped and staffed to receive and control 9-1-1 access calls. A Dispatch Center, Alarm Room, and Police Department are examples of facilities that may host the PSAP. Information coming into the PSAP may be processed at the PSAP, or the PSAP may route the call to an appropriate agency for processing. The PSAP dispatcher is trained to route the call to the appropriate local emergency medical, fire, and law enforcement agencies. Although EMS is usually activated by dialing 9-1-1, other methods of activating an emergency response include emergency alarm boxes, citizen band radios, and wireless telephones.

Enhanced 9-1-1, or E9-1-1, is a system that routes an emergency call to the 9-1-1 center closest to the caller and automatically displays the caller's phone number and address. E9-1-1 speeds up the transfer of information from the caller to the call taker and helps decrease the number of false alarms. It also assists in callbacks to obtain more complete information. Most 9-1-1 systems that exist today are E9-1-1 systems.

The FCC has established a program that requires wireless telephone carriers to provide E9-1-1 services. Wireless E9-1-1 provides the precise location of a 9-1-1 call from a wireless phone, within 50-100 meters in most cases. Wireless E9-1-1 is not yet available in all areas.

Voice over Internet Protocol (VoIP, also known as *Internet Voice*) is technology that allows users to make telephone calls by means of a broadband Internet connection instead of a regular telephone line. Companies offering this service have different features. Some services allow you to call only other people using the same service. Others allow you to call anyone who has a telephone number. Some services do not work during power outages and may not offer backup power. Some services offer E9-1-1 support as an optional service. Subscribers register and pay a fee for E9-1-1. With their subscription, an emergency call is automatically routed to the PSAP that handles 9-1-1 emergencies. If the subscriber is unable to speak, the PSAP operator will know the subscriber's location and be able to dispatch emergency personnel. If the user declines E9-1-1 service, he does not have direct access to emergency personnel via Internet Voice.

You Should Know

If a 9-1-1 caller does not speak English, the 9-1-1 call taker can add an interpreter from an outside service to the line. Communications centers that answer 9-1-1 calls also have special telephones for responding to 9-1-1 calls from deaf or hearing- and speech-impaired callers.

Dispatch

When an emergency occurs, a bystander frequently recognizes the event and activates the EMS system by calling 9-1-1 or another emergency number. The EMS dispatcher (Figure 10-5) gathers information and activates ("tones out") an appropriate EMS response based on the information received.

Emergency Medical Dispatchers

Formal emergency medical dispatch protocols and training began in the 1980s. Before this time, medical dispatchers averaged less than 1 hour of medical

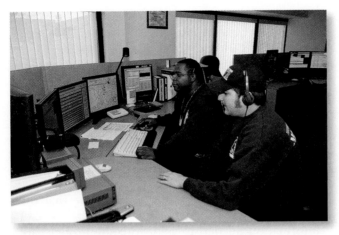

FIGURE 10-5 ▲ Example of an EMS dispatch center.

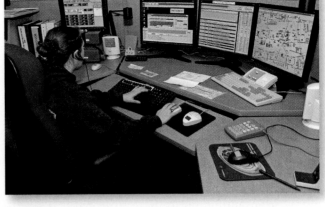

FIGURE 10-6 ▲ Computer-aided dispatch is used in many EMS systems.

You Should Know

Telephone conversations with the caller and telephone and radio transmissions between the dispatch center and police, fire, and EMS personnel are recorded. Courts have forced dispatch centers to release tapes of 9-1-1 calls in response to lawsuits by the media, attorneys, or other involved parties. 9-1-1 tapes may subsequently be heard on radio and television news. With this in mind, always be professional when communicating with others in the workplace and on an emergency call.

training. The Emergency Medical Dispatch program has been developed to certify personnel as Emergency Medical Dispatchers (EMDs). An EMD is knowledgeable about the geography of the area, the EMS system's capabilities, and the activities of other public service agencies. An EMD is responsible for:

- Verifying the address of the incident
- Asking questions of the caller
- Assigning responders to the incident
- Alerting/activating responders to the incident
- Providing prearrival instructions to the caller
- Communicating with responders
- Recording incident times

You Should Know

Emergency medical dispatchers are trained to provide prearrival instructions to the caller by phone when necessary. How to provide cardiopulmonary resuscitation (CPR), emergency care for choking, and bleeding control techniques are among the most common prearrival instructions provided by EMDs.

Computer-aided dispatch (CAD) is used in many EMS systems (Figure 10-6). When a call comes into a PSAP that uses CAD, the address and phone number of the caller are automatically entered into the CAD system. The dispatcher types a description of the emergency into the computer and then assigns a priority level to the call. As a result, an "event" is created for which many activities related to it can be tracked, retrieved, and evaluated. The software used by the CAD system can connect dispatchers with local, state, and national computer database systems. Important times pertaining to an emergency call that are tracked and evaluated in most EMS systems include the following:

- Call received
- EMS crew dispatched
- EMS crew vehicle en route
- EMS crew on the scene
- EMS crew makes patient contact
- EMS crew en route to receiving facility
- EMS crew arrival with patient at receiving facility
- EMS crew returning from the hospital
- EMS crew available for service
- EMS crew arrival at the station/quarters

Objective 1

When the dispatcher has enough information about an EMS call to determine the type of response needed and the proper unit to send, a signal is sent to begin the activation process. The crew may receive a signal by pager, radio, or cell phone. General guidelines to ensure effective radio communication during the activation and response phase of a typical EMS call are listed in the following *Making a Difference* box.

Making a Difference

Guidelines for Effective Radio Communication

- Make sure you have checked that your equipment is available and in good working order at the start of your shift.
- Before speaking into the radio:
  - —Make sure the radio is on and the volume is properly adjusted.
  - —Reduce background noise as much as possible.
  - —Listen to the frequency that you will be transmitting on to make sure that it is clear before speaking.
  - —Hold the radio's microphone about 2-3 inches away from your mouth.
  - —Locate and press the "push to talk" (PTT) button. To make sure your first words are not cut off, pause (with the PTT button depressed) for about one to two seconds before speaking.
- Using a normal tone of voice, address the unit being called by its name and number. Then identify the name of your unit (and number, if appropriate) as determined by your local protocols.
- Wait for the unit being called to signal you to begin your transmission by saying, "Go ahead," or some other term standard in your area. A response of "Stand by" means, "Wait until further notice."
- When the unit being called has acknowledged your call (and has stopped speaking), relay your message. Speak clearly, keeping your transmissions brief.
- At the end of your message, the unit being called may repeat back the pertinent information from your message to make sure that the unit has received the information correctly. If the information is verified as correct, acknowledge the unit's transmission and announce that you are clear.
- Use plain English in your radio communications. Avoid the use of "ten codes" and slang.
- Avoid meaningless phrases, such as "Be advised."
- Do not use profanity on the air. (The FCC may impose substantial fines.)
- Avoid words that are hard to hear like "yes" and "no;" use "affirmative" and "negative."
- Courtesy is assumed; there is no need to say "please," "thank you," and "you're welcome."

- When transmitting a number that might be confused with another, give the number, then give the individual digits. For example, do not say "fifty one." Instead, say "five one."
- Do not offer a diagnosis of the patient's complaint or injury. Remain objective and impartial in describing patients.

You Should Know

Many EMS personnel incorrectly assume that the call taker in the dispatch center has every piece of information needed to assist with the proper care of your patient. The reality is that in some cases the caller is too excited, frightened, confused, or reluctant to deliver the needed information.

En Route to the Call

Objective 1

The format for your radio report may be determined by local or state protocols. The following "script" may help you understand a typical call. The script below begins with the electronic or tone activation of a radio or pager. We will use "Medic 51" to indicate your communication with dispatch.

Dispatch Center: "Medic 51 (five, one), respond code 3 to 4321 (four, three, two, one) East Main Street for a report of difficulty breathing. Call number 987 (nine, eight, seven). Time out 1402 (fourteen, zero, two)."

Medic 51: "Dispatch, Medic 51 (five, one) received. Responding to report of difficulty breathing at four, three, two, one East Main Street."

Dispatch Center: "Medic 51 (five, one), dispatch received, you are responding. Caller reports your patient is 70-year-old female in the kitchen of this address. The door will be unlocked. 1403 (fourteen, zero, three)."

Medic 51: "Dispatch, Medic 51 (five, one), received. 70-year-old female in the kitchen and the door will be unlocked."

Arrival at the Scene

Objective 9

Additional radio contact with the dispatch center will be needed on your arrival at the scene.

Medic 51: "Dispatch, Medic 51 (five, one). We are on scene."

Dispatch Center: "Medic 51 (five, one), Received, on scene at 1406 (fourteen, zero, six)."

You Should Know

When to Notify Dispatch

- Receiving the call
- Responding to the call
- Arriving at the scene
- Leaving the scene for the receiving facility
- Arriving at the receiving facility
- Leaving the hospital for the station
- Arriving at the station

Making a Difference

Your patients are individuals of varying ages with a wide range of life experiences, knowledge, reasoning abilities, skills, and medical needs.

Communicating with the Patient

Objectives 5, 7, 8

When communicating with a patient, begin by identifying yourself and establishing your role. Explain that you are there to provide assistance. Recognize the patient's need for privacy, preserve the patient's dignity, and treat the patient with respect. Address the patient by proper name, Mr. __ or Mrs. __. Ask the patient what he wishes to be called, and then ask for permission to use this name. Do not use words such as "hon," "dear," or "sweetheart" when speaking to a patient. Phrases such as these are disrespectful and unprofessional.

While talking with the patient, family members, or bystanders, look at the person with whom you are talking instead of looking at your chart (Figure 10-7). Although this takes practice, nothing conveys a greater sense of your understanding and control of the situation.

Be confident and remain calm. Know what you are going to say before you say it. Have all of the information you need before you start talking. Speak clearly and at an appropriate speed or pace, not too rapidly and not too slowly. Avoid the tendency to get excited. Speaking in a calm and professional manner will give the impression that you are in control of the situation.

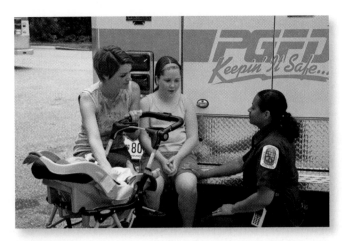

FIGURE 10-7 ▲ When talking with a patient, family members, or bystanders, be confident, calm, and respectful.

Listen carefully to what your patient is telling you. Do not interrupt your patient before she has finished telling you what the problem is. Do not anticipate what the patient is going to say and finish her sentences for her. Allow the patient time to explain what is wrong in her own words.

Help ease your patient's fears by explaining what you are about to do, how you will do it, and why it must be done. Use common terms (not medical terminology) when asking questions and explaining the care you will provide.

Be aware of your body position. Most patients find it intimidating if you are standing over them. Be truthful. Patients have a legal right to know about their condition. This does not mean you have to be brutal, but do not lie to the patient about their medical condition.

The following "script" is an example of possible communication between you and a patient as you enter the patient's home.

> **Medic 51:** (As you enter the home.) "Hello, ambulance (or fire department) here. Did someone call 9-1-1?"
>
> **Patient:** "Yes! In here."
>
> **Medic 51:** (As you approach and kneel next to patient.) "Hi! My name is Joe. I am an Emergency Medical Technician with the ambulance (or fire department). I am here to help you. Can you tell me about the emergency today?"
>
> **Patient:** "Hard to breathe."
>
> **Medic 51:** "My partner and I will be glad to take care of you. Could you please tell me your name and what you prefer to be called?"
>
> **Patient:** "Mrs. Jones. Call me Linda."
>
> **Medic 51:** "Linda, when did your trouble breathing start?"

Patient: "Yesterday."

Medic 51: "I would like to give you some oxygen to help your breathing."

Patient: "OK."

Medic 51: "I am going to put this oxygen mask on your face. I want you to breathe normally. The oxygen will help your breathing."

Elderly Patients

An elderly patient may have difficulty hearing and poor vision. Assume a position directly in the patient's line of vision and speak directly toward him. Begin speaking to the patient in a normal tone of voice. If the patient has difficulty hearing, speak a little more loudly until he can hear you. Speak slowly and say each word clearly. Be careful not to "talk down" to the patient. Ask the patient one question at a time and allow the patient time to respond. If it is necessary to repeat the question, phrase it exactly as it was asked the first time. Provide reassurance with a soothing voice and calm manner.

Children

Young infants (birth to 6 months of age) are unafraid of strangers and have no modesty. Older infants (6 months to 1 year of age) do not like to be separated from their caregiver (separation anxiety). They may be threatened by direct eye contact with strangers. If possible, assess the baby on the caregiver's lap. Avoid loud noises, bright light, and quick, jerky movements. Smile and use a calm, soothing voice. Allow the baby to suck on a pacifier for comfort, if appropriate and if the child is willing to take it. Do not force the pacifier if the child does not want it.

A toddler (1 to 3 years of age) responds appropriately to an angry or a friendly voice. When separated from their primary caregiver, most toddlers experience strong separation anxiety. A toddler can answer simple questions and follow simple directions. However, you cannot reason with a toddler. A toddler is likely to be more cooperative if he is given a comfort object like a blanket, stuffed animal, or toy.

Remember This!

Toddlers understand "soon," "bye-bye," "all gone," and "uh-oh." A toddler's favorite words are "no" and "mine," so avoid asking questions that can be answered with a yes or no. If you ask questions that begin with "May I," "Can I," or "Would you like to," a toddler will probably say no. If you then do whatever you asked him anyway, you will immediately lose the toddler's trust and cooperation.

Toddlers are distrustful of strangers. They are likely to resist examination and treatment. When touched, they may scream, cry, or kick. Toddlers do not like having their clothing removed and do not like anything on their face. Encourage the child's trust by gaining the cooperation of her caregiver. By talking with the caregiver first, the child may be more at ease if she sees that the adult is not threatened (Figure 10-8). When possible, allow an infant or young child to remain on the caregiver's lap. If this is not possible, try to keep the caregiver within the child's line of vision. Approach the child slowly and address her by name. Talk to her at eye level, using simple words and short phrases. Speak to her in a calm, reassuring tone of voice. Although a young child may not understand your words, she will respond to your tone.

Remember This!

Do not threaten a child if he is uncooperative.

Preschoolers (4 to 5 years of age) are afraid of the unknown, the dark, being left alone, and adults who look or act mean. They may think their illness or injury is punishment for bad behavior or thoughts. Approach the child slowly and talk to him at eye level. Use simple words and phrases and a reassuring tone of voice. Assure the child that he was not bad and is not being punished.

A preschooler may feel vulnerable and out of control when lying down. Assess and treat the child in an upright position when possible. Preschoolers are

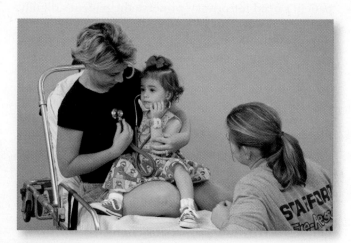

FIGURE 10-8 ▲ Encourage the trust of a young child by gaining the cooperation of her caregiver. By talking with the caregiver first, the child may be more at ease if she sees that the adult is not threatened.

modest. They do not like being touched or having their clothing removed. When assessing a child, keep in mind that he has probably been told not to let a stranger touch him. Remove clothing, assess the child, and then quickly replace clothing. Allow the caregiver to remain with the child whenever possible.

Preschoolers are curious and like to "help." Encourage the child to participate. Tell the child how things will feel and what is to be done just before doing it. For example, a preschooler may fear being suffocated by an oxygen mask. It may be helpful to use a doll or a stuffed animal to explain the procedure. The child may want to hold or look at the equipment first.

Preschoolers are highly imaginative. When talking with a preschooler, choose your words carefully. Avoid baby talk and frightening or misleading terms. For example, avoid words such as "take," "cut," "shot," "deaden," or "germs." Instead of saying, "I'm going to take your pulse," you might say, "I'm going to see how fast your heart is beating."

When caring for a school-age child (6 to12 years of age), approach in a friendly manner and introduce yourself. Talk directly to the child about what happened, even if you also obtain a history from the caregiver. Explain procedures before carrying them out. Allow the child to see and touch equipment that may be used in his care.

Remember This!

Honesty is very important when interacting with school-age children. If you are going to do something to the child that may cause pain, warn the child just before you do it. Give a simple explanation of what will take place and do it just before the procedure so that he does not have long to think about it. For example, if a child has a possible broken leg and you must move the leg to apply a splint, warn the child just before you move the leg.

Adolescents (13 to 18 years of age) expect to be treated as adults. Talk to an adolescent in a respectful, friendly manner, as if speaking to an adult. If possible, obtain a history from the patient instead of a caregiver. Expect an adolescent to have many questions and want detailed explanations about what you are planning to do or what is happening to him. Explain things clearly and honestly. Allow time for questions. Do not bargain with an adolescent in order to do what you need to do. Recognize the tendency for adolescents to overreact. Do not become angry with an emotional or hysterical adolescent.

Non–English-Speaking Patients

Communication with non–English-speaking patients may require the use of an interpreter. Explain to the interpreter the type of questions that will be asked. Avoid interrupting a family member (or bystander) and interpreter when they are communicating. If an interpreter is not present at the scene, contact dispatch or medical direction. Telephone companies often have interpreters who are available 24 hours a day.

You Should Know

Not all hearing-impaired people hear the same sounds in the same way.

Hearing-Impaired Patients

Because a patient has a hearing impairment does not mean that he lacks mental intelligence. Many deaf patients do not consider a lack of hearing a disability. In fact, they often resent being treated as if they have a disability. A common mistaken belief of some healthcare professionals is that you must speak more slowly and loudly for the patient to understand you. Not only does this not work, it may actually confuse the patient. When you speak more slowly than normal, you have a tendency to overemphasize the way you move your mouth when you speak. This can lead to a greater misunderstanding if the patient is trying to read your lips. Try not to drastically change the way you speak. Use your normal tone of voice and speak at your normal speed—as if you were carrying on a conversation with any other patient (Figure 10-9). If the patient has a sound amplification device or hearing aid, you may need to help him put it in place.

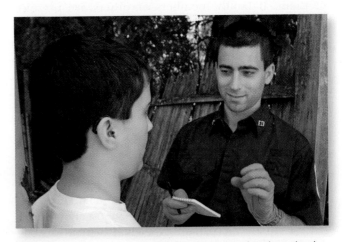

FIGURE 10-9 ▲ When speaking to a hearing-impaired patient, use your normal tone of voice and speak at your normal speed—as if you were carrying on a conversation with any other patient.

You may have to get your patient's attention with a gentle touch on the shoulder. Face your patient directly so that he can see your face and mouth. Make sure that there is adequate lighting so the patient can see your face and mouth clearly. When speaking, do not move your head around. Doing so makes it difficult for the patient to follow what you are saying. If the patient has some limited ability to hear, try to reduce any unnecessary background noise. For example, shut off televisions, radios, dishwashers, or other noisy appliances while talking with the patient. You may even resort to the use of paper and pen to communicate.

When questioning your patient about his condition, think about the questions you want to ask. Then ask him short, direct questions that require a very specific answer. Make sure to actually speak or say every word in your question. Ask one question at a time and follow up on the answer before starting another line of questioning. Doing so will allow you and the patient to focus on one problem at a time. It can even lead to a better interview. Avoid the use of sign language unless you are very skilled.

Remember to explain any procedure before providing care. Be sure to inform the staff at the receiving facility of the patient's hearing impairment.

Visually-Impaired Patients

The term *visual impairment* applies to a variety of vision disturbances. Visual impairments range from blindness and lack of usable sight to low vision. **Low vision** is a visual impairment that interferes with a person's ability to perform everyday activities.

If the patient is visually impaired, approach the patient from the front and introduce yourself. Identify any persons with you. Speak in a normal voice. Most blind persons are not hearing impaired so there is no need to raise your voice or shout when talking to them. If family members or others are present, address the patient by name so that it is clear to whom you are talking. Clearly explain any care you are going to provide before doing so. In this way, you do not surprise or startle the patient. Be sure to talk directly to the patient, not through a family member. Do not avoid the use of words such as "see" and "blind." These words are parts of normal speech.

You Should Know

When walking with a visually impaired patient, make sure that the pathway is free of clutter. Offer the patient your arm and let him hold on just above your elbow. Guide the patient by leading him. It can be very helpful to "verbalize" the location of your equipment. When giving directions, indicate left and right according to the way the patient is facing.

A very strong bond can form between a visually impaired patient and his guide dog. Make every attempt to keep them together if at all possible. Do not pet or otherwise distract a guide dog. A blind person's safety depends on the animal's full attention.

Speech-Impaired Patients

Many patients experience speech difficulties caused by a brain injury or a lack of oxygen to the brain that do not affect other cognitive abilities. For example, a stroke patient may be unable to speak but may be able to understand your questions. You may be able to establish some other means of communication, such as a hand squeeze or even eye blinks. If your patient appears to understand your questions but is unable to answer, stop asking the questions but continue to talk to the patient. Let him know that you understand he is unable to talk. It may be comforting to the patient to know that you are aware of his situation.

Making a Difference

Never assume that a person who cannot speak clearly lacks mental intelligence. A severe speech deficit can be completely unrelated to intelligence.

Children and adults may have language problems that stem from a hearing impairment, a congenital learning disorder, a speech delay, or cerebral palsy. Other speech problems may occur when a patient has difficulty with his speech pattern, such as stuttering. A patient who has cancer of the larynx may have a hoarseness or harshness in his voice. These patients may have only a limited ability to respond to your questions. Try to keep your questions short and to the point. In some situations, it may be helpful to ask questions that can be answered with a yes or no. Allow the patient time to respond and in his own way. Rushing the patient to answer may only increase his anxiety and frustration. Pay attention and listen carefully to what the patient has to say. He may even use hand gestures or a notepad to communicate his needs.

Communicating with Family Members and Bystanders

Objective 8

When talking with family members and bystanders, avoid interrupting when they are talking. Speak clearly and use common words (avoid using medical terms). Speak at an appropriate speed or pace, not too rapidly and not too slowly.

Assume a helpful posture and face the person speaking. Maintain eye contact while listening carefully. Clarify information that is unclear.

Communicating with Individuals from Other Agencies

Objective 8

Communications with individuals from other agencies should be organized, concise, thorough, and accurate. When receiving a report from others at the scene (such as bystanders or Emergency Medical Responders [EMRs]), listen carefully to their report (Figure 10-10). Ask questions if any information is unclear. Be professional and thank them for their efforts.

In some EMS systems, you may be required to give a verbal report to an Advanced Life Support (ALS) professional arriving on the scene where you have been providing care. Keeping your report brief and pertinent, you will need to relay the following information:

- Patient's name (if known)
- Patient's age and gender
- Chief complaint
- Pertinent history of present illness or problem
- Major pertinent past illnesses
- Mental status
- Vital signs
- Pertinent physical examination findings
- Emergency medical care given
- Patient's response to emergency medical care
- Orders received from medical direction (if applicable)

Communicating with Medical Direction

You may need to contact medical direction for advice, if a patient refuses care, during difficult patient management situations, or to obtain orders to give medications. When communicating with medical direction, it is very important that your radio or telephone communication be professional, organized, concise, and pertinent (Figure 10-11). The information that you give to the physician must be accurate because the physician will use this information to determine whether to order medications and procedures.

After receiving an order for a medication or procedure (or denial of such a request), use the "echo" procedure. This means that you must repeat the order back to the physician, word for word. Be sure to document any orders received and question any orders that are unclear or appear to be inappropriate.

En Route to the Receiving Facility

Objective 9

Contact your dispatch center as you begin patient transport to the receiving facility.

> **Medic 51:** "Medic 51 (five, one) to Dispatch."
>
> **Dispatch Center:** "Dispatch. Medic 51 (five, one) go ahead."
>
> **Medic 51:** "Dispatch, Medic 51 (five, one) is transporting one patient to Anytown Medical Center—non-emergent."
>
> **Dispatch Center:** "Received, Medic 51 (five, one). Transporting one patient to Anytown Medical Center, non-emergent. Time: 1426 (fourteen, two, six)."

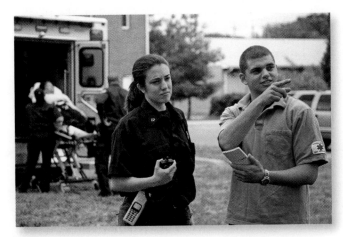

FIGURE 10-10 ▲ When receiving a report from others at the scene (such as an EMR), listen carefully to his report.

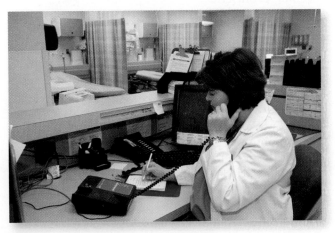

FIGURE 10-11 ▲ When communicating with medical direction, it is very important that your radio or telephone communication be professional, organized, concise, and pertinent.

In most EMS systems, EMS personnel are required to notify any receiving facility of the condition of the patient they are transporting to that facility. The essential elements of this type of report and the order in which they should occur are as follows:

- Identify the unit and the level of the care provider (such as BLS, ALS)
- Estimate time of arrival at facility
- Patient's age and gender
- Chief complaint
- Brief, pertinent history of present illness or problem
- Major past illnesses
- Mental status
- Vital signs
- Pertinent physical exam findings
- Emergency medical care given
- Response to emergency medical care

Your ability to communicate effectively with the receiving facility directly affects the care that the patient receives. This report is your chance to paint a very clear picture in the minds of the receiving facility staff. The clearer you paint the picture, the better prepared they will be for your arrival and the subsequent treatment of your patient. If you do not use the standard reporting format, you run the risk of omitting essential information. Patient care may be delayed while the hospital attempts to get the information they need. This could negatively affect your patient's health.

A sample radio report simulating communication with a receiving facility is shown below. You will need to practice a radio report like this one many times to become proficient.

> **Medic 51:** "Anytown Medical Center, Medic 51 (five, one)"
>
> **Anytown Medical Center:** "Anytown Medical Center. Go ahead Medic 51 (five, one)."
>
> **Medic 51:** "Anytown Medical Center, EMT Smith on Medic 51 (five, one). We are en route to your facility. Expected arrival time: 10 minutes. The patient is a 70-year-old woman with a chief complaint of difficulty breathing that started yesterday. Patient denies any past medical history or medications. Patient is awake and oriented to person, place, time, and event. Baseline vital signs follow: respirations 20, pulse 80, blood pressure of 130/78. Exam reveals crackles in the bases of both lungs. There is swelling of both of the patient's legs to the level of her calves. We have placed the

patient in a semi-Fowler's position and put her on oxygen by nonrebreather mask at 15 L/min. The patient reports feeling 'a little better.' Any questions or orders?"

> **Anytown Medical Center:** "Medic 51 (five, one), Anytown Medical Center report received (your report may be repeated to ensure accuracy). No orders or questions. Contact us if there is any change in patient condition before arrival. Anytown Medical Center clear."
>
> **Medic 51:** "Medic 51 (five, one) clear."

Arrival at the Receiving Facility

Notify dispatch as soon as you arrive at the receiving facility.

> **Medic 51:** "Dispatch, Medic 51 (five, one). Arrival at Anytown Medical Center."
>
> **Dispatch Center:** "Received, Medic 51 (five, one). Arrival at Anytown Medical Center at 1448. (fourteen, four, eight)"

On arrival at the receiving facility, the staff expects a verbal report that follows a specific format. The verbal report (sometimes called a *hand-off report*) is essentially a summary of the information that you gave over the radio. Give your verbal report to a healthcare professional of equal or higher medical skills. Begin the verbal report by introducing the patient by name (if known). Summarize the information already provided by radio or telephone to the receiving facility:

- Patient's chief complaint
- Pertinent patient history that was not previously given
- Emergency medical care given en route and the patient's response to the treatment given
- Vital signs taken en route
- Any additional information collected en route but not transmitted to the receiving facility

Give your verbal report in a polite and respectful manner (Figure 10-12). The receiving facility staff may ask you questions to clarify information or may have additional questions about the patient or your observations at the scene. Effective communication with the receiving facility staff is important. It can make the difference between prompt, efficient care for the patient's injury or illness and problems and confusion that may delay patient care.

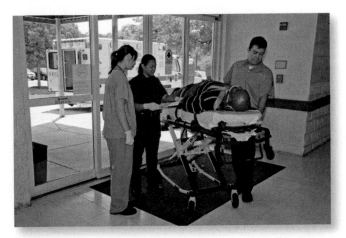

FIGURE 10-12 ▲ Give a verbal report to the receiving facility staff in a polite and respectful manner.

En Route to the Station

Objective 9

Notify dispatch when you are leaving the receiving facility and are en route to the station.

> **Medic 51:** "Medic 51 (five, one) to Dispatch."
>
> **Dispatch Center:** "Dispatch. Go ahead Medic 51 (five, one)."
>
> **Medic 51:** "Dispatch, Medic 51 (five, one) is leaving Anytown Medical Center en route to our station."
>
> **Dispatch Center:** "Received, Medic 51 (five, one). En route to your station. Time: 1510 (fifteen, one, zero)."

Contact dispatch again on arrival at the station or earlier, when you enter your service area, per your agency's guidelines.

> **Medic 51:** "Medic 51 (five, one) to Dispatch."
>
> **Dispatch Center:** "Dispatch. Medic 51 (five, one), go ahead."
>
> **Medic 51:** "Dispatch, Medic 51 (five, one) is back at our station and in service."
>
> **Dispatch Center:** "Received, Medic 51 (five, one). In station and available for service. Time: 1518 (fifteen, one, eight)."

Legal Considerations

Objective 6

Your interaction with a patient should always be direct, polite, and honest. There are legal limits to the information that you may share with others about your patient. These legal limitations are found in the Health Insurance Portability and Accountability Act (HIPAA) (see Chapter 3). Generally, you may only share medical information about your patient with those healthcare professionals who will have direct contact with your patient. These legal limitations extend to the radio report given to the receiving facility. Do not use any patient "identifiers" beyond the age and gender of your patient over the radio. Individuals who disobey HIPAA privacy rules face criminal and civil penalties.

On the Scene Wrap-Up

While you were interviewing the patient, your partner has calmed the patient's husband and learned that the patient is suffering from a brain illness that causes her to not remember her family. The phone call to the dispatch center was made without his knowledge by the patient. Further conversations with the patient's husband reveals that he has medical power of attorney for this patient and does want her transported for evaluation by the hospital. Because you have treated the patient and her husband with respect and listened to what they had to say, your patient transport is uneventful. Your verbal report to the hospital contains all of the needed information to allow the hospital staff to begin giving appropriate patient care on your arrival. ■

Sum It Up

▶ Communication is the process of sending and receiving information. As an EMT, you must be able to communicate effectively with crewmembers, emergency dispatchers, medical direction, and other healthcare professionals; law enforcement personnel and other public safety workers; the patient; and the patient's family.

▶ The Federal Communications Commission (FCC) is the U.S. government agency responsible for the development and enforcement of rules and regulations pertaining to radio transmissions.

▶ Very High Frequency (VHF) radio frequencies can be subdivided into low band and high band. Low-band frequencies generally have a greater range than high-band VHF frequencies. Radio waves in the low-band frequency range bend and follow the curvature of the Earth, allowing radio transmission over long distances. Radio waves in the high-band frequency range travel in a straight line. This straight-line quality means that the radio wave is easily blocked by topography such as a hill, mountain, or large building.

▶ Ultra-High Frequency (UHF) radio waves travel in a straight line but do have an ability to reflect or bounce around buildings. 800-megahertz frequencies are UHF radio signals that use computer technology to make transmissions more secure than the other types of radio transmission.

▶ A base station is a transmitter/receiver at a stationary site such as a hospital, mountaintop, or public safety agency. A radio signal generated by the base station may be sent directly to a receiving unit or to a repeater as needed. A mobile two-way radio is a vehicular-mounted communication device. A portable radio is a handheld communication device. A repeater is a device that receives a transmission from a low-power portable or mobile radio on one frequency and then retransmits it at a higher power on another frequency so it can be received at a distant location.

▶ Mobile data computers (MDCs) (also called mobile data terminals or MDTs) are computers mounted in emergency vehicles that display information pertaining to the calls for which EMS personnel are dispatched. The computer is also used to send and receive text messages between the EMS crew and the dispatch center.

▶ An EMS communications network must provide a means by which a citizen can reliably access the EMS system (usually by dialing 9-1-1). To ensure adequate EMS system response and coordination, there must also be a means for dispatch to emergency vehicle communication, communication between emergency vehicles, communication from the emergency vehicle to the hospital, hospital-to-hospital communication, and communication between agencies, such as between EMS and law enforcement personnel.

▶ 9-1-1 is the official national emergency number in the United States and Canada. When the numbers 9-1-1 are dialed, the caller is quickly connected to a single location called a Public Safety Answering Point (PSAP). Although EMS is usually activated by dialing 9-1-1, other methods of activating an emergency response include emergency alarm boxes, citizen band radios, and wireless telephones.

Enhanced 9-1-1, or E9-1-1, is a system that routes an emergency call to the 9-1-1 center closest to the caller and automatically displays the caller's phone number and address. Voice over Internet Protocol (VoIP, also known as Internet Voice) is technology that allows users to make telephone calls by means of a broadband Internet connection instead of using a regular telephone line.

▶ Emergency Medical Dispatchers (EMDs) are trained professionals who are responsible for verifying the address of the incident, asking questions of the caller, assigning responders to the incident, alerting/activating responders to the incident, providing prearrival instructions to the caller, communicating with responders, and recording incident times.

▶ Dispatch should be notified when receiving the call, responding to the call, arriving at the scene, leaving the scene for the receiving facility, arriving at the receiving facility, leaving the hospital for the station, returning to service, and arriving at the station.

▶ When communicating with a patient, identify yourself and explain that you are there to provide assistance. Recognize the patient's need for privacy, preserve the patient's dignity, and treat the patient with respect.

▶ When talking with family members and bystanders, avoid interrupting when they are talking. Speak clearly and use common words (avoid using medical terms). Speak at an appropriate speed or pace, not too rapidly and not too slowly. When communicating with individuals from other agencies, be organized, concise, thorough, and accurate.

▶ It may be necessary to contact medical direction for advice, obtain orders to give medications, or receive other orders. The information given to the physician must be accurate because the physician will use this information to determine whether to order medications and procedures. Repeat orders back to the physician, word for word.

▶ Use a standardized reporting format when relaying a verbal report to medical direction or to the staff of the receiving facility.

▶ The Health Insurance Portability and Accountability Act (HIPAA) limits the medical information that may be shared about an individual.

11 Documentation

By the end of this chapter, you should be able to:

Knowledge Objectives ▶
1. Explain the components of the written report and list the information that should be included on the written report.
2. Identify the various sections of the written report.
3. Describe what information is required in each section of the prehospital care report and how it should be entered.
4. Define the special considerations concerning patient refusal.
5. Describe the legal implications associated with the written report.
6. Discuss all state and/or local record and reporting requirements.

Attitude Objectives ▶
7. Explain the rationale for patient care documentation.
8. Explain the rationale for the Emergency Medical Services system's gathering data.
9. Explain the rationale for using medical terminology correctly.
10. Explain the rationale for using an accurate and synchronous clock so that information can be used in trending.

Skill Objectives ▶
11. Complete a prehospital care report.

On the Scene

It's the end of a very busy shift and you are tired. You and your partner have run a record number of calls in a short period. Your last patient of the shift is complaining of chest pain. He has a handwritten list of medications that seems to cover a full page and then some. Rather than write down all of the medications on the list, you decide to "scan" the list for what you believe to be the important medications and just record those on your prehospital care report. You then hand this information to the charge nurse at the receiving hospital. When she asks for information about the patient's medications, you refer her to a copy of your report.

You walk outside of the Emergency Department to help your partner restock and clean the ambulance. As you are finishing these tasks, you hear an announcement over the Emergency Department loudspeaker asking for your crew to report to the room where you left your patient. As you enter the room, you see members of the Emergency Department staff performing cardiopulmonary resuscitation (CPR) on the patient that you just brought in. A doctor looks around and asks if anyone has information about this patient. ■

THINK ABOUT IT

As you read this chapter, think about the following questions:

● What information should have been given to the Emergency Department staff during your verbal report?
● Is there any danger to your patient because of your omission of information on the prehospital care report?

Introduction

A prehospital care report (PCR) is known by many names (see the following *You Should Know* box). No matter what its name in your area, a PCR is a legal record that documents the patient care delivered in the field. Healthcare professionals use the information in the PCR to begin appropriate treatment after the patient arrives at the receiving facility. Inaccurate, illegible, or incomplete information on the prehospital care report regarding the patient's condition, assessment, and care can have grave consequences. Every Emergency Medical Technician (EMT) must learn to document accurately, legibly, and completely (Figure 11-1).

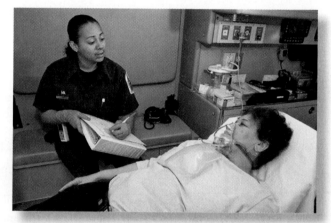

FIGURE 11-1 ▲ An EMT must document accurately, legibly, and completely.

You Should Know

The prehospital care report may also be called the:
● Patient care report
● Run report
● Encounter form
● EMS form
● Run sheet
● Trip sheet
● Incident report
● Ambulance report

Characteristics of Good Documentation

An EMT is a healthcare professional. A healthcare professional's documentation is a reflection of his professionalism and credibility. Just as you must prac-

tice to become skilled at assessing a patient, writing a good report is also a skill that requires practice. Characteristics of good documentation are shown in the following *Making a Difference* box.

Making a Difference

Characteristics of Good Documentation

● Complete
● Clear
● Concise
● Objective
● Timely
● Accurate (including spelling)
● Legible

Accurate and complete documentation tells a story about what happened while the patient was in your care. This includes the patient's condition on arrival at the scene, your assessment findings, the emergency care performed, and the patient's response to the care given. Your documentation should contain facts that are supported by what you see, hear, feel, and smell. It should not contain jargon, slang, bias, opinions, or impressions. Do not use phrases like, "I felt," or "I thought." Subjective information that can be documented includes what the patient says that pertains to his current illness or complaint.

Remember This!

When completing a PCR, *never* "label" a patient. Examples of labeling include using words such as "rude," "confrontational," or "frequent flyer." Words such as these can give the impression that the care you provide to these patients differs from the care you provide to patients who are friendlier or whom you see less often.

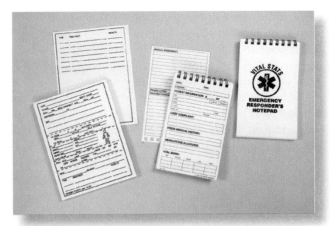

FIGURE 11-2 ▲ You may find it convenient to use a preprinted pocket-sized form to jot down notes while you are interviewing a patient. This information can then be used when writing a complete report when the call is over.

When completing a paper report, use a ballpoint pen with black or blue waterproof ink. Since paper PCRs usually consist of multiple pages, you will need to press firmly to make sure the information you write appears on the last page of the form. Use a strong card or separator to assure that you are not writing through to the next set of report forms. Write neatly and in a manner that is easy to read. Print if necessary. Spelling is important. Many medical terms are spelled similarly but have completely different meanings. If you do not know how to spell a specific word, either look it up or use a different phrase. If you find medical terms confusing, it is generally better to use common words to describe or explain something in your report than to use medical terms incorrectly.

The story that you write in the PCR about a call should be clear and to the point. It is not necessary to write a novel to describe what happened. However, you must include enough detail that you will be able to recall events that occurred two weeks previously and even five years previously. In addition, the story should be clearly written so that the healthcare professionals who assume responsibility for your patient will be able to read the report and know what happened on the basis of what you wrote.

Remember This!

Two guidelines you should remember about documentation are: "If it is not written down, it was not done," and "If it was not done, do not write it down."

Although EMS calls are usually very busy scenes, you must make it a habit to document the care you give in a timely manner. Since your ability to recall details will usually begin to fade with time, it is a good idea to make notes throughout a call and then use them to write a complete report when the call is over. Some EMS professionals use preprinted pocket-sized forms to jot down notes while they are interviewing a patient (Figure 11-2). You will need to develop a system that works for you and then use it consistently.

Advances in technology have led to the availability and use of mobile and pen-based reporting systems. Electronic prehospital care reports are called ePCRs. Some electronic systems can interface with EMS equipment, such as an automated external defibrillator (AED). This allows data recorded from the AED to be sent to the electronic reporting system. Some electronic systems provide anatomical templates that allow EMS personnel to easily document medical or trauma body system findings by patient gender and age. Although this technology will affect the manner in which you complete your prehospital care reports, you are still expected to document the same basic information.

Uses of the Prehospital Care Report

Medical Uses

One of the most important necessities of giving prehospital medical care is the thorough, honest, and complete documentation of that care. Your accurate observation and documentation of the patient's vital signs, medical history, mental status, medications, allergies, and related patient information is very important to the Paramedics, physicians, and nurses who will assume the care of your patient.

The PCR may be the only source of information for hospital personnel to refer to later for important information about the scene, the patient's condition on EMS arrival at the scene, emergency medical care provided or attempted, and changes in the patient's condition.

Legal Uses

The PCR is an official record of the care given by EMS. When you transfer patient care to another healthcare professional, you are expected to give a verbal report of what occurred while the patient was in your care. You are also expected to provide that individual with a completed PCR. Your completed PCR becomes part of the patient's medical record.

Because a PCR is a legal document, it must accurately reflect the events that occurred and the time they occurred. When skills are performed, accurately document who performed them and the time they were done. For example, if oxygen is given, document the device used, the time it was applied, who applied it, the liter flow used, and the patient's response to the care given. At a minimum, the patient's response should include a description of his mental status, skin color, and oxygen saturation level (if available).

Remember This!

Pay attention to time intervals when documenting.

A patient's attorney will often request a copy of a PCR when researching a patient's complaint about his care. A poorly documented PCR is more likely to cause a jury to find liability against an EMT than a well-documented report. PCRs that contain "red flags" cause individuals who read the report to question the facts about the emergency care given to a patient. Examples of documentation "red flags" that must be avoided are shown in the following *Remember This!* box.

Administrative Uses

A PCR not only provides an accurate record of the circumstances of the patient encounter, but it also enables the billing department to honestly and accu-

Remember This!

Documentation "Red Flags"

- Incomplete
- Vague
- Opinions
- Labeling
- Late
- Inaccurate
- Illegible
- Altered
- Report missing

rately bill the appropriate agency or individual for your services. The PCR may also be used to collect agency or service statistics. Examples of statistics that are often assessed in an EMS system include response times, number of calls in which a lights and siren response was used, number of interfacility transports, and the number of calls to 9-1-1 for which the patient subsequently refused transport.

Monitoring and evaluating data allows administrative staff to measure the agency's performance, determine if additional resources are required, and compare their performance with similar agencies. Careful analysis of your response times may show that your agency needs additional staffing and units at certain times of day and in specific locations. This makes the use of accurate and synchronous clocks very important to the appropriate and timely response to calls for help.

You Should Know

Failing to obtain a signature from the patient at the time of service is a common reason for billing errors. If you are unable to obtain a signature from the patient, be sure to document why the patient was unable to sign. If another person signs the form instead of the patient, document the identity of the signer and the relationship of the signer to the patient.

Educational and Research Uses

PCRs may be used to show employees examples of good documentation. A patient's refusal of treatment and/or transport is an example of a situation that requires careful documentation. EMS agencies often hold continuing education sessions with their personnel to discuss patient refusals and show examples of proper documentation in these situations.

Data obtained from the PCR may be collected and used for research purposes. The medical information that you gather about your patient is intended to help you give the most appropriate care possible. In many instances the protocols or treatments that you use have been developed with information from the research of similar types of calls. Careful study of your patient's response to currently recommended care may reveal a better way to treat this type of problem. Your careful documentation may assist with the care of more than just the patients you treat.

The PCR may also be used to determine the frequency with which an EMT performs specific patient care procedures and determine continuing education needs. For instance, the training officer in your EMS agency may notice that the EMS unit to which you are assigned responds to many trauma calls but not to many pediatric calls. The training officer may schedule a continuing education session for you and your partner to review pediatric assessment and vital signs to make sure that you remain competent in performing these skills.

Quality Management

The information contained in your PCR can and will be used to assess the quality of emergency medical care given to the patient. Most EMS agencies have developed standards for documentation that they expect you to use when completing your report. Completed reports are typically evaluated for:

- Adequacy of documentation
- Compliance with local rules and regulations
- Compliance with agency documentation standards
- Appropriateness of medical care

Elements of the Prehospital Care Report

The National Highway Traffic Safety Administration (NHTSA), the Trauma/EMS Systems program of the Health Resources and Services Administration's (HRSA), and the National Association of State EMS Directors have been working together to develop a national EMS database. The National Emergency Medical Services Information System (NEMSIS) is the database that will be used to store EMS data from every state in the nation (see the following *You Should Know* box).

You Should Know

Components of the National EMS Information System:

- Dispatch data
- Incident data
- Patient data
  —Demographics
  —Medical history
  —Assessment
  —Medical device data
  —Treatment/medications
  —Procedures
  —Disposition
- Injury/trauma data
- Cardiac arrest data
- Financial data
- EMS system demographic data
- EMS personnel demographic data
- Quality management indicators
- Outcome indicators
- Domestic terrorism data
- Linkage data

The information collected will be useful in the following:

- Developing nationwide EMS training curricula
- Evaluating patient and EMS system outcomes
- Facilitating research efforts
- Determining national fee schedules and reimbursement rates
- Addressing resources for disaster and domestic preparedness
- Providing valuable information on other issues or areas of need related to EMS care.

The recommended minimum information that should be included in a PCR is called the **minimum data set** (see the following *Remember This!* box).

Remember This!

Minimum Data for a Prehospital Care Report

Administrative information

- Time incident reported to 9-1-1
- Time unit notified
- Time of arrival at patient
- Time unit left scene
- Time of arrival at destination
- Time of transfer of care

Patient information

- Chief complaint
- Mechanism of injury or nature of illness
- Level of consciousness (AVPU)
- Breathing rate and effort
- Heart rate
- Skin perfusion (capillary refill) for patients less than 6 years of age
- Skin color and temperature
- Systolic blood pressure for patients older than 3 years of age

Administrative or Dispatch Information Section

Objectives 1, 2, 3

Statistical information pertaining to an EMS call is known by many names (see the following *You Should Know* box).

You Should Know

The statistical portion of a PCR may also be called:
- Run data
- Alarm information
- Alarm history
- Call information
- Dispatch information
- Administrative information
- Statistical data
- Incident information

Examples of additional statistical information that may be required by some EMS agencies is shown in the following *You Should Know* box. Table 11-1 gives

You Should Know

Additional Statistical Information

- Shift
- Type of incident
- En route to hospital
- Arrival at hospital
- Hospital destination
- Time unit available for service
- Total number of patients
- Extrication time
- Additional EMS units on the scene
- Transport type (ground ambulance, air ambulance)
- Transport mode (with or without lights/siren)
- Mileage to the scene, to the hospital, and total mileage
- Employee numbers of the responding EMS unit

You Should Know

When mileage is recorded for billing purposes, it must include four digits and must be accurate to the tenth of a mile. Your agency must establish the appropriate guidelines for this information per federal requirements. Inappropriate documentation or falsification of this information has severe consequences.

examples of how to complete the administrative section of the PCR. The administrative section of a sample PCR is shown in Figure 11-3.

Patient and Scene Information

The patient and scene information section of the PCR requires the entry of patient information, including the patient's name, age, address, gender, and weight (Figure 11-4). If the patient is stable, this information is usually obtained while taking the patient's SAMPLE history. If the patient is unstable, the minimum information necessary is obtained (such as name and age) on the scene. The rest is obtained on arrival at the receiving facility. This information should be collected from each patient, even if your agency does not perform any billing for EMS services. Table 11-2 gives examples of how to complete the patient and scene information portion of a PCR.

TABLE 11-1 Completing the Administrative Section of a Prehospital Care Report

Form Field	Explanation	Example
Alarm number	All calls should have a unique number for tracking purposes. In most cases, this number will be provided by your dispatch center.	2008-12857
Alarm date	Enter the date the call was received, using the date format MMDDYY (unless specified otherwise by your EMS agency). If the call *originated* twelve minutes before midnight on 01/01/08 but was completed at 0043 on 01/02/08, the date entered as the *dispatch date* would be 01/01/08.	01/01/08
Unit number or name	Enter your unit's designated radio call sign or unit descriptor.	Medic 51
Alarm time	This is the time that the dispatch center received the call. All times are generally entered as military time. Note: All times should be recorded from accurate and synchronous clocks.	2348
Dispatch time	This is the time that your unit is notified of the call by the dispatch center.	2349
Unit en route	This is the time that your unit begins travel to the scene.	2350
Arrival time	This entry is the time that your unit arrives at or on the scene.	2354
Patient contact	This entry is the time that you make contact with the patient. In some cases, the arrival time and patient contact time may be the same if the patient is waiting for EMS arrival. But in many cases, the arrival time and patient contact time differ. This is because the EMS crew must park the vehicle and then make entry into the patient's home or other location. Additional delays may occur if the scene is not safe to enter and the EMS crew must stage (wait at a safe distance) for law enforcement personnel to secure the scene.	2357
Time unit left scene	If the patient is not transported (or if the patient is transported but your EMS unit is not the transport vehicle), this is the time that your unit leaves the scene. If the patient is transported in your unit, this is the time your unit leaves with the patient toward the destination. (It is not when the patient is placed in the back of the ambulance.)	0015
Time of arrival at destination	This is the time your unit arrives on the grounds of the receiving facility or helicopter landing zone.	0025
Time of transfer of care	This is the time that you transfer care to the receiving facility.	0038
Time unit available	This is the time that your unit is back in service and available for another call.	0043

EMS ENCOUNTER FORM

CALL NUMBER	ALARM DATE	ALARM TIME	DISPATCH TIME	UNIT RPT	ARRIVAL TIME	PT CONTACT
0 8 1 2 8 5 7	0 1 0 1	2 3 4 8	2 3 4 9	M 5 1	2 3 5 4	2 3 5 7

PT#	TOTAL PTS	LEFT SCENE	DEST ARRIVAL	TRANSFER CARE	AVAILABLE		
0 1	0 1	0 0 1 5	0 0 2 5	0 0 3 8	0 0 4 3		

BLOCK NUMBER	DIR	STREET NAME	CITY	ZIP
1 2 3	W	M A I N S T	A N Y T O W N	7 6 1 2 3

FIGURE 11-3 ▲ The administrative section of a sample PCR.

TABLE 11-2 Completing the Patient Information Section of a Prehospital Care Report

Form Field	Explanation	Example
Scene location	This is the location of the patient or scene. This address may differ from the patient's address information. Include street address, city, state, and zip code.	123 W Main Street Anytown, TX 76123
Number of patients	This number is typically noted as 1 of ___. The first number represents the patient for whom you are filling out the form, and the second number represents the total number of patients at the scene (such as 1 of 3). Each patient will require an additional report completed in its entirety. You may not list multiple patients on the same report.	1 of 3
Patient name	Print the patient's complete first name, middle initial and last name. Do not use nicknames or abbreviations. It is very important to confirm spelling and include Sr., Jr., or II after the last name, if appropriate.	Thomas R. Nixon
Patient gender	Mark whether the patient is male or female.	Male
Patient mailing address	This is the patient's mailing address and may differ from the scene location information. Include street address, city, state, and zip code.	123 W Main Street Anytown, TX 76123
Patient weight (in kilograms)	Enter the patient's current weight in kilograms. If you do not calculate the weight in kilograms, then enter the patient's weight in pounds (lbs) and note it on your chart.	80 kg
Patient age	Enter the patient's date of birth and calculate his age. Use months or days as needed for patients less than two years of age.	75 years
Social Security Number	If needed for billing purposes, enter the patient's Social Security Number. You may need to inform the patient that all information gathered as part of his care is confidential and may only be released to other healthcare providers.	123-45-6789
Patient phone number	Enter the patient's phone number, including the area code.	(123) 456-7890

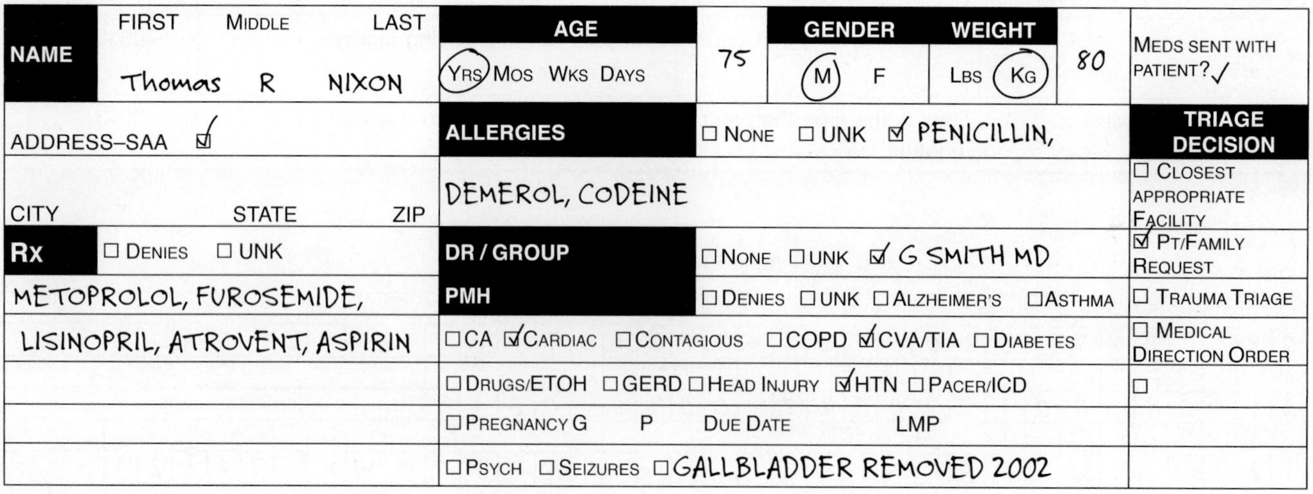

FIGURE 11-4 ▲ The patient information section of a sample PCR.

TIME	PULSE (RATE/QUALITY)	BP	RESP RATE	BREATH SOUNDS / RESP EFFORT		PUPILS	SKIN	SPO2
2359	92, S/R	178/94	24		1.CLEAR ☑NONLABORED	PERL	W/P/D	96 ☑RA ☐O2
0004	88, S/R	170/90	20		2.CRACKLES ☐LABORED 3.RHONCHI ☐RETRACTIONS	PERL	W/P/D	99 ☐RA ☑O2
0009	84, S/R	166/84	18		4.WHEEZES ☐NASAL FLARE 5.DIMISHED ☐GRUNTING	PERL	W/P/D	99 ☐RA ☑O2
								☐RA ☐O2

LOC U/A ☑AWAKE ☑ALERT ORIENTED: ☑PERSON ☑PLACE ☑TIME ☑EVENT ☐VERBAL ☐PAIN ☐UNRESP

LOSS OF CONSCIOUSNESS ☐YES ☑NO ☐UNK **PEDS** AGE–APPROPRIATE? ☐YES ☐NO CAP REFILL:

CHIEF COMPLAINT CHEST PRESSURE/WEAKNESS

U/A crew found pt standing lying on couch. Pt appears anxious. States watching TV when suddenly felt weak and had a "pressure-type" feeling in the center of his chest. Denies nausea, vomiting. Pt states he feels "a little" short of breath, but speaks in complete sentences. Describes pressure as constant. Hx of heart failure and HTN, but denies prior episodes of chest discomfort. Took daily aspirin dose with dinner.

Head / Face / Airway	Airway open; nose & ears clear; no trauma or STI	
Neck	Trachea midline, no JVD, no trauma, deformity, or STI	
Chest	Lungs clear bilat; chest intact with no trauma, deformity, STI, or pain on palp;	O 2-3 HRS.
	equal chest rise & fall; good tidal volume	P AT REST
Abd	SNT; no masses or pain on palp; old surgical scar from gallbladder surg	Q "PRESSURE"
Pelvis	No trauma, deformity, STI, or pain on palp	R LEFT ARM
Back	No trauma, deformity, STI, or pain on palp	S 6/10
Ext	Moves all on command; left grip weaker than right due to CVA n 1996; strong and = pulses; no trauma or STI; moderate swelling of feet and ankles bilat	T NO PRIOR HX

FIGURE 11-5 ▲ The patient assessment section of the PCR is also called the narrative section of the form.

Patient Assessment Section

The patient assessment section of the PCR is also called the *narrative section* of the form (Figure 11-5). Some EMS forms (both paper and electronic) consist of check boxes to record patient assessment information. Other EMS forms have a combination of boxes and blank lines on which you are expected to write a short story (narrative), using information gathered from the patient interview and your assessment findings. Some EMS systems, such as those in Maryland and North Carolina, use web-based electronic reporting (Figure 11-6). Some electronic systems will ask you to check boxes and then will create a short narrative based on those entries. No matter what form of documentation you use, it is your responsibility as an EMS professional to be sure that all documentation is accurate and complete.

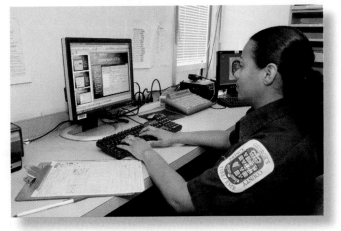

FIGURE 11-6 ▲ Some EMS systems use web-based electronic reporting.

ALS Assist

In most instances it will be the EMT who assesses and documents a patient's vital signs. Your honest reporting of this information to the Paramedic *will* make a difference in the care that the patient receives.

Documentation

General Guidelines

Some important points to keep in mind when writing a PCR include the following:

- Document important observations about the scene such as the presence of empty pill bottles, suicide note, or weapons.
- Document the events of a call in chronological order.

- Document pertinent negatives. A **pertinent negative** is a finding expected to accompany the patient's chief complaint but not found during the patient assessment. For instance, clear lung sounds in a patient complaining of difficulty breathing is a pertinent negative.
- Use abbreviations only if they are standard and approved by your EMS system. A list of common abbreviations is provided later in this chapter.
- When documenting information of a sensitive nature (such as a communicable disease), note the source of that information, such as the patient, family member, or bystander. For example, if a patient's wife tells you that her husband has "infectious hepatitis" but the patient does not relay this information, you would document, "Patient's wife states patient has infectious hepatitis."
- Document the emergency care delivered. Document the time of each intervention, who performed it, and the patient's response to the intervention.
- Document any orders received from medical direction and the results of carrying out the orders.
- Document changes in the patient's condition throughout the call.
- Do not intentionally leave spaces blank; use "N/A" if information does not apply.

Confidentiality

Objective 5

The PCR and the information on it are considered confidential. Do not show the form or discuss the information contained on it with unauthorized persons. Violation of patient confidentiality laws can lead to serious consequences. Your report and the information it contains can be distributed only to other healthcare providers who will provide care to your patient and to members of your agency who perform billing or quality management functions.

Local and state protocol and procedures will determine where the different copies of the PCR should be distributed. Know your state laws and local protocols.

Patient Refusals

Objective 4

As discussed in Chapter 3, all competent adults have the right to refuse emergency care. If your patient is a child or mentally incompetent adult, only a parent or legal guardian can refuse care on behalf of the patient. A patient's refusal of care may not always be in his best interest, but you cannot and should not force any competent patient to accept your care.

You Should Know

Most EMS systems in the United States require phone or radio contact with a base hospital or physician for field refusals. Research, understand, and follow your local protocol.

If a patient refuses treatment or transport, call advanced medical personnel to the scene as soon as possible to evaluate the patient or contact medical direction. Document any telephone or radio advice given by medical direction.

Make multiple attempts to try to convince the patient to accept care. If a patient refuses treatment or transport and medical direction agrees that the patient can be allowed to refuse care, you must inform the patient of the following:

- The nature of his illness or injury
- The treatment that needs to be performed
- The benefits of that treatment
- The risks of not providing that treatment
- Any alternatives to treatment
- The dangers of refusing treatment (including transport)

A refusal of care does not release you from liability if you know that the patient's condition will worsen without care and you do not attempt to inform your patient of the risks of refusing care. A sample refusal form is shown in Figure 11-7. Your chart should reflect that fact that you tried to reason with your patient and informed him of the risks of not receiving care. In those instances in which the patient is adamantly refusing, you should ask the patient to read, understand, and sign your agency's refusal form. If the patient refuses to sign the refusal form, then attempt to have a family member sign as a witness that the patient would not sign the form. You may also have law enforcement personnel or other healthcare providers at the scene act as witnesses that the patient would not sign the refusal. Inform the patient of (and document) your willingness to return should his condition change or should he change his mind (Figure 11-8).

In some instances, a patient who is refusing transport may allow you to perform an assessment. If so, perform an assessment and document your findings and the patient's refusal of transport in the proper fashion.

REFUSAL OF SERVICES AGAINST MEDICAL ADVICE – RELEASE OF RESPONSIBILITY

CALL NUMBER

☐☐☐☐☐☐☐

REFUSAL CRITERIA

The patient meets all of the following: (check all that apply)

☐ Is an adult (18 or over), or if under 18, is being released to a parent, guardian, responsible party, or law enforcement personnel.

☐ Is oriented to person, place, time, and event.

☐ Exhibits no evidence of: ☐ Altered level of consciousness ☐ Alcohol or drug ingestion that impairs judgment

☐ Understands the nature of his/her medical condition, as well as the risks and consequences of refusing care.

PATIENT/ GUARDIAN/ POWER OF ATTORNEY HAS BEEN ADVISED: (check all that apply)

☐ That it is the preference of the attending EMT/Paramedic to arrange for transport to the closest appropriate medical facility for further evaluation and treatment.

☐ That an ambulance is available for transportation to the closest appropriate medical facility for treatment.

☐ That transport by means other than by ambulance could be hazardous and is not recommended based upon current condition/complaint, specific injury, or medical illness.

☐ That significant risk(s) could be involved with refusal of EMS treatment and/or transportation, related from, but not limited to; exacerbation of present complaint / condition / injuries, or the possibility of significant disability and/or death occurring from refusal of emergent medical care or transportation.

☐ Patient has been informed of their right to refuse prehospital treatment and/or offer of transport to an appropriate medical facility (after being advised of potential complications) and understands the consequences of his/her decision.

☐ Should the patient change his/her mind or if his/her condition changes, he/she has been advised to contact the healthcare provider of his/her choice (9-1-1, personal physician, emergency department, or urgent care center in his/her area) to address his/her medical needs.

The following section must be signed by the patient, nearest relative, legal guardian, or responsible party/authority in the case of a minor or when the patient is physically or mentally incompetent.

It is my choice and at my own insistence, I _____ elect not to receive ☐Assessment ☐Treatment ☐Transportation against the advice of the attending EMT/Paramedic(s) and the _____ (EMS Agency) and, when applicable, the base hospital physician. The potential risks associated with my refusal have been explained to me before my signature on this document, which includes risk of serious illness, injury, and death. I hereby release the attending Emergency Medical Technician/Paramedic, _____ (EMS Agency) and its employees, officials, agents, volunteers, and when applicable, the base hospital and the base hospital physician from further responsibility for my well-being. I understand there may be injuries or complications not known to EMS personnel at this time, but which may result in further illness, injury, permanent disability, or death. I further deny being physically or mentally impaired by the use of drugs or alcohol. If I change my mind or if my condition changes, I have been advised to contact the healthcare provider of my choice (9-1-1, personal physician, emergency department or urgent care center in my area) to address my medical needs. I also acknowledge that I have been provided with a copy of the _____ (EMS Agency) Notice of Privacy Practices that describes how my health information is used and shared.

I have received and read the above information and am voluntarily signing this release without undue stress, duress, and without pressure.

_____   _____   _____
Patient / Responsible Party Signature   Witness   Witness
Firma del Paciente / Persona Responsable   Testigo   Testigo

Relationship: ☐ Self   ☐ _____

If released in care of custody of relative of friend: _____   _____
                                      Name   Relationship

If released in custody of law enforcement agency: _____   _____
                                  Officer's Signature   Agency

FIGURE 11-7 ▲ Sample EMS refusal form.

TIME	PULSE (RATE/QUALITY)	BP	RESP RATE	BREATH SOUNDS / RESP EFFORT		PUPILS	SKIN	SPO 2
								☐RA ☐O2
PT REFUSED ALL VITAL SIGNS X3 ATTEMPTS				☐ ☐	1.CLEAR ☑NONLABORED 2.CRACKLES ☐LABORED 3.RHONCHI ☐RETRACTIONS			☐RA ☐O2
				☐ ☐	4.WHEEZES ☐NASAL FLARE 5.DIMISHED ☐GRUNTING			☐RA ☐O2
								☐RA ☐O2

LOC U/A ☑AWAKE ☑ALERT ORIENTED: ☑PERSON ☑PLACE ☑TIME ☑EVENT ☐VERBAL ☐PAIN ☐UNRESP

LOSS OF CONSCIOUSNESS ☐YES ☑NO ☐UNK **PEDS** AGE–APPROPRIATE? ☐YES ☐NO CAP REFILL:

CHIEF COMPLAINT MOTOR VEHICLE CRASH

U/A PT found standing outside vehicle in street next to a 2-car MVC with moderate damage. Pt stated no need for ambulance. Pt states husband was driving when car pulled in front of them making a U-turn and they broadsided a 4-door car. Estimated speed 25-35 mph. Pt was restrained passenger. Airbag deployed. Pt denies alcohol or drugs. Pt states in no physical distress. Pt states she has soreness in both knees and lower back. Denies head, neck, upper back, abdominal, or pelvic pain/soreness. Denies headache, dizziness, loss of consciousness, SOB, CP, and n/v. Pt ambulatory w/o assistance. Pt repeatedly refused assessment including vital signs on scene.

Head / Face / Airway	Pt advised that ambulance on scene and transport for	
Neck	evaluation recommended. Pt declined stating that if pain she would go to MD later. Pt told to go to	
Chest	MD or call 9-1-1 if sudden increase in pain in areas of complaint or sudden onset of pain in	O
	any area. Contacted G Smith MD @ 2210. Orders: Review refusal form with pt.	P
Abd	OK to refuse treatment/transport. Refusal form	Q
Pelvis	reviewed with pt. Pt verbalized understanding of risks of refusal. Pt and witness signatures obtained.	R
Back		S
Ext		T

FIGURE 11-8 ▲ Sample of an actual EMS refusal narrative for a patient involved in a motor vehicle crash.

You Should Know

Documentation of a patient's refusal should include the following:

- Patient name, age
- Date of birth
- Medical history
- Two sets of vital signs
- Chief complaint
- Mental status exam findings (speech, gait, appropriate behavior, level of cooperation, ability to follow instructions/commands, etc.)
- Physical exam findings
- Reason for refusal
- Signed refusal form
- Advice given
- Patient understands risks of refusal
- Patient understands possible outcome if advice is not followed
- Any telephone or radio advice given by medical direction

Falsification

Falsification of information on the PCR may lead to suspension or revocation of the EMT's certification/ license and other legal action. Falsifying information may harm the patient because false information may mislead other healthcare professionals about the patient's condition, assessment, and care. Specific areas of difficulty in EMS documentation include vital signs and treatments given. Never attempt to make up vital signs that were not taken or document care that was not given. For example, if an intervention such as oxygen was overlooked, do not chart that the patient was given oxygen.

Error Correction

As previously noted, the PCR is considered a legal document and may be used as evidence in a court preceding. In most instances, your reports will be written in a very busy and hectic atmosphere. The potential for errors is quite high. Mistakes can and do occur. Your response to a mistake should be honest and very straightforward.

If an error is discovered while the report form is being written, draw a single horizontal line through the error, initial it, and write the correct information beside it (Figure 11-9). Do not erase or try to obliterate the error. Erasures may be interpreted as an attempt to cover up a mistake.

If an error is discovered after the report form is submitted, draw a single line through the error, initial and date it, and add a note with the correct

TIME	PULSE (RATE/QUALITY)	BP	RESP RATE	BREATH SOUNDS / RESP EFFORT		PUPILS	SKIN	SPO2
2359	92, S/R	178/94	24	1.CLEAR 2.CRACKLES 3.RHONCHI 4.WHEEZES 5.DIMISHED	☑NONLABORED ☐LABORED ☐RETRACTIONS ☐NASAL FLARE ☐GRUNTING	PERL	W/P/D	96 ☑RA ☐O2
0004	88, S/R	170/90	20			PERL	W/P/D	99 ☐RA ☑O2
0009	84, S/R	166/84	18			PERL	W/P/D	99 ☐RA ☑O2
								☐RA ☐O2

LOC U/A ☑AWAKE ☑ALERT ORIENTED: ☑PERSON ☑PLACE ☑TIME ☑EVENT ☐VERBAL ☐PAIN ☐UNRESP

LOSS OF CONSCIOUSNESS ☐YES ☑NO ☐UNK **PEDS** AGE–APPROPRIATE? ☐YES ☐NO CAP REFILL:

CHIEF COMPLAINT CHEST PRESSURE/WEAKNESS

U/A crew found pt ~~standing~~ lying on couch. Pt appears anxious. States watching TV when suddenly felt weak and had a "pressure-type" feeling in the center of his chest. Denies nausea, vomiting. Pt states he feels "a little" short of breath, but speaks in complete sentences. Describes pressure as constant. Hx of heart failure and HTN, but denies prior episodes of chest discomfort. Took daily aspirin dose with dinner.

Head / Face / Airway	Airway open; nose & ears clear; no trauma or STI		
Neck	Trachea midline, no JVD, no trauma, deformity, or STI		
Chest	Lungs clear bilat; chest intact with no trauma, deformity, STI, or pain on palp;	O	2-3 HRS.
	equal chest rise & fall; good tidal volume	P	AT REST
Abd	SNT; no masses or pain on palp; old surgical scar from gallbladder surg	Q	"PRESSURE"
Pelvis	No trauma, deformity, STI, or pain on palp	R	LEFT ARM
Back	No trauma, deformity, STI, or pain on palp	S	~~6/10~~ 8/10
Ext	Moves all on command; left grip weaker than right due to CVA n 1996; strong and = pulses; no trauma or STI; moderate swelling of feet and ankles bilat	T	NO PRIOR HX

FIGURE 11-9 ▲ If you make an error while writing a report, draw a single horizontal line through the error, initial it, and write the correct information beside it.

information. If information was omitted, or if additional information comes to your attention after you have written the original report, add a supplemental narrative (addendum) on a separate report form with the correct information, the date, and your initials and attach it to the original.

Documentation Formats

Effective documentation requires an organization approach. Although there are several formats to choose from, three of the more commonly used are discussed here. You will need to determine which method works for you, modify it if needed, and then use it consistently to ensure that no important information is omitted when documenting patient care.

SOAP

The SOAP method of documentation is one of the most commonly used. SOAP is a memory aid that stands for *S*ubjective findings, *O*bjective findings, *A*ssessment, and *P*lan.

- *Subjective findings.* Subjective findings include information told to you by the patient, family members, or bystanders. Examples include the patient's chief complaint, history of the present illness, related symptoms, and SAMPLE and OPQRST history.

- *Objective findings.* Objective findings include information that can be seen, heard, smelled, measured, or felt. Information contained in this portion of your report includes your primary and secondary survey findings and the patient's vital signs (if they are not recorded elsewhere on the report).

- *Assessment.* The information that should be documented here is your field impression of the patient's illness or injury based on the subjective and objective findings found during your interaction with the patient.

- *Plan.* Document the emergency care given, the patient's response to each intervention, mode of patient transport, transportation destination, and ongoing assessment findings.

The following is an example of documentation using the SOAP format.

S Chief complaint: 44-year-old woman complaining of pain in hip and lower back.

SAMPLE: Allergies: hydrocodone. Takes no medications, no pertinent PMH. Breakfast at 0700. Patient was climbing stairs in bank building because elevator wasn't working. Slipped and fell about 6 steps. Rates hip and lower back pain 6 on 0 to 10 scale.

O Fall injury. Patient found between floors 7 and 8 in stairwell of bank building.

Head/face/airway: Awake, alert, and oriented to person, place, time, event. Denies hitting head during fall or loss of consciousness. DCAP-BTLS negative; denies pain on palpation. PERL. No drainage from ears or nose.

Neck: DCAP-BTLS negative, trachea midline

Chest: DCAP-BTLS negative, breath sounds clear/equal bilaterally

Abdomen: soft, nontender; DCAP-BTLS

Pelvis: complains of left hip pain on palpation, femoral pulses strong and equal

Back: complains of lumbar pain on palpation

Extremities: DCAP-BTLS negative; equal pulses, movement, sensation

A Fall injury with hip and lower back trauma

P Oxygen by nonrebreather mask at 15 L/min. Patient refused spinal stabilization (cervical collar, spider straps, head blocks, backboard). Transported down remaining stairs on backboard and then placed in position of comfort on stretcher. Transported code 2 by ground ambulance to XYZ hospital.

CHART

CHART is another commonly used documentation format. CHART stands for *C*hief complaint, *H*istory, *A*ssessment, *R*x (treatment), and *T*ransport. The main difference between the SOAP and CHART formats is that the subjective information in SOAP is separated into two parts in CHART (chief complaint and history).

- *Chief complaint.* The chief complaint is the patient's description of his illness or injury. If the patient is unresponsive or has an altered mental status, this information is usually obtained from family members, bystanders, or your evaluation of the scene.
- *History.* Document the patient's history of the present illness (including OPQRST if appropriate) and SAMPLE history.
- *Assessment.* Document objective findings from your primary and secondary surveys that can be seen, heard, smelled, measured, or felt. Include vital signs if they are not recorded elsewhere on the report.
- *Rx (treatment).* Document any treatment the patient received before your arrival, as well as the emergency care you provided. Document the patient's response to each intervention.
- *Transport.* Document the mode of patient transport, transportation destination, ongoing assessment findings, any treatment provided en route, and the patient's response to the treatment given.

The following is an example of documentation using the CHART format.

Chief complaint: 44-year-old woman complaining of pain in hip and lower back.

History: Fall injury. Patient found between floors 7 and 8 in stairwell of bank building. Patient was climbing stairs in bank building because elevator wasn't working. Slipped and fell about 6 steps. Rates hip and lower back pain 6 on 0 to 10 scale. Allergies: hydrocodone. Takes no medications, no pertinent PMH. Breakfast at 0700.

Assessment:

Head/face/airway: awake, alert, and oriented to person, place, time, event. Denies hitting head during fall or loss of consciousness. DCAP-BTLS negative; denies pain on palpation. PERL. No drainage from ears or nose.

Neck: DCAP-BTLS negative, trachea midline

Chest: DCAP-BTLS negative, breath sounds clear/equal bilaterally

Abdomen: soft, nontender; DCAP-BTLS

Pelvis: complains of left hip pain on palpation, femoral pulses strong and equal

Back: complains of lumbar pain on palpation

Extremities: DCAP-BTLS negative; equal pulses, movement, sensation

Rx: Oxygen by nonrebreather mask at 15 L/min. Patient refused spinal stabilization (cervical collar, spider straps, head blocks, backboard). Transported down remaining stairs on backboard and then placed in position of comfort on stretcher.

Transport: Transported code 2 by ground ambulance to XYZ hospital.

Narrative

The narrative documentation format is like writing a short story about the events of the call. Documentation includes assessment findings, pertinent historical information, treatment, patient responses, and transport data in chronological order. Although this method of documentation is easy to learn, locating specific information is often difficult.

The following is an example of documentation using the narrative format. Please note that explanations for some abbreviations are provided in parentheses for clarity. This would not be done in an actual report because it would defeat the purpose of using the abbreviations.

R/T (respond to) fall injury. 44-year-old woman found between floors 7 and 8 in stairwell of bank building. Patient was climbing stairs in bank building because elevator wasn't working. Slipped and fell about 6 steps. C/O (complains of) hip and lower back pain; rates pain 6 on 0 to 10 scale. Allergies: hydrocodone. Takes no medications, no pertinent PMH. Breakfast at 0700.

Head/face/airway: Awake, alert, and oriented to person, place, time, event. Denies hitting head during fall or loss of consciousness. DCAP-BTLS negative; denies pain on palpation. PERL. No drainage from ears or nose.

Neck: DCAP-BTLS negative, trachea midline

Chest: DCAP-BTLS negative, breath sounds clear/equal bilaterally

Abdomen: soft, nontender; DCAP-BTLS

Pelvis: complains of left hip pain on palpation, femoral pulses strong and equal

Back: complains of lumbar pain on palpation

Extremities: DCAP-BTLS negative; equal pulses, movement, sensation

Rx: Oxygen by nonrebreather mask at 15 L/min. Patient refused spinal stabilization (cervical collar, spider straps, head blocks, backboard). Transported down remaining stairs on backboard and then placed in position of comfort on stretcher. Transported code 2 by ground ambulance to XYZ hospital.

Special Situations

Objective 6

Mass Casualty Incidents

In a mass casualty incident (MCI), comprehensive documentation must often wait until after the casualties are triaged and transported. You must know and follow local procedures for documentation in these situations. The local MCI plan should include a means of temporarily recording patient information (such as using triage tags) that can be used later to complete the PCR (Figure 11-10).

Special Reports

Most state and local jurisdictions have reporting requirements that you must be aware of. Special reports may be required for infectious disease exposure, body fluid exposure, work-related injury, and reportable incidents such as elder and child abuse.

Reporting requirements for abuse situations vary among states. Some states (such as Alaska, Oregon, Massachusetts, Nevada, and Maine) have strict reporting requirements for EMS professionals. Some states allow telephone reports, whereas others require written reports. In many states, reporting suspected abuse to emergency department staff does not satisfy the reporting requirements under state law. Contact your state EMS agency for guidance about mandatory reporting requirements.

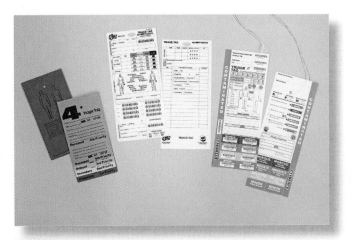

FIGURE 11-10 ▲ In a mass casualty incident, triage tags are often used to record patient information.

Common Medical Abbreviations

ABBREVIATION	MEANING
<	less than
>	more than
=	equal
~	approximately, about
↑	increased
↓	decreased
→	going to or leading to
△	change
♀ or F	female
♂ or M	male
$\bar{a}$	before
AAA	abdominal aortic aneurysm
ABD, abd	abdomen
ABG	arterial blood gas
AC	antecubital (vein)
ACE	angiotensin converting enzyme
ACS	acute coronary syndrome
Afib	atrial fibrillation
AIDS	acquired immunodeficiency syndrome
A & O	alert and oriented
A & O × 4	alert and oriented to person, place, time, and event

ABBREVIATION	MEANING	ABBREVIATION	MEANING
A & P	anterior and posterior; anatomy and physiology	COPD	chronic obstructive pulmonary disease
AMA	against medical advice	CP	chest pain
AMI	acute myocardial infarction	CPh	cellular phone
Amt	amount	CPR	cardiopulmonary resuscitation
Ant	anterior	C-spine	cervical spine
ARDS	adult respiratory distress syndrome	CSF	cerebrospinal fluid
ASA	aspirin	CT	computed tomography
ASHD	atherosclerotic heart disease	CVA	cerebrovascular accident
AV	arteriovenous, atrioventricular	D/C	discontinue
		DCAP-BTLS	*d*eformities, *c*ontusions, *a*brasions, *p*unctures, *b*urns, *t*enderness, *l*acerations, *s*welling
BBO$_2$	blow by oxygen		
BCP	birth control pills		
Bilat	bilateral	Defib	defibrillation
Bld	blood	D/T	dispatched to
BLS	basic life support	DKA	diabetic ketoacidosis
BM	bowel movement	DM	diabetes mellitus
BOW	bag of waters	DNP	did not patch
BP	blood pressure	DO	doctor of osteopathy
bpm	beats per minute	DOA	dead on arrival
BS	breath sounds, blood sugar	DOE	dyspnea on exertion
BSA	body surface area	DPT	diphtheria, pertussis, and tetanus
BM	bag-mask		
BW	birth weight	D50	50% dextrose
c/m	cool and moist	D5W	5% dextrose in water
CA, Ca, ca	cancer, carcinoma	DX, Dx, dx	diagnosis
CABG	coronary artery bypass graft	ECG	electrocardiogram
		ED	Emergency Department
CAD	coronary artery disease	EDC	expected date of confinement (due date)
caps	capsules		
CC, C.C.	chief complaint	ENT	ear, nose, and throat
cc	cubic centimeter	Epi	epinephrine
C/O	complains of	ETA	estimated time of arrival
CCU	coronary care unit	ETOH	ethyl alcohol
CHF	congestive heart failure	Exam	examination
Clr	clear	Ext	extremities
cm	centimeter	F/U	follow-up
CMS	circulation, motor, sensory	FDA	Food and Drug Administration
CN	courtesy notification		
CNS	central nervous system	FSI	full spinal immobilization
CO	carbon monoxide, cardiac output	ft	foot, feet
		FUO	fever of undetermined origin
CO$_2$	carbon dioxide		
Conc	conscious	Fx	fracture
Cond	condition	g, gm	gram

ABBREVIATION	MEANING
Gx	gravida
GB	gallbladder
GI	gastrointestinal
GLF	ground level fall
GSW	gun shot wound
GU	genitourinary
GYN, gyn	gynecology
h/d	hot/dry
h/m	hot/moist
H/A	headache
HEENT	*h*ead, *e*yes, *e*ars, *n*ose, *t*hroat
Hgb	hemoglobin
HIV	human immunodeficiency virus
HPI	history of present illness
HR	heart rate
Hr	hour
HTN	hypertension
Hx	history
ICS	intercostal space
ICU	intensive care unit
IDDM	insulin-dependent diabetes mellitus
inf	inferior
inj	injection
IUD	intrauterine device
IV	intravenous
JVD	jugular vein distention
K+	potassium
kg	kilogram
KO	keep open
KVO	keep vein open
l	liter
LAD	left anterior descending (coronary artery)
lat	lateral
lb	pound
lt	left
LMP	last menstrual period
LOC	loss of consciousness, level of consciousness
LR	Lactated Ringer's
LUQ	left upper quadrant
LV	left ventricle
m	meter
MAE	moves all extremities

ABBREVIATION	MEANING
MD	medical doctor, muscular dystrophy
mm	millimeter
mEq	millequivalent
Mg	magnesium
mg	milligram
mcg	microgram
MDI	metered dose inhaler
MI	myocardial infarction
mL	milliliter
mm	millimeter
MOI	mechanism of injury
MRI	magnetic resonance imaging
MS	multiple sclerosis, morphine sulfate
MVA	motor vehicle accident
MVC	motor vehicle crash, motor vehicle collision
N/A	not applicable
N/C	nasal cannula, no charge
NIDDM	non-insulin-dependent diabetes mellitus
n/v	nausea/vomiting
n/v/d	nausea/vomiting/diarrhea
Na$^+$	sodium
NaCl	sodium chloride
NFO	no further orders
NG, N/G	nasogastric
NKA	no known allergies
NKDA	no known drug allergies
NPA	nasopharyngeal airway
No △	no change
NPO	nothing by mouth
NS	normal saline
NTG	nitroglycerin
OB	obstetrics
OB/GYN	obstetrics and gynecology
OD	overdose
OPA	oropharyngeal airway
OTC	over-the-counter
oz	ounce
p̄	after
P	phosphorus, pulse
PCN	penicillin
Peds	pediatrics
PERL	pupils equal, round, reactive to light

ABBREVIATION	MEANING	ABBREVIATION	MEANING
PERLA	pupils equal, round, reactive to light and accommodation	Sz	seizure
pH	hydrogen ion concentration	T	temperature
PI	present illness	Tabs	tablets
PID	pelvic inflammatory disease	TB	tuberculosis
PMH	past medical history	temp.	temperature
PMS	premenstrual syndrome; *p*ulses, *m*ovement (motion), *s*ensation	TKO	to keep open
		TIA	transient ischemic attack
		TMJ	temporomandibular joint
P.O.	by mouth	TPR	temperature, pulse, respirations
POV	privately owned vehicle	TRX, x-port	transport
ppm	parts per million	tsp	teaspoon
p.r.n.	as needed, as necessary	TV	tidal volume
PSVT	paroxysmal supraventricular tachycardia	Tx	treatment
		UA	urinalysis
PT	physical therapy	U/A	upon arrival
PTA	prior to arrival	URI	upper respiratory infection
PTCA	percutaneous transluminal coronary angioplasty	UTI	urinary tract infection
		VF/VFib	ventricular fibrillation
PVC	premature ventricular complex	VS	vital signs
		VT	ventricular tachycardia
q	every	w/d	warm/dry
q.h.	every hour	w/m	warm/moist
R	respirations	w/d/p	warm/dry/pink
RBC	red blood cell	W/O	without
RLQ	right lower quadrant	WBC	white blood cell
RN	registered nurse	x-fer	transfer
R/O	rule out	y.o./YO	year old
ROM	range of motion		
ROS	rate of speed		
RP	reporting or responsible party		
R/T	respond to		
RUQ	right upper quadrant		
Rx	prescription, treatment		
SQ, SubQ	subcutaneous		
sec	second		
SIDS	sudden infant death syndrome		
SNT	soft nontender		
SO	standing order		
SOB	shortness of breath		
S&S, S/S	signs and symptoms		
stat	immediately		
STD	sexually transmitted disease		
SVN	small volume nebulizer		
Sx	symptom		

On the Scene   Wrap-Up

A doctor looks around the room and asks if anyone knows if the patient had taken any Viagra in the last 24 hours. You realize that you did not note this medication on the PCR because you did not think it was pertinent to the care of this patient. You immediately respond to the doctor's question by informing him that the patient told you that he did take Viagra 14 hours ago.

You now realize that your verbal report to the hospital staff should have included this important information in order to allow the hospital staff to begin giving appropriate care to the patient on your arrival. Your documentation should also have included a complete list of the patient's medications.

The patient recovers because of the hard work of the Emergency Department staff. The doctor takes the time to explain why it is so important to ask patients if they have used medications for erectile problems 24 to 48 hours before giving nitroglycerin. You leave the hospital with a new understanding of how the smallest part of your care may have the greatest impact. ∎

Sum It Up

▶ Good documentation is complete, clear, concise, objective, timely, accurate, and legible.

▶ A PCR has many important functions.
- *Continuity of care.* The PCR may be used by receiving facility staff to help determine the direction of treatment following the EMS treatments given.
- *Legal document.* Good documentation reflects the emergency medical care provided, status of the patient on arrival at the scene, and any changes upon arrival at the receiving facility.
- *Education and research.* The PCR can be used to show proper documentation and how to handle unusual or uncommon situations, as well as identify training needs for the EMS providers.
- *Administrative.* The PCR is used for billing and EMS service statistics.
- *Quality management.* Completed reports are typically evaluated for adequacy of documentation, compliance with local rules and regulations, compliance with agency documentation standards, and appropriateness of medical care.

▶ A PCR generally consists of an administrative section, patient and scene information section, and patient assessment (narrative) section.
- The administrative section includes data pertaining to the EMS call, such as the date, times, service, unit, and crew information.
- The patient and scene information section includes data such as the patient's name, age, gender, weight, address, date of birth, and insurance information.
- The patient assessment section includes the patient's chief complaint, mechanism of injury/nature of illness, location of the patient, treatment given before arrival of EMS, patient signs and symptoms, care given, vital signs, SAMPLE history, and changes in condition.

▶ The PCR form and the information on it are considered confidential. Local and state protocols and procedures determine where the different copies of the PCR should be distributed.

▶ Mentally competent adults have the right to refuse care and transport. You must make sure that the patient fully understands your explanation and the consequences of refusing treatment or transport. Call advanced medical personnel to the scene as soon as possible to evaluate the patient or contact medical direction.

▶ Falsification of information on the PCR may lead not only to suspension or revocation of the EMT's certification/license but also to poor patient care because other healthcare professionals have a false impression of which assessment findings were discovered or what treatment was given.

▶ When a documentation error occurs, do not try to cover it up. Instead, document what did or did not happen, and time, date, and initial your entry.

Medical-Behavioral Emergencies and Obstetrics and Gynecology

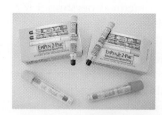
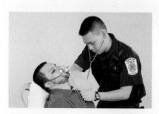
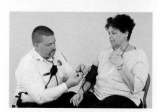

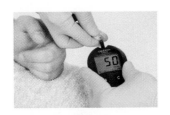
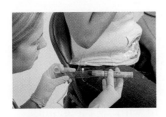
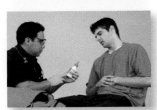
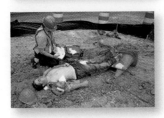
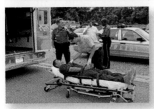
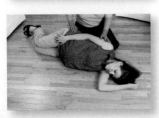

12 Pharmacology

By the end of this chapter, you should be able to:

Knowledge Objectives ▶
1. Identify which medications will be carried on the unit.
2. State the medications carried on the unit by the generic name.
3. Identify the medications with which the Emergency Medical Technician (EMT) may assist the patient with administering.
4. State the medications the EMT can assist the patient with by the generic name.
5. Discuss the forms in which the medications may be found.

Attitude Objectives ▶
6. Explain the rationale for administration of medications.

Skill Objectives ▶
7. Demonstrate general steps for assisting the patient with self-administration of medications.
8. Read the labels and inspect each type of medication.

On the Scene

While performing a standby at a local grade school soccer game, you notice one of the players slap at her leg and cry out in pain. The player runs to the sidelines and starts talking with the coach. A parent runs from the sidelines to be with the player. Her parent helps her lie down on the ground as other parents huddle around her. You and your partner are flagged over. As you approach, you notice that the patient seems to be having trouble breathing. As you kneel at the patient's side, the child's mother introduces herself. She tells you that her daughter has just been stung by a bee and is allergic to them. In addition, she says that she is unable to find her daughter's "sting kit." ■

THINK ABOUT IT

As you read this chapter, think about the following questions:

• What do you need to know about this scene?
• What questions will you ask?

- Is there any danger to you or your partner?
- How will you get help if it is needed?
- What pharmacological intervention is needed to help this patient?
- Do you have the training, knowledge, and ability to help?
- What information will need to be relayed to the hospital if you transport this patient?

Introduction

Pharmacology is the study of drugs or medications and their effect on living systems. This chapter will introduce you to a basic understanding of pharmacology and the concepts of medication administration. You must be familiar with medications carried on the Emergency Medical Services (EMS) unit and physician-prescribed medications that medical direction will authorize you to assist patients in taking. Although drugs may be lifesaving when properly given, they may be fatal if improperly administered. You must be knowledgeable about each medication that you administer. This chapter includes information about the very important responsibilities that you will have to your patients when giving a medication.

Remember This!

The drug dosing and administration information in this chapter should be viewed as guidelines. It is not intended to take the place of your local or state protocols or scope of practice.

Drug Legislation and Federal Regulatory Agencies

From the very earliest recorded history, humankind has used herbs, plants, and minerals to ease pain and treat diseases. The realization that these plants, herbs, and minerals had an effect on the body was the beginning of the science of pharmacology. This science continues to advance every day with the use of chemical compounds that help in the fight against illnesses and disease. The medications that we consider as a part of everyday life have developed with time. In addition, the safety and regulation of the medications that we use has also changed.

Drug Legislation in the United States

Drug legislation in the United States has been put in place to protect the public from contaminated or mislabeled drugs. Important events and laws pertaining to the purchasing, distribution, dispensing, and giving of drugs are shown in Table 12-1. Controlled substances are listed in Table 12-2.

Federal Regulatory Agencies and Services

The Drug Enforcement Agency (DEA) is a division of the Justice Department. It became the sole legal drug enforcement agency in July 1973 and replaced the Bureau of Narcotics and Dangerous Drugs (BNDD).

The Food and Drug Administration (FDA) is a part of the U.S. Department of Health and Human Services. It enforces the Federal Food, Drug, and Cosmetic Act by means of seizure and criminal prosecution as necessary.

Drug Sources, Names, and References

Drug Sources

Drugs can be obtained from many sources. Morphine, a commonly used drug for pain relief, is an example of a drug obtained from a plant. Some drugs are obtained from minerals or mineral products, such as iron. Advances in technology have enabled drug companies to make many of the drugs formerly obtained from animals and humans (such as insulin and some vaccines) in the laboratory. Drugs that are made in a laboratory are called **synthetic drugs. Semi-synthetic drugs** are naturally occurring substances that have been chemically altered, such as antibiotics.

TABLE 12-1 Landmarks in Food and Drug Legislation in the United States

Year	Legislation/Event	Notes
1848	Drug Importation Act	Required U.S. Customs Service inspectors to stop entry of contaminated drugs from overseas
1862	President Lincoln appointed a chemist to serve in the new Department of Agriculture	Beginning of the Bureau of Chemistry, the predecessor of the Food and Drug Administration
1902	Biologics Control Act	Passed to ensure purity and safety of serums, vaccines, and similar products used to prevent or treat diseases in humans
1906	Pure Food and Drug Act	Prohibited interstate commerce in misbranded and impure foods, drinks, and drugs
1912	Shirley Amendment	Prohibited labeling medicines with false therapeutic claims intended to defraud the purchaser
1914	Harrison Narcotic Act	• Established the word "narcotic" • Required prescriptions for products exceeding the allowable limit of narcotics • Required increased record keeping for physicians and pharmacists who dispense narcotics
1927	Bureau of Chemistry reorganized into two separate entities	• Regulatory functions located in the Food, Drug, and Insecticide Administration • Nonregulatory research located in the Bureau of Chemistry and Soils
1930	Name of the Food, Drug, and Insecticide Administration shortened to Food and Drug Administration (FDA)	Name shortened as a result of an agricultural appropriations act
1937	Elixir of Sulfanilamide kills 107 persons, many of whom were children	Elixir of Sulfanilamide was a liquid that contained a poison; the deaths that resulted emphasized the need to establish drug safety before marketing
1938	Federal Food, Drug, and Cosmetic Act of 1938	• Required that new drugs be shown to be safe before marketing • Established the FDA's responsibility for supervising and regulating drug safety • Authorized factory inspections • Required that drugs contain a label listing all of the ingredients and directions for use
1951	Durham-Humphrey Amendment	Required that prescription drugs (also called *legend drugs*) must carry the following label: "Caution: Federal law prohibits dispensing without a prescription."
1962	Kefauver-Harris Drug Amendments	• Thalidomide, a sleeping pill, found to have caused birth defects in thousands of babies born in western Europe • 1962 drug amendments passed to ensure drug effectiveness and greater drug safety • Drug manufacturers required to prove to FDA the effectiveness of their products before marketing them

Continued

TABLE 12-1 Landmarks in Food and Drug Legislation in the United States *Continued*

Year	Legislation/Event	Notes
1970	Comprehensive Drug Abuse Prevention and Control Act (Controlled Substances Act)	• Consolidated over 50 federal narcotic, marijuana, and dangerous drug laws into 1 law • Designed to regulate the manufacture, importation, possession, and distribution of certain drugs in the United States • Established five schedules (classifications) of drugs based on their accepted medical use in the United States, abuse potential, and potential for addiction
1983	Orphan Drug Act	Enabled FDA to promote research and marketing of drugs needed for treating rare diseases
1988	Food and Drug Administration Act of 1988	Officially established FDA as an agency of the Department of Health and Human Services
1990	Anabolic Steroid Act	Identified anabolic steroids as a class of drugs and specified over two dozen items as controlled substances

TABLE 12-2 Schedule of Controlled Substances

Schedule	Description
1	• No acceptable medical use in United States • Used for research, analysis, or instruction only • High abuse potential • May lead to severe dependence • Examples: heroin, peyote, marijuana (cannabis), lysergic acid diethylamide (LSD), Ecstasy, XTC
2	• Acceptable medical use in United States • High abuse potential • May lead to severe physical and/or psychological dependence • Examples: morphine, meperidine (Demerol), codeine, oxycodone (OxyContin, Percocet, Tylox, Roxicodone, Roxicet), methadone, propoxyphene (Darvon), amphetamines, cocaine, opium
3	• Acceptable medical use in United States • Less abuse potential than drugs in Schedules I and II • May lead to moderate/low physical or high psychological dependence • Examples: anabolic steroids ("body-building" drugs); preparations containing limited narcotic quantities or combined with one or more active ingredients that are noncontrolled substances, such as acetaminophen with codeine (Tylenol #3), acetaminophen with hydrocodone (Vicodin)
4	• Acceptable medical use in United States • Lower abuse potential compared with drugs in Schedule III • May lead to limited physical or psychological dependence • Examples: alprazolam (Xanax), diazepam (Valium), lorazepam (Ativan), midazolam (Versed), phenobarbital
5	• Acceptable medical use in United States • Low abuse potential compared with drugs in Schedule IV • May lead to limited physical or psychological dependence • Examples: narcotic-containing preparations to suppress cough (Robitussin A-C) or control diarrhea (Lomotil)

TABLE 12-3 Examples of Drug Names

Generic Name	Trade Name	Chemical Name
albuterol	Proventil, Ventolin	alpha1[(tert-Butylamino)methyl]-4-hydroxy-*m*-xylene-alpha, alpha'-diol sulfate
ibuprofen	Motrin, Advil	(±)-2-(p-isobutylphenyl) propionic acid
sildenafil citrate	Viagra	1-[4-ethoxy-3-(6,7dihydro-methyl-7-oxo-3-propyl-1H-pyrazolo [4,3-d]pyrimidin-5-yl)phenylsulfonyl]-4-methylpiperazine citrate

Drug Names

Chemical Name

A drug's **chemical name** is a description of its composition and molecular structure. This name is useful for determining the effects of a drug on the body.

Generic Name

The **generic name** (also called the *nonproprietary name*) is the name given to a drug by the company that first manufactures it. It is often a simplified version of the drug's chemical name or structure. Generic names are printed in lowercase letters.

Trade Name

A drug's **trade name** is also known as its *brand name* or *proprietary name*. Trade names are capitalized. When a company makes a new drug, the manufacturer patents the drug and its trade name. The patent usually lasts 20 years. During that time, the drug company that holds the patent has the sole right to make, market, and sell the drug. When the patent expires, other drug companies can make and sell generic versions of the drug, but they cannot use the drug's original trade name. As a result, a drug may have several different trade names if it is made and sold by different manufacturers (see Table 12-3).

Making a Difference

In the field, the generic and trade names are the names most often used to identify a drug or medication. An informed Emergency Medical Technician (EMT) is able to recognize both of these names.

Sources of Drug Information

Before giving *any* medication, you have a responsibility to the patient to know as much as you can about the drug you will be giving or assisting the patient in taking. There are many sources of drug information available to help you find out more about a drug before giving it.

The United States Pharmacopeia (USP) is an official publication that contains information about drugs marketed in the United States. It lists approved drugs and gives directions for their general use.

The American Hospital Formulary Service (AHFS) is published by the American Society of Hospital Pharmacists. It is available in hospital pharmacies and most Emergency Departments. It contains information about drugs for FDA-approved uses as well as some investigational uses of medications.

The *Physician's Desk Reference* (PDR) is well known to healthcare professionals. This publication contains a collection of package inserts provided by drug manufacturers. The information includes the accepted use, dosages, and side effects for commercially available drugs. It lists specific drugs for FDA-approved uses. The PDR also contains a product identification guide showing actual sizes and color pictures of commonly prescribed drugs.

Patient package inserts are published by drug companies. They are required by law, and their content is approved by the FDA. Other sources of information include pharmacists, poison centers, and drug references produced by medical publishers.

Drug Forms and Routes of Drug Administration

Drug Forms

Objective 5

Every drug is supplied in a specific form by the drug's manufacturer. This is done to allow properly controlled concentrations of the drug to enter the bloodstream where the drug has an effect on the target body system.

TABLE 12-4 Liquid Drug Forms

Liquid Drug Form	Description	Example
Elixir	Clear liquids made with alcohol, water, flavors, or sweeteners	Terpin hydrate, Nyquil
Emulsion	Mixture of two liquids, one distributed throughout the other in small globules	Cold cream
Gel	Clear or transparent semisolid substances that liquefy when applied to the skin or a mucous membrane	Glucose
Lotion	Preparation applied to protect the skin or treat a skin disorder	Calamine lotion
Solution	Liquid preparation of one or more chemical substances, usually dissolved in water	5% dextrose in water, 0.9% normal saline
Spirits	Volatile substances dissolved in alcohol	Spirit of ammonia
Suspension	Drug particles mixed with, but not dissolved in, a liquid	Oral antibiotics (amoxicillin), activated charcoal
Syrups	Drugs suspended in sugar and water	Cough syrup
Tincture	Alcohol solution prepared from an animal or vegetable drug or chemical substance	Tincture of iodine

A drug's effects may be local or systemic. A **local effect** of a drug usually occurs only in a limited part of the body (usually at the site of drug application). For instance, if you apply calamine lotion to a rash on your arm or leg, the effects of the drug are limited to the extremity to which the drug was applied.

Drugs with **systemic effects** are absorbed into the bloodstream and distributed throughout the body. For example, when you go to see the dentist to have a cavity fixed, he often gives you an injection in the mouth where the dental work will be done. The drug used is often a combination of lidocaine and epinephrine. Lidocaine numbs the area (a local effect). Epinephrine constricts the blood vessels in the area to limit bleeding (a local effect). However, another effect of epinephrine is an increase in heart rate (a systemic effect).

Gas Forms

Drugs that are in a gas form are breathed in and absorbed through the respiratory tract. Oxygen is an example of a drug that you will be giving in gas form.

Liquid Drugs

Liquid drugs contain medication that is ground into a powder and °mixed with a substance, such as water.

Table 12-4 shows examples of different types of liquid drug forms.

Solid Drugs

A drug that is in solid form is usually swallowed. In some cases (such as when a patient takes aspirin for chest pain), the drug is chewed first and then swallowed. Although solid drugs are generally easy to administer, the patient must be responsive and cooperative and have an intact gag reflex. Table 12-5 shows examples of different types of solid drug forms.

Routes of Drug Administration

The route of drug administration is one of the most important factors influencing the effects of a drug and the rate at which the onset of drug action occurs. Although some drugs can be used both locally and systemically, most drugs are given via a single route of administration.

Oral

The oral route of drug administration is used infrequently in the prehospital setting. Commonly used oral dosage forms include liquids, tablets, and capsules. Activated charcoal may be given by this route (Figure 12-1).

TABLE 12-5 Solid Drug Forms

Solid Drug Form	Description	Example
Caplet	An oval-shaped tablet that has a film-coated covering	Tylenol caplets
Capsule	Small gelatin container containing a medication dose in powder or granule form	Actifed
Enteric-coated tablets	Tablets that have a special coating so that they break down in the intestines instead of the stomach	Aspirin
Gelcap	Small gelatin container containing a liquid medication dose	Dayquil Gelcaps
Powders	Drugs ground into fine particles	Calcium carbonate
Suppositories	Drugs mixed in a firm base such a cocoa butter that, when placed into a body opening, melt at body temperature	Glycerin, aspirin
Tablets	Powdered drugs, molded or compressed into a small form	Nitroglycerin

Stop and Think!

Patients who are unresponsive, uncooperative, have no gag reflex, or are vomiting should *not* be given drugs orally.

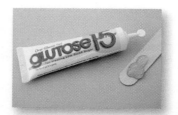

FIGURE 12-2 ◀ Oral glucose.

Buccal

Buccal means, "pertaining to the cheek." To give a drug by this route, a drug is placed in the mouth against the mucous membranes of the cheek until the drug is dissolved. The drug may act locally on the mucous membranes of the mouth or systemically when swallowed in the saliva. Buccal drugs are rapidly

absorbed into the bloodstream. Oral glucose may be given by this route (Figure 12-2).

Sublingual

Sublingual drugs are given under the tongue. The drug must remain under the tongue until it is dissolved and absorbed. The drug is absorbed rapidly into the bloodstream because of the rich blood supply under the tongue. The patient should not swallow the drug or take it with water. If swallowed, the drug may be inactivated by gastric juice in the stomach. Nitroglycerin (NTG) may be given by this route (Figure 12-3).

Inhalation

Drugs given by the inhalation route have a rapid onset of action because of the large surface area and blood supply of the lungs. To make sure that normal gas exchange of oxygen and carbon dioxide is continuous in the lungs, drugs given by inhalation must be in the form of a gas (such as oxygen) or fine mist (such as an aerosol). Oxygen is given for its systemic effects. A metered-dose inhaler (MDI) such as albuterol is given for its localized effect on the lungs (Figure 12-4).

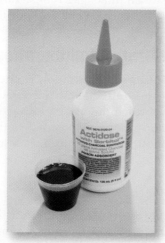

FIGURE 12-1 ▲ Activated charcoal is a suspension. It contains drug particles that are mixed with, but not dissolved in, a liquid.

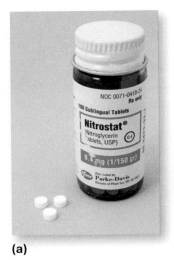

(a)

(b)

FIGURE 12-3 ▲ Sublingual nitroglycerin is available in **(a)** tablet and **(b)** spray form.

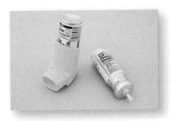

FIGURE 12-4 ◄ Metered dose inhaler.

Subcutaneous

Drugs given by the **subcutaneous (SubQ) route** are given by means of a needle inserted underneath the skin into the subcutaneous tissue. The onset of action of SubQ drugs is faster than the oral route but slower than the intramuscular route. Absorption is delayed in circulatory collapse, such as shock. Only a small volume of drug can be given by this route.

Intramuscular

When a drug is given by the **intramuscular route,** a medication in a liquid form is injected into a large mass of skeletal muscle (Figure 12-5). Sites commonly used in prehospital care include the arm (deltoid muscle) and mid-lateral thigh (vastus lateralis muscle). The injection is usually made with a longer needle than that used with a SubQ injection. Larger volumes can be given by the intramuscular route than the subcutaneous route. The onset of action is faster than the SubQ route because of the muscle's blood supply and large absorbing surface. Epinephrine is an example of a drug that may be given by this route (Figure 12-6). Epinephrine is discussed in more detail in Chapter 20.

You Should Know

In some states, EMTs are permitted to give naloxone in cases of narcotic overdose. With an order from medical direction, the EMT gives naloxone to the patient by means of an atomizer that is connected to a syringe. The atomizer is placed a short distance (about 1.5 cm) into the patient's nose. When the EMT pushes the plunger on the syringe, the atomizer disperses a mist-like spray onto the inner surface of the patient's nostril, where the drug is quickly absorbed.

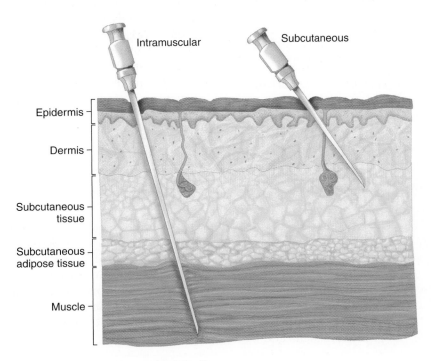

Intramuscular

Subcutaneous

Epidermis

Dermis

Subcutaneous tissue

Subcutaneous adipose tissue

Muscle

FIGURE 12-5 ▲ Subcutaneous and intramuscular injections.

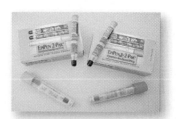

FIGURE 12-6 ◀ Epinephrine auto-injectors are available for adults and children.

Stop and Think!

An EMT is responsible for his own actions when giving drugs. Although drugs may be life saving when given properly, they may cause death if they are improperly given.

Drug Administration

General Guidelines

Before giving any drug, you must assess the patient. The extent of the physical examination you perform will depend on the patient's illness or present condition. The physical exam provides baseline information by which you will be able to evaluate the effectiveness of the medications given. Obtain a medication history from the patient including the following:

- Prescribed medications (name, strength, daily dosage)
- Over-the-counter medications
- Allergies to medications

You must be knowledgeable about each drug you give, including the following:

- **Mechanism of action:** how the drug exerts its effect on body cells and tissues

Stop and Think!

Many patients use herbal and nontraditional medications. Always ask your patient for information about any herbs and herbal remedies that they may have used (or routinely take) before giving any medication. In these situations, you must consider the possibility of a negative interaction between the drug you are about to give and the substances the patient has already taken. If the patient has taken any herbal or nontraditional medications, consult medical direction before giving any medication.

- **Indications:** the condition(s) for which the drug has documented usefulness
- **Dose:** the amount of the drug that should be given to the patient
- **Route of administration:** the route and form in which the drug should be given to the patient
- **Contraindications:** condition(s) for which a drug should not be used because it may cause harm to the patient or offer no improvement of the patient's condition or illness
- **Side effects:** expected (and usually unavoidable) effects of the drug

Administration of Medications Carried in the Emergency Medical Services Unit

Objectives 1, 2

The medications that are most commonly found in EMS units include activated charcoal (see Table 12-6), oral glucose (see Table 12-7), and oxygen (see Table 12-8). This list may vary from state to state and even EMS system to EMS system.

You Should Know

Activated charcoal is given in doses according to the patient's body weight. The recommended dose is 1 gram (g) of activated charcoal per kilogram (kg) of the patient's body weight. One kg is equal to 2.2 pounds (lb). An *estimate* of the patient's weight in kg can be made by dividing by the patient's weight in pounds by 2 and then subtracting 10%.

Example: Patient weight = 200 lb
$$200/2 = 100$$
$$100 \times 10\% = 10$$
$$100 - 10 = 90 \text{ kg}$$

In this example, a 200-lb patient weighs about 90 kg. The patient would receive about 90 g of activated charcoal. This is not an acceptable conversion method for a pediatric patient. For children, the preferred method is the actual calculation of the conversion in most cases. When obtaining authorization to give the medication from medical direction, request a dose amount from the physician (be prepared to give the patient's weight).

TABLE 12-6 Activated Charcoal

Generic name	activated charcoal
Trade name	Liqui-Char, Actidose, InstaChar, SuperChar, and others
Mechanism of action	Activated charcoal acts as an adsorbent and will bind with many (but not all chemicals) and slow down or block the absorption of the chemical by the body.
Indications	Poisoning by mouth
Dosage	• Adults and children: 1gram activated charcoal per kilogram of body weight • Usual adult dose: 25 to 50 grams • Usual infant/child dose: 12.5 to 25 grams
Side effects	• Black stools • Some patients, particularly those who have ingested poisons that cause nausea, may vomit. • If the patient vomits, consider repeating the dose once (check with medical direction).
Contraindications	• Medical direction does not give permission • Altered mental status • Ingestion of acids or alkalis • Inability to swallow
Special considerations	• Obtain an order from medical direction either on line or off line to give the medication. • Grasp the container in your hand and shake thoroughly. Since charcoal looks like mud, the patient may need to be persuaded to drink it. Place a straw in the container or pour the activated charcoal into a glass and ask the patient to drink it. • If the patient does not drink all of the medication in the first drink, shake the container before the second dose because the activated charcoal will settle to the bottom of the container or glass.

Stop and Think!

Always observe BSI precautions when giving any medication.

Remember This!

- Before giving activated charcoal, you must determine if your patient can follow directions and swallow safely.
- Activated charcoal looks like tar, stains any material with which it comes in contact, and doesn't taste good. Be prepared for the patient to spit out the medication.

Assisting with Prescribed Medications

Objectives 3, 4

After consulting with medical direction, an EMT can give some medications to patients who fit established criteria. An EMT can give, or assist a patient in taking, the following physician-prescribed medications when authorized by medical direction:

- Prescribed metered-dose inhaler (MDI) (see Table 12-9)
- NTG (see Table 12-10)
- Epinephrine (see Table 12-11)

Since the Department of Transportation EMT curriculum was written, many states have passed legislation to include aspirin as a medication that can be carried on an EMS unit and given by EMTs

TABLE 12-7 Oral Glucose

Generic name	oral glucose
Trade name	Glutose, Insta-glucose
Mechanism of action	Increases the amount of sugar available for use as energy by the body
Indications	Patients with altered mental status who have a known history of diabetes controlled by medication and can swallow
Dosage	One tube
Side effects	• None when given properly • May be aspirated by the patient without a gag reflex
Contraindications	• Medical direction does not give permission • Unresponsiveness • Inability to swallow
Special considerations	• Obtain order from medical direction either on line or off line. • Confirm signs and symptoms of altered mental status with a known history of diabetes. • Make sure the patient is responsive, can swallow, and can protect his airway. • Squeeze the glucose from the tube onto a tongue depressor. Place the tongue depressor between the patient's cheek and gum. • Although the body readily absorbs glucose, keep in mind that it is also rapidly metabolized and your patient will need additional care

TABLE 12-8 Oxygen

Generic name	oxygen
Mechanism of action	Oxygen is a molecule that is needed for body metabolism. Giving oxygen increases the amount available in the bloodstream for use by the body's cells.
Indications	• Cardiac or respiratory arrest • Suspected low oxygen levels from any cause (seizures, diabetic emergency, altered mental status) • Any suspected cardiopulmonary emergency, especially complaints of shortness of breath or chest pain
Dosage	• Nasal cannula (1 to 6 L/min) • Nonrebreather mask (15 L/min) • Cardiac or respiratory arrest: positive-pressure ventilation with 100% oxygen

TABLE 12-9 Prescribed Metered-Dose Inhaler

Generic (trade) name	albuterol (Proventil, Ventolin), isoetharine (Bronkosol)
Mechanism of action	Albuterol dilates bronchioles, reducing airway resistance.
Indications	An EMT can assist a patient in taking a prescribed inhaler if *all* of the following criteria are met: • The patient has signs and symptoms of a respiratory emergency. • The patient has a physician-prescribed handheld inhaler. • There are no contraindications to giving the medication. • The EMT has specific authorization by medical direction.
Dosage	Number of inhalations based on medical direction's order or physician's order based on consultation with the patient
Side effects	• Increased heart rate • Shaking or tremors • Nervousness
Contraindications	• Medical direction does not give permission. • Patient is unable to use device. • Inhaler is not prescribed for the patient. • Patient has already met maximum prescribed dose before EMT arrival.
Special considerations	• An MDI automatically delivers a specific dose of medication each time it is activated. • Contact medical direction for an order to assist with giving this medication. • Assist the patient in finding his MDI if it is not readily available. • Help the patient direct the spray into his mouth just as he attempts to take a breath. Wait at least three minutes before assisting with another dose from the MDI. • Recheck the patient's vital signs and reassess the patient's degree of breathing difficulty.

(see Table 12-12). Check your state and local protocols for the appropriate use of this drug.

Remember This!

- NTG is a frequently "shared" medication. Make sure that the medication belongs to the patient and that you have contacted medical direction before giving it.
- NTG is heat and light sensitive. If the patient has been carrying this medication in a pocket, it may no longer be effective.

- Be watchful for a change in the patient's level of responsiveness after giving this medication.
- Because NTG relaxes blood vessels, it has the potential to significantly decrease the patient's blood pressure. Reassess the patient's vital signs after *each dose* of this drug.
- You will need to ask the patient if he has taken any drugs for erectile problems, such as Viagra or Cialis. Giving NTG to a patient who has taken these drugs within 24 to 48 hours may lead to irreversible hypotension and death.

TABLE 12-10 Nitroglycerin

Generic name	nitroglycerin
Trade name	Nitrostat, Nitrobid, Nitrolingual, Nitroglycerin Spray
Mechanism of action	• Relaxes blood vessels • Decreases the workload of the heart
Indications	An EMT can assist a patient in taking nitroglycerin if *all* of the following criteria are met: • The patient has signs and symptoms of chest discomfort suspected to be of cardiac origin. • The patient has physician-prescribed sublingual tablets or spray. • There are no contraindications to giving nitroglycerin. • The EMT has specific authorization by medical direction.
Dosage	Dosage is 1 tablet or 1 spray under the tongue. This dose may be repeated in 3 to 5 minutes (maximum of three doses) if: • The patient experiences no relief • The patient's systolic blood pressure remains above 100 mm Hg systolic • The patient's heart rate remains between 50 and 100 beats per minute • There are no other contraindications • The EMT is authorized by medical direction to give another dose of the medication
Side effects	Hypotension is a common and significant side effect. Other side effects include tachycardia, bradycardia, headache, palpitations, and fainting.
Contraindications	• Medical direction does not give permission • Medication is not prescribed for the patient • Patient has already taken maximum prescribed dose before EMT arrival • Hypotension or blood pressure below 100 mm Hg systolic • Heart rate <50 beats/minute or >100 beats/minute • Head injury (recent) or stroke (recent) • Infants and children • Patient has taken a medication for erectile dysfunction within the last 24 to 48 hours
Special considerations	• Ask the patient to lift his tongue while you place the tablet or spray dose under the tongue (while wearing gloves), or have the patient place the tablet or spray under the tongue. • Have the patient keep his mouth closed with the tablet under the tongue (without swallowing) until it is dissolved and absorbed. • Recheck the patient's vital signs within 2 minutes. • Reassess the patient's degree of discomfort.

TABLE 12-11   Epinephrine

Generic name	epinephrine
Trade name	Adrenalin
Mechanism of action	Epinephrine works by relaxing the passages of the airway and constricting the blood vessels. The opening of the airway allows the patient to move more air into and out of the body, which will increase the amount of oxygen in the bloodstream. Constriction of the blood vessels slows the leakage of fluid from the blood vessels into the space around the cells of the body.
Indications	An EMT can assist a patient in using an epinephrine auto-injector if *all* of the following criteria are met: • The patient has signs and symptoms of an allergic reaction. • The patient has a physician-prescribed epinephrine auto-injector. • The EMT has specific authorization by medical direction.
Dosage	Adult—one adult auto-injector Infant and child—one infant/child auto-injector
Side effects	Rapid heart rate Chest pain or discomfort Anxiety Headache Excitability Dizziness Nausea, vomiting
Contraindications	There are no contraindications when used in a life-threatening situation.
Special considerations	• Give the patient oxygen by nonrebreather mask before giving epinephrine. • Assist the patient with removing the Epi-Pen from its container. Next, remove the "safety" cap from one end of the auto-injector. • Help the patient to press the auto-injector against the outside portion of one thigh. • Have the patient press the Epi-Pen into his thigh until you hear it release. The auto-injector will propel a spring-driven needle into the patient's thigh and then inject the drug into the muscle of the outer thigh. This will cause pain, and the patient may move very suddenly. • After the drug has been delivered, the needle will be exposed and must be disposed of properly in an appropriate container. • Note any changes in patient condition and vital signs. • The patient will need to be transported for additional care.

You Should Know

In most EMS systems, an EMS dispatcher will ask a few precautionary screening questions and then instruct a patient who is experiencing a possible heart attack to take aspirin (if there are no contraindications).

Drug Administration Procedure

Before giving a medication, consult with medical direction. An EMT can give medications only by the order of a licensed physician. The physician's order may be a written protocol (standing order) or a verbal order. When speaking with medical direction, be sure to relay relevant information about the patient, including the following:

- Patient's age
- Chief complaint
- Vital signs
- Signs and symptoms
- Allergies
- Current medications
- Pertinent past medical history

TABLE 12-12   Aspirin

Generic name	acetylsalicylic acid
Trade name	Bayer, Ecotrin, Empirin
Mechanism of action	Blocks a part of the clotting process in the bloodstream and may reduce the risk of a heart attack
Indications	Chest pain or discomfort that is suspected to be of cardiac origin
Dosage (adult)	Two to four 81-mg tablets (baby aspirin), chewed and swallowed
Side effects	• Rapid pulse • Dizziness • Flushing • Nausea, vomiting • Gastrointestinal bleeding
Contraindications	• Known allergy or sensitivity to aspirin • Bleeding ulcer or bleeding disorders • Stroke • Children and adolescents
Special considerations	• If ordered by medical direction, aspirin should be given as soon as possible after the patient's onset of chest discomfort. • Aspirin should be used with caution in a patient who has a history of asthma, nasal polyps, or nasal allergies. Severe allergic reactions in sensitive patients have occurred.

The physician's order will include the name, dose, and route of the drug to be given. Make sure you clearly understand the orders received from medical direction. Repeat the orders back to the physician, including the name of the drug, dose, and route of administration. If an order received from medical direction is unclear or seems incorrect, ask the physician to repeat the order.

Before giving a drug, use the five "rights" of drug administration (see the following *You Should Know* box).

1. *Right patient.* If assisting a patient in taking his own medication, make sure that the medication is prescribed for *that* patient.
2. *Right drug.* Select the right medication. Use only medications that are in a clearly labeled container. If the label is unclear or blurred, do not give the drug. Carefully read the label and check it three times before administering:
   (1) when removing the drug from the drug box,
   (2) when preparing the drug for administration,

and (3) before actually giving the drug to the patient. Check the drug's expiration date.
3. *Right dose.* Check and recheck the dose ordered against the dose to be given.
4. *Right route.* You must know the route(s) by which a drug is to be given.

You Should Know

The "Five Rights" of Drug Administration

Once a drug enters the patient's body it cannot be removed. You must be right the first time!

Always ask yourself these five questions before you give a patient a medication:

1. Do I have the right patient?
2. Is this the right medication?
3. Is this the right dose?
4. Is this the right route?
5. Is this the right time?

5. *Right time (frequency)*. Although many drugs are ordered for one-time administration, some may be repeated. Determine from medical direction the frequency with which a drug may be given.

After giving a drug:

- Document the time you gave the drug
- Document the patient's response to the drug
- Monitor the patient for possible adverse (harmful) effects, as well as expected results
- Reassess and record the patient's vital signs

On the Scene   Wrap-Up

Because you work in an area that allows EMTs to carry and give an EpiPen auto-injector, you are able to assist the patient with the use of this lifesaving drug. Your knowledge of the indications, contraindications, side effects, and appropriate dose of the medications found in this chapter can and will help you to save lives.

Sum It Up

▶ A drug's chemical name is a description of its composition and molecular structure. The generic name (also called the nonproprietary name) is the name given to a drug by the company that first manufactures it. A drug's trade name is also known as its brand name or proprietary name.

▶ A local effect of a drug usually occurs only in a limited part of the body (usually at the site of drug application). Drugs with systemic effects are absorbed into the bloodstream and distributed throughout the body.

▶ Each drug is in a specific medication form to allow properly controlled concentrations of the drug to enter the bloodstream where the drug has an effect on the target body system.

▶ Before giving a drug, an EMT must know the following:
- The drug's mechanism of action: the desired effects the drug should have on the patient
- Indications for the drug's use, including the most common uses of the drug in treating a specific illness
- Contraindications: situations in which the drug should not be used because it may cause harm to the patient or offer no possibility of improving the patient's condition or illness
- Correct dose (amount) of the drug to be given
- The proper route by which the drug is given
- Side effects: the actions of a drug other than those desired. Some side effects may be predictable.

▶ Medications that are typically carried on the EMS unit and may be given by EMTs include activated charcoal, oral glucose, and oxygen. Some EMS systems also include aspirin.

▶ Medications an EMT can assist a patient in taking with approval by medical direction include a prescribed inhaler, NTG, and an epinephrine auto-injector.

▶ Before giving a drug, use the five "rights" of drug administration: Right drug, right patient, right dose, right route, and right time (frequency).

▶ After giving a drug, document the time you gave the drug, document the patient's response to the drug, monitor the patient for possible adverse (harmful) effects, and reassess and record the patient's vital signs.

13 Respiratory Emergencies

By the end of this chapter, you should be able to:

Knowledge Objectives ▶
1. List the structures and functions of the respiratory system.
2. State the signs and symptoms of a patient with breathing difficulty.
3. Describe the emergency medical care of the patient with breathing difficulty.
4. Recognize the need for medical direction to assist in the emergency medical care of the patient with breathing difficulty.
5. Describe the emergency medical care of the patient with breathing distress.
6. Establish the relationship between airway management and the patient with breathing difficulty.
7. List signs of adequate air exchange.
8. State the generic name, medication forms, dose, administration, action, indications, and contraindications for each prescribed inhaler.
9. Distinguish between the emergency medical care of the infant, child and adult patient with breathing difficulty.
10. Differentiate between upper airway obstruction and lower airway disease in the infant and child patient.

Attitude Objectives ▶
11. Defend Emergency Medical Technician (EMT) treatment regimens for various respiratory emergencies.
12. Explain the rationale for administering an inhaler.

Skill Objectives ▶
13. Demonstrate the emergency medical care for breathing difficulty.
14. Perform the steps in facilitating the use of an inhaler.

You are working as an EMT on a Basic Life Support (BLS) ambulance with a BLS partner. At 2:00 a.m. you are dispatched to a call for a child in respiratory distress. Although you use lights and siren en route to the call, your response time to the scene is eight minutes. You make a mental note that you are 20 minutes from the nearest hospital.

Upon arrival, you find a 3-year-old girl in moderate respiratory distress. Her parents are very anxious. They tell you that their daughter has been diagnosed with reactive airway disease and has been prescribed an inhaler to be given every four hours with a spacer. They filled the prescription today, but are not sure they are using it correctly.

The child's color is pink and she is coughing frequently. She is breathing 22 times per minute. Her heart rate is 120. When you listen to her lungs, you hear slight expiratory wheezing that is scattered throughout both lung fields. ■

THINK ABOUT IT

As you read this chapter, think about the following questions:

- What emergency care can you give to help this child?
- Could you set up a metered-dose inhaler with a spacer and instruct the parents and patient on the appropriate technique?

Introduction

As an Emergency Medical Technician (EMT), you will often encounter patients with respiratory emergencies. You must be able to recognize the signs of breathing difficulty, determine if the patient's breathing is adequate or inadequate, and deliver appropriate patient care based on these findings.

When authorized by medical direction, you may assist a patient in taking a prescribed inhaler. Before assisting with the administration of any medication, you must know the generic and trade names, medication forms, dose, administration, action, indications, and contraindications for the medication to ensure patient safety.

The Respiratory System

Function of the Respiratory System

Objective 1

The major functions of the respiratory system are to deliver oxygen from the atmosphere to the blood where it gets distributed to body cells and remove carbon dioxide produced by the body cells to the atmosphere. As an EMT, you must make sure this happens by main-taining an open airway. Maintaining an open airway allows a free flow of air into and out of the lungs.

When we breathe in, the air entering the body from the atmosphere is rich in oxygen and contains little carbon dioxide. Carbon dioxide is the waste product exchanged when breathing. The oxygen-rich air enters the alveoli in the lungs and passes through the walls of capillaries into the bloodstream. Carbon dioxide passes from the blood through the capillary walls into the alveoli. It leaves the body in the air we breathe out.

Anatomy Review
Nose and Nasal Cavity

The nose warms, humidifies, and filters the air before it enters the lungs (Figure 13-1). A wall of tissue called the septum separates the right and left nostrils. The nose is lined with a mucous membrane that is fragile. When the nose is subjected to trauma, it is prone to bleed and become inflamed, which can cause an airway obstruction. The nose is prone to trauma because of its location on the face. The nasal cavity is separated from the cranium by a thin bone that can become fractured as a result of head trauma.

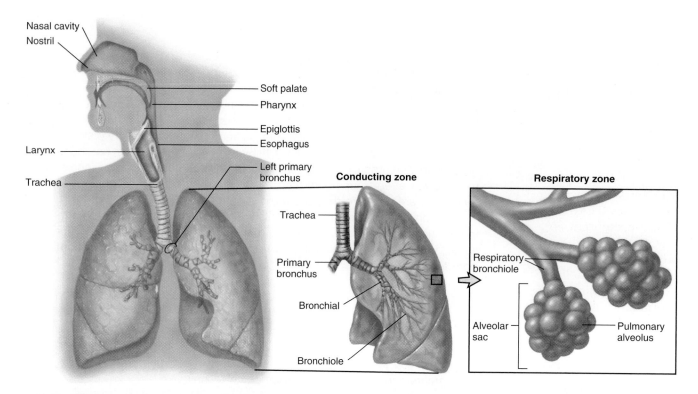

FIGURE 13-1 ▲ Anatomy of the respiratory system.

The Mouth and Oral Cavity

The mouth and its structures serve many functions. The most important function is its ability to move fresh air in and out of the lungs. Air enters the body through the mouth or nose and passes down the pharynx (throat), past the epiglottis, down the trachea, and into the lungs. Air entering the mouth is not filtered or warmed as efficiently as air entering the nostrils.

Remember This!

You must be able to recognize signs of an airway obstruction and act quickly to remove it in order for the patient to survive.

The upper airway is the most common place for an airway obstruction to occur. When a patient becomes unresponsive, the tongue falls back into the rear of the mouth. This can cause a complete airway obstruction. Other common causes of upper airway obstruction include teeth, blood, and other secretions.

The epiglottis is a piece of cartilage that protects the lower airway from aspiration. When we swallow, the epiglottis closes off the trachea and prevents food from entering. Choking may result if the epiglottis fails to close, allowing food or liquids to enter the airway. When a patient becomes unresponsive, he may lose his gag reflex and this protective response. Placing an unresponsive, uninjured patient on his side (recovery position) while suctioning out the airway will allow material to flow from the mouth by gravity and reduce the risk of aspiration.

Trachea and Lower Airway

The larynx contains the vocal cords. This is the narrowest part of an adult's airway. The vocal cords are responsible for sound production. An airway obstruction at or below this level will affect the ability to produce sound. The space between the vocal cords is called the glottis (also called the glottic opening). The largest cartilage of the larynx is the thyroid cartilage, also called the Adam's apple. The cricoid cartilage is the most inferior (lowest) of the cartilages of the larynx.

The windpipe (trachea) extends to the level of the upper and middle portion of the breastbone (sternum). The trachea is protected and supported by C-shaped rings of cartilage. This allows for some expansion during breathing and coughing. At about the middle of the breastbone, the trachea divides into two main branches. One branch, the right mainstem bronchus, allows air in and out of the right lung. The other, the left mainstem bronchus, allows air in and out of the left lung.

You Should Know

The glottic opening is located directly behind the thyroid cartilage and is the narrowest part of an adult's airway. In infants and children younger than 10 years of age, the narrowest part of the airway is at the level of the cricoid cartilage.

Lungs

The lungs are very elastic and are made up of many tiny air sacs. The lungs are divided into three separate lobes on the right and two lobes on the left. Even a tiny blockage in the lower airways can completely collapse a segment of the lung, making breathing much more difficult. Collapse can also occur because of a penetrating injury to the lung, as in stabbing or gunshot wounds. If open communication occurs between the outside atmosphere and the lung, it will collapse the lung, requiring emergency care.

Diaphragm

The major muscle used for breathing is a dome-shaped muscle known as the diaphragm. The diaphragm divides the chest cavity from the abdominal cavity.

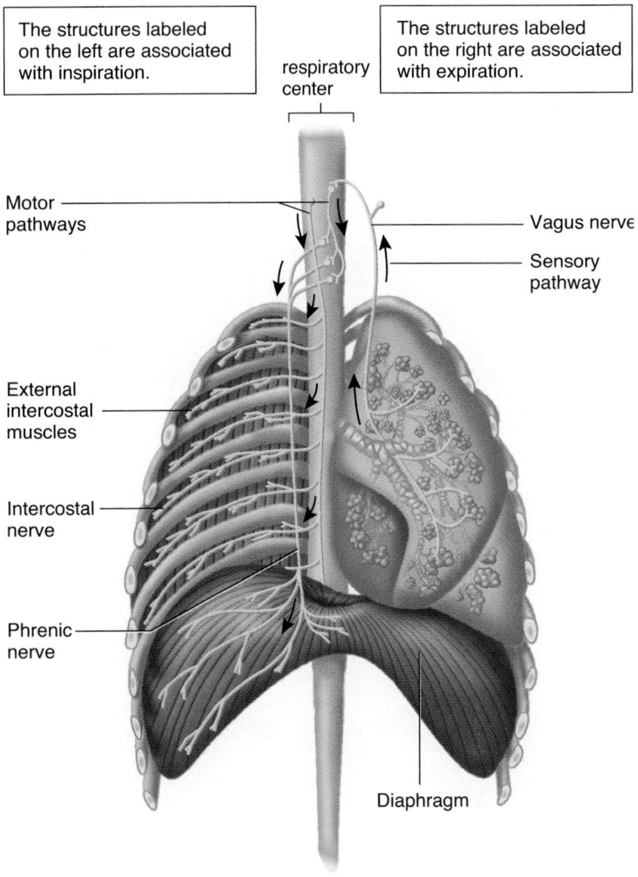

FIGURE 13-2 ▲ Muscles used in breathing and nervous control of breathing.

Mechanics of Breathing

Breathing (also called *pulmonary ventilation*) is the mechanical process of moving air into and out of the lungs. Inhalation is the process of breathing in and moving air into the lungs. Exhalation is the process of breathing out and moving air out of the lungs. Respiration is the exchange of gases between a living organism and its environment.

The breathing process consists of four phases:

- The movement of room air into and out of the lungs (pulmonary ventilation)
- The diffusion of oxygen and carbon dioxide in the alveoli (external respiration). **Diffusion** is the movement of gases or particles from an area of higher concentration to an area of lower concentration.
- The transport of oxygen to the cells and carbon dioxide away from the cells (internal respiration)
- The regulation of ventilation

Muscles of Breathing

Normal breathing involves two primary muscles: the diaphragm and the external intercostal muscles between the ribs. Inhalation is an active process (requires muscle contraction). The diaphragm and external intercostal muscles contract (Figure 13-2). As the diaphragm moves down and the chest wall moves upward and outward, the thoracic (chest) cavity pressure decreases, allowing for the movement of air into the lungs (inspiration). After inhalation, the tiny air sacs (alveoli) are inflated while oxygen and carbon dioxide cross an alevolar membrane. Oxygen enters the circulation, while carbon dioxide is exhaled into the atmosphere. The chest cavity enlarges and fills with air. Inhalation continues until the pressure between the lungs and atmosphere equalizes.

Exhalation is normally a passive process. The diaphragm and external intercostal muscles relax (Figure 13-3). The chest cavity becomes smaller, and the diaphragm returns to its resting state, pushing air from the lungs. Air is forced out of the lungs and into the atmosphere.

Normal breathing is quiet, painless, and occurs at a regular rate. Both sides of the chest rise and fall equally. Normal breathing does not require excessive use of the muscles between the ribs, above the collarbones, or in the abdomen during inhalation or exhalation. These muscles are called accessory muscles for breathing. Accessory muscles are used during periods of respiratory distress. This use is particularly common

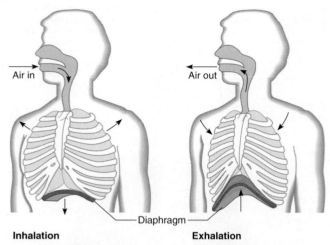

Inhalation
- Rib cage moves up and out
- Diaphragm contracts and moves downward
- Lungs expand

Exhalation
- Rib cage moves down and in
- Diaphragm relaxes and moves upward
- Lungs recoil

FIGURE 13-3 ▲ The mechanism of breathing.

in patients with chronic obstructive pulmonary disease (COPD) and in infants and children. The muscles of the diaphragm and neck are used to assist in inspiration. The internal intercostal muscles and abdominal muscles may be used during forceful exhalation.

Gas Exchange

The tissues of the body depend on a continuous supply of oxygen to maintain metabolism. Interruption of the body's oxygen supply and/or removal of carbon dioxide can lead to shock and death.

Air entering the alveoli from the atmosphere during inspiration is rich in oxygen (oxygen-rich) and contains little carbon dioxide. During alveolar/capillary exchange, oxygen-rich air enters the alveoli during inhalation (Figure 13-4). Oxygen is then passed from the alveoli into the capillaries to enrich the oxygen-poor blood. This oxygen-rich blood is distributed to the cells of the body where the oxygen is passed from

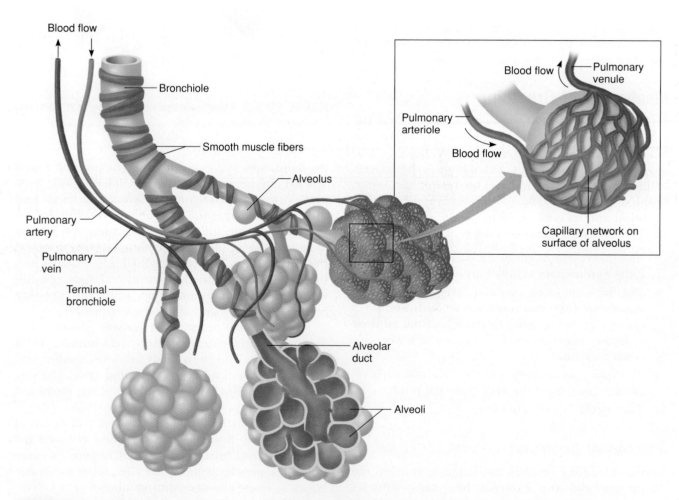

FIGURE 13-4 ▲ During alveolar/capillary exchange, oxygen-rich air enters the alveoli during each inhalation. Oxygen-poor blood in the capillaries passes into the alveoli. During capillary/cellular exchange, cells give up carbon dioxide to the capillaries.

the capillaries to the cells of the body. The capillary blood then collects the waste carbon dioxide from the cells and transports it to the lungs where the carbon dioxide is passed from the capillaries to the alveoli and exhaled from the body.

Control of Respiration

Respiration is controlled by nerve, reflex, and chemical responses in different parts of the body (Figure 13-5). The medulla of the brain stem generates impulses that travel along nerves to the respiratory muscles. The respiratory muscles are stimulated to contract, resulting in inhalation.

The walls of the bronchi and bronchioles contain stretch receptors. As the lungs inflate, the stretch receptors sense the stretching and generate impulses to depress the medulla. Depression of the medulla limits the extent of inspiration, preventing overinflation of the lungs.

The main stimulus for breathing is the level of carbon dioxide in the blood. A buildup of carbon dioxide in the blood causes an increase in the rate and depth of ventilation. An unusually low level of carbon dioxide in the blood results in a decrease in the rate and depth of ventilation.

Chronic respiratory diseases may alter the normal respiratory drive over time because of the prolonged high levels of carbon dioxide. Instead of an increase in carbon dioxide levels stimulating breathing, low levels of oxygen in the blood become the breathing stimulus. This kind of breathing stimulus is called hypoxic drive.

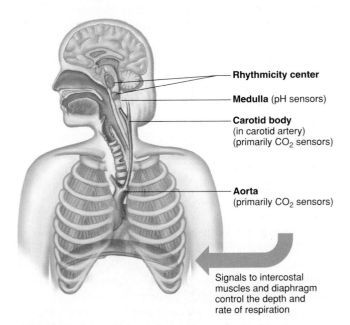

Rhythmicity center

Medulla (pH sensors)

Carotid body
(in carotid artery)
(primarily CO_2 sensors)

Aorta
(primarily CO_2 sensors)

Signals to intercostal muscles and diaphragm control the depth and rate of respiration

FIGURE 13-5 ▲ Receptors (sensors) in the medulla of the brain (and to some extent those in the aorta and carotid arteries) monitor the level of carbon dioxide in the blood.

Giving high concentration oxygen for prolonged periods to patients with this kind of breathing may depress respirations and result in respiratory arrest.

Remember This!

Never withhold oxygen from a patient who needs it. Be prepared to assist ventilations if necessary.

Infant and Child Anatomy Considerations

A child's nasal passages are very small, short, and narrow. It is easy for children to develop obstruction of these areas with mucus or foreign objects. If an infant or child is having difficulty breathing, you may see nasal flaring. Nasal flaring refers to widening of the nostrils when the patient breathes in. This sign is the body's attempt to increase the size of the airway and increase the amount of available oxygen.

Objective 9

Newborns are primarily nose breathers. A newborn will not automatically open his mouth to breathe when his nose becomes obstructed. As a result, any obstruction of the nose will lead to respiratory difficulty. You must make sure the newborn's nose is clear to avoid breathing problems. **Head bobbing** is an indicator of increased work of breathing in infants. When the baby breathes out, the head falls forward. The baby's head comes up when the baby breathes in and its chest expands.

Although the opening of the mouth is usually small, a child's tongue is large in proportion to the mouth. The tongue is the most common cause of upper airway obstruction in an unconscious child because the immature muscles of the lower jaw allow the tongue to fall to the back of the throat.

In children, the opening between the vocal cords (glottic opening) is higher in the neck and more toward the front than in an adult. As we grow older, our neck gets longer and the glottic opening drops down. The flap of cartilage that covers this opening, the epiglottis, is larger proportionally and floppier in children. Therefore, any injury to or swelling of this area can block the airway.

In children, the trachea is softer, more flexible, and has a smaller diameter and shorter length than in adults. The trachea has rings of cartilage that keep the airway open. In children, this cartilage is soft and collapses easily, which can then obstruct the airway. Extending or flexing the neck too far can result in crimping of the trachea and a blocked airway. To avoid blocking the airway, place the head of an infant or young child in a neutral or "sniffing" position. This may require slight elevation of the shoulders.

A child's ribs are soft and flexible because they are made up mostly of cartilage. The muscles between the ribs (intercostal muscles) help lift the chest wall during breathing. Because these muscles are not fully developed until later in childhood, the diaphragm is the primary muscle of breathing. As a result, the abdominal muscles move during breathing. During normal breathing, the abdominal muscles should move in the same direction as the chest wall. If they are moving opposite each other, this is called **seesaw breathing** and is abnormal. A child's respiratory rate is normally faster than an adult's and decreases with age. Because the muscles between the ribs are not well developed, a child cannot keep up a rate of breathing that is more rapid than normal for very long.

The stomach of an infant or child often fills with air during crying. Air can also build up in the stomach if rescue breathing is performed. As the stomach swells with air, it pushes on the lungs and diaphragm. This action limits movement and prevents good ventilation. Because infants and young children depend on the diaphragm for breathing, breathing difficulty results if movement of the diaphragm is limited.

The skin of an infant or child will more reliably show changes related to the amount of oxygen in the blood. Pale (whitish) skin may be seen in shock, fright, or anxiety. A bluish (cyanotic) tint, often seen first around the mouth, suggests inadequate breathing or poor perfusion. This is a critical sign that requires immediate treatment.

Assessing the Patient with Breathing Difficulty

Scene Size-Up

When you are called for a patient with breathing difficulty, determine if it is caused by trauma or a medical condition. If the scene suggests trauma might be a cause, determine the mechanism of injury from the patient, family members, or bystanders and your inspection of the scene. If trauma is suspected, be sure to maintain spinal stabilization while you assess the patient. If the scene suggests a medical cause, determine the nature of the illness from the patient, family members, or bystanders. Observe the patient's environment for clues to the cause of the patient's breathing difficulty.

Primary Survey

After making sure that the scene is safe, form a general impression before approaching your patient. You should use this method when evaluating all respiratory emergencies.

Assess the patient's appearance (mental status and body position), work of breathing, and skin color. If the patient looks agitated or limp or appears to be asleep, approach him immediately and begin the primary survey. Observe the patient's position. Patients with dyspnea often sit or stand to inhale adequate air. In a tripod position, the patient prefers to sit up and lean forward, with the weight of his upper body supported by his hands on his thighs or knees. Orthopnea is breathlessness when lying flat that is relieved or lessened when the patient sits or stands. **Paroxysmal nocturnal dyspnea** is a sudden onset of difficulty breathing that occurs at night. It occurs because of a buildup of fluid in the alveoli or pooling of secretions during sleep.

Remember that normal breathing is quiet, painless, and occurs at a regular rate. Approach the patient immediately and begin the primary survey if the patient:

- Looks as if he is struggling (laboring) to breathe
- Has noisy breathing
- Is breathing faster or more slowly than normal
- Looks as if his chest is not moving normally

Approach the patient immediately and begin your primary survey if the patient's skin looks flushed (red), pale (whitish color), gray, or blue (cyanotic). As a patient's respiratory distress increases, he will typically have a decrease in oxygenated blood. This causes the patient's skin, nail beds, and mucous membranes to look bluish-grey in color. This is a late sign of hypoxia. **Hypoxia** is a condition in which there is a lack of oxygen. This could be generalized in the body or limited to a particular area of the body (tissue hypoxia). Earlier indications of hypoxia include confusion, anxiety, irritability, restlessness, an increased respiratory rate, increased heart rate, and mild respiratory distress. Oxygen should be given when a patient presents with respiratory distress.

After forming a general impression, assess the patient's mental status. As the amount of oxygen in the blood decreases, the patient may become anxious, restless, confused, and combative. As the amount of carbon dioxide in the blood increases, the patient may become increasingly difficult to arouse.

Assess the patient's airway and breathing. Observe how many words the patient can speak before he needs to take a breath. Can the patient answer questions in full sentences? Or can he speak only a few words before needing to take a breath? If your patient is awake but appears to have trouble breathing, ask, "Can you speak?" "Are you choking?" If he is able to speak or make noise, air is moving past his vocal cords. If a complete airway obstruction is present, you may initially see rise and fall of the chest but you will not hear or feel air movement. If the patient's heart stops, you may see irregular, gasping breaths (agonal respirations) just after this occurs. Do not confuse gasping respirations with adequate breathing.

When assessing the patient's breathing, note the rise and fall of the chest. Estimate the respiratory rate. The patient with breathing difficulty often has a respiratory rate outside the normal limits for his age. The normal respiratory rate for an adult is 12 to 20 breaths/min. If the rate is below 12, it is called **bradypnea.** If the rate is above 20, it is called **tachypnea.** If the respiratory rate falls out of the normal range, look for possible causes for this abnormal vital sign. An increase in a patient's respiratory rate is an early sign of respiratory distress. Agonal (slow, gasping) respirations may be observed just before death. The patient with agonal respirations requires immediate positive-pressure ventilation with 100% oxygen. Possible causes of changes in respiratory rate are shown in Table 13-1.

Note the depth/equality of the patient's breathing. In an adult, a normal breath is about 7 to 8 mL per kilogram of patient weight. This amount is called the tidal volume. Minute volume is the total amount of air breathed in and out in one minute. Minute volume = tidal volume × respiratory rate. Think of tidal volume as the depth of a patient's breathing. When a patient has a tube inserted into his trachea, tidal volume can be measured directly. When a patient is not intubated (does not have an airway

tube in his trachea), we must learn to assess the patient's tidal volume using our eyes and ears. You can indirectly assess tidal volume by watching the rise and fall of the patient's chest. Assess whether the chest rise and fall appears normal, increased, or decreased. The patient with difficulty breathing often has inadequate or shallow respirations. Place your stethoscope on the patient's chest and listen closely. You should hear air movement during the whole time the chest expands, as well as while it contracts. This is important to note because it is possible to see rise and fall of a patient's chest with little or no air exchange. For example, shallow respirations, even in the presence of an increased respiratory rate, may be inadequate to ventilate the patient. Comparing from side to side, determine if breath sounds are present or absent, equal or unequal, clear or noisy. The patient with inadequate breathing requires immediate positive-pressure ventilation with 100% oxygen. Table 13-2 lists common abnormal breath sounds and their significance.

Note the rhythm of the patient's respirations. Conditions that may cause irregular breathing include a head injury, drug overdose, and diabetic emergency. Note any signs of increased work of breathing (respiratory effort). A patient who is having difficulty breathing is working hard (laboring) to breathe. He may be gasping for air. You may see him use the muscles in his neck to assist with inhalation. He may use his abdominal muscles and muscles between the ribs to assist with exhalation. You may see retractions, "sinking in" of the soft tissues between and around the ribs or above the collarbones. Indentations of the skin above the collarbones (clavicles) are called **supraclavicular retractions.** Indentations of the skin between the ribs are called **intercostal retractions.** Indentations of the skin below the rib cage are called **subcostal retractions.**

Note if the patient's respirations are quiet, absent, or noisy. Normal breathing is quiet. However, quiet breathing is not always a good sign. Breathing becomes quiet when a partial airway obstruction becomes a complete obstruction. Quiet breathing in a patient with asthma may indicate a decrease in air movement. Noisy breathing is usually abnormal breathing and a sign that the patient is in distress. Noisy breathing is indicated by stridor, snoring, wheezing, gurgling, or grunting (see Chapter 7).

Assess the patient's circulation and perfusion. While feeling the patient's pulse, estimate the heart rate. Note its regularity and strength. Note the color, temperature, and condition (moisture) of the patient's skin. Observe the nail beds, earlobes or tops of the ears, lips, base of the tongue, and the area around the mouth for pallor or cyanosis. Cyanosis is a very late finding in infants and children. If cyanosis is present,

TABLE 13-1 Possible Causes of Changes in Respiratory Rate

Decreased Respiratory Rate	Increased Respiratory Rate
Drug overdose	Fever
Respiratory distress	Pain
Respiratory failure	Anxiety
Head injury	Respiratory distress
Hypothermia	Respiratory failure
	Certain drugs
	Increased metabolic rate
	Hypoxia
	Trauma
	Diabetic ketoacidosis

TABLE 13-2 Abnormal Breath Sounds and What They Mean

Breath Sound	Description	What It Means
Crackles (rales)	• Short popping or crackling sounds • Heard more often on inhalation than on exhalation	Movement of air through moisture or fluid
Wheezes	• High- or low-pitched whistling sounds • Usually heard at the end of inhalation or on exhalation	Movement of air through narrowed lower airways

the child may require positive-pressure ventilation. In infants and children younger than 6 years of age, assess capillary refill. If appropriate, evaluate for possible major bleeding.

Establish patient priorities. Priority patients include the following:

• Those in whom an open airway cannot be established or maintained
• Those who are experiencing difficulty breathing or who exhibit signs of respiratory distress
• Those with absent or inadequate breathing and who require continuous positive-pressure ventilation

Objective 2

A summary of the signs and symptoms of breathing difficulty is shown in the following *You Should Know* box.

You Should Know

Signs and Symptoms of Breathing Difficulty

• Shortness of breath
• Restlessness, anxious appearance, concentration on breathing
• Possible altered mental status (with fatigue or obstruction)
• Breathing rate too fast or slow for age
• Irregular breathing pattern
• Depth of breathing unusually deep or shallow
• Noisy breathing
• Sitting upright, leaning forward to breathe
• Unable to speak in complete sentences
• Pain with breathing

• Retractions, use of accessory muscles
• Abdominal breathing (diaphragm only)
• Coughing
• Increased pulse rate
• Unusual anatomy (barrel chest)
• Skin that looks flushed, pale, gray, or blue and feels cold or sweaty

Remember This!

When a patient experiences a respiratory emergency, Advanced Life Support (ALS) assistance should be requested as soon as possible. If ALS personnel are not available, the patient should be transported promptly to the closest appropriate facility.

Secondary Survey

If your patient is responsive, find out his medical history first before performing the physical examination. Remember to use OPQRST to recall important questions to ask when obtaining the history of the present illness. The patient should be your primary source of information. Additional sources of information include the scene, family members, friends, and bystanders. The information you collect will help guide where you look and what you are looking for in the focused physical exam. Examples of questions to ask a patient who is having breathing difficulty are shown in the following *Making a Difference* box.

After the primary survey, an unresponsive medical patient (or a patient with an altered mental status) needs a rapid medical assessment. This quick head-to-toe physical exam will help you identify the patient's problem. Treat problems as you find them.

Possible Questions to Ask a Patient with Difficulty Breathing

SAMPLE:

- Can you tell me why you called us today?
- Do you have any allergies to medications, dust, pollen, pets, perfume, or foods?
- Do you have a prescribed inhaler? What is the name of the medication? How many times per day do you use it? When did you last use it? Do you take any other medications? Has the dosage of any of your medications been changed recently?
- Do you have a history of asthma? How often do you have asthma attacks? Compared with other attacks, would you describe this one as mild, moderate, or severe?
- Do you have a history of congestive heart failure or chronic obstructive pulmonary disease (COPD)?
- Have you had a recent cold, flu, bronchitis, pneumonia, or other infection?
- Do you smoke? How many packs per day?
- Have you ever been hospitalized or had a tube inserted into your airway for your breathing difficulty?
- When did you last have anything to eat or drink?
- What were you doing when your symptoms began?

OPQRST:

- *O*nset: How long ago did your symptoms begin?
- *P*rovocation/Palliation: What makes the problem better or worse? Does anything you do relieve your symptoms?
- *Q*uality: Can you describe your discomfort? [If the patient is having pain, ask him what it feels like (dull, burning, sharp, stabbing, shooting, throbbing, pressure, or tearing)].
- *R*egion/Radiation: Do you have any pain associated with your breathing? Where is the pain? Is the pain in one area or does it move? Is the pain located in any other area?
- *S*everity: On a scale of 0 to 10, with 0 being the least and 10 being the worst, what number would you give your breathing difficulty? (If the patient is having pain, ask him to rate his pain using the 0 to 10 scale).
- *T*ime: How long has your breathing difficulty been present? Did your symptoms begin suddenly or gradually? Have you ever had these symptoms before? When? How long did it last?

Determining the Patient's Level of Respiratory Distress

When determining the patient's level of respiratory distress, find out as much patient information as possible and apply the most appropriate interventions and treatments. This needs to be done rapidly and accurately. The patient should be placed in one of four categories:

1. No breathing difficulty or shortness of breath
2. Mild breathing difficulty
3. Moderate breathing difficulty
4. Severe breathing difficulty

Remember This!

Ask the patient with breathing difficulty to count to 10. This will give you an idea of the patient's level of respiratory distress. For example, the person with no breathing difficulty can count to 10 easily. A person who is having severe breathing difficulty will usually be unable to count to 10.

No Breathing Difficulty

Objective 7

A patient who has no breathing difficulty has no signs of respiratory distress. The patient appears relaxed and denies shortness of breath. Breathing is quiet and unlabored. The patient is able to speak in full sentences without pausing to catch his breath. Breathing is regular and at a rate within normal limits for his age. The patient's breathing pattern is smooth and regular. There is equal rise and fall of the chest with each breath. The patient may have occasional sighing respirations. The patient's depth of breathing (tidal volume) is adequate. The color of the patient's skin and the mucous membranes of his mouth are normal. They do not appear pale, flushed, or bluish-gray.

Mild Breathing Difficulty

Objectives 2, 3, 5

A patient who has mild breathing difficulty may be hypoxic but can move an adequate amount of air. His heart rate and respiratory rate may be increased. He is alert and can answer your questions in complete sentences. This patient should be given high-concentration oxygen by nonrebreather mask. If indicated, start to treat the underlying cause of the patient's breathing difficulty with the patient's prescribed metered-dose inhaler (MDI).

Remember This!

Always have resuscitation equipment within arms reach when caring for a patient who presents with respiratory distress. Examples of equipment that should be available include oxygen, oral and nasal airways, bag-mask (BM) device, suction unit and suction catheters, and an automated external defibrillator (AED).

Stop and Think!

Do not insert a nasal airway into the nose of a patient with trauma to the nose or mid-face.

Moderate Breathing Difficulty

Objective 2

A patient who has moderate breathing difficulty may be hypoxic, but he can still move an adequate amount of air (although his tidal volume may be decreased). The patient may be awake but is restless and irritable. Hypoxia and an increase in carbon dioxide levels can cause this response. Look for cyanosis.

Objectives 3, 5

The patient with moderate breathing difficulty will have an increased heart rate and respiratory rate. He will have difficulty answering questions and will be unable to speak in complete sentences. With this in mind, ask questions that require only a short answer. Try to keep the patient calm and relaxed. Give high-concentration oxygen by nonrebreather mask. Pulse oximetry should be used on all patients receiving oxygen—especially on ALL respiratory patients, not just those with moderate to severe difficulty breathing. Check vital signs, level of responsiveness, and the patient's response to your treatment.

Making a Difference

Respiratory distress is very frightening for the patient. If you remain calm and appear to have a plan of action, this can be very comforting to the patient in respiratory distress.

If the patient's condition does not improve, prepare to assist ventilations. Assisted ventilation requires skill. The patient with moderate breathing difficulty may resist your attempts to assist his breathing. Explain to the patient that you are going to help his breathing. Match squeezing the bag with the patient's breathing—do not try to take over. Ask the patient to try and breathe with you. As the patient starts to breathe in, gently squeeze the bag. Stop squeezing as the chest starts to rise. Interpose extra ventilations, if necessary. Some patients may require only an extra breath or a slightly larger volume. Allow the patient to exhale before giving the next breath. Feel for changes in the patient's lung compliance with the BM device. Signs of adequate and inadequate artificial ventilation are listed in Table 13-3.

Attempt to treat the underlying cause of the patient's breathing difficulty. If the patient has a prescribed inhaler, have the patient try to use it if possible. The patient's ability to use the inhaler will depend on the level of respiratory distress. Assisting a patient with a prescribed inhaler is discussed later in this chapter.

TABLE 13-3 Signs of Adequate and Inadequate Artificial Ventilation

Signs of Adequate Artificial Ventilation	Signs of Inadequate Artificial Ventilation
• Chest rise and fall is seen with each artificial ventilation.	• Chest does not rise and fall with artificial ventilation.
• Rate of ventilation is sufficient, about once every three to five seconds for an infant or child, once every 5 to 6 seconds for an adult.	• Rate of ventilation is too slow or too fast.
• Heart rate improves with artificial ventilation.	• Heart rate does not return to normal with artificial ventilation.

Severe Breathing Difficulty

Objective 2

A patient who has severe breathing difficulty may be sleepy or unresponsive. The patient may have been wild and combative but now appears quiet. This is a sign of respiratory failure. The patient is wearing out. If the patient is responsive, he may be unable to speak or may only be able to speak in short phrases of 1 to 2 words. The patient may assume a tripod position and may need support to maintain a sitting position as he tires. His breathing rate may initially be rapid with periods of slow breathing. As he tires and his condition worsens, his breathing rate will slow and then become agonal (gasping) respirations. As his breathing muscles tire, his breathing will become shallow. The patient's skin may appear blue or mottled despite being given oxygen.

Objectives 3, 5, 6

Remember:

- An unresponsive patient is unable to protect his own airway.
- Do not try to insert an oral airway in a semiresponsive patient. This can cause gagging and vomiting.
- If necessary, assist an unresponsive patient's breathing by using a BM device connected to 100% oxygen.

Common Respiratory Disorders

Dyspnea is a common chief complaint that you will encounter. **Dyspnea** is a sensation of shortness of breath or difficulty breathing. The patient may express his breathing difficulty in different ways. For example, the patient may say that he is "short of breath"; "short-winded"; or "can't get my breath." Causes include trauma (see Chapter 25) and medical conditions, such as those listed in Table 13-4.

Croup

Objective 10

Croup is an infection, usually caused by one of the same viruses responsible for common colds. The virus affects the larynx and the area just below it (Figure 13-6). It is spread from person to person by droplets from coughing and sneezing. Although there are many types of viruses responsible for croup, one cause is respiratory syncytial virus (RSV). Some viruses that cause croup are most widespread in late fall and early winter. Croup caused by RSV usually peaks in the middle of winter, although some cases occur in the spring.

Signs and Symptoms

Viral croup most commonly occurs in children between the ages of 6 months and 3 years, although it can occur in older children. The child's caregiver

TABLE 13-4 Possible Causes of Difficulty Breathing

Trauma Condition	Medical Condition
• Flail chest	• Croup
• Inhalation injury	• Epiglottitis
• Drowning incident	• Reactive airway disease
• Pulmonary contusion	• Allergic reaction
• Diaphragm injury	• Heart attack
• Tracheobronchial tree injury	• Partial airway obstruction
• Simple pneumothorax	• Chronic obstructive pulmonary disease
• Open pneumothorax	• Chronic bronchitis
• Tension pneumothorax	• Emphysema
• Traumatic asphyxia	• Abnormal heart rhythm
• Scapula fracture	• Lung cancer
• Rib fractures	• Congestive heart failure/acute pulmonary edema
	• Pneumonia
	• Foreign body airway obstruction
	• Acute pulmonary embolism

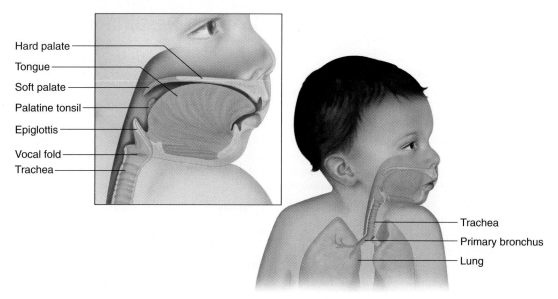

FIGURE 13-6 ▲ Croup affects the larynx and the area just below it.

usually relays symptoms of a cold for two to three days, such as a fever and a stuffy or runny nose. The virus that causes croup causes the walls of the trachea and larynx to become inflamed and swell. Inflammation and swelling in this area narrow the upper airway passages. As the upper airway passages narrow, the child may develop stridor, hoarseness, and a loud cough that sounds like the barking of a seal. Signs and symptoms of croup often worsen at night. Episodes of mild croup often break when air the child breathes is cooler than body temperature and humid but less than 100% saturated with water vapor. This cools the mucous membranes and constricts blood vessels in the affected area, decreasing swelling. Signs and symptoms are listed in the following *You Should Know* box.

You Should Know

Signs and Symptoms of Croup

- Gradual onset, usually over 2 to 3 days
- Stridor
- Barking cough
- Hoarse voice
- Low-grade fever (usually less than 102.2°F)

Emergency Care

Allow the child to assume a position of comfort. Avoid agitating the child. Allow the child to have his favorite blanket, doll, stuffed animal, or toy to help him feel secure. If possible, allow the caregiver to hold the child while giving supplemental oxygen. If the child will not tolerate a mask, give blow-by oxygen. If the child shows signs of respiratory failure or respiratory arrest, assist his breathing by using a BM device with 100% oxygen. Transport to the hospital for further evaluation.

Remember This!

In general, a patient who is having difficulty breathing instinctively assumes a position of comfort to improve his breathing. Do not force the patient to lie down. This may compromise the airway and cause immediate obstruction.

Epiglottitis

Objective 10

Epiglottitis is a bacterial infection of the epiglottis (Figure 13-7). It most commonly occurs in children between 3 and 7 years of age, but it may occur at any age. The onset of symptoms is usually sudden, developing over a few hours. Respiratory arrest may occur because of a complete airway obstruction or a combination of partial airway obstruction and fatigue.

Signs and Symptoms

A child who has epiglottitis is and looks very sick. Signs and symptoms are listed in the next *You Should Know* box. A comparison of croup and epiglottitis is shown in Table 13-5.

throat. This may agitate the child and worsen his respiratory distress. If respiratory arrest occurs, give positive-pressure ventilations with 100% oxygen. Rapidly transport the child to the closest appropriate medical facility.

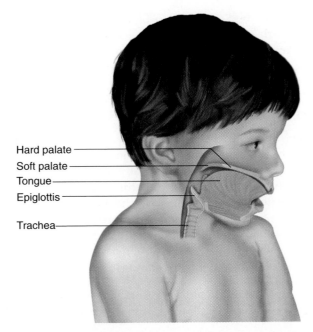

Hard palate
Soft palate
Tongue
Epiglottis
Trachea

FIGURE 13-7 ▲ Epiglottitis is a bacterial infection of the epiglottis.

You Should Know

Signs and Symptoms of Epiglottitis

- Restlessness
- Tripod position, unwilling to lie down
- Sudden onset of high fever, usually 102° to 104°F
- Sore throat
- Muffled voice
- Drooling
- Difficulty swallowing
- Dyspnea
- Stridor

Emergency Care

A child with suspected epiglottitis must be observed closely at all times. Avoid upsetting the child. Allow the child to assume a position of comfort with his favorite toy or blanket, if available. Allow the caregiver to hold the child while you give supplemental oxygen. If the child will not tolerate a mask, give blow-by oxygen. Do not attempt to look into the child's mouth or

Asthma

Objective 10

Asthma is widespread, temporary narrowing of the air passages that transport air from the nose and mouth to the lungs. Asthma may be triggered by many allergens or irritants. Asthma that is triggered by an allergic reaction is called **allergic asthma**. Asthma that is

TABLE 13-5 **Comparison of Croup and Epiglottitis**

	Croup	Epiglottitis
Age	6 months to 3 years	3 to 7 years
Cause	Viral	Bacterial
Onset	Gradual	Sudden
Signs/symptoms	• Stridor • Barking cough • Hoarse voice • Low-grade fever (usually less than 102.2°F)	• Stridor • Restlessness • Sore throat, drooling • Muffled voice • High fever (usually 102°F to 104°F) • Tripod position, unwilling to lie down • Difficulty swallowing • Dyspnea

triggered by factors not related to allergies is called **non-allergic asthma.** Possible asthma triggers are shown in the following *You Should Know* box and Figure 13-8. After exposure to the trigger, the smooth muscles surrounding the bronchioles spasmodically contract (bronchospasm) and swell, and mucus secretion increases. The mucus secreted is abnormally thick. Airway passages are narrowed because of smooth muscle contraction, excessive mucus secretion, or a combination of both. This results in the trapping of air in the bronchioles. Exhalation becomes prolonged as the patient tries to exhale the trapped air. This has

been described as trying to blow air through a straw filled with cotton.

At present, there is no cure for asthma. However, symptoms can be managed with proper prevention and treatment.

Signs and Symptoms

Wheezing is the most common asthma symptom. However, in the asthmatic patient, an absence of wheezing is a serious sign. An absence of wheezing in the asthmatic patient with breathing difficulty suggests that airflow is so diminished (the patient is moving too little air) that wheezing is not produced. Children with asthma will often have spells of frequent coughing, rather than wheezing. Other signs and symptoms associated with asthma are shown in the following *You Should Know* box.

You Should Know

Possible Triggers of Asthma

- Allergens such as dust mites, cockroaches, pollens, molds, pet dander, dust, shellfish, some medications
- Environmental irritants such as smoke, dust, paint fumes, smog, aerosol sprays, perfumes
- Weather factors such as extremes of heat, cold, humidity
- Exercise
- Colds, flu, sore throat, sinus infection
- Emotional stress

You Should Know

Signs and Symptoms of Asthma

Wheezing	Rapid breathing
Restlessness	Increased heart rate
Dry cough	Retractions
Dyspnea	Use of accessory muscles
Chest tightness	

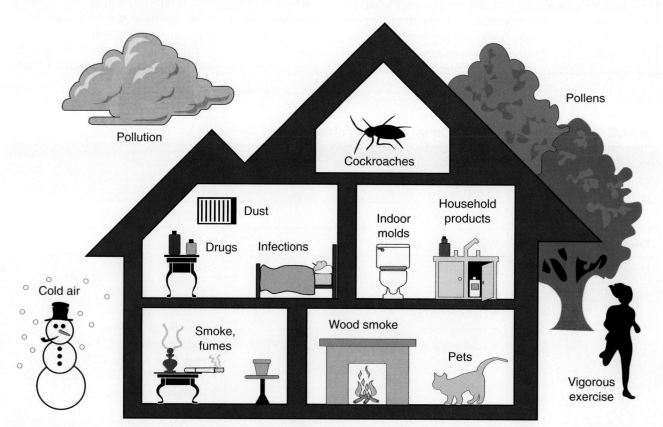

FIGURE 13-8 ▲ Possible asthma triggers.

Emergency Care

Objective 4

Allow the patient to assume a position of comfort. Give 100% oxygen, preferably by nonrebreather mask. Provide calm reassurance to help reduce the patient's anxiety. Encourage the patient to cough and breathe deeply to assist in the removal of secretions. If instructed to do so by medical direction, assist the patient in using his prescribed inhaler. Transport to the closest appropriate medical facility for further evaluation.

You Should Know

Patients with reactive airway disease have problems with air trapping. In these patients, positive-pressure ventilation can trigger further bronchoconstriction. It can also cause complications such as breath stacking and barotrauma. **Barotrauma** is injury to tissue caused by excess pressure. Breath stacking can lead to excessive inflation, tension pneumothorax, and low blood pressure. As a result, a slower respiratory rate (6 to 10 breaths/min) and smaller tidal volume (6 to 8 mL/kg) should be used for positive-pressure ventilation than that used for nonasthmatic patients. Be sure to allow the patient time to exhale before giving the next breath. The patient should have at least twice as long to exhale as he does to inhale. A slow, assisted ventilation may be all he can tolerate.

Chronic Bronchitis

Chronic bronchitis is defined as sputum production for 3 months of a year for at least 2 consecutive years. The major cause of chronic bronchitis is cigarette smoking. Respiratory irritants, such as smoke, irritate the airways and cause an increase in mucus production (Figure 13-9). Prolonged exposure to respiratory irritants eventually causes distortion and scarring of the bronchial wall, decreasing the size of the airway opening. Excessive mucus production in the bronchi causes a chronic or recurrent productive cough (sometimes of colored sputum). Because the size of the airway opening is decreased, some secretions are trapped in the alveoli and smaller air passages.

Some individuals with chronic bronchitis retain carbon dioxide. In healthy persons, the main stimulus to increase ventilation is an increase in carbon dioxide. Over time, patients with chronic bronchitis adapt to the retention of carbon dioxide and their main stimulus to breathe becomes a decrease in oxygen (hypoxic drive). The term *blue bloater* has been used to describe these individuals because the patient is often obese with a cyanotic complexion.

Signs and Symptoms

Signs and symptoms depend on severity of the disease and whether or not there are other problems in addition to the chronic bronchitis. Common signs and symptoms are shown in the following *You Should Know* box.

You Should Know

Signs and Symptoms of Chronic Bronchitis
- Productive cough
- Cyanosis
- Labored breathing
- Use of accessory muscles
- Increased respiratory rate
- Peripheral edema
- Inability to speak in complete sentences without pausing for a breath

Emergency Care

Objective 4

Allow the patient to assume a position of comfort. If signs of breathing difficulty are present, give oxygen by nonrebreather mask at 15 L/min or as ordered by medical direction. If no signs of respiratory distress are evident, give oxygen by nasal cannula at 2 L/min or as ordered by medical direction. Monitor the patient closely, reassessing every 5 minutes, and be prepared to assist ventilations as necessary. Provide calm reassurance to help reduce the patient's anxiety. Encourage the patient to cough and breathe deeply to help in the removal of secretions. If instructed to do so by medical direction, help the patient use his prescribed inhaler. Transport to the closest appropriate medical facility for further evaluation.

Emphysema

Emphysema is an irreversible enlargement of the air spaces distal to the terminal bronchioles. This disease leads to destruction of the walls of the alveoli, distention of the alveolar sacs, and loss of lung elasticity. The patient with emphysema may be called a *pink puffer* because he can often increase his respiratory rate to maintain a relatively normal amount of oxygen (pink color), although his work of breathing is increased during exhalation (puffer). Carbon dioxide levels are often normal in patients with emphysema because they hyperventilate to maintain normal oxygen levels.

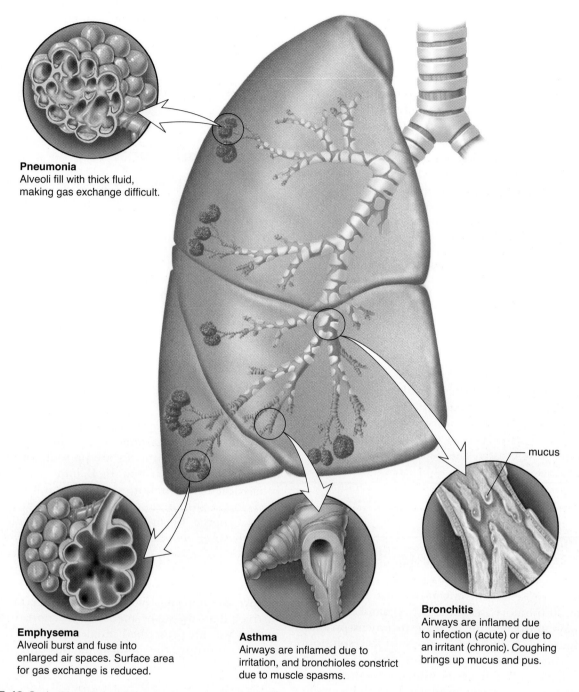

Pneumonia
Alveoli fill with thick fluid, making gas exchange difficult.

mucus

Bronchitis
Airways are inflamed due to infection (acute) or due to an irritant (chronic). Coughing brings up mucus and pus.

Emphysema
Alveoli burst and fuse into enlarged air spaces. Surface area for gas exchange is reduced.

Asthma
Airways are inflamed due to irritation, and bronchioles constrict due to muscle spasms.

FIGURE 13-9 ▲ Disorders of the lower respiratory tract.

Signs and Symptoms

In emphysema, the lungs inflate easily, but air becomes trapped in the lungs because of the lack of elastic recoil. The volume of air in the chest increases, giving the patient a barrel-chest appearance. The loss of elasticity causes exhalation to become an active (rather than passive) process, increasing the work of breathing. Signs and symptoms of emphysema are shown in the following *You Should Know* box.

You Should Know

Signs and Symptoms of Emphysema
- Barrel chest
- Use of accessory muscles
- Pursed-lip breathing
- Chronic cough
- Prolonged exhalation
- Increased respiratory rate
- Dyspnea with exertion

If signs of breathing difficulty are present, give oxygen by nonrebreather mask at 15 L/min or as ordered by medical direction. If no signs of respiratory distress are evident, give oxygen by nasal cannula at 2 L/min or as ordered by medical direction. Monitor the patient closely, reassessing every 5 minutes. Be prepared to assist ventilations as necessary. Provide calm reassurance to help reduce the patient's anxiety. Encourage the patient to cough and breathe deeply to assist in the removal of secretions. If instructed to do so by medical direction, assist the patient in using his prescribed inhaler. Transport to the closest appropriate medical facility for further evaluation.

Pneumonia

Pneumonia is an infection that often affects gas exchange in the lung. It may involve the lower airways and alveoli, part of a lobe, or an entire lobe of the lung. Pneumonia is most often caused by bacteria and viruses, although it may also be caused by fungi and parasites. Bacterial pneumonia can occur in any part of the lung. It usually causes inflammation and swelling of the alveoli. Viral pneumonia often begins in the bronchioles and then spreads to the alveoli.

Signs and Symptoms

Signs and symptoms of pneumonia include:

- Fever
- Chills
- Increased respiratory rate
- Increased heart rate
- Possible cough
- Shortness of breath
- Malaise
- Possible pleuritic (sharp, stabbing) chest pain

Emergency Care

Allow the patient to assume a position of comfort. Give oxygen by nonrebreather mask at 15 L/min. Transport to the hospital for further evaluation and treatment.

Pulmonary Embolism

A **pulmonary embolus** is usually the result of a clot that forms in the deep veins in the leg and then travels through the veins to the heart and then to the pulmonary circulation. The clot becomes trapped in the smaller branches of the pulmonary arteries, causing partial or complete blood flow obstruction. As a result, a portion of the lung is ventilated but not perfused. To compensate, the patient's respiratory rate increases. If the area involved is large, respiratory failure will occur.

Factors that increase the risk for pulmonary embolism include the following:

- Obesity
- Prolonged bed rest or immobilization
- Recent surgery, particularly of the legs, pelvis, abdomen, or chest
- Leg or pelvic fractures or injuries
- Use of high-estrogen oral contraceptives
- Pregnancy
- Chronic atrial fibrillation (a heart rhythm disorder)

Signs and Symptoms

Signs and symptoms depend on the:

- Size and location of the embolus
- Number of emboli
- Presence or absence of underlying cardiac and pulmonary disease

Signs and symptoms include:

- Sudden onset of dyspnea
- Apprehension, restlessness
- Possible pleuritic chest pain
- Possible cough
- Increased respiratory rate
- Increased heart rate
- Possible blood-tinged sputum
- Possible hypotension

Emergency Care

Allow the patient to assume a position of comfort unless hypotension is present. If the patient is alert but showing signs of breathing difficulty, give oxygen by nonrebreather mask at 15 L/min. Provide positive-pressure ventilation with 100% oxygen as necessary. Reassess the patient frequently. Transport promptly to the closest appropriate medical facility.

Acute Pulmonary Edema

Pulmonary edema is most commonly caused by failure of the left ventricle of the heart. When the left ventricle fails, fluid is forced into the lung tissue as the right ventricle continues to pump blood into the pulmonary circulation. The alveoli fill with fluid, limiting their ability to effectively exchange oxygen and carbon dioxide. Other (noncardiac) conditions can result in pulmonary edema, including:

- Drowning
- Narcotic overdose
- Trauma
- High altitude
- Poisonous gases

Signs and Symptoms

Signs and symptoms of acute pulmonary edema include the following:

- Restlessness, anxiety
- Dyspnea on exertion
- Orthopnea
- Paroxysmal nocturnal dyspnea
- Frothy, blood-tinged sputum
- Cool, moist skin
- Use of accessory muscles
- Jugular venous distention
- Wheezing
- Crackles
- Rapid, labored breathing
- Increased heart rate
- Increased or decreased blood pressure (depending on severity of edema)

Emergency Care

Help the patient sit up (unless hypotension is present) to promote lung expansion. If breathing is adequate, administer oxygen by nonrebreather mask at 15 L/min. If breathing is inadequate, provide positive-pressure ventilation with 100% oxygen. Reassess frequently, monitoring vital signs at least every 5 minutes. Be prepared to assist ventilations as necessary. Provide calm reassurance to help reduce the patient's anxiety. Transport promptly to the closest appropriate medical facility.

Metered-Dose Inhalers

Objective 8

An MDI is used to deliver inhaled respiratory medications. A patient who has a prescribed MDI typically has reversible constriction of his airways. An MDI is small and consists of two parts, the medication canister and a plastic dispenser with a mouthpiece. Because some patients find it hard to coordinate breathing in and pressing the inhaler at the same time, a physician will often prescribe a "spacer" to be used with the MDI. The spacer increases the amount of medication delivered into the respiratory tract. The patient squeezes the MDI into a plastic holding chamber, then inhales the medication from the chamber. The use of spacers is very common in children and older adults. The spacer can also be attached to a resuscitation mask to aid medication delivery for a young child (Figure 13-10).

You Should Know

An MDI is also called an *aerosol inhaler* or *puffer*.

Medication Actions

Medications contained in an MDI are usually beta-2 agonists. This means that the drug stimulates beta-2 receptor sites in the lungs. When these receptor sites are stimulated in the bronchioles, the smooth muscle tissue relaxes (dilates), reducing airway resistance. This makes it easier for the patient to move air in and out. Table 13-6 lists important information about prescribed MDIs that you should know.

You Should Know

Inhaled steroids are another type of medication that may be given by means of an MDI. Inhaled steroids help decrease inflammation in the airways. Advair (fluticasone and salmeterol) is an example of a drug that is both a bronchodilator and inhaled steroid. Fluticasone is a steroid. It helps reduce inflammation. Salmeterol is a bronchodilator. It relaxes bronchial smooth muscle to improve breathing.

Indications

As an EMT, you can assist a patient in taking a prescribed inhaler if *all* of the following criteria are met:

- The patient has signs and symptoms of a respiratory emergency.
- The patient has a physician-prescribed handheld inhaler.
- There are no contraindications to giving the medication.
- You have specific authorization by medical direction.

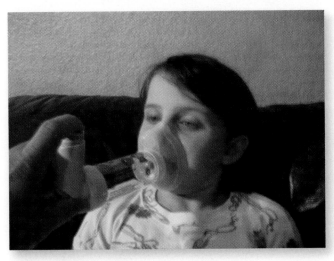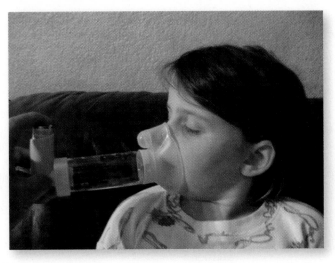

FIGURE 13-10 ▲ MDI use by children is very common. Children will often have a spacer available for use with the device. A spacer used for a young child may be equipped with a mask, such as the one shown here. In these photos, the child's father (a paramedic and respiratory therapist) is assisting her with a dose from her inhaler.
© *Randy Budd, RRT, CEP, City of Mesa Fire Department.*

TABLE 13-6 **Prescribed Metered-Dose Inhaler**

Generic (trade) name	• albuterol (Proventil, Ventolin) • isoetharine (Bronkosol) • metaproterenol (Alupent, Metaprel) • fluticasone and salmeterol (Advair)
Mechanism of action	Dilates bronchioles, reducing airway resistance
Indications	An EMT can assist a patient in taking a prescribed inhaler if *all* of the following criteria are met: • The patient has signs and symptoms of a respiratory emergency. • The patient has a physician-prescribed handheld inhaler. • There are no contraindications to giving the medication. • The EMT has specific authorization by medical direction.
Dosage	An MDI automatically delivers a specific dose of medication each time it is activated. The usual dosage is 2 puffs every 3 to 4 hours as needed for shortness of breath, associated with asthma and COPD. The number of inhalations is based on medical direction's order or the patient's physician order.
Side effects	• Increased heart rate • Shaking or tremors • Nervousness
Contraindications	• Medical direction does not give permission. • Patient is unable to use device. • Inhaler is not prescribed for the patient. • Patient has already met maximum prescribed dose before EMT arrival.

Assisting a Patient with a Metered-Dose Inhaler

STEP 1 ▶
- Contact medical direction for an order to assist with giving this medication.
- Make sure that you have the right medication, right patient, right route of administration, and that the patient is alert enough to use the medication.
- Check the expiration date of the inhaler.
- Check to see when the last dose was taken by the patient.
- Make sure the inhaler is at room temperature or warmer.
- Shake the inhaler, vigorously, several times.
- If the patient is wearing an oxygen mask, remove it now.

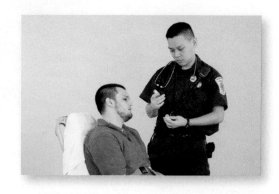

STEP 2 ▶ Have the patient exhale deeply and then have him put his lips around the mouthpiece of the inhaler.

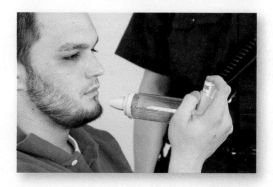

STEP 3 ▶ If the patient has a spacer device for use with his inhaler, it should be used. If a spacer is used, have the patient depress the inhaler to inject the dose into the chamber of the spacer. This is done before placing the mouthpiece of the spacer in the mouth.

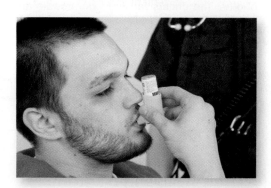

STEP 4 ▶
- Have the patient depress the MDI as he begins to inhale deeply. Help the patient direct the spray into his mouth as he attempts to take a breath.
- Instruct the patient to hold his breath as long as he comfortably can. (This helps with medication absorption.)

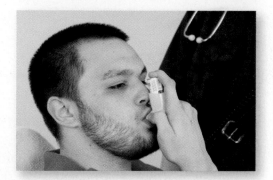

STEP 5 ▶ • If the patient is using a spacer, have him depress the inhaler, breathe in and hold his breath, breathe out, and then take another deep breath through the mouthpiece of the spacer and hold his breath.
• A patient who is using a spacer should try to take two deep breaths from the spacer and hold them for each puff from his inhaler.

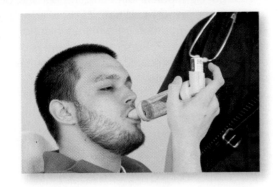

STEP 6 ▶ • Replace the previously removed oxygen mask. Recheck the patient's vital signs and reassess the patient's degree of breathing difficulty.
• Repeat the dose after 1-3 minutes per instructions from medical direction.
• When finished with the inhaler, wipe off the mouthpiece with an alcohol swab and replace the cap.
• After using an MDI, have the patient rinse his mouth out with water. This will decrease the possibility of side effects from the medication.

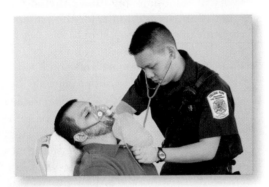

Remember This!

Not all respiratory emergencies will benefit from the use of an MDI. The patient should have symptoms that would benefit from giving an MDI.

Contraindications

Assisting a patient with the use of an MDI is contraindicated if any of the following conditions exists:

• The patient is unable to use the device. (This may be a result of the level of the patient's respiratory distress).
• The inhaler is not prescribed for the patient.
• Permission is not received from medical direction.
• The patient has already met the maximum prescribed dose before your arrival.

Procedure

Skill Drill 13-1 shows the procedure for assisting a patient with his prescribed MDI.

On the Scene Wrap-Up

Whenever you are dealing with patients in respiratory distress, remain calm and professional. This will help calm the patient and family members and decrease the patient's level of distress. Remember that any patient in respiratory distress will benefit from oxygen. Give oxygen by any means tolerated by the patient.

This child will benefit from oxygen and an MDI given appropriately. Teach the patient and parents that the spacer increases the amount of medication delivered into the respiratory tract. Have the patient depress the inhaler to inject the medication dose into the chamber of the spacer. Have the patient do this before placing the mouthpiece of the spacer in her mouth. Ask the patient to depress the inhaler, breathe in and hold her breath, breathe out, and then take another deep breath through the mouthpiece of the spacer and hold her breath. Explain to the patient (and parents) that a patient who is using a spacer should try to take two deep breaths from the spacer and hold them for each puff from the inhaler.

Reapply oxygen, recheck the patient's vital signs, and reassess the patient's degree of breathing difficulty. If ordered by medical direction, repeat the dose after one to three minutes. When finished with the inhaler, wipe off the mouthpiece with an alcohol swab and replace the cap. To decrease the possibility of side effects from the medication, have the patient rinse her mouth out with water. ∎

Sum It Up

▶ Signs of adequate breathing include a breathing rate within normal limits for the patient's age. The rhythm of breathing should be regular, breath sounds should be present and equal, chest expansion should be adequate and equal, and the depth of respirations (tidal volume) should be adequate.

▶ Signs of inadequate breathing include a rate outside the normal range for the patient's age, an irregular rhythm of breathing, diminished or absent breath sounds, and chest expansion that is unequal or inadequate. The patient shows signs of increased effort of breathing through the use of accessory muscles. His depth of respirations (tidal volume) may be inadequate. His skin may be pale or cyanotic (blue) and cool and clammy. There may be retractions above the clavicles, between the ribs and below the rib cage, especially in children. Nasal flaring may be present, especially in children. Seesaw breathing may be seen in infants. Agonal breathing (occasional gasping breaths) may be seen just before death.

▶ Signs of adequate artificial ventilation include:
  • The chest rises and falls with each artificial ventilation
  • The rate is sufficient, about 10 to 12 per minute for adults and 12 to 20 times per minute for children and infants
  • Heart rate improves with successful artificial ventilation

▶ Artificial ventilation is inadequate when:
  • The chest does not rise and fall with artificial ventilation

  • The rate is too slow or too fast
  • Heart rate does not improve with artificial ventilation

▶ Signs and symptoms of breathing difficulty include shortness of breath, restlessness, increased pulse rate, increased or decreased breathing rate, skin color changes, noisy breathing, inability to speak caused by breathing efforts, retractions, use of accessory muscles, altered mental status, abdominal breathing, coughing, irregular breathing rhythm, tripod position, and unusual anatomy (barrel chest).

▶ An MDI is used to deliver inhaled respiratory medications. A patient who has a prescribed MDI typically has reversible constriction of his airways. An MDI is small and consists of two parts, the medication canister and a plastic dispenser with a mouthpiece. A physician will often prescribe a "spacer" to be used with the MDI. The spacer increases the amount of medication delivered into the respiratory tract. The patient squeezes the MDI into a plastic holding chamber, then inhales the medication from the chamber. The use of spacers is very common in children and older adults. The spacer can also be attached to a resuscitation mask to aid medication delivery for a young child.

▶ As an EMT, you can assist a patient in taking a prescribed inhaler if *all* of the following criteria are met:
  • The patient has signs and symptoms of a respiratory emergency.
  • The patient has a physician-prescribed handheld inhaler.
  • There are no contraindications to giving the medication.
  • You have specific authorization by medical direction.

▶ Assisting a patient with the use of an MDI is contraindicated if any of the following conditions exists:
  • The patient is unable to use the device. (This may be caused by the level of the patient's respiratory distress).
  • The inhaler is not prescribed for the patient.
  • Permission is not received from medical direction.
  • The patient has already met the maximum prescribed dose before your arrival.

14 Cardiovascular Emergencies

By the end of this chapter, you should be able to:

Knowledge Objectives ▶

1. Describe the structure and function of the cardiovascular system.
2. Describe the emergency medical care of the patient experiencing chest pain/discomfort.
3. List the indications for automated external defibrillation.
4. List the contraindications for automated external defibrillation.
5. Define the Emergency Medical Technician's (EMT's) role in the emergency cardiac care system.
6. Explain the impact of age and weight on defibrillation.
7. Discuss the position of comfort for patients with various cardiac emergencies.
8. Establish the relationship between airway management and the patient with cardiovascular compromise.
9. Predict the relationship between the patient experiencing cardiovascular compromise and Basic Life Support.
10. Discuss the fundamentals of early defibrillation.
11. Explain the rationale for early defibrillation.
12. Explain that not all patients with chest pain will experience cardiac arrest, nor do all patients with chest pain need to be attached to an automated external defibrillator (AED).
13. Explain the importance of prehospital Advanced Cardiac Life Support (ACLS) intervention if it is available.
14. Explain the importance of urgent transport to a facility with ACLS if it is not available in the prehospital setting.
15. Discuss the various types of AEDs.
16. Differentiate between the fully automated and the semi-automated defibrillator.
17. Discuss the procedures that must be taken into consideration for standard operations of the various types of AEDs.
18. State the reasons for assuring that the patient is pulseless and apneic when you are using the AED.
19. Discuss the circumstances that may result in inappropriate shocks.
20. Explain the considerations for interruption of cardiopulmonary resuscitation when you are using an AED.
21. Discuss the advantages of AEDs.
22. Summarize the speed of operation of automated external defibrillation.

23. Discuss the use of remote defibrillation through adhesive pads.

24. Discuss the special considerations for rhythm monitoring.

25. List the steps in the operation of the AED.

26. Discuss the standard of care that should be used for a patient with persistent ventricular fibrillation and no available ACLS.

27. Discuss the standard of care that should be used for a patient with recurrent ventricular fibrillation and no available ACLS.

28. Differentiate between the single rescuer and multi-rescuer care with an AED.

29. Explain the reason for pulses not being checked between shocks with an AED.

30. Discuss the importance of coordinating ACLS-trained providers with personnel using AEDs.

31. Discuss the importance of post-resuscitation care.

32. List the components of post-resuscitation care.

33. Explain the importance of frequent practice with the AED.

34. Discuss the need to complete the Automated Defibrillator: Operator's Shift Checklist.

35. Discuss the role of national organizations such as the American Heart Association, American Safety & Health Institute, and others in the use of automated external defibrillation.

36. Explain the role medical direction plays in the use of automated external defibrillation.

37. State the reasons why a case review should be completed following the use of the AED.

38. Discuss the components that should be included in a case review.

39. Discuss the goal of quality improvement in automated external defibrillation.

40. Recognize the need for medical direction of protocols to assist in the emergency medical care of the patient with chest pain.

41. List the indications for the use of nitroglycerin (NTG).

42. State the contraindications and side effects for the use of NTG.

43. Define the function of all controls on an AED, and describe event documentation and defibrillator battery maintenance.

Attitude Objectives ▶ 44. Defend the reasons for obtaining initial training in automated external defibrillation and the importance of continuing education.

45. Defend the reason for maintenance of AEDs.

46. Explain the rationale for administering NTG to a patient with chest pain or discomfort.

Skill Objectives ▶ 47. Demonstrate the assessment and emergency medical care of a patient experiencing chest pain/discomfort.

48. Demonstrate the application and operation of the AED.

49. Demonstrate the maintenance of an AED.

50. Demonstrate the assessment and documentation of patient response to the AED.

51. Demonstrate the skills necessary to complete the Automated Defibrillator: Operator's Shift Checklist.

52. Perform the steps in facilitating the use of NTG for chest pain or discomfort.

53. Demonstrate the assessment and documentation of patient response to NTG.

54. Practice completing a prehospital care report for patients with cardiac emergencies.

Your quiet shift at the casino ends abruptly when you see an elderly woman slump forward onto a nickel slot machine. "Code 99, slot machines," you radio to the other EMTs. Donning your gloves, you move quickly to the patient. She doesn't respond to your voice or a shoulder shake, so you lower her limp body gently onto her back on the floor. "Call 9-1-1," you tell the next arriving officer. Carefully tilting her head back, you lower your ear above her nose and mouth and look to see if her chest rises. She is not breathing, so you deliver two breaths with just enough volume to make her chest rise. Then, sliding your fingers into the groove beside her trachea, you feel for a carotid pulse. There is none, so you place your hands over her breastbone and begin chest compressions. You scan the room, hoping another EMT will arrive quickly with the AED. ■

THINK ABOUT IT

As you read this chapter, think about the following questions:

- What could have caused the patient's heart to stop beating?
- What ratio of compressions to breaths will you provide?
- Why is it important for the AED to arrive quickly?
- How will you know if her circulation resumes?

Introduction

Cardiac emergencies are the most common type of medical emergency in the United States. As an Emergency Medical Technician (EMT), you must know the signs and symptoms of cardiac compromise and give appropriate patient care based on your assessment findings. When authorized by medical direction, an EMT may assist a patient in taking prescribed nitroglycerin (NTG). EMTs and automated external defibrillators (AEDs) are important links in the successful resuscitation of a patient in cardiac arrest outside the hospital.

Review of Circulatory System Anatomy and Physiology

Circulatory System

Components

Objective 1

The circulatory system is made up of the cardiovascular and lymphatic systems. The cardiovascular system is made up of three main parts: a pump (the heart), fluid (blood), and a container (the blood vessels). If there is a problem within this system, the problem will stem from one of these three parts.

The lymphatic system consists of lymph, lymph nodes, lymph vessels, tonsils, the spleen, and the thymus gland. The spleen, liver, and bone marrow are also associated with the circulatory system because they form and store blood.

Function

- *Transport.* Blood carries oxygen, food, hormones, minerals, and other essential substances to all parts of the body. Blood carries carbon dioxide and other waste material from the body's cells to the lungs, kidneys, or skin for elimination.
- *Maintenance of body temperature.* Blood vessels narrow (constrict) and widen (dilate) as needed to retain or dissipate heat at the skin's surface.
- *Protection.* The blood and lymphatic system protect the body against invasion by foreign microorganisms through the immune (defense) system.

The Cardiovascular System

The Heart

The heart lies in the chest cavity (mediastinum) behind the sternum and between the lungs. The heart has four chambers (Figure 14-1). The two upper

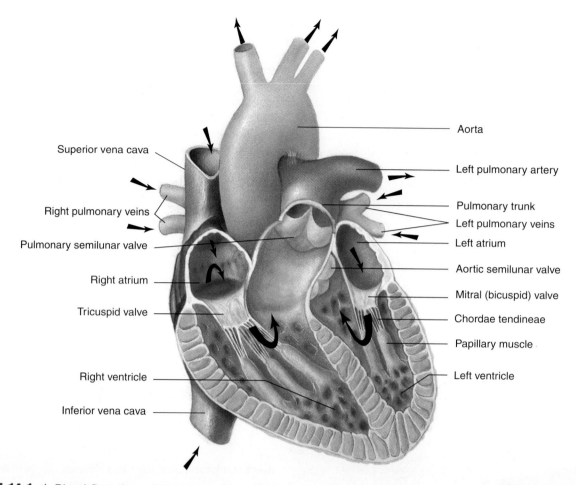

Superior vena cava

Right pulmonary veins

Pulmonary semilunar valve

Right atrium

Tricuspid valve

Right ventricle

Inferior vena cava

Aorta

Left pulmonary artery

Pulmonary trunk

Left pulmonary veins

Left atrium

Aortic semilunar valve

Mitral (bicuspid) valve

Chordae tendineae

Papillary muscle

Left ventricle

FIGURE 14-1 ▲ Blood flow through the heart. The right atrium receives blood that is low in oxygen from the body. Blood passes through the tricuspid valve into the right ventricle. The right ventricle pumps blood through the pulmonary valve to the lungs. The left atrium receives blood rich in oxygen from the lungs. Blood passes through the mitral valve into the left ventricle. The left ventricle pumps blood through the aortic valve to the aorta and out to the body.

chambers are the right and left atria. The atria are thin-walled chambers that receive blood from the systemic circulation and lungs. The two lower chambers are the right and left ventricles. The ventricles pump blood to the lungs and systemic circulation (body). The right ventricle pumps blood to the lungs. The left ventricle pumps blood to the body. The ventricles are larger and have thicker walls than the atria.

Four heart valves prevent the backflow of blood and keep blood moving in one direction (Figure 14-2). The tricuspid and mitral (bicuspid) valves are called **atrioventricular (AV) valves** because they lie between an atrium and ventricle. The **tricuspid valve** is located between the right atrium and right ventricle. The **mitral (bicuspid) valve** is located between the left atrium and left ventricle.

The pulmonic and aortic valves are called **semilunar valves** because they are shaped like half-moons. The **pulmonic valve** is located at the junction of the right ventricle and pulmonary artery. The **aortic valve** is located at the junction of the left ventricle and aorta (see the following *You Should Know* box).

You Should Know

Heart Valves

Atrioventricular valves

- Tricuspid
- Mitral (bicuspid)

Semilunar valves

- Aortic
- Pulmonic

The heart is more than a muscle. It contains specialized contractile and conductive tissue that allows the generation of electrical impulses. Unlike other cells of the body, specialized electrical (pacemaker) cells in the heart can produce an electrical impulse without being stimulated by another source, such as a nerve. This property is called **automaticity.** The electrical (pacemaker) cells in the heart are arranged in a system of pathways called the *conduction system* (Figure 14-3). Normally, an impulse begins in the sinoatrial

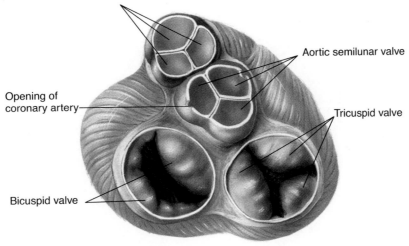

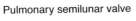
Pulmonary semilunar valve

Aortic semilunar valve

Opening of
coronary artery

Tricuspid valve

Bicuspid valve

FIGURE 14-2 ▲ The valves of the heart.

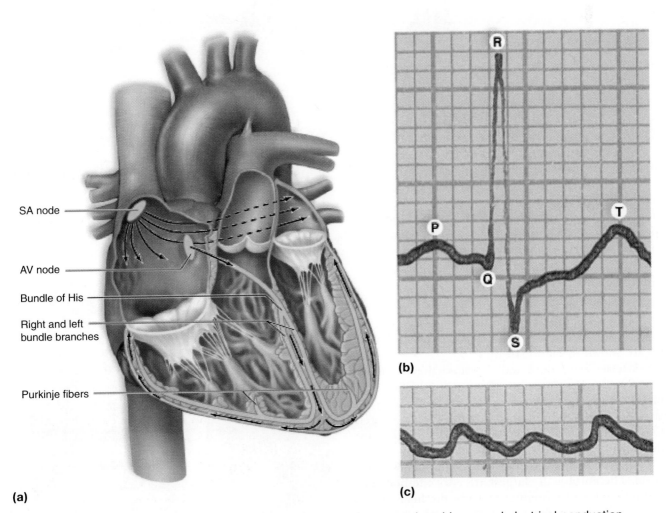

SA node

AV node

Bundle of His

Right and left
bundle branches

Purkinje fibers

(a)

(b)

(c)

FIGURE 14-3 ▲ **(a)** The heart's conduction system. **(b)** Waveforms produced by normal electrical conduction through the heart. **(c)** This is an example of ventricular fibrillation (VF). A patient in VF is unresponsive, not breathing, and has no pulse.

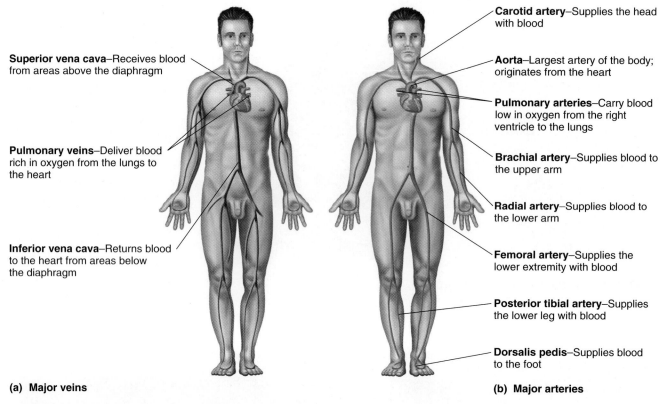

Superior vena cava–Receives blood from areas above the diaphragm

Pulmonary veins–Deliver blood rich in oxygen from the lungs to the heart

Inferior vena cava–Returns blood to the heart from areas below the diaphragm

(a) Major veins

Carotid artery–Supplies the head with blood

Aorta–Largest artery of the body; originates from the heart

Pulmonary arteries–Carry blood low in oxygen from the right ventricle to the lungs

Brachial artery–Supplies blood to the upper arm

Radial artery–Supplies blood to the lower arm

Femoral artery–Supplies the lower extremity with blood

Posterior tibial artery–Supplies the lower leg with blood

Dorsalis pedis–Supplies blood to the foot

(b) Major arteries

FIGURE 14-4 ▲ **(a)** Major veins and **(b)** major arteries.

(SA) node. The SA node is the heart's primary pacemaker. The impulse leaves the SA node and travels through the atrial muscle, and down to the atrioventricular (AV) node. The impulse spreads from the AV node to the bundle of His, to the right and left bundle branches, and then to the Purkinje fibers. The Purkinje fibers penetrate the ventricular muscle and cause the ventricles to contract. Blood is then pumped to the lungs and through the aorta to the body.

Major Blood Vessels

Blood flow from the heart through the body moves through the following vessels: arteries → arterioles → capillaries → venules → veins. Major veins and arteries are shown in Figure 14-4.

Arteries have thick walls because they transport blood under high pressure (Figure 14-5). They carry blood away from the heart to the rest of the body. All arteries, except the pulmonary arteries, carry oxygen-rich blood. Arteries help maintain blood pressure through vasoconstriction and vasodilation.

All arteries are direct or indirect branches of the aorta. The aorta is the largest artery of the body and is the major artery originating from the heart. It lies in front of the spine in the chest and abdominal cavities. It divides at the level of the navel into the iliac arteries.

Like the other organs of the body, the heart must have its own source of oxygen-rich blood. The heart depends on two coronary arteries and their branches for its supply of oxygenated blood (Figure 14-6). Most arteries receive blood when the left ventricle contracts. However, the valve leaflets cover the openings to the coronary arteries when the left ventricle

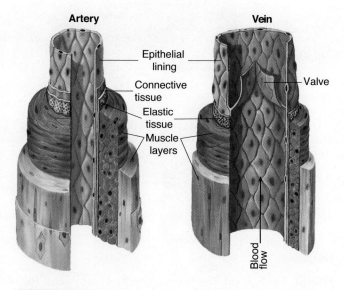

Artery

Vein

Epithelial lining

Connective tissue

Elastic tissue

Muscle layers

Valve

Blood flow

FIGURE 14-5 ▲ The walls of arteries are much thicker than the walls of veins.

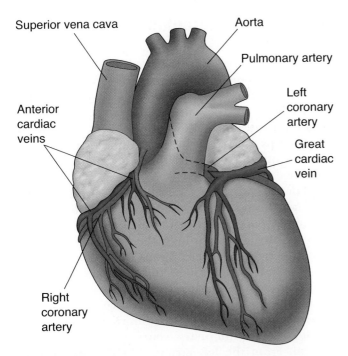

FIGURE 14-6 ▲ The heart depends on two coronary arteries and their branches for its supply of oxygenated blood.

depends on widening (dilation) of the arteries to increase blood flow through the coronary arteries.

The carotid arteries arise from the top of the aorta (aortic arch) and are the major arteries of the neck (Figure 14-7a). They supply the head and neck with oxygen-rich blood. The pulsations of these arteries can be felt on either side of the larynx in the grooves created by the large neck muscles.

The only arteries in the body that do not carry oxygen-rich blood are the pulmonary arteries. They arise out of the right ventricle where they deliver oxygen-poor blood to the lungs for gas exchange.

The brachial artery supplies the upper arm with blood. A brachial pulse can be felt on the inside of the arm between the elbow and the shoulder. This artery is used when determining a blood pressure (BP) with a blood pressure cuff and stethoscope (Figure 14-7b). The radial artery is the major artery of the lower arm. A radial pulse can be felt on the thumb side of the wrist (Figure 14-7c).

contracts. As a result, blood flows into the coronary arteries when the left ventricle is relaxed. During times of stress, the heart needs more oxygen and

Remember This!

The right and left carotid arteries should never be felt at the same time. Doing so can cause severe lowering of the heart rate and decrease blood flow to the brain.

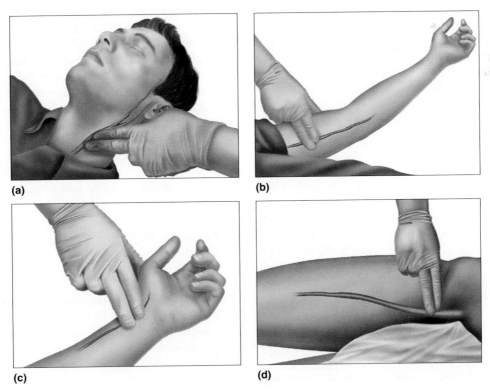

FIGURE 14-7 ▲ Major arteries and pulses: (a) Neck, or carotid, pulse. (b) Arm, or brachial, pulse. (c) Wrist, or radial, pulse. (d) Groin, or femoral, pulse.

The femoral arteries are the major arteries of the thigh. They supply the upper leg with blood. A femoral pulse can be felt in the groin area (the crease between the abdomen and thigh) (Figure 14-7d). The posterior tibial artery supplies the lower leg with blood. The posterior tibial pulse is located just behind the ankle bone (medial malleolus). The dorsalis pedis artery is an artery in the foot. A pedal pulse can be felt on the top surface of the foot.

Arterioles are the smallest branches of arteries leading to the capillaries. Capillaries are microscopic vessels whose walls are one cell thick. They serve as vessels for exchange of wastes, fluids, and nutrients between the blood and tissues. They connect arterioles and venules. All tissues except cartilage, hair, nails, and the cornea of the eye contain capillaries.

Venules are the smallest branches of veins leading from the capillaries. Veins are low-pressure vessels that collect blood for transport back to the heart. The major veins of the body include the pulmonary veins and the superior and inferior vena cavae (see Figure 14-4). Veins contain valves to prevent backflow of blood. All veins, except the pulmonary veins, carry deoxygenated (oxygen-poor) blood. The pulmonary veins deliver blood rich in oxygen from the lungs to the left atrium of the heart. The superior vena cava receives blood from areas above the diaphragm, such as the head and upper extremities. The inferior vena cava returns blood to the heart from areas below the diaphragm, such as the torso and lower extremities. Both the superior and inferior vena cava drain into the right atrium of the heart.

Blood

Formed elements of the blood include red blood cells (erythrocytes), white blood cells (leukocytes), and platelets (thrombocytes). Plasma is the liquid part of blood.

Red blood cells transport oxygen to body cells. Each red blood cell contains hemoglobin, an iron-containing protein. Hemoglobin carries oxygen from the lungs to the tissues and gives blood its red color. Red blood cells also transport carbon dioxide away from body cells. White blood cells defend the body from microorganisms, such as bacteria and viruses that have invaded the bloodstream or tissues of the body. Platelets are essential for the formation of blood clots. They function to stop bleeding and repair ruptured blood vessels.

Plasma is the clear, straw-colored liquid component of blood (blood minus its formed elements). Plasma carries nutrients to the cells and waste products from the cells.

Physiology of Circulation

The heart has two very important jobs. It must pump blood low in oxygen to the lungs, where the blood gives up carbon dioxide and takes on oxygen. It must also pump oxygen-rich blood to all of the body's cells. To understand how the heart achieves these tasks, think of the heart as a double pump. The pumps are the right heart (lung or pulmonary circuit) and the left heart (body or systemic circuit) (Figure 14-8).

For the purposes of understanding blood flow through the body, let's use the right atrium as our reference point. Blood low in oxygen enters the right atrium, flows through the tricuspid valve and into the right ventricle. From the right ventricle, blood is pumped through the pulmonic valve into the pulmonary arteries (pulmonary circuit) and then to the lungs where red blood cells are oxygenated. From the lungs, oxygen-rich blood flows through the pulmonary veins and into the left atrium. From the left atrium, blood flows through the mitral (also called the *bicuspid*) valve and into the left ventricle. From the left ventricle, blood is pumped through the aortic valve and into the aorta (systemic circuit). From the aorta, blood flows to the rest of the body through arteries, arterioles, capillaries, venules, and veins. Cells use the oxygen, along with nutrients from food, to make energy. Then, veins carry the blood (now low in oxygen) from the body cells back to the right heart. The superior and inferior vena cavae deliver oxygen-poor blood from the body to the right atrium. Understanding the concept of blood flow and how the cardiovascular system operates will help your assessment of a patient experiencing a cardiovascular emergency.

When the left ventricle contracts, a wave of blood is sent through the arteries, causing them to expand and recoil. A pulse is the regular expansion and recoil of an artery caused by the movement of blood from the heart as it contracts. A pulse can be felt anywhere an artery simultaneously passes near the skin surface and over a bone. Central pulses are located close to the heart and include the carotid and femoral pulses. Peripheral pulses are located farther from the heart and include the radial, brachial, posterior tibial, and dorsalis pedis pulses.

Blood pressure is the force exerted by the blood on the inner walls of the heart and blood vessels. Systolic blood pressure is the pressure exerted against the walls of the arteries when the left ventricle contracts. Diastolic blood pressure is the pressure exerted against the walls of the arteries when the left ventricle is at rest.

Perfusion is the circulation of blood through an organ or a part of the body. **Shock** (hypoperfusion) is

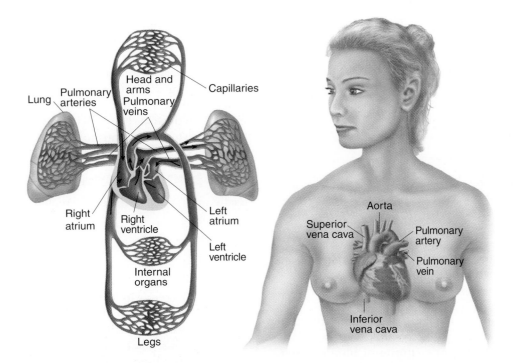

FIGURE 14-8 ▲ The heart works as a double pump. The right heart (pulmonary circuit) pumps blood to the lungs. The left heart (systemic circuit) pumps blood to the cells of the body. Red represents oxygen-rich blood and blue oxygen-poor blood.

inadequate circulation of blood through an organ or a part of the body. It is a state of profound depression of the vital processes of the body. Signs and symptoms of shock are listed in the following *You Should Know* box.

You Should Know

Signs and Symptoms of Shock

- Restlessness, anxiety, or altered mental status
- Pale, cyanotic, cool, clammy skin
- Rapid, weak pulse
- Rapid, shallow breathing
- Nausea and vomiting
- Reduction in total blood volume
- Low or decreasing blood pressure

Cardiovascular Disease

The American Heart Association estimates that more that 70 million Americans suffer from some sort of cardiovascular disease. **Cardiovascular disease** is disease of the heart and blood vessels. **Coronary heart disease** (CHD) is disease of the coronary arteries and the complications that result, such as angina pectoris or a heart attack. **Coronary artery disease** (CAD) is a term used for diseases that slow or stop blood flow through the arteries that supply the heart muscle with blood.

Acute Coronary Syndromes

The heart depends on two coronary arteries and their branches for its supply of oxygen-rich blood. During relaxation (diastole) of the left ventricle, blood flows into the coronary arteries, supplying oxygen and nutrients to the heart. During times of stress, the heart requires more oxygen and depends on widening (dilation) of the arteries to increase blood flow through the coronary arteries.

Acute coronary syndromes (ACSs) are conditions caused by temporary or permanent blockage of a coronary artery as a result of coronary artery disease. ACSs include unstable angina pectoris and myocardial infarction. These conditions will be described in more detail later. Common causes of CAD include arteriosclerosis and atherosclerosis. **Arteriosclerosis** means hardening (-*sclerosis*) of the walls of the arteries (*arterio*-). As the walls of the arteries become hardened, they lose their elasticity. Arteriosclerosis usually begins early in life and progresses slowly with age. In **atherosclerosis,** the inner lining (endothelium) of the walls of large and medium-size arteries becomes narrowed and thickens. Narrowing of the vessel occurs because of a buildup of plaque (Figure 14-9). Plaque is usually made up of calcium, fats (lipids), cholesterol, and other substances. Although it is not known for certain how atherosclerosis starts, researchers think that

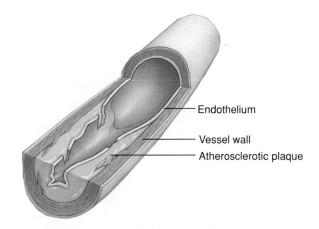

— Endothelium

— Vessel wall

— Atherosclerotic plaque

FIGURE 14-9 ▲ In atherosclerosis, the inner lining (endothelium) of the walls of large and medium-size arteries become narrowed and thicken. Narrowing of the vessel occurs because of a buildup of plaque.

inflammation causes damage to the inner lining of an artery. For example, tobacco smoke causes inflammation, damaging the inner lining of blood vessels. This speeds up the process of atherosclerosis.

When atherosclerosis affects a coronary artery, angina or a heart attack may result. When it affects the carotid arteries that supply the brain, a transient ischemic attack (TIA) or stroke may result. When atherosclerosis affects arteries that supply the arms, legs, and feet, the condition is called **peripheral artery disease (PAD).** When it affects arteries that supply the kidneys, kidney failure may result.

Conditions that may increase a person's chance of developing a disease are called **risk factors.** While some risk factors can be changed, others cannot. Risk factors that can be changed are called **modifiable risk factors.** Risk factors that cannot be changed are called **non-modifiable risk factors.** Factors that can be part of the cause of a person's risk of heart disease are called **contributing risk factors.** Heart disease risk factors are shown in Table 14-1.

When a coronary artery becomes narrowed or blocked, the part of the heart muscle it supplies is starved for oxygen and nutrients (becomes ischemic). **Ischemia** is decreased blood flow to an organ or tissue. Ischemia can result from narrowing or blockage of an artery or spasm of an artery. Atherosclerosis is a common reason for narrowing of a coronary artery. Body cells that lack oxygen (are ischemic) produce lactic acid. Lactic acid irritates nerve endings in the affected area, causing pain or discomfort.

You Should Know

Ischemia can be reversed if treated promptly.

Angina Pectoris

Angina pectoris (literally, "choking in the chest") is a symptom of CAD that occurs when the heart's need for oxygen exceeds its supply. Examples of conditions that may increase the heart's demand for oxygen include physical exertion and emotional upset. In these situations, the coronary arteries normally widen to allow more blood to reach the heart muscle. When a person has CAD, the affected artery (or arteries) is unable to widen adequately because of narrowing, thickening, or blockage of the blood vessel.

You Should Know

Angina most often occurs in patients who have disease involving one or more coronary arteries. However, it can also occur in persons who have other cardiac problems.

A person is said to have **stable angina pectoris** when his symptoms are relatively constant and predictable in terms of severity, signs and symptoms, precipitating events, and response to therapy. A person who has **unstable angina pectoris** has angina that is progressively worsening, occurs at rest, or is brought on by minimal physical exertion. A person with

TABLE 14-1   Heart Disease Risk Factors

Modifiable Factors	Non-modifiable Factors	Contributing Factors
Diabetes mellitus	Family history	Stress
High blood pressure	Gender	Depression
Elevated blood cholesterol	Race	Heavy alcohol intake (three or more drinks per day)
Tobacco smoke	Increasing age	
Lack of exercise		
Obesity		

unstable angina has episodes of chest discomfort that occur with increased frequency or are different from his typical pattern of angina. The person's discomfort usually lasts longer than stable angina (up to 30 minutes) and may radiate more widely. Examples of situations that may lead to ischemia of the heart muscle and anginal discomfort are shown in the following *You Should Know* box.

You Should Know

Angina Pectoris: Possible Triggers

- Physical exertion
- Emotional upset
- Eating a heavy meal
- Exposure to extreme hot or cold temperatures
- Cigarette smoking
- Sexual activity
- Stimulants, such as caffeine or cocaine

Acute Myocardial Infarction

An **acute myocardial infarction** (acute MI; "also called *heart attack*") occurs when a coronary artery becomes severely narrowed or is completely blocked, usually by a blood clot (thrombus). When the affected portion of the heart muscle (myocardium) is deprived of oxygen long enough, the area dies (infarcts) (Figure 14-10). Death of portions of the heart muscle may occur as early as 20 minutes after the onset of symptoms. The blockage within the affected coronary artery must be

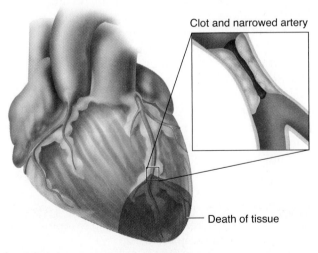

Clot and narrowed artery

Death of tissue

FIGURE 14-10 ▲ A heart attack (myocardial infarction) occurs when a coronary artery becomes severely narrowed or is completely blocked, usually by a blood clot (thrombus). When the affected portion of the heart muscle (myocardium) is deprived of oxygen long enough, the area dies (infarcts).

removed as soon as possible to prevent ischemic tissue from becoming dead tissue. If too much of the heart muscle dies, shock and cardiac arrest will result.

Patients who experience an ACS may receive treatment to open the blocked or partially blocked coronary artery. Clot-busting drugs (fibrinolytics) are sometimes used for this purpose. In some Emergency Medical Services (EMS) systems, Paramedics can give clot-busting drugs. In others, these drugs are given in the hospital. Some patients may undergo angioplasty to open the affected coronary artery. During **angioplasty,** a balloon–tipped catheter is inserted into a partially blocked coronary artery. When the balloon is inflated, plaque is pressed against the walls of the artery, improving blood flow to the heart muscle. About 20-30% of the time, the artery closes up again within six months and another angioplasty needs to be done. Drug-coated stents are now used to help decrease the rate in which a vessel re-narrows. A **stent** is a small plastic or metal tube that is inserted into a vessel or duct to help keep it open and maintain fluid flow through it. In some cases, the patient's cardiologist may recommend bypass surgery. A **coronary artery bypass graft (CABG)** (pronounced "cabbage") is a surgical procedure. When a CABG is performed, a graft is created from a healthy blood vessel from another part of the patient's body. One end of the graft may be attached to the aorta and the other end to the coronary artery beyond the blockage. In this way, the graft reroutes blood flow around the diseased coronary artery.

When caring for a patient who may be having a heart attack, keep in mind that "time is muscle." Studies have shown that the risk of death from a heart attack is related to the time elapsed between the onset of symptoms and start of treatment. The earlier the patient receives emergency care, the greater the chances of preventing ischemic heart tissue from becoming dead

Making a Difference

Because the benefits of treatment for a heart attack lessen quickly over time, it is important that patients seek medical attention as soon as possible after the onset of symptoms. Most patients experiencing an ACS do not seek medical care for two hours or more. When patients recognize that they are having an acute coronary syndrome, fewer than 60% use EMS for treatment and transportation to the hospital. Most patients are driven by someone else or drive themselves to the hospital.

Take the time to teach your patients, family, friends, and community how to recognize signs and symptoms associated with acute coronary syndromes. Teach them the importance of calling 9-1-1 as soon as they recognize these signs.

heart tissue. The American College of Cardiology and the American Heart Association recommend that eligible heart attack patients should receive treatment with clot-busting drugs within 30 minutes or angioplasty within 90 minutes from the time they present to EMS personnel or the Emergency Department.

Congestive Heart Failure

When a person has **congestive heart failure (CHF)**, one or both sides of the heart fail to pump efficiently. When the left ventricle fails as a pump, blood backs up into the lungs (**pulmonary edema**). When the right ventricle fails, blood returning to the heart backs up and causes congestion in the organs and tissues of the body. Swelling of the feet and ankles is often one of the first visible signs of CHF in patients who can walk. In patients confined to bed, swelling is seen around the lower back. Distention of the veins of the neck (jugular venous distention [JVD]) may also be seen.

Patient Assessment

When the heart muscle lacks oxygen (becomes ischemic), lactic acid and carbon dioxide build up. This usually results in chest pain or discomfort that starts in the center of the chest, behind the breastbone. The patient may describe the discomfort as an ache, heaviness, pressure, squeezing, constriction, or pain. Anginal discomfort may be accompanied by difficulty breathing, sweating, nausea, vomiting, weakness, and palpitations. The discomfort associated with stable angina typically lasts 2 to 5 minutes. It is usually quickly relieved (less than 5 minutes) by rest and/or drugs, such as nitroglycerin (NTG). Episodes of unstable angina are usually more severe and prolonged.

Remember This!

Because their signs and symptoms are similar, you will not be able to tell the difference between unstable angina and a heart attack in the field. Treat a patient with unstable angina with the same urgency as a patient with a possible heart attack.

Signs and symptoms of a heart attack vary. Typical signs and symptoms are shown in the following *You Should Know* box. Although chest discomfort is the most common symptom of a heart attack, studies have shown than about 20% of patients who are diagnosed as having a heart attack never have chest pain. When chest discomfort is present, the patient usually describes it as located under the breastbone (substernal), but it may be present across the chest or in the upper abdomen (epigastric pain). It may radiate to the neck, jaw,

You Should Know

Typical Heart Attack Signs and Symptoms

- Uncomfortable squeezing, ache, dull pressure, or pain in the center of the chest lasting more than a few minutes
- Discomfort in one or both arms, the back, neck, jaw, or stomach
- Anxiety, dizziness, irritability
- Abnormal pulse rate (may be irregular)
- Abnormal blood pressure
- Nausea, vomiting
- Lightheadedness
- Fainting or near-fainting
- Breaking out in a cold sweat
- Weakness
- Shortness of breath
- Difficulty breathing (dyspnea)
- Palpitations
- Feeling of impending doom

teeth, back, shoulders, arms, elbows, wrists, and, occasionally, to the back between the shoulder blades. Pain usually radiates down the left arm. The patient may describe symptoms of discomfort (rather than pain) such as "pressing," "tight," "squeezing," "viselike," "aching," "heaviness," "dull," "burning," "crushing," "smothering," or indigestion-type symptoms.

As with angina, a patient who is having a heart attack may have associated symptoms such as palpitations, fainting, sweating, shortness of breath, or nausea. **Palpitations** are an abnormal awareness of one's heart beat. Patients may describe palpitations as, "My heart is racing," "My heart is pounding," or "My heart skipped a beat." The patient may experience fainting (syncope) or near-fainting (near-syncope). **Fainting** is a sudden, temporary loss of consciousness that occurs when one or both sides of the heart do not pump out a sufficient amount of blood, resulting in inadequate blood flow to the brain.

Older adults, diabetic individuals, and women have heart attacks with signs and symptoms that differ from those of a "typical" patient. This is called an *atypical presentation* or *atypical signs and symptoms*. See Table 14-2 for examples of signs and symptoms that may be seen in these patients.

Patient assessment begins with a scene size-up and putting on appropriate personal protective equipment (PPE). Form a first impression and perform a primary survey. Assess the patient's mental status, airway, breathing, and circulation. Note the rate and rhythm of respirations and any signs of increased work of

TABLE 14-2 Atypical Signs and Symptoms of a Heart Attack

Older Adults	Diabetic Individuals	Women
Unexplained new onset or worsened difficulty breathing with exertion	Change in mental status	Pain or discomfort in the chest, arms, back, shoulders, neck, jaw, or stomach
Unexplained nausea, vomiting	Weakness	Anxiety, dizziness
Sweating	Fainting	Shortness of breath
Unexplained tiredness	Lightheadedness	Weakness
Change in mental status	Shoulder/back pain	Unusual tiredness
Weakness		Cold sweats
Fainting		Nausea, vomiting
Abdominal discomfort		

breathing (respiratory effort). Listen for air movement and note if respirations are quiet, absent, or noisy. If the patient is responsive, allow the patient to assume a position of comfort. Give 100% oxygen, preferably by nonrebreather mask. Provide calm reassurance to help reduce the patient's anxiety.

Assess the patient's pulse. If the patient has no pulse, begin cardiopulmonary resuscitation (CPR) unless there are signs of obvious death or the patient has an advance directive. If a pulse is present, estimate the heart rate. Assess pulse regularity and strength. A weak pulse may indicate a decrease in the amount of blood pumped out by the left ventricle as a result of a heart attack or CHF. An absent pulse in an extremity may indicate blockage of an artery in the extremity or severely low blood pressure.

Assess perfusion. Note the color, temperature, and condition (moisture) of the patient's skin. Cool extremities may occur from blood vessel narrowing (constriction). Sweating may indicate pain, anxiety, or shock. Pale or cyanotic (blue) skin may indicate a decrease in the amount of blood pumped out by the left ventricle as a result of a heart attack. If appropriate, evaluate for possible major bleeding.

Objectives 13, 14

If you have not already done so, establish patient priorities, determine the need for additional resources, and make a transport decision. Is there time to provide on-scene care, or should the patient be loaded into the ambulance and rapidly transported? Priority cardiac patients include those with severe chest pain with a systolic blood pressure of less than 100 millimeters of mercury (mm Hg), those with severe respiratory distress, and pulseless patients. Additional resources for any patient experiencing an ACS include activation of Advanced Life Support (ALS) assistance. ALS personnel will apply a cardiac monitor to the patient and look for signs of ischemia or injury to the patient's heart muscle. They will also start an intravenous line and give drugs for pain and abnormal heart rhythms, if present. Care should be taken to evaluate the time it will take for an ALS unit to arrive and the time that it would take to load the patient into the ambulance and transport rapidly to the closest appropriate hospital. Another consideration is meeting the ALS unit to transfer care to ALS before arrival at the hospital. In rural areas, this is often the safest way to initiate ALS care. Remember: Time is muscle.

Once you have made a transport decision, obtain a SAMPLE history from the patient if he is responsive. Remember to use the OPQRST tool if he is complaining of pain or discomfort. Examples of questions to ask a patient who is experiencing an acute coronary syndrome are shown in the next *Making a Difference* box. If the patient is unresponsive or has an altered mental status, quickly size up the scene, form a general impression, perform a primary survey, and then proceed to the rapid medical assessment.

Patients who have heart problems are often prescribed medications. Diuretics ("water pills") may be prescribed for high blood pressure or CHF. Drugs that widen (dilate) blood vessels, such as NTG, may be prescribed to relieve chest pain and reduce the heart's workload. Antiarrhythmics ("heart pills") may be prescribed to control abnormal heart rates or rhythms. Find out if the patient takes his medications regularly and his usual response to them. Ask if there have been any recent changes in medications (additions, deletions, or change in dosages).

Find out the patient's pertinent past medical history. Patients who smoke are at an increased risk for diseases of the heart and blood vessels. Patients with a family history of heart or blood vessel disease are at increased risk for developing these conditions. Provide all information obtained to the Paramedics who arrive on the scene or to the staff at the receiving facility.

- *O*nset: How long ago did your symptoms begin? Did your symptoms begin suddenly or gradually? What were you doing when your symptoms began? Were you resting, sleeping, or doing some type of physical activity?

- *P*rovocation/Palliation: What have you done to relieve the pain or discomfort? Does the discomfort disappear with rest? Have you taken any medications (such as nitroglycerin) to relieve the problem before we arrived? Is there anything that makes the pain worse?

- *Q*uality: What does the pain/discomfort feel like? (Ask the patient to describe the pain or discomfort in his own words [dull, burning, sharp, stabbing, shooting, throbbing, pressure, or tearing].)

- *R*egion/Radiation: Where is your discomfort? Is it in one area or does it move? Is it located in any other area? Is your discomfort worsened when you take a deep breath in or does it stay the same? Does it get better or worse when you change positions, or does it stay the same?

- *S*everity: On a scale of 0 to 10, with 0 being the least and 10 being the worst, what number would you give your discomfort?

- *T*ime: How long has the discomfort been present? Have you ever had these symptoms before? When? How long did it last? Compared with other episodes, would you describe this one as mild, moderate, or severe?

Additional questions:

- Do you have any allergies?

- Do you have high blood pressure, diabetes, or high cholesterol? Do you have a history of any heart problems? For example, have you ever had a heart attack, angina, congestive heart failure, or an abnormal heart rhythm? Have you ever had angioplasty, bypass surgery, or a heart transplant? Do you have a pacemaker or implanted defibrillator?

- Do you have a history of lung, liver, or kidney disease, or other medical condition?

- What medicines do you take? Do you take any medicines for your blood pressure or cholesterol? Do you take any water pills or medicines for your heart? When did you last take them? Do you take aspirin? When did you last take it? Do you take nitroglycerin? When did you last use it? Has the dose of any of your medications been changed recently? Do you take any medications for erectile dysfunction?

- When did you last have anything to eat or drink?

- Do you smoke? How many packs per day?

- Are you having any other symptoms? For example, do you feel nauseated, more tired than usual, lightheaded, or weak? Do you feel short of breath? Have you vomited?

If the patient is responsive, perform a focused physical examination. Remember, the focused exam is guided by the patient's chief complaint and presenting signs and symptoms. When a patient is complaining of chest discomfort, important body areas to assess include the neck, chest, abdomen, and extremities. If the patient is complaining of shortness of breath or difficulty breathing, assess the head, neck, chest, and lower extremities.

Look at the patient's face for signs of distress. Look at his neck for JVD. Look at his chest for use of accessory muscles, retractions, and equal rise and fall. Note the presence of secretions from the mouth and nose. If present, note if the secretions are blood tinged and/or foamy. These signs suggest pulmonary edema.

Observe the patient's position. The patient may place a clenched fist against his chest to indicate the location of his discomfort. The patient with CHF often sits upright with the legs in a dependent position, laboring to breathe. Assess the patient's extremities for swelling.

Listen to breath sounds. Wheezes or crackles may indicate failure of the left ventricle. If the patient can speak, note if he can speak in full sentences.

Obtain baseline vital signs. Assess the patient's pulse, respirations, and blood pressure. Assess oxygen saturation by using a pulse oximeter. An increased heart rate may suggest anxiety, pain, CHF, or an abnormal heart rhythm. A decreased heart rate may suggest an abnormal heart rhythm or the effect of some heart medications. The patient's respiratory rate may be increased as a result of anxiety, pain, or CHF. An elevated blood pressure may be the result of anxiety, emotional stress, or pain or may indicate preexisting high blood pressure. A fall in blood pressure may indicate shock or the effect of some heart medications.

Emergency Care
Objectives 2, 7

Allow the patient to assume a position of comfort. Most patients will prefer a semi-Fowler's position. Provide calm reassurance to help reduce the patient's anxiety.

Remember This!

Do not allow any patient who has a heart or breathing-related complaint to perform activities that require exertion, such as walking to the stretcher. Asking the patient to walk to a stretcher or ambulance *increases* the heart's need for oxygen. When providing emergency care to these patients, your goal is to *decrease* oxygen demand. Bring the stretcher to the patient—not the patient to the stretcher.

MONA is a memory aid used to recall the initial treatments often used by healthcare professionals when caring for patients experiencing an acute coronary syndrome. MONA stands for:

- M = *Morphine*
- O = *Oxygen*
- N = *Nitroglycerin*
- A = *Aspirin*

Although morphine is given only by ALS personnel in the field, EMTs can begin treating the patient with the remaining three drugs (in most EMS systems). Start by giving 100% oxygen, preferably by nonrebreather mask. If the patient's breathing is inadequate, give positive-pressure ventilation with 100% oxygen. Assess the adequacy of the ventilations delivered.

Objective 40

Many states have passed legislation to include aspirin as a medication that can be carried on an EMS unit and given by EMTs (see Table 14-3). Check your state and local protocols for the appropriate use of this drug. In some EMS systems, emergency medical dispatchers will ask the patient to chew aspirin while emergency personnel are en route to the scene. If ordered by medical direction (and there are no contraindications), aspirin should be given as soon as possible after the patient's onset of chest discomfort. Be sure to first verify that the patient is not allergic to aspirin. It should be used with caution in a patient who has a history of asthma, nasal polyps, or nasal allergies. Severe allergic reactions in sensitive patients have occurred.

Find out if the patient has been prescribed NTG. If the patient does have prescribed NTG, find out if the medication is with the patient and when the last dose was taken. Contact medical direction. If instructed to do so, assist the patient with its use and then continue with the focused exam. If the patient does not have prescribed NTG, continue the focused exam. Transport promptly if:

- The patient has signs of cardiac compromise and no prior history of cardiac problems

TABLE 14-3 Aspirin

Generic name	acetylsalicylic acid
Trade name	Bayer, Ecotrin, Empirin
Mechanism of action	Blocks a part of the clotting process in the bloodstream and may reduce the risk of a heart attack
Indications	Chest pain or discomfort that is suspected to be of cardiac origin
Dosage (adult)	Two to four 81-mg tablets (baby aspirin), chewed and swallowed
Side effects	• Rapid pulse • Dizziness • Flushing • Nausea, vomiting • Gastrointestinal bleeding
Contraindications	• Known allergy or sensitivity to aspirin • Bleeding ulcer or bleeding disorders • Stroke • Children and adolescents

- The patient has a history of cardiac problems but does not have NTG
- The patient has a systolic blood pressure of less than 100 mm Hg

Perform ongoing assessments until patient care is turned over to ALS personnel or medical personnel at the receiving facility.

You Should Know

Many patients consider most over-the-counter pain remedies to be the same as aspirin and may use the terms interchangeably. Acetaminophen (Tylenol) and aspirin are not the same, and cannot be interchanged in the care of chest pain or discomfort that is suspected to be of cardiac origin.

Assisting the Patient with Prescribed Nitroglycerin

Objectives 40, 41, 42

NTG is used to treat chest discomfort that is believed to be cardiac in origin. Until 2004, patients were told to take 1 NTG tablet, 5 minutes apart, for up to 3 doses when they had a sudden onset of chest pain/discomfort before calling 9-1-1. This was changed to encourage earlier contacting of EMS by patients with symptoms suggestive of ACSs. Patients are now taught that if their pain/discomfort does not improve (or worsens) within 5 minutes of taking one dose, the patient or a family member should call 9-1-1 right away. Patients are also taught to take a dose of the drug immediately before chest discomfort is expected to occur (such as before physical exertion) to prevent anginal symptoms. Table 14-4 summarizes important information about sublingual NTG that you should know.

Medication Actions

NTG causes relaxation (dilation) of the smooth muscle of blood vessel walls. Relaxation of the veins results in pooling of blood in the dependent portions of the body as a result of gravity. This effect reduces the amount of blood returning to the heart, decreasing the heart's workload. NTG causes some relaxation of the walls of arteries, including the coronary arteries. This helps reduce the resistance the heart must overcome to pump blood out to the body, thus decreasing the heart's workload. NTG

relaxes normal and atherosclerotic coronary arteries on the outer surface of the heart. This helps to improve blood flow and the delivery of oxygen to the heart.

Because NTG relaxes blood vessels, it has the potential to significantly decrease the patient's blood pressure. Reassess the patient's vital signs after *each dose* of this drug.

Indications

As an EMT, you can assist a patient in taking prescribed NTG if *all* of the following criteria are met:

- The patient has signs and symptoms of chest pain or discomfort.
- The patient has physician-prescribed NTG.
- There are no contraindications to giving the medication.
- You have specific authorization by medical direction (off line or on line).

Contraindications

Assisting a patient in taking prescribed NTG is contraindicated if any of the following conditions exists:

- Medical direction does not give permission
- Medication is not prescribed for the patient
- Patient has already taken the maximum prescribed dose before EMTs arrival
- Hypotension (blood pressure below 100 mm Hg systolic)
- Heart rate less than 50 beats/min or more than 100 beats/min
- Head injury (recent) or stroke (recent)
- Infants and children
- Patient who has taken a medication for erectile dysfunction within the last 24 to 48 hours

Remember This!

Before giving NTG, it is very important to ask the patient if he has taken any medications for erectile problems. Examples of oral medications that are used for this purpose include sildenafil (Viagra), tadalafil (Cialis), and vardenafil (Levitra). Giving NTG to a patient who has taken any of these drugs within 24 to 48 hours may lead to irreversible hypotension and death.

TABLE 14-4 Nitroglycerin

Generic name	nitroglycerin
Trade name	Nitrostat, Nitrobid, Nitrolingual, Nitroglycerin Spray
Mechanism of action	• Relaxes blood vessels thus increasing the flow of oxygenated blood to the heart muscle • Decreases the workload of the heart
Indications	An EMT can assist a patient in taking nitroglycerin if *all* of the following criteria are met: • The patient has signs and symptoms of chest discomfort suspected to be of cardiac origin. • The patient has physician-prescribed sublingual tablets or spray. • There are no contraindications to giving nitroglycerin. • The EMT has specific authorization by medical direction.
Dosage	Dosage is 1 tablet or 1 spray under the tongue. This dose may be repeated in 3 to 5 minutes (maximum of three doses) if: • The patient experiences no relief • The patient's systolic blood pressure remains above 100 mm Hg • The patient's heart rate remains between 50 and 100 beats/min • There are no other contraindications • The EMT is authorized by medical direction to give another dose of the medication
Side effects	Hypotension is a common and significant side effect. Other side effects include tachycardia, bradycardia, headache, palpitations, and fainting.
Contraindications	• Medical direction does not give permission • Medication is not prescribed for the patient • Patient has already taken maximum prescribed dose before EMT arrival • Hypotension (blood pressure below 100 mm Hg systolic) • Heart rate less than 50 beats/min or more than 100 beats/min • Head injury (recent) or stroke (recent) • Infants and children • Patient who has taken a medication for erectile dysfunction within the last 24 to 48 hours

Special Considerations

- Before giving any medication, make sure you have the right patient, right drug, right dose, right route, and right time.
- NTG works quickly. Its effects last about 5 to 7 minutes. Relief of chest pain or discomfort may occur within 1 to 2 minutes of administration.
- If authorized by medical direction, NTG can be repeated every 5 minutes for up to 3 tablets or sprays (provided the patient's vital signs remain stable). Ask the patient to rate his discomfort after each dose so you can detect any changes in the patient's condition.

- Monitor the patient's heart rate and blood pressure closely before and after administration. Compare the patient's blood pressure after each dose of NTG with his baseline blood pressure. Do not give another dose of NTG if the patient's blood pressure drops below 100 mm Hg systolic or is 30 mm Hg or more below the patient's baseline systolic blood pressure. If the blood pressure is below 100 mm Hg systolic, elevate the patient's legs and reassess the blood pressure.

Procedure

Skill Drills 14-1 and 14-2 show the procedure for assisting a patient with his prescribed NTG.

Assisting the Patient with Prescribed Nitroglycerin Tablets

STEP 1 ▶
- Put on appropriate personal protective equipment.
- Confirm that the patient has signs or symptoms of chest pain/discomfort.

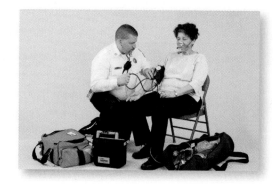

STEP 2 ▶
- Confirm that the patient has physician-prescribed nitroglycerin. Make sure that the nitroglycerin is not expired and that the patient is alert.
- Determine if the patient has already taken any doses. If so, find out the time of the last dose and the effects of the medication.
- Assess the patient's vital signs to make sure that the patient's systolic blood pressure is >100 mm Hg and her heart rate is 50 beats/minute and <100 beats/minute.
- If there are no contraindications, obtain an order from medical direction (either on line or off line) to assist the patient in taking the medication.

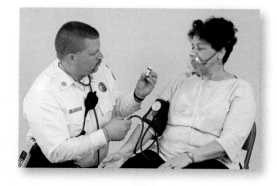

STEP 3 ▶
- Remove the oxygen mask from the patient.
- Pour one nitroglycerin tablet into the bottle cap. Ask the patient to lift her tongue while you place the tablet under the tongue (while wearing gloves), or have the patient place the tablet under the tongue.
- Have the patient keep her mouth closed with the tablet under the tongue (without swallowing) until it is dissolved and absorbed.

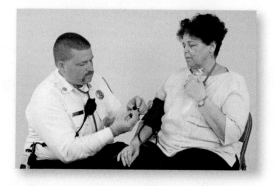

STEP 4 ▷
- Replace the oxygen mask on the patient.
- Recheck the patient's vital signs within 2 minutes. Reassess the patient's degree of discomfort.
- Document the patient's name, drug name and dose given, time of administration, and the patient's response to the drug.
- If an on-line order was received by medical direction, document the name of the physician giving the order.
- Perform ongoing assessments every 5 minutes, continuously monitoring the patient's airway and breathing.

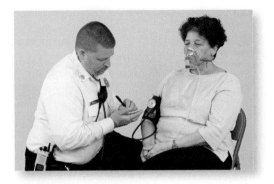

Cardiac Arrest

If the heart stops beating, no blood will flow. If no blood flows, oxygen cannot be delivered to the body's cells. When the heart stops, the patient is said to be in **cardiac arrest.** The signs of cardiac arrest include sudden unresponsiveness, absent breathing, and no signs of circulation. Possible causes of a cardiac arrest are shown in the following *You Should Know* box.

You Should Know

Possible Causes of Cardiac Arrest
- Heart and blood vessel diseases, such as heart attack and stroke
- Choking or respiratory arrest
- Seizures
- Diabetic emergency
- Severe allergic reaction
- Severe electrical shock
- Poisoning or drug overdose
- Drowning
- Suffocation
- Trauma
- Severe bleeding
- Abnormalities present at birth

Because the organs of the body must have oxygen, organ damage begins quickly after the heart stops. Brain damage begins 4 to 6 minutes after the patient suffers a cardiac arrest. Brain damage becomes irreversible in 8 to 10 minutes. Chest compressions are used to circulate blood any time that the heart is not beating. Chest compressions are combined with rescue breathing to oxygenate the blood. The combination of rescue breathing and external chest compressions is called **cardiopulmonary resuscitation (CPR).**

You Should Know

When a cardiac arrest occurs, CPR must be started as early as possible. However, even when performed expertly, CPR provides only about one third of the normal blood flow to the heart and brain.

Sudden cardiac death (SCD) is the unexpected death from cardiac causes early after symptom onset (immediately or within 1 hour) or without the onset of symptoms. About two thirds of sudden cardiac deaths take place outside the hospital, usually in a private or residential setting.

Assisting the Patient with Prescribed Nitroglycerin Spray

STEP 1 ▶
- Put on appropriate personal protective equipment.
- Confirm that the patient has signs or symptoms of chest pain/discomfort.

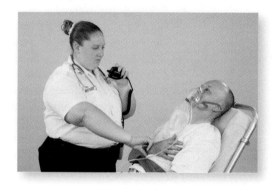

STEP 2 ▶
- Confirm that the patient has physician-prescribed nitroglycerin. Make sure that the nitroglycerin is not expired and that the patient is alert.
- Determine if the patient has already taken any doses. If so, find out the time of the last dose and the effects of the medication.
- Assess the patient's vital signs to make sure that the patient's systolic blood pressure is > 100 mm Hg and his heart rate is 50 beats/minute and < 100 beats/minute.
- If there are no contraindications, obtain an order from medical direction (either on line or off line) to assist the patient in taking the medication.

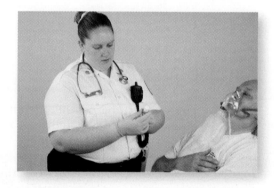

STEP 3 ▶
- Remove the oxygen mask from the patient.
- Ask the patient to lift his tongue while you spray the medication under his tongue (while wearing gloves), or have the patient self-administer the drug under his tongue.
- Have the patient keep his mouth closed (without swallowing) until the drug is absorbed.

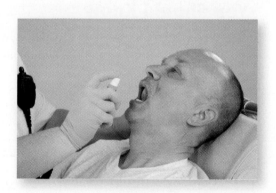

STEP 4 ▶
- Replace the oxygen mask on the patient.
- Recheck the patient's vital signs within two minutes. Reassess the patient's degree of discomfort.
- Document the patient's name, drug name and dose given, time of administration, and the patient's response to the drug.
- If an on-line order was received by medical direction, document the name of the physician giving the order.
- Perform ongoing assessments every five minutes, continuously monitoring the patient's airway and breathing.

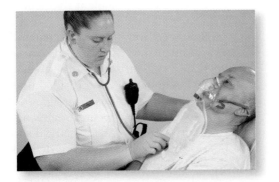

Fundamentals of Early Cardiopulmonary Resuscitation and Defibrillation

Objectives 10, 11

Survival of cardiac arrest depends on a series of critical actions called the *Chain of Survival.* The **Chain of Survival** is the ideal series of events that should take place immediately after recognition of an injury or the onset of sudden illness (Figure 14-11). The chain consists of four crucial steps:

1. *Early access (recognition of an emergency and calling 9-1-1).* The public must be educated to recognize the early warning signs of a heart attack. Many patients do nothing and hope their symptoms will go away. The average time between the onset of symptoms and admission to a medical facility is about 3 hours. Some patients may delay seeking help for more than 24 hours. A patient's collapse must be identified by a person who can activate the EMS system. CPR training teaches citizens how to contact the EMS system, decreasing the time to defibrillation. EMS personnel must arrive rapidly to the scene with all necessary equipment.

2. *Early CPR.* Bystander CPR is the best treatment the patient can receive until arrival of a defibrillator and advanced cardiac life support (ACLS) personnel.

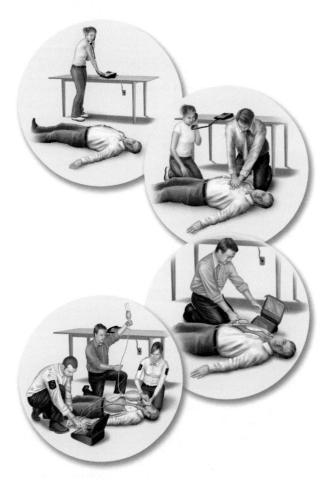

FIGURE 14-11 ▲ The Chain of Survival.

3. *Early defibrillation.* **Defibrillation** is the delivery of an electrical shock to a patient's heart to end an abnormal heart rhythm, such as **ventricular fibrillation (VF or VFib).** When the heart is in VF, the electrical impulses are completely disorganized. As a result, the heart cannot pump blood effectively. If you were able to look at the heart while it is in VF, you would see it quivering like a bowl of gelatin. For every minute that the patient's heart is in VF, his chances of surviving the cardiac arrest decrease by about 10% without bystander CPR. When bystander CPR is provided, the decline in survival is more gradual, averaging 3–4% per minute. The only effective treatments for VF are CPR and the delivery of electrical shocks to the heart with a machine called a **defibrillator.** The shock attempts to stop VF and allow the patient's normal heart rhythm to start again. CPR can keep oxygen-rich blood flowing to the heart and brain until the arrival of an **automated external defibrillator (AED)** and advanced care.

4. *Early ACLS.* Early advanced care provided by Paramedics at the scene is a critical link in the treatment of cardiac arrest. Paramedics combine rapid defibrillation by first-responding units with airway management and intravenous medications by the ALS units. If ACLS units are not available, the patient should be transported rapidly to a facility for definitive ACLS care.

Time is critical when dealing with a victim of cardiac arrest. A break in any of the links in the chain can reduce the patient's chance of survival, despite excellence in the rest of the chain.

Objective 5

You are an important part of the chain of survival. As an EMT, you will rarely perform one-rescuer CPR while on duty. However, you may need to perform CPR alone while your EMT partner is preparing equipment or your partner is driving to a receiving facility. When providing care for a patient in cardiac arrest, you must know:

- Appropriate use of body substance isolation precautions
- How to use an AED
- When to request available ALS backup
- How to suction the patient's airway
- How to use airway adjuncts
- How to use a bag-mask (BM) device with oxygen attached
- How to use a flow-restricted, oxygen-powered ventilation device
- Techniques for safe lifting and moving patients in cardiac arrest

- Techniques for interviewing bystanders and family members to obtain facts related to a cardiac arrest
- Techniques of effective CPR
- How to assist ALS personnel when requested (and allowed by state and regional authorities)

When you arrive at the scene of a cardiac arrest, you should start CPR immediately if the patient is unresponsive, breathless (apneic), and without a pulse. The steps for CPR are shown in Appendix A at the back of the book. However, you should not perform CPR if there is a valid Do Not Resuscitate (DNR) order or in cases of obvious death. If you arrive on the scene of a cardiac arrest and the DNR paperwork is unclear, the validity of the DNR order is questionable, or a written DNR order is not present, begin resuscitation efforts and call additional medical help to the scene.

Patient Assessment and Emergency Care

After determining that the scene is safe, form a general impression of the patient. A patient in cardiac arrest appears unresponsive and does not appear to be breathing. His skin color is usually pale, gray, or blue.

Assess Responsiveness

Begin the primary survey. Use the AVPU scale to quickly check the patient's level of responsiveness (mental status). Gently squeeze the patient's shoulders and shout, "Are you all right?" If the patient does not respond, shout for help. If you are alone and there is no response to your shout for help, contact your dispatcher and request additional resources, including an AED (if you do not have an AED with you).

A = Airway

If the patient is unresponsive and you do not suspect trauma, open his airway by using the head tilt–chin lift maneuver. If you suspect trauma, open the airway by using the jaw thrust without head tilt maneuver. If trauma is suspected but you are unable to maintain an open airway by using the jaw thrust without head tilt maneuver, open the airway by using the head tilt–chin lift maneuver. If the patient is an unresponsive infant or child, do not hyperextend the neck when opening the airway. Suction any blood, vomit, or other fluid that may be present from the patient's airway.

B = Breathing

After you have made sure that the patient's airway is open, assess his breathing. Place your face near the patient and look for the rise and fall of the chest. Listen and feel for air movement from the patient's nose or mouth. The assessment of breathing should take at least 5 seconds but no more than 10 seconds. If the patient's breathing is not adequate, begin rescue breathing by using a pocket mask, mouth-to-barrier device, or BM device. If the patient has dentures and they fit well, leave them in place to help provide a good mask seal. If the dentures are loose, remove them so they do not fall back into the throat and block the airway. Give two breaths (each breath over 1 second) with just enough force to make the chest rise with each breath.

Making a Difference

If the patient is breathing very slowly or has occasional, gasping breaths (agonal breathing), his breathing is inadequate. Provide emergency care as if the patient were not breathing at all.

Watch the patient's chest while you breathe into the patient. If your breaths are going in, you should see the chest rise with each breath. Be sure to pause between breaths. This pause allows you to take another breath. It also allows the patient's lungs to relax and air to escape. If the patient is unresponsive, insert an oral airway to help keep the patient's airway open. Continue breathing for the patient until he begins to breathe adequately on his own or another trained rescuer takes over.

If your first breath does not go in, gently reposition the patient's head and breathe for him again. If the breaths still do not go in, you must assume the airway is blocked. If the patient is unresponsive, check for a pulse.

Remember This!

Ventilate the patient with just enough pressure to make the chest rise with each breath. If you give breaths too quickly or too forcefully, you will push air into the stomach. This causes the stomach to distend (swell) with air and the patient may vomit. If the patient vomits, roll the patient onto his side until the vomiting stops. Suction the vomitus from the patient's mouth. Then roll the patient onto his back and resume rescue breathing if needed.

C = Circulation

Once you have made sure that the patient's airway is open and have started rescue breathing, assess circulation. Use the carotid artery to check the pulse of an unresponsive adult or child older than year of age. Feel for a brachial pulse in an unresponsive infant. Feel for a pulse for at least 5 seconds but no more than 10 seconds. If you definitely feel a pulse, give 1 breath every 5 to 6 seconds for an adult. Give 1 breath every 3 to 5 seconds for an infant or child. Reassess the patient's pulse about every 2 minutes. If you do not definitely feel a pulse within 10 seconds, or if you are uncertain, begin chest compressions.

Remember This!

For chest compressions to be effective, the patient must be positioned on a firm, level surface. If you find the patient in bed, move him to the floor. Place his arms at his sides. If the patient is found face down, ask your partner to help you carefully roll the patient, so that his head, shoulders, and chest move together as a unit without twisting. Once the patient is lying face up, position yourself at the patient's side so that you can provide rescue breathing and chest compressions if necessary.

Chest Compressions—Adult

Kneel beside the patient's chest. Place the heel of one hand in the center of the patient's chest, between the nipples. Place your other hand on top of the first. Interlock the fingers of both hands to keep your fingers off the patient's ribs. If you have arthritis in your hands or wrists, give compressions by grasping the wrist of the hand that is on the patient's chest with your other hand and push down with both.

Position yourself directly above the patient's chest so that your shoulders are directly over your hands. With your arms straight and your elbows locked, press down about 1½ to 2 inches on the adult patient's breastbone with the heels of your hands. Release pressure (let up) after each compression to allow the patient's chest to recoil. Releasing pressure on the patient's chest allows blood to flow into the chest and heart. When performing adult CPR, deliver 30 compressions at a rate of about 100 compressions per minute. One cycle consists of 30 chest compressions and 2 rescue breaths. After 5 cycles (which is about 2 minutes), check for a pulse. If the patient has a pulse, check breathing. If the patient has a pulse but is not breathing, give rescue breaths at a rate of 1 breath every 5 to 6 seconds. If there is still no pulse, continue CPR. Check for a pulse again every few minutes.

Because performing chest compressions is tiring, rescuers should switch roles about every 2 minutes or 5 cycles of CPR. The "switch" should ideally take place in 5 seconds or less. Two-rescuer CPR is discussed in more detail in Appendix A.

Chest Compressions—Child

For the general public, CPR guidelines for a child pertain to a child from 1 to about 8 years of age. For healthcare professionals, a child is considered 1 year to about the start of puberty (about 12 to 14 years of age). For children between the ages of 1 and 12 to 14, perform chest compressions if there is no pulse. You should also perform compressions if a pulse is present but the heart rate is less than 60 beats/min with signs of poor perfusion (pale, cool, mottled skin). A child's chest may be compressed using the heel of 1 hand or the same technique as for an adult. Press down on the breastbone about 1/3 to 1/2 the depth of the chest. Give chest compressions at a rate of about 100 compressions per minute. After every 30 compressions, give 2 rescue breaths.

Chest Compressions—Infant

For an infant, perform chest compressions if there is no pulse. You should also perform compressions if a pulse is present but the heart rate is less than 60 beats/min with signs of poor perfusion (pale, cool, mottled skin). Compress the infant's chest with two fingers. Press down on the breastbone about 1/3 to 1/2 the depth of the chest. Give chest compressions at a rate of about 100 compressions per minute. After every 30 compressions, give 2 rescue breaths.

When two healthcare professionals are available to perform CPR on an infant, the two-thumb technique is preferred for performing chest compressions. Place your thumbs side by side or one on top of the other over the lower half of the infant's breastbone. Your thumbs should be placed about one finger's width below the nipple line (Figure 14-12). Encircle the infant's chest with the fingers of both hands. Use your thumbs to compress the chest about 1/3 to 1/2 the depth of the chest.

CPR guidelines for adults, children, and infants are presented in Table 14-5.

D = Defibrillation

Types of Defibrillators

A **defibrillator** is a device that delivers an electrical shock to a patient's heart to stop an abnormal heart rhythm. **Defibrillation** is the technique of administering the electrical shock. A **manual defibrillator** requires the rescuer to analyze and interpret the patient's cardiac rhythm (Figure 14-13). If the rhythm requires defibrillation, the rescuer applies paddles or adhesive pads to the patient's chest to deliver the shock. This type of defibrillator is used by ALS and hospital personnel.

An **implantable cardioverter-defibrillator (ICD)** is a device that is surgically placed below the skin surface in the patient's chest wall (usually under the skin beneath the shoulder) or upper abdomen (Figure 14-14). A person who has an ICD has had, or is at high risk of having, heart rhythm problems. An ICD is programmed to recognize heart rhythms that are too fast or life threatening (such as VF). When an ICD recognizes a too-fast rhythm or VF, it delivers a shock to the heart to "reset" it. Because an ICD is in direct contact with the heart muscle by using wires, much less energy is needed to deliver a shock than when an external defibrillator is used.

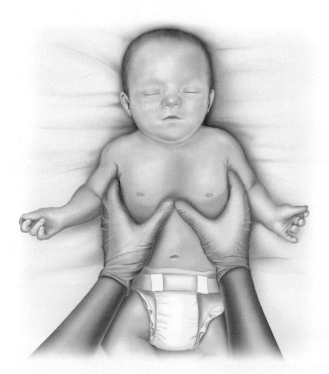

FIGURE 14-12 ▲ The two-thumb method of performing CPR on an infant. This method is used when two rescuers are available.

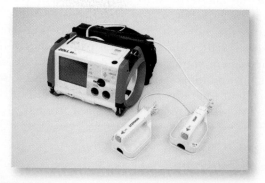

FIGURE 14-13 ▲ A manual defibrillator requires a healthcare professional to interpret the patient's heart rhythm.

TABLE 14-5 Cardiopulmonary Resuscitation Guidelines

	Adult	Child	Infant
Patient Age	More than 12 to 14 years	1 to 12 to 14 years	Under 1 year
Rescue Breaths	About 10-12 breaths/min 1 breath every 5-6 sec	About 12-20 breaths/min 1 breath every 3-5 sec	About 12-20 breaths/min 1 breath every 3-5 sec
Location of Pulse Check	Carotid	Carotid	Brachial
Method of Chest Compressions	Heel of one hand, other hand on top	Heel of 1 hand or same as for adult	2 fingers (1 rescuer) *or* 2 thumbs with the fingers of both hands encircling the chest (2 rescuers)
Depth of Chest Compressions	$1\frac{1}{2}$ to 2 inches	$\frac{1}{3}$ to $\frac{1}{2}$ the chest depth	$\frac{1}{3}$ to $\frac{1}{2}$ the chest depth
Rate of Chest Compressions	About 100/minute		
Ratio of Chest Compressions to Rescue Breaths (One Cycle)	1 or 2 rescuers: 30 compressions to 2 breaths (30:2)	1 rescuer: 30 compressions to 2 breaths (30:2) 2 rescuers: 15 compressions to 2 breaths (15:2)	1 rescuer: 30 compressions to 2 breaths (30:2) 2 rescuers: 15 compressions to 2 breaths (15:2)

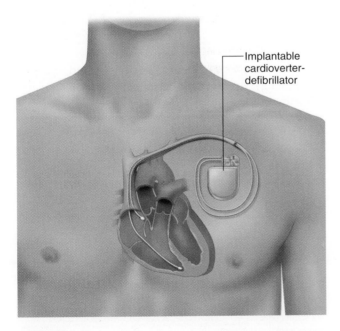

Implantable cardioverter-defibrillator

FIGURE 14-14 ▲ An ICD is surgically placed below the skin surface in the patient's chest wall (usually under the skin beneath the shoulder) or upper abdomen.

An AED contains a computer programmed to recognize heart rhythms that should be shocked, such as VF (Figure 14-15). The accuracy of AEDs in rhythm analysis is high both in detecting rhythms needing shocks and rhythms that do not need shocks. Accurate rhythm analysis is dependent on properly charged defibrillator batteries and proper defibrillator maintenance.

An AED is attached to the patient by means of connecting cables and two disposable adhesive pads. The adhesive pads have a thin metal pad covered by a thick layer of adhesive gel. The pads record the patient's heart rhythm and, if appropriate, deliver a shock. When the pads are placed on the patient's bare chest, the AED examines the patient's heart rhythm for any abnormalities.

Objectives 15, 16, 17

There are many AED manufacturers. As a result, there are slight differences in AED screen layouts, controls, and the location to plug in the adhesive pads. There are also differences in color, weight, and voice instructions. It is essential that you understand and be familiar with the operation of the AED used by your EMS agency.

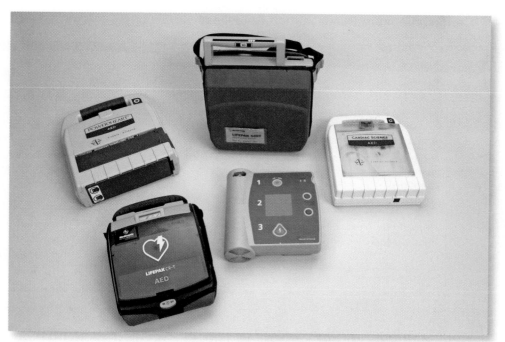

FIGURE 14-15 ▲ Examples of AEDs.

You must also know the difference between a fully automated external defibrillator and a semi-automated external defibrillator (SAED). When a fully automated external defibrillator is used, the pads are attached to the patient and the power turned on. The AED then performs all of the necessary steps to defibrillate the patient. A fully automated machine analyzes the patient's heart rhythm, warns everyone to stand clear of the patient if it recognizes a shockable rhythm, and then delivers a shock through the pads that were applied to the patient's chest.

An SAED is also called a *shock-advisory defibrillator*. When an SAED is used, the adhesive pads are attached to the patient and the power turned on. Some AEDs require the rescuer to press an "analyze" control to begin analyzing the patient's cardiac rhythm while others automatically begin analyzing the patient's cardiac rhythm when the adhesive pads are attached to the patient's chest. The SAED "advises" the rescuer of the steps to take based on its analysis of the patient's heart rhythm by means of a voice or visual message. For example, if an SAED detects a shockable rhythm, it will advise the rescuer to press the shock control to deliver a shock.

Objective 6

A standard AED is used for a patient who is unresponsive, not breathing, pulseless, and greater than or equal to 8 years of age (about 55 pounds or more than 25 kg). A special key or pad-cable system is available for some AEDs so that the machine can be used on children between 1 and 8 years of age. The key or pad-cable system decreases the amount of energy delivered to a dose appropriate for a child (Figure 14-16). If a child is in cardiac arrest and a key or pad-cable system is not available, use a standard AED.

Remember This!

Children who weigh more than 55 pounds (more than 25 kg) or are older than 8 years of age are defibrillated as adults.

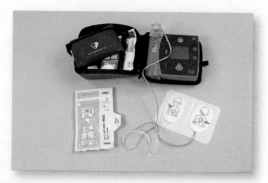

FIGURE 14-16 ▲ Special pads and cables are available for some AEDs for use on children between 1 and 8 years of age.

Emergency Medical Technicians and Automated External Defibrillators

Objectives 3, 4, 8, 9, 12

Not all patients who have chest pain experience a cardiac arrest. A patient who has chest pain or discomfort does not need to be attached to an AED. However, a patient who has signs of cardiac compromise is at increased risk of sudden cardiac death. With this in mind, make sure that you have oxygen, an oral airway, a BM device, suction equipment, and an AED within arm's reach in case of cardiac arrest.

Under current resuscitation guidelines, an AED should only be applied to an adult or child who is unresponsive, apneic, and pulseless. Although AEDs exist for use in infants, current resuscitation guidelines make no recommendation for or against AED use in infants.

When an adult experiences a cardiac arrest caused by VF, prompt defibrillation is the most important treatment you can provide from the time of the arrest to about 5 minutes following the arrest. For example, if you arrive on the scene and see an adult collapse (witness a cardiac arrest), assess the patient's airway, breathing, and circulation, and then quickly apply an AED. Perform CPR until the AED is ready. Survival rates from witnessed cardiac arrest are highest when immediate CPR is provided and defibrillation occurs within 3 to 5 minutes.

When EMS personnel arrive more than 4 to 5 minutes after an adult cardiac arrest, studies have shown increased survival rates when CPR is performed for about two minutes before attempting defibrillation. Check with your medical director about what your EMS agency's standard operating procedure is in these situations. Your medical director may recommend that if you arrive at the scene of an adult cardiac arrest, did not witness the patient's collapse, and your response time is more than 4 to 5 minutes, your operating procedure should be to provide 5 cycles of CPR (about 2 minutes) and then analyze the patient's rhythm with an AED.

Advantages of Automated External Defibrillators

Objectives 21, 22, 23, 24

- Learning to use and operate an AED is easy. The AED provides voice and visual prompts to the user. During training, rescuers learn to recognize a cardiac arrest [unresponsive, breathless (apneic), pulseless patient], learn how to properly attach the AED to the patient, and memorize the treatment sequence.

- Less training is required to operate and maintain skills using an AED than with a manual defibrillator.

- Studies comparing the use of manual defibrillators and AEDs have shown that the first shock can be delivered sooner with the AED than with manual defibrillators.

- AEDs use adhesive pads attached to the patient by connecting cables to deliver shocks to the patient. This helps ensure rescuer safety because the rescuer is not in direct contact with the patient when the AED is analyzing the patient's rhythm or during the shock phase of AED operation. This feature permits what is called *remote, hands-free,* or *hands-off* defibrillation. The adhesive pads used cover a larger surface area than the paddles of manual defibrillators, delivering more effective shocks.

- Some AEDs are equipped with a screen that allows rescuers to view the patient's heart rhythm. This is often useful to ALS personnel because they can select specific drugs to give the patient on the basis of the rhythm seen. They can also continue monitoring the patient's heart rhythm with the AED after resuscitation.

- In some areas, studies have shown high (49-74%) survival rates for witnessed cardiac arrests outside of a hospital when CPR and AEDs are used. Examples of areas showing improved survival rates include casinos, airports, and commercial passenger planes.

Medical Direction and Quality Management

Objectives 36, 37, 38, 39

Just as for the other skills you perform as an EMT, you will operate an AED under the authorization of a medical director. To ensure delivery of the best quality patient care possible, the medical director (or designated representative) carefully reviews every call in which an AED is used. Quality management involves the performance of individuals using AEDs, the effectiveness of the EMS system in which AEDs are used, and data collection and review.

AEDs are equipped with memory modules that record important information for later review by medical direction. The data from the AED can be downloaded to a computer or pocket PC. Examples of information recorded by an AED include the patient's heart rhythm, number of shocks delivered, time of each shock delivered, and the energy level used for each shock. Some AEDs also document CPR compression data. Some AEDs have an audio recording feature that is voice activated so that conversation during the call is recorded.

In addition to the data from the AED, the medical director will also review the prehospital care report pertaining to the call, voice recordings (if the AED is so equipped), and magnetic tape recordings stored in the AED (if so equipped). Each call is reviewed to determine if the patient was treated according to professional standards and local standing orders. Other areas that may be evaluated include:

- Scene command
- Safety
- Efficiency
- Speed
- Professionalism
- Ability to troubleshoot
- Completeness of patient care
- Interactions with other professionals and bystanders

By reviewing each call in which an AED is used, problems within the EMS system can be identified, each link in the Chain of Survival can be evaluated, and EMS personnel can learn from their successes and mistakes.

Special Considerations

- Before using the AED, make certain all personnel are clear of the patient, stretcher, and defibrillator.
- Before applying the AED pads, quickly look at the patient's chest and upper abdomen for a small lump under the skin that suggests the presence of a permanent pacemaker or ICD. Do not hesitate to apply an AED if the patient is in cardiac arrest and has a pacemaker or ICD in place. In these situations, place the AED pads at least 1 inch from the pacemaker or ICD.
- When applying AED pads to the patient's chest, make sure there are no air pockets between the pads and the patient's skin. Press from one edge of the pad across the entire surface to remove all air.
- If the patient has a hairy chest, the AED pads may not stick to the patient's chest. The AED will be unable to analyze the patient's heart rhythm and will give a "check electrodes" message. Try pressing down firmly on each AED pad and see if that corrects the problem. If the "check electrodes" message from the AED persists (and you have a second set of AED pads available), quickly remove the AED pads. This will remove some of the patient's chest hair. Quickly look at the patient's chest. If a lot of chest hair remains, quickly shave the areas of the chest where the AED pads will be placed. Put on a second set of AED pads. Follow the prompts by the AED.

- Before using an AED, familiarize yourself with the manufacturer's recommendations regarding the use of the device around water. If the patient is lying on a metal surface, remove the patient from contact with the surface before attaching the AED.
- If a medication patch is present on the patient's chest, make sure you are wearing gloves and then remove the patch. Do not place an AED pad over the medication patch and try to defibrillate through it. Examples of medications that may be worn in patch form by patients include NTG; nicotine; hormone replacement therapy; and medications for nausea, vomiting, dizziness, blood pressure, and pain control. After removing the patch, wipe the area clean with a dry cloth before applying the AED pads. Do not use alcohol or alcohol-based cleansers.
- Before delivering a shock with an AED, make sure that oxygen is not flowing over the patient's chest. Fire can be ignited by sparks from poorly applied AED pads in an oxygen-enriched atmosphere.

Operation of the Automated External Defibrillator

Objectives 25, 26, 28, 29, 43

Follow these steps to operate an AED:

1. *Power.* Be sure the patient is lying face up, on a firm, flat surface. Start CPR if the AED is not immediately available. Place the AED next to the rescuer who will be operating it. Turn on the power. Depending on the brand of AED, this is done by either pressing the "on" button or lifting up the AED screen or lid.

2. *Pads.* Open the package containing the AED pads. Connect the pads to the AED cables (if not preconnected). Then apply the pads to the patient's bare chest. The correct position for the pads is usually shown on the package containing the pads. Alternately, it may be shown in a diagram on the AED itself. If the patient's chest is wet, quickly dry it before applying the pads. Briefly stop CPR to allow pad placement on the patient's chest. Connect the cable to the AED.

3. *Analyze.* Analyze the patient's heart rhythm. Some AEDs require you to press an "analyze" button. Other defibrillators automatically start to analyze when the pads are attached to the patient's chest. Do not touch the patient while the AED is analyzing the rhythm.

4. *Shock.* If the AED advises that a shock is indicated, check the patient from head to toe to make sure no one is touching the patient (including you) before pressing the shock

control. Make sure oxygen is not flowing over the patient's chest. Remove oxygen-delivery devices, such as a BM device, from around the patient and stretcher. Shout, "Stand clear!" Press the shock control once it is illuminated and the machine indicates it is ready to deliver the shock. Resume CPR, beginning with chest compressions, immediately after delivery of the shock. Do not stop to check the patient's pulse. After 5 cycles of CPR, reanalyze the rhythm. Continue this sequence until the patient regains a pulse or ALS personnel take over patient care. The decision to remain on scene for ALS personnel, transport and rendezvous with ALS, or transport directly to a medical facility depends on local protocol, transport time, and medical direction.

The adult AED sequence is shown in Skill Drill 14-3.

Inappropriate Delivery of Shocks

Objectives 18, 19

In some cases, an AED may deliver inappropriate shocks. In all cases, it can be attributed to one of two things: mechanical or human error. Mechanical error, such as low batteries, can cause an inappropriate delivery of shocks. This is because accurate rhythm analysis is dependent on properly charged defibrillator batteries.

Human error, such as failure to follow the manufacturer's instructions in the use of an AED, can result in the delivery of inappropriate shocks. To avoid delivering inappropriate shocks:

- Attach an AED only to unresponsive, apneic, pulseless patients
- Place an AED in the "analyze" mode *only* when cardiac arrest has been confirmed and all movement, including the movement of patient transport, has stopped. When transporting a patient, the AED may remain attached to the patient. However, do not press the "analyze" button while the patient is being moved. For example, if you are en route to the hospital with the patient in an ambulance, the vehicle must be brought to a stop before you press the "analyze" button.
- Avoid using cell phones, radios, or other devices that emit electrical signals during rhythm analysis. Signal "noise" may interfere with the AED's analysis of the patient's cardiac rhythm.

Interruption of Cardiopulmonary Resuscitation

Objective 20

Movement caused by CPR can cause the AED to stop its analysis of the patient's rhythm. No one should be touching the patient when the patient's cardiac rhythm is being analyzed and when shocks are delivered. Chest compressions and positive-pressure ventilations must be stopped when the rhythm is being analyzed and when shocks are delivered. This prevents accidental shocks to rescuers and allows accurate rhythm analysis. Resume CPR immediately after delivering a shock or when the AED advises that no shock is indicated.

When chest compressions are stopped for even a few seconds (such as to give rescue breaths or perform other procedures), blood flow to the heart and brain drops quickly and drastically. To help improve your patient's chances of surviving a cardiac arrest, make sure that interruptions in chest compressions are kept to a minimum when performing CPR.

Postresuscitation Care

Objectives 30, 31, 32

If the patient begins moving, check the patient's pulse and breathing. If the patient is breathing adequately, apply oxygen by nonrebreather mask at 15 L/min and transport. If the patient is not breathing adequately, provide positive-pressure ventilation with 100% oxygen. Secure the patient to a stretcher. Depending on local protocol, you may be expected to remain on scene for ALS personnel, begin transport and rendezvous with ALS personnel, or transport directly to a medical facility. Remember to use proper lifting and moving techniques when transferring the patient to the ambulance. Keep the AED attached to the patient during transport. En route, perform a focused physical exam and then perform ongoing assessments every 5 minutes.

Cardiac Arrest During Transport

Objective 27

If you are transporting a patient who stops breathing and becomes pulseless, stop the vehicle. Start CPR and apply the AED. Analyze the rhythm as soon as the AED is ready. Deliver a shock, if indicated. Immediately resume CPR. Continue resuscitation (and transport) according to your local protocol.

Support of the Family

Any emergency involving a cardiac arrest is a stressful situation, regardless of the cause of the arrest. Family members, friends, or bystanders at the scene may be anxious, angry, sad, hysterical, demanding, or impatient. Allow them to have and express their emotions. However, do not let others distract you from treating the patient. Accept their concerns and recognize that their behavior stems from grief.

Adult Automated External Defibrillator Sequence

STEP 1 ▶
- Be sure the patient is lying face up, on a firm, flat surface.
- Place the AED next to the rescuer who will be operating it. Turn on the power of the AED.
- If more than one rescuer is present, one rescuer should continue CPR while the other readies the AED for use.
- One rescuer should apply the AED pads to the patient's bare chest.

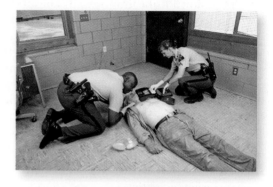

STEP 2 ▶
- Analyze the patient's heart rhythm. Do not touch the patient while the AED is analyzing the rhythm.
- If the AED advises that a shock is indicated, check the patient from head to toe to make sure no one is touching the patient (including you) before pressing the shock control. Make sure oxygen is not flowing over the patient's chest.
- Shout, "Stand clear!"

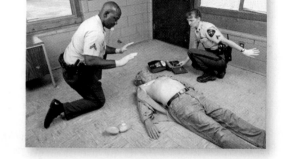

STEP 3 ▶ Press the shock control once it is illuminated and the machine indicates it is ready to deliver the shock.

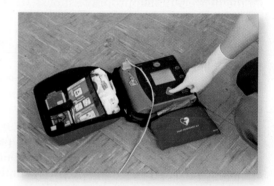

STEP 4 ▶
- After delivery of the shock, quickly resume CPR, beginning with chest compressions.
- After 5 cycles of CPR, reanalyze the rhythm.

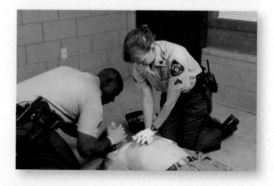

Identify yourself and, using a gentle but firm tone of voice, let them know that everything that can be done to help will be done. Allow family members to be present, unless they are emotionally distraught and interfere with your efforts to resuscitate the patient. Comfort them by being sympathetic and listening with empathy, but do not give false hope or reassurance.

When to Stop Cardiopulmonary Resuscitation

You should stop CPR only if:

- Effective breathing and circulation have returned
- The scene becomes unsafe
- You are too exhausted to continue
- You transfer patient care to a healthcare professional with equal or higher certification
- A physician assumes responsibility for the patient

Automated External Defibrillator Maintenance

Objective 34

Maintenance procedures for an AED should be performed according to the manufacturer's recommendations. Little maintenance is needed with newer AEDs because they perform automated self-tests. Some AEDs perform daily self-tests whereas others occur weekly. An AED self-tests when it is powered on. It may also self-test when batteries are installed. When an AED self-tests, it examines its internal circuitry, battery status, electronics used in heart rhythm analysis, defibrillator electronics, and microprocessor electronics. A manual AED self-test can be performed at any time. Check the policies of your EMS agency regarding requirements for regular maintenance schedules.

Failure of an AED is most often related to improper device maintenance, commonly battery failure. No defibrillator can work properly without properly functioning batteries. Always have extra batteries on hand.

Training and Sources of Information

Objectives 33, 35

Many organizations publish materials about CPR and automated external defibrillation, including the American Heart Association, American Safety and Health Institute, American Red Cross, and National Safety Council.

To maintain skill proficiency, most EMS systems permit a maximum of 90 days between practice drills to reassess proficiency in AED usage; many systems practice skills as often as once a month.

On the Scene   Wrap-Up

Another EMT arrives with the AED and turns it on. After the large electrode patches are applied, he tells you to stop CPR so that the machine can analyze the patient's heart rhythm. The machine's monotone voice states, "Shock advised, stand clear." The other EMT commands "Stand clear!" and scans the patient to be sure no one is touching her as he depresses the flashing shock button. You see her body twitch as the electric shock travels through your patient's heart. After the shock, you resume CPR for about 2 minutes and then wait anxiously as the machine again analyzes her heart rhythm. As the machine says, "No shock advised," you see her chest heave with a sudden intake of breath. You can feel a carotid pulse, weak at first, but stronger with each beat.

You carefully roll the patient onto her side. Your partner then takes a moment to explain the situation to the patient's husband. When the Paramedics arrive, you give a brief report. You cannot believe how exhilarated you feel as you help the Paramedics wheel her out to the ambulance. ∎

Sum It Up

▶ The circulatory system consists of the cardiovascular and lymphatic systems. The cardiovascular system is made up of the heart, blood, and blood vessels. The lymphatic system consists of lymph, lymph nodes, lymph vessels, the tonsils, the spleen, and the thymus gland. The circulatory system is responsible for transporting oxygen, water, and nutrients (such as sugar and vitamins) throughout the body. It also carries away wastes produced by body cells (such as carbon dioxide) to the lungs, kidneys, or skin for removal from the body.

▶ The heart is divided into four chambers. The two upper chambers are the right and left atria. The atria receive blood from the body and lungs. The right atrium receives blood that is low in oxygen from the body. The left atrium receives blood rich in oxygen from the lungs. The two lower chambers of the heart are the right and left ventricles. The ventricles are larger and have thicker walls than the atria because their function is to pump blood to the lungs and body. The right ventricle pumps blood to the lungs. The left ventricle pumps blood to the body.

▶ Four heart valves prevent the backflow of blood and keep blood moving in one direction. The tricuspid and mitral (bicuspid) valves are called atrioventricular (AV) valves because they lie between the atria and ventricles. The aortic and pulmonic valves are called semilunar valves because they are shaped like half-moons.

▶ The liquid portion of the blood is called plasma. Plasma carries blood cells throughout the body. The formed elements of the blood include red blood cells, white blood cells, and platelets.

▶ Blood vessels that carry blood away from the heart to the rest of the body are called arteries. Arteries have thick walls because they transport blood under high pressure. Vessels that return blood to the heart are called veins. The walls of veins are thinner than arteries. Capillaries are the smallest and most numerous of the blood vessels.

▶ Acute coronary syndromes (ACS) are conditions caused by temporary or permanent blockage of a coronary artery as a result of coronary artery disease (CAD). ACSs include unstable angina pectoris and myocardial infarction.

▶ Arteriosclerosis means hardening (-sclerosis) of the walls of the arteries (arterio-). As the walls of the arteries become hardened, they lose their elasticity. In atherosclerosis, the inner lining (endothelium) of the walls of large and medium-size arteries become narrowed and thicken.

▶ Conditions that may increase a person's chance of developing a disease are called risk factors. While some risk factors can be changed, others cannot. Risk factors that can be changed are called modifiable risk factors. Risk factors that cannot be changed are called non-modifiable risk factors. Factors that can be part of the cause of a person's risk of heart disease are called contributing risk factors.

▶ Ischemia is decreased blood flow to an organ or tissue. Ischemia can result from narrowing or blockage of an artery or spasm of an artery. Atherosclerosis is a common reason for narrowing of a coronary artery.

▶ Angina pectoris (literally, "choking in the chest") is a symptom of CAD that occurs when the heart's need for oxygen exceeds its supply. A person is said to have stable angina pectoris when his symptoms are relatively constant and predictable in terms of severity, signs and symptoms, precipitating events, and response to therapy. A person who has unsta-

ble angina pectoris has angina that is progressively worsening, occurs at rest, or is brought on by minimal physical exertion.

▶ An acute myocardial infarction (acute MI; "heart attack") occurs when a coronary artery becomes severely narrowed or is completely blocked, usually by a blood clot (thrombus). When the affected portion of the heart muscle (myocardium) is deprived of oxygen long enough, the area dies (infarcts). If too much of the heart muscle dies, shock (hypoperfusion) and cardiac arrest will result.

▶ The risk of death from a heart attack is related to the time elapsed between the onset of symptoms and start of treatment. The earlier the patient can receive emergency care, the greater the chances of preventing ischemic heart tissue from becoming dead heart tissue.

▶ When a person has congestive heart failure (CHF), one or both sides of the heart fail to pump efficiently. When the left ventricle fails as a pump, blood backs up into the lungs. When the right ventricle fails, blood returning to the heart backs up and causes congestion in the organs and tissues of the body.

▶ Signs and symptoms of a heart attack vary. Although chest discomfort is the most common symptom of a heart attack, some patients never have chest pain. Older adults, diabetic individuals, and women who have a heart attack are more likely to present with signs and symptoms that differ from those of a "typical" patient. This is called an atypical presentation or atypical signs and symptoms.

▶ Many states have passed legislation to include aspirin as a medication that can be carried on an EMS unit and given by EMTs. Check your state and local protocols for the appropriate use of this drug.

▶ As an EMT, you can assist a patient in taking prescribed NTG if the patient has signs and symptoms of chest pain or discomfort, the patient has physician-prescribed NTG, there are no contraindications to giving the medication, and you have specific authorization by medical direction (off line or on line).

▶ If the heart stops beating, no blood will flow. If no blood flows, oxygen cannot be delivered to the body's cells. When the heart stops, the patient is said to be in cardiac arrest. The signs of cardiac arrest include sudden unresponsiveness, absent breathing, and no signs of circulation. Brain damage begins 4 to 6 minutes after the patient suffers a cardiac arrest. Brain damage becomes irreversible in 8 to 10 minutes. Chest compressions are used to circulate blood any time that the heart is not beating. Chest compressions are combined with rescue breathing to oxygenate the blood. The combination of rescue breathing and external chest compressions is called cardiopulmonary resuscitation (CPR).

- Sudden cardiac death (SCD) is the unexpected death from cardiac causes early after symptom onset (immediately or within 1 hour) or without the onset of symptoms. Survival of cardiac arrest depends on a series of critical actions called the Chain of Survival. The Chain of Survival is the ideal series of events that should take place immediately after recognizing an injury or the onset of sudden illness. The chain consists of 4 steps:

  1. Early access
  2. Early CPR
  3. Early defibrillation
  4. Early advanced cardiac life support

- An automated external defibrillator (AED) contains a computer programmed to recognize heart rhythms that should be shocked (defibrillated), such as ventricular fibrillation (VF or Vfib). A standard AED is used for a patient who is unresponsive, not breathing, pulseless, and greater than or equal to 8 years of age (about 55 pounds or more than 25 kg). A special key or pad-cable system is available for some AEDs so that the machine can be used on children between 1 and 8 years of age. The key or pad-cable system decreases the amount of energy delivered to a dose appropriate for a child. If a child is in cardiac arrest and a key or pad-cable system is not available, use a standard AED.

- When an adult experiences a cardiac arrest as a result of VF, prompt defibrillation is the most important treatment you can provide from the time of the arrest to about 5 minutes following the arrest. If you witness a cardiac arrest, assess the patient's airway, breathing, and circulation, and then quickly apply an AED. Perform CPR until the AED is ready.

- To ensure delivery of the best-quality patient care possible, the medical director (or designated representative) carefully reviews every call in which an AED is used. Each call is reviewed to determine if the patient was treated according to professional standards and local standing orders.

- If the patient has a pacemaker or implantable cardioverter-defibrillator (ICD) in place, place the AED pads at least 1 inch from the device.

- Before using an AED, familiarize yourself with the manufacturer's recommendations regarding the use of the device around water. If a medication patch is present on the patient's chest, make sure you are wearing gloves and then remove the patch.

- To operate an AED, place the AED next to the rescuer who will be operating it. Turn on the power. Connect the AED pads to the AED cables (if not preconnected). Then apply the pads to the patient's bare chest in the locations indicated on the pads. Connect the cable to the AED. Analyze the patient's heart rhythm. If the AED advises that a shock is indicated, check the patient from head to toe to make sure no one is touching the patient (including you) before pressing the shock control. Make sure oxygen is not flowing over the patient's chest. Shout, "Stand clear!" Press the shock control once it is illuminated and the machine indicates it is ready to deliver the shock. Resume CPR, beginning with chest compressions, immediately after delivery of the shock.

- If you are transporting a patient who stops breathing and becomes pulseless, stop the vehicle. Start CPR and apply the AED. Analyze the rhythm as soon as the AED is ready. Deliver a shock, if indicated. Immediately resume CPR. Continue resuscitation (and transport) according to your local protocol.

- Maintenance procedures for an AED should be performed according to the manufacturer's recommendations. Failure of an AED is most often related to improper device maintenance, commonly battery failure.

- Many organizations publish materials about CPR and automated external defibrillation, including the American Heart Association, American Safety and Health Institute, American Red Cross, and National Safety Council.

15 Diabetes and Altered Mental Status

By the end of this chapter, you should be able to:

Knowledge Objectives ▶

1. Identify the patient with altered mental status who is taking diabetic medications and the implications of a diabetes history.
2. State the steps in the emergency medical care of the patient with altered mental status who is taking diabetic medications.
3. Establish the relationship between airway management and the patient with altered mental status.
4. State the generic and trade names, medication forms, doses, administration, action, and contraindications for oral glucose.
5. Evaluate the need for medical direction in the emergency medical care of the diabetic patient.

Attitude Objectives ▶

6. Explain the rationale for administering oral glucose.

Skill Objectives ▶

7. Demonstrate the steps in the emergency medical care of the patient with altered mental status who is taking diabetic medications.
8. Demonstrate the steps in the administration of oral glucose.
9. Demonstrate the assessment and documentation of patient response to oral glucose.

On the Scene

You are responding to a call to "Check welfare." A woman called 9-1-1. She says she is worried. Her elderly neighbor has not been seen in two days and his newspapers are stacked up on the front walk. Law enforcement personnel are on the scene and tell you it is safe to enter the residence. You see the patient, an elderly man, lying on the floor. You shake him gently as you say, "I'm an Emergency Medical Technician. Sir, are you all right?" There is no response. You place a hand on his forehead, lift his chin, and look, listen, and feel for breathing. He is breathing quietly, about 16 times per minute. When you reach to feel his radial pulse, you notice how cold and pale his skin is. His heart rate is 128 beats per minute. ■

THINK ABOUT IT

As you read this chapter, think about the following questions:

- What are some possible causes of this patient's altered mental status?
- What additional assessment should you perform?
- Is there more information that you should look for in his home?
- What treatment measures would be appropriate for this patient?

Introduction

A patient with an altered mental status can be challenging to care for because he usually cannot tell you what is wrong. You must obtain a careful history from the patient, family, or others to find out the underlying cause of the patient's altered mental status. An altered mental status should be treated as a medical emergency. Regardless of cause, emergency care of the patient with an altered mental status focuses on the patient's airway, breathing, and circulation.

Altered Mental Status

Altered mental status means a change in a patient's level of awareness. Altered mental status is also called an *altered level of consciousness* (ALOC). When using the AVPU scale to assess a patient's responsiveness, a patient has an altered mental status if he is rated a V, P, or U. The change in the patient's mental status may occur gradually or suddenly. A patient with an altered mental status may appear

You Should Know

Common Causes of Altered Mental Status

A-E-I-O-U TIPPS

- *A*lcohol, Abuse
- *E*pilepsy (seizures)
- *I*nsulin (diabetic emergency)
- *O*verdose, (lack of) oxygen (hypoxia)
- *U*remia (kidney failure)
- *T*rauma (head injury), Temperature (fever, heat- or cold-related emergency)
- *I*nfection
- *P*sychiatric conditions
- *P*oisoning (including drugs and alcohol)
- *S*hock, Stroke

confused, agitated, combative, sleepy, difficult to awaken, or unresponsive. The length of the patient's altered mental status may be brief or prolonged. Examples of conditions that can cause an altered mental status are shown in the preceeding *You Should Know* box.

Emergency Care of Patients with an Altered Mental Status

When assessing a patient who has an altered mental status, keep in mind that the patient's usual mental status may be different from that of the average person. It is important to ask the family if the patient's mental status appears different from what is normal for him or her. Regardless of the cause, emergency care of the patient with an altered mental status focuses on his airway, breathing, and circulation.

Objective 3

- A patient who has an altered mental status is at risk of an airway obstruction. As awareness decreases, muscle tone decreases. When this occurs, the tongue can fall back into the throat and cause an airway obstruction. The breathing muscles may not expand and contract as strongly as normal. This can result in inadequate breathing, low blood oxygen, and respiratory failure.

- Establish and maintain an open airway. Stabilize the cervical spine if there is any possibility of trauma. If the patient cannot maintain his own airway, insert an oral or nasal airway as needed. Suction as necessary.

- Give oxygen. If the patient's breathing is adequate, apply oxygen by mask at 15 L/min. If the patient's breathing is inadequate, assist his breathing with a bag-mask (BM) or mouth-to-mask device.

- Position the patient. If the patient is sitting or standing, help him to a position of comfort on a firm surface. If there is no possibility of trauma to the head or spine, place him in the recovery position.

- Remove or loosen tight clothing.
- Assess the patient's vital signs, including oxygen saturation if a pulse oximeter is available. Assess the patient's blood glucose level (per local protocol).
- Maintain body temperature.
- Comfort, calm, and reassure the patient and his family.
- Reassess for signs that the patient is responding to interventions.

Altered Mental Status with a History of Diabetes

Glucose, a sugar, is the basic fuel for body cells. The level of sugar in the blood (the "blood sugar") must remain fairly constant to ensure proper functioning of the brain and body cells. The brain must constantly be supplied with glucose because it cannot store it. The brain is very sensitive to changes in glucose levels. Changes in glucose levels can result in changes in the patient's behavior.

The body's blood glucose level is primarily regulated by the pancreas (Figure 15-1). Normal blood glucose levels generally range between 70 and 120 milligrams/deciliter (mg/dL). A rise in the blood glucose level (such as after a meal) stimulates beta cells in the pancreas to secrete the hormone insulin. Because glucose is a large molecule, it cannot easily enter the body's cells where it is needed. **Insulin** helps glucose enter the body's cells to be used for energy. As the blood glucose level drops toward normal, the release of insulin slows. Excess glucose is stored in the liver and muscles as glycogen. A drop in the blood glucose level stimulates the release of glucagon from alpha cells in the pancreas. **Glucagon** is a hormone

that stimulates cells in the liver to break down stores of glycogen into glucose. This increases the blood glucose level. As the blood glucose level rises toward normal, the release of glucagon slows. **Somatostatin** is a hormone that is released by delta cells in the pancreas. This hormone inhibits the release of insulin and glucagon (Table 15-1).

For cells to use sugar properly there must be an adequate supply of insulin. In a healthy person, insulin secretion increases after eating. Insulin helps transport glucose from the blood into cells, including muscle, liver, and fat cells where the glucose is stored or used as fuel.

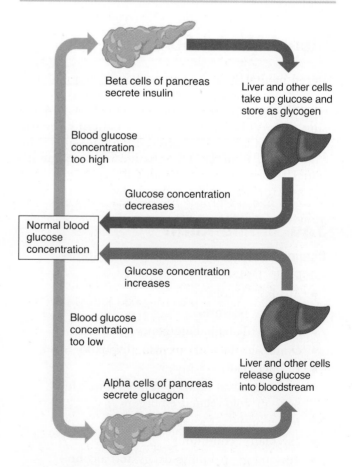

FIGURE 15-1 ▲ The body's blood glucose level is primarily regulated by the pancreas.

TABLE 15-1 Pancreatic Cell Function

Pancreatic Cells	Hormone Released	Hormone Function
Alpha	Glucagon	Stimulates cells in the liver to break down stores of glycogen into glucose; increases blood sugar
Beta	Insulin	Helps glucose enter body cells to be used for energy; decreases blood sugar
Delta	Somatostatin	Inhibits release of insulin and glucagon

TABLE 15-2 Major Types of Diabetes Mellitus

Diabetes Type	Other Names	Possible Causes
Type 1	Insulin-dependent diabetes mellitus (IDDM) Juvenile diabetes	Usually unknown Viral infection Injury to pancreas Immune system disorder
Type 2	Non-insulin-dependent diabetes mellitus (NIDDM) Adult-onset diabetes	Insulin resistance and relative insulin shortage
Gestational	Diabetes during pregnancy	Changes in body metabolism caused by pregnancy

Types of Diabetes

Diabetes mellitus is a disease involving the pancreas. There are three major types of diabetes mellitus (Table 15-2). The pancreas either produces too little insulin or stops producing it completely. Sugar builds up in the blood. The body's cells do not have enough sugar for energy and do not perform properly.

Type 1 Diabetes Mellitus

In **type 1 diabetes mellitus,** little or no insulin is produced by beta cells in the pancreas. This results in a buildup of glucose in the blood. Despite the buildup of glucose in the blood, the body's cells are starved for glucose because without insulin, glucose is unable to enter most body cells.

Although it may occur at any age, type 1 diabetes usually begins during childhood or young adulthood. Signs and symptoms vary widely and may develop suddenly or gradually over days to weeks. Common signs and symptoms are shown in the following *You Should Know* box. Because the patient's pancreas isn't producing insulin, the patient with type 1 diabetes mellitus requires treatment with insulin. Some patients also require treatment with oral medication to manage their blood glucose level.

You Should Know

Type 1 Diabetes: Common Signs and Symptoms

- "Three polys"
  - —**Polyuria** (increased urination)
  - —**Polydipsia** (increased thirst)
  - —**Polyphagia** (increased appetite)
- Abdominal pain with vomiting
- Fruity breath odor
- Blurred vision
- Tiredness

You Should Know

According to the American Diabetes Association, most Americans who are diagnosed with diabetes have type 2 diabetes.

Type 2 Diabetes Mellitus

Type 2 diabetes mellitus is the most common type of diabetes. It usually affects people older than 40 years of age, especially those who are overweight. Type 2 diabetes is caused by a combination of insulin resistance and relative insulin shortage. **Insulin resistance** refers to a condition in which the pancreas releases insulin, but the normal effect of insulin on the tissue cells of the body is diminished. In an attempt to counteract this resistance, the pancreas releases more insulin into the bloodstream. Insulin levels rise. In some cases, glucose builds up in the bloodstream despite the increased amount of insulin. This results in high blood glucose levels or type 2 diabetes. Major causes of insulin resistance include obesity, genetics, sedentary lifestyle, and stress. Type 2 diabetes mellitus can often be managed by diet, exercise, and oral medications that lower blood sugar levels (see Table 15-3). Some people require insulin.

Gestational Diabetes

When a woman develops diabetes during pregnancy, it is called **gestational diabetes.** Gestational diabetes does not include previously diabetic pregnant patients. According to the American Diabetes Association, gestational diabetes affects about 4% of all pregnant women. Hormones released during pregnancy can change the effectiveness of insulin. These changes usually begin in the fifth or sixth month of pregnancy. Diabetes develops if the pancreas cannot make enough insulin to control the level of glucose in the blood. Treatment for gestational diabetes includes a special diet; regular, moderate exercise (according to physician instructions); and daily blood glucose testing. Some patients require insulin injections.

Gestational diabetes usually goes away after the baby is born, but it may take several weeks. The mother is at increased risk for gestational diabetes in her next pregnancy and for type 2 diabetes later in life.

Complications of Diabetes Mellitus

If diabetes is not controlled, high glucose levels can cause complications, particularly to blood vessels and cells of the nervous system (see the following *You Should Know* box). One of the ways people can limit the progression of this disease is to regularly monitor their blood sugar and follow their doctor's instructions regarding diet, exercise, and prescribed medications to help regulate their blood sugar level.

You Should Know

Possible Complications of Diabetes Mellitus

- Changes in the retina that can lead to blindness
- Kidney damage
- Nerve damage that can lead to loss of sensation, numbness, and pain
- Circulatory disorders such as a heart attack, stroke, blood vessel damage, and slow wound healing

Hypoglycemia

Hypoglycemia is a lower-than-normal blood sugar level. In adults, hypoglycemia is a blood glucose level less than 70 mg/dL.

Hypoglycemia is the most common diabetic emergency. The onset of hypoglycemia symptoms is sudden (minutes to hours). Early signs and symptoms of hypoglycemia include signs of stimulation of the sympathetic division of the autonomic nervous system. For example, the presence of sweating, palpitations, increased heart rate, tremors, pale color, hunger, and nervousness serves as an early warning system.

Remember that the brain cannot store glucose. If hypoglycemia is not corrected, signs and symptoms reflecting the brain's lack of an adequate glucose

TABLE 15-3 Examples of Oral Diabetes Medications

Generic name	Trade name
tolbutamide	Orinase
chlorpropamide	Diabinese
tolazamide	Tolinase
glyburide	Micronase
glipizide	Glucotrol
glimepiride	Amaryl
repaglinide	Prandin
metformin	Glucophage
rosiglitazone maleate	Avandia
pioglitazone hydrochloride	Actos

supply will quickly follow. These signs and symptoms may include tiredness, irritability, visual disturbances, difficulty concentrating, confusion, combativeness, fainting, seizures, and loss of consciousness. Prolonged hypoglycemia can lead to irreversible brain damage. Common signs and symptoms of hypoglycemia are shown in Table 15-4.

Remember This!

Hypoglycemia is also called *insulin shock*. Keeping this in mind may help you remember the later signs and symptoms of hypoglycemia.

The blood sugar level may become too low if the diabetic patient:

- Has taken too much insulin
- Has not eaten enough food
- Has overexercised and burned off sugar faster than normal

- Experiences significant physical (such as an infection) or emotional stress

Remember This!

Many patients with serious medical conditions such as diabetes, a drug allergy, or a heart condition carry information with them about their condition. If your patient is unable to answer questions, look for a medical identification card or a medical identification (ID) necklace or bracelet so that you can provide proper emergency care.

Hyperglycemia

Hyperglycemia is a higher-than-normal blood sugar level. The onset of hyperglycemia symptoms is gradual (hours to days).

Normally, the body metabolizes carbohydrates for energy. As hyperglycemia worsens, body cells become starved for sugar. Although sugar is present in the blood, it cannot be transported into the body's cells

TABLE 15-4 Hypoglycemia and Hyperglycemia

	Hypoglycemia	Hyperglycemia
Onset	Sudden (minutes to hours)	Gradual (hours to days)
Signs and Symptoms	Altered mental status (varies from nervousness to coma) **Early signs** • Sweating • Palpitations • Increased heart rate • Tremors • Pale color • Hunger • Headache • Nervousness **Later signs** • Confusion, combativeness, irritability, difficulty concentrating • Tiredness • Staggering walk • Visual disturbances • Cool, pale, clammy skin • Fainting • Seizures • Coma	Altered mental status (varies from drowsiness to coma) Rapid, deep breathing (Kussmaul respirations) Sweet or fruity (acetone) breath odor Loss of appetite Thirst Dry skin Abdominal pain Nausea and/or vomiting Increased heart rate Normal or slightly decreased blood pressure Weakness

without insulin. The buildup of sugar causes the kidneys to increase urine output, which leads to dehydration. Signs of dehydration include warm, dry skin and a loss of skin elasticity (poor skin turgor). Increased urine output results in the loss of large amounts of sodium, potassium, and other electrolytes. This can result in abnormal heart rhythms, abdominal pain, vomiting, and muscle cramping. The body begins breaking down fats and proteins to provide energy. The breakdown of fats and proteins produces waste products, including acids. The patient begins breathing deeply and rapidly in an attempt to get rid of the excess acid by "blowing off" carbon dioxide. This breathing pattern is called **Kussmaul respirations.** The patient's breath may have a fruity (acetone) odor. It has been estimated that 25-30% of the population can't smell ketones on a patient's breath, so you cannot use the absence of this sign to rule out hyperglycemia. Signs and symptoms of hyperglycemia are shown in Table 15-4.

Diabetic ketoacidosis (DKA) is severe, uncontrolled hyperglycemia (usually over 300 mg/dL). DKA usually occurs in people who have type 1 diabetes but may also occur in those who have type 2 diabetes. DKA is also called *diabetic coma.*

The blood sugar level may become too high when the diabetic patient:

- Has not taken his insulin or oral diabetic medication, or has taken an incorrect dose
- Has eaten too much food that contains or produces sugar
- Has lost a large amount of fluid, such as through vomiting
- Experiences physical (such as infection, pregnancy, or surgery) or emotional stress that affects the body's insulin production

You Should Know

Family or friends who may be on the scene of a diabetic emergency can usually direct you to the location of any medications being taken by the patient. If the patient is taking insulin, it is usually stored in the refrigerator with the patient's name and dosage clearly marked on the container.

Patient Assessment

Objective 1

Observe the patient's environment for clues to the cause of the patient's altered mental status. Look for medical identification indicating a history of diabetes and current use of insulin or oral diabetic medication. Assess the patient's abdomen and belt for the presence of an insulin pump. If the patient is in a private residence, look in the refrigerator for insulin.

Perform a primary survey. Stabilize the spine if needed. Assess the patient's mental status, airway, breathing, and circulation. Identify any life-threatening conditions and provide care based on those findings. Establish patient priorities. Priority patients include:

- Patients who give a poor general impression
- Unresponsive patients with no gag reflex or cough
- Responsive patients who are unable to follow commands

Advanced Life Support (ALS) assistance should be requested as soon as possible. If ALS personnel are not available, the patient should be transported promptly to the closest appropriate facility.

Perform a physical examination. If the patient is unresponsive, perform a rapid medical assessment. Follow with evaluation of baseline vital signs and gathering of the patient's medical history. If the patient is responsive, gather information about the patient's medical history and then perform a focused medical assessment. Sources of information for a patient who has an altered mental status include the scene, family members, friends, and bystanders. Information obtained from the patient may be unreliable. Examples of questions to ask when caring for a patient who has an altered mental status are shown in the next *Making a Difference* box. Provide all information obtained to the receiving facility.

Emergency Care

Objectives 2, 3

- Stabilize the spine if trauma is suspected.
- Any patient who has an altered mental status is at risk of not being able to manage his own airway. It is critical for you to aggressively assess the need for an oral or nasal airway and to continuously monitor and reassess the patient's airway. Suction as necessary.
- Give oxygen. If the patient's breathing is adequate, apply oxygen by nonrebreather mask at 15 L/min if not already done. If the patient's breathing is inadequate, provide positive-pressure ventilation with 100% oxygen and assess the adequacy of the ventilations delivered.
- Position the patient. If there is no possibility of cervical spine trauma, place the patient

in a lateral recumbent (recovery) position to aid drainage of secretions. If the patient who is immobilized because of suspected trauma vomits, the patient and backboard should be turned as a unit and the patient's airway cleared with suctioning.

- Remove or loosen tight clothing. Maintain body temperature.
- Perform a blood glucose test (if permitted by state and local protocol).
- If the patient is responsive, determine if the patient is alert enough to swallow. Give oral glucose according to local or state medical direction or protocol.
- Transport. Perform ongoing assessments until patient care is turned over to ALS personnel or medical personnel at the receiving facility.

Making a Difference

Questions to ask about a patient experiencing a possible diabetic emergency:

- Does the patient have a history of diabetes?
- What time did the patient's symptoms begin? Did the patient's symptoms begin suddenly or gradually?
- What was the patient doing when his symptoms began?
- When was the patient's last meal or snack? How much did the patient eat (or drink)? Did the patient vomit after eating? Has the patient skipped any meals?
- Is the patient taking any medications (prescription and over the counter)?
- When did the patient last take his medications? For patients taking insulin, ask whether they have taken their insulin today and how much insulin was taken. Has the patient's insulin (or oral diabetic medication) dosage changed recently?
- Does the patient have any associated symptoms (such as nausea, vomiting, weakness)?
- Has the patient performed an unusual exercise or physical activity today?
- Has the patient had a recent infection or surgery?
- Has the patient experienced any psychological stress?
- Has the patient consumed any alcohol?
- What is the patient's normal blood glucose level? What was the patient's blood sugar level the last time it was measured?

Remember This!

Because a lack of glucose can cause permanent brain damage, any diabetic patient with an altered mental status should be considered to have hypoglycemia until proven otherwise.

Remember This!

Patients who have had diabetes for some time are often familiar with the EMS system. After receiving glucose for hypoglycemia, the patient's mental status usually quickly returns to normal. Some patients then refuse transport to the hospital. In these situations, you should contact medical direction for instructions about how to proceed. In specific cases, medical direction will allow the patient to refuse transport if you make sure that an adult is present and the patient eats a substantial meal. If these conditions are met and medical direction authorizes the patient's refusal, complete a refusal form. The patient's signature should be obtained on the form and a witness signature should be obtained at the same time. Ideally, this will be the person taking responsibility for the patient. Be sure to document the advice the patient was given, the patient's understanding of the risks of his refusal, and the patient's understanding of the possible outcome if the advice given is not followed.

Performing a Blood Glucose Test

Blood glucose testing is used to assist in the management of patients with specific signs and symptoms. The results obtained from the test helps determine if the patient's glucose level is too high, too low, or within normal limits. Patient care, treatment, and outcome may be improved with its use.

Indications

1. Unresponsive patient, cause unknown (any age group, including trauma)
2. Known diabetic patient with any of the following signs and symptoms:
   - Altered mental status (confusion, change in usual behavior)
   - Unresponsiveness
   - Slurred speech
   - Cold and clammy skin or hot, dry skin/mucous membranes
   - Pale or flushed color
   - Sweating

- Headache, dizziness
- Palpitations and/or abnormal heart rhythm seen on heart monitor
- Visual disturbances
- Shakiness or states "feels funny"
- Excessive urination/thirst
- Acetone (fruity) breath
- Rapid, deep breathing (Kussmaul respirations)
- Seizures

3. Patients with altered mental status, cause unknown (including trauma), especially if showing signs/symptoms listed above
4. Special situations
   - Infant or child having seizures or an altered mental status
   - Pregnancy with signs and symptoms listed previously or signs and symptoms of pregnancy-induced hypertension (see Chapter 20)
   - Older adults
   - Patients with a history of alcoholism
   - Overweight patients
   - Malnourished patients
   - Patients on long-term drug therapies, such as steroids or hormonal therapy

Procedure

To check a patient's glucose level, you will take a blood sample from the patient. In adults, the most common site used is the side of a finger. Pricking the side of a finger (or toe) is less painful than pricking the pad of a finger or toe. The device used to prick the patient's finger is called a **lancet.** Some lancets are adjustable, allowing you to change how deeply the lancet pierces the patient's skin. This is important if alternate sites are used, such as the fleshy part of the hand, base of the thumb, upper arm, thigh, and back of the calf.

You Should Know

If you use a site other than the fingertip to test a patient's blood glucose level, keep in mind that alternate sites will not show changes in blood glucose levels as quickly as the fingertips. If you suspect your patient has hypoglycemia, use the fingertip for glucose testing.

The device used to measure the amount of glucose in a blood sample is called a **blood glucose meter**

or **glucometer.** A drop of blood is placed on a patch on a test strip. The test strip is inserted into the glucometer. The glucometer analyzes the specimen and gives a digital display of the patient's glucose level. Many patients who have diabetes have a glucometer to regularly check their glucose levels. Physicians and diabetes educators usually tell their patients to check their glucose level before meals, before bed, and one to two hours after meals. If the patient has type 1 diabetes, the patient is usually asked to check his glucose level at 2 a.m. or 3 a.m. at least once a week. In addition to these "routine" tests, the patient may need to check his glucose level before exercising, if he shows signs or symptoms of low blood sugar, and when he is sick.

Skill Drill 15-1 shows how to perform a blood glucose test with a glucometer. Because the features of glucometers vary, be sure you are familiar with the devices approved for use in your EMS system.

You Should Know

Blood Glucose Testing: Equipment

- Blood glucose test strips
- Glucometer
- Disposable lancets
- Disposable gloves
- Gauze pads
- Alcohol swabs
- Small adhesive bandage
- Watch or clock with second hand (if using color-changing strips)
- Sharps container

Oral Glucose

Objectives 4, 5

If approved by medical direction (and your state and local EMS system), you may give oral glucose to a patient who has an altered mental status and a history of diabetes controlled by medication and is able to swallow. Oral glucose given to a patient with an altered mental status and a known history of diabetes can make a difference between development of coma (unconsciousness) and ability to maintain consciousness. If oral glucose is not available (and if approved by medical direction), other quick-sugar mixtures can be used. It has been estimated that quick-sugar food (see the next *Remember This!* box) can increase a person's blood sugar about 30 mg/dL in about 20 minutes.

Performing a Blood Glucose Test with a Glucometer

STEP 1 ▶
- Put on appropriate personal protective equipment.
- Identify the need for blood glucose testing on the basis of your assessment findings, the patient's chief complaint, and past medical history.

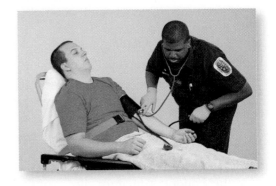

STEP 2 ▶
- Assemble and prepare the necessary equipment.
- Explain the procedure to the patient.

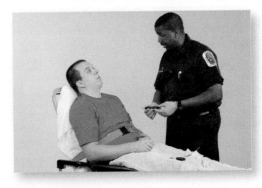

STEP 3 ▶
- Select and cleanse the puncture site. Be sure to allow the area to dry before pricking the skin. Any alcohol present on the skin will interfere with the test results.
- Prick the skin quickly with the lancet to get a small drop of blood. Apply a drop of blood on the test strip. Be sure to completely cover the patch on the test strip with blood.

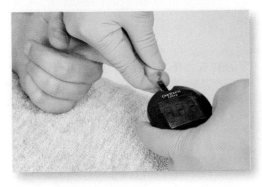

STEP 4 ▶
- Turn on the glucometer. Insert the test strip. (Some manufacturers have the test strip placed in the machine before the drop of blood is obtained. Follow the manufacturer's instructions).
- Wait for the glucometer to analyze the sample and display the patient's glucose reading.
- Apply a small adhesive bandage to the puncture site.

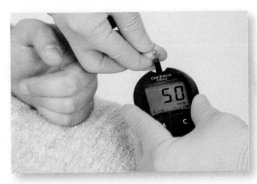

Quick-Sugar Foods

- Fruit juice, such as orange or apple juice (½ cup)
- Water mixed with 1 tablespoon of table sugar
- Jam or jelly (2 tablespoons)
- Honey or corn syrup (1 tablespoon)
- Regular (nondiet) soft drink (½ cup)

Before giving any medication, specific criteria must be met (Table 15-5). These criteria include making sure that the medication to be given is indicated for the patient. You must also make sure that the patient does not have any allergies to the medication. Even though you are giving glucose, it is possible that the patient may have an allergy to the way the drug is packaged or manufactured. If a drug contains any preservatives, it is possible the patient may have an adverse reaction to the preservative in the medication. Next, you must make sure that the patient is responsive, has an open airway, and can swallow. Because any patient who has an altered mental status has the potential to become unresponsive without warning, it is essential to make sure the patient has (and maintains) an open airway. If all of these criteria are met and medical direction has given the order to administer the drug, oral glucose can be given. Skill Drill 15-2 shows the steps in giving oral glucose.

Seizures

Seizures are another possible cause of altered mental status. A **seizure** is a temporary change in behavior or consciousness caused by abnormal electrical activity within one or more groups of brain cells. A seizure is a symptom (not a disease) of an underlying problem within the central nervous system.

The most common cause of adult seizures in a patient with a known seizure disorder is the failure to take anti-seizure medication. The most common cause of seizures in infants and young children is a high fever. **Epilepsy** is a condition of recurring seizures in which the cause is usually irreversible. Known causes of seizures are shown in the next *You Should Know* box. The cause of seizures is unknown in 30% of cases.

Types of Seizures

Although there are many different types of seizures, they can be categorized into two main areas—generalized seizures and partial seizures. Partial seizures can evolve into generalized seizures.

TABLE 15-5 Oral Glucose

Generic name	oral glucose
Trade name	Glutose, Insta-glucose
Mechanism of action	Increases the amount of sugar available for use as energy by the body
Indications	Patients with altered mental status who have a known history of diabetes controlled by medication and can swallow
Dosage	One tube
Side effects	• None when given properly • May be aspirated by the patient without a gag reflex
Contraindications	• Medical direction does not give permission • Unresponsive • Unable to swallow • Known allergy to the glucose preparation

Giving Oral Glucose

STEP 1 ▷
- Put on appropriate personal protective equipment.
- Obtain an order from medical direction either on line or off line.
- Confirm that the patient has an altered mental status, has a history of diabetes controlled by medication, and is able to swallow and protect his airway.

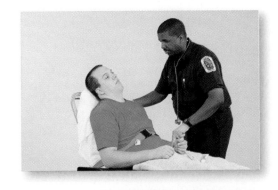

STEP 2 ▷ Squeeze the glucose from the tube onto a tongue depressor.

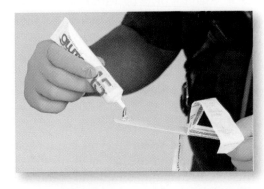

STEP 3 ▷
- Place the tongue depressor between the patient's cheek and gum.
- Remove the tongue depressor from the patient's mouth once the gel is dissolved or if the patient loses consciousness or seizes.

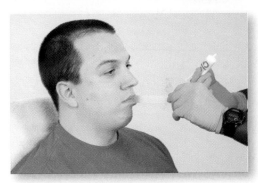

STEP 4 ▷
- Document the patient's name, drug name and dose given, time of administration, and response to the drug.
- If an on-line order was received by medical direction, document the name of the physician giving the order.
- Perform ongoing assessments every five minutes, continuously monitoring the patient's airway and breathing.

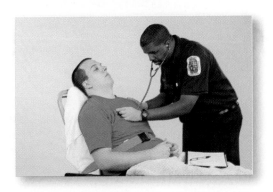

Known Causes of Seizures

- Failure to take anti-seizure medication
- Rapid rise in body temperature (febrile seizure)
- Infection
- Low oxygen level (hypoxia)
- Head trauma
- Brain tumor
- Poisoning
- Low blood sugar level (hypoglycemia)
- Seizure disorder
- Previous brain damage
- Electrolyte disturbances
- Alcohol or drug withdrawal
- Eclampsia (seizures associated with pregnancy)
- Abnormal heart rhythm
- Genetic and hereditary factors
- Stroke

Generalized Seizures

A **generalized seizure** begins suddenly and involves a period of altered mental status. In this type of seizure, nerve cells in both hemispheres of the brain begin firing abnormally. There are two main types of generalized seizures, tonic-clonic seizures and absence seizures.

Tonic-Clonic Seizures

When most people hear the word "seizure," they think of the kind of seizure that involves stiffening and jerking of the patient's body. This type of generalized seizure is called a **tonic-clonic seizure** and is very common. Tonic-clonic seizures are also called *generalized motor seizures* or *grand mal seizures*. A tonic-clonic seizure usually has four phases:

1. Aura
2. Tonic phase
3. Clonic phase
4. Postictal phase

An **aura** is a peculiar sensation that comes before a seizure. Not all seizures are preceded by an aura. Common auras are listed in the following *You Should Know* box. The aura is followed by a loss of consciousness. During the tonic phase, the body's muscles stiffen (Figure 15-2). The patient's breathing may be noisy, and he may turn blue. This phase usually lasts 15 to 20 seconds. During the clonic phase, alternating jerking and relaxation of the body occurs. The jerking movements during the clonic phase are often called **convulsions.** This is the longest phase of the seizure. It may last several minutes.

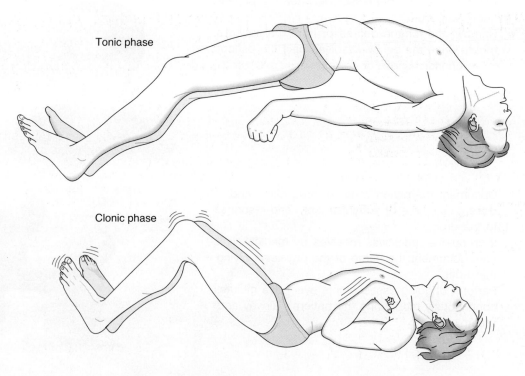

Tonic phase

Clonic phase

FIGURE 15-2 ▲ During the tonic phase of a seizure, the body's muscles stiffen. During the clonic phase, alternating jerking and relaxation of the body occurs.

The patient's heart rate and blood pressure are increased. His skin is usually warm, flushed, and moist. He may lose control of his bowels and bladder. Bleeding may occur if the patient bites his tongue or cheek.

The **postictal phase** is the period of recovery that follows a seizure. During this period, the patient often appears limp, has shallow breathing, and has an altered mental status. This altered mental status may appear as confusion, sleepiness, memory loss, unresponsiveness, or difficulty talking. During this phase the patient slowly awakens. He may complain of a headache and muscle soreness. This phase may last minutes to hours.

You Should Know

Common Auras
- Unusual taste
- Dreamy feeling
- Feeling of fear
- Visual disturbance such as a flashing or floating light
- Unpleasant odor
- Stomach pain
- Rising or sinking feeling in the stomach

Absence Seizures

Absence (petit mal) **seizures** are another type of generalized seizure. They usually occur in children older than 5 years of age and can occur in adults. An absence seizure is characterized by a brief loss of consciousness (for 5 to 10 seconds) without a loss of muscle tone. The patient may have a blank stare accompanied by slight head turning or eye blinking. This type of seizure does not cause muscle contractions and is not associated with an aura or postictal state.

Partial Seizures

In a **partial seizure,** nerve cells fire abnormally in one hemisphere of the brain. There are two main categories of partial seizures, simple partial seizures and complex partial seizures. A partial seizure may progress into a generalized seizure.

Simple Partial Seizures

A **simple partial seizure** (also called a *focal seizure* or *focal motor seizure*) involves motor or sensory symptoms with no change in mental status. This type of seizure usually lasts about 10 to 20 seconds. Examples of motor symptoms include stiffening or jerking of muscles in one part of the body. For instance, the patient's face or an extremity may begin to twitch or jerk. Sensory symptoms may include pain, numbness, or tingling that is localized to a specific area.

Complex Partial Seizures

A **complex partial seizure** (also called a *temporal lobe seizure* or *psychomotor seizure*) is a partial seizure in which the patient's consciousness, responsiveness, or memory is impaired. This type of seizure is often preceded by an aura and generally lasts for less than 30 minutes (averaging about 1 to 3 minutes). A complex partial seizure may be associated with repeat behaviors (**automatisms**) such as lip-smacking, chewing or swallowing movements, fumbling of the hands, or shuffling of the feet. Postictal confusion or sleep may follow the seizure.

Status Epilepticus

Status epilepticus is recurring seizures without an intervening period of consciousness. Status epilepticus is a medical emergency. It can cause brain damage or death if it is not treated. Complications associated with status epilepticus include the following:

- Aspiration of vomitus and blood
- Long-bone and spine fractures
- Dehydration
- Brain damage caused by a lack of oxygen or a depletion of glucose (sugar)

Remember This!

Brain damage can occur in as little as 5 minutes of sustained seizure activity; therefore, emergency ALS intervention should occur as quickly as possible. Do not delay transport for the seizure activity to abate in cases of prolonged seizures.

Patient Assessment

When you arrive on the scene, perform a scene size-up before starting emergency medical care. If the scene is safe, approach the patient and try to find out if the seizure is the result of trauma or an illness. Remember to put on appropriate personal protective equipment (PPE). Check for a medical ID. Look for evidence of burns or suspicious substances that might indicate poisoning or a toxic exposure. Are there signs of recent trauma? Perform a primary survey and a physical exam. Demonstrate a caring attitude when performing your assessment and providing care.

Depending on its severity, injuries can occur during a seizure. Because he may bite his tongue or cheek during a seizure, be sure to look in the patient's mouth for bleeding when the seizure is over. You may see scrapes on his head, face, or extremities because of the seizure. Fractures of the skull, arm, or leg can also occur.

When taking the patient's SAMPLE history, speak with kindness to the family members and friends of the patient. Show concern about the patient's condition and well-being. Find out if the patient has any allergies. Also find out if he is taking any medications (prescription and over the counter). Has there been any recent change in his medications (a new medication, a medication that he has stopped taking, or a change in dosage)? When finding out the patient's past medical history, ask the following questions:

- Is this the patient's first seizure?
- If the patient has a history of seizures, is he on a seizure medication? Did the patient take the prescribed medication today? How often do the seizures usually happen? Does this seizure look like those the patient has had before?
- Does the patient have a history of stroke or diabetes? (Low blood sugar can cause seizures.)
- Does he have a history of heart disease? (An irregular heart rhythm can cause a low oxygen level and lead to seizures.)
- Does the patient use or abuse alcohol or drugs? (Alcohol or drug withdrawal can result in seizures).

When finding out the events that led to the seizure, think about the questions in the following bulleted list. If the seizure has stopped by the time you arrive, be sure to ask what the seizure looked like. If the seizure is in progress when you arrive, keep these questions in mind while watching the patient. You will need to describe what you saw (or what the family or bystanders describe to you) to ALS personnel who arrive on the scene or to the staff at the receiving facility. Your description of the seizure may be important in finding the cause of the seizure.

- What was the patient doing at the time of the seizure? Did he hit his head or fall?
- Did the patient cry out or attract your attention in any way?
- What did the seizure look like? When did the seizure start? How long did it last?
- Did the seizure begin in one area of the body and progress to others?
- Did the patient lose bowel or bladder control?

- When the patient woke up, was there any change in his speech? Was he able to move his arms and legs normally?
- Did the patient exhibit any unusual behavior before, during, or after the seizure?

You Should Know

- Many cardiac arrests are called in to 9-1-1 as a seizure.
- More than 30% of new patients with epilepsy will never know what causes their seizures.

Emergency Care

Treating a patient experiencing a seizure can be difficult. If the patient is postictal, he is sometimes combative or confused. The patient may not let you perform the skills that are necessary. As a result, frustration can set in on both sides. Keep in mind that you are on the scene for a purpose. That purpose is to provide the best emergency care possible. It may take you several attempts to get answers to questions, put oxygen on the patient, or get the patient loaded into the ambulance. Remember that as a patient becomes conscious in the postictal phase, confusion and combativeness are normal. No matter what caused the seizure, your emergency care must focus on the patient's airway, breathing, and circulation.

- Protect the patient's privacy. Ask bystanders (except the patient's family or caregiver) to leave the area.
- Position the patient. If the patient is sitting or standing, help him to the floor.
- If the patient is actively seizing, protect the patient from harm by moving furniture and other objects away from the patient (Figure 15-3). Protect the patient's head with a pillow or other soft material. Do not insert anything into the patient's mouth. This includes your fingers, an oral airway, a padded tongue blade, or a bite block. Undo any tight clothing. Remove eyeglasses. Do not try to restrain body movements during the seizure.
- As soon as the seizure is over, make sure the patient's airway is open. Be sure to have suction available because the patient may vomit during or after the seizure. Gently suction the patient's mouth if secretions are present. If the patient's breathing is adequate, apply oxygen by mask at 15 L/min. If the seizure is prolonged or if the patient's breathing is inadequate, assist his breathing with a BM or mouth-to-mask device. If

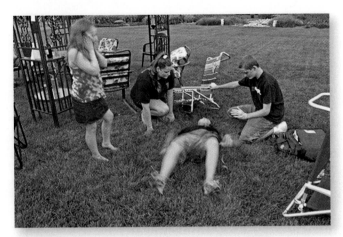

FIGURE 15-3 ▲ Protect a person who is having a seizure from harm by moving furniture and other objects away from him. If he is wearing eyeglasses, remove them. Undo any tight clothing.

the patient is confused or agitated, he may not tolerate an oxygen mask. In this case, blow-by oxygen is acceptable. When the patient is able to tolerate a mask, it should be applied. Place the patient in the recovery position if no trauma is suspected.

- Comfort, calm, and reassure the patient and his family. Watch the patient very closely for repeat seizures.

- When ALS personnel arrive at the scene (or when transferring patient care at the receiving facility), pass on any patient information that you have gathered. You should include what the patient looked like when you first arrived on the scene, the care you gave, and the patient's response to your care. You should also include in your report any background information obtained from friends and family about the nature and appearance of the seizure.

- Some patients are light sensitive (photophobic) after a seizure. Take care to reduce the patient's exposure to bright lights and loud noises. Although rapid transport may be the best course of action, take care not to stimulate the patient more than necessary.

Stroke

A **stroke** is caused by the blockage or rupture of an artery supplying the brain (Figure 15-4). A stroke is also called a *cerebrovascular accident* or *brain attack*. Strokes cause brain injury because the blood supply to the brain is reduced or cut off. The brain is deprived of necessary oxygen and nutrients, resulting in injury to the brain cells.

Types of Stroke

There are two main forms of stroke: ischemic and hemorrhagic. **Ischemic strokes** are caused by a blood clot that decreases blood flow to the brain. Eighty percent of all strokes are ischemic strokes. Ischemic strokes can be further classified as either thrombotic or embolic (Figure 15-5). In a thrombotic stroke, a blood clot (thrombus) forms in a blood vessel of, or

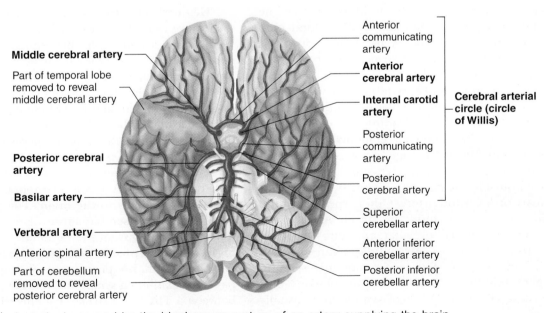

Middle cerebral artery

Part of temporal lobe removed to reveal middle cerebral artery

Posterior cerebral artery

Basilar artery

Vertebral artery

Anterior spinal artery

Part of cerebellum removed to reveal posterior cerebral artery

Anterior communicating artery

Anterior cerebral artery

Internal carotid artery

Posterior communicating artery

Posterior cerebral artery

Superior cerebellar artery

Anterior inferior cerebellar artery

Posterior inferior cerebellar artery

Cerebral arterial circle (circle of Willis)

FIGURE 15-4 ▲ A stroke is caused by the blockage or rupture of an artery supplying the brain.

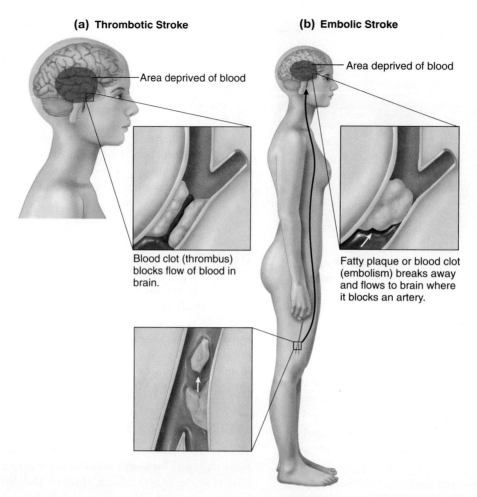

(a) Thrombotic Stroke

Area deprived of blood

Blood clot (thrombus) blocks flow of blood in brain.

(b) Embolic Stroke

Area deprived of blood

Fatty plaque or blood clot (embolism) breaks away and flows to brain where it blocks an artery.

FIGURE 15-5 ▲ Ischemic strokes are caused by a blood clot that decreases blood flow to the brain. The blood vessel may be partially or completely blocked by the blood clot. **(a)** Thrombotic stroke. **(b)** Embolic stroke.

leading to, the brain. The blood vessel may be partially or completely blocked by the blood clot. Symptom onset is gradual. A thrombotic stroke is the most common cause of stroke in persons over 50 years of age.

In an embolic stroke, a blood clot breaks up and travels through the circulatory system where it lodges in a vessel within or leading to the brain. The blood clot is now called an **embolus.** A cerebral embolus results from blockage of a vessel within the brain by a fragment of a foreign substance originating from outside the central nervous system, usually the heart or a carotid artery. Other types of emboli include tumor fragments, an air embolus (from injury to the chest), or a fat embolus (from an injury to a long bone). An embolism can occur in persons of any age, but it is commonly seen in young or middle-aged adults and in persons with preexisting diseases. Onset of symptoms is usually sudden.

Hemorrhagic strokes (also called *cerebral hemorrhages*) are caused by bleeding into the brain (Figure 15-6). They account for the remaining 20% of all strokes. There are two forms of hemorrhagic stroke. **Subarachnoid hemorrhage** is caused by a ruptured blood vessel in the subarachnoid space, usually caused by an **aneurysm** (an abnormal bulging of a blood vessel). **Intracerebral hemorrhage** is caused by a ruptured blood vessel within the brain itself (usually a result of chronic high blood pressure).

A **transient ischemic attack (TIA)** is sometimes called a *mini-stroke.* A TIA is a temporary interruption of the blood supply to the brain. The patient's signs and symptoms resemble those of a stroke but are temporary, lasting from a few minutes to several hours. Signs and symptoms completely resolve within 24 hours with no permanent damage. While the patient is exhibiting symptoms, it is not possible to tell between a TIA and a stroke. Patients who experience a TIA may be at increased risk for eventual stroke.

Subarachnoid hemorrhage

Intracerebral hemorrhage

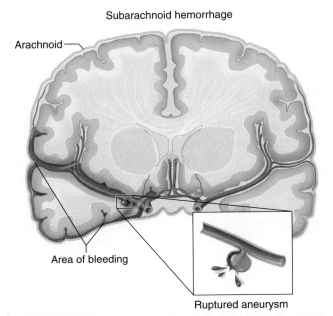

Arachnoid

Area of bleeding

Ruptured aneurysm

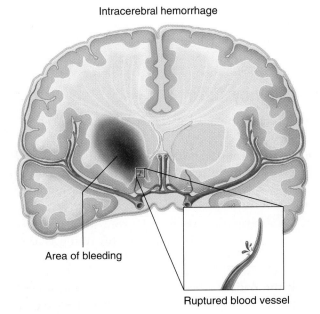

Area of bleeding

Ruptured blood vessel

FIGURE 15-6 ▲ A hemorrhagic stroke is caused by bleeding into the brain.

Making a Difference

The Cincinnati Prehospital Stroke Scale

If a person has an altered mental status, you can quickly assess three areas to find out if he might be having a stroke:

1. Ask the patient to smile. Both sides of the face should move equally. If one side droops, does not move at all, or does not move as well as the other side, request ALS personnel right away or begin transport to the closest appropriate facility.

2. Ask the patient to close his eyes and raise his arms out in front of him. Both arms should move the same or both arms should not move at all. If one arm either does not move or one arm drifts down compared with the other, request ALS personnel right away or begin transport to the closest appropriate facility.

3. Ask the patient to say a simple sentence, for example, "You can't teach an old dog new tricks" or "The sky is blue in Cincinnati." The patient should be able to say the right words without slurring or forgetting or substituting words. Request ALS personnel right away or begin transport to the closest appropriate facility if the patient is unable to speak, slurs words, or uses the wrong words.

This technique is called the *Cincinnati Prehospital Stroke Scale*. You may be able to recognize key signs of a stroke by using this simple test.

Risk Factors

Risk factors for stroke include:

- Hypertension
- Cigarette smoking
- Cardiovascular diseases, such as atherosclerosis, myocardial infarction (heart attack), and heart rhythm disorders (such as atrial fibrillation)
- Diabetes mellitus
- TIA

Signs and Symptoms

The patient's signs and symptoms are related to the artery affected and the part of the brain deprived of oxygen, glucose, and other nutrients. A stroke occurring on the right side of the brain will produce symptoms on the left side of the body. A stroke occurring on the left side of the brain will affect the right side of the body.

Warning signs of a stroke include:

- Sudden weakness or numbness of the face, arm, or leg on one side of the body
- Sudden dimness or loss of vision, particularly in one eye
- Loss of speech or trouble talking or understanding speech
- Sudden, severe headache with no known cause
- Unexplained dizziness, unsteadiness, or sudden falls, especially with any of the previous symptoms

- Confusion, agitation
- Seizures
- Inappropriate behavior, such as excessive laughing or crying

Emergency Care

- Maintain spinal stabilization if trauma is suspected.
- Establish and maintain an open airway. Remove ill-fitting dentures, if present. Insert an oral or nasal airway as needed. Have suction equipment readily available, and suction as necessary.
- Give oxygen as specified by your local protocol. In most areas, if the patient's breathing is adequate and his oxygen saturation is more than 93%, low-flow oxygen is given by nasal cannula. If the patient's breathing is inadequate, provide positive-pressure ventilation with 100% oxygen and assess the adequacy of the ventilations delivered.
- Position the patient. If the patient is unresponsive and there is no possibility of cervical spine trauma, place the patient in the recovery (lateral recumbent) position to aid drainage of secretions. If the patient is immobilized because of suspected trauma and vomits, the patient and backboard should be turned as a unit and the patient's airway cleared with suctioning.
- Protect paralyzed extremities from injury.
- Explain procedures to the patient. Although the patient may be unresponsive or responsive but unable to speak, he may still be able to hear and understand. This is called *expressive aphasia*. If the patient is unable to understand your words or speech, he may be experiencing *receptive aphasia*.
- Monitor mental status, blood pressure, pulse, and respirations often and document your findings.
- Do not give the patient anything to eat or drink.
- Attempt to find out from the patient, family members, friends, or bystanders:
  —If the patient sustained trauma to the head or neck
  —If the patient is taking any medications, including prescription, over-the-counter (such as aspirin), and illicit drugs.
  —When the patient's symptoms began
  —Whether the onset of symptoms was gradual or sudden
  —Whether the patient had any seizure activity

—Pertinent past medical history (such as a previous stroke, TIA, diabetes mellitus, angina, heart attack, heart rhythm disorder, smoking, and/or high blood pressure)

Syncope

Because the brain is unable to store important nutrients such as oxygen and glucose, disruption of the blood flow to the brain for more than 5 to 10 seconds will result in unresponsiveness. **Syncope** (fainting) is a brief loss of responsiveness caused by a temporary decrease in blood flow to the brain. Syncope is sometimes called a *blackout*. Common causes of syncope are listed in the following *You Should Know* box.

You Should Know

Syncope: Common Causes

- Low blood sugar
- Bearing down when urinating or having a bowel movement
- Strenuous coughing
- Breath holding or hyperventilation
- Blood drawing or the sight of blood
- Standing in one place too long
- Bleeding, dehydration
- Some drugs used for anxiety, high blood pressure, nasal congestion, and allergies
- Sudden drop in blood pressure
- Standing up suddenly from a lying position
- Head trauma
- Hot and humid conditions
- Crowded places
- Eating a heavy meal
- Fasting
- Heart rate that is too fast or too slow
- Stroke
- Witness to violence or other disturbing experiences

Before a person faints, he often has warning signs or symptoms (see the following *You Should Know* box). These warning signs and symptoms are called **near syncope** or **presyncope.** Syncope usually results within a few seconds of the onset of symptoms. The patient usually recovers shortly after lying down.

Near Syncope: Signs and Symptoms

- Dizziness
- Anxiety
- Lightheadedness
- Pale skin
- Sweating
- Weakness
- Nausea
- Thready pulse
- Low blood pressure
- Partial or complete loss of vision or hearing

Patient Assessment

Perform a primary survey. If there is any possibility of trauma, stabilize the spine. Assess the patient's mental status, airway, breathing, and circulation. Just before fainting, the patient's skin is often cool, pale, and moist. This is the sympathetic nervous system's attempt to restore blood flow to the brain. The patient's skin usually returns to normal color and temperature when he is placed in a lying position and his blood pressure returns to normal. Suspect hypovolemic shock or a heart problem if the patient's skin remains cool and clammy after he is placed in a lying position. Hot or warm, dry skin may indicate a fever. This can result in dehydration and hypovolemia. Look inside the patient's mouth and assess the elasticity of the patient's skin (skin turgor). Dry mucous membranes and poor skin turgor suggest dehydration and hypovolemia.

Perform a focused history and physical examination. If the patient is unresponsive, perform a rapid medical assessment. Follow with evaluation of baseline vital signs and gathering of the patient's medical history. If the patient is responsive, gather information about the patient's medical history and then perform a focused medical assessment. Examples of questions to ask the patient, family members, friends, and bystanders at the scene are shown in the following *Making a Difference* box. Provide all information obtained to the ALS personnel who arrive on the scene or to the staff at the receiving facility.

Remember This!

You can generally tell the difference between a seizure and syncope. With syncope, the patient regains consciousness within a couple of minutes and is completely alert after the event.

Questions to ask about a patient with near syncope or syncope

- When did the patient's symptoms begin?
- What was the patient doing when his symptoms began?
- Is this the first time the patient has fainted?
- Were there any symptoms before the event? For example, did the patient complain of weakness, lightheadedness, dizziness, visual disturbances, headache, chest pain, or pounding in his chest before he fainted?
- Did anyone see what happened? Did you see any jerking muscle movements? Did the patient lose control of his bowels or bladder?
- If the patient fainted, how long was the patient unresponsive? Did the patient appear confused after awakening?
- Did the patient fall? Are there any signs of trauma?
- What is the patient's past medical history? Does the patient have a history of diabetes, seizures, high blood pressure, heart problems, or any other condition?
- When was the patient's last meal or snack?
- Is the patient taking any medications (prescription or over the counter)? When did the patient last take his medications?

Emergency Care

- Establish and maintain an open airway. Stabilize the cervical spine if there is any possibility of trauma. If the patient cannot maintain his own airway, insert an oral or nasal airway as needed. Suction as necessary.
- Give oxygen. If the patient's breathing is adequate, apply oxygen by mask at 15 L/min. If the patient's breathing is inadequate, assist his breathing with a BM or mouth-to-mask device.
- Position the patient. If there are no contraindications, place the patient on his back with his feet elevated about 8-12 inches.
- Remove or loosen tight clothing.
- Assess the patient's vital signs, including oxygen saturation if a pulse oximeter is available. Assess the patient's blood glucose level (per local protocol). Treat for low blood sugar if indicated.
- Maintain body temperature.

- Comfort, calm, and reassure the patient and his family.
- Reassess for signs that the patient is responding to interventions.

On the Scene   Wrap-Up

By the time the Paramedic crew arrives, you have obtained the patient's blood pressure, applied oxygen by nonrebreather mask, and checked the patient's blood sugar. The patient's blood pressure is 96/54 and his blood sugar is normal. You did not find any other abnormal findings in your examination. The Paramedics start an IV and recheck the patient's vital signs. They notice that his breathing is now more labored, so they insert an oral airway and instruct you to assist the patient's breathing with a BM device while they prepare to insert an endotracheal tube. While the tube is inserted in the patient's airway, a police officer performs a quick search of his home and finds his prescribed medicines but nothing else that is unusual. The Paramedics leave the scene with lights and sirens on to hasten their arrival to the hospital.

You wonder what caused this patient's condition. Later, the Paramedics tell you that he had a stroke with bleeding in his brain. Apparently, the stroke happened a day or two ago. His body temperature was low from lying immobile on the floor for so long. Unfortunately, his condition rapidly worsened at the hospital and he died an hour after arrival. ■

Sum It Up

▶ As an EMT, you should assess every patient and determine his chief complaint as well as his signs and symptoms. Give emergency medical care based on the patient's signs and symptoms. Keep in mind that some patient complaints may apply to more than one illness.

▶ An altered mental status refers to a change in a patient's level of awareness. It is also called an altered level of consciousness (ALOC). A change in the patient's mental status may occur gradually or suddenly. It may last briefly or it may be prolonged. A patient with an altered mental status may appear confused, agitated, combative, sleepy, difficult to awaken, or unresponsive. An altered mental status should be treated as a medical emergency. Regardless of the cause, emergency care of the patient with an altered mental status focuses on his airway, breathing, and circulation.

▶ A seizure is a temporary change in behavior or consciousness caused by abnormal electrical activity within one or more groups of brain cells. A seizure is a symptom of an underlying problem within the central nervous system. The most common cause of adult seizures in patients with a known seizure history is the failure to take anti-seizure medication. The most common cause of seizures in infants and young children is a high fever. Epilepsy is a condition of recurring seizures; the cause is usually irreversible.

▶ The type of seizure that involves stiffening and jerking of the patient's body is called a tonic-clonic seizure (formerly called a grand mal seizure). This type of seizure typically has 4 phases:
- Aura—A peculiar sensation that comes before a seizure
- Tonic phase—The body's muscles stiffen, the patient's breathing may be noisy, and the patient may turn blue
- Clonic phase—Alternating jerking and relaxation of the body occurs
- Postictal phase—The period of recovery that follows a seizure; the patient often appears limp, has shallow breathing, and has an altered mental status

▶ Status epilepticus is recurring seizures without an intervening period of consciousness. Status epilepticus is a medical emergency. It can cause brain damage or death if it is not treated.

▶ A stroke is caused by the blockage or rupture of an artery supplying the brain. There are two main forms of stroke: ischemic and hemorrhagic.
- Ischemic strokes are caused by a blood clot that decreases blood flow to the brain. Ischemic strokes can be further classified as either thrombotic or embolic. In a thrombotic stroke, a blood clot (thrombus) forms in a blood vessel of, or leading to, the brain. In an embolic stroke, a blood clot breaks up and travels through the circulatory system where it lodges in a vessel within or leading to the brain.
- Hemorrhagic strokes (also called cerebral hemorrhage) are caused by bleeding into the brain. Subarachnoid hemorrhage is caused by a ruptured blood vessel in the subarachnoid space, usually a result of aneurysm (an abnormal bulging of a blood vessel). Intracerebral hemorrhage is caused by a ruptured blood vessel within the brain itself (usually a result of chronic high blood pressure).

▶ A transient ischemic attack (TIA) is a temporary interruption of the blood supply to the brain. Signs and symptoms completely resolve within 24 hours with no permanent damage.

▶ The Cincinnati Prehospital Stroke Scale is a useful tool that can be used to find out if a person who has an altered mental status might be having a stroke. The Scale assesses three main areas:

1. Ask the patient to smile. Both sides of the face should move equally.

2. Ask the patient to close his eyes and raise his arms out in front of him. Both arms should move the same or both arms should not move at all.

3. Ask the patient to say a simple sentence. The patient should be able to say the right words without slurring or forgetting or substituting words.

If the patient's response is not normal, request ALS personnel right away or begin transport to the closest appropriate facility.

By the end of this chapter, you should be able to:

Knowledge Objectives ▶

1. Recognize the patient experiencing an allergic reaction.
2. Describe the emergency medical care of the patient with an allergic reaction.
3. Establish the relationship between the patient with an allergic reaction and airway management.
4. Describe the mechanisms of allergic response and the implications for airway management.
5. State the generic and trade names, medication forms, dose, administration, action, and contraindications for the epinephrine auto-injector.
6. Evaluate the need for medical direction in the emergency medical care of the patient with an allergic reaction.
7. Differentiate between the general category of those patients having an allergic reaction and those patients having an allergic reaction and requiring immediate medical care, including immediate use of an epinephrine auto-injector.

Attitude Objectives ▶

8. Explain the rationale for administering epinephrine with an auto-injector.

Skill Objectives ▶

9. Demonstrate the emergency medical care of the patient experiencing an allergic reaction.
10. Demonstrate the use of an epinephrine auto-injector.
11. Demonstrate the assessment and documentation of patient response to an epinephrine injection.
12. Demonstrate proper disposal of equipment.
13. Demonstrate completing a prehospital care report for patients with allergic emergencies.

You and your partner are called to a local elementary school for a "possible allergic reaction." Upon your arrival, you find an anxious six-year-old girl. You can see that her face is swollen. She says she "can't breathe right" and had this same problem last week at lunch time. As you quickly assess the patient, your partner obtains the patient's vital signs. Her blood pressure is 100/64, pulse 110 (strong and regular). Her respirations are 20/min, shallow and labored. Her skin is flushed, warm, and dry. You can hear the patient wheezing with each breath. ■

THINK ABOUT IT

As you read this chapter, think about the following questions:

- What are some of the common causes of an allergic reaction?
- Are the patient's signs and symptoms consistent with an allergic reaction?
- Can you provide emergency care for this child if her parents are not present?

Introduction

Allergic reactions can range from a mild rash to life-threatening anaphylaxis. You must be able to recognize the signs and symptoms of these conditions and provide appropriate patient care. Your ability to recognize and manage anaphylaxis may be life-saving.

Causes of Allergic Reactions

An **allergic reaction** is an exaggerated response by the body's immune system to a substance. The substance that causes an allergic reaction can enter the body in four ways: ingestion, injection, inhalation, or absorption through the skin or mucous membranes (Figure 16-1). Common causes of allergic reactions are shown in Table 16-1.

One cause of allergic reactions deserves special mention. Latex allergy has become increasingly common among patients and healthcare professionals. Products that are commonly made of latex are shown in Table 16-2. The main source used to make natural rubber latex is the rubber tree. Several chemicals are added to the tree's milky fluid during the manufacture of commercial latex. Latex contains proteins that may be absorbed through the skin or inhaled. This can cause an allergic reaction in susceptible persons. Skin absorption may increase when perspiration collects under latex gloves or other clothing that contains latex. Some latex gloves contain powder to make the gloves easier to put on and take off. The glove powder acts as a carrier of latex protein, which can become airborne when the gloves are put on or removed. Latex proteins can cause an allergic reaction when inhaled by individuals allergic to latex.

Among those who have the greatest chance of developing a latex allergy are people who have had many dental or medical procedures or surgeries, people with spina bifida, people with urinary system abnormalities, and healthcare workers. Some foods contain proteins that are similar to rubber (see Table 16-3). These foods may cause an allergic reaction in highly sensitive people who have a latex allergy.

What Happens in an Allergic Reaction

An **antigen** is any substance that is foreign to an individual and causes antibody production. When the body's immune system detects an antigen, white blood cells respond by producing antibodies specific to that antigen. An **antibody** is a substance produced by white blood cells to defend the body against bacteria, viruses, or other antigens. The antibodies attach to mast cells, which are found in connective tissue. The formation of antigen-specific antibodies is called **sensitization** and occurs with the body's first exposure to the antigen. The mucous membranes of the respiratory and digestive tracts contain large numbers of mast cells.

When the body is re-exposed to the same antigen, the antigen attaches to the antibody on the sensitized

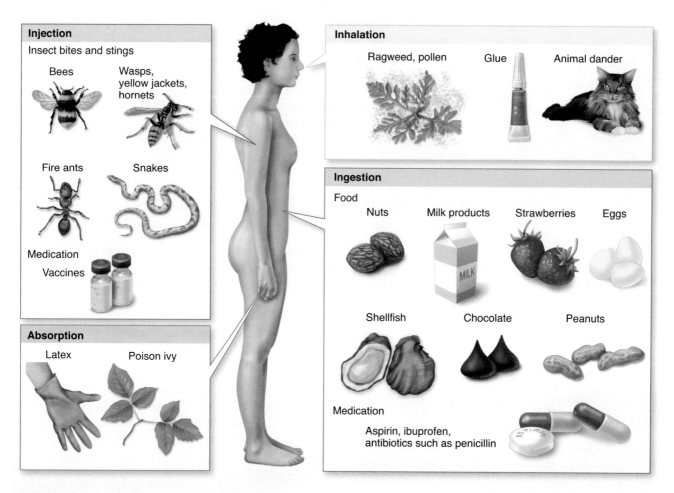

FIGURE 16-1 ▲ An allergen can enter the body in four ways: ingestion, injection, inhalation, or absorption through the skin or mucous membranes.

TABLE 16-1 Routes of Entry of Allergens and Possible Causes of Allergic Reactions

Ingestion	Injection	Inhalation	Surface Absorption
• Aspirin	• Bees	• Pollen	• Pollen
• Nonsteroidal anti-inflammatory drugs (Ibuprofen [Advil, Motrin])	• Wasps	• Mold	• Latex
	• Yellow jackets	• Dust	• Soap
• Insulin	• Hornets	• Grasses	• Cleansers
• Antibiotics	• Spiders	• Mildew	• Fertilizer
• Peanuts	• Fire ants	• Paint	• Poison ivy, oak, sumac
• Tree nuts	• Scorpion	• Perfume	
• Milk products	• Jellyfish	• Animal dander	
• Berries	• Snakes	• Bug spray	
• Eggs	• Antivenin	• Latex	
• Seafood	• Dyes used in diagnostic x-rays and scans		
• Chocolate	• Animal serum (vaccines)		
• Grains	• Transfusion of blood or blood products		
• Beans			
• Food preservatives (sulfites)			

TABLE 16-2 Products That Commonly Include Latex

Household Products	Healthcare Products
Erasers	Adhesive tape and bandages
Rubber bands	Latex rubber gloves
Dishwashing gloves	Blood pressure cuff tubing
Balloons	Stethoscope tubing
Condoms	Tourniquets
Diaphragms	Electrode pads
Baby bottle nipples	Oral and nasal airways
Pacifiers	Airway masks
Diapers	Thermometer probes
Sanitary pads	Suction tubing
Incontinence pads	Medication vial tops
Rubber toys and balls	Endotracheal tubes
Handles on tools, racquets	Syringe plungers
Tires	Bulb syringes
Hot water bottles	Urinary catheters
Shoe soles	Wound drains
Computer mouse pads	Ostomy pouches
Expandable fabric (waistbands)	Material used to fill root canals
Motorcycle and bicycle handgrips	Wheelchair cushions
Swimming goggles	Crutch pads
Some scuba diving suits	Mattresses on stretchers

TABLE 16-3 Foods That May Cause an Allergic Reaction in People Who Have a Latex Allergy

Association with Latex Allergy	Food
High	Banana, avocado, chestnut
Moderate	Apple, celery, kiwi, papaya, potato, tomato
Low or uncertain	Cherry, fig, hazelnut, mango, nectarine, peach, peanut, pear, pineapple, walnut

mast cell. This causes the release of substances that include histamine. The effects of histamine and the other substances released include vessel dilation and leakage of fluid and may be limited to one area of the body (localized) or affect multiple body systems (systemic). When an antigen causes signs and symptoms of an allergic reaction, the antigen is called an **allergen.**

Most allergic reactions happen soon after re-exposure to an allergen. Some reactions are mild, causing symptoms that are annoying but not life

threatening. For example, inhaling an antigen such as plant pollen can result in irritation of the eyes, nose, and respiratory tract. Signs and symptoms often include red, watery eyes; sneezing and a runny nose; and coughing. When an allergic reaction is severe and affects multiple body systems, it is called **anaphylaxis.** Anaphylaxis is a life-threatening emergency. Signs and symptoms of an allergic reaction may progress in minutes from mild to severe. In some cases, a severe reaction occurs without warning.

Remember This!

The more rapid the onset of symptoms after exposure to an allergen, the more severe the allergic reaction is likely to be.

After re-exposure to an allergen, the release of histamine and other chemicals cause serious signs and symptoms that affect many body systems. The initial symptoms of an allergic reaction usually include itching (**pruritus**) and swelling at the site of exposure to the allergen. Many patients also develop hives (**urticaria**) and a rash. Effects of histamine and other chemicals on the respiratory system can include swelling in the throat and narrowing of the lower airways. Swelling of the upper airway can result in hoarseness; stridor; and noisy, labored breathing. Narrowing of the lower airways results in wheezing that can sometimes be heard without the need of a stethoscope. Effects on the skin can include itching, hives, and a rash. Effects on the gastrointestinal system can include nausea, vomiting, diarrhea, and abdominal pain or cramps. The patient's heart rate may be irregular. Because one of the effects of histamine is widening (dilation) of the blood vessels, effects on the cardiovascular system can cause lightheadedness, weakness, and an increased heart rate. The patient's blood pressure can drop quickly and drastically. Signs and symptoms of an allergic reaction are shown in Tables 16-4 and 16-5.

Patient Assessment

Objective 1

When you are dispatched to a call for a possible allergic reaction, keep in mind that the patient's condition can worsen in minutes. When you arrive at the scene, perform a scene size-up. Be aware of possible hazards to yourself and your crew, such as bees or other insects, or other environmental hazards such as pool chemicals or cleaning fluids. Once the scene is determined to be safe to enter, quickly find out as much information as you can about the nature of the illness from the patient, family, or bystanders. Look at the patient's environment for clues about the cause of the patient's chief complaint.

Form a general impression of the patient. If your general impression indicates the patient has a decreased level of responsiveness or shows signs of respiratory distress or failure, move quickly. Perform a primary survey and identify any life-threatening conditions and provide care based on those findings.

Remember This!

Before touching the patient, ask about the possibility of latex allergy so that you do not inadvertently worsen the patient's current condition.

TABLE 16-4 Signs and Symptoms of an Allergic Reaction*

Mild Allergic Reaction	Moderate or Severe Allergic Reaction
Anxiety	Anxiety, fright, altered mental status, unresponsiveness
Runny nose	Feeling of impending doom
Stuffy nose	Swelling of the face, eyes, lips, tongue, or throat
Sneezing	Hoarseness
Red, watery eyes	Difficulty swallowing or talking
Red skin (flushing)	Stridor
Rash	Difficulty breathing
Hives	Weakness
Itching	Coughing
Feeling of fullness in mouth or throat	Wheezing
Swelling of hands, feet	Abdominal cramps, pain
Tingling of hands, feet	Nausea, vomiting
Coughing	Dizziness, lightheadedness, unexplained fainting
Abdominal cramps	Low blood pressure
Urgency to urinate	Chest discomfort or tightness

* Not all signs and symptoms are present in every case.

TABLE 16-5 Signs and Symptoms of an Allergic Reaction by Body System

Body System	Signs and Symptoms
Respiratory	Tightness in the throat ("lump in the throat") or chest Coughing Labored breathing Noisy breathing Hoarseness Stridor Difficulty talking Wheezing
Cardiovascular	Lightheadedness, fainting Weakness Increased heart rate Irregular heart rhythm Decreased blood pressure Circulatory collapse
Nervous	Restlessness Fear, panic, or a feeling of impending doom Headache Altered mental status, unresponsiveness Seizures
Skin (integumentary)	Warm, tingling feeling in the face, mouth, chest, feet, and hands Itching (pruritus) Rash Hives (urticaria) Red skin (flushing) Swelling of the face, neck, hands, feet and/or tongue
Gastrointestinal	Nausea Vomiting Abdominal cramps, pain Urgency to urinate Diarrhea
Generalized findings	Itchy, watery eyes Runny nose

Assess the patient's mental status. A patient experiencing an allergic reaction is often anxious. Provide calm reassurance to help reduce the patient's anxiety. If the patient has an altered mental status or his mental status is decreasing, move quickly. If the patient is unresponsive and there is any possibility of trauma, stabilize the patient's cervical spine.

Objective 3

Assess the patient's airway. The presence of stridor, hoarseness, difficulty swallowing, or swelling of the tongue suggests an impending airway obstruction. If any of these signs are present, request Advanced Life Support (ALS) assistance as soon as possible. If

ALS personnel are not available, complete your primary survey and then prepare the patient for prompt transport to the closest appropriate facility.

Assess the patient's breathing. Carefully assess for signs of respiratory distress or respiratory failure. A patient who is experiencing an allergic reaction may have coughing, wheezing, an increased respiratory rate, difficulty breathing, and/or a feeling of chest tightness. Assess the patient's circulation. The patient may complain of lightheadedness or weakness. He may have an increased heart rate, irregular heart rhythm, and/or low blood pressure. Respiratory and skin symptoms often appear earlier in children than in adults. Cardiovascular and gastrointestinal symptoms often occur earlier in adults than in children. Although most anaphylaxis patients present with typical symptoms, some may present with unexplained fainting, a cardiac-related event, or low blood pressure.

You Should Know

Although anaphylaxis can occur with antigens that are ingested, inhaled, or absorbed, it is more common when an antigen is injected (such as an insect sting or intravenous antibiotics).

If you have not already done so, establish patient priorities and make a transport decision. Is there time to provide on-scene care, or should the patient be loaded into the ambulance and rapidly transported? Priority patients include:

- Patients who give a poor general impression
- Patients experiencing difficulty breathing
- Patients with signs and symptoms of shock
- Unresponsive patients with no gag reflex or cough
- Responsive patients who are unable to follow commands

Request ALS personnel as soon as possible for a patient with signs and symptoms of anaphylaxis. Consider the time it will take for an ALS unit to arrive and the time that it will take to load the patient into the ambulance and transport rapidly to the closest appropriate hospital. If needed, contact medical direction for advice.

Once you have made a transport decision, obtain a SAMPLE history from the patient if he is responsive. Examples of questions to ask a patient who is experiencing an allergic reaction are shown in the following *Making a Difference* box. If the patient is unresponsive or has an altered mental status, quickly size up the scene, perform a primary survey, and then proceed to the rapid medical assessment. Follow with

Making a Difference

Questions to ask a patient who is experiencing an allergic reaction:

- When did your symptoms begin?
- How were you exposed?
- What were you doing when the symptoms began?
- How soon after exposure did your symptoms begin?
- Do you have any allergies to medications, foods, other substances or materials?
- Are you taking any medications (prescription and over the counter)? Do you take your medications regularly? Has there has been any recent change in medications (additions, deletions, or change in dosages)?
- Have you ever experienced an allergic reaction? Is so, what were you exposed to that caused the reaction? How serious was the reaction? Were you hospitalized? Have you ever been intubated or "needed a breathing tube" because of an allergic reaction?
- Do you have a physician-prescribed epinephrine auto-injector or anaphylaxis kit? If so, have you given yourself a dose before we arrived?
- Have you taken any medications to relieve your symptoms before we arrived?
- Do you have a history of asthma, heart disease, high blood pressure, or other illness?

evaluation of baseline vital signs and gathering of the patient's medical history. A family member, friend, coworker, or others at the scene may be able to provide important information about the cause of the patient's symptoms.

Quickly look to see if the patient is wearing medical identification that indicates the patient has an allergy. Patients who have known allergies usually know how to avoid whatever it is that triggers an allergic reaction. These patients are advised by their physician to wear medical identification that clearly identifies what they are allergic to.

Patients who have severe allergic reactions may be prescribed an anaphylaxis kit. An anaphylaxis kit contains an epinephrine auto-injector (Epi-Pen) (Figure 16-2). Some kits also contain a metered-dose inhaler. When the patient is exposed to something to which he has a severe allergic reaction, the patient self-administers the epinephrine by means of an automatic injectable needle and syringe. People who have an allergy to latex are advised to carry an epinephrine auto-injector, wear medical identification,

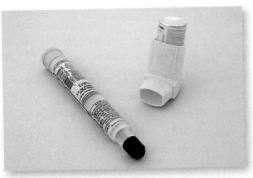

FIGURE 16-2 ▲ An anaphylaxis kit contains an epinephrine auto-injector. Some kits also contain a metered-dose inhaler.

and carry extra pairs of nonlatex gloves for emergency medical or dental care. In addition to looking for medical identification devices (such as a bracelet) indicating the patient has an allergy, also look for peel-and-stick plastic decals that may indicate a latex allergy (Figure 16-3). You may find decals such as this one at the entrance to a patient's home and on a car window or windshield, alerting Emergency Medical Services (EMS) personnel that someone inside is allergic to latex.

If the patient has a latex allergy, make a note of this on your prehospital care report. Write the words "LATEX ALLERGY" clearly on the report and include latex in the allergy section of the form. If your EMS agency has a latex-free kit, use latex-free supplies from the kit for patient care. Place a latex allergy wristband from the kit on the patient. If your EMS agency does not have a latex-free kit, wrap cotton gauze over blood pressure cuff tubing and stethoscope tubing to avoid contact with the patient. Wrap cotton gauze over the patient's upper arm before placing a blood pressure cuff on the patient. Remember to communicate the presence of the patient's latex allergy to ALS personnel arriving on the scene and/or to the staff at the receiving facility when transferring patient care.

Perform a focused physical exam and obtain baseline vital signs. Assess the patient's pulse, respirations,

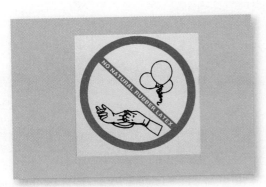

FIGURE 16-3 ▲ Latex allergy decal.

and blood pressure. Assess oxygen saturation by using a pulse oximeter. Provide all information obtained to the ALS crew arriving on the scene or to the receiving facility staff.

Emergency Care

Objectives 2, 4, 6, 7

If the patient has come in contact with a substance that is causing an allergic reaction without signs of respiratory distress or shock:

- Maintain an open airway
- Give oxygen
- Transport and perform ongoing assessments often while en route

A patient without wheezing or signs of respiratory compromise or hypotension should not receive epinephrine. However, keep in mind that the condition of a patient experiencing an allergic reaction can change rapidly. A patient who was initially stable can develop massive airway swelling and a possible airway obstruction in minutes. Remember that the presence of stridor, hoarseness, difficulty swallowing, or swelling of the tongue suggests an impending airway obstruction. Constant reassessment is essential.

If the patient has come in contact with a substance that caused a past allergic reaction and complains of respiratory distress or shows signs and symptoms of shock:

- Establish and maintain an open airway. The patient with an allergic reaction may initially present with airway/respiratory compromise, or airway/respiratory compromise may develop as the reaction progresses. Make sure suction equipment is within arm's reach.

- Give oxygen. If the patient's breathing is adequate, apply oxygen by nonrebreather mask at 15 L/min if not already done. If the patient's breathing is inadequate, provide positive-pressure ventilation with 100% oxygen and assess the adequacy of the ventilations delivered. Ventilation with a bag-mask device may be difficult because of narrowing of the patient's bronchioles.

- Find out if the patient has a prescribed epinephrine auto-injector available. In some EMS systems, Emergency Medical Technicians (EMTs) are authorized to carry epinephrine auto-injectors. In these situations, a physician-prescribed auto-injector (carried by the patient) is not necessary. Obtain an order from medical direction either on line or off line to give (or assist the patient in giving) epinephrine by means of an auto-injector. After administration, reassess the patient in 2 minutes. Record reassessment findings and prepare for transport. If the patient does not have a prescribed epinephrine auto-injector or you do not carry this medication, transport immediately.

- Perform ongoing assessments every 5 minutes. Transport promptly to the closest appropriate medical facility.

- If the patient's condition improves, provide supportive care. Continue to give oxygen and treat for shock.

- If the patient's condition worsens, contact medical direction for orders to give an additional dose of epinephrine, if available. Signs that indicate the patient's condition is worsening include decreasing mental status, increasing breathing difficulty, and decreasing blood pressure. Treat for shock. Be prepared to begin cardiopulmonary resuscitation (CPR) and use the automated external defibrillator (AED), if necessary.

Remember This!

When caring for a patient experiencing an allergic reaction, quickly determine if ALS personnel are needed. ALS personnel will apply a cardiac monitor to the patient, start an intravenous line, and give drugs that can quickly help decrease the severity of the patient's symptoms. They will also perform advanced airway techniques if the patient's condition warrants it. Evaluate the time it will take for an ALS unit to arrive and the time that it would take to load the patient into the ambulance and transport rapidly to the closest appropriate facility. Another consideration is meeting the ALS unit to transfer patient care to ALS personnel before arrival at the hospital.

Using an Epinephrine Auto-Injector
Medication Actions
Objective 5

Epinephrine works by relaxing the bronchial passages of the airway and constricting the blood vessels. The opening of the airway allows the patient to move more air into and out of the lungs, which will increase the amount of oxygen in the bloodstream. Constriction of the blood vessels slows the leakage of fluid from the blood vessels into the space around the cells of the body. Table 16-6 summarizes important information about epinephrine auto-injectors that you should know.

Indications

As an EMT, you can give epinephrine by means of an auto-injector if *all* of the following criteria are met:

- The patient exhibits signs and symptoms of a severe allergic reaction, including respiratory distress and/or signs and symptoms of shock.

- The medication is prescribed for the patient, or your EMS system authorizes EMTs to carry the medication.

- Medical direction has authorized use for the patient.

You Should Know

In some states, EMTs now carry Epi-Pens on their units and are not limited to administering the medication to patients who have been prescribed one. The EMT can give the medication to a patient when ordered by medical direction. Check your local protocol.

Contraindications

There are no contraindications when an epinephrine auto-injector is used in a life-threatening situation.

Special Considerations

- Before giving any medication, make sure you have the right patient, right drug, right dose, right route, and right time.

- Epi-Pens are available in two strengths (Figure 16-4). The Epi-Pen auto-injector (0.3 mg) is used for individuals weighing 66 pounds or more. The Epi-Pen Jr. auto-injector (0.15 mg) is for individuals weighing between 33 and 66 pounds. Both strengths deliver a single dose. Because a single

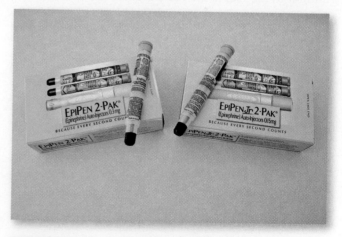

FIGURE 16-4 ▲ Epi-Pens are available in two strengths. Both strengths deliver a single dose of epinephrine.

TABLE 16-6 Epinephrine

Generic name	epinephrine
Trade name	Adrenalin
Mechanism of action	Epinephrine works by relaxing the bronchial passages of the airway and constricting the blood vessels. The opening of the airway allows the patient to move more air into and out of the lungs, which will increase the amount of oxygen in the bloodstream. Constriction of the blood vessels slows the leakage of fluid from the blood vessels into the space around the cells of the body.
Indications	An EMT can assist a patient in using an epinephrine auto-injector if *all* of the following criteria are met: • The patient shows signs and symptoms of a severe allergic reaction, including respiratory distress and/or signs and symptoms of shock. • The patient has a physician-prescribed epinephrine auto-injector, or your EMS system authorizes EMTs to carry the medication. • The EMT has specific authorization by medical direction.
Dosage	Adult—one adult auto-injector (0.3 mg) Infant and child—one infant/child auto-injector (0.15 mg)
Side effects	Rapid heart rate Anxiety Excitability Nausea, vomiting Chest pain or discomfort Headache Dizziness
Contraindications	There are no contraindications when used in a life-threatening situation.

dose of epinephrine may not completely reverse the effects of an anaphylactic reaction (even when the proper dose is given), the patient's physician may prescribe more than one auto-injector.

You Should Know

- If a physician prescribed a child an Epi-Pen Jr., he will switch and prescribe the Epi-Pen as the child grows and epinephrine dosage requirements increase.

- Sometimes a child will not use his prescribed Epi-Pen because he knows that using it will result in a potentially painful needlestick.

- Look closely at the auto-injector container. Make sure that the epinephrine is not expired (Figure 16-5). Look into the clear window of the Epi-Pen container. The solution should be clear. If the solution is discolored or contains solid particles

(precipitate), do not use the medication. If a red flag is present in the window of the auto-injector, the epinephrine has already been injected (Figure 16-6). Find out if the patient has already taken any doses before your arrival today or if the patient used the auto-injector in the past and forgot to get a new Epi-Pen.

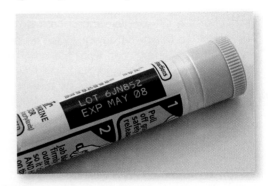

FIGURE 16-5 ▲ Look at the auto-injector container and make sure that the epinephrine is not expired.

Assisting the Patient with a Prescribed Epinephrine Auto-Injector

STEP 1 ▶ Put on appropriate personal protective equipment. Confirm that the patient has signs or symptoms of a severe allergic reaction. Confirm that the patient has a physician-prescribed epinephrine auto-injector (unnecessary if state/local protocols permit an EMT to carry and administer an auto-injector). Obtain an order from medical direction either on line or off line. Make sure that the epinephrine is not expired. Look into the clear window of the EpiPen container. The solution should be clear.

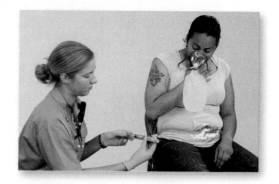

STEP 2 ▶ Remove (or assist the patient in removing) the EpiPen from its container by unscrewing the cap off of the EpiPen carrying case and removing the EpiPen from its storage tube.

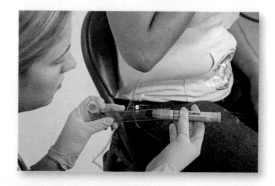

STEP 3 ▶ Grasp (or assist the patient in grasping) the EpiPen with the black tip pointing downward.

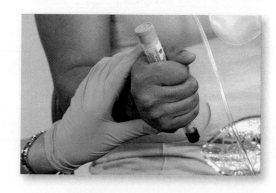

STEP 4 ▶ Form a fist (or have the patient do so) around the EpiPen (black tip down). With the other hand, pull off the "safety" cap from the other end of the auto-injector.

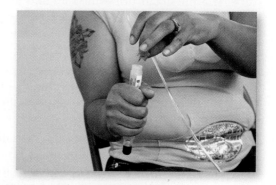

STEP 5 ▶ Press the auto-injector against the outside portion of one thigh (or assist the patient in doing so) for about 10 seconds until you hear it release. Hold the EpiPen perpendicular (at a 90° angle) to the thigh. It is designed to work through clothing. The auto-injector will propel a spring-driven needle into the patient's thigh and then inject the drug into the muscle of the outer thigh. This will cause pain, and the patient may move very suddenly.

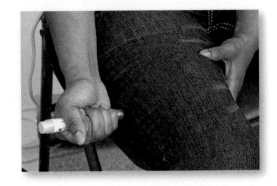

STEP 6 ▶ After the drug has been delivered, the window on the auto-injector will show red. Remove the EpiPen from the patient's thigh (or have the patient do so) and massage the injection area for 10 seconds. Remember that the needle will be exposed and must be disposed of properly in an appropriate container. Document the patient's name, drug name and dose given, time of administration, and the patient's response to the drug. If an on-line order was received by medical direction, document the name of the physician giving the order. The patient will need to be transported for additional care. Perform ongoing assessments every 5 minutes, continuously monitoring the patient's airway and breathing.

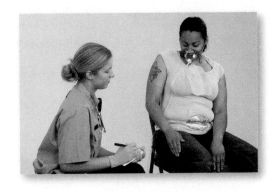

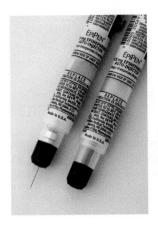

FIGURE 16-6 ◀ Look into the clear window of the EpiPen container. If a red flag is present in the window of the auto-injector, the epinephrine has already been injected.

- Place the patient on a pulse oximeter and give him oxygen by nonrebreather mask.
- Monitor the patient's breath sounds, heart rate, and blood pressure closely before and after administration. The effects of the epinephrine injected last about 10 to 20 minutes.

Procedure

Skill Drill 16-1 shows the procedure for using an epinephrine auto-injector.

You immediately recognize the child's signs and symptoms are consistent with an allergic reaction. The child tells you she is allergic to peanuts. The child's teacher tells you that the school has a signed consent form on file from the child's parents allowing the school to authorize care in an emergency.

While giving the child oxygen by nonrebreather mask, you learn that the patient traded her cookies for another child's cookies. It appears that the cookies she ate contained peanut butter. You ask the child if she has a prescribed epinephrine auto-injector. She nods that she does, but she forgot her kit and left it at home today. As you and your partner quickly load the patient into the ambulance, you notice that the patient's respiratory distress is worsening. Your partner asks the child's teacher to notify the child's parents of your destination and then begins rapid transport to the closest appropriate hospital. ■

Sum It Up

▶ An allergic reaction is an exaggerated immune response to any substance. The substance that causes an allergic reaction can enter the body in four ways: ingestion, injection, inhalation, or absorption through the skin or mucous membranes. Possible causes include insect bites/stings, food, plants, and medications, among others.

▶ An antigen is any substance that is foreign to an individual and causes antibody production. An antibody is a substance produced by white blood cells to defend the body against bacteria, viruses, or other antigens. The antibodies attach to mast cells, which are found in connective tissue. This process, called sensitization, occurs with the body's first exposure to the antigen. When an antigen causes signs and symptoms of an allergic reaction, the antigen is called an allergen. When an allergic reaction is severe and affects multiple body systems, it is called anaphylaxis. Anaphylaxis is a life-threatening emergency.

▶ Assessment findings pertaining to the respiratory system may include tightness in the throat ("lump in the throat") or chest, coughing, rapid breathing, labored breathing, noisy breathing, hoarseness, stridor, difficulty talking, and wheezing. Assessment findings pertaining to the cardiovascular system may include an increased heart rate, lightheadedness, fainting, weakness, irregular heart rhythm, decreased blood pressure, and circulatory collapse. Assessment findings pertaining to the nervous system may include restlessness, fear, panic or a feeling of impending doom, headache, an altered mental status, unresponsiveness, and seizures. Assessment findings pertaining to the skin may include itching (pruritus), hives (urticaria), red skin (flushing), and swelling to the face, neck, hands, feet, and/or tongue. The patient may state he has a warm tingling feeling in the face, mouth, chest, feet, and hands. Assessment findings pertaining to the gastrointestinal system may include nausea, vomiting, abdominal cramps/pain, an urgency to urinate, and diarrhea. Generalized findings may include itchy, watery eyes and a runny nose.

▶ Assessment findings that reveal shock (hypoperfusion) or respiratory distress indicate the presence of a severe allergic reaction.

▶ If the patient has come in contact with substance that caused past allergic reaction and complains of respiratory distress or shows signs and symptoms of shock, form a general impression, perform a primary survey, and perform a focused history and physical exam. Assess the patient's baseline vital signs and SAMPLE history. Give oxygen if not already done. Find out if the patient has a prescribed epinephrine auto-injector available. With approval from medical direction, help the patient with administration of the epinephrine auto-injector. Reassess in two minutes. Record reassessment findings. If the patient does not have an epinephrine auto-injector available, transport immediately.

▶ If the patient has contact with a substance that causes an allergic reaction without signs of respiratory distress or shock, continue with a focused assessment. A patient who is not wheezing or without signs of respiratory compromise or hypotension should not receive epinephrine.

▶ A patient experiencing an allergic reaction may initially present with airway/respiratory compromise, or airway/respiratory compromise may develop as the allergic reaction progresses.

▶ If the patient's condition improves, provide supportive care. Continue to give oxygen and treat for shock. If the patient's condition worsens, contact medical direction for orders to give an additional dose of epinephrine, if available. Signs that indicate the patient's condition is worsening include decreasing mental status, increasing breathing difficulty, and decreasing blood pressure. Treat for shock. Be prepared to begin CPR and use the AED, if necessary.

17 Poisoning and Overdose

By the end of this chapter, you should be able to:

Knowledge Objectives ▶
1. List various ways that poisons enter the body.
2. List signs and symptoms associated with poisoning.
3. Discuss the emergency medical care for the patient with possible overdose.
4. Describe the steps in the emergency medical care for the patient with suspected poisoning.
5. Establish the relationship between the patient suffering from poisoning or overdose and airway management.
6. State the generic and trade names, indications, contraindications, medication form, dose, administration, actions, side effects, and reassessment strategies for activated charcoal.
7. Recognize the need for medical direction in caring for the patient with poisoning or overdose.

Attitude Objectives ▶
8. Explain the rationale for administering activated charcoal.
9. Explain the rationale for contacting medical direction early in the prehospital management of the poisoning or overdose patient.

Skill Objectives ▶
10. Demonstrate the steps in the emergency medical care for the patient with possible overdose.

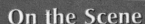

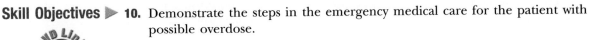

On the Scene

You and your Emergency Medical Technician partner are dispatched to a private residence for a "possible overdose." On arrival at the scene, an anxious family member ushers you into a bedroom where you find a 35-year-old woman lying in bed. Your first impression reveals that the patient's eyes are closed and she is unaware of your approach. She is breathing about 8 to 10 breaths/min. Her breathing does not appear labored. Her skin looks pink and dry. Her face looks swollen, as if she has been crying. An empty bottle of Percocet tablets is on the nightstand. After repeatedly calling her name, the patient slowly opens her eyes and then goes back to sleep. The family member at your side says that the patient and her husband "have been having problems." ■

As you read this chapter, think about the following questions:

- What is the route of toxic exposure in this situation?
- If the patient took the Percocet tablets on the nightstand, what other signs and symptoms can you anticipate finding during your patient assessment?
- In what types of poisonings is activated charcoal used?
- Should activated charcoal be given to this patient? Why or why not?

Introduction

Poisoning and substance abuse calls are common emergencies. Many children are poisoned every year as they explore their environments. Many adults overdose on medication, either accidentally or deliberately. In this chapter we will discuss the routes by which poisons may enter the body, signs and symptoms associated with poisoning and overdose, and the emergency medical care for these patients.

What Is a Poison?

A **poison** is any substance taken into the body that interferes with normal body function. **Poisoning** is exposure to a substance that is harmful in any dosage. A **toxin** is a poisonous substance. An **antidote** is a substance that neutralizes a poison.

You Should Know

- More than 80% of toxic exposures are accidental.
- More than 90% of toxic exposures occur in the home.
- More than 50% of poisonings occur in children younger than 6 years of age.
- More than 90% of poisonings involve only one substance.
- More than 75% of poisonings occur by ingestion.

A **Poison Control Center (PCC)** is a medical facility that provides free telephone advice to the public and medical professionals in case of exposure to poisonous substances. In the United States, the national telephone number is 1-800-222-1222 (toll-free). This number is staffed 24 hours a day, 7 days a week, 365 days a year by pharmacists, physicians, nurses, and poison information providers. A PCC is an excellent resource that is often used by Emergency Medical Services (EMS) personnel. When the substance involved is known, the medical professionals at a PCC can help determine the toxicity of the substance and give advice about the emergency care the patient should receive.

You Should Know

The ability to accept treatment orders/instructions from a PCC is based on local medical direction and local protocols. Be sure to check and find out if you are able to accept treatment orders from your local PCC.

Objective 1

A poison may be a solid, liquid, spray, or gas (Table 17-1). Toxins enter the body in four ways: ingestion, inhalation, injection, or absorption (Figure 17-1). Exposure to a toxin may be accidental or intentional. Most poisonings are accidental. Examples of accidental poisonings are shown in the following *You Should Know* box.

You Should Know

Examples of Accidental Poisonings

Bites and stings

Food poisoning

Medication taken/given more than once by mistake

Wrong medication taken/given

Someone else's medication taken/given

Medication doses given/taken too close together

Exposure through breast milk

Wrong dose/medication given by healthcare professional

TABLE 17-1 Examples of Common Poisons

Form of Poison	Examples
Solid	Medicines, plants, granulated detergent, granular pesticides, fertilizers, pool chemicals, disc batteries, chalk, clay, fabric softener, diaper pail deodorizer, toilet bowl deodorizer
Liquid	Syrup medicines, laundry soap, fabric softener, laundry bluing/brightening products, baby oil, bath oil/bubble bath, cream or lotion makeup, mouthwash, permanent wave solutions, hair removal products, rubbing alcohol, nail glue remover, furniture polish, lighter fluid, typewriter correction fluid, gasoline, kerosene, drain opener, disinfectants, toilet bowl cleaner, rust remover, pool chemicals, lamp oil, paint, antifreeze, windshield solution, brake fluid
Spray	Oven cleaner, glass cleaner, air freshener, insecticides, weed killer, spray paint, fabric softener, disinfectants
Gas	Carbon monoxide, automobile exhaust fumes, fumes from gas or oil burning stoves, tear gas, chlorine gas and pool chemicals, chemicals that workers are exposed to at industrial plants

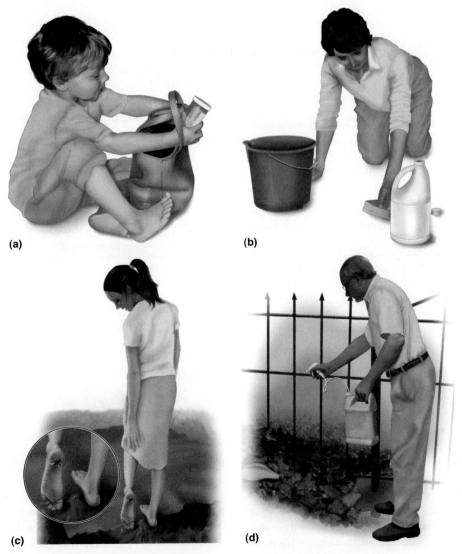

(a)

(b)

(c)

(d)

FIGURE 17-1 ▲ A toxin can enter the body in four ways: **(a)** ingestion, **(b)** absorption, **(c)** injection, or **(d)** inhalation through the skin or mucous membranes.

TABLE 17-2 Common Toxidromes

Toxidrome	Signs/Symptoms	Examples
Sympathomimetic (produces signs and symptoms like those of the sympathetic division of the autonomic nervous system)	Agitation, rapid breathing, increased heart rate, increased blood pressure, fever, seizures, sweating	Amphetamines, methamphetamines Cocaine Phencyclidine (PCP) Ecstasy Caffeine, pseudoephedrine (found in over-the-counter cold remedies)
Cholinergic	Altered mental status, decreased or increased heart rate, fever, seizures, "SLUDGEM": • *S*alivation • *L*acrimation (tearing) • *U*rination • *D*efecation • *G*astrointestinal distress • *E*mesis (vomiting) • *M*iosis (pupil constriction)	Organophosphate and carbamate insecticides (ant sprays, flea sprays, and insect sprays, powders, and liquids) Some mushrooms Nerve agents (Sarin gas)
Anticholinergic	Confusion, hallucinations, agitation, coma, blurred vision; warm, flushed, dry skin; dilated pupils	Antihistamines such as diphenhydramine (Benadryl) Jimson weed Tricyclic antidepressants such as amitriptyline (Elavil), desipramine (Norpramin), nortriptyline (Aventyl, Pamelor)
Opioid (narcotics)	Altered mental status, coma, slow or absent breathing, slow heart rate, low blood pressure, constricted pupils Note: Meperidine, propoxyphene, and diphenoxylate may cause *dilated* pupils.	morphine codeine heroin diphenoxylate (Lomotil) meperidine (Demerol) methadone (Dolophine) propoxyphene (Darvon)
Sedative/hypnotic (substances used to aid sleep, reduce anxiety, and treat depression, epilepsy, and high blood pressure)	Slurred speech, hallucinations, confusion, coma, respiratory depression, low blood pressure, pupil dilation or constriction, blurred vision, dry mouth, decreased temperature, staggering walk	Barbiturates (phenobarbital) Benzodiazepines (diazepam [Valium]) Alcohol GHB (a date rape drug or "liquid x")

Signs and symptoms of a toxic exposure can vary depending on the substance involved; the route of entry; the amount ingested, inhaled, injected, or absorbed; and the length of the exposure. Signs, symptoms, and characteristics that often occur together in toxic exposures are called **toxidromes** (Table 17-2). When the cause of a toxic exposure is unknown, knowing the "typical" signs and symptoms of certain toxic exposures can help you to identify the poison and allow you to give appropriate care.

Commonly Misused and Abused Substances

Intentional poisonings may occur because of suicide or homicide (murder), substance abuse or misuse, or acts of terrorism. **Substance abuse** is the deliberate, persistent, and excessive self-administration of a substance in a way that is not medically or socially approved. Recreational use of substances is considered intentional abuse. **Substance misuse** is the self-administration of a substance for unintended purposes, or for appropriate purposes but in improper amounts or doses, or without a prescription for the person receiving the medication. **Tolerance** occurs when an individual requires progressively larger doses of a drug to achieve the desired effect. **Addiction** is a psychological and physical dependence on a substance that has gone beyond voluntary control. **Withdrawal** is the condition produced when an individual stops using or abusing a drug to which he or she is physically or psychologically addicted. An **overdose** is an intentional or unintentional overmedication or ingestion of a toxic substance. Commonly misused and abused substances include stimulants, depressants, hallucinogens, and designer drugs.

Stimulants

Stimulants increase mental and physical activity. Examples include cocaine, amphetamines, methamphetamines, and phencyclidine (PCP). Common legal stimulants include caffeine and nicotine. Stimulants produce feelings of alertness and well-being. They may produce violent behavior. Other signs and symptoms of stimulant misuse or abuse are listed in the following *You Should Know* box. When the effects of the drug wear off, the user is often exhausted and sleeps. On awakening, the user may be confused, depressed, or suicidal.

You Should Know

Signs and Symptoms of Stimulant Misuse or Abuse

- Restlessness
- Irritability
- Combativeness
- Increased heart rate
- Increased respiratory rate
- Increased blood pressure
- Sweating
- Tremors
- Hallucinations
- Fever
- Headache
- Dizziness
- Moist or flushed skin
- Chest pain/discomfort
- Palpitations
- Nausea/vomiting
- Loss of appetite

Depressants

Depressants include alcohol, barbiturates, narcotics (opiates), and benzodiazepines. Signs and symptoms of depressant misuse or abuse are listed in the following *You Should Know* box.

You Should Know

Signs and Symptoms of Depressant Misuse or Abuse

- Drowsiness
- Slurred speech
- Decreased heart rate
- Decreased blood pressure
- Decreased respiratory rate
- Poor coordination
- Confusion

Alcohol

Alcohol slows mental and physical activity. It affects judgment, vision, reaction time, and coordination. When approaching the patient who has ingested alcohol, observe the scene for evidence of trauma. In large quantities, alcohol can cause death.

Making a Difference

Signs and symptoms of alcohol misuse or abuse can mimic those of other medical conditions such as a diabetic emergency, head injury, epilepsy, drug reaction, or central nervous system (CNS) infection. In addition, alcohol abuse can often mask potentially lethal conditions such as a head injury. Do not *assume* the patient is intoxicated. Carefully assess the patient for the presence of other injuries or illnesses. Perform a blood glucose test (if permitted by state and local protocol).

Disulfiram (Antabuse) is a medication prescribed for alcoholics to discourage them from drinking. When combined with alcohol or alcohol-containing foods, medications, or products (such as over-the-counter cough medications, mouthwash, and facial cleaning products) Antabuse produces unpleasant, and sometimes serious, reactions. Reactions last 30 minutes to 8 hours (usually 3 to 4 hours) and include nausea, vomiting, abdominal discomfort, chest discomfort, palpitations, headache, dizziness, and blurred vision. Although rare, seizures, heart failure, heart attack, and cardiac arrest have occurred.

Alcohol withdrawal syndrome occurs 6 to 48 hours after a chronic alcoholic reduces or stops his alcohol consumption. Signs and symptoms of alcohol withdrawal include tremors ("the shakes"), anxiety, irritability, inability to sleep, sweating, nausea, and vomiting. The patient must be monitored closely by healthcare professionals or **delirium tremens (DTs)** can occur. DTs usually begin 24 to 72 hours after a chronic alcoholic reduces or stops alcohol consumption. The diagnosis of DTs is made when symptoms of alcohol withdrawal progress beyond the usual symptoms of withdrawal. DTs are potentially fatal. Signs and symptoms of DTs include those of alcohol withdrawal plus altered mental status (confusion, visual and/or auditory hallucinations, severe agitation), seizures, increased heart rate, increased blood pressure, and elevated body temperature. Symptoms may be present for several days. In general, seizures associated with alcohol withdrawal occur 6 to 48 hours after the last drink.

Barbiturates

Barbiturates are prescribed to relieve anxiety, promote sleep, control seizures, and relax muscles. Examples of barbiturates include pentobarbital (Nembutal), secobarbital (Seconal), amobarbital (Amytal) and phenobarbital (Luminal). Street names for these drugs include yellow jackets, reds, blues, Amy's, rainbows, Barbs, downers, goof balls, and stumblers. Barbiturates are particularly dangerous when combined with alcohol. Overdose can produce respiratory depression, coma, and death. Withdrawal can cause anxiety, tremors, nausea, fever, convulsions, and death.

Narcotics

Narcotics are prescribed drugs used to relieve moderate to severe pain, control diarrhea, and suppress cough. Narcotics include opium, opium derivatives, and man-made compounds that produce opium-like effects (see the next *You Should Know* box). Overdose can result in respiratory depression, constricted (pinpoint) pupils, shock, and death. Withdrawal can cause tearing, nasal congestion, headache, joint pain, dilated pupils, abdominal cramps, increased heart rate, chills, fever, gooseflesh, tremors, loss of appetite, vomiting, diarrhea, sweating, confusion, and intense agitation.

Benzodiazepines

Benzodiazepines are prescribed medications used to control anxiety and stress, aid sleep, and relax muscles. They are also used for sedation and to control seizures. These drugs vary widely in their onset, indications, potency, and duration of effect. Table 17-3 lists common benzodiazepines. Overdose can result in

respiratory depression and death. Respiratory depression may be especially significant if benzodiazepines are taken in combination with alcohol or other drugs. Withdrawal can cause anxiety, tremors, nausea, fever, seizures, and death.

TABLE 17-3 Benzodiazepines

Generic Name	Trade Name
alprazolam	Xanax
chlordiazepoxide	Librium
clonazepam	Klonopin
clorazepate	Tranxene
diazepam	Valium
lorazepam	Ativan
midazolam	Versed
oxazepam	Serax

Hallucinogens

Hallucinogens include lysergic acid diethylamine (LSD), PCP (angel dust), and mescaline (street names include "buttons," "mess," and "peyote"). These drugs produce changes in mood, thought, emotional, and self-awareness. Signs and symptoms of hallucinogen misuse and abuse include flushed face, sudden mood changes, fear, and anxiety. They can also cause hallucinations, profound depression, and irrational and disruptive behavior that can make the user dangerous to himself and others.

Designer Drugs

Designer drugs are variations of federally controlled substances that have high abuse potential (such as narcotics and amphetamines). These drugs are produced by persons ranging from amateurs to highly skilled chemists (called "cookers") and sold on the street. Designer drugs can be injected, smoked, snorted, or ingested. Signs and symptoms of designer drug misuse and abuse are unpredictable and depend on the drug that is being chemically altered. Because designer drugs are often much stronger than the original form of the drug, overdose occurs frequently.

Fentanyl (Sublimaze), a narcotic analgesic, is one drug used to make designer narcotics. Street names include "china white," "synthetic heroin," "Persian white," and "Mexican brown." Signs and symptoms of misuse or abuse include respiratory depression and mental status depression.

Designer amphetamines include "Ecstasy." The chemical name for Ecstasy is MDMA—methylenedioxymethamphetamine. It is also called "Adam," "XTC," and "Love Drug." Signs and symptoms of misuse or abuse include increased heart rate, sweating, agitation, erratic mood swings, and increased blood pressure.

General Care for Poisoning and Overdose

Scene Size-Up

Objectives 3, 4

When responding to a call involving a possible toxic exposure, you may or may not know the substance(s) involved. For example, a 9-1-1 caller may tell the dispatcher that her toddler ate rat poison, or that a teenager took an overdose of sleeping pills. On the other hand, the 9-1-1 dispatcher may not have any information available from the caller other than an "unresponsive person" or a person who "is not acting

You Should Know

Toxic exposures that involve more than one substance (such as alcohol and recreational drugs) are often difficult to recognize and treat. In these situations, the patient will most likely not have signs and symptoms specific to only one toxidrome. In any case, do not delay providing emergency care in order to find the cause of the toxic exposure.

right." Remember scene safety in *all* circumstances. Protecting yourself and your crew must be your primary concern so that you are not injured or poisoned.

Use appropriate protection or have trained rescuers remove the patient from the poisonous environment. Call for additional resources if needed. On arrival at the scene, observe the patient's environment for clues as to the source of the poisoning, such as:

- Unusual odors
- Smoke or flames
- Open medicine cabinet
- Open or overturned containers
- Syringes or other drug paraphernalia

Primary Survey

As with all patients, form a general impression and then quickly assess the patient's mental status, airway, breathing, and circulation. Stabilize the patient's spine if needed.

Many toxic exposures result in mental status changes. For example, sedatives and alcohol cause CNS depression. Agitation or violent behavior may be caused by CNS stimulants, such as cocaine, amphetamines, and PCP. Some substances can cause CNS stimulation *or* depression depending on the dose ingested. Some toxins can cause visual or auditory hallucinations and personality changes. Seizures are a complication of toxic exposures and should be anticipated. Any toxic exposure that results in mental status changes increases the patient's risk of problems with his or her ABCs.

Objective 5

When assessing the patient's airway, look for burns around the mouth and blisters of the lips or mucous membranes. Note if the patient has trouble swallowing or is drooling. Excessive salivation is one of the signs associated with organophosphate insecticide exposure (see Table 17-2). Listen for stridor and hoarseness. If any of these signs are present, the patient is at risk of an airway obstruction. You may need to use airway adjuncts such as an oral or nasal airway to keep the patient's airway open. Because some substances increase airway secretions and others cause nausea and vomiting, have suction equipment within arm's reach while the patient is in your care.

You Should Know

Odors can provide clues about the possible cause of the patient's signs and symptoms. For example, cyanide exposure is associated with an odor of bitter almonds. Exposure to arsenic or organophosphate insecticides is associated with the smell of garlic.

Many toxic exposures affect breathing. For instance, substances that can cause a decreased respiratory rate include sedatives, narcotics, and depressants such as alcohol (see Table 17-2). Substances that can cause an increased respiratory rate include aspirin, amphetamines, methamphetamines, caffeine, cocaine, PCP, and carbon monoxide. Be prepared to provide positive-pressure ventilation. Narrowing of the lower airway because of swelling, mucus, or spasms of the bronchi may cause wheezing.

Toxic exposures can also affect the victim's heart rate and blood pressure. Drugs that stimulate the sympathetic division of the autonomic nervous system will result in an increased heart rate. For instance, expect to see an increased heart rate if the patient has been exposed to amphetamines, cocaine, and Ecstasy. When taken in excess, alcohol and some prescribed heart medications are examples of substances that can cause a decreased heart rate. Some plants such as lily of the valley, foxglove, and oleander contain substances that can slow the heart rate. An irregular heart rhythm and shock are complications of toxic exposures and should be anticipated.

Establish patient priorities. Priority patients include the following:

- Patients who give a poor general impression
- Patients experiencing difficulty breathing
- Patients with signs and symptoms of shock
- Unresponsive patients with no gag reflex or cough
- Responsive patients who are unable to follow commands

If a patient with a suspected toxic exposure has any of the previous findings, provide initial emergency care and transport immediately to the closest appropriate medical facility, with Advanced Life Support (ALS) backup if available.

Secondary Survey

Finding out as much information as you can about the circumstances surrounding a toxic exposure is important. In cases involving an intentional exposure, keep in mind that the history obtained from the patient may not be reliable. Relay all information you find out when transferring care to ALS personnel or the staff at the receiving facility. Examples of questions to ask include the following

- What poison was involved? Find out (and document) the exact name of the substance.
- How much was taken?
- When was it taken (or when did the exposure occur)? The answer to this question influences patient symptoms and the emergency care that will be provided by ALS personnel and at the hospital. If the patient is unresponsive, finding out the time of ingestion or exposure may be impossible unless someone witnessed the event. In such situations, an estimate of the time of ingestion or exposure can often be made by determining when the patient was last seen.
- Where was the patient found? Any witnesses?
- Over what period was the substance ingested (or did the exposure occur)?
- Why was it taken? Attempt to find out whether the ingestion was accidental, intentional, recreational, or a suicide attempt.
- What else was taken? For instance, did the patient ingest any alcohol or take any acetaminophen (Tylenol)? Although many intentional ingestions involve more than one substance, your patient may not volunteer this information.
- Was any seizure activity observed?
- Has a PCC been contacted? If so, what instructions were received? What has already been done to treat the poisoning?
- How much does the patient weigh? In cases of ingested poisons, this information is necessary to determine the dose of activated charcoal.
- Does the patient have any allergies to medications or other substances or materials?
- What medications (prescription and over the counter) is the patient currently taking? Has there been any recent change in medications (additions, deletions, or change in dosages)?
- Does the patient have any underlying illnesses (such as heart disease, high blood pressure, diabetes, kidney disease, liver disease, or seizures)? Many ingested substances are broken

down in the liver and prepared for removal from the body by the kidneys. Patients who have illnesses that affect these organs may receive a toxic dose without intentionally taking too much of a substance.

- Does the patient have a history of depression or mental health problems? Has the patient ever been treated at a mental health or rehabilitation facility? These questions are important in determining the possibility of a suicide attempt.

Remember This!

Ask questions using "Who, What, Where, When, Why, and How" as a memory aid.

Objective 2

The patient's vital signs and physical exam findings (toxidrome) can provide clues to help you identify the substance involved. For instance, if you find a patient unresponsive with pinpoint pupils and slow breathing, consider the possibility of a narcotic overdose. On the other hand, don't assume that all is well if the patient's vital signs are within normal limits. A poisoned patient's condition can change quickly.

A quick check of the patient's pupils can reveal important clues. Cocaine and amphetamines are examples of substances that can cause dilated pupils. Most narcotics, some sedatives, organophosphates, and PCP cause constricted pupils. Exposure to anticonvulsants, PCP, and sedatives can result in rapid, jerky eye movements (nystagmus).

Assess the patient's skin color, temperature, and moisture. Note any redness, blisters, or patient complaints of burning or itching. Look for liquids or powder on the patient's skin or clothing.

Common signs and symptoms of poisoning are shown in the following *You Should Know* box.

Emergency Care

Objective 7

- Have trained rescuers remove the patient from the source of the poison.
- Follow proper decontamination procedures, if necessary, and prepare the ambulance to receive the patient. Methods used for decontamination will depend on the toxin and type of exposure.

You Should Know

Common Signs and Symptoms of Poisoning

- Altered mental status
- Difficulty breathing
- Headache
- Nausea
- Vomiting
- Diarrhea
- Chest or abdominal pain
- Sweating
- Seizures
- Burns around the mouth
- Burns on the skin

- Establish and maintain an open airway. Remove pills, tablets, or fragments with gloves from the patient's mouth, as needed, without injuring oneself. Be alert for vomiting and have suction ready. Pills or fragments need to be transported to the hospital with the patient so that Emergency Department personnel can identify any unknown substances. Pills should be placed in a zip-closure bag and properly labeled.
- Give oxygen. If the patient's breathing is adequate, apply oxygen by nonrebreather mask at 15 L/min if not already done. If the patient's breathing is inadequate, provide positive-pressure ventilation with 100% oxygen and assess the adequacy of the ventilations delivered.
- Call a poison center for advice about decontamination procedures and patient care as needed. Do not delay transport to contact poison control.
- If the patient has ingested a poison (and is awake), consult medical direction about giving activated charcoal.
- If the patient is unresponsive or seizing, consult medical direction about checking the patient's blood sugar.
- If possible, bring all containers, bottles, labels, and other evidence of suspected poisons to the receiving facility.
- If the patient vomits, save the vomitus in a container (such as a portable suction unit) and transport it to the receiving facility for analysis.
- Anticipate complications, including:
  —Seizures
  —Vomiting
  —Shock
  —Agitation
  —Irregular heart rhythm

- When ALS personnel arrive at the scene (or when transferring patient care at the receiving facility), pass on any patient information that you have gathered. You should include what the patient looked like when you first arrived on the scene, the care you gave, and the patient's response to your care.
- If the patient is stable, perform ongoing assessments every 15 minutes while the patient is in your care. If the patient is unstable, perform ongoing assessments every 5 minutes.

Remember This!

When caring for a patient who intentionally exposed himself to a toxic substance, ensure the safety of yourself and your crew while on the scene *and* during patient transport. Watch for behavioral changes and unpredictability.

Ingested Poisons

Most toxic exposures that you will respond to are because of ingested poisons. In some cases, they will be the result of intentional overdoses. Examples of ingested poisons are shown in the following *You Should Know* box.

You Should Know

Examples of Ingested Poisons
- Heart, blood pressure medications
- Tranquilizers, nerve pills
- Antihistamines, cough and cold medicines
- Vitamins, iron pills
- Pain relievers, fever-reducers
- Diabetes medicines
- Miniature batteries
- Arts, crafts, and office supplies
- Food, alcoholic beverages
- Mothballs
- Cigarettes, tobacco products
- Pesticides
- Antifreeze, windshield solution
- Indoor and outdoor plants (wild mushrooms, philodendron, foxglove, castor bean, dieffenbachia, pokeweed, holly berries)
- Cleaning products (drain cleaner, toilet bowl cleaner, oven cleaner, rust remover, laundry detergent, automatic dishwasher detergent)
- Cosmetics and personal care products (artificial nail remover, perfume, aftershave, mouthwash, facial cleansers, hair tonics)
- Hydrocarbons (gasoline, kerosene, lamp oil, motor oil, lighter fluid, furniture polish, paint thinner)

Patient Assessment

Signs and symptoms of ingested poisons are listed in the following *You Should Know* box. Because the patient's signs and symptoms are related to the drug ingested, the amount ingested, and the length of time since the ingestion, try to find out this information as quickly as possible. For example, how many pills were in the bottle before they were ingested? How many are left in the bottle? If the patient took a prescription medication, when was the prescription last filled? Ingestions sometimes involve liquids. Attempt to obtain information about the product from the container's label. When possible, take the label with you to the hospital.

You Should Know

Signs and Symptoms of Ingested Poisons
- History of ingestion
- Nausea
- Vomiting
- Diarrhea
- Altered mental status
- Abdominal pain
- Chemical burns around the mouth
- Unusual breath odors

Emergency Care

- Using gloves, remove pills, tablets, or fragments from the patient's mouth, as needed, without injuring oneself.
- Establish and maintain an open airway. Be alert for vomiting; have suction ready. When indicated (and if trauma is not suspected), position the patient in the recovery position to reduce the risk of aspiration.
- Give oxygen. If the patient's breathing is adequate, apply oxygen by nonrebreather mask at 15 L/min if not already done. If the patient's breathing is inadequate, provide positive-pressure ventilation with 100% oxygen. Assess the adequacy of the ventilations delivered.

- Consult medical direction about giving activated charcoal.
- Bring all containers, bottles, labels, and other evidence of suspected poisons to the receiving facility.
- Transport the patient to the closest appropriate facility, keeping the patient warm.
- En route to the receiving facility, perform ongoing assessments (including vital signs) as often as indicated.
- Carefully document all patient care information on a PCR.

You Should Know

When ingestions cause death, the most common substances involved are pain relievers, antidepressants, stimulants and street drugs, sedatives, and cardiovascular medications.

Giving Activated Charcoal

Objective 6

If the patient is alert and cooperative, medical direction may instruct you to give the patient activated charcoal. Activated charcoal binds (adsorbs) with many (but not all) chemicals, slowing down or blocking absorption of the chemical in the gastrointestinal (GI) tract.

Activated charcoal is produced by heating wood pulp to high temperatures and then "activating" it with steam or strong acids. This process creates tiny pores on each particle of charcoal that increases its surface area. With this large surface area, activated charcoal will bind many ingested toxins. However, charcoal can only bind a drug that is *not yet absorbed* from the gastrointestinal (GI) tract.

Medication Actions

Activated charcoal binds many toxic substances in the GI tract to prevent them from being absorbed and then carries them out of the GI tract. Activated charcoal does not bind well to some substances such as some pesticides (malathion), cyanide, strong caustics (acids and bases), iron, mercury, ethanol, methanol, and petroleum products (such as gasoline, turpentine, and kerosene).

Indications and Dosage

If ordered by medical direction (and approved by your state and local EMS system), you may give activated charcoal for some ingested poisons. The dosage of activated charcoal for adults and children is 1 gram of activated charcoal per kilogram of body weight. The usual adult dose is 25 to 50 grams. The usual dose for an infant or child 12.5 to 25 grams. If the activated charcoal is not premixed, mix the appropriate dosage in a glass of water (8 ounces) to produce a thick slurry.

Contraindications

- Patient has an altered mental status.
- Patient is unable to swallow.
- Medical direction does not give authorization.
- Patient has ingested acids or alkalis. Examples of acids include rust removers, phenol, and battery acid. Examples of alkalis include ammonia, household bleach, and drain cleaner.

Special Considerations

- Obtain an order from medical direction either on line or off line to give the medication.
- Before giving any medication, make sure you have the right patient, right drug, right dose, right route, and right time.
- Activated charcoal can be harmful or fatal if the patient accidentally inhales it. Before giving this drug, you must make sure that the patient is awake, cooperative, has an open airway, and can swallow.
- Activated charcoal looks like mud. It is often helpful to put the medication in a cup, cover it with a lid, and have the patient drink the mixture through a straw.
- Do not give activated charcoal with ice cream, sherbet, milk, or other drinks. Because charcoal binds with whatever it is mixed with, flavoring with drinks impairs charcoal's capacity to bind with other substances.
- After giving charcoal, reassess the patient's airway, breathing, and circulatory status. Be prepared for the patient to vomit or for his condition to worsen. Signs of worsening of the patient's condition include decreasing mental status, increasing breathing difficulty, and decreasing blood pressure. If the patient's condition improves, give supportive care. Perform ongoing assessments every 5 minutes. Transport promptly to the closest appropriate medical facility.

Procedure

Skill Drill 17-1 shows the procedure for giving a patient activated charcoal. Information about activated charcoal appears in Table 17-4.

Giving Activated Charcoal

STEP 1 ▶ Put on appropriate personal protective equipment. Because charcoal will stain any clothing it contacts, take additional precautions as necessary. Obtain an order from medical direction either on line or off line. Make sure that the patient is awake, cooperative, has an open airway, and can swallow.

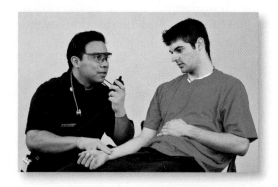

STEP 2 ▶ Make sure that the activated charcoal is not expired. Grasp the container in your hand and shake thoroughly.

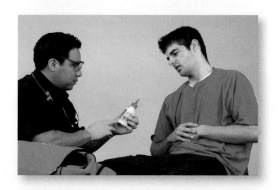

STEP 3 ▶ Cover the patient's lap or chest with old towels and have a large basin available should the patient vomit. Because charcoal looks like black mud, the patient may need to be persuaded to drink it. Place a straw in the container or pour the activated charcoal into a covered opaque container and ask the patient to drink it. If the patient does not drink all of the medication in the first drink, shake the container before the second dose because the activated charcoal will settle to the bottom of the container or glass. Some patients, particularly those who have ingested poisons that cause nausea, may vomit. Vomiting may also occur when charcoal is drunk either too slowly or too rapidly. If the patient vomits, consider repeating the dose once (check with medical direction).

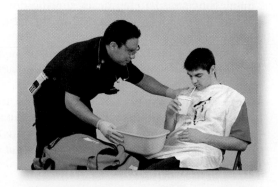

STEP 4 ▶ Document the patient's name, drug name and dose given, time of administration, and the patient's response to the drug. If an on-line order was received by medical direction, document the name of the physician giving the order. The patient will need to be transported for additional care. Perform ongoing assessments every five minutes.

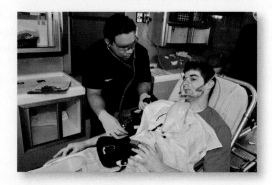

TABLE 17-4 Activated Charcoal

Generic name	activated charcoal
Trade name	Liqui-Char, Actidose, InstaChar, SuperChar, and others
Mechanism of action	Activated charcoal acts as an adsorbent and will bind with many (but not all chemicals) and slow down or block absorption of the chemical by the body.
Indications	Poisoning by mouth
Dosage	Adults and children: 1 gram activated charcoal/kilogram of body weight Usual adult dose: 25 to 50 grams Usual infant/child dose: 12.5 to 25 grams
Side effects	Nausea, vomiting, abdominal cramping, constipation, black stools
Contraindications	• Medical direction does not give permission • Altered mental status • Unable to swallow • Ingestion of acids or alkalis

Inhaled Poisons

A poison may be inhaled in the form of sprays, dust, droplets, vapors, gases, and fumes. Because the lungs have a large surface area and good blood supply, inhaled poisons can be quickly absorbed and distributed throughout the body. Some inhaled toxins cause significant and permanent damage to the lungs, brain, kidneys, liver, heart, blood, and bone marrow.

Some chemicals (such as ammonia and chlorine) produce fumes with a characteristic odor that can alert you to their presence. However, some gases have no odor. This makes them particularly dangerous because exposure to the poison can occur without the person even being aware of the exposure. Such is the case with many carbon monoxide poisonings. Carbon monoxide is a colorless, odorless gas that is the result of incomplete combustion. It is the most common cause of death from poisonous gas. Every year a story makes national news because someone, or a group of people, died as a result of carbon monoxide exposure when a fuel-burning appliance malfunctioned (such as an oil or gas furnace, gas water heater, gas range or oven, gas dryer, gas or kerosene space heater, or wood stove). Other sources of inhaled poisons include

- Designer drugs
- Wells, sewers
- Anesthetic gases
- Chemical warfare
- Water purification

- Fumes from sprays and liquid chemicals
- Cleaners, degreasing agents, fire extinguishers
- Solvents in dry cleaning fluid, electrical equipment
- Refrigerator and air conditioner gases in the home and in commercial ice-making plants
- Gases produced as by-products from fires, lightning, heating, and fuel exhausts

Inhalants are household and commercial products that can be abused by intentionally breathing the product's gas or vapors for its mind-altering effects. Inhalant use is called "huffing" or "sniffing." According to the National Institute on Drug Abuse (NIDA), **sudden sniffing death syndrome (SSDS)** can occur when a person sniffs highly concentrated amounts of the chemicals in solvents or aerosol sprays. Death occurs within minutes because of heart failure. This syndrome is particularly associated with the abuse of butane, propane, and chemicals in aerosols.

A thorough scene size-up on arrival at the scene is essential. Resist the temptation to immediately enter the scene and begin patient care. Without some knowledge of the substance involved, you could place yourself and your crew at unnecessary risk for exposure. Assess the situation for potential or actual danger. Precautions against fire and explosion may be necessary for some gases. If the scene is not safe to enter, move to a safe location. If you have been trained to do so (and are properly equipped), identify and establish safety zones. Contact dispatch for additional resources as necessary.

Examples of inhaled poisons are shown in the following *You Should Know* box.

You Should Know

Examples of Inhaled Poisons

Carbon monoxide

Carbon dioxide

Chlorine

Ammonia

Propane

Cyanide

Freon

Tear gas

Inhalants and fumes
- Hair spray
- Cleaning fluids
- Typewriter correction fluid
- Nail polish remover
- Glue, rubber cement
- Paint, paint thinner
- Lighter fluid
- Room deodorizers
- Felt marker pens

Patient Assessment

Signs and symptoms of an inhalation exposure depend on the substance inhaled, the amount inhaled, and the extent and duration of exposure. A person who experiences a toxic exposure in a confined space, such as a closed room or garage, is more likely to experience more severe signs and symptoms that a person exposed in an open area. In general, the longer and more concentrated the exposure, the more risk of the incident being fatal. Signs and symptoms of an inhalation exposure are listed in the following *You Should Know* box.

You Should Know

Signs and Symptoms of Inhaled Poisons

- History of inhalation of toxic substance
- Altered mental status
- Difficulty breathing
- Chest pain/discomfort
- Cough
- Hoarseness
- Dizziness
- Headache
- Confusion
- Seizures

Emergency Care

- Have trained rescuers remove the patient from the poisonous environment.
- After making sure the scene is safe to enter and you are properly equipped, remove the patient's contaminated clothing. Discard contaminated clothing in an appropriate container.
- Establish and maintain an open airway. Be alert for vomiting; have suction ready. When indicated (and if trauma is not suspected), position the patient in the recovery position to reduce the risk of aspiration.
- Give oxygen. If the patient's breathing is adequate, apply oxygen by nonrebreather mask at 15 L/min if not already done. If the patient's breathing is inadequate, provide positive-pressure ventilation with 100% oxygen. Assess the adequacy of the ventilations delivered.
- Contact medical direction or a poison center to help determine potential toxicity.
- If relevant, bring all containers, bottles, labels, and other evidence of suspected poisons to the receiving facility.
- Transport the patient to the closest appropriate facility. En route to the receiving facility, perform ongoing assessments (including vital signs) as often as indicated.
- Carefully document all patient care information on a PCR.

Injected Poisons

Poisons that can be injected include:

- Bee, wasp, and ant venom
- Spider, tick, and scorpion venom
- Snake venom
- Drugs

Patient Assessment

The patient's signs and symptoms are related to the substance injected, the amount injected, and the length of time since the exposure occurred. Be alert for signs and symptoms of anaphylaxis. Signs and symptoms of injected poisons are listed in the next *You Should Know* box.

Emergency Care

- Remove the patient (and rescuers) from the environment if repeated stings or bites are likely.

Signs and Symptoms of Injected Poisons

- Weakness
- Dizziness
- Chills
- Fever
- Abnormal heart rate or rhythm
- Nausea
- Vomiting

- Establish and maintain an open airway. Be alert for vomiting; have suction ready.
- Give oxygen. If the patient's breathing is adequate, apply oxygen by nonrebreather mask at 15 L/min if not already done. If the patient's breathing is inadequate, provide positive-pressure ventilation with 100% oxygen and assess the adequacy of the ventilations delivered.
- Contact medical direction/poison center to help determine potential toxicity.
- If applicable, bring all containers, bottles, labels, and other evidence of suspected poisons to the receiving facility.
- Monitor the patient closely for signs and symptoms of anaphylaxis. If the patient has severe respiratory distress or signs of shock and has been prescribed an epinephrine auto-injector (or if you are authorized to carry it), contact medical direction and request an order to give epinephrine or assist the patient in taking it.
- Transport the patient to the closest appropriate facility or rendezvous with an ALS unit en route. En route to the receiving facility, perform ongoing assessments (including vital signs) as often as indicated.
- Carefully document all patient care information on a PCR.

Absorbed Poisons

Toxins can enter the body by absorption through the eye, skin, or mucous membranes. Examples of poisons that can be absorbed include

- Toxins from plants such as poison ivy, poison oak, and poison sumac
- Pesticides
- Fertilizers
- Cocaine
- Chemical warfare agents

Patient Assessment

Absorbed poisons generally cause redness of the affected area. Signs and symptoms of absorbed poisons are listed in the following *You Should Know* box.

You Should Know

Signs and Symptoms of Absorbed Poisons

- History of exposure
- Liquid or powder on patient's skin
- Burns
- Itching
- Irritation
- Redness

Emergency Care

- Remove the patient from the source of the poison. Remove any powder or residue from the patient's skin carefully.
- While wearing chemical protective clothing and gloves, remove the patient's contaminated clothing and jewelry. Dispose of contaminated clothing in an appropriate container.
- Establish and maintain an open airway.
- Give oxygen. If the patient's breathing is adequate, apply oxygen by nonrebreather mask at 15 L/min if not already done. If the patient's breathing is inadequate, provide positive-pressure ventilation with 100% oxygen and assess the adequacy of the ventilations delivered.
- If the exposure involves the patient's skin and the poison is in powder form, brush the powder off the patient, then continue as for other absorbed poisons. Be careful not to brush the chemical onto unaffected areas. If the poison is in liquid form, irrigate the skin with clean water for at least 20 minutes (and continue en route to the receiving facility if possible). Pay particular attention to skin creases and fingernails. Do not apply grease or ointments to the affected area.
- If the exposure involves the patient's eye, flush the affected eye with clean water 2 or 3 inches from the eye for at least 20 minutes. Ask the patient to blink often while flushing. If only one eye is involved, be careful not to contaminate the unaffected eye. Do not allow the patient to rub his eyes. Continue en route to the receiving facility if possible. When flushing is complete, cover both eyes with moistened dressings or eye pads.

- Contact medical direction or a poison center to help determine potential toxicity.
- If applicable, bring all containers, bottles, labels, or other evidence of suspected poisons to the receiving facility.
- Transport the patient to the closest appropriate facility. En route to the receiving facility, perform ongoing assessments (including vital signs) as often as indicated.
- Carefully document all patient care information on a PCR.

On the Scene Wrap-Up

As you perform your primary and secondary surveys, you notice that the patient's breathing is shallow and slowly decreasing. She no longer responds when you call her name or apply a painful stimulus. A slow, weak pulse is present. Her blood pressure is 92/60. The patient's pupils are constricted. You recognize that these signs and symptoms are consistent with a toxic exposure to narcotics. Your partner inserts an oral airway and begins positive-pressure ventilation using a bag-mask device connected to 100% oxygen.

On arrival at the hospital, you quickly relay the patient's history and vital signs to the emergency department (ED) staff. An ED nurse takes over positive-pressure ventilation while another inserts an intravenous (IV) line and gives the patient naloxone IV. Within minutes the patient is awake and alert, and her respiratory rate, heart rate, and blood pressure have returned to normal. ■

Sum It Up

- A poison is any substance taken into the body that interferes with normal body function. Poisoning is exposure to a substance that is harmful in any dosage. A toxin is a poisonous substance. An antidote is a substance that neutralizes a poison.

- A Poison Control Center (PCC) is a medical facility that provides free telephone advice to the public and medical professionals in case of exposure to poisonous substances. Medical professionals at a PCC can help determine the toxicity of a substance and give advice about the emergency care the patient should receive.

- A poison may be a solid, liquid, spray, or gas. Toxins enter the body in four ways — ingestion, inhalation, injection, or absorption. Exposure to a toxin may be accidental or intentional.

- Signs and symptoms of a toxic exposure can vary depending on the substance involved, route of entry, the amount ingested, inhaled, injected, or absorbed, and the length of the exposure.

- Signs, symptoms, and characteristics that often occur together in toxic exposures are called toxidromes. When the cause of a toxic exposure is unknown, knowing the "typical" signs and symptoms of certain toxic exposures can help you to identify the poison and give appropriate care. Toxic exposures that involve more than one substance (such as alcohol and recreational drugs) are often difficult to recognize and treat. In these situations, the patient will most likely not have signs and symptoms specific to only one toxidrome.

- A thorough scene size-up on arrival at the scene of a toxic exposure is essential. Resist the temptation to immediately enter the scene and begin patient care. Without some knowledge of the substance involved, you could place yourself and your crew at an unnecessary risk for exposure. Assess the situation for potential or actual danger. Contact dispatch for additional resources as necessary.

- Finding out as much information as you can about the circumstances surrounding a toxic exposure is important. In cases involving an intentional exposure, keep in mind that the history obtained from the patient may or may not be reliable. Relay all information you obtained when transferring care to ALS personnel or the staff at the receiving facility.

- When caring for a patient exposed to a toxin, try to find out (and document) the exact name of the substance. If applicable, bring all containers, bottles, labels, and other evidence of poison agents to the receiving facility.

CHAPTER

18 Environmental Emergencies

By the end of this chapter, you should be able to:

Knowledge Objectives ▶
1. Describe the various ways that the body loses heat.
2. List the signs and symptoms of exposure to cold.
3. Explain the steps in providing emergency medical care to a patient exposed to cold.
4. List the signs and symptoms of exposure to heat.
5. Explain the steps in providing emergency care to a patient exposed to heat.
6. Recognize the signs and symptoms of water-related emergencies.
7. Describe the complications of drowning.
8. Discuss the emergency medical care of bites and stings.

Attitude Objectives ▶
There are no attitude objectives identified for this lesson.

Skill Objectives ▶

9. Demonstrate the assessment and emergency medical care of a patient with exposure to cold.
10. Demonstrate the assessment and emergency medical care of a patient with exposure to heat.
11. Demonstrate the assessment and emergency medical care of a near-drowning patient.
12. Demonstrate completing a prehospital care report for patients with environmental emergencies.

On the Scene

You and your Emergency Medical Technician partner are called for a 45-year-old woman who was bitten by a rattlesnake. Upon arrival at the scene, you find the patient sitting at her kitchen table. She points to her right index finger, which you notice is swollen. The patient states she was trying to kill a baby rattlesnake with a garbage can lid when it bit her. The patient is alert and oriented to person, place, time, and event, and denies any other injuries. ■

THINK ABOUT IT

As you read this chapter, think about the following questions:

• What additional information should you try to obtain from the patient?
• What treatment measures would be appropriate for this patient?
• How should the patient's injured extremity be positioned?

Environmental emergencies include exposure to heat and cold, water-related emergencies, and bites and stings. Medical conditions can be caused or worsened by the weather, terrain, atmospheric pressure, or other local factors. The keys to appropriate management of any environmental emergency are recognizing signs and symptoms of the emergency as early as possible and providing prompt, efficient emergency medical care.

You must be aware of the ways in which the body loses heat in order to effectively manage patients with temperature-related emergencies. Cold-related emergencies occur in many groups of individuals, including hunters, sailors, skiers, climbers, swimmers, and military personnel. A cold emergency may occur in the wilderness, as well as in rural and urban settings. It can also occur in the summer at night, in a cold building, or following a water exposure. Heat-related emergencies occur in many different settings and may occur during any season of the year. Heat emergencies range from minor effects to life-threatening conditions. Drowning is the most common type of water-related emergency you will encounter.

Because of differences in climates and terrain, not all species of spiders, snakes, insects, scorpions, or marine animals are present in all areas of the United States. Recognizing the signs and symptoms of poisonous bites and stings may help minimize the patient's risk of loss of life or limb.

Body Temperature

Body temperature is the balance between the heat produced by the body and the heat lost from the body. Body temperature is measured in heat units called degrees (°). The body is divided into two areas for temperature control: core temperature and peripheral (surface) temperature. The body core (the deep tissues of the body) includes the contents of the skull, vertebral column, chest, abdomen, and pelvis. Core temperature is the temperature that is essential for the body to convert food to energy (metabolism). The temperature of the periphery is not critical. The body core is normally maintained at a fairly constant temperature, usually within 1°F (approximately 0.6°C) of normal, unless a person develops a fever.

Body temperature remains constant if the heat produced by the body equals the heat lost. When the body produces too much heat, the temperature can temporarily rise to as high as 101°F to 104°F (38.3°C

to 40.0°C). This type of temporary rise in temperature can occur, for example, during strenuous exercise. When the body is exposed to cold, the temperature can often fall to below 96°F (35.6°C).

You Should Know

A rectal temperature is considered a measurement of the body's core temperature. When measured orally, the average normal temperature is between 98.0°F (Fahrenheit) and 98.6°F, which is about 37°C (Celsius). The temperature measured in the armpit (the axillary temperature) or orally is about 1°F (about 0.6°C) less than the rectal (core) temperature.

The peripheral area of the body includes the skin, subcutaneous tissue, and fat. The temperature of the body's extremities rises and falls in response to the environment. At room temperature, the temperature in the peripheral areas of the body is slightly below those of the body core.

Temperature Regulation

The skin plays a very important role in temperature regulation. Cold and warmth sensors (receptors) in the skin detect changes in temperature. These receptors relay the information to the hypothalamus. The hypothalamus (located in the brain) functions as the body's thermostat. It coordinates the body's response to temperature.

The cardiovascular system regulates blood flow to the skin. Blood vessels widen (dilate) and narrow (constrict) in response to messages from the hypothalamus. When high temperatures are sensed, blood vessels in the skin dilate. When low temperatures are sensed, blood vessels in the skin constrict (narrow). When these vessels narrow, sweating stops and the major body muscles shiver to increase heat.

You Should Know

The body regulates core temperature through vasodilation, vasoconstriction, sweating (which cools the body through evaporation), shivering, increasing or decreasing activity, and behavioral responses (such as applying or removing layers of clothing, which ultimately results in heat regulation).

Heat Production

Body heat is produced mainly by the conversion of food to energy (metabolism). Most of the heat produced in the body is made by the liver, brain, heart, and the skeletal muscles during exercise. The heat made by skeletal muscle is important in temperature control. This is because muscle activity can be increased to produce heat when needed.

The body begins a series of actions when its cold sensors are stimulated. These actions are designed to conserve heat and increase heat production. One action is to produce more epinephrine and other hormones. The increased production of epinephrine and other hormones increases the rate at which the body converts food to energy, which increases heat production. Another action is to constrict peripheral blood vessels. This decreases blood flow and heat loss through the skin. It also keeps warm blood in the body's core. Muscle activity also increases. Muscle activity may be voluntary (such as walking, running, or moving about) or involuntary (such as shivering).

Heat Loss

Objective 1

Knowing how the body loses heat will allow you to prevent further heat loss when treating patients with a cold-related emergency. The body loses heat to the environment in five ways (Figure 18-1):

1. Radiation
2. Convection
3. Conduction
4. Evaporation
5. Breathing

Most heat loss occurs when heat is transferred from the deeper body organs and tissues to the skin. From there it is lost to the air and other surroundings. Some heat loss occurs through the mucous membranes of the respiratory, digestive, and urinary systems.

More than half of the heat lost from the body occurs by radiation. **Radiation** is the transfer of heat, as infrared heat rays, from the surface of one object to the surface of another without contact between the two objects. The heat from the sun is an example of radiation. When the temperature of the body is more than the temperature of the surroundings, the body will lose heat. **Convection** is the transfer of heat by the movement of air current. Wind speed affects heat loss by convection (wind-chill factor). Conduction is the transfer of heat between objects that are in direct

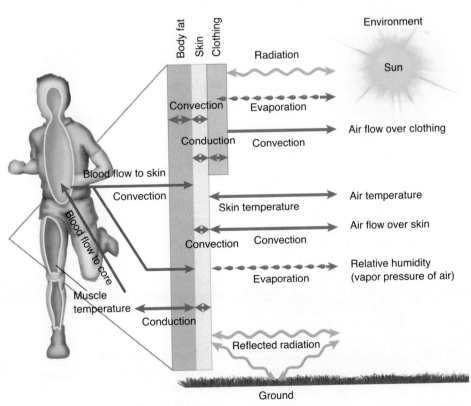

FIGURE 18-1 ▲ The body loses heat by radiation, convection, conduction, evaporation, and breathing.

contact. Heat flows from warmer areas to cooler ones. The amount of heat lost from the body by conduction depends on the following:

- The temperature difference between the body and the object
- The amount of time the body and the object are in contact
- The amount (surface area) of the body in contact with the object

Evaporation is a loss of heat by vaporization of moisture on the body surface. The body will lose heat by evaporation if the skin temperature is higher than the temperature of the surroundings. The body gains heat when the temperature of the surrounding air is higher than body temperature. As relative humidity rises, the effectiveness of body cooling by evaporation decreases.

The body also loses heat by breathing in cool air and exhaling the air that has become heated in the lungs. Additionally, the body continuously loses a relatively small amount of heat through the evaporation of moisture from within the lungs.

When the body's warmth sensors are stimulated, the body takes action to increase heat loss. Peripheral blood vessels dilate. Blood flow to the body surface increases. Heat escapes from the skin surface by radiation and conduction. When air currents pass across the skin, additional heat is lost by convection. This heat loss cools the body's core. The body's sweat gland secretion also increases. The sweat travels to the skin's surface. When air currents pass across the skin, heat is lost through evaporation.

Making a Difference

Consider a situation in which a patient is found lying on the ground or roadway after a motor vehicle crash. In cold climates, the patient may experience a cold-related emergency after lying on a cold surface. Taking a long time to assess the patient increases the amount of time he is exposed to the environment. In warm climates, patients have experienced severe burns from prolonged exposure to the hot ground or pavement. Even after being placed on a long backboard, patients have experienced burns on the back surfaces of their arms because they were left in contact with the pavement. Do not assume that a patient's complaints are related only to injuries from the crash. His complaints may also be related to the environment in which you found him. Be sensitive to these types of situations.

Exposure to Cold

Types of Cold Emergencies

There are two main types of cold emergencies: a generalized cold emergency (generalized hypothermia) and a local cold injury. A local cold injury is damage to a specific area of the body, such as fingers or toes. Local cold injury is discussed later in this chapter.

Hypothermia

Hypothermia is a core body temperature of less than 95°F (35°C). This condition results when the body loses more heat than it gains or produces. Hypothermia can be broken down into three stages: mild, moderate, and severe.

- Mild hypothermia (core body temperature 93.2°F to 96.8°F, or 34.0°C to 37.0°C)
- Moderate hypothermia (86.0°F to 93.1°F, or 30.0°C to 33.9°C)
- Severe hypothermia (less than 86.0°F, or less than 30.0°C)

It is important to realize that the stages of hypothermia are not a hard-and-fast rule for everyone. Some patients may show signs and symptoms at different temperatures. It is also important to understand that the temperatures shown here are core body temperatures. The usual methods for measuring temperature (oral and tympanic) may not accurately reflect the core temperature. A rectal temperature gives the most accurate measure of core temperature. However, obtaining a rectal temperature in the field often raises issues of patient sensitivity and welfare, such as exposure to cold by removing clothing. In most cases, you will need to make judgments about hypothermia based on your patient's signs and symptoms.

Remember This!

Temperatures below 95°F (35°C) are significant because at or below this temperature, the body typically does not generate enough heat to restore normal body temperature or maintain proper organ function.

Hypothermia may occur from exposure to conditions that result in excessive heat loss. Hypothermia can occur even in warm weather. For example, a person who remains in a cool environment, such as a swimming pool, can experience hypothermia. Hypothermia can also occur when the body loses its ability to maintain a normal body temperature. This situation can occur in patients who are in shock.

Some factors increase a person's risk of experiencing hypothermia (see the following *You Should Know* box). A person's age is one factor. Many hypothermia cases occur in urban settings and involve older adults. Older adults are at risk of hypothermia because of the following:

- Lack of heat in the home
- Poor diet or appetite
- Loss of subcutaneous fat for body insulation
- Lack of activity
- Delayed circulation
- Decreased efficiency of temperature control mechanisms

You Should Know

Factors That Contribute to Hypothermia

- Cold, windy weather conditions
- Prolonged exposure to a cool environment
- Immersion in water
- Improper, inadequate, or wet clothing
- Low body weight
- Poor physical condition
- Low blood sugar
- Recent trauma or burn injury
- Drug or alcohol intake
- Extremes in age (very young children, the elderly)
- Impaired judgment resulting from mental illness or Alzheimer's disease
- Preexisting medical conditions
- Previous cold exposure

Young children are at risk of hypothermia because they have less subcutaneous fat for body insulation. Their large surface area in relation to their overall size also results in a more rapid heat loss. Newborns are unable to shiver. Infants and very young children are unable to protect themselves from the cold. They cannot put on clothes and cannot move to warm surroundings without help.

Some illnesses and injuries increase a person's risk of hypothermia. These conditions include shock, head or spinal injuries, burns, generalized infection, and low blood sugar. The use of drugs or alcohol can affect a person's judgment, preventing him from taking proper safety measures. These safety measures might include wearing more clothing, increasing the room temperature, or coming in from the cold.

Alcohol dilates the body's peripheral vessels and depresses the central nervous system. Heat loss may occur quickly because of dilated vessels. Sedation from alcohol can cause the sedation that comes from cold exposure to go unrecognized.

Assessment of the Patient with a Cold-Related Injury

Objective 2

When you are called for a patient with a possible cold-related injury, carefully size up the scene on arrival. A cold environment requires special safety considerations because of the presence of ice, snow, or wind. You may need to wait on the scene until the necessary equipment or rescue personnel arrive.

Look at the patient's environment for signs of cold exposure. The signs of exposure may be very obvious or very subtle. Subtle signs of exposure include:

- Alcohol ingestion
- Underlying illness
- Overdose or poisoning
- Major trauma
- Outdoor recreation
- Decreased room temperature (such as in the home of an older adult)

Removing the patient from the environment must be your main concern. Use trained rescuers for this purpose when necessary. While you assess the need for additional resources, think about what your department or agency can handle safely. For example, can your department safely removing a person who is trapped in a freezing lake? In all cases of cold-related emergencies, you should request Advanced Life Support (ALS) personnel as soon as possible.

Stop and Think!

What equipment do you have in place right now to help you treat a cold-related emergency? Your answer to this question should be a reminder to check your seasonal equipment for use in an emergency setting.

After ensuring your safety, perform a primary survey. Approach the patient and form a general impression. Notice the clothing the patient is wearing. Is it adequate for the climate that you are in? What are the surroundings like? As you continue your assessment, keep in mind that you need to move the patient to a warm location as quickly and as safely as possible. Remove any cold or wet clothing. Protect the patient from the environment. This may include shielding the patient from the wind. Cover him to help preserve body heat. A lot of body heat is lost through the head. Covering the patient's head can help reduce heat loss. Stabilize his spine if needed.

Assess the patient's mental status, airway, breathing, and circulation. Remember that mental status decreases as the patient's body temperature drops. However, as the patient's body temperature drops, there may be no clear difference between the stages of hypothermia. The patient may show the following signs:

- Difficult (slow, slurred) speech
- Confusion
- Memory lapse (amnesia)
- Mood changes
- Combativeness
- Unresponsiveness
- Loss of motor skills and coordination
- Uncontrollable shivering; later, a lack of shivering

Remember This!

A patient who has severe hypothermia may be alive but may have such a weak pulse or shallow breathing that you are unable to feel it. Do not assume a patient is dead until he is warm and has no pulse. Take longer than usual to assess the breathing and heart rate of a patient who has been exposed to cold before starting cardiopulmonary resuscitation (CPR). Assess breathing for 30 to 45 seconds. Also, assess for a pulse for 30 to 45 seconds.

The patient's vital signs will also change as hypothermia worsens. The patient's breathing rate is initially increased, then slow and shallow, and finally absent. The heart rate is initially increased, then slow and irregular, and finally absent. Blood pressure may be normal at first and then low to absent. The pupils dilate and are slow to respond. The skin is initially red; then pale; then blue; and finally gray, hard, and cold to the touch. To assess the patient's general temperature, place the back of your hand between the patient's clothing and his abdomen. The patient experiencing a generalized cold emergency will have a cool or cold abdominal skin temperature.

The patient's motor and sensory functions also change with the degree of hypothermia. The patient may initially complain of joint aches or muscle stiffness. He may show a lack of coordination and a staggering walk. Shivering is usually present initially. As hypothermia worsens, shivering gradually decreases until it is absent. Shivering stops below 86.0°F to 89.6°F (30.0°C to 32.0°C). The patient loses sensation and his muscles become rigid. Be certain to assess the patient for other injuries. Identify any life-threatening conditions and provide care based on your findings. The signs and symptoms of hypothermia are listed in Table 18-1.

If the patient is responsive, or if family members or bystanders are available, try to obtain a SAMPLE history. Keep in mind that some illnesses or injuries increase a person's risk of hypothermia. Find out if the patient has a history of alcohol abuse; thyroid disorder; diabetes; stroke; or trauma to the head, neck,

TABLE 18-1 Signs and Symptoms of Hypothermia

Mild	Moderate	Severe
• Increased heart rate	• Shivering that may gradually decrease and become absent; shivering becomes replaced with rigid muscles	• Irrational attitude that changes to unresponsiveness
• Increased respiratory rate		• Rigid muscles
• Cool skin (to preserve core temperature)		• Cold skin
• Shivering	• Decreasing heart rate and respiratory rate	• Blue or mottled skin
• Difficulty talking, slurred speech	• Irregular heart rate	• Slow or absent breathing
• Difficulty moving	• Pale, blue (cyanotic), or mottled skin	• Slowly responding pupils
• Memory lapse (amnesia), mood changes, combative attitude	• Progressive loss of responsiveness	• A heart rate that is slow, irregular, or absent
• Joint aches, muscle stiffness	• Dilated pupils	• A pulse that is hard to feel or absent
• Altered mental status, confusion, or poor judgment (patient may actually remove clothing)	• Blood pressure that is difficult to obtain	• Low-to-absent blood pressure
		• Cardiopulmonary arrest

or spine. When finding out what events led to the patient's present situation, ask the following questions:

- How long has the patient been exposed to the cold?
- What was the source of the cold (for example, water or snow)? If the patient was exposed to water, what was the approximate water temperature?
- What was the patient doing when his symptoms began?

Remember This!

Moving water robs the body of heat even faster than still water.

Emergency Care of Patients with Hypothermia

Objective 3

The basic principles of rewarming a hypothermic patient involve conserving the heat he has and replacing the body fuel he is burning up to generate that heat. Remove the patient from the cold environment as quickly and as safely as possible to protect him from further heat loss. When moving the patient, keep in mind known or suspected injuries. Cut away cold or wet clothing rather than tugging and pulling at the patient's clothes. Protect the patient from the cold with available materials, such as blankets, a sleeping bag, newspapers, or plastic garbage bags (Figure 18-2).

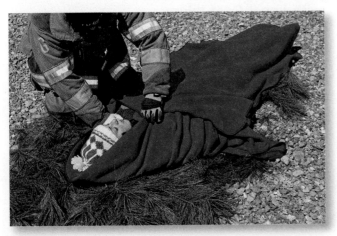

FIGURE 18-2 ▲ Protect the patient from the cold with available materials. Make sure to cover the patient's head, leaving her face exposed so that you can watch her airway. Place insulating material between the patient and the surface on which she is lying.

Make sure to cover the patient's head. However, leave her face exposed so that you can watch her airway. Place insulating material between the patient and the surface on which she is lying. Protect the patient from drafts.

Handle the patient gently. Avoid rough handling. Do not allow the patient to walk or exert herself. Rough handling or exertion may force cold blood in the periphery to the body's core. Make sure the patient's airway is open and that suction is within arm's reach. As the body cools, the cough reflex is depressed and respiratory secretions increase. Frequent suctioning may be necessary.

Give oxygen. If the patient's breathing is adequate, apply oxygen by mask at 15 L/min. If the patient's breathing is inadequate, assist her breathing with a bag-mask (BM) or mouth-to-mask device. Assess pulses for 30 to 45 seconds. If the patient has no pulse, begin CPR.

Stop and Think!

The decision to rewarm a hypothermic patient depends on your local protocol and the degree of hypothermia. Be sure to consult with medical direction before rewarming the patient.

There are two main types of rewarming: passive and active. **Passive rewarming** is the warming of a patient with minimal or no use of heat sources other than the patient's own heat production. Passive rewarming methods include placing the patient in a warm environment, applying clothing and blankets, and preventing drafts. Passive external rewarming is appropriate for all hypothermic patients.

Active rewarming involves adding heat directly to the surface of the patient's body. Active rewarming should not delay definitive care and may be used if the patient is alert and responding appropriately (follow local protocol):

- If the patient shows signs of mild hypothermia, apply warm blankets. Apply heat packs or hot water bottles to the groin, armpits, and the back of the neck. To prevent burns, place a towel or dressings between the heat pack or hot water bottle and the patient's skin.
- If the patient shows signs of moderate hypothermia, apply warm blankets. Apply heat packs or hot water bottles to the torso only. Take care to avoid burning the underlying tissue.
- If the patient shows signs of severe hypothermia, apply warm blankets. Active rewarming will need

to be done at the hospital. Alert the receiving facility of the patient's condition and your estimated time of arrival.

- Do not allow a patient to eat or drink stimulants (such as coffee, tea, or chocolate) or to drink alcohol. Do not rub or massage the patient's extremities. Doing so can cause cold blood to move from the extremities to the body core, causing a further decrease in temperature.

- During transport, turn the heat up in the patient area of the ambulance. En route to the receiving facility, perform ongoing assessments (including vital signs) as often as indicated. Carefully document all patient care information on a prehospital care report (PCR).

Remember This!

In general, chemical heat packs can provide 100°F heat for about 6 to 10 hours. Hot water bottles and warm rocks or towels are also good sources of heat. However, remember that a patient who has an altered mental status may not recognize when a heat source is too hot. No matter what heat source is used, careful monitoring is essential.

Local Cold Injury

When the body is exposed to cold, blood is forced away from the extremities to the body core. This puts the arms and legs at risk of local cold injury. **Local cold injury** (also called *frostbite*) involves tissue damage to a specific area of the body. It occurs when a body part, such as the nose, ears, cheeks, chin, hands, or feet, is exposed to prolonged or intense cold. Local tissue injury usually occurs when these areas are wet, poorly protected, or unprotected. Cold causes the blood vessels to narrow in the affected part. This narrowing decreases circulation to the involved area. Ice crystals form within the cells, which damages them. Hypothermia is often accompanied by frostbite.

Patients at risk of local cold injury include those with circulation problems, such as diabetics. Patients with a history of heart or blood vessel disease are also at risk. Alcohol, nicotine, and some medications decrease blood flow to the skin, increasing the risk of a local cold injury. Patients who have experienced a soft-tissue injury such as a burn or a previous cold injury are also at risk. Other factors that affect the risk of local cold injury include the following:

- Ambient temperature
- Windchill factor

- The length of exposure
- The type and number of clothing layers worn, including tight gloves and tight or tightly laced footwear
- Whether or not the patient is wet
- Whether or not the patient has had direct contact with cold objects

A local cold injury may be early (superficial frostbite) or late (deep frostbite). A superficial cold injury involves the uppermost skin layers. Early (superficial) local cold injury is also called *frostnip*. In a superficial cold injury, the skin of the exposed area first appears red and inflamed. With continued cooling, the area then becomes gray or white. When you press on the skin, normal color does not return (blanching). You may see a clear demarcation (a visible line of color change), although this sign may not be present at the scene. The patient may complain of a loss of feeling in the injured area. The skin beneath the affected area remains soft. If the area is rewarmed, the patient experiences tingling or burning. This is followed by a "pins-and-needles" sensation as the area thaws and circulation improves.

A deep cold injury involves more tissue layers. This type of injury is more serious than superficial frostbite. In a deep cold injury, the whitish skin color is followed by a waxy appearance. The affected area becomes frozen. It will feel stiff and solid when you touch it. The patient may complain of slight burning pain followed by a feeling of warmth and then numbness. Swelling may be present. Blisters may be present, usually appearing in 1 to 7 days. If the affected area has thawed or partially thawed, the skin may appear flushed, with areas that are blue, purple, pale, or mottled.

Emergency Care of Patients with Local Cold Injury

Complete a scene size-up before beginning emergency medical care. After making sure that the scene is safe, remove the patient from the cold environment. Protect the affected area from further injury. Give oxygen. If the patient's breathing is adequate, apply oxygen by nonrebreather mask at 15 L/min if not already done. If the patient's breathing is inadequate, provide positive-pressure ventilation with 100% oxygen and assess the adequacy of the ventilations delivered.

If the injury is *early* or *superficial*, gently remove any jewelry or wet or restrictive clothing. If clothing is frozen to the skin, leave it in place. Rewarm the affected part by placing it against a warm part of the body such as the stomach or armpit (Figure 18-3). Splint the affected extremity and apply soft padding. (Avoid pressure when applying the soft padding.) Loosely cover the affected area with dry sterile dressings or clothing. Do not rub or massage the affected area or re-expose

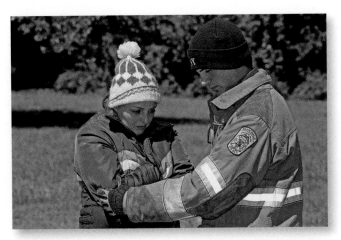

FIGURE 18-3 ▲ To care for an early (superficial) local cold injury, warm the affected part by placing it against a warm part of the body, such as the stomach or armpit.

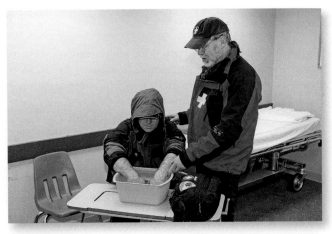

FIGURE 18-4 ▲ If you are instructed to do so, care for a late or deep local cold injury by placing the affected part in a warm (not hot) water bath.

the affected area to the cold. Doing so can cause damage to the skin and surrounding tissue.

If the injury is *late* or *deep*, gently remove any jewelry or wet or restrictive clothing. If clothing is frozen to the skin, leave it in place. Loosely cover the affected area with dry, sterile dressings or clothing. Take care to avoid doing any of the following:

- Breaking blisters
- Rubbing or massaging the affected area
- Applying heat to or rewarming the affected area
- Allowing the patient to walk on an affected extremity

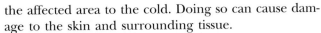

Remember This!

Check your local protocol about care for local cold injuries. Do not use dry sources of heat (such as heat packs, a heating pad, fire, or a radiator) for rewarming. These heat sources are difficult to control. The skin of the affected area will be numb and insensitive to the heat. Therefore, these heat sources can result in skin burns.

When an extremely long or delayed transport is certain, contact medical direction for instructions or follow your local protocol. Do not begin rewarming if there is a risk that the affected part will be exposed to the cold again. If you are instructed to begin active, rapid rewarming, be aware that the patient will complain of intense pain during thawing. Handle the affected area gently. Submerge the affected area in a warm water bath (100°F to 105°F or 37.8°C to 40.6°C) (Figure 18-4). Do *not* use hot water. If a thermometer is not available, test the water by pouring some of it over the inside of your arm. Check the temperature of

the water often, adding more warm water as needed. Continuously stir the water around the affected part to keep heat evenly distributed. Continue rewarming until the affected part is soft and color and sensation return (Figure 18-5). Gently dry the area after rewarming. Dress the area with dry, sterile dressings. If the affected area is a hand or foot, place dry sterile dressings between the fingers or toes. Elevate the affected extremity to decrease swelling. Protect against refreezing of the warmed part. En route to the receiving facility, perform ongoing assessments (including vital signs) as often as indicated. Carefully document all patient care information on a PCR.

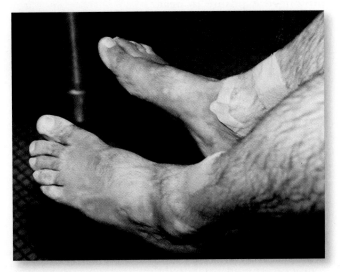

FIGURE 18-5 ▲ Thawed frostbite. This picture shows the typical appearance of frostbite soon after rewarming. The patient experienced deep frostbite as a result of wearing mountaineering boots that were too tight in extreme cold at high altitude. *Courtesy of James O'Malley, MD, from Knoop, et al., Atlas of Emergency Medicine, 2nd edition, McGraw-Hill Company, Inc.*

Exposure to Heat

Hyperthermia (a high core body temperature) results when the body gains or produces more heat than it loses. There are three main types of heat emergencies: heat cramps, heat exhaustion, and heat stroke. Heat cramps are the mildest form of heat-related emergencies. Heat stroke is the most severe.

Predisposing Factors

Although everyone is susceptible to heat illness, it affects people differently. The human body can adjust to heat stress if it is given several weeks to adapt to changes in temperature and humidity. This process is called *acclimation* or *acclimatization*. Physically fit, acclimatized, well-hydrated people are more likely to tolerate extremes of heat than older adults and children. The climate can increase a person's risk of hyperthermia. High ambient temperature reduces the body's ability to lose heat by radiation. High relative humidity reduces the body's ability to lose heat by the evaporation of sweat. Cooling of the body through the evaporation of sweat becomes ineffective as humidity rises, particularly if the humidity is above 50%. Exercise and strenuous activity can cause the loss of more than 1 liter (L) of sweat per hour. However, dehydration does not only occur when a person is exercising in the heat. A person can become dehydrated when doing other activities, such as spending a day at the beach, working in the yard, visiting a theme park, or any other activity that requires prolonged exposure to heat.

Older adults are at higher risk for heat emergencies for many reasons. Some reasons include the following:

- Medications
- Lack of mobility (the patient cannot escape the hot environment)
- Impaired ability to maintain a normal temperature
- Impaired ability to adapt to temperature changes
- Impaired sense of thirst

Newborns and infants are also at a higher risk for heat-related emergencies. This higher risk results from their impaired ability to maintain a normal temperature and their inability to remove their own clothing.

Some medications can increase the risk of hyperthermia. For example, amphetamines and cocaine increase muscle activity, which increases heat production. Alcohol impairs the body's ability to regulate heat. Tricyclic antidepressants and antihistamines

weaken the body's ability to lose heat. Illnesses and conditions that increase the risk of a heat-related emergency are shown in the following *You Should Know* box.

You Should Know

Conditions That Increase the Risk of a Heat-Related Emergency

- Heart disease
- Dehydration
- Obesity (because of increased insulation)
- Fever
- Fatigue
- Diabetes
- Thyroid disorder
- Parkinson's disease
- Previous history of a heat-related emergency

Types of Heat-Related Emergencies
Objective 4

Heat cramps usually affect people who sweat a lot during strenuous activity in a warm environment. Water and electrolytes are lost from the body during sweating. This loss leads to dehydration. The loss of water and electrolytes causes painful muscle spasms that usually occur in the shoulders, arms, abdomen, and muscles at the back of the lower legs. The cramps usually improve when the patient is moved to a cool environment, drinks water, and rests.

Heat exhaustion is also a result of too much heat and dehydration. It is the most common heat-related illness. The signs and symptoms of heat exhaustion are shown in the next *You Should Know* box. A patient who has heat exhaustion usually sweats heavily. His oral body temperature is usually normal or slightly elevated (up to 101-102°F, or 38.3-38.9°C). The patient's symptoms usually improve with a move to a cool environment, the removal of excess clothing, and rest. The patient may drink water if he is awake and alert and is not nauseated (and if approved by medical direction). Severe heat exhaustion often requires intravenous (IV) fluids. Heat exhaustion may progress to heat stroke if it is not treated.

Heat stroke is the least common but most serious form of heat-related illness. Heat stroke is a medical emergency. It occurs when the body can no longer regulate its temperature. In other words, the body's cooling system has completely shut down. Most patients have hot, flushed skin and many do not sweat. Athletes and firefighters who wear heavy

You Should Know

Signs and Symptoms of Heat Exhaustion

- Oral body temperature normal or slightly elevated (up to 101-102°F, or 38.3-38.9°C)
- Cool, pale, moist skin
- Muscle cramps
- Heavy sweating
- Fast heart rate
- Thirst
- Dizziness
- Tiredness
- Weakness
- Headache
- Nausea, vomiting
- Fainting

You Should Know

Signs and Symptoms of Heat Stroke

- Altered mental status
- Dry, hot, flushed skin
- A high body temperature (higher than 103°F, or 39.4°C, orally)
- A fast heart rate initially and then a slow heart rate
- Deep breathing followed by periods of shallow breathing
- Headache
- Dizziness
- Nausea
- Vision disturbances
- Muscle twitching, seizures
- Unresponsiveness

uniforms and perform strenuous activity for long periods in a hot environment are at risk for heat stroke. Military recruits, athletes, construction workers, and foundry and laundry workers are also at risk.

You Should Know

Some research shows that up to 50% of heat stroke patients still sweat. If you are caring for a patient who has a heat-related illness and are unsure if the patient has heat exhaustion or heat stroke, treat the patient for heat stroke.

A patient with heat stroke has a very high body temperature. He also has an altered mental status. He may have a seizure or become unresponsive. Fifty to eighty percent of patients who experience heat stroke die. You must act quickly to lower the patient's body temperature and increase his chances of survival. Prompt treatment may lower the death rate to between 15% and 20%. Call for ALS personnel as soon as possible. The patient will need IV fluids and further care at the hospital.

Emergency Care of Patients with Heat-Related Emergencies

Objective 5

The first step in the emergency care of a patient suffering from a heat-related illness is to remove him from the hot environment. Move the patient to a cool (air-conditioned) location.

Remember This!

Spray bottles filled with water are an excellent resource when trying to cool a patient who has been exposed to the heat.

Follow these guidelines if the patient has moist, pale, skin that is normal to cool in temperature:

- Consult medical direction or follow local protocol.
- Give oxygen. If the patient's breathing is adequate, apply oxygen by mask at 15 L/min. If the patient's breathing is inadequate, assist his breathing with a BM or mouth-to-mask device.
- Remove as much of the patient's outer clothing as possible. Loosen clothing that cannot be easily removed. Cool the patient by fanning (Figure 18-6). Do not cool the patient to the point of shivering because shivering generates heat. *Do not delay transport to cool the patient!*
- Place the patient in a supine position. If the patient's mental status worsens and you do not suspect trauma, place him in the recovery position.
- If the patient is awake and alert and is not nauseated, have him slowly drink water. (Consult medical direction or follow local protocol.) If the patient has an altered mental status, is nauseated, or is vomiting, do *not* give fluids. Place the patient in the recovery position.
- Comfort, calm, and reassure the patient. En route to the receiving facility, perform ongoing

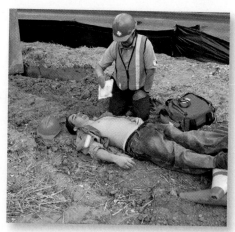

FIGURE 18-6 ▲ Place the patient on his back and remove as much of his outer clothing as possible. Cool the patient by fanning.

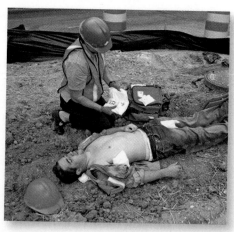

FIGURE 18-7 ▲ Place the patient on his back. Remove as much of the patient's outer clothing as possible. Cool the patient by applying cool packs to the back of the neck, armpits, and groin. Wet the patient's skin and keep it wet by applying water with a sponge or wet towels.

assessments (including vital signs) as often as indicated.

- Carefully document all patient care information on a PCR.

Follow these guidelines if the patient has hot and dry or moist skin:

- Consult medical direction or follow local protocol.
- Call for ALS personnel as soon as possible. If ALS personnel are not available, transport *immediately* to the closest appropriate facility. Alert the receiving facility of the patient's condition and your estimated time of arrival.
- Give oxygen. If the patient's breathing is adequate, apply oxygen by mask at 15 L/min. If the patient's breathing is inadequate, assist his breathing with a BM or mouth-to-mask device.
- Start cooling the patient. Remove as much of the patient's outer clothing as possible. Apply cool packs to the back of the neck, armpits, and groin. Make sure to place a towel or dressings between the cool pack and the patient's skin to prevent local cold injury. Wet the patient's skin and keep it wet by applying water with a sponge or wet towels (Figure 18-7). Alternately, you can cover the patient with a sheet and keep the sheet wet. Fan the patient aggressively to promote evaporation and convective cooling. Note that fanning may not be effective if the humidity is high. *Never* try to cool a patient by placing him in an ice water bath.
- Comfort, calm, and reassure the patient. En route to the receiving facility, perform ongoing assessments (including vital signs) every 5 minutes.
- Carefully document all patient care information on a PCR.

Water-Related Emergencies

Drowning is a process that results in harm to the respiratory system from submersion or immersion in a liquid. **Delayed drowning** (also called *secondary drowning*) occurs when a victim appears to have survived an immersion or submersion episode but later dies from respiratory failure or an infection. **Immersion** refers to covering of the face and airway in water or other fluid. In a **submersion** incident, the victim's entire body, including his airway, is under the water or other fluid.

Risk Factors

Drowning is associated with risk factors (see the next *You Should Know* box). The highest drowning rate occurs in children under 1 year of age. Drownings in this age group occur most often in bathtubs, buckets, or toilets. Among children 1 to 4 years of age, most drownings occur in residential swimming pools. Drownings involving older children tend to occur in open water areas such as ponds, lakes, and rivers. In the United States, drowning is second only to motor vehicle crashes (MVCs) as the most common cause of injury and death in children between the ages of 1 month and 14 years.

Drownings involve males more often than females. Studies suggest that males may be more at risk for drowning because of higher exposure rates to water-related activities, higher alcohol consumption while in or around water, and more risk-taking behavior.

There are racial differences in drowning rates between African Americans and white Americans, particularly in children. During 2002-2003, African-

Drowning Risk Factors

- Age
- Gender
- Race
- Inability to swim
- Use of drugs, alcohol
- Underlying illness or injury (low blood sugar, heart disease, irregular heart rhythm, seizures, fainting, depression, anxiety/panic disorder, severe arthritis, trauma [head or spinal injury])
- Child abuse, suicide, or homicide
- Hypothermia

American children ages 5 to 19 years fatally drowned at more than twice the rate of white children in this age group. Environmental factors may be a reason. Research shows that white children usually drown in a backyard swimming pool. African-American children tend to drown in lakes (unsupervised swimming) and unattended canals or quarries (accidental falls).

The children of parents who can swim are more likely to be strong swimmers than are children of parents who cannot swim. Reportedly, men of all ages, races, and educational levels are stronger swimmers than women are. However, as noted previously, white males have a higher incidence of drowning than white females.

The use of alcohol or drugs near water increases a person's risk of drowning. According to the National Center for Injury Prevention and Control, alcohol use is involved in about 25% to 50% of adolescent and adult deaths associated with water recreation. Alcohol affects judgment, balance, and coordination. Alcohol's effects are intensified with exposure to the sun and heat. Drugs such as phencyclidine (PCP), lysergic acid diethylamide (LSD), and marijuana alter the senses and affect judgment.

Consider the presence of an underlying illness or associated injury in all drowning incidents. For example, a person who has low blood sugar, heart disease, irregular heart rhythm, seizures, fainting, depression, anxiety/panic disorder, or severe arthritis is at increased risk of drowning. Because drowning is the most common cause of unintentional injury for persons with seizure disorders, a person with a seizure history should

Remember This!

Any breathless (apneic), pulseless patient who has been submerged in cold water should be resuscitated.

always be supervised when swimming or boating. Possible injuries that may be associated with drowning include head or spinal cord injury (from diving, falls, horseplay, surfing, water skiing, or jet skiing), cuts, bites, and stings. Child abuse, suicide, or homicide may be a factor in some drowning incidents. Carefully assess the patient for other signs of injury.

You Should Know

According to the National Center for Injury Prevention and Control, most boating deaths that occurred in 2004 were caused by drowning. The rest resulted from trauma, hypothermia, carbon monoxide poisoning, or other causes. Among those who drowned, 90% were not wearing life jackets.

Because water conducts heat 25 to 30 times more than air, drowning victims are at risk of hypothermia. Water colder than 91.4°F (33°C) will lead to ongoing heat loss. Children are at increased risk for hypothermia because they have less subcutaneous fat and a relatively greater body surface area than adults.

Effects of Drowning

The sequence of events that leads to drowning, particularly in cold water, begins with an initial period of panic as the victim realizes that he cannot make it to safety. Temperature receptors in the skin stimulate the conscious victim to take several deep breaths (hyperventilation) in an attempt to store oxygen before breath holding. The victim may swallow large amounts of water, causing the stomach to swell (distend). This increases the risk of vomiting. The victim holds the breath until breathing reflexes override the breath-holding effort. How long the victim is voluntarily able to hold his breath until breathing reflexes take over is determined by the levels of oxygen and carbon dioxide in the blood.

In some individuals, cold water stimulation of the temperature receptors in the skin triggers the **mammalian diving reflex.** This reflex is present in seals and other diving mammals. In humans, the diving reflex is strongest in infants less than 6 months old, and the effects decrease with age. The diving reflex triggers the shunting of blood to the brain and heart from the skin, gastrointestinal (GI) tract, and extremities. The victim's heart rate slows in response to the increased volume of blood in the body's core. These actions help the body conserve oxygen and may help the victim survive.

As carbon dioxide builds up as a result of breath holding, a decreased supply of oxygen is delivered to the body's tissues (hypoxia). The victim begins struggling violently and gasping for air. Without adequate oxygen, acid builds up in the blood and tissues. The buildup of acid is called **acidosis.** In about 85% of drownings, large amounts of water enter the trachea and lungs (aspiration). The entry of water into the trachea and lungs is called a **wet drowning.** The patient's chances of survival are affected by the amount and type of material taken into the lungs. Aspirating cold water may hasten the onset of hypothermia.

In about 15% of drownings, little water is aspirated. This occurs because the sensitive tissue near the vocal cords begins to spasm (**laryngospasm**). This protective reflex causes closing of the larynx to prevent the passage of water into the lungs. This is called a **dry drowning.** Although laryngospasm causes little fluid to enter the lungs, it also prevents the entry of air. As a result, hypoxia worsens and the victim suffocates.

Although many factors influence a drowning victim's chances for survival (see the following *You Should Know* box), the most important are the length of the immersion or submersion and the severity of the hypoxia.

You Should Know

Factors That Influence a Drowning Victim's Chances for Survival

- Length of immersion or submersion
- Duration of hypoxia
- Ability to swim
- Age of victim
- Cleanliness of the water
- Temperature of the water
- Victim signs and symptoms
- Preexisting medical conditions
- Presence of drugs and/or alcohol
- Presence of associated injuries (especially to the cervical spine and head)
- Response to initial resuscitation efforts

Assessment of the Drowning Victim

Study the scene and determine if approaching the patient is safe. Evaluate the mechanism of injury. Obtain additional help *before* contact with the patient(s). A cold environment requires special safety considerations because of the presence of ice, snow, or wind. Call for specially trained personnel as needed to remove the patient from the environment. Do not enter a body of water unless you have been trained in water rescue and have the proper safety equipment

and personnel with you. Do not enter fast-moving water or venture out on ice unless you have been trained in this type of rescue.

Remember This!

Professionals trained in water rescue are generally called for incidents that involve the removal of victim(s) from any body of water other than a swimming pool. This includes lakes, ponds, canals, washes, rivers, or any other body of water, whether still or moving.

Perform a primary survey. Stabilize the patient's spine as needed (see the following *You Should Know* box). If the patient is in the water and spinal injury is suspected, place the patient on a long board before removing the patient from the water.

You Should Know

Drowning: Special Considerations

Suspect neck injury:

- When the mechanism of injury is unknown
- When signs of facial trauma are present
- When signs of drug or alcohol use are present
- In incidents involving use of a water slide and swimming, boating, water-skiing, or diving accidents

Objectives 6, 7

Signs and symptoms of drowning vary. The most common signs and symptoms are reflected in changes in the nervous and respiratory systems. While assessing the patient, protect him from environmental temperature extremes.

Assess the patient's mental status. A drowning victim's mental status may range from awake and alert to confused, combative, difficult to arouse, or unresponsive. Some patients have seizures. These variations in mental status may be caused by an associated injury or by a lack of oxygen from immersion or submersion.

Hypoxia can result from fluid in the lungs and contaminants from the water and/or laryngospasm. Coughing, vomiting, choking, or signs of airway obstruction may be present. The drowning victim may have difficulty breathing or absent or inadequate breathing. Gastric distention may be present. The victim may cough up pink, frothy fluid. Respiratory failure and pneumonia are possible complications that can occur in victims who survive a drowning incident. The onset of symptoms can be delayed for as long as 24 to 36 hours after the incident. If water was inhaled into the lungs (aspirated), it may take days for normal lung function to return.

Hypoxia and acidosis can cause irregular heart rhythms. If the heart muscle is deprived of an adequate oxygen supply, damage to the heart muscle can occur. This can result in cardiogenic shock. In **cardiogenic shock,** the heart muscle fails to pump blood effectively to all parts of the body. Effects of an inadequate oxygen supply and acidosis on the cardiovascular system may include a fast or slow heart rate, an irregular heart rhythm, or even an absent pulse. The patient's skin is often cool, clammy, and pale or cyanotic. Possible signs and symptoms of drowning are listed in the following *You Should Know* box.

You Should Know

Signs and Symptoms of Drowning

- Altered mental status, seizures, unresponsiveness
- Coughing, vomiting, choking, or airway obstruction
- Absent or inadequate breathing
- Difficulty breathing
- Fast, slow, or absent pulse
- Cool, clammy, and pale or cyanotic skin
- Vomiting
- Possible abdominal distention

Identify any life-threatening conditions and provide care based on these findings. Establish patient priorities. Priority patients include:

- Patients who give a poor general impression
- Patients experiencing difficulty breathing
- Patients with signs and symptoms of shock
- Unresponsive patients with no gag reflex or cough
- Responsive patients who are unable to follow commands

Request ALS assistance as soon as possible. If ALS personnel are not available, transport the patient promptly to the closest appropriate facility.

Perform a secondary survey. If the patient is unresponsive, perform a rapid physical examination. Follow with evaluation of baseline vital signs and gathering of the patient's medical history. If the patient is responsive, gather information about the patient's medical history before performing a focused physical exam. When performing a physical examination, carefully assess the patient for other injuries.

When gathering a SAMPLE history, attempt to find out the following:

- When did the incident occur (length of submersion)?
- Where did the incident occur (such as near rocks, pool, bathtub)? Note the cleanliness of the water. Try to find out the temperature of the water.
- How did the incident occur?
- Did the patient experience any loss of responsiveness?
- Was the incident witnessed? This information is useful in determining possible head or spinal injury. Look for signs of abuse or neglect in infants, children, and older adults.

Emergency Care of the Drowning Victim

- Ensure the safety of all rescue personnel. Remove the patient from the water as quickly and safely as possible.
- If spinal injury is suspected and the patient is still in the water, stabilize the head and spine. Move and secure the patient onto a long backboard and then remove the patient from the water. If spine injury is not suspected, place the patient on the left side (recovery position) to allow water, vomitus, and secretions to drain from the upper airway. Suction as needed to remove debris, vomitus, or other foreign material from the upper airway.
- Rescue breathing is the most important initial care you can provide for a drowning victim. After making sure the scene is safe, start rescue breathing as soon as you can open the victim's airway. In most cases, rescue breathing is started when the victim is in shallow water or has been removed from the water. Do not use abdominal thrusts in an attempt to clear water from the patient's airway. This can cause injury, vomiting, and aspiration, and delay CPR.

Remember This!

Most drowning victims who require rescue breathing or chest compressions vomit. Be sure to always have suction equipment within arm's reach when caring for a drowning victim.

Drowning Prevention

- Take swimming lessons that include instruction in general water safety and emergency water survival training.
- Use properly fitted U.S. Coast Guard–approved personal flotation devices when on boats or participating in water sports.
- Avoid alcohol use around water.
- Obey warning signs in dangerous areas.
- Swim in areas with lifeguard coverage, when possible.
- Ask a lifeguard about water depth and conditions before entering the water. Be aware that weather conditions can change quickly.
- Make sure an adult is constantly watching children swimming or playing in or around water.
- Never swim alone or in unsupervised places. Always swim with a buddy.
- Know local weather conditions and the forecast before swimming or boating. Strong winds and thunderstorms with lightning strikes are dangerous to swimmers and boaters.
- Watch for dangerous waves and signs of rip currents (water that is discolored and unusually choppy, foamy, or filled with debris). If you are caught in a rip current, swim parallel to the shore. Once out of the current, swim toward the shore.

- Give oxygen. If the patient's breathing is adequate, apply oxygen by nonrebreather mask at 15 L/min if not already done. If the patient's breathing is inadequate, provide positive-pressure ventilation with 100% oxygen. Assess the adequacy of the ventilations delivered.
- It may be difficult to feel a pulse in a drowning victim, particularly if the victim is cold. If you cannot feel a central pulse, begin CPR after the patient has been removed from the water. Attach an automated external defibrillator (AED) and follow the AED prompts.
- After the patient has been removed from the water and is in a safe location, quickly remove wet clothing and dry the patient to prevent heat loss. Treat for hypothermia if indicated. The hypothermic drowning victim must be handled gently. As with all other hypothermic patients, remove wet clothing. Then dry and wrap the patient in blankets to maintain body heat.

- Transport promptly. Keep the patient warm during transport. En route to the hospital, perform ongoing assessments every 15 minutes if the patient is stable. If the patient is unstable, perform ongoing assessments every 5 minutes.
- Record all patient care information, including the patient's medical history and the emergency care provided, on a PCR.

Making a Difference

Because of the possibility of delayed complications, *all* victims of an immersion or submersion incident should be transported for physician evaluation.

Diving Emergencies

Barotrauma

Barotrauma is a diving-related injury caused by pressure. It can occur on ascent or descent. Barotrauma occurring on ascent is called *pulmonary overpressurization syndrome* (POPS) or *burst lung*. Barotrauma occurring on descent is called *lung squeeze* or *the squeeze*. Air pressure in the body's air-filled cavities increases, causing damage to the tissues within the cavity (such as the ear, sinuses, lungs, and GI tract).

Signs and symptoms of barotrauma include the following:

- Ear: bloody drainage from the ear, mild to severe pain in the ear, nausea, dizziness, disorientation
- Sinuses: mild to severe pain over the sinuses, bleeding from the nose
- Lungs: difficulty breathing, chest pain, cough, pulmonary edema
- GI tract: mild to severe abdominal pain

Emergency Care for Barotrauma

- Establish and maintain an open airway.
- Give oxygen at 15 L/min by nonrebreather mask. Some authorities do not recommend positive-pressure ventilation because of the risk of further injury. Consult with medical direction and check local protocol.
- Transport promptly.

Air Embolism

Air embolism may occur when divers ascend too rapidly or hold their breath during ascent. Onset is usually rapid and dramatic, often occurring within minutes of surfacing. As the diver ascends, air trapped in the lungs expands. If the air is not exhaled, the alveoli rupture, damaging adjacent blood vessels. Air bubbles are forced into the circulatory system through ruptured pulmonary veins. The air bubbles become lodged in small arteries, cutting off circulation. The size and location of the bubbles determines the patient's signs and symptoms. Signs and symptoms of an air embolism are listed in the following *You Should Know* box.

You Should Know

Signs and Symptoms of an Air Embolism

- Dizziness
- Confusion
- Shortness of breath
- Visual disturbances
- Weakness or paralysis in extremities
- Sudden unresponsiveness after surfacing (can occur before surfacing)
- Pink, frothy sputum
- Respiratory arrest
- Cardiac arrest

Emergency Care for Air Embolism

- Establish and maintain an open airway.
- Give oxygen. If the patient's breathing is adequate, apply oxygen by nonrebreather mask at 15 L/min if not already done. If the patient's breathing is inadequate, provide positive-pressure ventilation with 100% oxygen and assess the adequacy of the ventilations delivered.
- If neck or spine injury is not suspected, the patient should be placed on the left side with the head and chest tilted downward. Some authorities recommend placing the patient in a supine position because of the difficulty of maintaining the position described previously. Consult medical direction or follow local protocol regarding patient positioning.
- Maintain body temperature. Remove wet clothing. Dry the patient and cover with blankets, towels, or dry clothing.
- If possible, obtain all relevant information regarding the patient's dive and relay to the receiving facility.
- Consult medical direction about transport to a recompression facility.

Decompression Sickness

Decompression sickness (also called *the bends*) is a diving-related injury that results from dissolved nitrogen in the blood and tissues. As a diver descends, nitrogen and oxygen are dissolved in the blood. If the diver ascends rapidly, there is not enough time for the nitrogen to be reabsorbed from the blood. Nitrogen bubbles form in the bloodstream, interfering with tissue perfusion. The size and location of the bubbles determines the patient's signs and symptoms. Signs and symptoms of decompression sickness are listed in the following *You Should Know* box.

You Should Know

Signs and Symptoms of Decompression Sickness

- Fatigue
- Weakness
- Shortness of breath
- Skin rash
- Itching
- Joint soreness
- Dizziness
- Headache
- Paralysis
- Seizures
- Unresponsiveness

Emergency Care for Decompression Sickness

- Establish and maintain an open airway.
- Give oxygen. If the patient's breathing is adequate, apply oxygen by nonrebreather mask at 15 L/min if not already done. If the patient's breathing is inadequate, provide positive-pressure ventilation with 100% oxygen and assess the adequacy of the ventilations delivered.
- If neck or spine injury is not suspected, the patient should be placed on the left side with the head and chest tilted downward. Some authorities recommend placing the patient in a supine position because of the difficulty of maintaining the position described previously. Consult medical direction or follow local protocol regarding patient positioning.
- Maintain body temperature. Remove wet clothing. Dry the patient and cover with blankets, towels, or dry clothing.

- If possible, obtain all relevant information regarding the patient's dive and relay to the receiving facility.
- Consult medical direction about transport to a recompression facility.

Bites and Stings

Snakebites

Venomous snakes in the United States include pit vipers and coral snakes (see Table 18-2). In about 20%

TABLE 18-2 Poisonous North American Snakes

Species	Common Name
Crotalids	
• Large rattlesnakes	Eastern diamondback rattlesnake
	Western diamondback rattlesnake
	Mojave Desert sidewinder
	Timber/canebrake rattlesnake
	Rock rattlesnake
	Speckled rattlesnake
	Black-tailed rattlesnake
	Twin-spotted rattlesnake
	Mojave rattlesnake
	Tiger rattlesnake
	Western rattlesnake
	Prairie rattlesnake
	Grand Canyon rattlesnake
	Southern Pacific rattlesnake
	Great Basin rattlesnake
	Northern Pacific rattlesnake
	Ridge-nosed rattlesnake
• Smaller rattlesnakes	Massasauga
	Pygmy
• Moccasins	Southern copperhead
	Eastern/western cottonmouth
Elapidae	
	Sonoran (Arizona) coral snake
	Eastern coral snake
	Texas coral snake

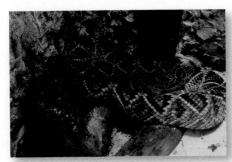

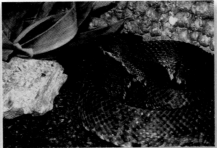

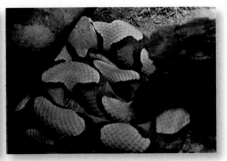

FIGURE 18-8 ▲ Rattlesnakes do not always "rattle" before striking. The eastern diamondback, the largest U.S. rattlesnake, is shown here. *Courtesy of Jason Thurman, MD, from Knoop, et al., Atlas of Emergency Medicine, 2nd edition, McGraw-Hill Company, Inc.*

FIGURE 18-9 ▲ A cottonmouth. *Courtesy of Jason Thurman, MD, from Knoop, et al., Atlas of Emergency Medicine, 2nd edition, McGraw-Hill Company, Inc.*

FIGURE 18-10 ▲ The head of a copperhead is reddish brown to copper in color; thus, the reason for its name. *Courtesy of Jason Thurman, MD, from Knoop, et al., Atlas of Emergency Medicine, 2nd edition, McGraw-Hill Company, Inc.*

of snakebites, venom is not injected ("dry bites"). Most snakebites:

- Occur in men between the ages of 17 and 27 years
- Occur on an arm (67%) or leg (33%)
- Occur between April and October
- Are associated with alcohol intoxication

Pit vipers (which include rattlesnakes, cottonmouths [water moccasins], and copperheads) are responsible for 98% of all venomous snakebites in the United States. Pit vipers have the following features:

- Infrared pit (heat sensor) between eye and nostril (used to determine the position of its prey by the relative intensity of heat noted by its heat sensors; also used to guide the direction of the strike)
- Catlike elliptical pupils
- Triangular head
- Two long fangs (each fang has a least three pairs of alternate fangs behind it)

Rattlesnakes may strike without warning (Figure 18-8). They do not always "rattle" before striking. Most deaths from rattlesnake bites are a result of envenomation by the eastern and western diamondback rattlesnakes. A cottonmouth can strike while under water (Figure 18-9). The inside of its mouth is pale white; thus, the reason for its name. The copperhead is often found in wooded mountains, abandoned buildings, and damp, grassy areas. Its head is reddish brown to copper in color; thus the reason for its name (Figure 18-10). A copperhead can climb low bushes and trees in search of food. The bites of copperheads are not as toxic as a rattlesnake or cottonmouth bite.

Signs and symptoms of most pit viper bites usually appear within 30 to 60 minutes. Signs and symptoms depend on the following:

- Location of the bite
- Amount and properties of the venom injected
- Victim's general health
- Size of the victim

Common characteristics of pit viper bites include one or more fang marks, swelling, and burning pain in the area of the bite. Pain usually begins within 5 minutes and swelling within 10 minutes of a bite, but these can be delayed for several hours. Discoloration is common, appearing over the bite site within 3 to 6 hours (Figures 18-11 and 18-12). Signs and symptoms of pit viper bites are listed in Table 18-3.

Coral snakes are shy, nocturnal, and seldom bite. The Sonoran (Arizona) coral snake is about 15 to 20 inches long. The eastern coral snake and Texas coral snake average 20 to 45 inches in length. Coral snakes have the following features:

- Black, red, and yellow (or cream) bands that completely encircle the snake's body (Figures 18-13 and 18-14)
- Black head
- Short, small fangs
- Round, black eyes
- No facial pits

Whereas pit vipers tend to strike and release their venom, coral snakes tend to hang on and inject their venom with a series of chewing movements. The venom of a coral snake primarily affects the nervous system. Signs and symptoms may be delayed

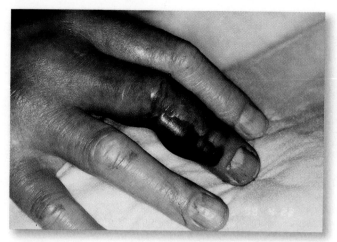

FIGURE 18-11 ▲ A rattlesnake bite six hours after the injury. *Courtesy of Sean P. Bush, from Knoop, et al., Atlas of Emergency Medicine, 2nd edition, McGraw-Hill Company, Inc.*

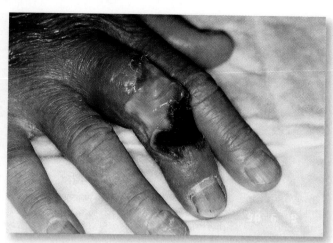

FIGURE 18-12 ▲ The same patient as in Figure 18-11, seven weeks after the rattlesnake bite. *Courtesy of Sean P. Bush, from Knoop, et al., Atlas of Emergency Medicine, 2nd edition, McGraw-Hill Company, Inc.*

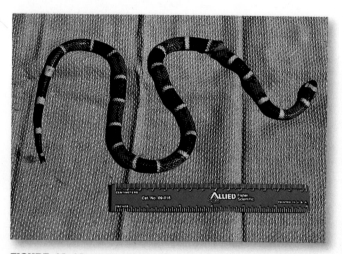

FIGURE 18-13 ▲ The bite of a coral snake is poisonous. A coral snake has black and red-on-yellow (or cream) bands that completely encircle the snake's body. *Courtesy of Steven Holt, MD, from Knoop, et al., Atlas of Emergency Medicine, 2nd edition, McGraw-Hill Company, Inc.*

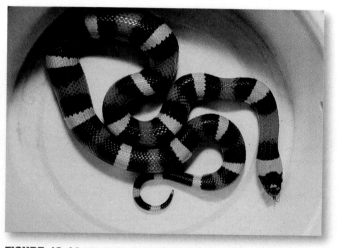

FIGURE 18-14 ▲ This is a picture of a Mexican milk snake. Its red-on-black rings indicate a nonvenomous snake. Unfortunately this "rule" applies only to snakes native to the United States. *Courtesy of Sean P. Bush, from Knoop, et al., Atlas of Emergency Medicine, 2nd edition, McGraw-Hill Company, Inc.*

up to 12 hours after the bite. Because of the snake's small mouth, scratch marks or tiny puncture marks may be visible at the injection site with little or no pain at the site. There is usually minimal to moderate swelling. Early signs and symptoms include slurred speech, difficulty swallowing, and dilated pupils. If the bite is not treated, paralysis can occur within 8 to 24 hours. Death occurs because of

TABLE 18-3 Signs and Symptoms of Pit Viper Bites

Local Signs and Symptoms	Systemic Signs and Symptoms
Fang marks or semicircle of teeth marks	Weakness
Burning pain	Sweating
Red and swollen area around the fang or teeth marks	Nausea and vomiting
Discoloration and blisters common	Shock

TABLE 18-4 Signs and Symptoms of Coral Snake Bites

Early Signs and Symptoms	Late Signs and Symptoms (may be delayed for up to 12 hours)
Scratch marks or tiny puncture marks	Nausea/vomiting
Little or no pain at the site	Difficulty breathing
Minimal to moderate swelling	Seizures
Slurred speech	Paralysis
Muscle weakness	Respiratory failure
Difficulty swallowing	
Dilated pupils	

respiratory failure secondary to paralysis of the respiratory muscles. Signs and symptoms of coral snake bites are shown in Table 18-4.

Remember This!

Coral snakes can be differentiated from other striped snakes by remembering, "Red on yellow, kill a fellow. Red on black, venom lack" or "Red on black is a friend of Jack's; red on yellow can kill a fellow."

Emergency Care for Snakebites
Objective 8

- Ensure the safety of all rescuers. Make sure that the patient and rescuers are beyond the snake's striking distance, which is about the same as its body length. *It is not necessary to capture the snake for identification.* If the snake is dead, transport it in a closed container to the hospital with the patient (if required by your local protocol).
- Establish and maintain an open airway.
- Give oxygen. If the patient's breathing is adequate, apply oxygen by nonrebreather mask at 15 L/min if not already done. If the patient's breathing is inadequate, provide positive-pressure ventilation with 100% oxygen and assess the adequacy of the ventilations delivered.
- Keep the patient calm. Limit the patient's physical activity to minimize circulation of venom.
- Remove rings, watches, and tight clothing from the injured area before swelling begins.
- The pressure immobilization technique should be used for situations involving a coral snake bite. This technique involves immediately wrapping the entire bitten extremity with an elastic

bandage or article of clothing as you would for a sprain (Figure 18-15). Wrapping the extremity slows lymph flow from the bite site, delaying toxicity. After the arm or leg is wrapped, the bandage should be snug, but loose enough to fit a finger under. After wrapping the extremity, follow by splinting with any available object. Position the splinted arm or leg slightly below the level of the patient's heart.

—Pit viper bites cause more local tissue injury and pain than coral snake bites. Since the pressure immobilization technique causes an increase in pressure within the wrapped area, this technique is not currently recommended for pit viper bites. Position the affected arm or leg slightly below the level of the patient's heart.

- Frequently reassess the presence of distal pulses in the affected extremity. If swelling is present, mark the outer edge of the swelling and the time with a pen or marker (Figure 18-16). This allows other healthcare professionals to monitor the swelling progression.
- Some authorities recommend washing the wound, and some do not. Those who do not recommend washing say that not washing the wound allows for identification of venom from the wound. Be sure to check your local protocol.
- If a tourniquet or constricting band was applied to the affected arm or leg before your arrival, and pulses are present in the extremity, leave it in place until the victim is evaluated at the hospital. If a tourniquet or constricting band was applied and pulses are absent in the extremity, consult medical direction for instructions.
- Observe the patient closely for the development of signs and symptoms of an allergic reaction; treat as needed.

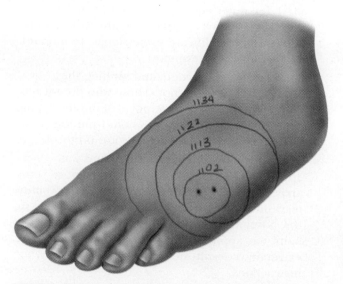

FIGURE 18-15 ◄ Pressure immobilization technique for coral snake bite.

- Because the onset of signs and symptoms can be delayed, all snakebite victims should be transported for physician evaluation. En route to the hospital, perform ongoing assessments as often as indicated.
- Carefully document all patient care information on a PCR.

Remember This!

When caring for snakebites, do not:

- Apply heat or cold to the bite site
- Cut the wound
- Attempt to suck out the venom
- Apply a constricting band or tourniquet

You Should Know

Typical signs and symptoms of an injection-related poisoning include the history of a bite (spider or snake) or sting (insect, scorpion, or marine animal), pain, redness, swelling, weakness, dizziness, chills, fever, nausea, vomiting, bite marks, or the presence of a stinger.

FIGURE 18-16 ▲ If swelling is present as a result of a bite or sting, mark the outer edge of the swelling and note the time with a pen or marker.

Spider Bites

Arthropods are animals that have a segmented body, jointed legs, a digestive tract and, in most cases, a hard outer shell. They have no backbone. Examples of arthropods are shown in the following *You Should Know* box.

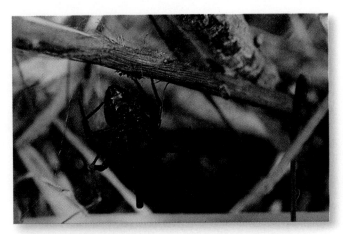

FIGURE 18-17 ▲ A black widow spider has a shiny, black body with a red hourglass figure on the abdomen. *Courtesy of Alan B. Storrow, MD, from Knoop, et al., Atlas of Emergency Medicine, 2nd edition, McGraw-Hill Company, Inc.*

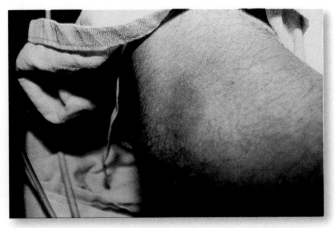

FIGURE 18-18 ▲ Black widow spider bite. *Courtesy of Gerald O'Malley, DO, from Knoop, et al., Atlas of Emergency Medicine, 2nd edition, McGraw-Hill Company, Inc.*

You Should Know

Examples of Arthropods

- Spiders
- Insects
- Crustaceans
- Scorpions
- Lice
- Fleas
- Ticks
- Bed bugs
- Horseshoe crabs
- Centipedes
- Millipedes
- Mites

A black widow spider has a shiny, black body with a red hourglass figure on the abdomen (Figure 18-17). The male is approximately half the size of the female, brown, and its venomous bite tends to be milder than envenomation by a female. The red or yellow-orange hourglass figure on the abdomen may be absent or hard to see in young female spiders. Black widow spiders spin irregular webs under rocks, logs, and vegetation and in woodpiles, barns, garages, trash piles, and outdoor structures.

The venom of a black widow spider primarily affects nerves and muscles. Signs and symptoms of a black widow spider bite include the following (Figure 18-18):

- Vague history of sharp pinprick followed by dull, numbing pain
- Tiny red marks at the point of entry of the venom
- Swelling
- Difficulty breathing
- Severe pain beginning 15 to 60 minutes after bite and increasing for 12 to 48 hours
- Lower extremity bite: localized pain followed by abdominal pain and rigidity

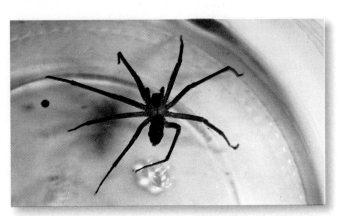

FIGURE 18-19 ▲ Brown recluse spider. *Courtesy of Alan B. Storrow, MD, from Knoop, et al., Atlas of Emergency Medicine, 2nd edition, McGraw-Hill Company, Inc.*

- Upper extremity bite: pain and rigidity in chest, back, and shoulders

Brown recluse spiders are small, brown or tan in color and have a dark band shaped like a violin on the head/thorax (Figure 18-19). Many victims of a brown recluse spider bite do not recall being bitten. However, shortly after the bite the victim experiences a mild stinging sensation. This soon changes to an aching feeling that is accompanied by itching. Swelling soon follows. Within 2 to 8 hours after the bite, the wound develops a reddish halo surrounding a violet-colored center (Figure 18-20). Large blisters may form within 1 to 2 days after the bite (Figure 18-21). The area often becomes larger over the next 24 to 72 hours. The tissue may die, resulting in a purple or black dry scab in the center of the area. Over a period of 2 to 5 weeks, the scab separates, leaving a deep, poorly healing ulcer (Figure 18-22). Signs and symptoms of a brown recluse spider bite are listed in the following *You Should Know* box.

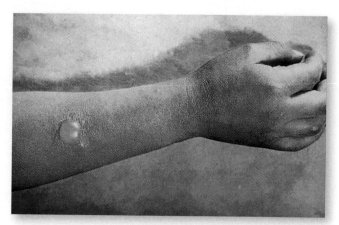

FIGURE 18-20 ▲ A brown recluse spider bite about eight hours after the bite. *Centers for Disease Control.*

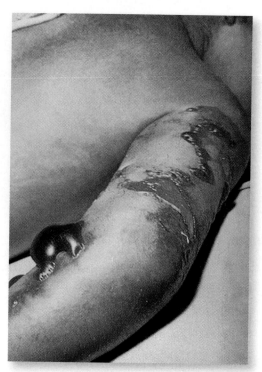

FIGURE 18-21 ▲ A brown recluse spider bite about 24 hours after the bite. *Center for Disease Control.*

You Should Know

Signs and Symptoms of a Brown Recluse Spider Bite

- Mild stinging sensation at the site of bite
- Local swelling
- Reddish ring appears around the bite within 2 to 8 hours after the bite
- Fever, chills
- Weakness
- Rash
- Nausea/vomiting
- Joint pain
- Redness and blister formation at site
- Open sore formation at site in 7 to 14 days

Emergency Care for Spider Bites

Objective 8

- Establish and maintain an open airway.
- Give oxygen. If the patient's breathing is adequate, apply oxygen by nonrebreather mask at 15 L/min if not already done. If the patient's breathing is inadequate, provide positive-pressure ventilation with 100% oxygen and assess the adequacy of the ventilations delivered.
- Gently wash the area.
- If possible, remove jewelry from the injured area before swelling begins.
- If swelling is present, mark the outer edge of the swelling and note the time with a pen or marker.
- If the bite is on an arm or leg, position the limb slightly below the level of the patient's heart.

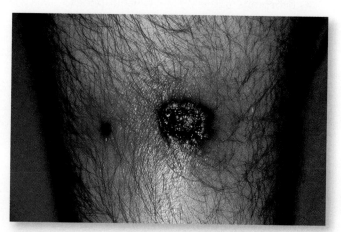

FIGURE 18-22 ▲ A deep, poorly healing sore from a brown recluse spider bite about two to five weeks after the bite. *Courtesy of Keven J. Knoop, MD, from Knoop, et al., Atlas of Emergency Medicine, 2nd edition, McGraw-Hill Company, Inc.*

- Observe the patient closely for the development of signs and symptoms of an allergic reaction; treat as needed.
- Transport promptly. En route to the hospital, perform ongoing assessments as often as indicated.
- Carefully document all patient care information on a PCR.

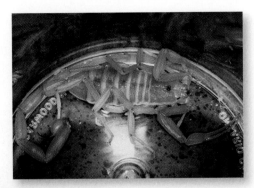

FIGURE 18-23 ▲ A bark scorpion is yellow to brown and usually less than 5 cm long. *Courtesy of Sean P. Bush, from Knoop, et al., Atlas of Emergency Medicine, 2nd edition, McGraw-Hill Company, Inc.*

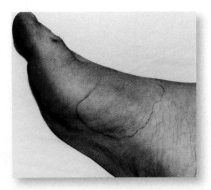

FIGURE 18-24 ▲ The bite of a bark scorpion typically produces pain, numbness or tingling, swelling, and redness at the sting site. *Courtesy of Stephen Corbett, MD, from Knoop, et al., Atlas of Emergency Medicine, 2nd edition, McGraw-Hill Company, Inc.*

Scorpion Stings

In North America, the sculptured or bark scorpion is the only species of scorpion that injects venom that is dangerous to humans (Figure 18-23). The scorpion injects venom by means of a stinger located on its tail. Scorpion venom is very rapidly absorbed. It can be lethal in very young children and in older adults who have chronic illnesses. Signs and symptoms of a scorpion sting include the following:

- Local pain, numbness or tingling, swelling, and redness at the sting site (Figure 18-24)
- SLUDGEM (*s*alivation, *l*acrimation [tearing], *u*rination, *d*iarrhea, *g*astric cramping, *e*mesis [vomiting], *m*iosis [pupil constriction])
- Slurred speech
- Blurred vision
- Restlessness, jerking, and involuntary shaking
- Wandering eye movements
- Difficulty breathing
- Trouble swallowing
- Increased heart rate
- Seizures

Signs and symptoms from a scorpion sting usually peak in about 5 hours. Numbness, tingling, and pain can last up to 2 weeks after the sting.

Emergency Care for Scorpion Stings

Objective 8

- Establish and maintain an open airway. Excessive oral secretions may require frequent suctioning.
- Give oxygen. If the patient's breathing is adequate, apply oxygen by nonrebreather mask at 15 L/min if not already done. If the patient's breathing is inadequate, provide positive-pressure ventilation with 100% oxygen and assess the adequacy of the ventilations delivered.
- Gently wash the area.
- If possible, remove jewelry from the injured area before swelling begins.
- If swelling is present, mark the outer edge of the swelling and note the time with a pen or marker.
- If the bite is on an arm or leg, position the limb slightly below the level of the patient's heart.
- Watch the patient closely for the development of signs and symptoms of an allergic reaction; treat as needed.
- Transport promptly. En route to the hospital, perform ongoing assessments as often as indicated.
- Carefully document all patient care information on a PCR.

Hymenoptera Stings (Bees, Wasps, and Ants)

Stings from bees, hornets, wasps, and fire ants usually result in local pain, mild redness, swelling, and itching. When a honeybee stings, the barb on its stinger serves to anchor it in its victim (Figures 18-25 and 18-26). A honeybee stings only once and then dies when the sac detaches from its body. The sac then rhythmically continues to squeeze while anchored in its victim. The stingers of wasps, yellow jackets, hornets, and ants are not barbed. As a result, these insects are capable of repeatedly stinging their victim.

Africanized honeybees (also known as *Africanized bees* or *killer bees*) have been present in the United States since the early 1990s. To date, they are present in Florida, Texas, New Mexico, Arizona, Nevada, and California. It is anticipated that they may eventually be distributed as far north and east as North Carolina.

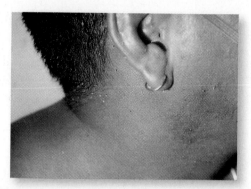

FIGURE 18-25 ▲ This patient's cheek, ear, and hairline show numerous stingers (barbs and venom sacs) from honeybees. *Courtesy of Alan B. Storrow, MD, from Knoop, et al., Atlas of Emergency Medicine, 2nd edition, McGraw-Hill Company, Inc.*

Although their venom is not known to be more toxic than typical honeybees, they are much more aggressive. Africanized bees may be agitated by everyday occurrences such as vibrations from passing vehicles, power equipment, and even people walking by on foot. Perceiving a threat to their nests, they have been known to attack in swarms of hundreds and chase their victims for long distances from the hive.

Signs and symptoms of hymenoptera stings vary. In many cases, the victim feels a stinging sensation at the site of the sting that is followed by local pain, redness, swelling, and itching. In sensitized individuals, anaphylaxis may occur within minutes in response to an insect sting and may cause death.

Emergency Care for Hymenoptera Stings

Objective 8

- Establish and maintain an open airway. Excessive oral secretions may require frequent suctioning.

- Give oxygen. If the patient's breathing is adequate, apply oxygen by nonrebreather mask at 15 L/min if not already done. If the patient's breathing is inadequate, provide positive-pressure ventilation with 100% oxygen and assess the adequacy of the ventilations delivered.

- If a stinger is present, remove it by scraping with a credit card other flat, straight edge. Avoid using tweezers or forceps as these can squeeze venom from the venom sac into the wound.

- Gently wash the area.

- If possible, remove jewelry from the injured area before swelling begins. If swelling is present, mark the outer edge of the swelling and note the time with a pen or marker.

- Watch the patient closely for the development of signs and symptoms of an allergic reaction; treat as needed.

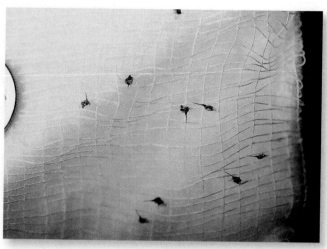

FIGURE 18-26 ▲ The barbs and attached venom sacs after removal from the patient. *Courtesy of Alan B. Storrow, MD, from Knoop, et al., Atlas of Emergency Medicine, 2nd edition, McGraw-Hill Company, Inc.*

- Transport promptly. En route to the hospital, perform ongoing assessments as often as indicated.

- Carefully document all patient care information on a PCR.

Marine Life Stings

Marine life envenomations usually occur when the creature is stepped on, swum into, or intentionally or accidentally picked up. In the United States, most marine life envenomations are caused by the stingray. Stingrays are found in the waters off coastal areas. They usually lie partially hidden in the sand and strike with their tail when disturbed. A stingray's tail can produce 1 to 4 venomous stings. The injury produced by the stingray's tail is a puncture wound (Figure 18-27). The lower

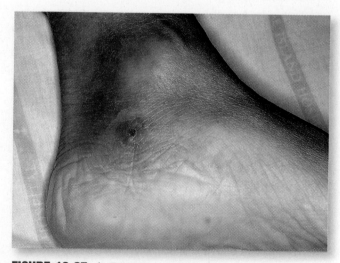

FIGURE 18-27 ▲ Puncture wound from a stingray. *Courtesy of Daniel L. Savitt MD, from Knoop, et al., Atlas of Emergency Medicine, 2nd edition, McGraw-Hill Company, Inc.*

extremities are the most common sites of injury, followed by the upper extremities, abdomen, and chest. Although the puncture wound is small, the sting is followed by immediate, excruciating localized pain. The pain usually reaches maximum intensity in about 90 minutes and takes several hours to resolve. Other signs and symptoms of stingray envenomation are listed in the following *You Should Know* box. Although a stingray injury is rarely fatal, wounds to the chest and abdomen are associated with an increased risk of death.

You Should Know

Signs and Symptoms of Stingray Envenomation

- Immediate, excruciating pain
- Swelling
- Nausea, vomiting
- Diarrhea
- Sweating
- Muscle cramps
- Weakness
- Headache
- Dizziness
- Fainting
- Paralysis
- Seizures
- Respiratory depression
- Low blood pressure
- Irregular heart rhythm
- Death

Emergency Care for Venomous Marine Injuries

Objective 8

- Establish and maintain an open airway. Excessive oral secretions may require frequent suctioning.
- Give oxygen. If the patient's breathing is adequate, apply oxygen by nonrebreather mask at 15 L/min if not already done. If the patient's breathing is inadequate, provide positive-pressure ventilation with 100% oxygen and assess the adequacy of the ventilations delivered.
- In the case of a stingray injury, flush the wound *immediately* and then immerse the injured part in hot water to patient tolerance (109-113°F [43-45°C]) for 30 to 90 minutes to inactivate the venom and provide pain control. Do *not* apply cool compresses or ice. Elevate the injured arm or leg. Cover the wound with a sterile dressing.

- If possible, remove jewelry from the injured area before swelling begins. If swelling is present, mark the outer edge of the swelling and note the time with a pen or marker.
- Transport promptly. En route to the hospital, perform ongoing assessments as often as indicated.
- Carefully document all patient care information on a PCR.

Dog and Cat Bites

Dog and cat bites are common. In fact, someone in the United States seeks medical attention for a dog bite–related injury every 40 seconds. Dog bites are more common than cat bites. Because a dog's jaw can exert more than 450 pounds of pressure per square inch, dog bites usually result in crushing-type injuries, cuts, scrapes, and puncture wounds (Figure 18-28). Injuries may involve bones, vessels, tendons, muscles, and nerves.

In adults, most dog bites occur on the extremities. In children four years of age and younger, most dog bites occur on the face, neck, and scalp. Children are at greater risk of injury and death from dog bites than adults are. This may be because of a child's small size and inability to fend off an attack and because many children do not know how to behave around a dog. Dog

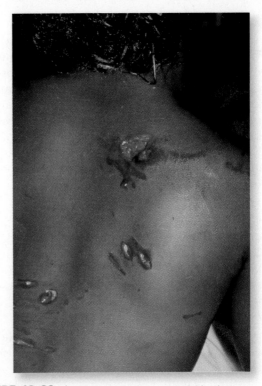

FIGURE 18-28 ▲ This dog bite occurred when an eight-year-old girl was attacked by several dogs.
Courtesy of Matthew D. Sztajnkrycer, MD, PhD.

bite–related injuries are highest for children 5 to 9 years of age. Males are bitten more often than females.

In the United States, most dog bites occur at home. The victim is often the dog's owner or a friend of the owner. In most cases, the attack involves an unrestrained dog on the owner's property. Deaths involving neonates (less than 30 days of age) usually occur on the dog owner's property and involve one dog and a sleeping child. Male and unspayed or unneutered dogs are more likely to bite than are female and spayed or neutered dogs.

According to the CDC, data pertaining to deadly dog attacks that occurred during the period 1979–1998 revealed that at least 25 breeds of dogs were involved in the fatal attacks. Pit bull–type dogs and Rottweilers were involved in more than half of the deaths for which the breed was known. However, since 1975, dogs belonging to more than 30 breeds have been responsible for fatal attacks on people, including Dachshunds, a Yorkshire terrier, and a Labrador retriever.

Cat bites occur more often in females. They usually happen in or near the victim's home. Because cats have narrower, sharper teeth than dogs, a cat bite is usually a puncture wound. Since infectious material is deposited deep in the tissue, most cat bites become infected.

Emergency Care for Dog and Cat Bites

Objective 8

- When obtaining a SAMPLE history, find out the type of animal involved and time elapsed since the injury. Find out when the patient last had a tetanus shot. Also, find out if the animal's shots are current. Be sure to relay this information to the receiving facility staff. Knowing this information helps the staff decide on an appropriate treatment plan for the patient.
- Establish and maintain an open airway.
- Give oxygen. If the patient's breathing is adequate, apply oxygen by nonrebreather mask at 15 L/min if not already done. If the patient's breathing is inadequate, provide positive-pressure ventilation with 100% oxygen and assess the adequacy of the ventilations delivered.
- Control bleeding, if present, with direct pressure and cover the wound with a sterile dressing. If there is no bleeding, gently wash the wound and then cover it with a sterile dressing.
- If possible, remove jewelry from the injured area before swelling begins. If swelling is

present, mark the outer edge of the swelling and note the time with a pen or marker.
- Because of the high risk of wound infection, the patient should be transported for physician evaluation. En route to the hospital, perform ongoing assessments as often as indicated.
- Carefully document all patient care information on a PCR.

Human Bites

Human bites in children usually occur while playing or fighting. In adults, bites are associated with alcohol use and clenched-fist injuries that occur during fights. Human bites can occur with child, elder, or spousal abuse. A human bite may or may not break the skin.

A **clenched-fist injury** (also called a *fight bite*) is the most serious human bite. In this type of injury, the fist of an individual strikes the teeth of another. The skin on the hand may or may not be broken. The underlying tissue and joints may be injured, even if the skin is not broken. If the skin is broken, tissue and joints may be injured, and the likelihood of infection is increased. When a bite is inflicted by an adult, infection is common because the human mouth contains many types of bacteria. Bites inflicted by children rarely become infected because they are usually superficial.

Emergency Care for Human Bites

Objective 8

- Establish and maintain an open airway.
- Give oxygen. If the patient's breathing is adequate, apply oxygen by nonrebreather mask at 15 L/min if not already done. If the patient's breathing is inadequate, provide positive-pressure ventilation with 100% oxygen and assess the adequacy of the ventilations delivered.
- Control bleeding, if present, with direct pressure and cover it with a sterile dressing. If there is no bleeding, gently wash the wound and then cover it with a sterile dressing.
- If possible, remove jewelry from the injured area before swelling begins. If swelling is present, mark the outer edge of the swelling and note the time with a pen or marker.
- Because of the high risk of wound infection, the patient should be transported for physician evaluation. En route to the hospital, perform ongoing assessments as often as indicated.
- Carefully document all patient care information on a PCR.

The patient assures you that the snake is dead out on the back porch. You quickly remove the patient's rings and watch from the injured hand and then position the affected arm slightly below the level of her heart. You use a pen to mark the outer edge of the swelling in her finger with the time. While your partner performs a focused physical examination, you obtain the patient's vital signs. Her blood pressure is 140/90, pulse 92 (strong and regular), and respirations 16. Lung sounds are clear bilaterally. The patient's skin is pink, warm, and dry. The patient states that she has a history of depression for which she takes Prozac, she is allergic to Lithium, and she last ate about 2 hours before your arrival. She denies any respiratory difficulty, chest discomfort, or other symptoms. Other than the swollen index finger, your partner did not find any other abnormal findings during his examination. Distal pulses in the affected extremity are strong and regular.

You apply oxygen by nonrebreather mask at 15 L/min and contact your Poison Control Center. The PCC asks you to provide them with a description of the snake and then transport the patient to the closest appropriate facility for physician evaluation. En route to the hospital, you reassess the patient's vital signs and the injured finger. Although distal pulses in the affected extremity remain strong and regular, the patient's index finger is swelling rapidly and she is becoming increasingly anxious. Once again, you mark the outer edge of the swelling in her finger with the time. After contacting medical direction with a brief report, you focus your attention on calmly reassuring the patient during the remainder of the short ride to the hospital. ■

Sum It Up

▶ The skin plays a very important role in temperature regulation. Cold and warmth sensors (receptors) in the skin detect changes in temperature. These receptors relay the information to the hypothalamus. The hypothalamus (located in the brain) functions as the body's thermostat. It coordinates the body's response to temperature.

▶ The body loses heat to the environment in 5 ways:

1. Radiation
   • Radiation is the transfer of heat from the surface of one object to the surface of another without contact between the two objects. When the temperature of the body is more than the temperature of the surroundings, the body will lose heat.

2. Convection
   • Convection is the transfer of heat by the movement of air current. Wind speed affects heat loss by convection (windchill factor).

3. Conduction
   • Conduction is the transfer of heat between objects that are in direct contact. Heat flows from warmer areas to cooler ones.

4. Evaporation
   • Evaporation is a loss of heat by vaporization of moisture on the body surface. The body will lose heat by evaporation if the skin temperature is higher than the temperature of the surroundings.

5. Breathing
   • The body loses heat through breathing. With normal breathing, the body continuously loses a relatively small amount of heat through the evaporation of moisture.

▶ Hypothermia is a core body temperature of less than 95°F (35°C). This condition results when the body loses more heat than it gains or produces.

   • A rectal temperature gives the most accurate measure of core temperature. However, obtaining a rectal temperature in the field often raises issues of patient sensitivity and welfare, such as exposure to cold by removal of clothing.

   • Your main concern in providing care should be to remove the patient from the environment. Use trained rescuers for this purpose when necessary. Perform an initial assessment, keeping in mind that you need to move the patient to a warm location as quickly and as safely as possible. Remove any cold or wet clothing. Protect the patient from the environment. Assess the patient's mental status, airway, breathing, and circulation. Keep in mind that mental status decreases as the patient's body temperature drops.

   • You may need to rewarm the patient. The two main types of rewarming are passive and active.

   —Passive rewarming is the warming of a patient with minimal or no use of heat sources other than the patient's own heat production. Passive rewarming methods include placing the patient in a warm environment, applying warm clothing and blankets, and preventing drafts.

—Active rewarming should be used only if sustained warmth can be ensured. Active rewarming involves adding heat directly to the surface of the patient's body. Warm blankets, heat packs, and/or hot water bottles may be used, depending on how severe the hypothermia is.

▶ Local cold injury (also called frostbite) involves tissue damage to a specific area of the body. It occurs when a body part, such as the nose, ears, cheeks, chin, hands, or feet, is exposed to prolonged or intense cold. When the body is exposed to cold, blood is forced away from the extremities to the body's core. A local cold injury may be early (superficial frostbite) or late (deep frostbite).

▶ When the body gains or produces more heat than it loses, hyperthermia (a high core body temperature) results. The 3 main types of heat emergencies are heat cramps, heat exhaustion, and heat stroke.

1. Heat cramps usually affect people who sweat a lot during strenuous activity in a warm environment. Water and electrolytes are lost from the body during sweating. This loss leads to dehydration and causes painful muscle spasms.

2. Heat exhaustion is also a result of too much heat and dehydration. A patient with heat exhaustion usually sweats heavily. His body temperature is usually normal or slightly elevated. Severe heat exhaustion often requires IV fluids. Heat exhaustion may progress to heat stroke if it is not treated.

3. Heat stroke is the most severe form of heat-related illness. It occurs when the body can no longer regulate its temperature. Most patients have hot, flushed skin and do not sweat. Individuals who wear heavy uniforms and perform strenuous activity for long periods in a hot environment are at risk for heat stroke.

▶ The first step in the emergency care of a patient suffering from a heat-related illness is to remove him from the hot environment. Move the patient to a cool (air-conditioned) location and follow treatment guidelines recommended for the patient's degree of heat-related illness.

▶ When providing emergency care for a drowning victim, ensure the safety of the rescue personnel. Suspect a possible spine injury if a diving accident is involved or unknown.

▶ Any breathless, pulseless patient who has been submerged in cold water should be resuscitated.

▶ Signs and symptoms of bites and stings typically include a history of a bite (spider, snake) or sting (insect, scorpion, marine animal), pain, redness, swelling, weakness, dizziness, chills, fever, nausea, and vomiting. Bite marks may be present.

▶ If a stinger is present, remove it by scraping the stinger out with the edge of card. Avoid using tweezers or forceps as these can squeeze venom from the venom sac into the wound.

▶ When caring for a victim of a bite or sting, watch closely for development of signs and symptoms of an allergic reaction; treat as needed.

19 Behavioral Emergencies

By the end of this chapter, you should be able to:

Knowledge Objectives ▶
1. Define behavioral emergencies.
2. Discuss the general factors that may cause an alteration in a patient's behavior.
3. State the various reasons for psychological crises.
4. Discuss the characteristics of an individual's behavior that suggest that the patient is at risk for suicide.
5. Discuss special medical and legal considerations for managing behavioral emergencies.
6. Discuss the special considerations for assessing a patient with behavioral problems.
7. Discuss the general principles of an individual's behavior that suggest that he is at risk for violence.
8. Discuss methods to calm behavioral emergency patients.

Attitude Objectives ▶
9. Explain the rationale for learning how to modify your behavior toward the patient with a behavioral emergency.

Skill Objectives ▶

10. Demonstrate the assessment and emergency medical care of the patient experiencing a behavioral emergency.
11. Demonstrate various techniques to safely restrain a patient with a behavioral emergency.

On the Scene

You and your Emergency Medical Technician partner are working an ambulance night shift in a busy section of the city. You are dispatched to a patient that is mildly combative and stating that he wants to commit suicide. The dispatcher advises you to "stage" for law enforcement. After waiting for a brief period, you get the all clear and enter the scene. As you enter, police officers advise that they were called for a person who had told his sister that he wanted to commit suicide by taking a bottle of pills. The officers tell you that they have the pills and it does not appear that the patient took any. While you are assessing him, the patient tells you he did not take any of the pills. He adds that the stresses in his life right now made him feel like he wanted to die. Your assessment reveals the patient is alert and oriented to person, place, time, and event. His vital signs are within normal limits. The patient repeatedly tells you that he does not want to go to the hospital. ■

THINK ABOUT IT

As you read this chapter, think about the following questions:

- What precautions should be taken at the scene of a behavioral emergency?
- Are the patient's actions considered a suicide attempt or a suicide gesture?
- Can this patient legally refuse transport to the hospital?

Introduction

You will respond to many situations involving behavioral emergencies. Some behavioral emergencies occur because of an injury or sudden illness. Others may be the result of mental illness or the use of mind-altering substances. You must be able to recognize the factors that can cause changes in a patient's behavior. When providing care for a patient experiencing a behavioral emergency, you must remember to ensure your own safety. You must be able to assess the patient and scene for signs of potential violence. You must also know methods to use to calm a patient experiencing a behavioral emergency and how to apply restraints if these methods are unsuccessful.

Behavior

Behavior is the way in which a person acts or performs. It includes any or all of a person's activities, including physical and mental activity. Abnormal behavior is a way of acting or conducting one's self that:

- Is not consistent with society's norms and expectations
- Interferes with the individual's well-being and ability to function
- May be harmful to the individual or others

Behavioral Change

Objective 1

A behavioral emergency is a situation in which a patient displays abnormal behavior that is unacceptable to the patient, family members, or community. A behavioral emergency can be the result of extremes of emotion that lead to violence or other inappropriate behavior. A behavioral emergency can also be caused by a psychological or physical condition such as mental illness, lack of oxygen, or low blood sugar.

Objectives 2, 3

Factors that may cause a change in a patient's behavior include alcohol or drugs, situational stressors, medical illnesses, or psychiatric illnesses or crises (Table 19-1). Psychological crises include panic, agitation, bizarre thinking and behavior, and destructive behavior. The patient who experiences a psychological crisis may be a danger to himself. He may show self-destructive behavior, such as suicidal gestures. He may also be a danger to others, acting in a threatening manner or even committing violence.

Remember This!

Do not assume that a patient has a psychiatric illness until you have ruled out possible physical causes for his behavior.

TABLE 19-1 Factors That May Cause Changes in Behavior

Mind-Altering Substances	• Alcohol, drugs	
Situational Stressors	• Rape • Loss of a job • Career change • Death of a loved one • Marital stress or divorce	• Physical or psychological abuse • Natural disasters (tornado, flood, earthquake, hurricane) • Man-made disasters (war, explosion)
Medical Illnesses	• Poisoning • Central nervous system infection • Head trauma • Seizure disorder • Lack of oxygen (hypoxia)	• Low blood sugar • Inadequate blood flow to the brain • Extremes of temperature (excessive cold or heat)
Psychiatric Illnesses or Crises	• Panic • Agitation • Bizarre thinking and behavior	• Self-destructive behavior, suicidal gesture (danger to self) • Threatening behavior, violence (danger to others)

Psychological Crises

Anxiety and Panic

Anxiety and fear are normal responses to a perceived threat. **Anxiety** is a state of worry and agitation that is usually triggered by a real or imagined situation. It's the person's response to the anxiety that determines its degree of impact. A person who is anxious is afraid of "losing control" or may feel that he will not be able to meet another's expectations. Some anxiety is good. To a point, it can increase awareness and performance. However, as one's level of anxiety increases, it drains energy, shortens one's attention span, and interferes with thinking and problem solving.

Fear is usually triggered by a specific object or situation, such as a fear of losing a job or being unable to pay the bills. Fear and anxiety bring on various symptoms:

- Worry
- Confusion
- Apprehension
- Helplessness
- Negative thoughts

People show anxiety at different levels of intensity, ranging from uneasiness to a panic attack. Anxiety can have a medical cause. Conditions that may cause anxiety are shown in the following *You Should Know* box.

You Should Know

Conditions Associated with Anxiety

- Asthma
- Diabetes
- Heart problems
- Thyroid disorder
- Seizure disorder
- Inner ear disturbances
- Premenstrual syndrome
- Withdrawal from alcohol, sedatives, or tranquilizers
- Reaction to cocaine, amphetamines, caffeine, aspartame, or other stimulants

An **anxiety disorder** is more intense than normal anxiety. Anxiety normally goes away after the stressful situation that caused it is over. An anxiety disorder lasts for months and can lead to phobias. Anxiety disorders are the most common mental illness in America. A patient with an anxiety disorder often has physical signs and symptoms that accompany the patient's intense worry. Common signs and symptoms include the following:

- Tiredness
- Headaches
- Muscle tension

- Muscle aches
- Difficulty swallowing
- Trembling
- Twitching
- Irritability
- Sweating
- Hot flashes

A **panic attack** is an intense fear that occurs for no apparent reason. Panic attacks can build gradually over several minutes or hours or occur suddenly. Most panic attacks do not last longer than one-half hour. Signs and symptoms that are often associated with a panic attack are shown in the following *You Should Know* box. The fear that accompanies a panic attack is very real to the patient. It is sometimes difficult for healthcare professionals to relate to that fear because there may be no obvious trigger. Do not minimize the patient's symptoms. Be supportive, calm, and reassuring.

You Should Know

Signs and Symptoms Common to Panic Attacks

- Numbness or tingling sensations (usually in the fingers, toes, or lips)
- Shortness of breath or a smothering sensation
- Heart palpitations (a rapid or irregular heartbeat)
- A fear of going crazy or being out of control
- Nausea or abdominal distress
- Choking
- Sweating
- Hot flashes or chills
- A feeling of detachment or being out of touch with one's self
- Trembling or shaking
- Dizziness or faintness
- Fear of becoming seriously ill or dying

Obsessive-Compulsive Disorder

Obsessive-compulsive disorder (OCD) is a type of anxiety disorder. **Obsessions** are recurring thoughts, impulses, or images that cause the person anxiety. Examples of common obsessions include a fear of dirt or germs, extreme need for neatness, and doubts about whether an appliance was turned off. **Compulsions** are recurring behaviors or rituals. The behavior is performed with the hope of preventing obsessive thoughts or making them go away. Examples of compulsions include the following:

- Excessive handwashing
- Checking and rechecking to see if a door is locked
- Touching things in a particular order
- Saying a name or phrase repeatedly
- Repeating a behavior several times

People with OCD often worry that something bad is going to happen to them or a loved one if they don't repeat a certain behavior. For example, they may think that a loved one will be hurt if they do not count to a certain number 5 times or flip a light switch on and off 48 times. Although some rituals are common in healthy people (such as handwashing), the obsessions and/or compulsions of a person with OCD take up at least 1 hour every day and interfere with the person's normal routine.

OCD usually begins gradually during adolescence or early adulthood. An adult who has OCD recognizes that his thoughts or behavior are excessive or unreasonable but is unable to control them. A person who has OCD often has another condition, such as depression, other anxiety disorder, or eating disorder.

Phobias

A **phobia** is an irrational and constant fear of a specific activity, object, or situation (other than a social situation). A **social phobia** is an extreme anxiety response in situations in which the individual may be seen by others. A person who has a social phobia fears that he will act in an embarrassing or shameful manner. Examples of common phobias are shown in Table 19-2.

A phobia is a type of anxiety disorder. Some phobias are common and usually do not create a problem because the person simply avoids the activity, object, or situation. For example, a person who is afraid of elevators or escalators usually avoids that situation or endures it with extreme anxiety. Although an adult recognizes that the fear associated with a phobia is excessive or unreasonable, a child may not recognize it as such. A child exposed to a phobic stimulus may express his anxiety by crying, tantrums, freezing, or clinging.

A phobic reaction resembles a panic attack. The signs and symptoms may include panic, sweating, difficulty breathing, and/or an increased heart rate.

Depression

Depression is a state of mind characterized by feelings of sadness, worthlessness, and discouragement. It often occurs in response to a loss. The loss may be losing a job, the death of a loved one, or the end of

TABLE 19-2 Common Phobias

Specific Phobias	Social Phobias
• Fear of animals (especially insects or spiders) • Thunder and/or lightning • Doctors or dentists • Germs, bacteria • Being alone • Blood, injection, or injury • Situations (heights, enclosed places, elevators, crossing bridges, driving or riding in vehicles, airplane travel)	• Public speaking • Eating in public • Using public restrooms • Writing while others are looking on • Performing publicly

a relationship. Signs of depression vary with age. Depressed children may be sad, irritable, or cry frequently. They may express anger by acting out toward parents, teachers, or other authority figures. Older children may have no appetite and may experience headaches or skin disorders. Depressed teens may behave unpredictably, run away, or change their physical and social activities. They may have no appetite, show no interest in their appearance, use alcohol or drugs excessively, or attempt suicide.

You Should Know

More Americans suffer from depression than from coronary heart disease, cancer, and AIDS combined.

Depressed adults show a lack of interest in their job, home, or appearance. They focus on the negative aspects of life, past events, and failures. They may attempt suicide. Depression in an older adult is often related to retirement. It may also be connected to the belief that he lacks control over his life, or it may result from a loss, such as the death of a spouse or other loved one. Older adults may feel useless or that they are a "burden." They may feel lonely as loved ones die or move away. A depressed older adult often withdraws, refuses to speak to anyone, and confines himself to bed. The signs and symptoms of depression are shown in the following *You Should Know* box.

You Should Know

Signs and Symptoms of Depression
- Loss of appetite
- Diarrhea or constipation
- Tiredness
- Difficulty sleeping or sleeping too much
- Muscle aches
- Vague pains
- Constant feelings of sadness, irritability, or tension
- Significant weight loss or gain
- A loss of interest in usual activities or hobbies
- Crying spells
- An inability to make decisions or concentrate
- Feelings of anger, helplessness, guilt, worthlessness, hopelessness, or loneliness
- Thoughts of suicide or death

Bipolar Disorder

Bipolar disorder (also known as *manic-depressive illness*) is a brain disorder that causes unusual shifts in a person's mood, energy, and ability to function. A person with bipolar disorder has alternating episodes of mood elevation (mania) and depression. When manic, the person often appears restless. He may be extremely energetic and enthusiastic. Typically, a manic person is easily distracted, requires little sleep, and develops unrealistic plans. A person with bipolar disorder will also usually experience periods of depression in which he feels worthless. He may consider suicide. The person's mood is often normal in between the periods of mania and depression.

Paranoia

Paranoia is a mental disorder characterized by excessive suspiciousness or delusions. **Delusions** are false beliefs that the patient believes are true, despite facts to the contrary. Common delusions of a paranoid patient include the following:

- Believing that people are following him, harassing him, plotting against him, reading his mind, or controlling his thoughts
- Believing that he possesses great power or special abilities
- Believing that he is a famous person

Remember This!

Hallucinations involve the senses. Delusions involve beliefs.

Paranoid patients may experience hallucinations. **Hallucinations** are false sensory perceptions. In other words, the patient sees, hears, or feels things others cannot. For example, a patient with visual hallucinations may think he sees worms or snakes crawling on the floor. An example of an auditory hallucination is hearing voices. An example of a tactile hallucination is feeling insects crawling on the skin.

Paranoid patients are suspicious, distrustful, and prone to conflict. They often feel as if they are being mistreated and misjudged. These patients tend to carry grudges, recalling wrongs done to them years earlier. They are excitable and unpredictable, with outbursts of bizarre or aggressive behavior.

Schizophrenia

Schizophrenia is a group of mental disorders. It is not the same as multiple personality disorder. Symptoms include hallucinations, delusions, disordered thinking, rambling speech, and bizarre or disorganized behavior. Schizophrenic patients are often reserved, withdrawn, and indifferent to the feelings of others. They prefer to be alone and have few, if any, close friends. They can become combative and are at high risk for suicidal and homicidal behavior. Your interpersonal interactions with the schizophrenic patient can either calm or escalate the situation, simply through eye contact and lines of questioning.

Suicide

Objective 4

A **suicide gesture** is self-destructive behavior that is unlikely to have any possibility of being fatal, for instance, threatening to kill oneself and then taking ten aspirin tablets. A suicide gesture is a conscious or subconscious attempt to call attention to their distress rather than to end life. A **suicide attempt** is self-destructive behavior for the purpose of ending one's life that, for unanticipated reasons, fails. For instance, an individual may have taken a sufficient number of aspirin tablets to cause death but was found by a family member before death occurred. A **completed suicide** is death by a self-inflicted, consciously intended action.

Most people who commit suicide express their intentions beforehand. You should take every suicide action seriously and arrange for patient transport for evaluation.

You Should Know

Risk Factors for Suicide

- Previous suicide attempt(s)
- History of mental disorders, particularly depression
- History of alcohol and/or substance abuse
- Family history of suicide
- Family history of child maltreatment
- Feelings of hopelessness
- Impulsive or aggressive tendencies
- Barriers to accessing mental health treatment
- Loss (relational, social, work, or financial)
- Physical illness
- Easy access to lethal methods
- Unwillingness to seek help because of the stigma attached to mental health and substance abuse disorders or suicidal thoughts
- Cultural and religious beliefs, for example, the belief that suicide is a noble resolution of a personal problem
- Local epidemics of suicide
- Isolation, a feeling of being cut off from other people

Depression is a factor that contributes to suicide. Arrest, imprisonment, or the loss of a job may be a source of depression. The risk of suicide is greatest in persons who have previously attempted suicide. The probability of successful suicide may increase with successive attempts, increasing the patient's risk. For example, a patient who ingested pills on his first attempt may slash his wrists on a second attempt.

Remember This!

Men commit suicide more frequently than women do, although women *attempt* suicide more frequently than men do.

The more well thought out the plan, the more serious the suicide risk. A patient who has chosen a lethal plan of action and told others about it is at an increased risk. An unusual gathering of articles that could be used to commit suicide increases the risk (such as the purchase of a gun or a large volume of pills). If you've been told that the patient is suicidal, ask him. For example, ask the patient, "Your family says you've thought about killing yourself. Can you tell me about it?" If the patient says he has had suicidal thoughts, ask if he has planned how he would carry it out. Then determine if he has a means to do it.

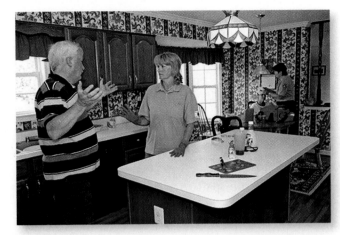

FIGURE 19-1 ▲ When you arrive on the scene of a possible behavioral emergency, carefully assess the scene for possible dangers, including the presence of weapons.

Assessment and Emergency Care for Patients with Behavioral Emergencies

Objective 6

Calls to a scene involving a behavioral emergency cause healthcare professionals anxiety because the scene is often unpredictable. Take steps to ensure your safety and that of other healthcare professionals responding to the scene. Start by considering the dispatch information you are given. Have you responded to this location in the past? If so, how many times? Were those calls violent in nature? Find out from your dispatcher if law enforcement personnel are already on the scene. If they are not, ask that they respond to the scene. Remember, your safety comes first.

Remember This!

If you suspect a dangerous situation, do *not* enter the scene until law enforcement personnel are present and the safety of the scene is assured.

When you arrive on the scene, complete a scene size-up before beginning emergency medical care. Carefully assess the scene for possible dangers. Start by visually locating the patient. Visually scan the area for possible weapons (Figure 19-1). Look for signs of violence and evidence of substance abuse. Does the patient have a method or the means of committing suicide? Is this a domestic violence situation? Are there multiple patients? Also, note the general condition of the environment. Look for signs of possible underlying medical problems, such as medications, home oxygen, or other medical equipment.

Objective 7

Check with the family and bystanders to see if the patient has threatened violence or has a history of violence, aggression, or combativeness. Patient postures that may indicate potential violence include:

- Standing or sitting in a position that threatens the self or others
- Inability to sit still, nervous pacing
- Clenched fists or jaw
- Having an unsafe object in his hands
- Eyes darting from one object to another

Remember This!

Throughout your assessment and care of the patient, maintain alertness to danger. *Never* turn your back on a violent or potentially violent patient, and always assure easy access to an exit from the room or area. Never corner yourself or the patient.

Speech patterns may indicate potential violence. Examples include erratic speech, yelling, shouting, cursing, or threats of harm to the self or others. Watch the patient's movements closely. Movements that may indicate potential violence include:

- Moving toward rescuers
- Carrying heavy or threatening objects
- Tense muscles
- Quick, irregular movements

Other signs of potential violence include a flushed face, agitation, turning away when spoken to, and avoiding eye contact.

When you are called to the scene of a behavioral emergency, be prepared to spend time at the scene. Limit the number of people around the patient. Take time to calm the patient. Start by approaching the patient slowly and purposefully. Do *not* make any quick movements. If the patient is lying down, it is safest to approach him from the head.

Remember This!

Do *not* place the patient between yourself and an exit.

Clearly identify yourself and try to build a connection with the patient. Explain who you are and what you are trying to do for him. As you talk with him, begin your assessment of the patient's mental status, airway, breathing, and circulation (ABC). Is he alert and oriented to person, place, time, and event? If the patient is confused, you will probably need to state more than once who you are and what you are doing. Respect the patient's personal space by limiting physical touch. Keep in mind that treating any life-threatening illness or injury that you find takes priority over the patient's behavioral problem.

Be aware of your position and posture when talking to your patient. Standing over him will immediately put him on the defensive. Face him and sit or stand at or below the patient's level while maintaining a comfortable distance from him. Maintain eye contact with the patient. Let him know what you expect and what he can expect from you. As you assess and provide care for your patient, keep him informed about what you are doing.

Note the patient's appearance, speech, and mood. Is he speaking normally or is his speech garbled? Does he seem anxious, depressed, excited, agitated, angry, hostile, or fearful? If the patient appears disturbed or agitated, try to provide a safe, nonthreatening environment in which you can assess him. Pay attention to the patient's thought process. Does it appear disordered? Is the patient hearing or seeing things that are not there? Does he have unusual worries or fears?

Methods to Calm Patients with Behavioral Emergencies

Objective 8

Do not assume you cannot talk with a patient with a behavioral problem until you have tried. Be polite and respectful when talking with the patient. Be careful not to talk down to him. Ask the patient open-ended questions, using a calm, reassuring voice. Open-ended questions require more than a "yes" or "no" answer.

For example, "Why were we called here today?" After asking a question, give the patient time to answer you. Allow him to tell you his story without being judgmental. Show you are listening by rephrasing or repeating part of what is said.

Be aware of your own reactions to the situation and to what the patient is saying. For example, an anxious patient may make you anxious. A hostile patient may make you angry. Be careful not to allow your personal feelings to get in the way of your professional judgment. Do not threaten, challenge, or argue with disturbed patients. Keeping your emotions in check when caring for these patients can be difficult. Monitor yourself. If your feelings and actions escalate, it is likely that the patient's feelings and actions will also escalate.

Give your patient honest reassurance. Answer his questions honestly—do not lie to him. However, do not make promises you cannot keep. If the patient is hearing or seeing things, do not "play along." In other words, do not tell the patient you are seeing or hearing the same things he is in an attempt to win his trust. Instead, let the patient know that you do not hear what he is hearing but are interested in knowing what it is that he is hearing.

Stop and Think!

Never leave a patient who is experiencing a behavioral emergency alone.

If possible, involve trusted family members or friends in the patient's care. However, if family members or bystanders are disruptive as you attempt to assess the patient, or if they interfere with your care of the patient, ask law enforcement personnel to remove them from the area.

Restraining Patients with Behavioral Emergencies

Avoid restraining a patient unless the patient is a danger to you, himself, or others. When using restraints, have police present, if possible, and get approval from medical direction. If you must use restraints, apply them with the help of law enforcement and other Emergency Medical Services (EMS) personnel.

Remember This!

Be aware that after a period of combativeness and aggression, some apparently calm patients may cause unexpected and sudden injury to you, themselves, or others.

Avoid the use of unreasonable force. **Reasonable force** is the amount of force necessary to keep a patient from injuring you, himself, or others. Use only the force necessary for restraint. You can determine what is reasonable by looking at all the circumstances involved. These circumstances include the following:

- The patient's size and strength
- The type of abnormal behavior
- The patient's body build and mental state
- The method of restraint

Making a Difference

Avoid acts or physical force that may cause injury to the patient.

When applying restraints, make certain you have enough assistance. You will need at least four healthcare or law enforcement personnel (one for each extremity). Have a plan. Decide who will do what before attempting to restrain the patient. It is extremely important that there is no confusion while you are applying restraints, as it will give the patient an opportunity to escape the restraints. Be sure to take body substance isolation (BSI) precautions for protection against body fluids.

Estimate the range of motion of the patient's arms and legs. Stay beyond that range until you are ready to restrain the patient. Once the decision has been made to restrain, act quickly.

When applying restraints, make certain you have enough assistance. You will need at least four healthcare or law enforcement personnel (one for each extremity) (Figure 19-2). Have a plan. Decide who will do what before attempting to restrain the patient. It is extremely important that there is no confusion while you are applying restraints, as it will give the patient an opportunity to escape the restraints. Be sure to take body substance isolation (BSI) precautions for protection against body fluids. Restrain on cue to gain rapid control of the patient.

One EMS professional should talk to the patient throughout the procedure. Tell the patient you are restraining him for his safety and for the safety of those around him. Secure the patient's extremities with restraints approved by medical direction, such as soft leather or cloth. Secure the patient on his back to the stretcher with chest, waist, and thigh straps (Figure 19-3). If the patient is spitting, cover the patient's face with a disposable surgical mask.

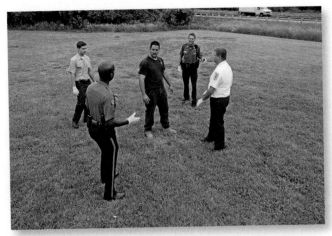

FIGURE 19-2 ▲ Once the decision has been made to restrain a patient, act quickly. One EMS professional should talk to the patient throughout the procedure. At least four persons should approach the patient, one assigned to each of the patient's extremities. Restrain on cue to gain rapid control of the patient.

Reassess the patient's airway, breathing, and circulation frequently. Suction as necessary. Chest straps should not hinder the patient's breathing. Reassess distal pulses in each extremity to make sure circulation is not impaired by the restraints. When using restraints, be careful to avoid doing any of the following:

- Inflicting unnecessary pain
- Using unreasonable force
- Leaving a restrained patient unattended
- Removing the restraints once they have been applied

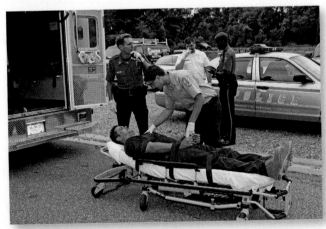

FIGURE 19-3 ▲ Secure the patient on his back to the stretcher with chest, waist, and thigh straps. Reassess the patient's airway, breathing, and circulation frequently.

You Should Know

Acceptable Restraints

- Soft leather straps
- Padded cloth straps
- Nylon restraints
- Velcro straps

Stop and Think!

A restrained patient must *never* be left alone. You must constantly monitor the status of his airway, breathing, and circulation while the patient is in your care.

It is important to document the use of restraints. Make sure to document your findings each time you reassess the patient while he is in restraints and in your care.

Remember This!

Documenting the Use of Restraints

When caring for a patient in restraints, document the following information:

- The reason for the restraints
- The number of personnel used to restrain the patient
- The type of restraint used
- The time the restraints were placed on the patient
- The status of the patient's ABCs and distal pulses before and after the restraints were applied
- Reassessment of the patient's ABCs and distal pulses

Medical and Legal Considerations

Objective 5

Emotionally disturbed patients may falsely accuse EMS and law enforcement personnel of unprofessional conduct, including sexual misconduct. To protect yourself against false accusations, it is very important that you document the patient's abnormal behavior. If possible, have witnesses present when you provide patient care. This is especially important during transport. When possible, use attendants of the same gender and involve third-party witnesses.

Emotionally disturbed patients will often resist treatment. To provide care against the patient's will, you must have a reasonable belief that the patient could harm you, himself, or others. If the patient is a threat to you, himself, or others, the patient may be transported without consent after you contact medical direction and receive approval to do so. Law enforcement personnel are usually required.

On the Scene   Wrap-Up

The patient stated that he wanted to commit suicide but did not actually take any pills. However, by making the statement that he intentionally wanted to harm himself, it became necessary for the patient to be transported and evaluated by a physician. In this case, the patient went to the hospital without incident. ∎

Sum It Up

▶ As an Emergency Medical Technician (EMT), you will likely encounter various behavioral emergencies. A behavioral emergency is a situation in which a patient displays abnormal behavior that is unacceptable to the patient, family members, or community. A behavioral emergency can be caused by extremes of emotion or by psychological or physical conditions. A number of factors can result in these emergencies, including mental illness, a lack of oxygen, low blood sugar, alcohol or drugs, situational stressors, medical illnesses, or psychiatric illnesses or crises.

▶ Anxiety is a state of worry and agitation that is usually triggered by a real or imagined situation. An anxiety disorder is more intense than normal anxiety.

▶ A panic attack is an intense fear that occurs for no apparent reason.

▶ Obsessive-compulsive disorder (OCD) is a type of anxiety disorder. Obsessions are recurring thoughts, impulses, or images that cause the person anxiety. Compulsions are recurring behaviors or rituals that are performed with the hope of preventing obsessive thoughts or making them go away.

▶ A phobia is an irrational and constant fear of a specific activity, object, or situation (other than a social situation). A social phobia is an extreme anxiety response in situations in which the individual may be seen by others. A phobic reaction resembles a panic attack.

- Depression is a state of mind characterized by feelings of sadness, worthlessness, and discouragement. It often occurs in response to a loss. The loss may be losing a job, the death of a loved one, or the end of a relationship.

- Bipolar disorder is a brain disorder that causes unusual shifts in a person's mood, energy, and ability to function. A person with bipolar disorder has alternating episodes of mood elevation (mania) and depression. The person's mood is often normal between the periods of mania and depression.

- Paranoia is a mental disorder characterized by excessive suspiciousness or delusions. Paranoid patients are suspicious, distrustful, and prone to argument. They are excitable and unpredictable, with outbursts of bizarre or aggressive behavior.
  - Delusions are false beliefs that the patient believes are true, despite facts to the contrary.
  - Hallucinations are false sensory perceptions. The patient sees, hears, or feels things that others cannot.

- Schizophrenia is a group of mental disorders. Symptoms include hallucinations, delusions, disordered thinking, rambling speech, and bizarre or disorganized behavior. These patients can become combative and are at high risk for suicidal and homicidal behavior.

- A suicide gesture is self-destructive behavior that is unlikely to have any possibility of being fatal. A suicide attempt is self-destructive behavior for the purpose of ending one's life that, for unanticipated reasons, fails. A completed suicide is death by a self-inflicted, consciously intended action.

- Most people who commit suicide express their intentions beforehand. You should take every suicide action seriously and arrange for patient transport for evaluation.

- When called to a scene that involves a behavioral emergency, remember that the scene may be unpredictable. Take steps to ensure your safety and that of other healthcare professionals responding to the scene. Complete a scene size-up before beginning emergency medical care. Carefully assess the scene for possible dangers. Start by visually locating the patient. Visually scan the area for possible weapons. Be prepared to spend time at the scene. Limit the number of people around the patient. Take time to calm the patient.

- Avoid restraining a patient unless the patient is a danger to you, himself, or others. When using restraints, have police present, if possible, and get approval from medical direction. If you must use restraints, apply them with the help of law enforcement and other EMS personnel.

By the end of this chapter, you should be able to:

Knowledge Objectives ▶

1. Identify the following structures: uterus, vagina, fetus, placenta, umbilical cord, amniotic sac, and perineum.
2. Identify and explain the use of the contents of an obstetrics kit.
3. Identify predelivery emergencies.
4. State indications of an imminent delivery.
5. Differentiate the emergency medical care provided to a patient with predelivery emergencies from a normal delivery.
6. State the steps in the predelivery preparation of the mother.
7. Establish the relationship between body substance isolation and childbirth.
8. State the steps to assist in a delivery.
9. Describe care of the baby as the head appears.
10. Describe how and when to cut the umbilical cord.
11. Discuss the steps in the delivery of the placenta.
12. List the steps in the emergency medical care of the mother after delivery.
13. Summarize neonatal resuscitation procedures.
14. Describe the procedures for the following abnormal deliveries: breech birth, prolapsed cord, limb presentation.
15. Differentiate the special considerations for multiple births.
16. Describe special considerations of meconium.
17. Describe special considerations of a premature baby.
18. Discuss the emergency medical care of a patient with a gynecological emergency.

Attitude Objectives ▶ 19. Explain the rationale for understanding the implications of treating two patients (mother and baby).

Skill Objectives ▶ 20. Demonstrate the steps to assist in the normal cephalic delivery.

21. Demonstrate necessary care procedures of the fetus as the head appears.
22. Demonstrate postdelivery care of an infant.
23. Demonstrate how and when to cut the umbilical cord.
24. Attend to the steps in the delivery of the placenta.

25. Demonstrate the postdelivery care of the mother.
26. Demonstrate the procedures for the following abnormal deliveries: vaginal bleeding, breech birth, prolapsed cord, limb presentation.
27. Demonstrate the steps in the emergency medical care of the mother with excessive bleeding.
28. Demonstrate completing a prehospital care report for patients with obstetrical or gynecological emergencies.

On the Scene

It is late in your shift when the emergency page goes out: "Emergency response teams, report to the warehouse." It's clear when you arrive that this is no ordinary emergency. A woman is squatting on the floor, grunting and screaming, "The baby's coming, the baby's coming!"

You can tell by the dark stain on her jeans that her bag of waters has broken. The plant supervisor tells you that the paramedics are en route, but about 20 minutes away. You put on your goggles, mask, and gloves, ask your partner to run back to ambulance to get the obstetrics kit, and you prepare to deliver a baby. ■

THINK ABOUT IT

As you read this chapter, think about the following questions:

• What questions should you ask the mother to determine if this will be a complicated delivery?
• What equipment will you need?
• How will you assist with the delivery of the baby?
• How will you assess the baby?

Introduction

Caring for Mother and Baby

You may be called to care for a woman in labor. Although childbirth is a natural process and most deliveries occur with no complications, these situations are often stressful for the patient, the patient's family, and emergency care providers. Once the mother delivers, you will be responsible for her care and for that of her baby. To provide the best possible care for both patients, you must know how to assist during childbirth and how to provide care for both mother and baby after delivery.

Anatomy and Physiology of the Female Reproductive System

Objective 1

The female reproductive organs are found in the pelvic cavity (Figure 20-1). The **ovaries** are paired, almond-shaped organs located on either side of the uterus. The ovaries perform two main functions: producing eggs and secreting hormones, such as estrogen and progesterone. Each ovary contains thousands of follicles. About once a month during a woman's reproductive years, a follicle matures to release an egg (**ovulation**). The fallopian tubes (also called *uterine tubes*) extend from each ovary to the uterus. They receive and transport the

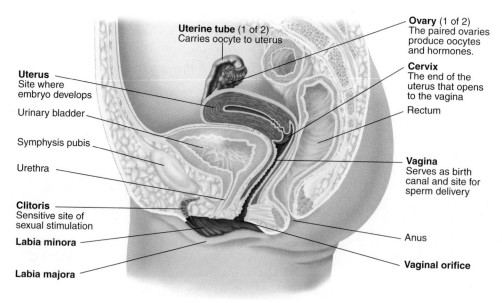

FIGURE 20-1 ▲ The structures of the female reproductive system.

egg to the uterus after ovulation. Fertilization normally takes place in the upper third of the fallopian tube.

The uterus (womb) is a pear-shaped, hollow, muscular organ located in the pelvic cavity. It prepares for pregnancy each month of a woman's reproductive life. If pregnancy does not occur, the inner lining of the uterus sloughs off and is discarded. This discharge of blood and tissue from the uterus is called **menstruation.** It is often referred to as a woman's *period.* If pregnancy does occur, the developing embryo implants in the uterine wall and develops there. The uterus stretches throughout pregnancy to adjust to the increasing size of the fetus. During **labor,** the uterus contracts powerfully and rhythmically to expel the infant from

the mother's body. After delivery of the infant, the uterus quickly clamps down to stop bleeding.

The **cervix** is the narrow opening at the distal end of the uterus. It connects the uterus to the vagina. During pregnancy, it contains a plug of mucus. The mucus plug seals the opening to the uterus, keeping bacteria from entering. When the cervix begins to widen during early labor, the mucus plug, sometimes mixed with blood (**bloody show**), is expelled from the vagina. The vagina is also called the birth canal. It is a muscular tube that serves as a passageway between the uterus and the outside of the body (Figure 20-2). It receives the penis during intercourse. It also serves as the passageway for menstrual flow and the delivery

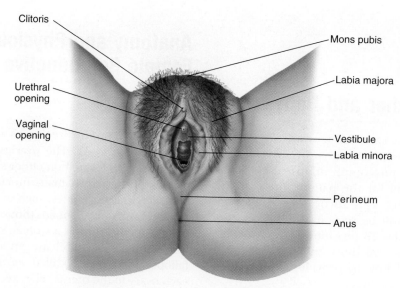

FIGURE 20-2 ▲ External female reproductive structures.

of an infant. The **perineum** is the area between the vaginal opening and anus. It is commonly torn during **childbirth.**

The Structures of Pregnancy

Pregnancy begins when an egg (ovum) joins with a sperm cell (fertilization). The **zygote** (fertilized egg) passes from the fallopian tube into the uterus. The zygote implants in the wall of the uterus (implantation) (Figure 20-3). During the first 3 weeks after fertilization, the developing structure is called a **blastocyst.** From the 3rd to the 8th week, the developing structure is called an **embryo.** From the 8th week until birth, the developing structure is called a **fetus.**

The **placenta** is a specialized organ through which the fetus exchanges nourishment and waste products during pregnancy (Figure 20-4). It is also called the

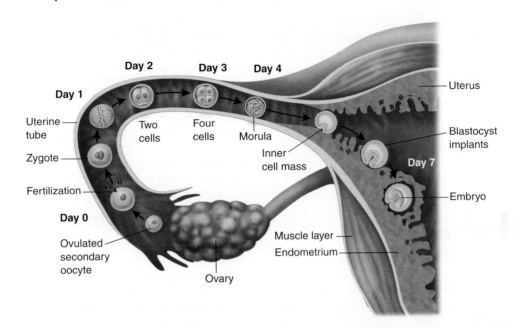

FIGURE 20-3 ▲ Pregnancy begins when an egg joins with a sperm cell (fertilization). The fertilized egg passes from the fallopian tube into the uterus. The egg implants in the wall of the uterus around day 7.

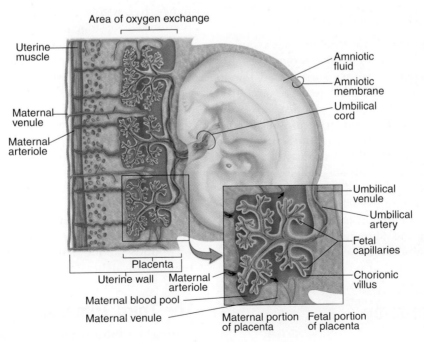

FIGURE 20-4 ▲ In the placenta, nutrients and oxygen pass from the maternal blood to the embryo while wastes pass in the opposite direction.

afterbirth because it is expelled after the baby is born. The placenta begins to develop about two weeks after fertilization occurs. It attaches to the mother at the inner wall of the uterus and to the fetus by the umbilical cord. The placenta is responsible for:

- The exchange of oxygen and carbon dioxide between the blood of the mother and fetus (the placenta serves the function of the lungs for the developing fetus)
- The removal of waste products from the fetus
- The transport of nutrients from the mother to the fetus
- The production of a special pregnancy hormone that maintains the pregnancy and stimulates changes in the mother's breasts, cervix, and vagina in preparation for delivery
- The maintenance of a barrier against harmful substances
- The transfer of heat from the mother to the fetus

You Should Know

Although the placenta is an effective protective barrier between the mother and fetus, it does not protect the baby from everything. Some medications and toxic substances (such as alcohol) pass easily from the mother's blood to the baby. It is very important for a pregnant woman to consult with her doctor before taking any medicine or herbal supplement.

The **umbilical cord** is the lifeline that connects the placenta to the fetus. It contains two arteries and one vein. The umbilical arteries carry blood low in oxygen from the fetus to the placenta. The umbilical vein carries oxygenated blood to the fetus. This is the opposite of normal circulation. The umbilical cord attaches to the umbilicus (navel) of the fetus.

The **amniotic sac** (also called the *bag of waters*) is a membranous bag that surrounds the fetus inside the uterus. It contains fluid (amniotic fluid) that helps protect the fetus from injury. The amniotic fluid provides an environment that is at a constant temperature. It also allows the fetus to move and functions much like a shock absorber. The amniotic sac contains about 1 liter (L) of fluid at term.

Normal Pregnancy

Pregnancy usually takes 40 weeks and is divided into three 90-day intervals called *trimesters*.

The First Trimester

During the first trimester (months 1-3), the mother stops menstruating (missed period). Her breasts become swollen and tender. She urinates more frequently and may sleep more than usual. Nausea and vomiting (usually called *morning sickness*) are usually at their worst during the second month. Despite its name, morning sickness can occur at *any* time of day. During the first weeks after conception, the mother's body begins to produce more blood to carry oxygen and nutrients to the fetus. Her heart rate increases by as much as 10 to 15 beats/min because her heart must work harder to pump this increased amount of blood. Normal weight gain during the first trimester is only about 2 pounds (about 907 grams or 0.907 kilograms).

During the first 13 weeks of pregnancy, the fetus is developing rapidly. Cells differentiate into tissues and organs. The arms, legs, heart, lungs, and brain begin to form. By the end of the first trimester, the fetus is about 3 inches long and weighs about half an ounce.

The Second Trimester

In the second trimester (months 4-6), the signs of pregnancy become more obvious. The uterus expands to make room for the fetus and can be felt above the pubic bone. The mother's abdomen also enlarges and her center of gravity often changes. As a result, she will often walk and move differently. The mother begins to feel the fetus move at about the 4th or 5th month. Her circulatory system continues to expand, which lowers her blood pressure. During the first 6 months of pregnancy, her systolic blood pressure may drop by 5-10 points. Her diastolic blood pressure may drop by 10-15 points. In her third trimester, her blood pressure gradually returns to its pre-pregnancy level. The mother may feel dizzy or faint when taking a hot bath or shower or in hot weather. This occurs because heat causes the capillaries in her skin to dilate, temporarily reducing the amount of blood returning to her heart and, thus, reducing the amount of blood pumped to her brain.

During the second trimester (about the 13th to 24th week of pregnancy), the fingers, toes, eyelashes, and eyebrows of the fetus are formed. At about the 5th month, the heartbeat of the fetus can be heard with a stethoscope. By the end of this trimester, the heart, lungs, and kidneys are formed. The fetus weighs about $1\frac{3}{4}$ pounds (about 794 grams or 0.794 kilograms) and is about 13 inches (about 33 centimeters) long.

The Third Trimester

During the third trimester (months 7-9), the mother may complain of a backache because of muscle strain. Stretch marks may appear (Figure 20-5). The mother

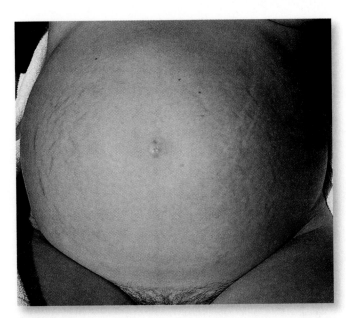

FIGURE 20-5 ▲ This woman is 39 weeks pregnant. Stretch marks are common in the third trimester of pregnancy.
Courtesy of Stephen Corbett, MD, from Knoop, et al., Atlas of Emergency Medicine, 2nd edition, McGraw-Hill Company, Inc.

urinates frequently because the weight of the uterus presses on the bladder. She may be short of breath as her uterus expands beneath the diaphragm.

During the third trimester (about the 25th to 40th week of pregnancy), the fetus continues to grow rapidly, gaining about one-half pound a week and reaching a length of about 20 inches. Fetal movement occurs often and is stronger. Normally, the head of the fetus settles in the pelvis in preparation for delivery. **Premature labor** (also called *preterm labor*) occurs when a woman has labor before her 37th week of pregnancy.

Complications of Pregnancy

Abortion

Objective 3

An **abortion** is the termination of pregnancy before the fetus is able to live on its own outside the uterus. A **therapeutic abortion** is an abortion performed for medical reasons, often because the pregnancy poses a threat to the mother's health. An **elective abortion** is an abortion performed at the request of the mother. A **threatened abortion** is a condition in which the cervix remains closed and the fetus remains in the uterus but the patient experiences vaginal spotting or bleeding and/or pain resembling menstrual cramps. A threatened abortion may progress to a complete abortion or may subside, and the pregnancy may continue

to term. An **incomplete abortion** is one in which part of the products of conception have been passed but some remain in the uterus. The cervix is open and the patient will bleed heavily until all of the products of conception are removed from the uterus.

A **spontaneous abortion,** also called a *miscarriage,* is the loss of a fetus because of natural causes. It usually occurs before the 20th week of pregnancy, most often between the 7th and 12th weeks of pregnancy. In most miscarriages, the fetus dies because of a genetic abnormality that is usually unrelated to the mother. During a miscarriage, the mother often experiences lower back pain or cramping abdominal pain, vaginal bleeding, and the passage of tissue or clot-like material from the vagina.

Not all abdominal pain or bleeding that occurs during the early weeks of pregnancy indicates a miscarriage. Bleeding sometimes occurs during early pregnancy, and the mother is still able to carry the fetus to full term. The patient needs to be evaluated by a physician. Prepare the patient for transport to the hospital. Give oxygen and treat the patient for shock if signs are present. Place bulky dressings against the vaginal opening if necessary, but do not pack any material into the vagina. Keep the patient warm. Collect any tissue or clot-like material passed from the vagina. A clean plastic container with a lid or a biohazard bag can be used for this purpose. Be sure the collected tissue accompanies the patient to the hospital. Perform ongoing assessments as often as indicated during transport. Record all patient care information, including the patient's medical history and all emergency care given, on a prehospital care report (PCR).

Making a Difference

Any situation that involves bleeding during pregnancy is likely to be a very emotional one. Most women associate bleeding during pregnancy with "losing the baby." This may or may not be the case and cannot be accurately determined in the field. Grief is a very normal reaction to the threatened loss of the pregnancy. While treating your patient's physical condition, remember to provide her with emotional support as well.

Ectopic Pregnancy

Once conception occurs, the fertilized egg normally travels through the fallopian tube to the uterus. The fertilized egg implants in the uterine lining and begins to grow. This process usually takes about 4 to 9 days. An **ectopic pregnancy** occurs when a fertilized egg implants outside the uterus. An ectopic pregnancy is a medical emergency. The most common

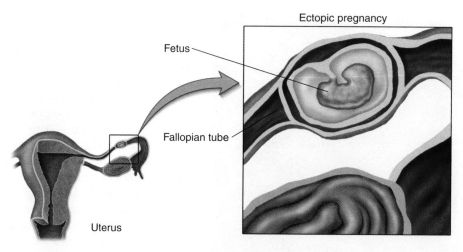

Ectopic pregnancy

Fetus

Fallopian tube

Uterus

FIGURE 20-6 ▲ An ectopic pregnancy occurs when a fertilized egg implants outside the uterus, usually inside a fallopian tube.

site where this occurs is inside a fallopian tube (Figure 20-6). An ectopic pregnancy that occurs in a fallopian tube is called a *tubal pregnancy*. Less commonly, the egg implants in the abdomen, cervix, or an ovary. In an ectopic pregnancy, the growing fetus bursts through the tissue in which it has implanted. Severe bleeding can occur as a result of ruptured blood vessels.

The initial signs and symptoms of an ectopic pregnancy include a missed menstrual period or small amounts of vaginal bleeding that occur irregularly over 6 to 8 weeks. The patient may complain of mild cramping on one side of the pelvis, nausea, lower back pain, and lower abdominal or pelvic pain.

If rupture occurs, the patient often complains of a sudden onset of severe pain on one side of the lower abdomen. Vaginal bleeding may or may not be present. The patient may feel faint or may actually faint. In addition, the patient may complain of severe pain in the back of the shoulder (referred pain). Severe internal bleeding may be present. The patient may have signs of shock, such as decreasing blood pressure, an increased heart rate, and cool, clammy skin.

Prepare for immediate transport to the closest appropriate facility. Keep on scene time to a minimum. Request an early response of Advanced Life Support (ALS) personnel to the scene or consider an ALS intercept while en route to the receiving facility. Do not delay transport for ALS arrival. Give oxygen by nonrebreather mask. Treat the patient for shock if signs are present. Keep the patient warm. Remember to provide emotional support for the patient and family. Perform ongoing assessments as often as indicated during transport. Record all patient care information, including the patient's medical history and all emergency care given, on a PCR.

Remember This!

Although there are many causes of abdominal pain, you must consider lower abdominal pain in any woman of childbearing age to be caused by an ectopic pregnancy until proven otherwise. An ectopic pregnancy is a medical emergency.

Preeclampsia and Eclampsia

Preeclampsia (also called *pregnancy-induced hypertension* or *toxemia of pregnancy*) is a disorder of pregnancy that causes blood vessels to spasm and constrict. Blood vessel constriction results in high blood pressure. It also decreases blood flow to the mother's organs, including the placenta. Less blood flow to the placenta usually means that less oxygenated blood and nutrients reach the baby. In some cases, the baby may need to be delivered early to protect the health of the mother. Preeclampsia also causes changes in the blood vessels. These changes cause the mother's capillaries to leak fluid into her tissues. This results in swelling.

The cause of preeclampsia is not known. It usually occurs during the 3rd trimester of pregnancy. It tends to occur in young mothers during their first pregnancy and in women whose mothers or sisters had preeclampsia. The risk of preeclampsia is higher in women older than age 40, in women carrying multiple babies, and in teenage mothers. Women who had high blood pressure, diabetes, or kidney disease before they became pregnant are also at risk of preeclampsia.

The signs and symptoms of preeclampsia include the following:

- Weight gain of more than 2 pounds per week or a sudden weight gain over 1 to 2 days
- Visual disturbances such as blurred vision, or the appearance of flashing lights or spots before the eyes
- Swelling of the face and hands that is present on arising from sleep
- Headaches
- Right-upper-quadrant abdominal pain
- Increased blood pressure (more than 140/90 mm Hg)

Remember This!

If your patient complains of blurred vision, nausea, a severe headache, and pain in the right upper quadrant of the abdomen, she may be very close to having a seizure (eclampsia). Because eclampsia is associated with a significant risk of death for the mother and fetus, move quickly and begin patient transport as soon as possible.

If untreated, preeclampsia may progress to eclampsia. Eclampsia is the seizure phase of preeclampsia. **Eclampsia** is associated with a significant risk of death for the mother and fetus. Keep on-scene time to a minimum. Request an early response of ALS personnel to the scene or consider an ALS intercept while en route to the receiving facility. Do not delay transport for ALS arrival. Be sure to have suction readily available. Give oxygen. If the patient's breathing is adequate, apply oxygen by nonrebreather mask at 15 L/min if not already done. If the patient's breathing is inadequate, provide positive-pressure ventilation with 100% oxygen. Assess the adequacy of the ventilations delivered. Keep the patient calm and position her on her left side. Avoid any stimulus that might trigger a seizure, such as bright lights and siren noise. Dim the lights. Prepare for immediate transport *without* lights or siren. If the patient has a seizure, protect her from injury and watch her breathing closely. When the seizure is over, make sure her airway is clear and give oxygen. Perform ongoing assessments as often as indicated during transport. Record all patient care information, including the patient's medical history and all emergency care given, on a PCR.

Vaginal Bleeding in Late Pregnancy

Vaginal bleeding may occur late in pregnancy (third trimester). It may or may not be accompanied by pain. The possible causes of vaginal bleeding in late pregnancy include placenta previa, abruptio placentae, and a ruptured uterus.

Placenta previa occurs when the placenta attaches low in the wall of the uterus instead of at its top or sides. In this position, the placenta may cover all or part of the cervix (the entrance to the birth canal) (Figure 20-7). If the placenta covers the cervical opening during the early months of pregnancy, it will often

Remember This!

All third-trimester bleeding should be considered a life-threatening emergency.

Remember This!

It is not necessary for you to determine the cause of vaginal bleeding. However, it is important for you to recognize that the patient needs immediate transport and evaluation by a physician.

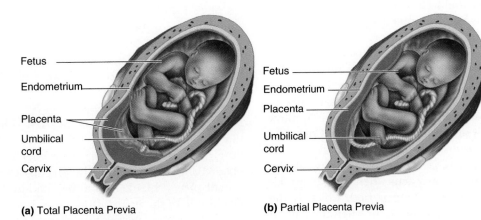

(a) Total Placenta Previa

(b) Partial Placenta Previa

FIGURE 20-7 ▲ Placenta previa. **(a)** In a total placenta previa, the placenta completely covers the cervix. **(b)** In a partial placenta previa, the placenta partially covers the cervix.

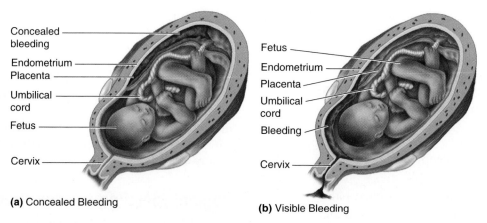

Concealed bleeding
Endometrium
Placenta
Umbilical cord
Fetus
Cervix

(a) Concealed Bleeding

Fetus
Endometrium
Placenta
Umbilical cord
Bleeding
Cervix

(b) Visible Bleeding

FIGURE 20-8 ▲ **(a)** Abruptio placentae occurs when a normally implanted placenta separates prematurely from the wall of the uterus (endometrium) during the last trimester of pregnancy. Vaginal bleeding may absent (concealed or hidden bleeding). **(b)** Vaginal bleeding that is visible may be moderate to severe and is usually dark red.

shift position as the uterus grows, moving away from the cervical opening. If the placenta does not shift from the cervical opening as the pregnancy progresses, then placenta previa exists.

You Should Know

Placenta previa is the cause of most cases of severe bleeding in the third trimester of pregnancy.

Normally, the cervix begins to widen and thin out in the latter part of pregnancy. This is the body's way of preparing for labor. If the mother has placenta previa, vaginal bleeding can occur because placental blood vessels that are implanted in the wall of the uterus are torn as the cervix widens and thins out. The more the placenta covers the cervical opening, the greater the risk of bleeding.

Abruptio placentae (also called *placental abruption*) occurs when a normally implanted placenta separates prematurely from the wall of the uterus (endometrium) during the last trimester of pregnancy. If the placenta begins to peel away from the wall of the uterus, bleeding occurs from the blood vessels that transfer nutrients to the fetus from the mother. The larger the area that peels away, the greater the amount of bleeding. The placenta may separate partially or completely (Figure 20-8). Partial separation may allow time for treatment of the mother and fetus. Complete separation often results in death of the fetus.

A ruptured uterus is the actual tearing of the uterus. Uterine rupture can occur when the patient has been in strong labor for a long period, which is the most common cause. It can also occur when the patient has sustained abdominal trauma, such as a severe fall or a sudden stop in a motor vehicle collision.

A patient with any of these conditions needs ALS care and immediate transport to the closest appropriate facility. Keep on-scene time to a minimum. Request an early response of ALS personnel to the scene or consider an ALS intercept while en route to the receiving facility. Do not delay transport for ALS arrival. Because exposure to blood is possible, be sure to wear appropriate personal protective equipment (PPE). Give oxygen and treat the patient for shock. Keep the patient warm. Perform ongoing assessments every 5 minutes during transport. Record all patient care information, including the patient's medical history and all emergency care given, on a PCR.

Table 20-1 lists some of the causes, signs, and symptoms of vaginal bleeding in late pregnancy.

Making a Difference

A woman late in her second trimester or in her third trimester of pregnancy should be positioned on her left side. When a woman in late pregnancy is placed on her back, the weight of the fetus compresses major blood vessels, such as the inferior vena cava and the aorta (Figure 20-9). This compression decreases the amount of blood returning to the mother's heart and lowers her blood pressure. As a result, the amount of oxygen and nutrients delivered to the fetus is decreased.

Positioning the patient on her left side shifts the weight of her uterus off the abdominal vessels. If the patient is immobilized to a backboard, tilt the board slightly to the left by placing a rolled towel, small pillow, blanket, or other padding under the right side of the board. Doing so will shift the weight of the patient's uterus and decrease the pressure on the abdominal blood vessels.

TABLE 20-1 Causes of Vaginal Bleeding in Late Pregnancy

Signs and Symptoms	Placenta Previa	Abruptio Placentae	Uterine Rupture
Vaginal bleeding	• Sudden • Bright red	• May be absent (concealed or hidden) • If seen, may be moderate to severe; usually dark red	• May or may not be present
Abdominal pain	• Usually none (**P**ainless = **P**revia)	• Sudden, severe	• Sudden, severe • Abdomen tender, rigid • Possible contractions
Signs of shock	• Likely	• Yes; may seem out of proportion to amount of blood loss seen	• Yes
Fetal movement	• Usually present	• Decreased • May be absent	• Absent

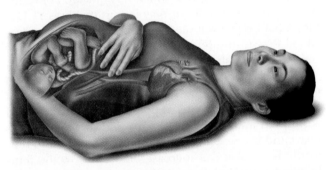

(a)

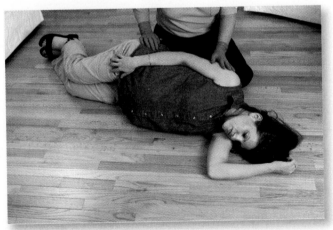

(b)

FIGURE 20-9 ▲ (a) When a woman in late pregnancy is placed on her back, the weight of the fetus compresses major blood vessels in the abdomen, such as the inferior vena cava and aorta. This decreases the amount of blood returning to the mother's heart and lowers her blood pressure. **(b)** To relieve pressure on the abdominal blood vessels, place the pregnant patient on her left side.

Trauma and Pregnancy

Direct or indirect trauma to a pregnant uterus can cause injury to the uterine muscle. This can cause the release of chemicals that cause uterine contractions, perhaps inducing premature labor.

Trauma is more likely to cause the death of the mother than any other complication of pregnancy. The effects of trauma on the fetus depend on:

• The length of the pregnancy (the age of the fetus)
• The type and severity of the trauma
• The severity of blood flow and oxygen disruption to the uterus

You Should Know

Causes of Trauma in Pregnancy
• Motor vehicle crashes
• Gunshot wounds
• Stabbings
• Domestic violence
• Falls
• Burns

Motor vehicle crashes (MVCs) are the most common cause of serious blunt trauma in pregnancy (Figure 20-10). Abruptio placentae, placenta previa, and uterine rupture are often seen in MVCs. These conditions increase the risk of fetal distress or death. Gunshot wounds and stab wounds to the abdomen of

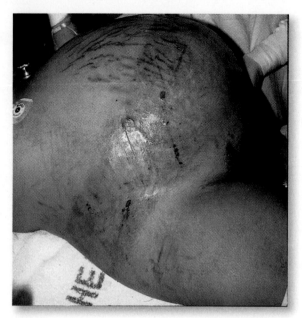

FIGURE 20-10 ▲ This woman experienced significant blunt trauma to the abdomen during in her third trimester of pregnancy. *Courtesy of John Fildes, MD, from Atlas of Emergency Medicine, 2nd edition, McGraw-Hill Company, Inc.*

a pregnant patient do not usually result in the mother's death. However, the likelihood of fetal death is high.

For some women, pregnancy is a time when physical abuse starts. It is estimated that 25-45% of women who are battered are battered during pregnancy. Physical abuse can result in the following conditions:

- Blunt trauma to the abdomen
- Severe bleeding
- Uterine rupture
- Miscarriage
- Premature labor
- Premature rupture of the amniotic sac

One in four pregnant women experiences a fall during pregnancy. A woman's center of gravity shifts as the size of her abdomen increases during pregnancy and her pelvic ligaments loosen. As a result, a pregnant patient must readjust her body alignment and balance, which increases her risk for falls and injury. Some of these falls are a result of slippery floors, hurrying, or carrying objects.

A thermal burn of more than 20% of the mother's body surface area increases the risk of fetal death. In cases of electrical burns, the likelihood of fetal death is high, even with a rather low electrical current. This is most likely because the fetus is floating in amniotic fluid and has a low resistance to the current.

Assessing the Pregnant Patient

Assessment of the pregnant patient is the same as that of other patients. However, because of the normal changes in vital signs that occur with pregnancy, the patient's vital signs may not be as diagnostically helpful as they are in a nonpregnant patient. For example, the pregnant patient's heart rate is normally slightly faster than usual. Her breathing rate is also slightly faster and more shallow than normal. Her blood pressure is often slightly lower than normal until the third trimester. It is important to take vital signs in all patients. However, you will need to pay special attention to the pregnant patient's history and look for other signs that may suggest a potential problem. For example, a patient with a history of vaginal bleeding for three hours who has cold, pale, clammy skin is probably in shock—even if her vital signs appear normal.

Despite a significant amount of internal or external bleeding, young, healthy pregnant patients can maintain relatively normal vital signs for a significant time and then develop signs of shock very quickly. For example, the pregnant patient may lose as much as $1\frac{1}{2}$ L of blood before you will see a decrease in blood pressure. Blood flow to the fetus may be significantly decreased before signs of shock are obvious in the mother.

The signs of early shock are difficult to detect in the pregnant patient. As blood is lost because of trauma or complications of pregnancy, available blood is shunted away from the uterus and to the mother's heart and brain. This change compromises blood flow to the fetus. You can increase blood flow to the fetus by placing the pregnant patient on her left side.

Obtaining a SAMPLE History

Obtain a SAMPLE history to gather information about the pregnant patient's medical history.

- *Signs and symptoms.* The signs and symptoms that may indicate a possible complication of pregnancy include:
  — Seizures
  — Weakness
  — Dizziness
  — Faintness
  — Signs of shock
  — Lightheadedness
  — Vaginal bleeding
  — Altered mental status
  — Passage of clots or tissue
  — Swelling of the face and/or extremities
  — Abdominal cramping or pain (may be constant or may come and go)

- *Allergies.* Ask if the patient has any allergies to medications or other materials, such as latex.
- *Medications.* If childbirth is likely while the patient is in your care, the patient's answers to your questions about drugs are *very* important. For example, if the patient admits to heroin use within the last 4 hours, you must anticipate that her baby will need resuscitation when it is delivered. Examples of questions to ask about medications include the following:
  —Do you take any prescription medications? What is the medication for? When did you last take it? Are you taking prenatal vitamins? Have you taken fertility medications?
  —Do you take any over-the-counter medications, such as aspirin, allergy medications, cough syrup, or vitamins? Do you take any herbs?
  —Have you recently started taking any new medications? Have you recently stopped taking any medications?
  —Do you use alcohol or any recreational drugs (crack, heroin, methadone, cocaine, marijuana)?
- *Pertinent past medical history.* Ask the patient the following questions:
  —Have you been seeing a doctor during your pregnancy?
  —Do you have a history of heart problems, respiratory problems, high blood pressure, diabetes, epilepsy, or any other ongoing medical conditions?
  —Do you smoke? Do you use alcohol?
- *Last oral intake.* When did you last have something to eat or drink?
- *Events leading to the injury or illness.* Find out about the events leading to the present situation by asking specific questions. If the patient is pregnant, ask the following questions:
  —Do you know your due date?
  —Is this your first pregnancy? Is there only one fetus, or are there multiples? If so, how many?
  —How many children do you have? Were your children delivered vaginally? Did you have any problems with any of those pregnancies (such as premature labor, large babies, hemorrhage, cesarean section, miscarriage, abortion)?
  —Have you had any prenatal care?
  —Have you had any problems with this pregnancy?
  —Do you know if the baby is head first or breech? (Has the baby turned?)

If the patient is having contractions, ask specific questions to determine if delivery is about to happen. These questions are covered later in this chapter. If the patient is complaining of abdominal pain,

remember to use OPQRST to help identify the type and location of the patient's pain. Examples of additional questions to ask include the following:

- When was your last menstrual period? Was it a normal period? Are your periods usually regular? Did you have any bleeding after that period?
- Where is your pain exactly? (Ask the patient to point to the location.) What is it like (constant, comes and goes, dull, sharp, cramping)?
- Have you had any vaginal bleeding or discharge? What color was it?

Perform a physical exam. Keep in mind that your patient may be anxious about having her clothing removed and having an examination performed by a stranger. Be certain to explain what you are about to do and why it must be done. Remember to properly drape or shield an unclothed patient from the stares of others. Conduct the examination professionally and efficiently, and talk with your patient throughout the procedure.

As an Emergency Medical Technician (EMT), you must not visually inspect the vaginal area unless major bleeding is present or you anticipate that childbirth is about to occur. In these situations, it is best to have another healthcare professional or law enforcement officer present. If possible, include a female attendant or rescuer in your examination. The vaginal area is touched *only* during delivery and (ideally) when another healthcare professional or law enforcement officer is present.

Remember This!

When caring for a pregnant patient, keep in mind that the well-being of the fetus is entirely dependent on the well-being of the mother.

Emergency Care of Pregnancy Complications

When you arrive at the scene, first consider your personal safety. During the scene size-up, evaluate the mechanism of injury or the nature of the illness before approaching the patient.

- An **obstetric emergency** (an emergency related to pregnancy or childbirth) is frequently associated with bleeding. Take body substance isolation (BSI) precautions and put on appropriate PPE. In addition to gloves, you should wear eye protection, a mask, and a gown. During childbirth, blood and amniotic fluid are expected and may splash.
- Determine the total number of patients. If a delivery is about to happen, there is going to be another patient. Call for additional help to the

scene to assist you in caring for both mother and baby.

- After the scene size-up, form a general impression by pausing a short distance from the patient to determine if the patient appears "sick" or "not sick." Determine the urgency of further assessment and care.

- Perform a primary survey to identify and treat any life-threatening conditions.

  —As with all patients, your initial attention must be directed at making sure the patient has an open airway, adequate breathing, and adequate circulation.

  —Manually stabilize the patient's head and neck if trauma is suspected.

  —Control obvious external bleeding, if present. If vaginal bleeding is present, apply external vaginal pads as necessary. As the pad becomes blood-soaked, replace it with a new one. Place all blood-soaked clothing and pads in a biohazard container and send them to the hospital with the patient. These items will be used to estimate the patient's blood loss.

  —Treat for shock if indicated. Give oxygen and maintain the patient's body temperature. Use blankets or sheets as needed to prevent heat loss.

- Perform a physical exam. Take the patient's vital signs and gather the patient's medical history.

- If a spinal injury is suspected, the patient should be immobilized on a long backboard. Remember to tilt the board slightly to the left by placing a rolled towel, small pillow, blanket, or other padding under the right side of the board.

- Prepare for transport to the nearest appropriate hospital. Provide emotional support to the patient on the scene and during transport.

- Perform ongoing assessments as often as indicated during transport. Record all patient care information, including the patient's medical history and all emergency care given, on a PCR.

Stop and Think!

If the mother suffers a cardiac arrest, continue cardiopulmonary resuscitation (CPR). If the mother is more than 24 weeks pregnant, the fetus may be able to be delivered and survive. Inform dispatch so that they can notify the hospital that will receive the patient. On arrival at the hospital, special equipment will be used to assess the condition of the fetus.

Normal Labor

Labor is the process in which the uterus repeatedly contracts to push the fetus and placenta out of the mother's body. It begins with the first uterine muscle contraction and ends with delivery of the placenta. **Delivery** is the actual birth of the baby at the end of the second stage of labor.

Stages of Labor

In the days or weeks leading up to the birth, the head of the fetus normally settles in the pelvis. The mother may feel she can "breathe easier," but she will also feel the need to urinate frequently. The cervix begins to open (dilate) and thin out (efface). In addition, the mucus plug may be expelled (bloody show). (Figure 20-11.)

The First Stage of Labor

The first stage of labor begins with the first uterine contraction. This stage ends with a complete thinning and opening (dilation) of the cervix. Contractions usually begin as regular cramp-like pains that gradually increase in strength. They usually last from 30 to 60 seconds and occur every 5 to 15 minutes. In a woman who has not previously given birth, this stage of labor lasts about 8 to 16 hours. It lasts about 6 to 8 hours in a woman who has previously given birth. The bag of waters (amniotic sac) often bursts during this stage.

You Should Know

Timing Contractions

You will need to know how far apart your patient's contractions are and how long each contraction lasts. Place the fingertips of one hand high on the patient's uterus. When you feel the patient's abdomen become hard under your fingers, the contraction has started. When the hardness is gone, the contraction has ended.

Using a watch that shows seconds, begin timing at the start of a contraction. End timing at the beginning of the next contraction. This measure tells you how far apart the contractions are. You will need to time a series of contractions, such as four or five contractions in a row, to see if they are regular or irregular.

To determine how long a contraction is, begin timing at the start of a contraction and end timing when the same contraction is over.

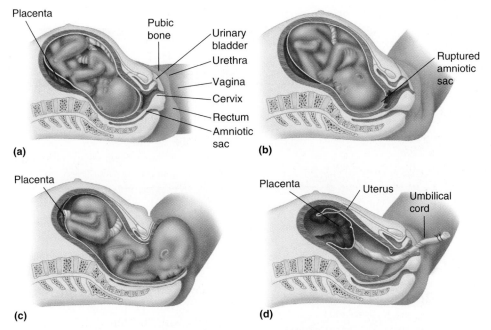

FIGURE 20-11 ▲ The stages of labor. **(a)** The relationship of the fetus to the mother. **(b)** Stage 1 begins with the onset of uterine contractions and ends with complete thinning out and opening of the cervix. **(c)** Stage 2 begins with full dilation of the cervix and ends with delivery of the baby. **(d)** Stage 3 begins with delivery of the baby and ends with delivery of the placenta.

The Second Stage of Labor

The second stage of labor begins with the opening of the cervix and ends with delivery of the infant. Contractions during this stage are stronger. They last from 45 to 60 seconds and occur every 2 to 3 minutes.

During this stage, the fetus begins its descent into the birth canal. The **presenting part** is the part of the infant that comes out of the birth canal first. Normally, the first part of the infant that descends into the birth canal is the head. This is called a **cephalic (head) delivery** or presentation. If the buttocks or feet descend first, it is called a **breech delivery** or presentation.

Toward the end of this stage of labor, the mother experiences an urge to bear down or push with each contraction. The presenting part will appear and disappear at the vaginal opening between contractions. As the presenting part presses on the rectum, the mother will feel an urge to move her bowels. Eventually, the presenting part will remain visible at the vaginal opening between contractions. This is called **crowning.** This stage of labor averages 1 to 2 hours in a woman who has not previously given birth. In a woman who has given birth in the past, this stage of labor lasts 20 to 30 minutes.

The Third Stage of Labor

The third stage of labor begins with delivery of the infant and ends with delivery of the placenta. This stage of labor normally lasts 5 minutes to an hour.

During this stage of labor, the placenta peels away from the wall of the uterus, leaving tiny blood vessels exposed. The uterus normally contracts to close these blood vessels. The placenta usually delivers within 15 to 30 minutes of the infant's birth.

Remember This!

The Stages of Labor

Stage 1. Begins with the onset of uterine contractions; ends with complete thinning and opening of the cervix

Stage 2. Begins with opening of the cervix; ends with delivery of the infant

Stage 3. Begins with delivery of the infant; ends with delivery of the placenta

You Should Know

False Labor

Women often have false labor pains about 2 to 4 weeks before delivery. False labor pains are called *Braxton-Hicks contractions.* These contractions help prepare the woman's body for delivery by softening and thinning her cervix. It is sometimes difficult to tell the difference between false labor and true labor. Table 20-2 lists the differences between the contractions of true and false labor.

TABLE 20-2 True and False Labor Contractions

True Labor Contractions	False Labor Contractions
• Occur regularly	• Are usually weak, irregular
• Get closer together	• Do not get closer together over time
• Become stronger as time passes; each lasts about 30 to 60 seconds	• Do not get stronger
• Continue despite the patient's activity	• May stop or slow down when the patient walks, lies down, or changes position

Normal Delivery

Predelivery Considerations

Objective 4

Generally, you should transport a woman in labor to the hospital unless delivery of the baby is expected within a few minutes. You must determine if there is time for the mother to reach the hospital or if preparations should be made for delivery at the scene. To make this decision, ask the patient the following questions:

- Is this your first pregnancy?
  —Labor with a first pregnancy is usually longer than that of subsequent deliveries.
- When is your due date?
  —Knowing the due date will help you determine if the baby is premature or full term.
- Has your bag of waters broken? When? What was the color of the water?
  —Labor usually begins shortly after the bag of waters breaks. The greater the length of time since the bag of waters has broken until the start of labor, the greater the risk of fetal infection. The fetus usually needs to be delivered within 18 to 24 hours after the bag of waters has ruptured. Some women may not be sure if their water has broken or not. Some will tell you there was a "big gush of water." Others will describe a steady trickle of water when their water breaks. In others, the bag of waters may not break until well into the labor process. The fluid from the amniotic sac should be clear. If the mother tells you that the color of the water was brownish-yellow or green (like pea soup), expect that the baby's airway may need special care after delivery. The discolored water is the result of **meconium,** which

is material that collects in the intestines of a fetus and forms the first stools of a newborn.

- Have you experienced any vaginal bleeding or discharge? How long ago? Did you have any pain with the bleeding?
  —A discharge of mucus mixed with blood (bloody show) is a sign that labor has begun. If excessive bleeding is present, the mother is at risk for shock, and the baby's well-being is also at risk.
- Are you having any contractions? When did they start? How close are they now?
  —Contractions that are strong and regular, last 45 to 60 seconds, and are 1 to 2 minutes apart indicate the delivery will happen soon.
- Do you feel the need to push or bear down?
  —The urge to push, bear down, or have a bowel movement occurs as the baby moves down the birth canal and presses on the bladder and rectum. Delivery will occur soon.
- How many babies are there?
  —If delivery is to occur at the scene, this information will help you determine the additional resources you may need to call to help you. It will also help you determine the equipment you need to gather to assist with the delivery.

Additional questions that are important to ask include:

- Have you taken any medications or drugs?
  —Some medications or drugs taken by the mother will affect her baby. If the mother has taken narcotics within 4 hours of delivery, the baby's breathing may be very slow at delivery.
- Has your doctor told you if the baby is coming head first or feet first?
  —Normally, the baby's head presents first in the birth canal. If the mother has been told that

her baby is coming feet first (breech delivery) and the baby will be delivered on the scene, call for additional help.

Signs of Imminent Delivery

Objective 4

Consider delivering at the scene in the following three circumstances:

1. Delivery can be expected in a few minutes.
   - A woman in late pregnancy feels the urge to push, bear down, or have a bowel movement.
   - Crowning is present. To determine if crowning is present, you will need to look at the patient's perineum (Figure 20-12). Take appropriate BSI precautions, such as gloves, mask, gown, and eye protection. Position the patient on her back and remove her undergarments. Place padding under the hips to elevate them. Ask the patient to bend her knees and spread her thighs apart. Look at the patient's perineum while the patient is having a contraction. If you see bulging or the baby's head beginning to emerge from the birth canal, prepare for immediate delivery. After visually examining the perineum, remember to cover the area with a towel or sheet to protect the patient's modesty.
   - Contractions are regular, last 45 to 60 seconds, and are 1 to 2 minutes apart.

2. No suitable transportation is available

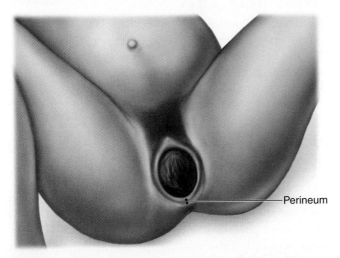

FIGURE 20-12 ▲ To check for crowning, look at the patient's perineum while the patient is having a contraction. If you see bulging or the baby's head beginning to emerge from the birth canal, prepare for immediate delivery.

3. The hospital cannot be reached because of heavy traffic, bad weather, a natural disaster, or a similar situation.

If there is time to transport the patient to the hospital, remove any undergarments that might obstruct delivery. Place the patient on her left side. Arrange for prompt transport.

Preparing for Delivery

Objective 8

If you make the decision that the delivery will occur on the scene, you will need to prepare yourself and the patient. As you make preparations for the delivery, keep in mind that the mother-to-be is doing all the work. Your job is to help the mother and newborn. For most women, the pain of labor and delivery is one of the things that worries them the most about having a baby. Although some women have labor with relatively little pain, most women experience considerable pain that worsens as labor progresses. The amount of pain experienced varies from woman to woman. Even if your patient has previously given birth, the pain she experiences may be different with each delivery.

Although you may be nervous about helping with the delivery, it is important that you appear calm and confident. Reassure the mother-to-be that you will not leave her alone and that you are there to help her. Because labor and delivery is very hard work, she may become tired and quite cranky. If she is irritable, do not take any comments she makes personally. Help her through her labor by offering words of support such as, "You're doing great!" Coach her to breathe slowly in through her nose and out through her mouth. As she tires, she may become less and less receptive to your instructions. You may need to repeat these instructions often. Repeat them as often as needed without appearing frustrated. As you prepare the patient and surroundings for the baby's arrival, remember to explain what you are doing to the patient and any family members that may be present.

Objectives 2, 7

Because blood and amniotic fluid are expected during childbirth and may splash, you must use BSI precautions, including gloves, mask, eye protection, and a gown. You will need a ready-made childbirth delivery kit (also called an *obstetrics* or *OB kit*). (Figure 20-13.) If a ready-made kit is not available, substitute the items in the list below with similar items that will serve the same purpose:

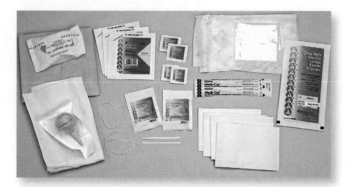

FIGURE 20-13 ▲ Contents of a ready-made childbirth delivery kit.

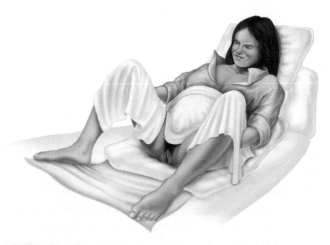

FIGURE 20-14 ▲ To prepare the mother for delivery, position her on her back with her head and back supported with pillows.

- Scissors (used to cut the umbilical cord)
- Hemostats or cord clamps (used to clamp the umbilical cord) or umbilical tape (used to tie the umbilical cord instead of clamping it)
  - —If these items are not available, you can use thick string, gauze, or clean shoelaces to tie off the umbilical cord.
- A bulb syringe (used to clear secretions from the infant's mouth and nose)
- Gauze sponges or towels (used to wipe and dry the infant)
- Sterile gloves (for protection from infection during delivery)
- A baby blanket (used to wrap and warm the infant)
- Sanitary pads (used to absorb vaginal drainage after delivery)
- A plastic bag or large plastic container with a lid (used to transport the placenta to the hospital)
- A sterile sheet, sterile towels, or barrier drapes (to create a sterile field around the vaginal opening).
  - —If these items are not available, you can use clean towels or clothing, a plastic sheet, or newspapers to provide a clean surface.

Objectives 5, 6, 8

Position your patient on her back with her head and back raised (Figure 20-14). Support her head and back with pillows. This position allows gravity to help when she pushes. Remove the patient's clothing and undergarments from the waist down. Gather clean, absorbent materials such as towels, sheets, blankets, clean clothing, or paper barriers. Place some of the absorbent material under the patient's buttocks. Make sure there is enough room in front of the mother's buttocks to provide a firm surface to support the infant after delivery. Have the patient bend her knees and spread her thighs apart. Place a towel, folded sheet, or paper barrier over the patient's abdomen and another across the inside of the patient's thighs. Remember not to touch the patient's vaginal area except during delivery and when another healthcare professional or law enforcement officer is present.

Your patient may tell you she feels as if she needs to have a bowel movement. Do not let her go to the bathroom. This sensation is caused by the presenting part of the infant in the birth canal pressing against the walls of the patient's rectum. If the mother urinates or has a bowel movement during a contraction, remove the material completely with a pad or washcloth and replace the soiled absorbent materials with clean ones. Do not hold the mother's legs together or attempt to delay or restrain delivery in any way.

Remember This!

Remember: Positioning the mother flat on her back compresses major blood vessels. This can lower her blood pressure and decrease blood flow to the uterus. It is also very hard for the patient to push well when lying flat.

Delivery Procedure

Objective 8

When the mother's cervix is completely open, she will feel an almost involuntary need to push. Pushing is done only with uterine contractions. When a contraction begins, tell the mother to take in a deep breath and blow it out. Have her take another deep breath, hold it while you or a family member quickly counts to 10, and bear down as if she is straining to have a bowel movement. Your patient will be holding her breath for about 6 seconds (not 10), but a quick count of 10 will be helpful to her. At the end of the count of 10, tell her to breathe out and quickly take another breath in, holding for another count of 10. Most contractions are long enough to permit two or three attempts at this. Once the contraction is over, she should blow out any remaining air and begin restful breathing. Encourage her to relax completely to conserve energy and recover for the next contraction.

At this point, it is common for your patient to say, "I just can't do this anymore." Offer her words of encouragement. Praise her on the progress she is making. You may notice more bloody show during this stage of labor. This is normal as the patient's cervix stretches open and some of the tiny blood vessels break.

Objective 9

When the infant's head appears, cup your gloved fingers over the bony part of the infant's crowning head. Apply very gentle pressure to prevent the baby's head from coming out too fast and tearing the perineum (an explosive delivery). (Figure 20-15.) Do not apply pressure to the infant's face or the soft spots on the baby's head (fontanelles). If the bag of waters does not break or has not broken, use your gloved fingertips in a pinching motion to break the bag. Push the sac away from the infant's head and mouth as they appear.

Objective 10

As the baby's head is being delivered, check the infant's neck to see if a loop of the umbilical cord is wrapped around the neck. If the cord is around the neck, gently loosen the cord and try to slip it over the baby's shoulder or head. If the umbilical cord is wrapped tightly around the baby's neck and cannot be loosened or is wrapped around the neck more than once, the cord must be removed. To do this, place two umbilical clamps

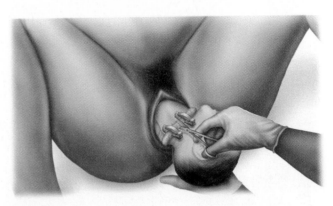

FIGURE 20-16 ▲ If the umbilical cord is wrapped tightly around the baby's neck and cannot be loosened, you will need to remove it. To do this, place two umbilical clamps or ties on the cord, approximately 3 inches apart. Carefully cut the cord between the two clamps. Remove the cord from the baby's neck.

or ties on the cord about 3 inches apart (Figure 20-16). Carefully cut the cord between the two clamps. Remove the cord from the baby's neck. Immediately notify dispatch and request an early response of ALS personnel to the scene (if not already done).

As the baby's head is delivered and before delivery of the shoulders, support the head with one hand and clear the infant's airway (Figure 20-17). Squeeze the bulb of a bulb syringe and then gently insert the narrow end of the syringe into the baby's mouth. Babies breathe mostly through their nose. Suction the baby's mouth first to be sure there is nothing for the baby to suck into his lungs if he should gasp when you suction his nose. To apply suction, slowly release pressure on the bulb. Remove the syringe from the baby's mouth and squeeze it several times to remove secretions from the syringe. Suction the mouth two to three times. Do not apply suction for more than 3 to 5 seconds per attempt. Be careful not to touch the back of the baby's throat with the bulb syringe. This can cause

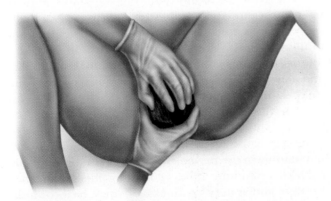

FIGURE 20-15 ▲ When the infant's head appears during crowning, cup your gloved fingers over the bony part of the infant's skull. Exert very gentle pressure to prevent the baby's head from coming out too fast and tearing the perineum.

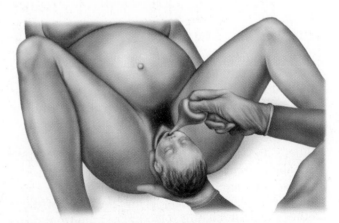

FIGURE 20-17 ▲ As the baby's head is delivered and before delivery of the shoulders, support the baby's head with one hand and clear the airway with a bulb syringe.

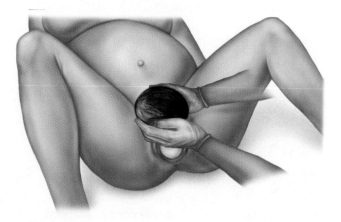

FIGURE 20-18 ▲ Gently guide the head upward to deliver the bottom shoulder.

severe slowing of the baby's heart rate. After clearing the mouth, suction each nostril. If a bulb syringe is not available, use a clean gauze pad or a cloth to wipe secretions from the baby's mouth and nose.

Once the baby's head is delivered, its head will usually turn to line up with its shoulders. This allows the baby's shoulders and the rest of the body to pass through the birth canal. Gently guide the head downward to deliver the top shoulder. Gently guide the head upward to deliver the bottom shoulder (Figure 20-18). Do not pull on the baby's head! Tell the mother not to push during this time.

After the shoulders are delivered, the rest of the baby's body should slip right out. Because the baby will be covered with blood and amniotic fluid, he will be wet and very slippery. You may find it helpful to use a clean towel to hold onto the baby. As the baby's chest and abdomen are born, support the newborn with both hands. As the feet are born, grasp the feet. Try to remember to note the time the baby was born. Keep the baby at or around the same level as the mother's vaginal opening until it is time to clamp the umbilical cord.

Remember This!

It is important to keep the baby at or around the same level as the mother's vaginal opening until the umbilical cord has been clamped. This is because blood can continue to flow between the newborn and the placenta. If you position the baby above the level of the mother's vaginal opening, such as on the mother's abdomen or chest, blood may drain from the baby's circulation into the placenta. This will decrease the amount of blood in the baby's circulation. If you place the baby below the level of the mother's vaginal opening, blood may drain from the placenta into the baby's circulation. This may cause thickening of the baby's blood.

Emergency Care of the Newborn and Mother

Once the baby is born, you will have two patients—the newborn and the mother. First provide care for the newborn. If possible, position the baby between you and the mother so that you can periodically observe the mother while providing care for her baby.

Caring for the Newborn

Objective 13

When the baby is born, look at the baby and ask yourself five questions at the time of birth:

1. Term gestation?
2. Clear of meconium?
3. Breathing or crying?
4. Good muscle tone?
5. Color pink?

If the answer to all of these questions is "Yes," proceed with providing warmth, clearing the baby's airway, and drying. If the answer to any question is "No," you will need to begin the initial steps of resuscitation.

Objective 16

Meconium forms the first stools of a newborn. It is thick and sticky in consistency and usually greenish to black in color. Meconium contains swallowed amniotic fluid, mucus, fine hair, blood, and other by-products of growth. In the newborn with a properly functioning gastrointestinal tract, the color and consistency of meconium changes after 3 or 4 days of feedings of breast milk or formula.

The presence of meconium in the amniotic fluid is an indication of possible fetal distress. Normally, meconium is not passed from the infant's rectum until after birth. However, during birth, if there is a low oxygen supply, the fetus's anal sphincter may relax and allow the passage of meconium into the amniotic fluid. A low oxygen supply may occur from compression of the umbilical cord, abruptio placentae, or maternal shock, among other causes. If inhaled, meconium may cause severe inflammation of the lungs and pneumonia in the newborn. Amniotic fluid is normally colorless. Amniotic fluid containing meconium may be thin and watery or thick and may be brownish-yellow or green in color.

If meconium is observed during delivery, be sure to suction the baby's mouth and nose as soon as the head is delivered. By suctioning the baby before the shoulders and chest are delivered and before the baby

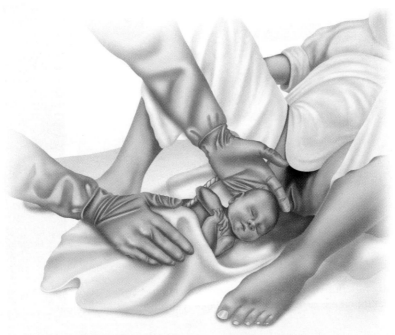

FIGURE 20-19 ▲ Keep the baby at or around the same level as the mother's vaginal opening until it is time to clamp the umbilical cord. Quickly dry the baby's body and head to remove blood and amniotic fluid.

begins breathing, you reduce the baby's risk of sucking the meconium into his lungs.

Quickly dry the baby's body and head to remove blood and amniotic fluid (Figure 20-19). Immediately remove the wet towel or blanket from the infant and then quickly wrap the baby in a clean, warm blanket. It is very important to keep a newborn warm. Newborns lose heat very quickly because they are wet and suddenly exposed to an environment that is cooler than that inside the uterus. Because most body heat is lost through the head as a result of evaporation, immediately dry the baby and cover its head as soon as possible. Wrap the baby's body and head in dry, warm blankets to prevent heat loss, keeping the face exposed.

Place the baby on his back or side with the neck in a neutral position. Wipe blood and mucus from the baby's mouth and nose. Suction the mouth and then the nose again. This suctioning will often cause the baby to begin crying and breathing.

Remember This!

Provide warmth, position the baby, clear the airway as necessary, dry, stimulate, and reposition. These actions should take 30 seconds or less to accomplish.

Airway and Breathing

You should begin to assess the newborn immediately after birth. Focus on the baby's breathing rate and effort, the heart rate, and skin color. Most babies will begin crying and breathing as a result of the stimulation provided during warming, suctioning, and drying. If the baby has not begun to breathe or is breathing very slowly, stimulate the baby. Do this by rubbing its back, chest, or extremities, or by tapping or flicking the bottom of the feet (Figure 20-20). These methods may be tried for 5 to 10 seconds to stimulate breathing.

If the baby's breathing is adequate, assess the heart rate. If the baby's breathing is not adequate and there is no improvement after 5 to 10 seconds, help the baby breathe by using mouth-to-mask breathing or an appropriately-sized bag-mask (BM) device connected to 100% oxygen. Breathe at a rate of 40 to 60 breaths per minute (slightly less than 1 breath per second). Use just enough pressure to see a gentle chest rise. If you use too much pressure, you will force air into the baby's stomach, which will compromise breathing.

Heart Rate

Assess the baby's pulse by feeling the brachial pulse on the inside of the upper arm. Count the heart rate for 6 seconds and multiply by 10 to estimate the beats per minute. Because a baby's heart rate is usually very fast, it may be helpful to tap out the heart rate as you count it. If the baby's heart rate is less than 100 beats per minute, immediately breathe for the baby by using mouth-to-mask breathing or a BM device. Reassess the baby's breathing, heart rate, and color after 30 seconds. If there is no improvement and the baby's heart rate is less than 60 beats per minute, begin chest compressions. If the baby's heart rate is more than 60 beats per minute but breathing is inadequate, continue

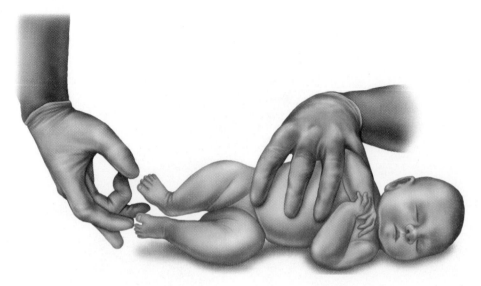

FIGURE 20-20 ▲ If the baby has not begun to breathe or is breathing very slowly, stimulate the baby by rubbing the baby's back, chest, or extremities, or by tapping or flicking the bottom of the feet.

breathing for the baby by using mouth-to-mask breathing or a appropriately sized BM device. Reassess in 30 seconds. If the baby's heart rate is more than 100 beats per minute, assess the baby's skin color.

You Should Know

A full-term baby's respiratory rate is normally between 30 and 60 breaths per minute and the heart rate is normally 100 to 180 beats per minute in the first 12 hours of life. After that, a newborn's normal respiratory rate is 30 to 50 breaths per minute and the heart rate is 120 to 160 beats per minute.

Skin Color

Look at the color of the baby's face, chest, or inside the mouth. A bluish tint in these areas is called *central cyanosis*. The skin of a newborn's extremities is often blue (acrocyanosis) immediately after delivery. This finding is common and requires no specific intervention. The baby's color should quickly improve if he is breathing adequately and is kept warm. If the baby is breathing adequately and has a heart rate of more than 100 beats per minute but central cyanosis is present, give blow-by oxygen if available (Figure 20-21). To do this, cup your hand around the oxygen tubing. Hold the tubing close to the baby's nose and mouth. Do not blow oxygen directly into the baby's face. The oxygen source should be set to deliver at least 5 L per minute.

Apgar Score

An Apgar score is used to assess an infant's condition at 1 and 5 minutes after birth. The Apgar score is used to assess 5 specific signs: *a*ppearance (color),

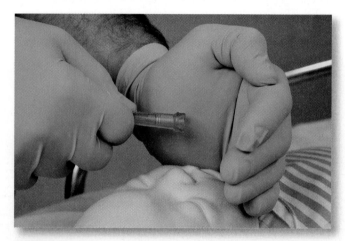

FIGURE 20-21 ▲ Giving blow-by oxygen.

*p*ulse (heart rate), *g*rimace (irritability), *a*ctivity (muscle tone), and *r*espirations. Each sign is assigned a value of either 0, 1, or 2 and added for a total Apgar score (Table 20-3). An Apgar score of 0 to 3 indicates a newborn in severe distress. A score of 4 to 6 indicates a newborn in moderate distress. A score of 7 to 10 indicates a newborn in mild distress or with no distress.

Caring for the Mother

Objectives 10, 12

When the umbilical cord stops pulsating, clamp or tie the umbilical cord in two places between the mother and the baby. The cord usually stops pulsating 3 to 5 minutes after delivery of the baby. Place the first clamp or tie approximately 4 to 6 inches from the baby's belly. Place the second clamp or tie about 2 to 3 inches

TABLE 20-3 Apgar Score

Sign	0	1	2
Appearance (color)	Blue or pale	Body pink Extremities blue	Completely pink
Pulse (heart rate)	Absent	Below 100/min	Above 100/min
Grimace (irritability)	No response	Grimace	Cough, sneeze, cry
Activity (muscle tone)	Limp	Some flexion of extremities	Active motion
Respirations (respiratory effort)	Absent	Slow, irregular	Good, crying

Remember This!

Do not delay resuscitation of a newborn to obtain an Apgar score.

Remember This!

Because it will tear easily, always handle the umbilical cord very gently.

distal to the first clamp (further away from the baby). If the clamps or ties are firmly in place, cut the cord between the two clamps with scissors (Figure 20-22). After the cord is cut, periodically check the cut ends for bleeding. If the cut end of the cord attached to the baby is bleeding, clamp (or tie) the cord proximal to the existing clamps or ties. Do not remove the first clamp or tie.

Objective 11

Gently wipe away any blood and amniotic fluid from the mother's perineum. Watch for delivery of the placenta. The placenta is usually delivered within 30 minutes of the baby. It is not necessary to wait for the placenta to deliver before transporting the mother and infant. The signs that indicate separation of the placenta from the uterus include:

* A gush of blood
* Lengthening of the umbilical cord
* Contraction of the uterus
* An urge to push

Encourage the mother to push to help deliver the placenta. Wrap the placenta in a towel. If the cord was cut, place the placenta in an appropriate biohazard container. If you clamped but did not cut the cord, place the wrapped placenta next to the baby.

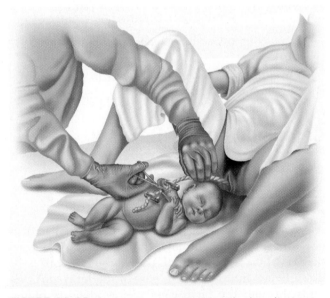

FIGURE 20-22 ▲ Cut the umbilical cord when it stops pulsating. Clamp or tie the umbilical cord in two places between the mother and the baby. Place the first clamp or tie approximately 4-6 inches from the baby's belly. Place the second clamp approximately 2-3 inches distal to the first. If the clamps/ties are firmly in place, cut the cord between the two clamps with scissors.

Stop and Think!

Never pull on the umbilical cord to speed delivery of the placenta. Pulling or tugging on the cord can cause the uterus to turn inside out. Uncontrollable bleeding and shock often follow.

After delivery of the placenta, check the mother's perineum for bleeding. When looking at the mother's vaginal area for bleeding, keep in mind that it is normal for the mother to lose up to 500 mL ($\frac{1}{2}$ L) of blood during childbirth. This amount of blood loss will not negatively affect most healthy young women. If the mother appears alarmed or concerned about the amount of blood, reassure her that this is normal. Place a sanitary pad over the vaginal opening, lower the mother's legs, and help her hold them together. While the patient is in your care, reassess her often to be sure she does not lose too much blood.

During delivery, the perineum can tear as it stretches to make room for the baby's head and body. Although most tears are usually small, they can be very large and extend from the vaginal opening to the rectum. Use a sanitary pad or pads to apply pressure to any bleeding tears. Be careful not to touch the side of the pad that will be placed against the patient. Do not place anything inside the vagina.

If vaginal bleeding appears excessive, give oxygen to the mother by nonrebreather mask. Stimulate the uterus to contract by performing uterine massage. With your fingers fully extended, place one hand horizontally across the abdomen, just above the pubic bone (Figure 20-23). This positioning is very important. It helps prevent downward shifting of the uterus during the massage. Cup your other hand around the uterus. Massage the area using a gentle kneading motion. Continue massaging until the uterus feels

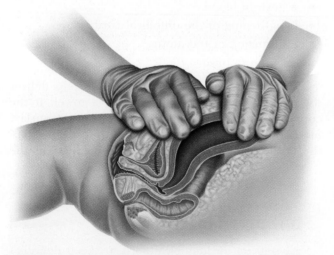

FIGURE 20-23 ▲ Stimulate the uterus to contract by performing uterine massage. With the fingers fully extended, place one hand horizontally across the abdomen, just above the pubic bone. Doing so helps prevent downward displacement of the uterus during the massage. Cup your other hand around the uterus. Massage the area, using a kneading motion. Continue massaging until the uterus feels firm, like a ball.

firm, like a ball. Bleeding should lessen as the uterus becomes firm. Recheck the patient every 5 minutes. If bleeding continues to appear excessive, reassess your massage technique and treat the patient for shock. If you have not already done so, record the time of delivery.

Making a Difference

Uterine massage is painful. Try to understand your patient's complaints of pain if you must perform this procedure. Explain what you are doing and why.

Encourage the mother to breastfeed her baby. Breastfeeding stimulates the uterus to contract. When the uterus contracts, blood vessels within the walls of the uterus constrict, decreasing bleeding. Make sure that the placenta is transported to the hospital with the mother. Hospital staff will look closely at the placenta for completeness. If pieces of the placenta stay in the uterus, the mother will have ongoing bleeding.

En route to the hospital, continue to provide supportive care. This care should include the following:

- Taking the patient's vital signs often
- Helping the mother to a position of comfort
- Keeping her warm
- Rechecking the amount of vaginal bleeding; replacing sanitary pads with clean ones as needed
- Replacing any soiled sheets and blankets with fresh ones
- Carefully placing all soiled items in an appropriate biohazard container

Complications of Delivery

Prolapsed Cord

Objective 14

A prolapsed cord is a serious emergency that endangers the life of the unborn fetus. A prolapsed cord occurs when a portion of the umbilical cord falls down below the presenting part of the fetus and presents through the birth canal before delivery of the head. With each contraction of the uterus, the cord is compressed between the presenting part and the mother's bony pelvis (Figure 20-24). Without blood flowing through the cord, the baby will suffocate. The pressure on the cord must be reduced or relieved as quickly as possible.

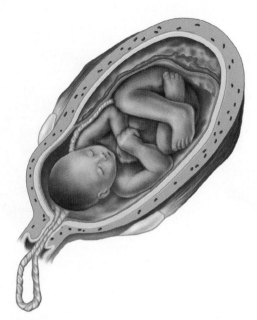

FIGURE 20-24 ▲ Prolapsed umbilical cord.

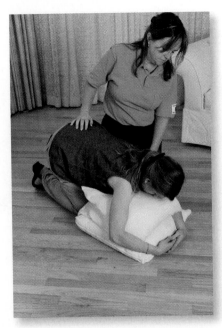

FIGURE 20-25 ▲ The knee-chest position. The mother is positioned on her hands and knees. Her head and chest are then lowered to the floor.

Quickly request an early response of ALS personnel to the scene or consider an ALS intercept while en route to the receiving facility. Place the mother in the knee-chest position. To do this, position her on her hands and knees. Then ask her to lower her head and chest to the floor (Figure 20-25). This will help lessen pressure on the cord in the birth canal. Insert a sterile gloved hand into the vagina and push the presenting part of the fetus away from the cord. Apply only enough pressure to the presenting part so that a pulse returns in the cord. A pulsating umbilical cord indicates the fetus is alive. Once this has been accomplished, leave your hand in place. Do *not* attempt to push the cord back into the vagina. With a wet gauze pad or cloth, cup the cord against the mother's body to keep it moist. Give oxygen to the mother. Transport rapidly to the closest appropriate medical facility. Keep pressure off the cord and monitor the cord pulsations during transport. Do not remove your hand until relieved by healthcare staff at the receiving facility. Perform ongoing assessments as often as indicated during transport. Record all patient care information, including the patient's medical history and all emergency care given, on a PCR.

Breech Birth

Objective 14

A breech birth occurs when the baby's buttocks or feet come out of the uterus first (Figure 20-26). A breech presentation is dangerous for the fetus because of the increased likelihood of delivery trauma or suffocation caused by a prolapsed cord. A breech presentation is best managed in the hospital. As soon as you recognize the presenting part is the baby's buttocks or leg, request an early response of ALS personnel to the scene or consider an ALS intercept while en route to the receiving facility. Give oxygen to the mother and place her in the knee-chest position or on her left side with her hips and legs elevated. These positions allow gravity to pull the baby away from the mother's cervix.

If delivery is about to occur, use BSI precautions, including gloves, mask, eye protection, and a gown. Prepare the mother in the same way as for a head-first delivery. Position the mother, give her oxygen, and prepare the OB kit. Allow the buttocks and trunk of the baby to deliver on their own. *Do not pull on the baby.* Pulling may cause the mother's cervix to clamp down tighter on the baby's head. Once the legs are clear, support (*do not pull or lift*) the baby's legs and trunk. Support the baby's body on your forearm or gently grasp the bony part of the baby's pelvis. Be careful not grasp the baby's abdomen to avoid injury to its internal organs. The head should deliver on its own.

If the head does not deliver within 3 minutes of the time the trunk was delivered, place a gloved hand into the vagina with your palm toward the baby's face. Spread your fingers and form a V with

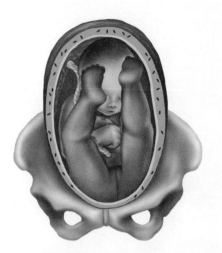
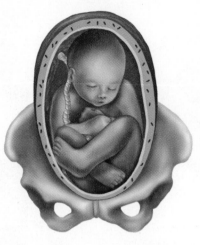
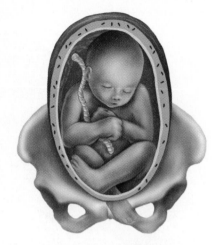

FIGURE 20-26 ▲ A breech presentation occurs when the baby's buttocks or feet come out of the uterus first.

your index and middle finger on either side of the baby's nose (Figure 20-27). Bend your fingers slightly and push the vaginal wall away from the baby's face. Hold the baby's mouth open slightly with your finger. This may allow air to enter the baby's mouth and nose. You must continue this position until the baby's head is delivered. If possible, give blow-by oxygen to the area near the baby's nose. For transport, place the patient on her left side. Perform ongoing assessments as often as indicated during transport. Record all patient care information, including the patient's medical history and all emergency care given, on a PCR.

Limb Presentation

Objective 14

A **limb presentation** occurs when an arm or leg of the baby protrudes from the vagina before the head (Figure 20-28). This situation is a medical emergency because the baby cannot be delivered in this position. Prepare for immediate transport as soon as you recognize a limb presentation. Give oxygen to the mother and place her in the knee-chest position or on her left side with her hips and legs elevated to decrease pressure on the umbilical cord.

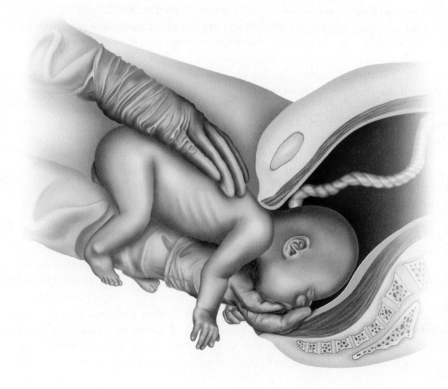

FIGURE 20-27 ◄ If the head does not deliver within three minutes of the time the trunk was delivered, place a gloved hand into the vagina with your palm toward the baby's face. Spread your fingers and form a V with your index and middle finger on either side of the baby's nose. Push the vaginal wall away from the baby's face and hold the baby's mouth open slightly with your finger. This may allow air to enter the baby's mouth and nose. You must continue this position until the baby's head is delivered.

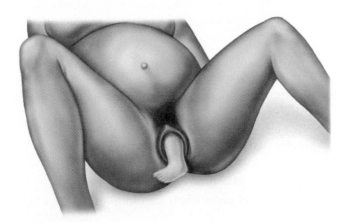

FIGURE 20-28 ▲ A limb presentation occurs when an extremity of the infant protrudes from the vagina before the head.

Multiple Births

Objective 15

A woman pregnant with twins (or more babies) usually goes into labor during or before her 37th week of pregnancy. A normal pregnancy is considered 40 weeks. The more babies a woman is expecting, the higher the risk of having a premature delivery. If the mother has been seeing a doctor regularly, she will usually know if she is expecting more than one baby.

Multiple birth babies are usually smaller than a single full-term baby and, if they are delivered vaginally, are easier for the mother to push out. However, complications can occur during delivery. For example, the umbilical cord may be compressed by one or more of the babies because the uterus is crowded. The first baby is often born head first, but the babies after that may be in a breech, transverse (sideways), or head-first position when they enter the birth canal.

Anticipate multiple births if:

- The mother's abdomen appears unusually large
- The mother's abdomen remains large after the first infant is delivered
- Contractions continue after delivery of the first infant

If multiple births are expected, request an early response of ALS personnel to the scene or consider an ALS intercept while en route to the receiving facility. Be prepared to resuscitate more than one baby. The steps for delivery and care of multiple babies, the mother, and placentas are the same as with the delivery of one baby. Each baby may be attached to its own placenta, or they may all be attached to the same one. Clamp or tie the umbilical cord after the first baby is born and then cut the cord.

If the second baby is not delivered within 10 minutes of the first, the mother and baby must be transported immediately for delivery of the second baby. If delivery of the second baby begins during transport, the ambulance should be pulled over to the side of the road for the delivery. Remember to note the times of birth for each baby. Clearly label and identify each baby. Perform ongoing assessments as often as indicated during transport. Record all patient care information, including the patient's medical history and all emergency care given, on a PCR.

Premature Birth

Objective 17

A **premature infant** is one born before the 37th week of gestation or weighing less than 5.5 pounds (2.5 kilograms). Premature babies (also called *preemies*) can have many health challenges, including serious infections and respiratory distress caused by underdeveloped lungs. They are also at increased risk for hypothermia and low blood sugar. Premature infants often require resuscitation. Care for a premature infant as you would for a term baby with the following special considerations:

- Keep the infant warm to reduce heat loss. Wrap the infant in dry, warm blankets. Cover the infant's body and head (keep the face exposed). Wrap the bundled baby in aluminum foil or a survival blanket to help preserve body heat. The foil should not be directly against the baby's skin but only around the bundled blankets.

- Keep the mouth and nose clear of fluid and mucus.

- Give blow-by oxygen. Do not allow cold oxygen to blow directly into the infant's face. Provide positive-pressure ventilation if breathing is inadequate.

- Prevent bleeding from the umbilical cord. Frequently check the cut end of the umbilical cord to be sure it is not bleeding. Premature infants cannot tolerate the loss of even small amounts of blood.

- Protect the infant from contamination. Premature infants are highly susceptible to infection. Do not breathe directly into the infant's face.

- Perform ongoing assessments as often as indicated during transport. Record all patient care information, including the patient's medical history and all emergency care given, on a PCR.

Gynecological Emergencies

Vaginal Bleeding with No History of Trauma

Objective 18

Gynecology is the study of the female reproductive system. Gynecological emergencies are conditions that affect the female reproductive organs. Obtain a SAMPLE history to gather relevant medical information.

- *Signs and symptoms.* Ask the patient if she has had these same symptoms before. Common signs and symptoms associated with gynecological emergencies are shown in the next *You Should Know* box.
- *Allergies.* Ask if the patient has any allergies to medications or other materials, such as latex.
- *Medications.* Ask if the patient takes any prescription or over-the-counter medications. Also ask her about the use of alcohol or any recreational drugs (crack, heroin, methadone, cocaine, marijuana).
- *Pertinent past medical history.* Ask if the patient has a history of heart problems, respiratory problems, high blood pressure, diabetes, epilepsy, or any other ongoing medical conditions. Does she have a history of:
  —Urinary tract infections?
  —Gallbladder problems?
  —**Endometriosis** (a condition in which uterine tissue is located outside the uterus, causing pain and bleeding)?
  —Kidney stones?
- *Last oral intake.* Find out when the patient last had something to eat or drink.
- *Events leading to the injury or illness.* Ask about the events leading to the present situation by asking specific questions.

If the patient is complaining of abdominal pain, use OPQRST to identify the type and location of the patient's pain. Examples of additional questions to ask include the following:

- Are you sexually active? Is it possible that you are pregnant?
- Do you use birth control?
- When was your last menstrual period? Was it a normal period? Are your periods usually regular? Did you have any bleeding after that period?
- Where is your pain exactly? (Ask the patient to point to the location.) What is it like (constant, comes and goes, dull, sharp, cramping)?

If the patient is having vaginal bleeding, ask the following questions (in addition to those listed previously):

- How long have you been bleeding?
- Is the blood dark red (like menstrual blood) or bright red?
- Is the bleeding heavier or lighter than a normal menstrual period? How many sanitary napkins have you used?
- Have you passed any clots?
- Do you feel dizzy when standing?

Stop and Think!

You must consider the possibility of pregnancy in any woman of childbearing age—especially if the patient is complaining of abdominal pain.

You Should Know

Common Signs and Symptoms of Gynecological Emergencies

- Abdominal pain of sudden or gradual onset
- Abdominal tenderness
- Vaginal discharge
- Abnormal vaginal bleeding
- Fever, chills
- Fainting
- Sweating
- Increased heart rate
- Nausea, vomiting
- Pain during intercourse
- Pain that worsens with coughing or urination
- Pain in the tip of the shoulder (may be seen in ectopic pregnancy)

Perform a physical exam. Keep in mind that your patient may be anxious about having her clothing removed and having an examination performed by a stranger. Be certain to explain what you are about to do and why it must be done. Remember to properly drape or shield an unclothed patient from the stares of others. Conduct the examination professionally and efficiently, and talk with your patient throughout the procedure.

As an EMT, you must not visually inspect the vaginal area unless major bleeding is present or you anticipate that childbirth is about to occur. In these situations, it is best to have another healthcare professional or law enforcement officer present. If possible, include a female attendant or rescuer in your examination. The vaginal area is touched only during delivery and (ideally) when another healthcare professional or law enforcement officer is present.

Assess baseline vital signs and provide emergency care. Take appropriate BSI precautions. Provide specific treatment based on the patient's signs and symptoms. Establish and maintain an open airway. Give oxygen. If the patient's breathing is adequate, apply oxygen by nonrebreather mask at 15 L/min if not already done. If the patient's breathing is inadequate, provide positive-pressure ventilation with 100% oxygen and assess the adequacy of the ventilations delivered. Treat for shock, if indicated. Keep the patient warm. Apply external vaginal pads as necessary. As the pad becomes blood-soaked, replace it with a new one. All blood-soaked garments and pads should accompany the patient to the hospital. Transport and provide ongoing assessments as often as indicated en route. Record all patient care information, including the patient's medical history and all emergency care given, on a PCR.

Vaginal Bleeding with a History of Trauma

Objective 18

Trauma to the external genitalia may occur from straddle injuries, blunt trauma, childbirth, or sexual assault. Take appropriate BSI precautions. Ensure and maintain an open airway. Give oxygen. Control bleeding with local pressure to the area, using trauma dressings or sanitary napkins. Do not pack or place dressings inside the vagina. Monitor the patient's vital signs and treat for shock if indicated. Provide additional care based on the patient's signs and symptoms. Provide reassurance and privacy. Transport to an appropriate medical facility for further care. Perform ongoing assessments as often as indicated during transport. Record all patient care information, including the patient's medical history and all emergency care given, on a PCR.

Apparent Sexual Assault

Criminal assault situations require initial and ongoing assessment and management, as well as psychological care. Take appropriate BSI precautions. When possible, have an EMT of the same gender assess the sexual assault victim. Ensure and maintain an open airway. Maintain a nonjudgmental attitude during the SAMPLE history and focused assessment. Protect the crime scene and document any pertinent findings. Discourage the patient from bathing, douching, urinating, or

cleaning wounds until after transport and evaluation at the receiving facility. It is very important to explain that these things remove evidence that can be helpful in the criminal or civil investigation. Do *not* allow the patient to do these things. Also, advise the patient to bring additional clothing to the hospital (if appropriate to wait on scene long enough for this to happen) or to advise a family member or friend to bring additional clothing along, as the clothing will be removed as evidence. Do not allow the patient to comb her hair or clean her fingernails.

Handle the patient's clothing as little as possible. Bag all items separately in paper bags, and seal with evidence tape (if available). Do not use plastic bags for bloodstained articles. Plastic holds in moisture, which can promote the growth of bacteria. Bacterial growth can contaminate evidence. Examine the genitalia only if profuse bleeding is present. Transport to an appropriate medical facility for further care. Perform ongoing assessments as often as indicated during transport. Record all patient care information, including the patient's medical history and all emergency care given, on a PCR.

You Should Know

Become familiar with your state's procedures and protocols regarding evidence handling.

On the Scene   Wrap-Up

The woman tells you that she already has seven children and that the last one came in 30 minutes. You place a hand on her abdomen and can tell that her contractions last about a minute with only 2 minutes between them. As you open the OB kit, she begins to grunt and her eyes bulge as she strains. The supervisor clears the area. When you remove the patient's jeans, you can see the baby's head protruding from her vagina. "Pant," you tell her as you grab a blanket and a bulb syringe. With the next contraction, the baby's head is delivered. You quickly suction its mouth and nose. One more push and the baby's body is guided out, one shoulder at a time into your waiting hands.

You carefully hang on to the slippery little infant and suction the little boy. You smile when you see the baby's face scrunch into a grimace and hear a hearty cry. You note the time as you glance at your watch to check his pulse. The baby's pulse is fine at 160 beats per minute. After drying him off, you place a dry blanket around him, taking care to cover his head. When the pulsation in the cord stops, you apply the clamps securely and then carefully cut it. You note that the baby's hands are a little blue, but the rest of his body is pink. He is crying and moving around.

You partner assumes care of the baby while you turn your attention to the mother. You can see the umbilical cord move up and down slightly and hear her moan. A moment later there is a small gush of blood and the placenta is delivered. Moments later you wheel your patients toward the ambulance. On arrival at the hospital, mom and baby are doing fine. The Emergency Department nurse commends both of you for doing a great job. ■

Sum It Up

▶ The vagina is also called the birth canal. It is a muscular tube that serves as a passageway between the uterus and the outside of the body.

▶ The placenta is a specialized organ through which the fetus exchanges nourishment and waste products during pregnancy.

▶ The umbilical cord is the lifeline that connects the placenta to the fetus. It contains two arteries and one vein. The umbilical vein carries oxygen-rich blood to the fetus. The umbilical cord attaches to the umbilicus (navel) of the fetus.

▶ The amniotic sac is a membranous bag that surrounds the fetus inside the uterus. It contains fluid (amniotic fluid) that helps protect the fetus from injury.

▶ An abortion is the termination of pregnancy before the fetus is able to live on its own outside the uterus. A spontaneous abortion, also called a miscarriage, is the loss of a fetus as a result of natural causes. It usually occurs before the 20th week of pregnancy.

▶ An ectopic pregnancy occurs when a fertilized egg implants outside the uterus.

▶ Preeclampsia is a disorder of pregnancy that causes blood vessels to spasm and constrict. Preeclampsia usually occurs during the third trimester of pregnancy. Eclampsia is the seizure phase of preeclampsia.

▶ Placenta previa occurs when the placenta attaches low in the wall of the uterus instead of at its top or sides. In this position, the placenta may cover all or part of the cervix (the entrance to the birth canal). Placenta previa can cause sudden, painless, bright red vaginal bleeding.

▶ Abruptio placentae occurs when a normally implanted placenta separates prematurely from the wall of the uterus (endometrium) during the last trimester of pregnancy. If the placenta begins to peel away from the wall of the uterus, bleeding occurs from the blood vessels that transfer nutrients to the fetus from the mother. The placenta may separate partially or completely. Partial separation may allow time for treatment of the mother and fetus. Complete separation often results in death of the fetus.

▶ A ruptured uterus is the actual tearing (rupture) of the uterus. Uterine rupture can occur when the patient has been in strong labor for a long period, which is the most common cause. It can also occur when the patient has sustained abdominal trauma, such as a severe fall or a sudden stop in an MVC.

▶ A pregnant patient's heart rate is normally slightly faster than usual. Her breathing rate is also slightly faster and more shallow than normal. Her blood pressure is often slightly lower than normal until the third trimester. It is important to take vital signs in all patients. However, you will need to pay special attention to the pregnant patient's history and look for other signs that may suggest a potential problem.

▶ You must not visually inspect the vaginal area unless major bleeding is present or you anticipate that childbirth is about to occur. In these situations, it is best to have another healthcare professional or law enforcement officer present.

▶ An obstetric emergency is an emergency related to pregnancy or childbirth. It is frequently associated with bleeding. During childbirth, blood and amniotic fluid are expected and may splash. Therefore, in caring for a patient with an obstetric emergency, you should take BSI precautions and put on appropriate PPE. In addition to gloves, you should wear eye protection, a mask, and a gown.

▶ Labor is the time and process in which the uterus repeatedly contracts to push the fetus and placenta out of the mother's body. It begins with the first uterine muscle contraction and ends with delivery of the placenta. Delivery is the actual birth of the baby at the end of the second stage of labor.

▶ Women often have false labor pains about 2 to 4 weeks before delivery. False labor pains are called Braxton-Hicks contractions. These contractions help prepare the woman's body for delivery by softening and thinning her cervix.

▶ A woman in labor should be transported to the hospital unless delivery of the baby is expected within a few minutes. You must determine if there is time for the mother to reach the hospital or if preparations should be made for delivery at the scene.

► Meconium is material that collects in the intestines of a fetus and forms the first stools of a newborn. The presence of meconium in amniotic fluid results in fluid that is greenish or brownish-yellow rather than clear. It is an indication of possible fetal distress during labor.

► The steps for delivery and care of multiple babies, the mother, and placentas are the same as with the delivery of one baby.

► A premature infant is one born before the 37th week of gestation or weighing less than 5.5 pounds (2.5 kilograms). Premature babies are at increased risk for hypothermia and low blood sugar.

► Complicated deliveries include a prolapsed cord, breech birth, and limb presentation. A prolapsed cord is a condition where the cord presents through the birth canal before delivery of the head. It presents a serious emergency that endangers the life of the unborn fetus. A breech presentation occurs when the buttocks or lower extremities are low in the uterus and will be the first part of the fetus delivered. The newborn is at great risk for delivery trauma. A limb presentation occurs when a limb of the infant protrudes from the birth canal.

► Trauma to the external genitalia should be treated as other bleeding soft tissue injuries. Alleged sexual assault situations require initial and ongoing assessment and management, as well as psychological care.

Division 5

Trauma

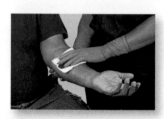
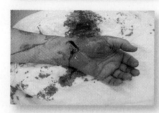
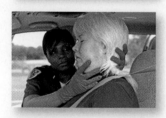
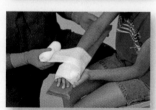
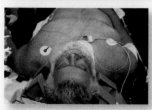

21 Bleeding and Shock

By the end of this chapter, you should be able to:

Knowledge Objectives ▶

1. List the structures and functions of the circulatory system.
2. Differentiate between arterial, venous, and capillary bleeding.
3. State methods of emergency medical care of external bleeding.
4. Establish the relationship between body substance isolation and bleeding.
5. Establish the relationship between airway management and the trauma patient.
6. Establish the relationship between mechanism of injury and internal bleeding.
7. List the signs of internal bleeding.
8. List the steps in the emergency medical care of the patient with signs and symptoms of internal bleeding.
9. List signs and symptoms of shock (hypoperfusion).
10. State the steps in the emergency medical care of the patient with signs and symptoms of shock.

Attitude Objectives ▶

11. Explain the sense of urgency to transport patients that are bleeding and show signs of shock (hypoperfusion).

Skill Objectives ▶

12. Demonstrate direct pressure as a method of emergency medical care of external bleeding.
13. Demonstrate the use of diffuse pressure as a method of emergency medical care of external bleeding.
14. Demonstrate the use of pressure points and tourniquets as a method of emergency medical care of external bleeding.
15. Demonstrate the care of the patient exhibiting signs and symptoms of internal bleeding.
16. Demonstrate the care of the patient exhibiting signs and symptoms of shock (hypoperfusion).
17. Demonstrate completing a prehospital care report for patient with bleeding and/or shock (hypoperfusion).

It is 7:30 p.m. when you and your partner are dispatched for an "ill woman." On arrival at the scene, you find an 85-year-old woman sitting outside a local restaurant. As you approach, you note that the patient is awake and breathing at a rate slightly faster than normal. Her skin looks pale. The patient states she feels weak, dizzy, and is slightly short of breath. She also complains of a dull pain in the middle of her abdomen that radiates to her back. As you count the patient's radial pulse, you notice that her skin is cold and clammy. The patient's initial vital signs reveal the following: blood pressure 70/46, pulse 138, respirations 24. The patient states that she has not eaten since lunch earlier today. A focused physical examination reveals that the patient's abdomen is distended, rigid, and tender. She denies any recent trauma. ■

THINK ABOUT IT

As you read this chapter, think about the following questions:

- What findings suggest that you need to move quickly and begin providing emergency care for this patient?
- What emergency care will you provide?

Introduction

Managing Bleeding and Treating Shock

Traumatic injuries and bleeding are some of the most dramatic situations you will encounter. Understanding the mechanism of injury and relevant signs and symptoms of bleeding and shock are important when dealing with the traumatized patient. Your first steps will be to perform a scene size-up and make sure the scene is safe. After assessing and managing the patient's airway and breathing, you must control bleeding from an artery or vein, if it is present. Bleeding that is uncontrolled or excessive will lead to shock. If shock is not corrected, it will lead to inadequate tissue perfusion and eventual cell and organ death. Treatment of shock and internal bleeding is performed immediately after the primary survey and before patient transport.

Perfusion

Objective 1

The structure and function of the cardiovascular system was presented in Chapter 4. Recall that perfusion is the circulation of blood through an organ or a part of the body. In order to have adequate perfusion, the heart, vessels, and the flow of blood must function properly. When the body's tissues are adequately perfused, oxygen and other nutrients are carried to the cells of all organ systems and waste products are removed. Shock is the inadequate circulation of blood through an organ or a part of the body. Shock is also called *hypoperfusion.* Uncontrolled bleeding that leads to depleted blood volume is one cause of shock.

Bleeding

A **wound** is an injury to the soft tissues. A **closed wound** occurs when the soft tissues under the skin are damaged but the surface of the skin is not broken. A bruise is an example of a closed wound. When the skin surface is broken, it is called an **open wound.** Cuts and scrapes are examples of open wounds.

If a blood vessel is torn or cut, bleeding occurs. Bleeding can occur from capillaries, veins, or arteries. The larger the blood vessel, the more blood flows through it. Therefore, the larger the blood vessel, the greater the bleeding and blood loss if the vessel is injured. **Hemorrhage** (major bleeding) is an extreme loss of blood from a blood vessel. It is a life-threatening condition that requires *immediate* attention. Hemorrhage may be internal or external. If it is not controlled, hemorrhage can lead to shock and, possibly, to death.

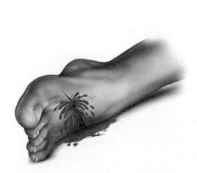
Arterial bleeding

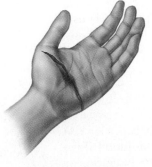
Venous bleeding

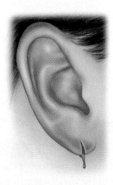
Capillary bleeding

FIGURE 21-1 ▲ Arterial bleeding, venous bleeding, and capillary bleeding.

When a blood vessel is cut or torn, the body's normal response is an immediate contraction (spasm) of the wall of the blood vessel. This action slows the flow of blood from the injured vessel by reducing the size of the hole. Next, platelets rush to the area to plug the torn vessel. Layers upon layers of platelets stick to each other like glue to fill the hole. Usually within seconds of the injury, a clot begins to form at the site of the torn vessel. This process is activated by substances from the wall of the injured vessel and from the platelets at the injury site. Clotting is usually complete within 6 to 10 minutes.

Some conditions may affect blood clotting. For example, **hemophilia** is a disorder in which the blood does not clot normally. A person with hemophilia may have major bleeding from minor injuries and may bleed for no apparent reason. Some medications, such as aspirin and Coumadin (a blood thinner), can interfere with blood clotting. A serious injury may also prevent effective clotting.

Types of Bleeding

Objective 2

The three types of bleeding are arterial, venous, and capillary (Figure 21-1). The characteristics of these types of bleeding are noted in Table 21-1.

Arterial Bleeding

Arterial bleeding is the most serious type of bleeding. The blood from an artery is bright red, oxygen-rich blood. When an artery bleeds, blood spurts from the wound because the arteries are under high pressure. Each spurt represents a heartbeat. Because a bleeding artery can quickly lead to the loss of a large amount of blood, arterial bleeding is life-threatening. This type of bleeding can be difficult to control because of high pressure within the artery.

Venous Bleeding

Bleeding occurs more often from veins than arteries because veins are closer to the skin's surface. Blood lost from a vein flows as a steady stream and is dark red or maroon because it is oxygen-poor blood. Venous bleeding is usually easier to control than arterial bleeding because it is under less pressure. Bleeding from deep veins (such as those in the thigh) can cause major bleeding that is hard to control. Bleeding from a vein is more serious than capillary bleeding.

Capillary Bleeding

Capillary bleeding is common because the walls of the capillaries are fragile and many are close to the skin's surface. When a capillary is torn, blood oozes slowly

TABLE 21-1 **Types of Bleeding**

	Arterial	Venous	Capillary
Color	Bright red	Dark red, maroon	Dark red
Blood Flow	Spurts with each heartbeat	Flows steadily	Oozes slowly
Bleeding Control	Difficult to control	Usually easier to control than arterial bleeding; bleeding from deep veins may be hard to control	Often clots and stops by itself within a few minutes

from the site of the injury because the pressure within the capillaries is low. Bleeding from capillaries is usually dark red. Capillary bleeding is usually not serious. This type of bleeding often clots and stops by itself within a few minutes.

External Bleeding

External bleeding is bleeding that you can see. You can see this type of bleeding because the blood flows through an open wound, such as a cut, scrape, or puncture. Capillary bleeding is the most common type of external bleeding. Clotting normally occurs within minutes. However, external bleeding must be controlled with your gloved hands and dressings until a clot is formed and the bleeding has stopped.

Remember This!

External bleeding may be hidden by clothing.

Emergency Care of External Bleeding
Objectives 3, 4

When you arrive at the scene of an emergency, first consider your personal safety. During the scene size-up, evaluate the mechanism of injury or the nature of the illness before approaching the patient. Personal protective equipment (PPE) *must* be worn when an exposure to blood or other potentially infectious material can be reasonably anticipated. HIV and the hepatitis virus are examples of diseases to which you may be exposed that can be transmitted by exposure to blood. Remember to put on disposable gloves before physical contact with the patient. Additional PPE, such as eye protection, mask, and gown, should be worn if there is a large amount of blood. PPE should also be worn when the splashing of blood or body fluids into your face or eyes is likely.

After the scene size-up, perform a primary survey. Bleeding may be obvious when you approach the patient. However, remember that making sure the patient has an open airway and adequate breathing

Stop and Think!

- *Never* touch blood or body fluids with your bare hands.
- *Always* wear PPE during *every* patient contact.
- Wash your hands immediately after exposure to blood and/or body fluids and after removing disposable gloves.
- If you were not wearing gloves and had contact with blood or body fluids, wash your hands with soap and water for at least two minutes.
- Remember to throw away contaminated gloves and other PPE in clearly labeled biohazard bags or containers.
- Report all exposures to your supervisor or Risk Management Department immediately.

takes priority over other care. Stabilize the cervical spine if needed. During your assessment of the patient's circulation, look for the presence of major (severe) bleeding. If it is present, you will need to control it during the primary survey.

If the patient is bleeding, keep in mind that the sight of blood is frightening for many patients. Conduct your examination professionally and efficiently. Remember to talk with your patient while you are providing care. Because clothing can hide and absorb large amounts of blood, cut or remove your patient's clothing as needed to see where the bleeding is coming from. Remember that your patient will often be anxious about having his clothing removed and having an exam performed by a stranger. Ease your patient's fears by explaining what you are doing and why it must be done. As you remove the patient's clothing, remember to properly drape or shield him from view of others not providing care.

An average adult man has a normal blood volume of about 5 to 6 L (5000 to 6000 mL). In a previously healthy patient, a sudden episode of blood loss will usually not produce vital sign changes until the patient has lost 15-30% of his blood volume (Table 21-2)

TABLE 21-2 Measures of Severe Blood Loss

Patient Type	Normal Blood Volume	Severe Blood Loss
Adult	5000-6000 mL	Loss of 1000 mL or more
Child (8-year-old)	2000 mL	Loss of 500 mL or more
Infant	800 mL	Loss of 100-200 mL or more

Therefore, estimate the severity of blood loss on the basis of the patient's signs and symptoms. If the patient shows signs and symptoms of shock, consider the bleeding severe.

Control bleeding by using direct pressure, elevation, pressure points, splints, or, a tourniquet. If bleeding is severe, give oxygen by nonrebreather mask. If signs of shock are present, treat the patient for shock. These techniques are described in the next section.

After completing the primary survey, decide whether the patient needs on-scene stabilization or immediate transport with additional emergency care en route to a hospital.

Making a Difference

Although covering a bleeding wound is important for any patient, it is especially important if your patient is a young child. A young child may fear that "all of my blood will leak out" if the wound is not covered quickly.

Controlling External Bleeding

Six methods may be used to control external bleeding:

1. Applying direct pressure to the wound
2. Elevating the affected extremity
3. Applying pressure to an arterial pressure point
4. Applying a splint to immobilize the extremity
5. Applying a pressure splint (air splint)
6. Applying a tourniquet (if the bleeding is severe and cannot be controlled with direct pressure)

Direct Pressure

To control external bleeding, begin by applying **direct pressure** to the bleeding site. Most bleeding can be controlled with direct pressure. Applying direct pressure slows blood flow and allows clotting to take place. Place a sterile **dressing** (such as a gauze pad) or a clean cloth (such as a towel or washcloth) over the wound. If you do not have a dressing or clean cloth available, use your gloved hand to apply firm pressure to the bleeding site until a dressing can be applied (Figure 21-2). Use your gloved fingertips if the bleeding site is small. If the patient has a large, open wound, you may need to apply direct pressure to the site with the palm of your gloved hand. Hold continuous, firm pressure to the bleeding site while the body works to plug the wound with a clot. If the bleeding does not stop within 10 minutes, press more firmly over a wider area.

If the bleeding site is on an extremity, continue direct pressure by applying a pressure bandage. A **pressure bandage** is a bandage with which enough pressure is applied over a wound site to control bleeding. Wrap roller gauze snugly over the dressings to hold them in place on the wound (Figure 21-3). Make sure that the pressure bandage is not so tight that it impedes blood flow past the dressing. For example, if you applied a pressure bandage to a wound on a patient's lower arm, you should be able to feel a pulse at his wrist if the bandage has been applied properly.

Remember This!

A pressure bandage that is wrapped too loosely will not be effective in controlling bleeding. A bandage that is applied too tightly can cause tissue damage.

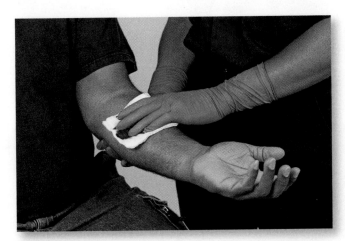

FIGURE 21-2 ▲ Apply direct pressure to a bleeding wound.

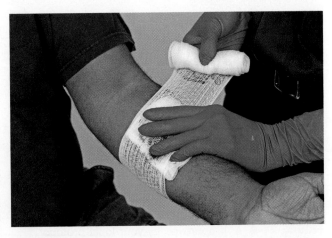

FIGURE 21-3 ▲ Continue direct pressure by applying a pressure bandage.

If blood soaks through the dressings, do not remove them. Removing the original dressings could disturb any blood clots that may be forming and cause more bleeding. Add another dressing on top of the first and continue to apply direct pressure.

Stop and Think!

If PPE is not available and you must provide care for a bleeding patient, use whatever materials are readily available to help protect yourself against disease. For example, use a plastic bag, plastic wrap, or other waterproof material to apply direct pressure to the wound. If the patient is able to help you, ask him to apply direct pressure to the wound with his own hand. When you have finished providing care, be sure to wash your hands with soap and water for at least 2 minutes.

Elevation

If bleeding continues from an arm or leg, direct pressure and elevation can be used together to help control the bleeding, if approved by your local protocol (Figure 21-4). If possible, elevate the extremity above the level of the heart while continuing to apply direct pressure. Raising the extremity above the heart reduces pressure at the wound site by reducing blood flow to it. This action allows blood to pool and clot. Do not elevate the extremity if pain, swelling, or deformity is present.

Pressure Points

If bleeding continues from an arm or leg, pressure points (also called *pulse points*) may be used to slow severe bleeding, if approved by your local protocol

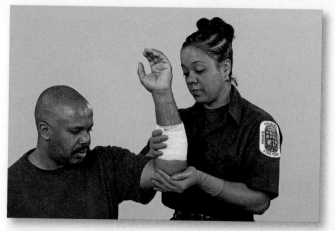

FIGURE 21-4 ▲ If approved by your local protocol, elevation may be used with direct pressure to control bleeding.

You Should Know

The use of elevation and pressure points has been taught to help control extremity bleeding for many years. However, according to the 2005 Resuscitation Guidelines, "There is insufficient evidence to recommend for or against the first aid use of pressure points or extremity elevation to control hemorrhage. The efficacy, feasibility, and safety of pressure points to control bleeding have never been subjected to study, and there have been no published studies to determine if elevation of a bleeding extremity helps in bleeding control or causes harm. Using these unproven procedures has the potential to compromise the proven intervention of direct pressure." Be sure to check your local protocols and learn about the approved methods of bleeding control in your area.

(Figure 21-5). When applying pressure at a pressure point, continue to apply direct pressure to the bleeding site. To slow bleeding in the lower arm, locate

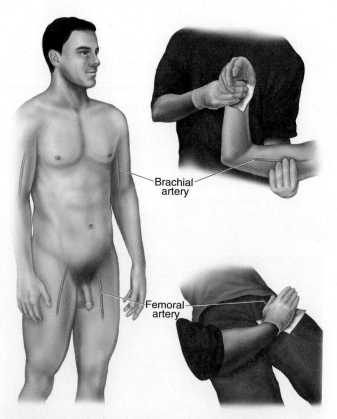

FIGURE 21-5 ▲ Pressure points may be used to slow severe bleeding from an arm or leg, if approved by your local protocol. To slow bleeding in the lower arm, press the brachial artery firmly against the humerus. To slow bleeding in the leg, press the femoral artery firmly against the pelvic bone with the palm of your hand.

the brachial artery in the upper arm. Use your first three fingers and press the brachial artery firmly against the upper arm bone (the humerus). To slow bleeding in the leg, use your fingers to locate the femoral artery in the groin. Press the femoral artery firmly against the pelvic bone with the heel of your hand.

Splints

The sharp ends of broken bones can pierce the skin and cause major bleeding. A broken bone that penetrates the skin is called an **open** or **compound fracture.** Unless a broken bone is immobilized, the movement of bone ends or bone fragments can damage soft tissues and blood vessels, which results in more bleeding. Dress and bandage the wound and then apply a splint. A **splint** is a device used to limit the movement of an injured arm or leg and reduce bleeding. After applying the splint, be sure to check the patient's fingers (or toes) often for color, warmth, and feeling. Dressing and bandaging are discussed in more detail in Chapter 22.

Pressure Splints

A pressure splint (also called an *air* or *pneumatic splint*) may help control bleeding associated with soft-tissue injuries or broken bones. It can also help to stabilize a broken bone. An air splint acts as a pressure bandage, applying even pressure to the entire arm or leg (Figure 21-6). Dress and bandage the wound before applying an air splint. After applying any splint, be sure to check the patient's fingers (or toes) often for color, warmth, and feeling. Direct pressure can be applied with an air splint in place. This may be necessary to control arterial bleeding from an arm or leg. Use a pressure splint only if approved by your local protocol.

The pneumatic antishock garment (PASG) is used in some Emergency Medical Services (EMS) systems. This garment is also called *Military Antishock Trousers* (MAST). If approved by your local protocol, this device can be used as a pressure splint to help

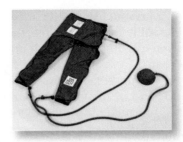

FIGURE 21-7 ▲ The pneumatic antishock garment (PASG) is used in some EMS systems to help control suspected severe bleeding in the abdomen or pelvis that is accompanied by hypotension.

control suspected severe bleeding in the abdomen or pelvis that is accompanied by hypotension (Figure 21-7). The PASG has three separate compartments that can be inflated: the abdomen, left leg, and right leg. All three compartments are inflated if there is an injury to the abdomen or pelvis. The abdominal compartment is *never* used without inflating both leg compartments. When the PASG is positioned on the patient, the top edge of the garment must be below the patient's lowest ribs. If the garment is positioned higher on the patient, the pressure caused by inflating the abdominal compartment could hamper the patient's breathing. The PASG is contraindicated in the following situations:

- Pulmonary edema
- Pregnancy
- Traumatic cardiac arrest
- Impaled objects in the abdomen
- Protruding abdominal organs
- Penetrating chest trauma
- Splinting of lower extremity fractures

Tourniquets

A **tourniquet** is a tight bandage that surrounds an arm or a leg. It is used to stop the flow of blood in an extremity. A tourniquet is rarely needed to control bleeding. In fact, studies have shown that direct pressure controls bleeding more effectively than a

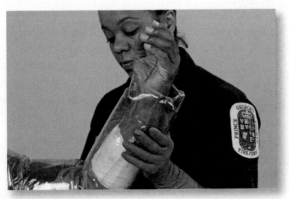

FIGURE 21-6 ▲ An air splint acts as a pressure bandage, applying even pressure to the entire arm or leg.

Stop and Think!

A tourniquet may be considered when direct pressure has failed to control hemorrhage. When you apply a tourniquet, you stop arterial and venous blood flow to the affected extremity. Be absolutely sure that you are authorized to apply a tourniquet per local protocol and have exhausted all other methods of bleeding control before considering the use of a tourniquet.

tourniquet. A tourniquet should be used *only* as a last resort to control life-threatening bleeding in an arm or leg when you absolutely cannot control the bleeding by any other means. A tourniquet can cause permanent damage to nerves, muscles, and blood vessels, resulting in the loss of the affected extremity.

To apply a tourniquet, use the following steps:

- Use a bandage at least 4 inches wide and 6 to 8 layers deep.
- Wrap the bandage around the extremity twice. Choose an area above the bleeding but as close to the wound as possible (Figure 21-8a).
- Tie a single knot in the bandage and place a stick or rod on top of the knot (Figure 21-8b).
- Tie the ends of the bandage over the stick in a square knot. Twist the stick until the bleeding stops (Figure 21-8c). Note the exact time the tourniquet is applied.

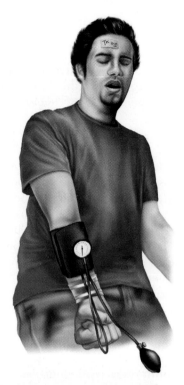

FIGURE 21-9 ▲ A blood pressure cuff may be used as a tourniquet. Place the cuff above the bleeding area. Inflate the cuff just enough to stop the bleeding.

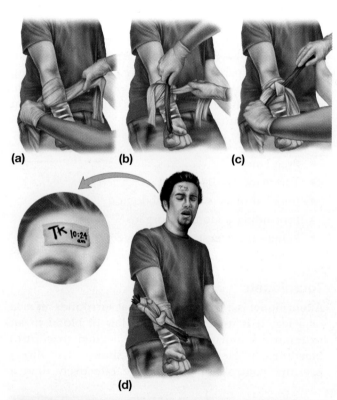

FIGURE 21-8 ▲ **(a)** To apply a tourniquet, use a bandage at least 4 inches wide and six to eight layers deep. Wrap the bandage around the extremity twice. Choose an area above the bleeding but as close to the wound as possible. **(b)** Tie a single knot in the bandage and place a stick or rod on top of the knot. **(c)** Tie the ends of the bandage over the stick in a square knot. Twist the stick until the bleeding stops. Note the exact time the tourniquet is applied. **(d)** Write *TK* on a piece of adhesive tape and the time the tourniquet was applied. Place the adhesive tape on the patient's forehead.

- After the bleeding has stopped, secure the stick or rod in place.
- Write the initials *TK*, for tourniquet, on a piece of adhesive tape and the time the tourniquet was applied. Place the adhesive tape on the patient's forehead. The information must be clearly visible to all who provide care to the patient (Figure 21-8d).
- When transferring patient care, be sure to notify the receiving personnel that you have applied a tourniquet.

Remember This!

A blood pressure cuff may be used as a tourniquet, if approved by your local protocol. Place the cuff above the bleeding area. Inflate the cuff just enough to stop the bleeding (Figure 21-9). Check the gauge on the cuff often to make sure there is no drop in pressure in the cuff.

Internal Bleeding

The body contains hollow and solid organs. Hollow abdominal organs include the stomach, intestines, gallbladder, and urinary bladder. When hollow abdominal organs rupture, they empty their contents into the abdominal cavity. This rupture irritates the abdominal lining and causes pain. Solid abdominal organs include the liver, spleen, and kidneys. These organs are protected by bony structures and do not move around much. Solid organs bleed when injured and can result in a large amount of blood loss. **Internal bleeding** is bleeding that occurs inside body tissues and cavities. It can result in blood loss severe enough to cause shock and death. A **bruise** is a collection of blood under the skin caused by bleeding capillaries. A bruise is an example of internal bleeding that is not life threatening.

Objective 6

Internal bleeding may result from blunt or penetrating trauma. It can also be caused by medical conditions, such as an ulcer. The two most common causes of internal bleeding are (1) injured or damaged internal organs and (2) fractures, especially fractures of the femur and pelvis. Internal bleeding may occur in any body cavity. However, major bleeding is most likely to occur in the abdominal cavity, chest cavity, digestive tract, or the tissues surrounding broken bones. An injury to the liver or spleen can result in a loss of massive amounts of blood into the abdominal cavity in a short time. A fracture of a long bone can result in a loss of 500-1000 mL of blood into the surrounding tissues. A femur fracture can produce a blood loss of 1000-2000 mL. The only signs of internal bleeding may be localized swelling and bruising.

Internal bleeding can cause blood to pool in a body cavity. This buildup of blood can cause pressure on vital organs. For example, a stab wound to the chest may hit a chamber of the heart. If bleeding escapes from the heart's chamber into the sac around the heart (the pericardial sac), the heart's ability to pump decreases. As blood fills the sac, the pressure in the sac increases and does not allow the heart muscle to expand during relaxation. If a blood vessel in the chest is torn, as much as 1500 mL of blood can build up in the pleural cavity of each lung. Breathing may be compromised as the blood builds up, crushing the air-filled lung.

Emergency Care of Internal Bleeding

Objective 6

Internal bleeding is difficult to assess because you cannot see it. However, you should suspect it when the mechanism of injury or the nature of the illness, as well as your patient's signs and symptoms, indicates that it is likely. Suspect internal bleeding when the mechanism of injury suggests that the patient's body was affected by severe force (Figure 21-10). Examples include penetrating trauma and blunt trauma such as falls, motorcycle crashes, pedestrian impacts, automobile collisions, and blast injuries.

Trauma is a common cause of internal bleeding. Internal bleeding may also occur in patients with medical emergencies. For example, it may occur because of a problem in the digestive tract, such as an ulcer. A patient with bleeding in the digestive tract may vomit blood or have bloody diarrhea. A patient with bleeding in the urinary tract may have blood in his urine.

Objective 7

Depending on the amount of bleeding, the signs and symptoms of internal bleeding may develop quickly or

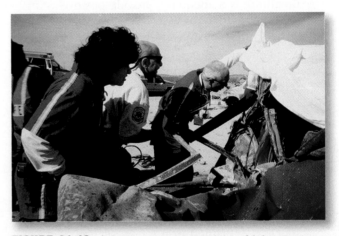

FIGURE 21-10 ▲ When the mechanism of injury suggests that the patient's body was affected by severe force, suspect internal bleeding. © *The McGraw-Hill Companies, Inc./Carin Marter, photographer.*

may take hours or days to develop. The signs and symptoms of internal bleeding include the following:

- Pain, tenderness, swelling, or discoloration of the skin (bruising) in the injured area
- A weak, rapid pulse
- Pale, cool, moist skin
- Broken ribs or bruising on the chest
- Vomiting or coughing up bright red blood or dark, "coffee-ground" blood
- A tender, rigid, and/or swollen abdomen
- Bleeding from the mouth, rectum, vagina, or other body opening
- Black (tarry) stools or stools with bright red blood

Objectives 5, 8

To provide emergency care to a patient with the signs and symptoms of internal bleeding, use the following steps:

- Conduct a scene size-up and ensure your safety. Evaluate the mechanism of injury or the nature of the illness before approaching the patient. Put on appropriate PPE.
- Perform a primary survey to identify and treat any life-threatening conditions. Manage the patient's airway and breathing. Stabilize the cervical spine if needed.
- Perform a physical examination. Identify the signs and symptoms of internal bleeding. Take the patient's vital signs, gather the patient's medical history, and document the information.
- Give oxygen. If the patient's breathing is adequate, apply oxygen by nonrebreather mask at 15 L/min if not already done. If the patient's breathing is inadequate, provide positive-pressure ventilation with 100% oxygen. Assess the adequacy of the ventilations delivered.
- A patient with internal bleeding may vomit. Watch the patient closely to make sure his airway remains clear. Make sure that you have suction within arm's reach at all times. Suction as needed.
- A patient with internal bleeding is a priority patient and needs rapid transport to the closest appropriate hospital. En route to the hospital, make the patient as comfortable as possible, provide reassurance, and keep him warm. Perform ongoing assessments every 5 minutes. If signs of shock develop, treat the patient for shock as explained in the next section.
- Record all patient care information, including the patient's medical history and the emergency care provided, on a PCR.

Stop and Think!

Never give a patient who may have internal bleeding or who may be in shock anything to eat or drink. The patient may need surgery and should not have anything in his stomach.

Shock

Shock (hypoperfusion) is the inadequate flow of blood through an organ or a part of the body. Shock is a life-threatening condition. It requires *immediate* emergency care. Shock can be caused by failure of the body's pump (the heart), fluid (blood), or container (the blood vessels).

- *Pump failure.* The amount of blood the heart pumps throughout the body depends on how many times the heart beats and the force of the contractions. Cardiogenic shock can result if the heart beats too quickly or too slowly or if the heart muscle does not have enough force to pump blood effectively to all parts of the body. This type of shock can occur because of a heart attack, a heart rhythm that is too fast or too slow, an injury to the heart, or other conditions that affect the heart's ability to pump.
- *Fluid loss.* Shock can result if there is not enough blood for the heart to pump through the cardiovascular system. Shock caused by severe bleeding is called **hemorrhagic shock.** The bleeding may be internal, external, or both. However, blood is not the only type of fluid that may be lost from the body. For example, body fluid may be lost because of vomiting or diarrhea. Plasma may be lost as a result of a burn. Fluid also may be lost because of excessive sweating or urination. Shock caused by a loss of blood, plasma, or other body fluid is called **hypovolemic shock.**
- *Container failure.* Normally, blood vessels work with the nervous system to increase or decrease the amount of blood sent to different areas of the body. When an area needs more blood, the vessels expand to provide it with more blood and constrict in areas that do not need it. When shock caused by container failure occurs, the blood vessels lose their ability to adjust the flow of blood. Instead of expanding and constricting as needed, the blood vessels remain enlarged. The amount of fluid in the body remains constant (there is no actual loss of fluid), but blood pools in the outer areas of the body. As a

result, there is an inadequate amount of blood to fill the enlarged vessels, and the vital organs are not perfused. The four major causes of this type of shock are:

1. Injury to the spinal cord (neurogenic shock)
2. Severe infection (**septic shock**)
3. Severe allergic reaction (**anaphylactic shock**)
4. Severe drug reaction

Regardless of the type of shock, cells are starved for enough oxygen-rich blood. When the body's cells and organs are not supplied with oxygen and nutrients, they begin to break down, and waste products build up. Unless adequate perfusion is quickly restored, death may soon follow. It is not important that you be able to determine the cause of the patient's shock. What is important is that you can promptly recognize the signs and symptoms of shock. Promptly recognizing and treating shock is critical to your patient's survival.

You Should Know

Cardiogenic shock is a pump problem. Hypovolemic shock is the most common type of shock. Hypovolemic shock is a volume problem. Neurogenic, septic, and anaphylactic shock, as well as some severe drug reactions, can cause container failure. Container failure is a pipe problem. Without an adequate supply of oxygen-rich blood:

- The brain, heart, and lungs will suffer damage after 4 to 6 minutes.
- The kidneys and liver will suffer damage after 45 to 90 minutes.
- The skin and muscles will suffer damage after 4 to 6 hours.

The Stages of Shock

Shock occurs in stages: early (compensated), late (decompensated), and irreversible (terminal).

Early Shock

Objective 9

Early (compensated) shock is sometimes called *shock with a normal blood pressure*. In early shock, the body's defense mechanisms attempt to protect the vital organs (the brain, heart, and lungs). (Figure 21-11.) You can recognize signs of early shock by assessing the patient for the following:

- *Mental status.* Some of the earliest signs of shock can be seen as changes in the patient's mental status. A patient in early shock will appear anxious and restless. Some patients are combative. These changes occur because the brain is not receiving an adequate supply of oxygenated blood.
- *Breathing.* As the body attempts to draw in more oxygen, the bronchioles expand to draw in more air and the patient's breathing rate increases.
- *Skin color, temperature, and condition (moisture).* As blood is shunted from the skin and muscles to the patient's vital organs, the patient's skin will look pale and feel cool and moist. You may notice that the patient's face appears pale, especially around the mouth and nose. During shock, the body diverts blood to the areas that are most dependent on a continuous, rich supply of oxygen. The patient's skin appears pale because the body diverts blood from the skin first. You may see beads of sweat on the patient's skin. Sweating is usually first visible on the upper lip and around the hairline.

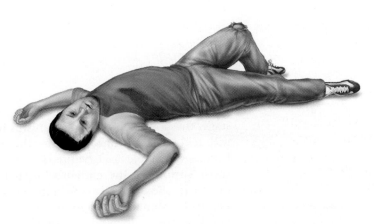

Anxiety, restlessness

Thirst

Nausea/vomiting

Increased respiratory rate

Slight increase in heart rate

Pale, cool, moist skin

Blood pressure in normal range

FIGURE 21-11 ▲ The signs and symptoms of early (compensated) hypovolemic shock.

- *Heart rate.* The patient's pulse will feel slightly faster than normal because the heart picks up its pace to pump oxygenated blood throughout the body.
- *The strength of the peripheral pulses.* Pulses in the arms and legs often feel weak because blood is being shunted away from them to protect the body's vital organs.
- *Capillary refill* (in children younger than 6 years of age). Delayed capillary refill (3 to 5 seconds) may indicate poor perfusion or exposure to cool temperatures. A capillary refill time longer than 5 seconds is markedly delayed and suggests shock.

Remember This!

It may be difficult to determine pale skin color in a dark-skinned person. In these situations, look at the patient's nail beds, the mucous membranes of his eyes, or inside his mouth. If these areas are pale, consider possible shock.

Early shock is often difficult to recognize. Remember to look for it and to consider the patient's mechanism of injury or the nature of the illness when assessing your patient. For example, an increased heart rate may be caused by many things. Fever, fear, pain, anxiety, stress, and exercise can all increase a person's heart rate. However, an increased heart rate accompanied by pale, cool skin and anxiety in a victim of a motorcycle crash should make you immediately think of shock. The sooner shock is recognized and appropriate treatment is begun, the better your patient's chance for survival. Early shock is usually reversible if it is recognized and the patient receives

You Should Know

Signs and Symptoms of Early (Compensated) Shock

- Anxiety, restlessness
- Thirst
- Nausea, vomiting
- An increased respiratory rate
- A slight increase in the heart rate
- Pale, cool, moist skin
- Delayed capillary refill (greater than 2 or 3 seconds) in an infant or young child
- Blood pressure in the normal range

emergency care to correct the cause of the shock. If early shock is not recognized or corrected, it will progress to the next stage.

Late Shock

Objective 9

When an ill or injured adult patient's systolic blood pressure drops to less than 90 mm Hg, late (decompensated) shock is present. The presence of a low blood pressure is the main difference between early (compensated) shock and late (decompensated) shock. In late shock, the body's defense mechanisms lose their ability to make up for the lack of oxygenated blood. A patient in late shock looks very sick (Figure 21-12). He is usually slow to respond, confused, or may even be unresponsive. His breathing is shallow, labored, and irregular. The patient's skin is cool and moist and may be pale, blue, or mottled. His pulse is fast and hard to feel (thready) or may be absent in his arms and legs. The signs of late shock are more obvious than early shock, but late shock is more difficult to treat. It is still reversible if the cause of the problem is quickly corrected.

You Should Know

Signs and Symptoms of Late Shock

- Slowness to respond, or confusion or unresponsiveness
- Extreme thirst (if the patient is awake)
- Nausea, vomiting
- Shallow, labored, irregular breathing
- A rapid heart rate
- Cool, moist skin that is pale, blue, or mottled
- Delayed capillary refill (greater than 2 or 3 seconds) in an infant or young child
- Low blood pressure

Irreversible Shock

Objective 9

Irreversible shock is also called *terminal shock.* At this stage, the body's defense mechanisms have failed. You will feel an irregular pulse as the patient's heart becomes irritable and begins to beat irregularly. As shock continues, the patient's heart rhythm becomes more chaotic and it can no longer effectively pump blood. Permanent damage occurs to the vital organs because the cells and organs have been without oxygenated blood for too long. Eventually, the heart stops, breathing stops, and death results.

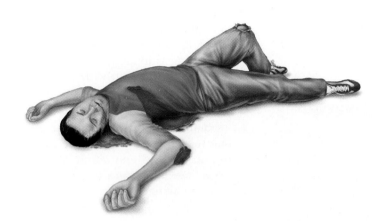

Slow to respond, confused
or unresponsive

If awake,
extreme thirst

Nausea/vomiting

Shallow, labored,
irregular breathing

Rapid heart rate

Cool, moist skin that
is pale, blue, or mottled

Low blood pressure

FIGURE 21-12 ▲ The signs and symptoms of late (decompensated) hypovolemic shock.

You Should Know

You will not know the point at which the patient moves from late to irreversible shock. Your goal should be to treat the patient as early as possible for shock to prevent the development of this lethal stage.

Infants and Children

Infants and children can maintain a normal blood pressure until more than half their blood volume is gone. By the time their blood pressure drops, they are close to death. Although children in shock tend to compensate longer than adults, they also get worse faster when their compensatory mechanisms fail. To spot signs of shock in a child, pay particular attention to the child's mental status and capillary refill (Figure 21-13 a-b). Also pay special attention to the child's skin temperature, color, and moisture (Figure 21-14) and to the strength of the child's pulses.

Remember This!

Suspect shock in an infant or child who is very listless and whose muscle tone appears floppy.

Emergency Care of Shock

Objective 10

To treat a patient in shock, use the following steps:

- Conduct a scene size-up and ensure your safety. Evaluate the mechanism of injury or the nature of the illness before approaching the patient. Put on appropriate PPE.

- Perform a primary survey to identify and treat any life-threatening conditions. Manage the patient's airway and breathing. Stabilize the cervical spine if needed.

- The heart can pump only the blood that it receives. Therefore, there must be an adequate

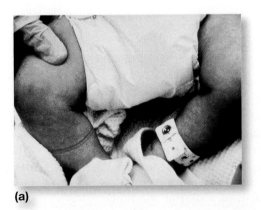

(a)

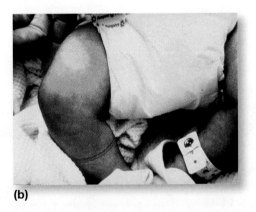

(b)

FIGURE 21-13 ▲ **(a)** Assess capillary refill in children younger than six years of age. **(b)** Delayed capillary refill in an infant. *EMSC Slide Set (CD-ROM). 1996. Courtesy of the Emergency Medical Services for Children Program, administered by the U.S. Department of Health and Human Service's Health Resources and Services Administration, Maternal and Child Health Bureau.*

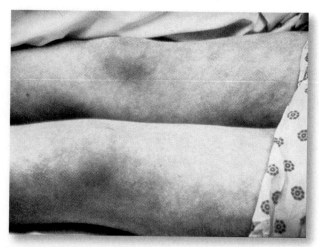

FIGURE 21-14 ▲ Mottled skin in a child. *EMSC Slide Set (CD-ROM). 1996. Courtesy of the Emergency Medical Services for Children Program, administered by the U.S. Department of Health and Human Service's Health Resources and Services Administration, Maternal and Child Health Bureau.*

volume of blood in the system and a steady volume of blood returning to the right side of the heart. One way to increase the amount of blood returning to the right side of the heart is to raise the patient's legs. If you suspect shock, place the patient on his back and raise his legs about 8-12 inches (shock position). Elevate the patient's legs only if he has no injuries to his head, spine, chest, abdomen, pelvis, or legs, and this procedure is approved by your medical director (Figure 21-15). A woman in late pregnancy should be positioned on her left side instead of on her back. When a woman in late pregnancy is placed on her back, the weight of the fetus compresses major blood vessels, such as the inferior vena cava and aorta. This compression decreases the amount of blood returning to the mother's heart and lowers her blood pressure. Positioning the patient on her left side shifts the weight of her uterus off the abdominal vessels.

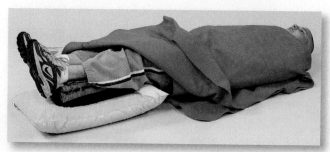

FIGURE 21-15 ▲ If you suspect shock, have the patient lie down and raise his legs about 8-12 inches. Do not elevate the patient's legs if there is an injury to his head, spine, chest, abdomen, pelvis, or legs.

- Give oxygen. If the patient's breathing is adequate, apply oxygen by nonrebreather mask at 15 L/min if not already done. If the patient's breathing is inadequate, provide positive-pressure ventilation with 100% oxygen and assess the adequacy of the ventilations delivered.
- Prevent heat loss by placing blankets under and over the patient. A patient in shock often has an altered mental status. Many patients are also nauseated and may vomit. Watch the patient closely to make sure his airway remains clear. Suction as needed.
- Control all obvious external bleeding, if present.
- Perform a physical exam. Take the patient's vital signs and gather the patient's medical history.
- A patient in shock is a priority patient and needs rapid transport to the closest appropriate hospital. Splint any bone or joint injuries en route.
- En route to the hospital, comfort, calm, and reassure the patient. Perform ongoing assessments every 5 minutes.
- Record all patient care information, including the patient's medical history and the emergency care provided, on a PCR.

On the Scene   Wrap-Up

The patient's complaint of abdominal pain, her vital signs, and her rigid, distended abdomen suggest that internal bleeding may be present. Her vital signs and cold, clammy skin are consistent with decompensated shock. Place the patient in a supine position and elevate her legs (shock position). Give 100% oxygen by nonrebreather mask and begin transport to the closest appropriate facility. En route to the hospital, make the patient as comfortable as possible, provide reassurance, and keep her warm. Perform ongoing assessments every 5 minutes. ■

Sum It Up

▶ Perfusion is the circulation of blood through an organ or a part of the body. Shock (hypoperfusion) is the inadequate circulation of blood through an organ or a part of the body.

▶ A wound is an injury to soft tissues. A closed wound occurs when the soft tissues under the skin are damaged but the surface of the skin is not broken (for example, a bruise). An open wound results when the skin surface is broken (for example, a cut or scrape).

▶ Hemorrhage (also called major bleeding) is an extreme loss of blood from a blood vessel. It is a life-threatening condition that requires *immediate* attention. If it is not controlled, hemorrhage can lead to shock and potentially to death.

▶ Hemophilia is a disorder in which the blood does not clot normally. A person with hemophilia may have major bleeding from minor injuries and may bleed for no apparent reason. Some medications or a serious injury may also prevent effective clotting.

▶ Arterial bleeding is the most serious type of bleeding. The blood from an artery is bright red, oxygen-rich blood. A bleeding artery can quickly lead to the loss of a large amount of blood.

▶ Venous bleeding is usually easier to control than arterial bleeding because it is under less pressure. Blood lost from a vein flows as a steady stream and is dark red or maroon because it is oxygen-poor blood.

▶ Capillary bleeding is common because the walls of the capillaries are fragile and many are close to the skin's surface. Bleeding from capillaries is usually dark red. When a capillary is torn, blood oozes slowly from the site of the injury because the pressure within the capillaries is low. Capillary bleeding often clots and stops by itself within a few minutes.

▶ External bleeding is bleeding that you can see. Clotting normally occurs within minutes. However, external bleeding must be controlled with your gloved hands and dressings until a clot is formed and the bleeding has stopped.

▶ You *must* wear PPE when you anticipate exposure to blood or other potentially infectious material. HIV and the hepatitis virus are examples of diseases to which you may be exposed that can be transmitted by exposure to blood.

▶ Six methods may be used to control external bleeding. You must know the methods of external bleeding control that are approved by medical direction and your local protocol.

  • Applying direct pressure slows blood flow and allows clotting to take place.

  • Elevating a bleeding arm or leg may help control the bleeding. Do not elevate the extremity if pain, swelling, or deformity is present.

  • If bleeding continues from an arm or leg, pressure points (also called *pulse points*) may be used to slow severe bleeding.

  • A splint is a device used to limit the movement of an injured arm or leg and reduce bleeding. After applying the splint, make sure to check the patient's fingers (or toes) often for color, warmth, and feeling.

  • A pressure splint (also called an air or pneumatic splint) can help control bleeding from soft-tissue injuries or broken bones. It can also help stabilize a broken bone.

  • A tourniquet is a tight bandage that surrounds an arm or leg. It is used to stop the flow of blood in an extremity. A tourniquet should be used to control life-threatening bleeding in an arm or leg when you cannot control the bleeding with direct pressure.

▶ Internal bleeding is bleeding that occurs inside body tissues and cavities. A bruise is a collection of blood under the skin caused by bleeding capillaries. A bruise is an example of internal bleeding that is not life threatening.

▶ Shock is the inadequate flow of blood through an organ or a part of the body. Shock can be caused by failure of the body's pump (the heart), fluid (blood), or container (the blood vessels).

  • Cardiogenic shock can result if the heart beats too quickly or too slowly or if the heart muscle does not have enough force to pump blood effectively to all parts of the body.

  • Shock caused by severe bleeding is called hemorrhagic shock. The bleeding may be internal, external, or both.

  • Shock caused by a loss of blood, plasma, or other body fluid is called hypovolemic shock.

▶ Early (compensated) shock is often difficult to recognize. Remember to look for it and to consider the patient's mechanism of injury or the nature of the illness when assessing your patient. Early shock is usually reversible if it is recognized and the patient receives emergency care to correct the cause of the shock.

▶ Late (decompensated) shock results when the patient's systolic blood pressure drops to less than 90 mm Hg. In this phase of shock, the body's defense mechanisms lose their ability to make up for the lack of oxygenated blood. The signs of late shock are more obvious than early shock, but late shock is more difficult to treat.

▶ Irreversible shock is also called terminal shock. You will feel an irregular pulse as the patient's heart becomes irritable and begins to beat irregularly. Permanent damage occurs to the vital organs because the cells and organs have been without oxygenated blood for too long. Eventually, the heart stops, breathing stops, and death results.

CHAPTER

22 Soft-Tissue Injuries

By the end of this chapter, you should be able to:

Knowledge Objectives ▶

1. State the major functions of the skin.
2. List the layers of the skin.
3. Establish the relationship between body substance isolation and soft-tissue injuries.
4. List the types of closed soft-tissue injuries.
5. Describe the emergency medical care of the patient with a closed soft-tissue injury.
6. State the types of open soft-tissue injuries.
7. Describe the emergency medical care of the patient with an open soft-tissue injury.
8. Discuss the emergency medical care considerations for a patient with a penetrating chest injury.
9. State the emergency medical care considerations for a patient with an open wound to the abdomen.
10. Differentiate the care of an open wound to the chest from an open wound to the abdomen.
11. List the classifications of burns.
12. Define superficial burn.
13. List the characteristics of a superficial burn.
14. Define partial-thickness burn.
15. List the characteristics of a partial-thickness burn.
16. Define full-thickness burn.
17. List the characteristics of a full-thickness burn.
18. Describe the emergency medical care of the patient with a superficial burn.
19. Describe the emergency medical care of the patient with a partial-thickness burn.
20. Describe the emergency medical care of the patient with a full-thickness burn.
21. List the functions of dressing and bandaging.
22. Describe the purpose of a bandage.
23. Describe the steps in applying a pressure dressing.
24. Establish the relationship between airway management and the patient with chest injury, burns, blunt and penetrating injuries.

25. Describe the effects of improperly applied dressings, splints, and tourniquets.

26. Describe the emergency medical care of a patient with an impaled object.

27. Describe the emergency medical care of a patient with an amputation.

28. Describe the emergency care for a chemical burn.

29. Describe the emergency care for an electrical burn.

Attitude Objectives ▶ There are no affective objectives identified for this lesson.

Skill Objectives ▶

30. Demonstrate the steps in the emergency medical care of closed soft-tissue injuries.

31. Demonstrate the steps in the emergency medical care of open soft-tissue injuries.

32. Demonstrate the steps in the emergency medical care of a patient with an open chest wound.

33. Demonstrate the steps in the emergency medical care of a patient with open abdominal wounds.

34. Demonstrate the steps in the emergency medical care of a patient with an impaled object.

35. Demonstrate the steps in the emergency medical care of a patient with an amputation.

36. Demonstrate the steps in the emergency medical care of an amputated part.

37. Demonstrate the steps in the emergency medical care of a patient with superficial burns.

38. Demonstrate the steps in the emergency medical care of a patient with partial-thickness burns.

39. Demonstrate the steps in the emergency medical care of a patient with full-thickness burns.

40. Demonstrate the steps in the emergency medical care of a patient with a chemical burn.

41. Demonstrate completing a prehospital care report for patients with soft tissue injuries.

On the Scene

The call went out: "House fire, people trapped." You can see the dark smoke curling up over the hill before you even arrive on the scene. You are on the third unit arriving at the fire; the nearest ambulance will be another 20 minutes. A firefighter crawls out through the gray smoke belching out of the front door, pulling an elderly man behind him. The Incident Commander tells you to take the patient. His clothes are smoldering slightly so you roll him on the ground and then quickly remove them. The patient moans as you douse his obvious burns with a bottle of water from your truck. "Call for a helicopter," you order, knowing that he will need to be taken to a burn center. As you apply oxygen, you assess him and can see that he has blistered burns over his face and singed eyebrows. The front of his chest and abdomen are covered with burns. Some burns are yellow, others are waxy white, and scattered charred areas are present. His right arm is burned completely around. ■

As you read this chapter, think about the following questions:

- What depth of burns does this patient have?
- How can you calculate the percentage of his body that has been burned?
- Is there any evidence that he has an inhalation injury?
- Why will he need the specialized resources of a burn center?
- What additional assessment and care will you need to perform?

Introduction

Managing Soft-Tissue Injuries

Soft tissues are the layers of the skin and the fat and muscle beneath them. Soft-tissue injuries range from bruises, cuts, and scrapes to amputations and full-thickness burns. Although soft-tissue injuries are common and impressive to look at, they are rarely life-threatening. You must be able to recognize the different types of soft-tissue injuries and give appropriate emergency care. This care includes controlling bleeding, preventing further injury, and reducing contamination.

Anatomy Review

Functions of the Skin

Objective 1

The skin is the body's first line of defense against bacteria and other organisms, ultraviolet rays from the sun, harmful chemicals, and cuts and tears. The skin helps regulate body temperature. It senses heat, cold, touch, pressure, and pain; nerves in the skin transmit this information to the brain and spinal cord. The skin is the site where vitamin D is produced. Sweat glands in the skin excrete excess water and some wastes.

Layers of the Skin

Objective 2

The epidermis is the outermost skin layer. It consists of four or five layers. New cells are continuously formed in the deeper layers of the epidermis. Older cells are pushed upward and sloughed off. The epidermis contains keratin, a waterproofing protein. The dermis is the deeper and thicker layer of skin containing sweat and sebaceous glands, hair follicles,

blood vessels, and nerve endings. The subcutaneous (fatty) layer helps conserve body heat. Fat can be used as an energy source when adequate food is not available. Accessory structures of the skin include the hair, nails, sweat glands, and oil (sebaceous) glands.

Soft-Tissue Injuries

Soft-tissue injuries damage the layers of the skin and the fat and muscle beneath them. The skin can be damaged by sharp or blunt objects, falls, or impacts with motionless objects. Chemicals, radiation, electricity, and extreme hot or cold temperatures can also cause injury to the skin.

Objective 3

Soft-tissue injuries may be open or closed. A soft-tissue injury that is associated with a break in the skin surface is an open wound. A closed wound is one in which the skin surface remains intact. The signs of a soft-tissue injury are usually obvious. Do not allow the appearance of a soft-tissue injury to distract you from performing an initial assessment and treating any life-threatening injuries. These injuries may be impressive to look at. However, you must remember that soft-tissue injuries are usually not the patient's most serious injuries unless they compromise the airway or are associated with severe bleeding. Because of the risk of exposure to blood and body fluids, personal protective equipment (PPE) must always be worn when dealing with soft-tissue injuries.

Closed Wounds

Objective 4

A **closed soft-tissue injury** occurs when the body is struck by a blunt object. There is no break in the skin, but the tissues and vessels beneath the skin surface are crushed or ruptured. Because there is no break in the skin, there is no external bleeding.

When assessing a closed wound, look carefully at the surface damage on the patient's skin and consider the mechanism of injury. With your knowledge of anatomy and how the injury occurred, try to visualize the possible damage to the organs and blood vessels beneath the area that was struck. For example, injuries to the upper abdomen can injure the liver, spleen, or pancreas. An injury to the lower abdomen can injure the bladder. An injury to the middle of the back can damage the kidneys. An injury to the neck can damage large blood vessels, the windpipe (trachea), and the spinal cord.

A contusion (bruise) is the most common type of closed wound (Figure 22-1). A contusion results when an area of the body experiences blunt trauma. In blunt trauma, a forceful impact occurs to the body, but there is no break in the skin. Examples of blunt force include a kick, fall, or blow. The outer skin layer, the epidermis, remains intact. However, the tissue layers and small blood vessels beneath it are damaged. The blunt force causes a small amount of internal bleeding in the area that was struck. Swelling, pain, and discoloration of the skin (ecchymosis) occur as blood leaks from the torn vessels into the surrounding tissue. At first, a contusion usually appears as a red area or as tiny red dots or splotches on the skin. The color changes to purple or blue within 2 to 5 days. After 5 to 10 days, the color changes to green and then yellow. It becomes brownish-yellow in color 10 to 14 days after the injury and then gradually disappears. Most contusions heal and disappear within 2 to 3 weeks.

If large blood vessels are torn beneath a bruised (contused) area, a **hematoma** forms (see Figure 22-1). A hematoma is a localized collection of blood beneath the skin caused by a tear in a blood vessel. Hematomas often occur with trauma of enough force to break

bones. Although similar to a contusion, a hematoma involves a larger amount of tissue damage. The patient may lose 1 or more liters of blood under the skin.

Crush injuries are caused by a compressing force applied to the body (see Figure 22-1). Crush injuries are also called *compression injuries*. Crush injuries may be open or closed injuries. An example of a minor crush injury is a hammer striking a thumb. Localized swelling and bruising are often present. In a severe crush injury, such as a car running over the chest and abdomen of a toddler, the extent of the injury may be hidden. You may see only minimal bruising, yet the force of the injury may have caused internal organ rupture. Internal bleeding may be severe and lead to shock. Crush injuries can result in compartment syndrome or crush syndrome.

Compartment Syndrome

Muscles of the body are covered by a tough sheet of fibrous tissue called **fascia** (Figure 22-2). Muscles in the arms and legs are separated from each other by fascia, forming compartments. Each compartment contains muscle cells and fibers, nerves, and blood vessels. When a compression injury occurs, the muscle

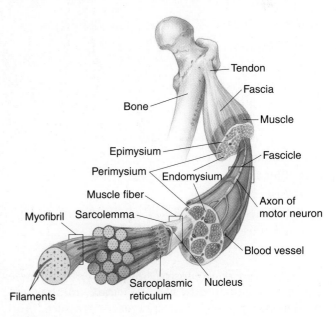

FIGURE 22-2 ▲ Fascia is a tough sheet of fibrous tissue that covers muscles and some organs of the body.

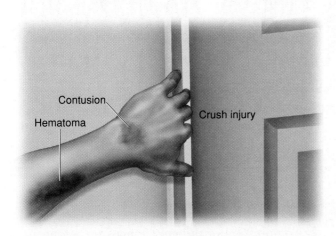

FIGURE 22-1 ▲ A contusion, a hematoma, and a crush injury without a break in the skin are examples of closed wounds.

is damaged, and swelling and/or bleeding results. Since fascia does not expand, swelling or bleeding causes an increase in pressure within the compartment. Increasing pressure compresses the muscle cells and fibers, nerves, and capillaries. When the pressure in the compartment becomes greater than the blood pressure within the capillaries, the capillaries collapse. This results in a decreased flow of blood (which contains oxygen and nutrients) to muscle and nerve cells. If the pressure in the compartment gets too high, blood flow stops. Without an adequate blood supply, the tissue within the compartment begins to die.

Compartment syndrome develops when the pressure within a compartment causes compression and abnormal function of nerves and blood vessels. Unless the pressure is relieved within 6 to 8 hours, permanent nerve and muscle damage can result, leading to paralysis, loss of the limb, or even death. To relieve the pressure within the compartment and attempt to save the affected limb, a physician will perform a fasciotomy. A **fasciotomy** is a surgical procedure in which the fascia is cut. By cutting the fascia, the pressure within the affected compartment is relieved.

Possible causes of compartment syndrome are listed in the following *You Should Know* box. Locations where compartment syndrome can occur include the arms, hands, legs, feet, and buttocks. The most common areas affected by compartment syndrome are the lower leg secondary to tibial fractures and the forearm secondary to fracture of the ulna or radius (see Figure 22-3).

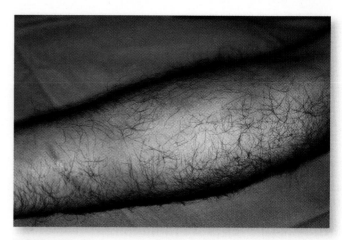

FIGURE 22-3 ▲ Compartment syndrome of the left leg. *Courtesy of Kevin J. Knopp, MD, from Atlas of Emergency Medicine, 2nd edition, McGraw-Hill Company, Inc.*

may seem out of proportion to the injury. The pain is worsened with passive stretching of the muscle. Weakness or paralysis of the affected extremity will be present. **Paresthesias** are abnormal sensations, such as tingling, burning, numbness, or a "pins-and-needles" feeling. Paresthesias are an early sign of nerve damage. **Anesthesia** means without sensation and refers to a loss of feeling in the affected limb. The affected area is usually swollen. It feels tight or full when touched because of increased pressure. Diminished peripheral pulses are a late sign of compartment syndrome.

You Should Know

The "5 Ps" of Compartment Syndrome

*P*ain on passive stretching of the muscle
*P*aralysis (or weakness)
*P*aresthesias
Increased *p*ressure
Diminished peripheral *p*ulses

Crush Syndrome

Crush syndrome can occur when a large amount of skeletal muscle is compressed for a long period. Examples of situations in which this type of injury occurs are listed in the following *You Should Know* box. Crush syndrome should be considered when three criteria exist:

1. Involvement of a large amount of muscle
2. Compression of the muscle mass for a long period (usually 4 to 6 hours, although it may be as little as 1 hour)
3. Compromised local blood flow

You Should Know

Possible Causes of Compartment Syndrome

- Compression injury
- Strenuous exercise
- Circumferential burns
- Frostbite
- Constrictive bandages, splints (including the pneumatic antishock garment), casts
- Animal/insect bites
- Bleeding disorders
- Arterial bleeding
- Soft-tissue injury
- Fracture

Signs and symptoms of compartment syndrome can be remembered by five "Ps": *p*ain, *p*aralysis (or weakness), *p*aresthesias, increased *p*ressure, and diminished peripheral *p*ulses. The earliest and most common symptom is severe, intense pain. The pain

Compression of the muscles causes damage to the muscle cells. Blood flow to the nerves, muscles, and tissues in the affected area(s) is compromised, resulting in muscle ischemia. Movement and sensation in the affected areas is also compromised. Damaged cells begin to leak toxic substances into the bloodstream. At the same time, large amounts of fluid build up in the compressed limbs. Hypovolemic shock develops because there is an inadequate volume of circulating blood. (Hypovolemic shock is the most common cause of death during the first few days after a crush injury.) Compartment syndrome develops because of increased pressure within the compressed limbs.

When the compressive force is removed, blood flow is restored to the muscles that were ischemic. Crush syndrome is called a *reperfusion injury* because although blood flow is restored to the muscles when the compressive force is removed, the toxic substances contained within the crushed areas are released into the circulation. The release of these toxins has many damaging effects. Kidney failure may occur within the first 60 hours of removal of the compressive force. Electrolyte abnormalities can cause irregular heart rhythms.

Emergency Care of Closed Wounds

Objective 5

To treat a patient with a closed wound, perform the following steps:

- Conduct a scene size-up and ensure your safety. Evaluate the mechanism of injury before approaching the patient. Put on appropriate PPE. If the mechanism of injury suggests a crushing injury, take extra care to evaluate the scene for hazards.
- Perform a primary survey to identify and treat any life-threatening conditions. Stabilize the

cervical spine if needed. If signs of shock are present or if internal bleeding is suspected, treat for shock (see Chapter 21).

- Perform a physical exam. Take the patient's vital signs and gather the patient's medical history.
- Splint any bone or joint injuries (see Chapter 23).
- If an extremity is injured, raise it above the level of heart unless there are signs or symptoms of a possible fracture, such as pain, swelling, or deformity. Apply an ice bag or cold pack. Place a cloth or bandage between the patient's skin and the cold source. Applying cold to the wound helps to reduce pain, constrict injured blood vessels (thereby reducing bleeding), and reduce swelling.
- Comfort, calm, and reassure the patient. En route to the hospital, perform ongoing assessments as often as indicated.
- Record all patient care information, including the patient's medical history and all emergency care given, on a prehospital care report (PCR).

Remember This!

- Never apply ice, an ice bag, or a cold pack directly to the skin. Doing so can cause tissue damage by freezing the tissue. Always use an insulating material such as a towel between the cold source and the skin.
- When applying ice, an ice bag, or a cold pack to a soft-tissue injury, limit the application of the cold source to 20 minutes or less to prevent cold injury.

Special Situations

- If signs of compartment syndrome are present, do not apply ice or elevate the extremity. Applying ice increases blood vessel constriction in an already compromised limb. Stabilize the extremity in the position found or place it in a position of comfort.
- If signs of compartment syndrome are present, splint the affected extremity for comfort and protection only when necessary, such as for a long transport.
- If the patient is trapped, try to find out how long the patient has been trapped. This information is very important. After finding out this

information, contact medical direction for instructions. In general, if the patient has been trapped for less than an hour (and adequate personnel and equipment are on the scene), the patient can be removed from the area and treatment begun. However, if the patient has been trapped for an hour or more, you should suspect crush syndrome. Contact dispatch and request Advanced Life Support (ALS) personnel to the scene. Before removing the patient from the area, ALS personnel will insert intravenous (IV) lines and begin infusing fluids. In situations like this, your time on the scene is likely to be much longer than usual. When ALS personnel have infused an adequate amount of IV fluid, they will most likely need your assistance in safely removing the patient from the area.

Open Wounds

Objective 6

In an **open soft-tissue injury,** a break occurs in the skin. Because of the break in the skin, open wounds are at risk of external bleeding and infection. Properly dressing the wound helps protect against infection and will help control bleeding.

An abrasion is a scrape. It is the most common type of open wound. An abrasion occurs when the outermost layer of skin (epidermis) is damaged by rubbing or scraping (Figure 22-4). Little or no oozing of blood (capillary bleeding) occurs. Although an abrasion is superficial, it can be very painful. Because the pain associated with the injury is like that of a second-degree burn, an abrasion is often called *road rash,* a *rug burn,* or a *friction burn.* Dirt and other foreign material can become ground into the skin with this type of

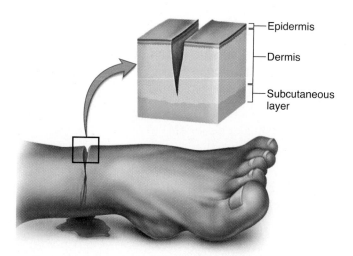

FIGURE 22-5 ▲ Any cut or tear in the skin is called a *laceration.*

injury. This greatly increases possible infection in a wound that is not properly cleansed with warm, soapy water or a fluid such as normal saline.

A laceration is a cut or tear in the skin of any length, shape, and depth (Figure 22-5). A laceration may occur by itself or with other types of soft-tissue injury. This type of injury can be made by a blunt object tearing the skin. It can also be made by a sharp instrument cutting through the skin, such as a knife, razor blade, or broken glass. This type of laceration is said to be linear, or regular. A stellate laceration is irregularly shaped. It is usually caused by forceful impact with a blunt object. Bleeding may be severe if a laceration is in an area of the body where large arteries lie close to the skin surface, such as in the wrists (Figure 22-6). You must control bleeding from

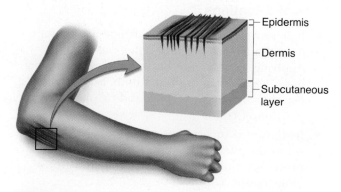

FIGURE 22-4 ▲ An abrasion results when the outermost layer of skin (epidermis) is damaged by rubbing or scraping.

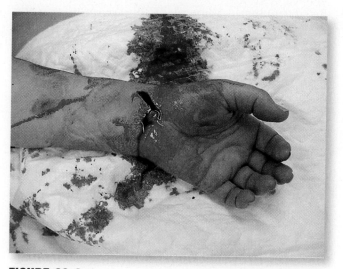

FIGURE 22-6 ▲ Laceration of the radial artery.
Trauma.org Image.

a laceration and cover the wound with a dressing to reduce the risk of infection.

A penetration, or **puncture wound,** results when the skin is pierced with a sharp, pointed object (Figures 22-7 and 22-8). Common objects that cause puncture wounds include nails, needles, pencils, splinters, darts, ice picks, pieces of glass, bullets, or knives. Some animal bites, such as those from cats, typically leave a deep puncture wound. An object that remains embedded in an open wound is called an **impaled object** (Figure 22-9). The severity of a puncture wound depends on where the injury is located. It also depends on how deep the wound is, the size of the penetrating object, and the forces involved in creating the injury. There is an increased risk of infection with this type of injury because the penetrating object may carry dirt and germs deep into the tissues. There may be little or no external bleeding with a puncture wound. However, internal bleeding may be severe. Assess the patient closely for signs and symptoms of shock if the puncture wound is in the chest or abdomen.

Gunshot and stab wounds are types of puncture wounds that can go completely through the body or body part. This creates both an entrance and an exit wound. An entrance wound from a bullet usually looks like a puncture wound. A bullet's exit wound is typically larger and more irregular. If a bullet breaks apart, it may create several exit wounds or none at all. Carefully examine your patient to find all wounds.

An **avulsion** is an injury in which a piece of skin or tissue is torn loose or pulled completely off

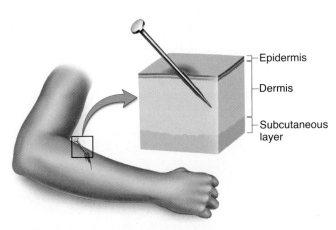

FIGURE 22-7 ▲ A penetration or puncture wound results when the skin is pierced with a sharp, pointed object.

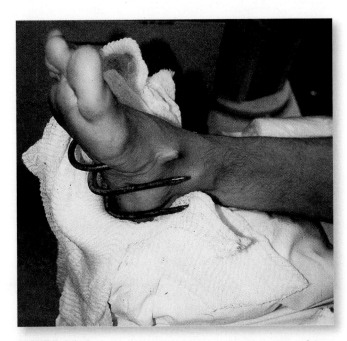

FIGURE 22-8 ▲ This patient has a puncture wound to the foot caused by a gardening tool. Foot x-rays revealed no associated bony injuries. *Courtesy of Matthew D. Sztajnkrycer, MD, PhD, from Knoop, et al., Atlas of Emergency Medicine, 2nd edition, McGraw-Hill Company, Inc.*

Stop and Think!

- Assume that any penetrating injury to the chest has involved the abdomen. Assume that a penetrating abdominal wound has involved the chest.

- A bullet that enters the body can travel in many directions. Suspect a possible spinal injury in every patient who has suffered a gunshot wound to the head, neck, chest, or abdomen.

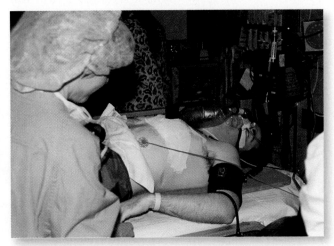

FIGURE 22-9 ▲ An object that remains embedded in an open wound is called an *impaled object.* © *The McGraw-Hill Companies, Inc./Carin Marter, photographer.*

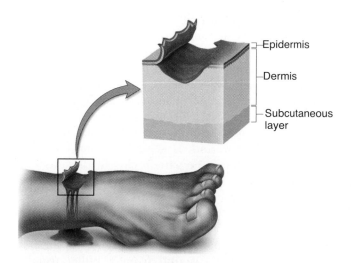

FIGURE 22-10 ▲ In an avulsion, a flap of skin or tissue is torn loose or pulled completely off. If the tissue is not totally torn from the body, it often hangs loose, like a flap.

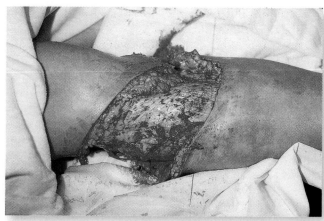

FIGURE 22-11 ▲ This degloving injury occurred after the patient's lower leg became tangled in a rope while she was water-skiing. *Courtesy of Alan B. Storrow, MD, from Knoop, et al., Atlas of Emergency Medicine, 2nd edition, McGraw-Hill Company, Inc.*

Remember This!

At a crime scene, disturb the patient and his clothing as little as possible while performing your assessment and during treatment. Cut around rather than through the areas penetrated by the weapon.

(Figure 22-10). If the tissue is not totally torn from the body, it often hangs loose, like a flap. The amount of bleeding varies with the extent and depth of the injury. A common avulsion injury is an avulsion of the forehead. This type of injury can occur when an unrestrained motor vehicle occupant is thrown through the windshield. In a degloving avulsion injury, the skin and fatty tissue are stripped away from an extremity like a glove (Figure 22-11).

Remember This!

Care for completely avulsed tissue like an amputated part.

A crush injury occurs when a part of the body is caught between two compressing surfaces. In an open crush injury, broken bone ends may stick out through the skin (Figure 22-12). Internal bleeding may be present and can be severe enough to cause shock. An example of an open crush injury is shown in Figure 22-13.

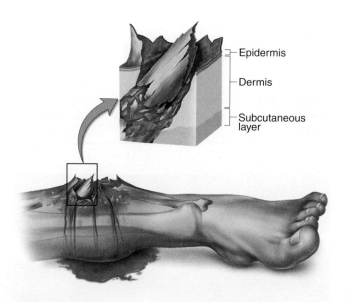

FIGURE 22-12 ▲ In an open crush injury, fractured bone ends may stick out through the skin.

An **amputation** is the separation of a body part from the rest of the body. If the body part is forcefully separated from the body, the edges of the wound are usually ragged (Figure 22-14). The remaining tissue may look shredded, with bones or tendons exposed. Massive bleeding may be present. Alternately, bleeding may be limited because blood vessels normally constrict and pull in at the point of injury when damaged. Bleeding can usually be controlled with direct pressure applied to the stump. Be sure to send the severed body part to the hospital with the patient.

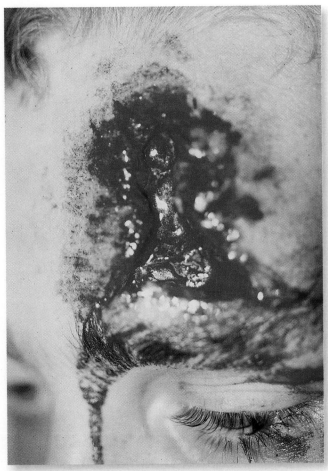

FIGURE 22-13 ▲ A fall from a bicycle resulted in this open crush injury. *Courtesy of Matthew D. Sztajnkrycer, MD, PhD, from Knoop, et al., Atlas of Emergency Medicine, 2nd edition, McGraw-Hill Company, Inc.*

You Should Know

Types of Open Wounds

- Abrasion
- Laceration
- Penetration, puncture wound
- Avulsion
- Open crush injury
- Amputation

Emergency Care of Open Wounds

Objective 7

To treat a patient with an open wound, perform the following steps:

- Conduct a scene size-up and ensure your safety. Evaluate the mechanism of injury before approaching the patient. Put on appropriate PPE.

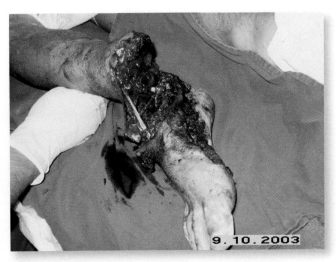

FIGURE 22-14 ▲ A 22-year-old with a traumatic amputation caused by a gear. *Trauma.org Image.*

- Perform a primary survey to identify and treat any life-threatening conditions. Stabilize the cervical spine if needed. If major bleeding is present from an open wound, expose the wound to assess the injury. You may need to remove and cut away clothing. Control bleeding. If signs of shock are present or major external bleeding is present, treat for shock.
- Once major bleeding is controlled, apply a sterile dressing to prevent further contamination of the wound. Bandage the dressing securely in place.
- Perform a physical exam. Take the patient's vital signs and gather the patient's medical history.
- Splint any bone or joint injuries.
- Comfort, calm, and reassure the patient. Perform ongoing assessments as often as indicated.
- Record all patient care information, including the patient's medical history and all emergency care given, on a PCR.

Special Considerations

The following soft-tissue injuries require special consideration:

- Penetrating chest injuries
- Eviscerations
- Impaled objects
- Amputations
- Neck injuries
- Eye injuries
- Mouth injuries
- Ear injuries
- Nosebleeds

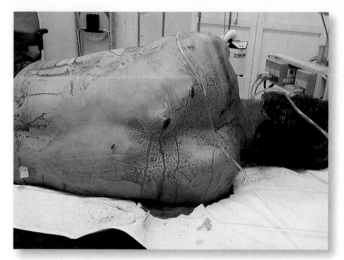

FIGURE 22-15 ▲ The front of this patient's chest showed visible bleeding, but no obvious injury. When the patient's back is examined, multiple wounds are found. Remember, the back is part of the chest. *Always* remember to check the back. *Trauma.org Image.*

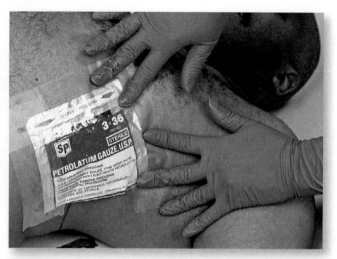

FIGURE 22-16 ▲ Cover an open chest wound with an airtight dressing taped on three sides.

Penetrating Chest Injuries

A **penetrating** (open) **chest injury** is a break in the skin over the chest wall (Figure 22-15). This type of injury results from penetrating trauma, such as gunshot wounds, stabbings, blast injuries, or an impaled object. The severity of an open chest injury depends on the size of the wound. If the chest wound is more than two thirds the diameter of the patient's windpipe, air will enter the chest wound rather than move through the trachea with each breath. You may hear a sucking or gurgling sound escaping from the wound when the patient breathes in. This sound occurs as air moves into the pleural cavity through the open chest wound. This type of injury is called a **sucking chest wound.** It is a life-threatening injury because the open wound can cause the lung on the injured side to collapse, affecting the patient's breathing.

Objectives 8, 10

You should consider *any* open chest wound a sucking chest wound. If an open chest wound is present, apply an occlusive (airtight) dressing to the wound. Examples of occlusive dressings include petroleum gauze, aluminum foil, or a piece of plastic wrap. Tape the dressing on three sides (Figure 22-16). The dressing will be sucked over the wound as the patient breathes in, preventing air from entering his chest. The open end of the dressing allows air that is trapped in the chest to escape as the patient breathes out. After covering the wound, give oxygen. Place the patient in a position of comfort if no spinal injury is suspected. If spinal injury is suspected, the patient should be placed on a long backboard and secured to the board.

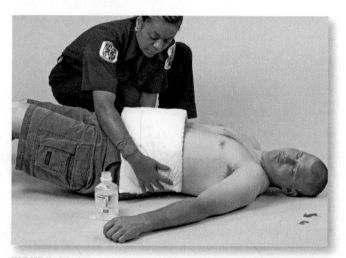

FIGURE 22-17 ▲ Cover the exposed organs and wound by applying a thick, moist dressing lightly over the organs and wound. Secure the dressing in place with a large bandage to retain moisture and prevent heat loss.

Eviscerations

Objective 9

An **evisceration** occurs when an organ sticks out through an open wound. In an abdominal evisceration, abdominal organs stick out through an open wound in the wall of the abdomen (Figure 22-17). Do not touch or try to place the exposed organ back into the body. Carefully remove clothing from around the wound. Lightly cover the exposed organs and wound with a thick, moist dressing. Secure the dressing in place with a large bandage to keep moisture in and prevent heat loss. Place the patient in a position of comfort if no spinal injury is suspected. Keep the patient warm. Assess for signs of shock and treat if present.

Impaled Objects

Objective 26

An impaled object is an object that remains embedded in an open wound. An impaled object is also called an *embedded object*. Do not remove an impaled object unless it interferes with cardiopulmonary resuscitation (CPR) or is impaled through the cheek and interferes with care of the patient's airway. After removing an object from the cheek, apply direct pressure to the bleeding by reaching inside the patient's mouth with gloved fingers.

Leave the object in the wound and manually secure it to prevent movement. Shorten the object only if necessary. Any movement of the object can cause further damage to nerves, blood vessels, and other surrounding tissues. Expose the wound area and control bleeding. Stabilize the object with bulky dressings and bandage them in place. Assess the patient for signs of shock and treat if present.

Amputations

Objective 27

In the case of an amputated body part, control bleeding at the stump. In most cases, direct pressure will be enough to control the bleeding. While providing care for the patient, ask an assistant to find the amputated part. The amputated part may be able to be reattached at the hospital. Because reattaching an amputated part is attempted only in very limited situations, do not suggest to the patient that it will be done.

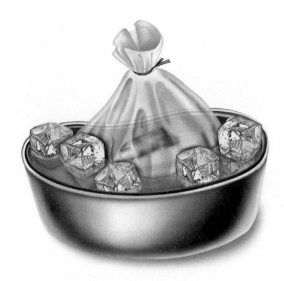

FIGURE 22-18 ▲ Place an amputated part in a dry plastic bag or waterproof container. Seal the bag or container and place it in water that contains a few ice cubes.

Put the amputated part in a dry plastic bag or waterproof container. Carefully seal the bag or container and place it in water that contains a few ice cubes (Figure 22-18). Immobilize the injured area to prevent further injury. Treat the patient for shock and keep him warm. Comfort, calm, and reassure the patient. Perform ongoing assessments every 5 minutes. Transport the amputated part with the patient to an appropriate facility.

Neck Injuries

Possible causes of a neck injury include the following:

- A hanging
- Impact with a steering wheel
- "Clothesline" injuries, in which a person runs into a stretched wire or cord that strikes his throat
- Knife or gunshot wounds

The neck contains many important blood vessels and airway structures. Swelling can cause an airway obstruction. A penetrating injury to the neck can result in severe bleeding (Figures 22-19). The signs and symptoms of a neck injury include shortness of breath, difficulty breathing, and a hoarse voice.

If a blood vessel is torn and exposed to the air, air can be sucked into the vessel and travel to the heart, lungs, brain, or other organs. This condition is called an *air embolism*. The air displaces blood and prevents tissue perfusion. Sometimes if a neck injury has damaged the airway, air will leak into the tissues. If this happens, there may be obvious swelling. When you palpate the skin, you will feel a "popping" as if there were crisped rice cereal trapped beneath it. This is called *subcutaneous emphysema* and is a very important finding to report to other healthcare professionals.

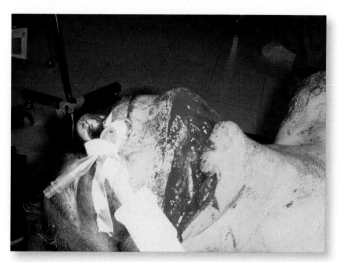

FIGURE 22-19 ▲ This patient is a 33-year-old man involved in a motor vehicle crash. He wore no seat belt and hit the windshield of the car he was driving. Despite the appearance of the injury, there were no injuries to the major blood vessels, trachea, or esophagus. The patient underwent surgery and was sent home 72 hours later. *Trauma.org Image.*

To care for an open neck wound:

- Immediately place a gloved hand over the wound to control bleeding.
- Cover the wound with an airtight (occlusive) dressing.
- Apply a bulky dressing over the occlusive dressing. To control bleeding, apply pressure over the dressing with a gloved hand. Compress the carotid artery only if absolutely necessary to control bleeding. When applying pressure, make sure not to press on the trachea or you may cause an airway obstruction. Do not press on both carotid arteries at the same time. Doing so can slow blood flow to the brain. It can also slow the patient's heart rate.
- Apply a pressure bandage. Wrap it across the injured side of the neck and under the opposite armpit (Figure 22-20). *Never apply a circular bandage around a patient's neck.* Strangulation can occur.
- Treat the patient for shock.

Remember This!

Consider an injury to the neck an injury to the spine. Immobilize the patient accordingly.

Eye Injuries

Eye injuries are common and often result from blunt and penetrating trauma. Causes of eye injuries are shown in the following *You Should Know* box. Swelling,

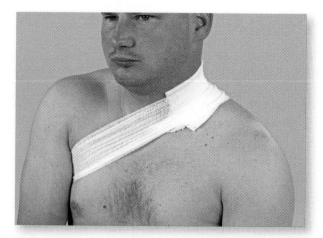

FIGURE 22-20 ▲ To care for an open neck wound, control bleeding and cover the wound with an airtight dressing. Apply a pressure bandage. Wrap it across the injured side of the neck and under the opposite armpit.

bleeding, or the presence of a foreign object in the eye are common signs of an eye injury and are easily seen. A foreign body, such as dirt, sand, and metal or wood slivers may enter the eye and cause severe pain.

You Should Know

Causes of Eye Injuries

- Motor vehicle crashes
- Sports and recreational activities
- Violence
- Chemical exposure from household and industrial accidents
- Foreign bodies
- Animal bites and scratches

If a foreign body is in the eye, try flushing it out of the affected eye. Do not exert any pressure on the eye. Hold the patient's eyelid open and gently flush the eye with warm water. Flush from the nose side of the affected eye toward the ear, away from the unaffected eye. It is important to flush *away* from the uninjured eye so that foreign bodies or chemicals are not transferred into the uninjured eye. Make sure to use a gentle flow of water when flushing the eye. A bulb or irrigation syringe, nasal cannula, or a bottle can be used for this purpose (Figure 22-21). Alternately, IV tubing connected to an IV bag of normal saline can be used. If none of these devices is available, try placing the patient's head under a gently running faucet and rinse the eye. Flush the eye for at least 5 minutes. If you are unable to remove the foreign body, cover both eyes and transport to the nearest appropriate medical facility.

If a foreign body is protruding from the eye, stabilize the object and transport as quickly as possible.

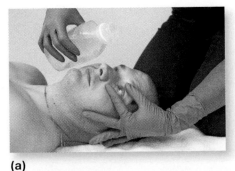
(a)

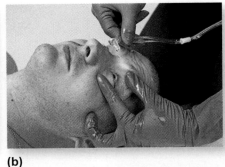
(b)

FIGURE 22-21 ◀ (a) To flush a foreign body from the eye, hold the patient's eyelid open and gently flush the eye with warm water. (b) Flush from the nose side of the affected eye toward the ear, away from the unaffected eye.

Do not attempt to remove the object. If the object is long, stabilize it with bulky gauze. Then cover the eye with a paper or Styrofoam cup secured with tape to keep the object from moving (Figure 22-22). If the object is short, make a doughnut-shaped base from roller gauze or a triangular bandage and place it around the eye. Be careful not to bump the object. Because both eyes normally move together, you will also need to cover the unaffected eye with a dressing. If you cover both eyes, be sure to tell the patient everything that you are doing. The patient may be frightened when he cannot anticipate movements and other procedures.

A chemical burn is the most urgent eye injury. The damage to the eye depends on the type and concentration of the chemical. The length of exposure and the elapsed time until treatment also affect the extent of damage. Early signs and symptoms of a chemical burn to the eye include:

- Pain
- Redness
- Irritation
- Tearing
- An inability to keep the eye open

- A sensation of "something in my eye"
- Swelling of the eyelids
- Blurred vision (usually caused by pain or tearing of the eye) or loss of vision

Alkali burns are more dangerous than acid burns because they penetrate more deeply and rapidly. Common household substances that contain alkalis include lye, cement, lime, and ammonia. Sulfuric acid is found in automobile batteries. It is one of the most common chemicals associated with acid burns of the eye. These exposures usually occur because of an automobile battery explosion.

Ask the patient if he is wearing contact lenses. If he is, have him remove them as soon as possible. If the lenses are left in, the irrigating solution will not be able to reach parts of the eye. If the patient does not wear contact lenses or if the lenses have been removed, immediately flush the eye with water or normal saline. Continue flushing the eye for at least 20 minutes. Flush away from the unaffected eye (as previously described). Transport immediately. Irrigation should be continued throughout transport.

You Should Know

Pepper spray is an irritant that causes significant pain when sprayed into the eyes. Vision is not usually affected, and the spray rarely causes eye damage. Flushing the affected eye for 5 minutes with warm water will generally stop further irritation.

A nonchemical burn to the eye can be caused by heat, radiation, lasers, infrared rays, and ultraviolet light (such as sunlight, arc welding, and bright snow). The patient will complain of severe pain in the eyes 1 to 6 hours after the exposure. Emergency care for a nonchemical burn to the eye includes covering both eyes with moist pads. Darken the room to protect the patient from further exposure to light. Transport the patient for further care.

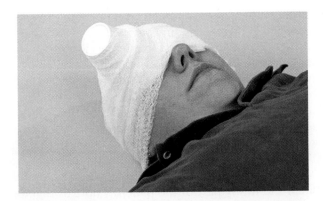

FIGURE 22-22 ▲ If a foreign body is protruding from the eye, stabilize it with bulky gauze. Then cover the eye with a paper or Styrofoam cup secured with tape to keep the object from moving. Cover the unaffected eye to limit movement of the affected eye.

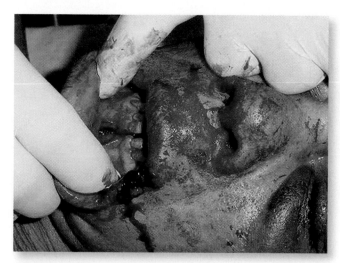

FIGURE 22-23 ▲ Jaw fracture resulting from direct frontal trauma. *Trauma.org Image.*

Mouth Injuries

An injury to the mouth can result in severe swelling or bleeding that causes an airway obstruction. Because the tongue is attached to the lower jaw (mandible), a lower-jaw fracture may allow the tongue to fall against the back of the throat, blocking the airway. The signs and symptoms depend on the area of the jaw affected. Tenderness, bruising, and swelling are common (Figure 22-23).

You Should Know

If the patient is unable to open his mouth or move his lower jaw side to side without pain, suspect a fracture.

The upper jawbone (maxilla) is often fractured in high-speed crashes. The patient's face is thrown forward into the windshield, steering wheel, and dashboard. A fracture of the maxilla is often accompanied by a black eye. The patient's face may appear unusually long. Swelling and pain are usually present.

A patient with a jaw fracture should receive spinal immobilization because of the mechanism of injury. Carefully look in the patient's mouth for teeth, blood, vomitus, and other potential obstructions. Suction as necessary. Look in the mouth for broken or missing teeth. If dentures or missing teeth are found, they should be transported with the patient. If a knocked-out (avulsed) tooth is found, handle the tooth by the crown. Do not handle the tooth by the root (the part that was embedded in the gum). Rinse the tooth (do not scrub it) in water. Place the tooth in milk or in a Save-a-Tooth™ kit (or similar product) if it is available. Control bleeding

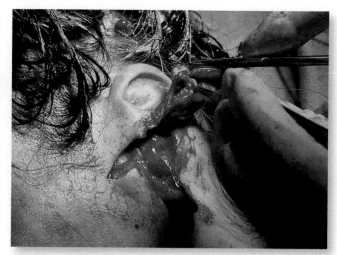

FIGURE 22-24 ▲ Ear laceration. *Trauma.org Image.*

and treat for shock if indicated. Transport the tooth with the patient to the hospital. *Trauma.org Image.*

Ear Injuries

A blow to the ear can result in bruising of the outer (external) portion of the ear. A severe blow can result in damage to the eardrum, with pain, bleeding, or both. Suspect a possible skull fracture if you see blood or fluid draining from a patient's ear. Place a sterile dressing loosely over the ear to absorb the drainage and bandage it in place. Never put anything into the ear to control bleeding. If the ear is avulsed, collect the avulsed part and care for it as you would an amputated part. Make sure that the avulsed part is transported with the patient to the hospital. An ear laceration is treated like any other soft-tissue injury (Figure 22-24).

Nosebleeds

Most nosebleeds come from a bleeding blood vessel in the front of the nose. This type of nosebleed is called an *anterior nosebleed*. It is usually easy to control. Tell the patient with a nosebleed not to blow his nose or sniffle. Doing so can prevent clots from forming or can break clots that have already developed. Do not put anything in the nose to try to control bleeding. If the patient can help you, have him sit up and lean his head forward. This position helps to keep blood from draining into the back of the patient's throat. Blood that is swallowed often makes a person feel sick to his stomach, increasing the chance of vomiting. If the patient cannot sit up, have him lie down with his head raised. Tell the patient to breathe through his mouth. Pinch the fleshy part of the patient's nostrils together with your thumb and two fingers for 15 minutes (Figure 22-25).

Some nosebleeds come from a bleeding blood vessel in the back of the nose. This type of nosebleed is called a *posterior nosebleed*. A posterior nosebleed

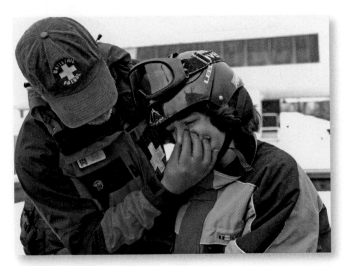

FIGURE 22-25 ▲ To stop a nosebleed, have the patient sit up, with the patient's head tilted forward. Pinch the fleshy part of the patient's nostrils together with your thumb and two fingers for 15 minutes.

occurs most often in older adults. This type of nosebleed is difficult to control, and the patient can develop shock. A patient with a posterior nosebleed needs rapid transport to the hospital. Treat for shock if present.

Burns

Burns may occur because of exposure to heat (thermal burn), chemicals, electricity, or radiation. Most burns are thermal burns that result from flames, scalds, or contact with hot substances. Chemical burns are caused by substances that produce chemical changes in the skin, resulting in tissue damage on contact. Acids and alkalis are substances that are commonly associated with a chemical burn. An electrical burn occurs when a person comes into contact with a source of electricity, including lightning. Body organs may be injured from the heat generated as the electrical current enters the body and travels through the tissues. Burns may also result from a high level of radiation exposure. Radiation burns are the least common type of burn.

The skin is the body's largest organ. Remember that the skin:

- Helps regulate body temperature
- Senses heat, cold, touch, pressure, and pain
- Helps maintain fluid balance
- Protects underlying tissues from injury

When the skin is disrupted because of a burn, many of these functions are affected. The body loses fluid, and the skin becomes less effective in helping to maintain body temperature. Because the skin surface is no longer intact, the body is at an increased risk of infection.

Determining the Severity of a Burn

The severity of a burn is determined by a number of factors:

- The depth of the burn (how deeply the burn penetrates the skin)
- The extent of the burn (how much of the body surface is burned)
- The location of the burn
- The patient's age
- Medical or surgical conditions present before the burn
- Associated factors (such as the mechanism of injury)

The Depth of the Burn

Objective 11

Burns are classified by how deeply the body's skin layers are affected. There are three categories of burns:

- Superficial (first-degree) burn
- Partial-thickness (second-degree) burn
- Full-thickness (third-degree) burn

You Should Know

A burn wound continues to change up to 24 hours after the injury.

Superficial Burns

Objectives 12, 13

A **superficial** (first-degree) **burn** affects only the epidermis. It results in only minor tissue damage (Figure 22-26). A sunburn is an example of a superficial burn. The skin is red, tender, and very painful (Figure 22-27). Blistering does not occur with a superficial burn. This type of burn does not usually require medical care and heals in 2 to 5 days with no scarring.

Partial-Thickness Burns

Objectives 14, 15

A **partial-thickness** (second-degree) **burn** involves the epidermis and dermis. The hair follicles and sweat glands are spared in this degree of burn (Figure 22-28). These burns commonly result from contact with hot liquids or flash burns from gasoline flames. A partial-thickness burn produces intense pain and some

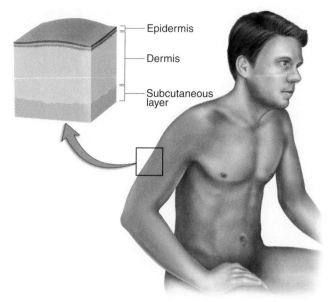

FIGURE 22-26 ▲ A superficial (first-degree) burn affects only the epidermis.

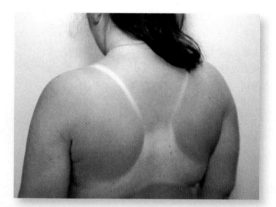

FIGURE 22-27 ▲ Superficial (first-degree) burn.

swelling. Blistering may be present (Figure 22-29). The skin appears pink, red, or mottled, and is sensitive to air current and pressure. This type of burn usually heals within 5 to 35 days. Scarring may or may not occur, depending on the depth of the burn.

You Should Know

Not all partial-thickness burns blister. However, if blistering is present, it is a partial-thickness burn.

Full-Thickness Burns

Objectives 16, 17

A **full-thickness** (third-degree) **burn** destroys both the epidermis and dermis and may include subcutaneous tissue, muscle, and bone (Figure 22-30). The color of the patient's skin may vary from yellow or pale to

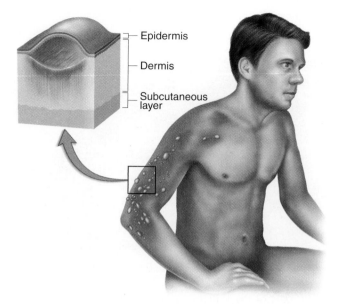

FIGURE 22-28 ▲ A partial-thickness (second-degree) burn affects the epidermis and dermis.

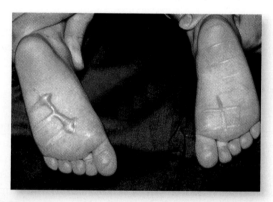

FIGURE 22-29 ▲ Partial-thickness (second-degree) burn. *EMSC Slide Set (CD-ROM). 1996. Courtesy of the Emergency Medical Services for Children Program, administered by the U.S. Department of Health and Human Service's Health Resources and Services Administration, Maternal and Child Health Bureau.*

black. The skin has a dry, waxy, or leathery appearance (Figure 22-31). A full-thickness burn is numb because the burn destroys nerve endings in the skin. However, many full-thickness burns are surrounded by areas of superficial and partial-thickness burns, which are painful. A large full-thickness burn requires skin grafting. Small areas may heal from the edges of the burn after weeks. Because the skin is so severely damaged in this type of burn, it cannot perform its usual protective functions. Rapid fluid loss often occurs. Be ready to treat the patient for shock.

The Extent of the Burn

When determining the seriousness of a burn, the extent of the burned area is important to determine. The depth of the burn must also be considered, although superficial burns are not included in the

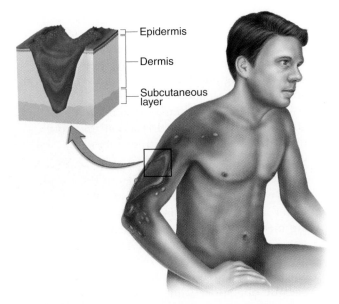

Epidermis

Dermis

Subcutaneous layer

FIGURE 22-30 ▲ A full-thickness (third-degree) burn causes damage to all layers of the epidermis and dermis and may include subcutaneous tissue, muscle, and bone.

FIGURE 22-31 ▲ Full-thickness (third-degree) burn. *EMSC Slide Set (CD-ROM). 1996. Courtesy of the Emergency Medical Services for Children Program, administered by the U.S. Department of Health and Human Service's Health Resources and Services Administration, Maternal and Child Health Bureau.*

TABLE 22-1   The Rule of Nines

Body Area	Adult	Child	Infant
Head and neck	9%	18%	18%
Front of trunk	18%	18%	18%
Back of trunk	18%	18%	18%
Each arm (shoulder to fingertips)	9%	9%	9%
Each leg (groin to toe)	18%	13.5%	13.5%
Genitals	1%	1%	1%

calculation of the extent a burn. The **rule of nines** is a guide used to estimate the affected body surface area (BSA). The rule of nines divides the adult body into sections that are 9% or are multiples of 9% (Figure 22-32). The rule of nines has been modified for children and infants (Table 22-1). To use the rule of nines to estimate the extent of a burn, add the percentages of the areas burned. For example, if an adult burned the front of the trunk (18%), the front and back of one arm (9%), and the front and back of one leg (18%), 45% of his BSA is burned.

You Should Know

Only partial-thickness and full-thickness burns are included when calculating the extent of a burn.

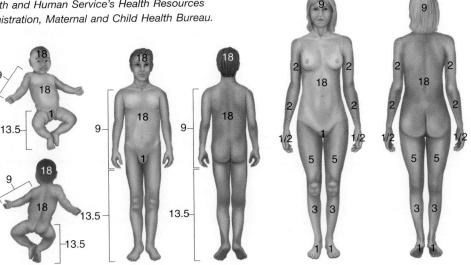

FIGURE 22-32 ▲ The rule of nines for an infant, a child, and an adult.

The "rule of palms" can be used for small or irregularly shaped burns, or burns that are scattered over the patient's body. The palm of the *patient's* hand equals 1% of the patient's BSA. If the patient's palm would fit over the burned area 8 times, the extent of the burn is 8% of the BSA.

Other Factors Related to Burn Severity

The Location of the Burn

The location of a burn is an important factor when determining burn severity. Burns to the face can cause breathing difficulty. Burns of the face and neck can interfere with the ability to eat or drink. Burns of the hands and feet can interfere with the patient's ability to walk, work, feed themselves, and perform other daily activities. Burns of the genitalia are prone to infection.

Preexisting Medical Conditions

A preexisting medical problem may increase a patient's risk of death or complications following a burn injury. A burn is considered severe if the patient is younger than 5 years of age or older than 55 years of age. The skin of infants, young children, and elderly people is thin. Burns in these patients may be more severe than they initially appear.

Burn Considerations for Infants and Children

- Children have a larger BSA than adults in relationship to the total body size. This larger surface area results in greater fluid and heat loss.
- Children who are burned are more likely than adults to develop shock or airway problems.
- Consider the possibility of child abuse when treating a burned child. A common burn associated with child abuse is caused by dipping the child in scalding water. "Stocking-like" burns with no associated splash marks are often present on the buttocks, genitalia, or extremities (Figure 22-33). Report all suspected cases of abuse to law enforcement and Emergency Department personnel in accordance with your state's regulations.

Burn Considerations for Older Adults

- Many older adults have thin skin and poor circulation. These factors affect the depth of a burn and slow the healing process.

- In older adults, the mechanisms and severity of burn injury are related to living alone. Older adults also tend to wear loose-fitting clothing while cooking and fall asleep while smoking. In addition, these patients tend to have declining vision, hearing, and sense of smell. Older adults may have a slowed reaction time and problems with balance and/or memory.
- Burns in older adults most often occur in the home. Scalds and flame burns are the most common type of burns in this age group.
- Older adults are more likely to have a preexisting medical condition, which increases their risk of complications after a burn. In some cases, the preexisting condition may be the cause of the burn. For example, an older adult may collapse because of a stroke while smoking or cooking.

Burns Best Treated in a Burn Center

Although most burns are minor, some types of burns are best treated in a burn center. A burn center offers specialized care—including services, equipment, and staff who are trained to treat serious burn injuries. A patient with any of the following types of burns should be transported to a burn center:

- Partial-thickness (second-degree) burns involving more than 10% of the total body surface area (TBSA) in adults or 5% of the TBSA in children

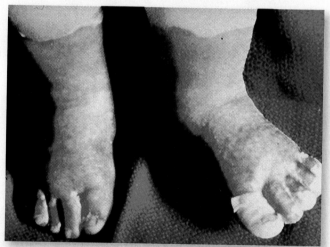

FIGURE 22-33 ▲ "Stocking-like" burns with no associated splash marks are caused by dipping a child in scalding water. This type of injury is usually seen in children younger than two years of age. The child's caregiver punishes the child, for example, for an "accident" when he is being potty trained. *EMSC Slide Set (CD-ROM). 1996. Courtesy of the Emergency Medical Services for Children Program, administered by the U.S. Department of Health and Human Service's Health Resources and Services Administration, Maternal and Child Health Bureau.*

- Chemical burns
- All burns involving the hands, face, eyes, ears, feet, or genitalia
- Circumferential burns of the torso or extremities
- Any full-thickness (third-degree) burn in a child
- All inhalation injuries
- Electrical burns, including lightning injuries
- All burns complicated by fractures or other trauma
- All burns in high-risk patients, including older adults; the very young; and those with preexisting conditions, such as diabetes, asthma, and epilepsy

Emergency Care of Thermal Burns
Objectives 18, 19, 20

To treat a patient with a thermal burn, perform the following steps:

- Conduct a scene size-up and ensure your safety. Evaluate the mechanism of injury before approaching the patient. Put on appropriate PPE.
  - If the patient is still in the area of the heat source, remove the patient from the area. If the patient's clothing is in flames, "stop, drop, and roll." Place the patient on the floor or ground. Roll him in a blanket to smother the flames.
  - Remove smoldering clothing and jewelry. If the patient's clothing is stuck to the burned area, do not attempt to remove it. Instead, cut around the clothing, leaving the burn untouched.
- Perform a primary survey to identify and treat any life-threatening conditions. Manage the patient's airway and breathing. Stabilize the cervical spine if needed.

Objective 24

- If the patient was in a confined space and was exposed to smoke, flames, or steam, you should be alert for potential airway problems. Examples of confined spaces include a room, vehicle, silo, pit, vessel, or vault. The signs and symptoms that suggest a possible airway problem are shown in the following *You Should Know* box. Patients who have signs of an inhalation injury will likely have inhaled poisonous gases such as carbon monoxide or cyanide. These gases are produced as a by-product of the substances that burn. High-flow oxygen is always indicated in these situations.
- Check the pulses in all extremities. Burn swelling that encircles an extremity (a **circumferential burn**) can act as a tourniquet.

You Should Know

Signs and Symptoms of Possible Inhalation Injury

- Facial burns
- Soot in the nose or mouth
- Singed facial or nasal hair
- Swelling of the lips or the inside of the mouth
- Coughing
- An inability to swallow secretions
- A hoarse voice

- After all immediate life threats have been managed, care for the burn itself. Perform a physical exam. Quickly determine the severity of the burn. Take the patient's vital signs and gather the patient's medical history.
  - Consider the following questions about to the burn:
    - How long ago did the burn occur?
    - How did it occur?
    - What was done to treat the burn before you arrived?
- Keep in mind that even after being removed from the heat source, burned tissue will continue to burn. You can help limit the progression of a surface burn injury if you can rapidly cool the burn shortly after it happens. Stop the burning process with clean, room temperature water for no more than 1 to 2 minutes. *Cooling the burn for more than 2 minutes can cause a critical loss of body heat and shock.*
- Cover the burned area with a dry dressing or sheet. If blisters are present, leave them intact and cover them loosely with a sterile dressing. Cover the patient with clean, dry sheets and blankets to keep him warm. Because burned tissue loses its ability to regulate temperature, cover the patient even when the outside temperature is warm. The sheet does not have to be sterile.
- Remove all jewelry as soon as possible. Swelling of the hands and fingers may occur soon after a burn.
- Look for other injuries and signs of shock. Treat and immobilize possible fractures. Treat soft-tissue injuries if present. Treat shock if present.
- Keep burned extremities elevated above the level of the heart.
- Transport to the closest appropriate facility. Comfort, calm, and reassure the patient. Perform ongoing assessments as often as indicated.

- Record all patient care information, including the patient's medical history and all emergency care given, on a PCR.

Remember This!

- Do not apply ice, butter, oils, sprays, lotions, or ointments to a burn.
- If a blister has formed, do not break it.
- Do not place ice or wet sheets on a burn.
- Do not transport a burn patient on wet sheets, wet towels, or wet clothing.

Chemical Burns

It has been estimated that more than 25,000 chemicals currently in use are capable of burning the skin or mucous membranes. Chemical burns can result from contact with wet or dry chemicals. The degree of injury in a chemical burn is based on the following:

- The mechanism of action of the chemical
- The strength of the chemical
- The concentration and amount of the chemical
- How long the patient was in contact with the chemical
- The body part in contact with the chemical
- The extent of tissue penetration

In some cases, the damage caused by the chemicals is not limited to the skin. Some chemicals, such as hydrofluoric acid, can be absorbed into the body and cause damage to internal organs.

Emergency Care of Chemical Burns

Objective 28

To treat a patient with a chemical burn, use the following steps:

- Conduct a scene size-up. As in all situations, your personal safety must be your primary concern. Evaluate the mechanism of injury before approaching the patient. Take the necessary scene safety precautions to protect yourself from exposure to hazardous materials. Wear gloves, eye protection, and other PPE as necessary. Additional resources, such as law enforcement, the fire service, the state or local hazardous materials team, and special rescue personnel, may be needed to secure the scene before you can safely enter the area.

- Perform a primary survey to identify and treat any life-threatening conditions.
  - Manage the patient's airway and breathing. Stabilize the cervical spine if needed.
  - Remove the patient's jewelry and clothing, including shoes and socks, which can trap concentrated chemicals. Do not remove clothing over the patient's head. Instead, cut his clothing as needed. Place the items in plastic bags to limit the exposure of others to the chemical.

- Perform a physical exam. Take the patient's vital signs and gather the patient's medical history.

- Stop the burning process by removing the chemical. Wet chemicals can be flushed with large amounts of water. Brush away dry chemicals before flushing.
  - Brush off dry chemicals from the patient's skin with towels, sheets, or your gloved hands. Brush the chemical *away* from the patient.
  - Flush the burn with large amounts of room temperature water at low pressure. If the burn covers a large area, put the patient in the shower or use a garden hose, if available. Chemical burns should be flushed for at least 20 minutes.

- Treat other injuries, if present.

- The patient should be decontaminated before transport to the hospital. If the patient is not fully decontaminated before transport, the receiving facility should be notified as soon as possible. This notification will allow them time to prepare to decontaminate the patient when he arrives at the facility.

- Comfort, calm, and reassure the patient. Perform ongoing assessments as often as indicated.

- Record all patient care information, including the patient's medical history and all emergency care given, on a PCR. Constantly check for status of scene safety, as it can change rapidly in a contamination scene.

Stop and Think!

The severity of a chemical burn can be misleading. The skin may not appear to be significantly damaged, yet a severe injury may be present. You may be contaminated by the chemical if you do not use appropriate precautions.

Electrical Burns

The severity of an electrical injury is related to the following:

- Amperage (the flow of the current)
- Voltage (the current's force)
- The type of current (alternating current or direct current)
- The current's pathway through the body
- The resistance of tissues to the current
- The duration of contact with the current

Normally, the skin is a resistor to the flow of electric current into the body. When electricity enters the body, it is converted to heat. Inside the body, the current follows the paths of blood vessels, nerves, and muscles. This results in major damage to the body's internal organs. The skin may show no signs or only minimal signs of injury despite massive internal damage.

Emergency Care of Electrical Burns

Objective 29

To treat a patient with an electrical burn, perform the following steps:

- Conduct a scene size-up and make sure the scene is safe before entering. Evaluate the mechanism of injury before approaching the patient. Take the necessary scene safety precautions to protect yourself from exposure to electrical hazards. Wear gloves, eye protection, and other PPE as necessary. If the patient is still in contact with the electrical source, you may need to contact appropriate resources before approaching the patient. These resources may include law enforcement, fire service, and utility company personnel (Figure 22-34). Do not attempt to remove the patient from the electrical source unless you have been trained to do so. If the patient is still in contact with the electrical source or you are unsure, do not touch the patient.
- Perform a primary survey to identify and treat any life-threatening conditions. Manage the patient's airway and breathing. Stabilize the cervical spine if needed. Monitor the patient closely for respiratory and cardiac arrest. Make sure an automated external defibrillator is immediately available to you. Cardiac arrest caused by an electrical injury usually responds to treatment if defibrillation is performed quickly.
- Perform a physical exam (Figure 22-35). Take the patient's vital signs and gather the patient's medical history. Provide oxygen.

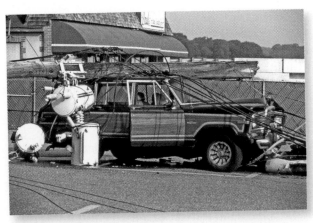

FIGURE 22-34 ▲ In situations involving electricity, additional resources, such as law enforcement, fire service, and utility company personnel, may be needed to secure the scene before you can safely enter the area.

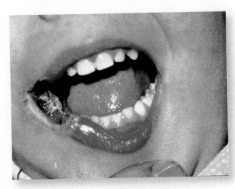

FIGURE 22-35 ▲ Electrical burn. *EMSC Slide Set (CD-ROM). 1996. Courtesy of the Emergency Medical Services for Children Program, administered by the U.S. Department of Health and Human Service's Health Resources and Services Administration, Maternal and Child Health Bureau.*

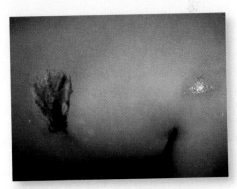

FIGURE 22-36 ▲ Electrical burn showing typical entrance and exit wounds. *Trauma.org Image.*

- Look for and treat other injuries if present. The patient may have fallen or been thrown from the electrical source. Treat the soft-tissue injuries associated with the burn.
- Look for both an entrance and an exit wound. The entrance wound may look dry and leathery. The exit wound is usually much larger (Figure 22-36).

- *All* electrical burns should be evaluated by a physician. Transport the patient to the hospital.
- Comfort, calm, and reassure the patient. Perform ongoing assessments as often as indicated.
- Record all patient care information, including the patient's medical history and all emergency care given, on a PCR.

Remember This!

Because electrical burns do more damage on the inside of the body than they do on the outside, it will be impossible for you to tell how bad an electrical burn really is. All electrical burns need to be evaluated at a hospital.

Emotional Support

Bleeding and soft-tissue injuries are dramatic injuries. The emergency care that you provide for bleeding and soft-tissue injuries is very important. It is also important to consider the psychological impact of these injuries. The patient and/or his family may experience many different emotions because of the injury. Remember that although grief is most often associated with death, *any* change of circumstance can cause a person to experience grief. A patient who has suffered a massive soft-tissue injury or major burn often goes through the stages of the grief process. You may see the emotions of fear, anger, guilt, and depression. Provide emotional support for the patient and family.

Some of the injuries you will care for will be the result of a suicide attempt. After an unsuccessful suicide attempt, the patient may want to talk with you about it or he may deny the attempt. Other injuries you will care for may be the result of abuse involving a child, spouse, or older adult. If you suspect abuse, share your concerns privately with the healthcare professional to which you transfer patient care. Follow your local protocol regarding reporting suspected cases of abuse. In addition to notifying the person to whom you transfer care, you may also be required to notify law enforcement or Emergency Department personnel. Although these situations may be difficult, you must not be confrontational with the patient, family members, or others at the scene.

When providing care for bleeding and soft-tissue injuries, you may experience anger, anxiety, frustration, fear, grief, and feelings of helplessness, especially if you are unable to relieve a patient's suffering or if a patient dies despite your care. You may feel sick at the sight of these injuries. These emotions are common and expected. You should not feel embarrassed or ashamed when these situations affect you. Seek the help of a peer counselor, mental health professional, social worker, or member of the clergy when you need assistance coping with these situations.

Making a Difference

The physical care you provide for a patient's illness or injury is very important. Good emergency care involves attending to the patient's physical and emotional needs in a professional, caring, concerned, and sensitive way. Always place the interests of the patient first when making patient care decisions.

Dressing and Bandaging

Objective 21

A dressing is an absorbent material placed directly over a wound. A **bandage** is material used to secure a dressing in place. The functions of dressing and bandaging wounds include:

- Helping to stop bleeding
- Absorbing blood and other drainage from the wound
- Protecting the wound from further injury
- Reducing contamination and the risk of infection

Dressings

When choosing a dressing, select one that is lint-free and large enough to cover the wound. A dressing of the right size should extend beyond the edges of the wound. If it is available, use a sterile dressing whenever possible because the dressing will be in direct contact with the open wound. When applying the dressing to the wound, wear gloves and hold the dressing by a corner. Place the dressing right over the wound—do not slide it in place.

Types of Dressings

The types of dressings commonly used in emergency care are sterile gauze pads, trauma dressings, occlusive dressings, and nonadherent pads.

Sterile Gauze Pads

Sterile gauze pads are the most common dressing used (Figure 22-37). They come in different shapes and sizes and are made of loosely woven material. This woven material allows blood and fluids to pass through the material and be absorbed.

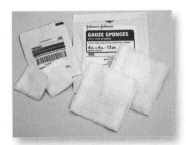

FIGURE 22-37 ▲ Sterile gauze pads come in different shapes and sizes.

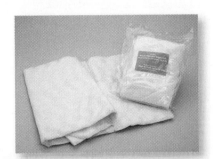

FIGURE 22-38 ▲ Trauma dressings are thick dressings that are used for large wounds. They are available in different sizes.

Small gauze pads are classified by their size in inches. For example, a "2 by 2" refers to a small dressing that is 2 inches long and 2 inches wide.

Remember This!

If blood soaks through a dressing, do not remove it. Apply more dressings and another bandage.

Trauma Dressings

Trauma dressings are thick dressings available in various sizes (Figure 22-38). This type of dressing is made of two layers of gauze with absorbent cotton in the center. A trauma dressing is used for large wounds. It can also be used to pad an injured arm or leg inside a splint.

Occlusive Dressings

An occlusive dressing is a special type of dressing made of nonporous material. This type of dressing is used to cover an open wound of the chest or neck and create an airtight seal. Although commercially-made occlusive dressings are available, plastic wrap or aluminum foil may also be used (Figure 22-39).

Nonadherent Pads

Nonadherent pads are special gauze pads that have a special coating. They are used to cover an open wound that is leaking fluid, such as a scrape or burn, but not

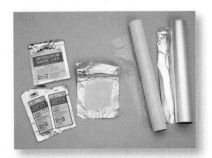

FIGURE 22-39 ▲ An occlusive dressing is used to cover an open wound and create an airtight seal. This type of dressing is made of nonporous material. Although commercially made occlusive dressings are available, plastic wrap or aluminum foil may also be used.

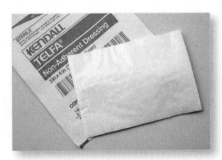

FIGURE 22-40 ▲ Nonadherent pads are used to cover an open wound but not stick to it.

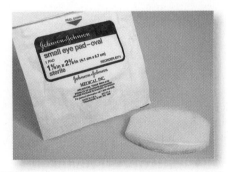

FIGURE 22-41 ▲ Eye pads are used to cover the eyes after a minor eye injury.

stick to it (Figure 22-40). Eye pads are nonadherent pads that used to cover the eyes after a minor eye injury (Figure 22-41). They may also be used to cover a small wound, such as a puncture. Adhesive strips, such as Band-Aids, are a combination of a nonadherent sterile dressing and a bandage.

Bandages

Objective 22

A bandage is applied to keep a dressing in place. Because a dressing separates the wound and the bandage, the bandage does not have to be sterile. Before applying a bandage on an extremity, remove the patient's jewelry and check the pulse distal to the wound. Tape is used to secure most dressings in place. Most tape used in first aid and Emergency Medical Services (EMS) kits today is made of silk, paper, or plastic because some patients are allergic to adhesive tape.

Types of Bandages

Fingertip and knuckle bandages are adhesive strips that are a sterile dressing and bandage combination. A knuckle bandage is made of cloth and shaped like an H. This type of bandage is useful for covering minor cuts or abrasions on a knuckle, elbow, heel, or chin.

Roller gauze (often called by the brand name *Kling*) is wrapped around and around a dressing to secure it in place. This type of bandage comes in different widths and lengths (Figure 22-42). Pick a roller bandage width that is appropriate for the body part to be bandaged. A 1-inch roll is used to bandage fingers, and a 2-inch roll is used for wrists, hands, and feet. A 3-inch roll is can be used for elbows and upper arms. A 4- to 6-inch roll is used for ankles, knees, and legs.

A roller bandage (often called by the brand name *Kerlix*) is made of soft, slightly elastic material and is available in various widths (Figure 22-43).

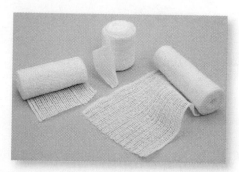

FIGURE 22-42 ▲ Roller gauze.

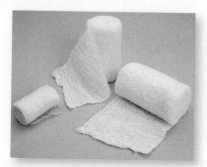

FIGURE 22-43 ▲ Roller bandage.

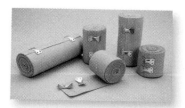

FIGURE 22-44 ▲ Elastic bandage.

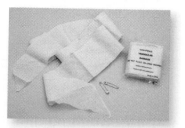

FIGURE 22-45 ▲ Triangular bandage.

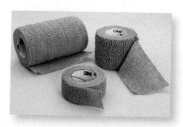

FIGURE 22-46 ▲ Coban is a self-adherent elastic wrap.

Elastic bandages (such as an Ace bandage or elastic wrap) should not be used to secure a dressing in place (Figure 22-44). If the injured area swells, the elastic bandage may act as a tourniquet. A triangular bandage is a large piece of muslin that can be folded and used as a bandage or sling (Figure 22-45). A triangular bandage that has been folded is called a *cravat*.

Coban and Kimberly-Clark Self-Adherent Wrap are elastic wraps coated with a self-adhering material that functions like tape (Figure 22-46). No pins or clips are required to hold the bandage in place. This type of bandage is often used as a pressure bandage.

Objectives 23, 25

A pressure bandage is a bandage with which enough pressure is applied over a wound site to control bleeding. To apply a pressure bandage:

- Cover the wound with several sterile gauze dressings or a bulky dressing.
- Apply direct pressure to the wound until bleeding is controlled.
- Secure the dressing firmly in place with a bandage. Assess the patient's pulse distal to the bandage.

- If possible, do not cover fingers or toes so you can determine if the bandage is too tight. A bandage may be too tight if the fingers or toes become cold to the touch, the fingers or toes begin to turn pale or blue, or the patient complains of numbness in the extremity.

Skill Drill 22-1 shows the steps used to apply a roller bandage. Figures 22-47 through 22-52 show the bandaging techniques for different soft-tissue injuries.

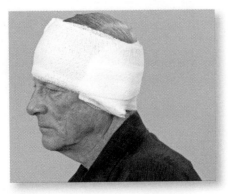

FIGURE 22-47 ▲ Head or ear bandage.

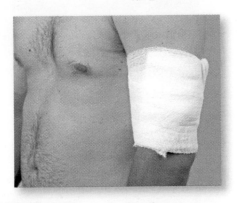

FIGURE 22-48 ▲ Upper-arm bandage.

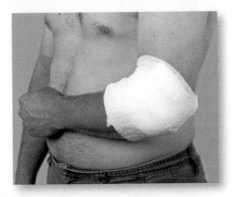

FIGURE 22-49 ▲ Elbow bandage.

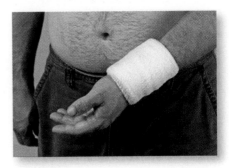

FIGURE 22-50 ▲ Wrist or forearm bandage.

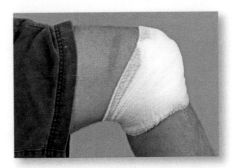

FIGURE 22-51 ▲ Knee bandage.

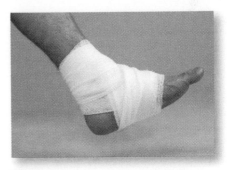

FIGURE 22-52 ▲ Foot or ankle bandage.

Applying a Roller Bandage

STEP 1 ▶ Start below the wound and work upward, applying the bandage directly over the sterile dressing on the wound.

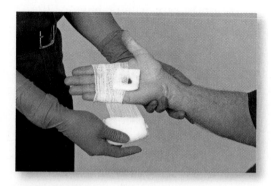

STEP 2 ▶ Using overlapping turns, cover the dressing completely. Unless the fingers are injured, leave them exposed so that you can assess circulation.

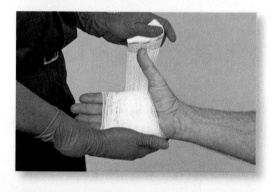

STEP 3 ▶ Tape or tie the bandage in place.

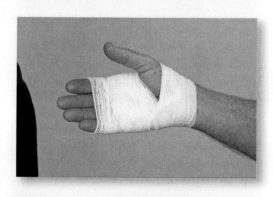

STEP 4 ▶ To make sure the bandage is not too tight, check a pulse distal to the wound site, the color of the fingers, and the temperature of the skin.

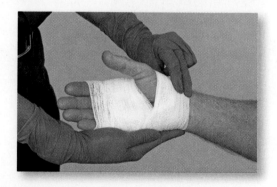

The estimated time of arrival for the helicopter is 5 minutes. You cover the patient with a clean sheet and then a warm blanket. He is responsive to painful stimulus only. His vital signs are blood pressure 104/70, pulse 128, respirations 24. As you continue your assessment, you can hear wheezing in his lungs. You are worried about his right arm because his fingers are pale and cold and you cannot feel a radial pulse in that arm. As the aircraft lands, the patient's breathing rate increases. He is using neck muscles to breathe and he is making a high-pitched noise with each inhalation. The flight crew springs into action. They start an IV, give him some drugs, and place a breathing tube before they move him to the helicopter. As they lift off, your partner shakes his head, commenting, "When will people learn that they can't smoke in bed?" ■

Sum It Up

▶ The skin is the body's first line of defense against bacteria and other organisms, ultraviolet rays from the sun, harmful chemicals, and cuts and tears.

▶ Closed soft-tissue injuries occur because of blunt trauma. In blunt trauma, a forceful impact occurs to the body, but there is no break in the skin. In a closed soft-tissue injury, there is no actual break in the skin, but the tissues and vessels may be crushed or ruptured. When assessing a closed soft-tissue injury, it is important to evaluate surface damage and consider possible damage to the organs and major vessels beneath the area of impact.

▶ Closed soft-tissue injuries include contusions, hematomas, and crush injuries. A contusion is a bruise. In a contusion, the epidermis remains intact. Cells are damaged and blood vessels torn in the dermis. Localized swelling and pain are typically present. A buildup of blood causes discoloration (ecchymosis). A hematoma is the collection of blood beneath the skin. A larger amount of tissue is damaged compared with a contusion. Larger blood vessels are damaged. Hematomas frequently occur with trauma sufficient to break bones. Crush injuries are caused by a crushing force applied to the body. These injuries can cause internal organ rupture. Internal bleeding may be severe and lead to shock.

▶ Compartment syndrome is a compression injury. It develops when the pressure within a compartment causes compression and abnormal function of nerves and blood vessels. Unless the pressure is relieved within 6 to 8 hours, permanent nerve and muscle damage can result, leading to paralysis, loss of the limb, or even death.

▶ Crush syndrome can occur when a large amount of skeletal muscle is compressed for a long period. Crush syndrome should be considered when three criteria exist:

1. Involvement of a large amount of muscle
2. Compression of the muscle mass for a long period (usually 4 to 6 hours, although it may be as little as 1 hour)
3. Compromised local blood flow

▶ In open soft-tissue injuries, a break occurs in the continuity of the skin. Because of the break in the skin, open injuries are susceptible to external hemorrhage and infection. In an abrasion, the outermost layer of skin (epidermis) is damaged by shearing forces (e.g., rubbing or scraping). A laceration is a break in the skin of varying depth. A laceration may be linear (regular) or stellate (irregular). Lacerations may occur in isolation or with other types of soft-tissue injury. A puncture results when the skin is pierced with a pointed object such as a nail, pencil, ice pick, splinter, piece of glass, bullet, or a knife. An object that remains embedded in the open wound is called an impaled object. In an avulsion, a flap of skin or tissue is torn loose or pulled completely off. In a degloving avulsion injury, the skin and fatty tissue are stripped away. In an amputation, extremities or other body parts are severed from the body. In an open crush injury, soft-tissue and internal organs are damaged. These injuries may cause painful, swollen, deformed extremities. Internal bleeding may be severe.

▶ An evisceration occurs when an organ sticks out through an open wound. In providing care, do not touch or try to place the exposed organ back into the body. Carefully remove clothing from around the wound. Lightly cover the exposed organs and wound with a thick, moist dressing. Secure the dressing in place with a large bandage to keep moisture in and prevent heat loss.

▶ An impaled object is an object that remains embedded in an open wound. Do not remove an impaled object unless it interferes with CPR or is impaled through the cheek and interferes with care of the patient's airway. Control bleeding and stabilize the object with bulky dressings, bandaging them in place. Assess the patient for signs of shock and treat if present.

- In the case of an amputated body part, control bleeding at the stump. In most cases, direct pressure will be enough to control the bleeding. Ask an assistant to find the amputated part, as it may be able to be reattached at the hospital. Put the amputated part in a dry plastic bag or waterproof container. Carefully seal the bag or container and place it in water that contains a few ice cubes.
- There are three categories of burns:
  - A superficial (first-degree) burn affects only the epidermis. It results in only minor tissue damage (such as sunburn). The skin is red, tender, and very painful. This type of burn does not usually require medical care and heals in 2 to 5 days with no scarring.
  - A partial-thickness (second-degree) burn involves the epidermis and dermis. The hair follicles and sweat glands are spared in this degree of burn. A partial-thickness burn produces intense pain and some swelling. Blistering may be present. The skin appears pink, red, or mottled and is sensitive to air current and pressure. This type of burn usually heals within 5 to 35 days. Scarring may or may not occur, depending on the depth of the burn.
  - A full-thickness (third-degree) burn destroys both the epidermis and dermis and may include subcutaneous tissue, muscle, and bone. The color of the patient's skin may vary from yellow or pale to black. The skin has a dry, waxy, or leathery appearance. Because the skin is so severely damaged in this type of burn, it cannot perform its usual protective functions. Rapid fluid loss often occurs. Be ready to treat the patient for shock.
- The rule of nines is a guide used to estimate the affected body surface area. The rule of nines divides the adult body into sections that are 9% or are multiples of 9%. This guideline has also been modified for children and infants. To estimate the extent of a burn by using the rule of nines, add the percentages of the areas burned.
- A dressing is an absorbent material placed directly over a wound. A bandage is used to secure a dressing in place. A pressure bandage is a bandage applied with enough pressure over a wound site to control bleeding. Dressings and bandages serve the following functions:
  - Help to stop bleeding
  - Absorb blood and other drainage from the wound
  - Protect the wound from further injury
  - Reduce contamination and the risk of infection

By the end of this chapter, you should be able to:

Knowledge Objectives ▶

1. Describe the function of the muscular system.
2. Describe the function of the skeletal system.
3. List the major bones or bone groupings of the spinal column, the thorax, the upper extremities, and the lower extremities.
4. Differentiate between an open and a closed painful, swollen, deformed extremity.
5. State the reasons for splinting.
6. List the general rules of splinting.
7. List the complications of splinting.
8. List the emergency medical care for a patient with a painful, swollen, deformed extremity.

Attitude Objectives ▶

9. Explain the rationale for splinting at the scene versus load and go.
10. Explain the rationale for immobilization of the painful, swollen, deformed extremity.

Skill Objectives ▶

11. Demonstrate the emergency medical care of a patient with a painful, swollen, deformed extremity.
12. Demonstrate completing a prehospital care report for patients with musculoskeletal injuries.

On the Scene

It must be the tenth time you have glanced at your watch, hoping your relief will arrive, when the alarm tones sound. The dispatch speaker crackles, "Respond to 22 St. Louis Lane. Person has fallen." When you get there, your 80-year-old patient is lying in a crumpled heap at the bottom of ten steps. Her husband says she was carrying a load of laundry, lost her footing, and fell from the top step. She is alert but is moaning. She says she has pain in her arms and leg. Your partner maintains in-line stabilization of her head as you continue your exam. Her skin is pink and warm, but she is grimacing and there are beads of sweat on her forehead. Her vital signs are blood pressure 168/100, pulse 116, and respirations 20. When you touch the back of her neck, she says that it hurts. She has no pain or obvious injury in her chest, abdomen, or pelvis. Her left leg has obvious swelling between the knee and hip. That same leg seems to be rotated slightly. Her left upper arm is very tender and swollen between her shoulder and her elbow. Her right wrist is angled strangely, and she groans loudly when you touch the area. "We're going do a few things to help your pain, Mrs. Brown," you tell your patient as your partner heads back to your rescue truck for supplies. ∎

THINK ABOUT IT

As you read this chapter, think about the following questions:

- Why did your partner maintain in-line stabilization of the patient's head before you knew that the patient had neck pain?
- What bones are likely to be injured as evidenced by the information that you have now?
- How will you splint her injuries?
- What additional assessments should you perform?
- Which injuries could cause the patient to develop shock?

Introduction

Managing Musculoskeletal Injuries

Injuries to the musculoskeletal system are some of the most common traumatic injuries you will encounter. Most of these injuries are not life threatening, but they may be very dramatic. Although an injury may not be life threatening, it may have a sudden impact on a patient physically, as well as emotionally and socially. You must be able to recognize a musculoskeletal injury and provide appropriate emergency care. This care includes preventing further injury, reducing pain, and decreasing the likelihood of permanent damage.

The Musculoskeletal System

Objective 1

The musculoskeletal system:

- Gives the body its shape
- Provides a rigid framework that supports and protects internal organs
- Provides for body movement
- Maintains posture
- Helps stabilize joints
- Produces body heat

The human skeleton provides the support for the body, much like the internal framework of a house. The skeleton provides a frame for other parts of the musculoskeletal system to attach to, including ligaments, tendons, and muscles. All parts of the musculoskeletal system work together to enable movement.

The Skeletal System

Objective 2

The skeletal system:

- Gives the body shape, support, and form
- Works with muscles to provide for body movement
- Stores minerals such as calcium and phosphorus
- Produces red blood cells
- Protects vital internal organs:
  —The skull protects the brain
  —The rib cage protects the heart and lungs
  —The lower ribs protect most of the liver and spleen
  —The spinal canal protects the spinal cord

Bones are living, growing tissues that are made up mostly of collagen and calcium. Collagen is a protein that provides a soft framework. Calcium is a mineral that strengthens and hardens the framework. New bone is constantly added to the skeleton, and old bone is removed. Bones become large, heavy, and thick during childhood and teenage years because new bone is added faster than old bone is removed.

You Should Know

Maximum bone strength and thickness is reached at about age 30. After age 30, the rate at which old bone is removed slowly begins to exceed the rate at which new bone is formed. **Osteoporosis** is a condition that develops when the rate of old bone removal occurs too quickly or when old bone replacement occurs too slowly. As a result, the bones of a person with osteoporosis become brittle and tend to break easily. Too little calcium over a person's lifetime is thought to play a major role in contributing to the development of osteoporosis.

Objective 3

The skeletal system is divided into the axial and appendicular skeletons (Figure 23-1). The axial skeleton includes the skull, spinal column, sternum, and ribs (Table 23-1). The appendicular skeleton is made up of the upper and lower extremities (arms and legs), the shoulder girdle, and the pelvic girdle (Table 23-2). The axial skeleton is made up of 80 bones. The appendicular skeleton consists of 126 bones.

The shoulder girdle is the bony arch formed by the collarbones (clavicles) and shoulder blades (scapulae). The pelvic girdle is made up of bones that enclose and protect the organs of the pelvic cavity. It

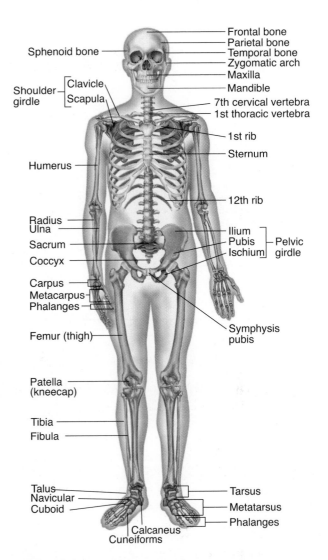

FIGURE 23-1 ▲ The human skeleton is made up of the axial skeleton, which consists of the skull, vertebral column, sternum, and ribs. The appendicular skeleton (blue) is attached and includes the shoulder and pelvic girdles as well as the limb bones.

TABLE 23-1 The Axial Skeleton

Bone	Purpose
Skull (cranium)	Houses and protects the brain Serves as a rigid container
Facial bones (eye sockets, cheeks, upper nose, and upper and lower jaw)	Houses and protects the brain and sensory organs (the structures that provide sight, smell, and taste) Provides shape and unique features
Spinal column	Protects the spinal cord Provides a center axis of support
Sternum (breastbone) and ribs	Protects the heart, lungs, and major blood vessels in the chest

TABLE 23-2 The Appendicular Skeleton

Bone	Purpose
Upper Extremities	
Shoulder girdle (collar bone and shoulder blade)	Provides structural support and movement/leverage
Upper arm bone (humerus)	
Forearm bones (radius and ulna)	
Wrist bones (carpals)	
Hand bones (metacarpals)	
Fingers (phalanges)	
Lower Extremities	
Pelvic girdle	Protects the bladder, female reproductive organs, and major blood vessels Provides a point of attachment for the legs and major muscles of the trunk Supports the weight of the upper body
Thigh (femur)	Provides structural support
Kneecap (patella)	Provides joint protection and support
Shin (tibia and fibula)	Provides structural support
Ankle (tarsals)	Provides structural support and movement/leverage
Foot (metatarsals)	Provides structural support and movement/leverage
Toes (phalanges)	Provides structural support and movement/leverage

provides a point of attachment for the lower extremities and the major muscles of the trunk. It also supports the weight of the upper body.

The skull is made up of the cranial bones, which house and protect the brain, and the facial bones, including the upper jaw (the maxilla), the lower jaw (the mandible), and the cheekbones (zygomatic bones). The skull is supported by the neck, which receives its strength from the vertebrae.

The vertebral column is made up of 7 cervical (neck) vertebrae, 12 thoracic vertebrae, 5 lumbar vertebrae, 5 fused vertebrae that form the sacrum, and 3 to 4 fused vertebrae that form the coccyx (tailbone). The vertebral column gives rigidity to the body while allowing movement. It also encloses the spinal cord. It extends from the base of the skull to the coccyx.

The chest (thorax) is made up of the 12 thoracic vertebrae, 12 pairs of ribs, and the breastbone (sternum). These structures form the thoracic cage,

which protects the organs within the thoracic cavity (for example, the heart, lungs, and major blood vessels). All of the ribs are attached posteriorly by ligaments to the thoracic vertebrae.

The sternum (breastbone) consists of three sections:

1. The manubrium is the uppermost (superior) portion; it connects with the clavicle and the first rib.
2. The body is the middle portion.
3. The xiphoid process is a piece of cartilage that makes up the lowermost (inferior) portion.

The uppermost portion of the sternum is attached to the clavicles, which joins the axial skeleton to the appendicular skeleton.

The upper extremities are made up of the bones of the shoulder girdle, the arms, the forearms, and the hands. The humerus is the upper arm bone. The

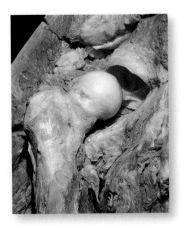

FIGURE 23-2 ◄ The hip joint is an example of a ball-and-socket joint. © *The McGraw-Hill Companies, Inc./Rebecca Gray, photographer/Don Kincaid dissections.*

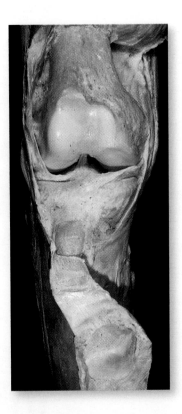

FIGURE 23-3 ◄ The knee joint is an example of a hinge joint. © *The McGraw-Hill Companies, Inc./Rebecca Gray, photographer/Don Kincaid dissections.*

biceps and triceps muscles are attached here, allowing the shoulder to rotate, flex, and extend. The forearm contains two bones: the radius (lateral/thumb side) and the ulna (medial side). The elbow is the joint where the humerus connects with the radius and the ulna. The forearm is connected to the wrist (carpals) and then to the hand (metacarpals) and fingers (phalanges).

The lower extremities are made up of the bones of the pelvis, the upper legs, the lower legs, and the feet. The pelvis is a bony ring formed by three separate bones that fuse to become one bone in an adult. The lower extremities are attached to the pelvis at the hip joint. The hip joint is formed by the socket of the hip bone and the upper end of the thighbone (femur).

The knee is protected anteriorly by the kneecap (patella) and attaches the femur to the two lower leg bones, the tibia (shinbone) and fibula. The lower leg attaches to the foot by the ankle. The tarsal bones make up the back part of the foot and heel. The metatarsals make up the main part of the foot. The toes (phalanges) are the foot's equivalent to the fingers.

The skeletal system includes many joints. A **joint** is a place where two bones come together. Some bone ends are covered with cartilage. Cartilage provides cushioning between bones. Joints are held in place by ligaments. Ball-and-socket joints allow movement in all directions (Figure 23-2). The only ball-and-socket joints in the body are the hip joint (pelvic bone and femur) and shoulder joint (scapula and humerus). A hinge joint allows only flexion and extension. Examples include the elbow (humerus and ulna) and knee (femur and tibia) (Figure 23-3.)

The Muscular System

The human body has over 600 muscles (Figure 23-4). Muscles are bundles of tiny fibers that expand and contract. Muscle fibers shorten (contract) when stimulated. They shorten by converting energy obtained from food (chemical energy) into movement (mechanical energy).

Skeletal muscles produce movement of the bones to which they are attached. Skeletal muscles also produce heat, which helps maintain a constant body temperature, and maintain posture. Skeletal muscles have a rich supply of blood vessels and nerves. In most cases, an artery and at least one vein accompany each nerve in a skeletal muscle. Skeletal muscle fibers are surrounded by connective tissue. The connective tissue covering supports and protects the delicate fibers. It also provides a pathway through which blood vessels and nerves can pass. A skeletal muscle fiber must receive a signal from a nerve before it can contract. When the signal is received, skeletal muscles produce rapid, forceful contractions.

Most skeletal muscles are attached to bones by means of tendons. Tendons create a pull between bones when muscles contract. The tendons of many muscles cross over joints, which contributes to the stability of the joint. Tendons can be damaged from overextension or overuse. Ligaments connect bone to bone.

A skeletal muscle has three main parts (Figure 23-5):

* The **origin** is the stationary attachment of the muscle to a bone.
* The **insertion** is the movable attachment to a bone.
* The **body** is the main part of the muscle.

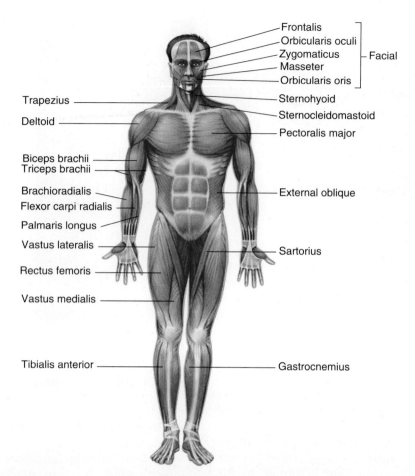

FIGURE 23-4 ▲ The human body has more than 600 skeletal muscles. A few of them are identified here.

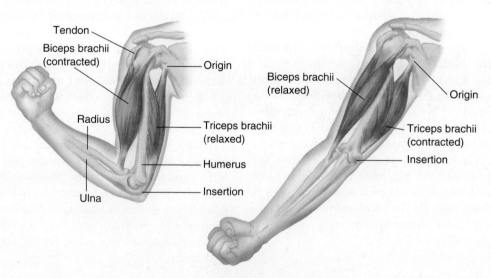

FIGURE 23-5 ▲ The origin of a skeletal muscle is the stationary attachment of the muscle to a bone. The insertion is the movable attachment to a bone. The body is the main part of the muscle.

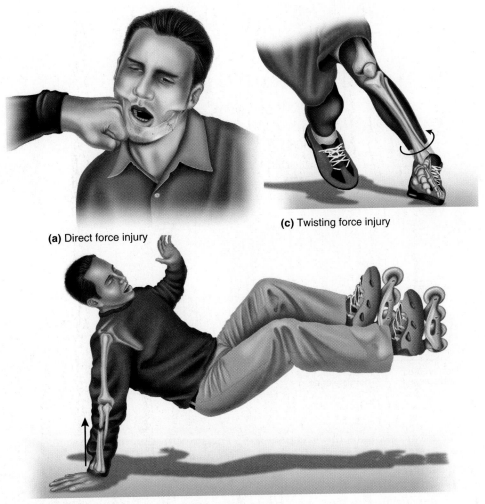

(a) Direct force injury

(c) Twisting force injury

(b) Indirect force injury

FIGURE 23-6 ▲ **(a)** Direct force injury. **(b)** Indirect force injury. **(c)** Twisting force injury.

Musculoskeletal Injuries

Mechanism of Injury

Injuries to bones and joints can be caused by direct forces, indirect forces, and twisting forces (Figure 23-6). A direct force causes injury at the point of impact, such as being struck in the face by a baseball. Indirect forces cause injury at a site other than the point of impact. For example, if your hand strikes the ground (direct force) during a fall, the energy travels up your arm and may result in an injury near your elbow, shoulder, or clavicle (indirect force). A twisting force causes one part of an extremity to remain in place while the rest twists, such as an ankle twisted while a person is playing basketball. Twisting injuries commonly affect the joints, such as ankles, knees, and wrists. Twisting forces cause ligaments to stretch and tear.

Types of Musculoskeletal Injuries

Objective 4

Injuries to bones and joints may be open or closed. In an open injury, the skin surface is broken. The bone may protrude through the wound or may pull back inside the body from muscle contraction. These injuries can result in serious blood loss. An open injury also increases the risk of contamination and infection. In closed bone and joint injuries, the skin surface is not broken. In any case, an open or closed bone or joint injury is often painful, swollen, and deformed.

A **fracture** is a break in a bone. If a bone is broken, chipped, cracked, or splintered, it is said to be fractured. Figure 23-7 shows some types of fractures. The bones of a child are more flexible than those of an adult and tend to bend more without

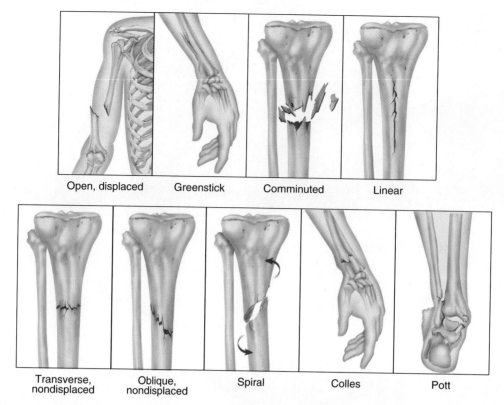

Open, displaced	Greenstick	Comminuted	Linear

Transverse, nondisplaced	Oblique, nondisplaced	Spiral	Colles	Pott

FIGURE 23-7 ▲ Some types of fractures.

breaking. This characteristic explains the greenstick fracture that is seen in children. A **greenstick fracture** occurs when the bone breaks on one side but not the other, like bending a green tree branch. In children and adolescents, an area of growing tissue called the **growth plate** (epiphyseal plate) can be found near each end of a long bone (Figure 23-8). During adolescence, the growth plates are replaced by solid bone when growth is complete. In a child, the growth plate is the weakest part of the skeleton.

The growth plate is even weaker than the surrounding ligaments and tendons. An injury to the growth plate is a fracture. Most growth plate injuries are caused by falls. Growth of the bone can be affected if a fracture in or around the growth plate causes the blood supply to the bone to be cut off. The healing of this type of injury is watched closely by the child's doctor.

An open fracture may result from bone ends or fragments tearing out through the skin (Figure 23-9).

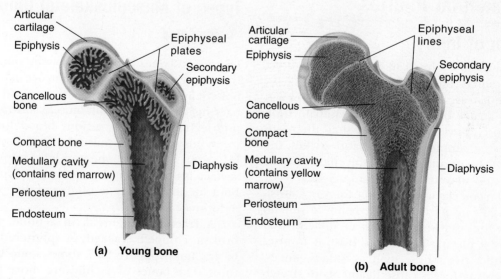

FIGURE 23-8 ▲ **(a)** The femur (thigh bone) of a child showing the growth plate (epiphyseal plate). **(b)** Adult long bone.

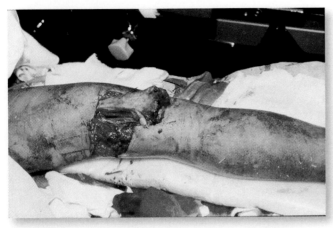

FIGURE 23-9 ▲ An open femur fracture. *Trauma.org Image.*

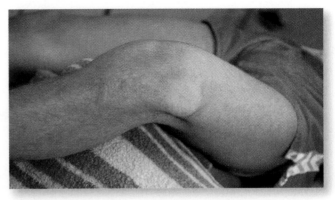

FIGURE 23-11 ▲ Knee dislocation. *Trauma.org Image.*

It may also be caused by a penetrating injury that has damaged a bone and the surrounding soft tissues, such as a gunshot wound. Closed fractures have no opening through the skin but can result in serious internal bleeding. For example, a broken femur (thighbone) can result in the loss of up to 1 L of blood. If the fracture is closed, the blood will have no place to go except to the surrounding tissue. As bleeding continues, the blood vessels and tissues of the thigh become compressed, reducing blood flow throughout the leg. Whether a fracture is open or closed, the movement of sharp bone ends can cause damage to arteries, muscles, and nerves. A suspected fracture should be immobilized to prevent further injury and pain.

A **dislocation** occurs when the end of a bone is forced from its normal position in a joint (Figure 23-10).

A partial dislocation (**subluxation**) means the bone is partially out of the joint. A complete dislocation means it is all the way out. Dislocations and subluxations usually result in temporary deformity of the affected joints and may result in sudden and severe pain. The surrounding muscles often spasm from the disruption, which worsens the pain. The pain stops almost immediately once the bone is back in place.

Dislocations most often occur in major joints such as the shoulder, hip, knee, elbow, or ankle (Figure 23-11). They can occur in smaller joints such as the finger, thumb or toe. Dislocations are usually caused by trauma, such as a fall. They can also be caused by an underlying disease, such as rheumatoid arthritis.

Dislocations and subluxations are dangerous because the change of position of the bone or bones involved can compress or damage the joint and its surrounding muscles, ligaments, nerves, or blood

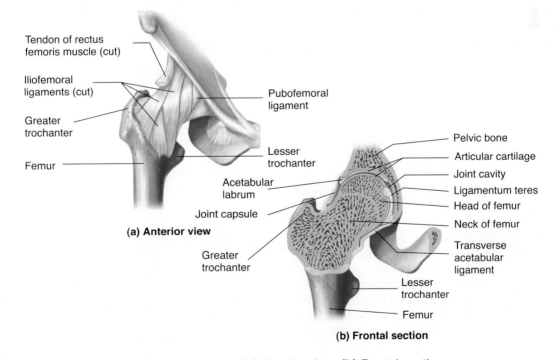

(a) Anterior view

(b) Frontal section

FIGURE 23-10 ▲ Dislocation of the right hip joint. **(a)** Anterior view. **(b)** Frontal section.

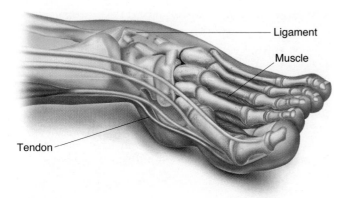

FIGURE 23-12 ▲ A sprain is a stretching or tearing of a ligament. Pain and bruising are usually present with all types of sprains.

vessels. Severe damage to nerves and blood vessels can occur if a joint is not put back in place properly. For this reason, you should not try to reduce (put back into place) a dislocation. A dislocation or subluxation may go back into place by itself. Be sure to let the healthcare professional to whom you are transferring patient care know if this occurs.

Remember This!

Remember: Ligaments "sprain"; muscles "strain."

A **sprain** is a stretching or tearing of a ligament, the connective tissue that joins the end of one bone with another (Figure 23-12). Sprains are classified as mild, moderate, and severe. Pain and bruising are usually present with all categories of sprains. When a sprain occurs, the patient will usually feel a tear or pop in the joint. A severe sprain produces excruciating pain at the moment of injury as the ligaments tear completely or separate from the bone. Tearing or separation loosens the joint and makes it nonfunctional. A moderate sprain partially tears the ligament, loosens the joint, and produces some swelling. A ligament is stretched in a mild sprain, but there is no joint loosening.

A **strain** is a twisting, pulling, or tearing of a muscle (Figure 23-13). Muscle injuries are more common than bone injuries. A muscle strain usually occurs when a muscle is stretched beyond its limit. A strain often occurs near the point where the muscle joins the tough connective tissue of the tendon. For example, muscles of the lower back may be strained when improper lifting or moving techniques are used. The signs and symptoms of a strain include pain with movement, little or no swelling, and a limited ability to bear weight on the affected extremity. The area around the injury may be tender to the touch. Bruising may be present if blood vessels are broken.

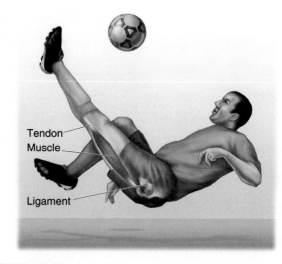

FIGURE 23-13 ▲ A strain is a twist, pull, or tear of a muscle or tendon.

Remember This!

Because they are treated in the same way, it is not important for you to know if an injury is a particular type of fracture or if the injury involves a muscle or bone. Treat any injury to an arm or leg as if a fracture exists.

Signs and Symptoms of Musculoskeletal Injuries

The signs and symptoms of musculoskeletal injuries vary depending upon the severity and type of injury. The three most common signs and symptoms of a musculoskeletal injury are pain, deformity, and swelling.

You Should Know

Signs and Symptoms of Musculoskeletal Injuries

- Pain or tenderness over the injury site
- Swelling
- Deformity, angulation (abnormal position of an extremity)
- Crepitation (grating sensation or sound)
- Limited movement
- Joint locked into position
- Exposed bone ends
- Bruising
- Bleeding
- Difference in length, shape, or size of one extremity compared with the other
- Loss of pulse or sensation below the injury site

Emergency Care of Musculoskeletal Injuries

To treat a patient with musculoskeletal injuries, perform the following steps:

- Conduct a scene size-up and ensure your safety. Assess the mechanism of injury before approaching the patient. Put on appropriate personal protective equipment (PPE).

- Perform a primary survey to identify and treat any life-threatening conditions. Stabilize the cervical spine if needed. If signs of shock are present or if internal bleeding is suspected, treat for shock.

- Perform a physical examination. Remember the DCAP-BTLS memory aid to recall what to look and feel for during the physical exam:
  —**D**eformities
  —**C**ontusions (bruises)
  —**A**brasions (scrapes)
  —**P**unctures/penetrations
  —**B**urns
  —**T**enderness
  —**L**acerations (cuts)
  —**S**welling

- Look for deformities, open injuries, and swelling. Note if signs of compartment syndrome are present (see Chapter 22). Feel along the length of the extremity for deformities, tenderness, and swelling. Feel and listen for crepitus, which is the grating of broken bone ends against each other. Check the *pulse, movement,* and *sensation* (PMS) in each extremity. Compare each extremity to the opposite extremity.
  —Assess the dorsalis pedis pulse (on top of the foot) in each lower extremity. Assess the radial pulse in each upper extremity.
  —If the patient is awake, assess movement of the lower extremities by asking if he can push his feet into your hands. Assess movement of the upper extremities by asking the patient to squeeze your fingers. Compare the strength of his grips and note if they are equal or if one side appears weaker.
  —If the patient is awake, assess sensation by touching the fingers and toes of each extremity and asking him to tell you where you are touching. Assess the patient's thumb or pinky (or great toe or baby toe) to avoid the confusion of having to describe which "middle" digit is being touched. If the patient is unresponsive, assess movement and sensation by gently pinching each foot and hand. See if the patient responds to pain with facial movements or movement of the extremity being pinched.

- Take the patient's vital signs and gather the patient's medical history.

- Cover open wounds with a sterile dressing. If bone ends are visible, do not intentionally reposition or replace them.

- Splint any bone or joint injuries. This technique is explained in detail in the next section.
  —Before applying a splint, you should manually stabilize the injured extremity. This will require another person, who will use his hands to gently support the extremity. To stabilize an injured bone, support the joints above and below the injury. For example, if a bone in the lower leg is broken, your assistant should use his hands to stabilize both the ankle and the knee. When a splint is applied, the splint must be long enough to stabilize both of these joints. To stabilize an injured joint, support the bones above and below it. Additional support may be needed underneath the injured area so that it does not sag. Do not release manual stabilization until the injured area has been properly immobilized.
  —Pad a rigid or semi-rigid splint before applying it. Padding helps lessen patient discomfort caused by pressure, especially around bony areas. After the extremity is splinted, apply an ice bag or cold pack. Place a cloth or bandage between the patient's skin and the cold source.

- Most sprains and strains can be treated with the RICE technique. RICE stands for *r*est, *i*ce, *c*ompression, and *e*levation.
  —*Rest.* Using a body part increases blood flow to that area and can increase swelling. Tell the patient to avoid using the injured area while it heals. The length of rest is determined by how severe the injury is.
  —*Ice.* Use a cold pack or place ice in a plastic bag and remove the excess air. Do not apply ice or a cold pack directly to the skin. Wrap the cold source in a cloth. Apply the ice to the injured area for 20 minutes and then remove it for 40 minutes. Follow this rotation hourly. Ice reduces blood flow into the affected area, which in turn reduces swelling.

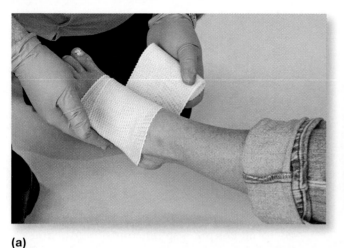

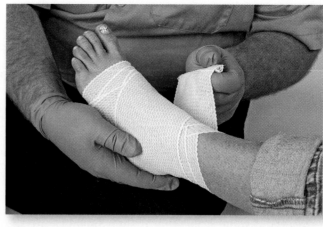

(a)   **(b)**

FIGURE 23-14 ▲ (a) When applying a compression bandage, begin wrapping below the injured area. **(b)** As you wrap the injured area, move toward the heart. Each wrap should overlap about one half the bandage's width.

—*Compression.* Apply an elastic bandage to the injured area. Compression reduces swelling and supports the injured area. It also allows for minor weight bearing and limited function. Use a 2-inch bandage for an injury to the wrist or hand. A 3-inch bandage should be used for the elbow and arm. Use a 4- or 6-inch bandage for an injury to the ankle, knee, or leg. When applying a compression bandage, begin wrapping the bandage below the injury (from the point farthest from the heart) (Figure 23-14). Wrap the injured area in an upward direction (toward the heart), overlapping about one half of the bandage's width. Make sure that the bandage is not wrapped too tightly. It must be tight enough to provide support but loose enough to allow circulation to the area. Assess pulses, movement, and sensation after applying the bandage. Be sure to document your findings.

—*Elevation.* To reduce swelling, keep the injured extremity higher than the patient's heart. This also helps remove waste products from the injured area.

Remember This!

- **D**eformities
- **C**ontusions (bruises)
- **A**brasions (scrapes)
- **P**unctures/ penetrations
- **B**urns
- **T**enderness
- **L**acerations (cuts)
- **S**welling
- **R**est
- **I**ce
- **C**ompression
- **E**levation
- **P**ulse
- **M**ovement
- **S**ensation

- Comfort, calm, and reassure the patient, family members, and friends of the patient. Perform ongoing assessments as often as needed.
- Record all patient care information, including the patient's medical history and all emergency care given, on a prehospital care report.

Stop and Think!

- If you are not sure whether a musculoskeletal injury is present, manually stabilize the injured area and then apply a splint. If no life-threatening conditions are present, splint an injured extremity before moving the patient.
- *Always* assess pulses, movement, and sensation in an extremity before and after care of the injury. Compare your assessment with an assessment of the opposite extremity. Be sure to document your findings.
- Make sure to remove any jewelry or tight clothing distal to an extremity injury. Doing so will allow for easy removal without cutting. It will also prevent injury from tissue compression once swelling increases.

Splinting

Objectives 5, 7

A splint is a device used to limit movement of (immobilize) a body part to prevent pain and further injury. The following *You Should Know* box lists the reasons for splinting. It also lists the hazards associated with improper splinting.

You Should Know

Reasons for Splinting

- To limit the motion of bone fragments, bone ends, or dislocated joints
- To lessen the damage to muscles, nerves, or blood vessels caused by broken bones
- To help prevent a closed injury from becoming an open injury
- To lessen the restriction of blood flow caused by bone ends or dislocations compressing blood vessels
- To reduce bleeding resulting from tissue damage caused by bone ends
- To reduce pain associated with the movement of the bone and the joint
- To reduce the risk of paralysis caused by a damaged spine

In some situations, the patient will have already splinted the injury by holding the injured part close to his body in a comfortable position. For example, you may find a patient with an injured wrist holding his arm close to his chest. With this type of injury, the patient will usually support the injured arm with his uninjured arm. Using the body as a splint is called an **anatomic splint,** also called a *self-splint*.

Many types of ready-made splints are available. If a ready-made splint is not available, a splint can be made. Materials commonly used include rolled-up magazines, branches, newspapers, umbrellas, boards, canes, cardboard, broom handles, wooden spoons, or a foam sleeping pad. An injured body part is usually secured to a splint with wide bandages or straps. If these materials are not available, you can substitute bandannas, climbing webbing, or torn pieces of clothing. Do not use narrow pieces of material because they can act like a tourniquet. A bandage or strap should never be tight enough to impede blood flow.

General Rules of Splinting

Objective 6

Follow these general guidelines when splinting a musculoskeletal injury:

- Take body substance isolation (BSI) precautions and wear appropriate PPE. In most situations, the patient should not be moved before splinting unless he is in danger.

Remember This!

Hazards of Improper Splinting

- The compression of nerves, tissues, and blood vessels from the splint
- A delay in transport of a patient with a life-threatening injury
- Distal circulation that is reduced as a result of the splint's being applied too tightly to the extremity
- Aggravating the musculoskeletal injury
- Causing or aggravating tissue, nerve, vessel, or muscle damage from excessive bone or joint movement

- If possible, remove or cut away clothing to expose the injury. Remove jewelry from the injured area.
- Assess pulses, movement, and sensation distal to the injury before and after applying a splint. You may find it helpful to lightly mark the pulse location with a pen to save time when rechecking pulses. Assess pulses, movement, and sensation every 15 minutes and document your findings.
- Cover open wounds with a sterile dressing.
- Before applying a rigid or semi-rigid splint, pad it to reduce patient discomfort caused by pressure, especially around bony areas.
- Splint the area above and below the injury. If a bone is injured, immobilize the joint above and below the injury. If a joint is injured, immobilize the bones above and below the injury.
- Before splinting an injured hand or foot, place it in the **position of function** (Figure 23-15). The natural position of the hand at rest looks as if you were gently grasping a small object, such as a baseball. Use a roll of tape, roller gauze, or a rolled up sock or glove as the "ball" and place it in the patient's palm before splinting his hand. Do not place the hand or foot in a position of function if you find it in an abnormal position and meet resistance or cause pain when you attempt to place it in the position of function.
- Pad the hollow areas (voids) between the splint and the extremity.
- Do not intentionally replace protruding bones. During the splinting process, bone ends may be drawn back into the wound. This is to be expected and is acceptable.

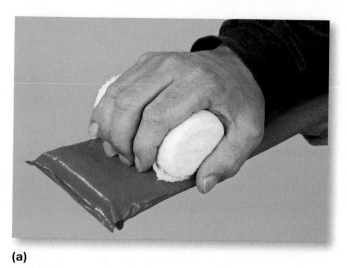

(a)

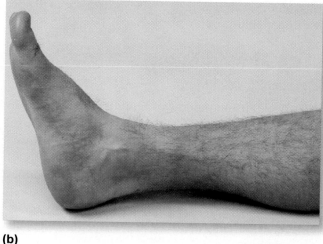

(b)

FIGURE 23-15 ▲ **(a)** Position of function for the hand. **(b)** Position of function for the foot.

- Avoid excessive movement of the injured area when applying a splint.
- When securing the splint to the injured area, avoid placing ties or straps directly over the injury.
- Splint the injury before moving the patient unless he is in danger or life-threatening conditions exist.
- When in doubt about whether a musculoskeletal injury is present, splint the injury.
- If the patient shows signs of shock, align him in the anatomical position on a long backboard. Treat the patient for shock and arrange for transport.

Stop and Think!

If your patient does not have a pulse in an extremity or has lost sensation or the ability to move the fingers or toes of the injured extremity after you applied a splint, the splint is too tight. Manually immobilize the injured area, loosen the splint, and adjust it. Reassess often and be sure to notify the healthcare professional who assumes responsibility for the patient when you transfer care.

Types of Splints

A variety of materials and techniques can be used for splinting. You may have to improvise because of the limited availability of splinting materials and/or the patient's position. Remember: The splint must be long enough to immobilize the area above and below the injury.

Remember This!

Warning Signs That a Splint is Too Tight

- The patient's fingers or toes become cold to the touch in the splinted extremity.
- The patient's fingers or toes begin to turn pale or blue in the splinted extremity.
- The patient is unable to move fingers or toes in the splinted extremity.
- The patient experiences increased pain in the splinted extremity.
- The patient experiences increased swelling below the splint.
- The patient complains of numbness or tingling in the extremity.
- The patient complains of burning or stinging in the splinted extremity.

Rigid Splints

Rigid splints are made of hard material, such as wood, strong cardboard, or plastic (Figure 23-16). They are available in different sizes. Some are preformed to fit certain body areas. Some rigid splints are padded, but others must be padded before they are applied to the patient. This type of splint is useful for immobilizing injuries that occur to the middle portion (midshaft) of a bone. The SAM Splint and aluminum ladder splints are examples of semi-rigid (flexible) splints. These splints can be molded to the shape of the extremity and are very useful for immobilizing joint injuries (Figure 23-17). They can be used in combination with other splints, such as a sling and swathe.

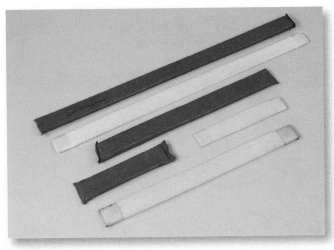

FIGURE 23-16 ▲ Rigid splints.

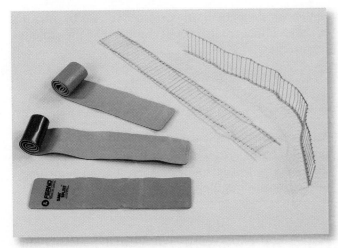

FIGURE 23-17 ▲ Semi-rigid splints.

Soft Splints

Soft splints are flexible and useful for immobilizing injuries of the lower leg or forearm. Examples of soft splints include a sling and swathe, blanket rolls, pillows, and towels (Figure 23-18). A sling and swathe is used to immobilize injuries to the shoulder (scapula), collarbone (clavicle), or upper arm bone (humerus). A triangular bandage is often used to make a sling. A **swathe** is a piece of soft material used to secure the injured extremity to the body. Roller gauze can also be used as a swathe.

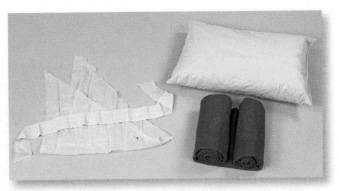

FIGURE 23-18 ▲ Soft splints.

- To make a swathe, unwrap a triangular bandage and place it on a flat surface. Grab the point of the shorter end of the triangle and fold it toward the longer end, like a bandanna.
- The swathe must be tight enough to limit movement of the arm but not so tight that chest movement is restricted. The patient may have difficulty breathing if chest movement is restricted. Make sure the patient's fingers remain exposed so that you can assess the pulse, movement, and sensation.

Traction Splints

A **traction splint** is a device used to immobilize a closed fracture of the femur (thighbone) (Figure 23-19). When applied, this type of splint maintains a constant, steady pull (traction) on the femur. A traction splint decreases muscle spasm and pain. It also keeps broken bone ends in a near-normal position. A unipolar traction splint has one pole that provides external support for the injured leg. A bipolar traction splint uses two external poles, one on each side of the injured leg, to provide external support. Two emergency care professionals are needed to apply a traction splint. Contraindications to the use of a traction splint are shown in the next *You Should Know* box.

Pneumatic Splints

A pneumatic splint requires air to be pumped in or suctioned out of it. The pressure within a pneumatic splint can vary with temperature and altitude. An air

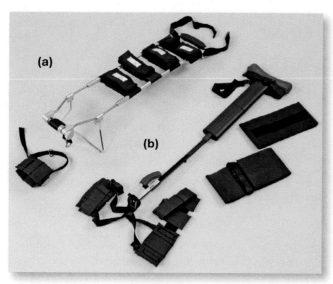

FIGURE 23-19 ▲ Traction splints. **(a)** Bipolar traction splint. **(b)** Unipolar traction splint.

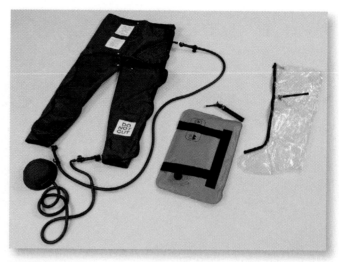

FIGURE 23-20 ▲ Pneumatic splints.

splint, vacuum splint, and the pneumatic anti-shock garment (PASG) are examples of pneumatic splints (Figure 23-20). A pneumatic splint is placed around the injured area and is inflated (air splint or PASG) or deflated (vacuum splint) until it becomes firm. When using an air splint, inflate it until you can make a slight dent in the splint with your fingers.

If permitted by local protocol, a PASG may be used to help control suspected severe bleeding in the abdomen or pelvis that is accompanied by hypotension. Remember that the PASG has three separate compartments that can be inflated: the abdomen, left leg, and right leg. All three compartments are inflated if there is an injury to the abdomen or pelvis. The abdominal compartment is *never* used without inflating both leg compartments. When the PASG is positioned on the patient, the top edge of the garment must be below the patient's lowest ribs. If the garment is positioned higher on the patient, the pressure caused by inflating the abdominal compartment can hamper the patient's breathing.

Care of Specific Musculoskeletal Injuries

Upper-Extremity Injuries

Upper-extremity injuries include injuries to the shoulder (clavicle, scapula, and humerus), upper arm (humerus), elbow, forearm (radius and ulna), wrist, and hand.

Injuries to the Shoulder

A shoulder injury typically involves three bones: the collarbone (clavicle), shoulder blade (scapula), and the upper arm bone (humerus). The patient will usually hold his arm in a position of comfort. Immobilize the injury in this position. Because the entire upper extremity must be immobilized to limit shoulder movement, a sling and swathe is usually used for this type of injury (Skill Drill 23-1). The sling forms a pouch and is used to support the weight of the arm. The swathe is used to immobilize the injury by securing the patient's arm to his chest.

Immobilizing a Shoulder Injury

STEP 1 ▶
- Immobilize a shoulder injury by using a sling and swathe. After assessing for a pulse, movement, and sensation in the injured arm, drape one end of a triangular bandage under the injured arm.
- Drape the other end over the opposite shoulder and around the patient's neck.

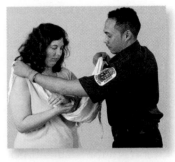

STEP 2 ▶ Pull the end of the bandage that is under the injured arm up to the patient's neck.

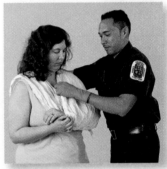

STEP 3 ▶
- Tie the two ends of the bandage to one side of the patient's neck.
- Twist and tuck the corner of the sling at the elbow.

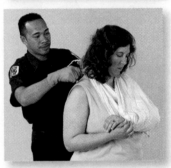

STEP 4 ▶ Use another bandage as a swathe and secure the arm to the chest.

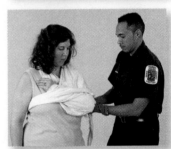

STEP 5 ▶ Reassess pulse, movement, and sensation in the injured arm.

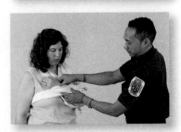

If ready-made materials are not available, fold up the bottom of the patient's shirt and pin or tape it in place for a sling. The arms of a long-sleeved shirt can be tied to one side of the patient's neck and the rest of the shirt used as a sling. A jacket that is zipped closed or wide strips cut from a sheet (or from the bottom of the patient's shirt) can be used as a swathe.

If the patient is holding his arm away from his body, provide support for the injured area, using a pillow, rolled towels, or similar material to fill the gap between the patient's arm and his chest. Secure the patient's arm and any support material to the patient's chest with a swathe. Ask the patient to hold his uninjured arm out to the side. Wrap the swathe around his chest and the injured extremity. Secure the swathe in place with a knot.

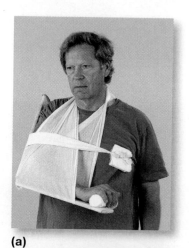

(a)

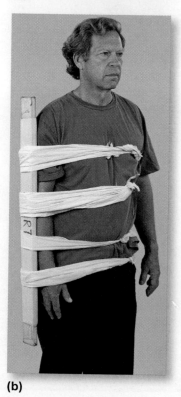

(b)

FIGURE 23-21 ◄ An upper-arm injury is usually best immobilized with a sling and swathe. A padded splint can be used to provide additional support. **(a)** Humerus injury immobilized with the elbow bent. **(b)** Humerus injury immobilized with the elbow straight.

Injuries to the Upper Arm (Humerus)

The upper arm bone (humerus) extends from the shoulder to the elbow. It is most often fractured at its upper end near the shoulder or in the middle of the bone. Fractures of the upper end of the bone typically occur in elderly patients who fall on an outstretched hand. The middle of the bone is more often fractured in young adults. An upper-arm injury should be immobilized from the shoulder (the joint above) to the elbow (the joint below). This type of injury is usually best immobilized with a sling and swathe. The swathe should not be placed directly on top of the injury. It should be positioned either above or below the fracture site. A padded splint or a SAM Splint formed around the upper arm and held in place with roller gauze can be used to provide additional support (Figure 23-21). The following *Making a Difference* box lists the steps used to immobilize a long-bone injury.

Making a Difference

Splinting a Long Bone

Follow these steps to immobilize a closed, nonangulated fracture of the humerus, radius, ulna, femur, tibia, or fibula:

- Take BSI precautions and wear appropriate PPE. Remove or cut away clothing to expose the injury. Remove jewelry from the injured limb.
- Ask an assistant to manually support the injured extremity, using one hand above the injury and one hand below the injury.
- Assess pulses, movement, and sensation below the injured area.
- Select a splint and measure it for proper length against the uninjured extremity. Make sure that the joint above and below the injured area will be immobilized. Pad a rigid or semi-rigid splint.
- Apply the splint, immobilizing the injured bone as well as the joint above and below the injury. When possible, immobilize the injured hand or foot in a position of function. Avoid excessive movement of the injured area when applying the splint.
- Pad the hollow areas between the extremity and the splint. Avoid placing ties or straps directly over the injury. Secure the entire injured extremity.
- Assess pulses, movement, and sensation every 15 minutes and document your findings.

Injuries to the Elbow

The elbow is formed by the joining of the upper arm bone (humerus) and the two forearm bones (radius and ulna). Because there are many nerves and blood vessels in the elbow area, consider an elbow injury a serious injury. Splinting an elbow injury requires immobilizing the humerus (the bone above the injury) and the radius and ulna (the bones below the injury). Many patients will not allow an injured elbow to be moved.

If you find the patient with his elbow in a bent position, consider using a semi-rigid or vacuum splint to immobilize the injury. These splints will conform to the shape of the arm, despite its odd position. You might also use a padded splint. After you have applied a splint, use a sling and swathe to further limit movement if the patient's condition allows him to be placed in a sitting or semi-sitting position.

If the arm is straight, use a soft or rigid splint that extends from the armpit to the wrist. Secure the injured arm to the body to prevent movement (Figure 23-22). Prepare for immediate transport. The following *Making a Difference* box lists the steps used to immobilize a joint injury.

Making a Difference

Splinting a Joint

Follow these steps to immobilize a closed, nonangulated injury to the elbow or knee:

- Take BSI precautions and wear appropriate PPE. Remove or cut away clothing to expose the injury. Remove jewelry from the injured limb.
- Ask an assistant to manually support the injured extremity with one hand above and one hand below the injury.
- Assess pulses, movement, and sensation below the injured area.
- Select a splint and measure it for proper length against the uninjured extremity. Make sure that the bones above and below the injured area will be immobilized. Pad a rigid or semi-rigid splint.
- Apply the splint, immobilizing the injured joint and the bones above and below the injury. When possible, immobilize an injured hand or foot in a position of function. Avoid excessive movement of the injured area when applying the splint.
- Pad the hollow areas between the extremity and the splint. Secure the entire injured extremity.
- Assess pulses, movement, and sensation every 15 minutes and document your findings.

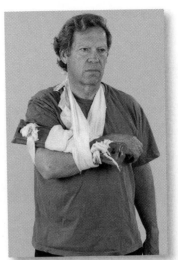

FIGURE 23-22 ◄
(a) Elbow injury immobilized with the elbow bent. **(b)** Elbow injury immobilized in a straight position.

(a)

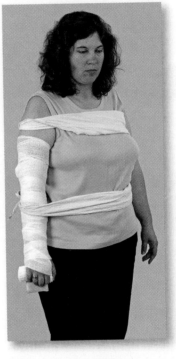

(b)

Injuries to the Forearm, Wrist, and Hand

The forearm, wrist, and hands contain many bones and are commonly injured. These areas can sustain serious injury with or without any visible deformity. The forearm extends from the elbow to the wrist. Some wrist fractures may present with gross deformity and hand displacement. Immobilize the extremity in the position found with a soft, rigid, or pneumatic splint.

When immobilizing an injury of the forearm, wrist, or hand with a rigid, semi-rigid, or soft splint, place the splint underneath the forearm. Remember that the joints above and below the injury site must be immobilized. Therefore, the splint must extend from the elbow (the joint above) to beyond the hand (the joint below). An injured forearm or wrist

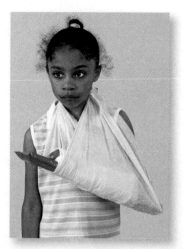

FIGURE 23-23 ▲ Immobilization of an injury to the forearm or wrist.

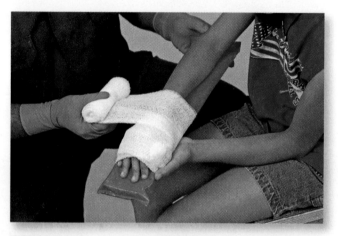

FIGURE 23-24 ▲ Immobilization of an injured hand.

should be placed in a sling and secured to the body with a swathe (Figure 23-23). A hand injury can be immobilized by using a variety of materials. Before applying the splint, place the hand in a position of function unless there is gross deformity or displacement (Figure 23-24). When possible, remember to leave the fingers exposed to check color, movement, and sensation.

If a finger is injured, you can use an anatomic splint by taping the injured finger to an uninjured finger next to it. Taping fingers (or toes) together is also called *buddy taping*. Provide additional support for the injured finger by placing padding between it and the finger next to it (Figure 23-25). If more than one finger is injured, immobilize the entire hand.

Lower-Extremity Injuries

Lower-extremity injuries involve the pelvis, hip, thigh (femur), knee, lower leg (tibia and fibula), ankle, foot, and toes.

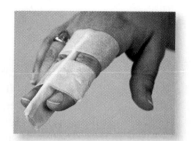

FIGURE 23-25 ▲ Immobilization of a finger injury.

Remember This!

The patient who has an isolated arm injury is often most comfortable in a sitting or semi-sitting position. If the patient's condition requires that he be positioned on his back, the weight of the patient's arm and splint on his chest and upper abdomen can hamper chest movement. If the patient *must* be positioned on his back and the arm must be immobilized with the elbow bent, try to splint the patient's arm so that the weight of the arm and splint will be supported on the patient's upper legs, rather than on his chest or abdomen. Using a soft pillow under the injured extremity will help alleviate and distribute the weight more evenly across the chest and allow better lung expansion if the patient must absolutely be transported flat on his back.

Injuries to the Pelvis and Hip

An injury to the pelvis can result in massive, life-threatening internal bleeding. Swelling and obvious deformity may not be easy to see because the pelvis is protected by many muscles and soft tissues. Call for Advanced Life Support (ALS) personnel immediately. Keep in mind that a force strong enough to cause an injury to the pelvis demands spinal stabilization as well. Treat the patient for shock if an injury to the pelvis is present.

The hip joint is formed by the socket of the hip bone and the upper end of the thighbone (femur). In a hip dislocation, the upper end of the thighbone is popped out of its socket. As the bone is pushed out of its socket, blood vessels and nerves can be damaged. The patient usually complains of severe pain and is unable to move the affected leg. If nerve damage is present, the patient may not have any feeling in the foot or ankle area. You may see that one leg is shorter than the other, and the affected leg may be turned inward or outward. When present, these signs suggest a hip fracture; however, they are not always present. About 50% of patients with a hip dislocation have other injuries, such as injuries to the pelvis, legs, back, or head.

In most hip dislocations, the head of the thighbone is pushed out and back (a posterior dislocation). This most often occurs during a motor vehicle crash (MVC) when a front seat occupant strikes the dashboard with his knees. The energy from the impact is transmitted along the femur to the hip joint. In a posterior dislocation, the hip is in a fixed position, bent and twisted in toward the middle of the body.

In an anterior hip dislocation, the upper end of the thighbone slips out of its socket and moves forward. With this type of injury, the hip is usually only slightly bent and the leg twists out and away from the middle of the body. An anterior dislocation is much less common than a posterior dislocation.

Immobilizing the pelvis or hip requires the use of a splint that extends from the level of the lower back and past the knee on the affected side. A long backboard is usually used for this purpose. A blanket or similar padding is placed between the patient's legs. The injured leg is secured to the uninjured leg and the patient's entire body is secured to the backboard (Figure 23-26). When splinting the legs together, move the good leg to the injured leg. If possible, *do not move the injured leg to the good leg.* Secure the legs together with straps, triangular bandages, or roller gauze secured in four places on the legs—two above the knee and two below. Ties are usually placed just above the ankles, at the calves, just above the knees, and at the thighs. Make sure the knots are secured over the padded material between the patient's legs so that they do not rub against the patient. Additional straps or triangular bandages should be used around the pelvis to secure it to the backboard and limit movement.

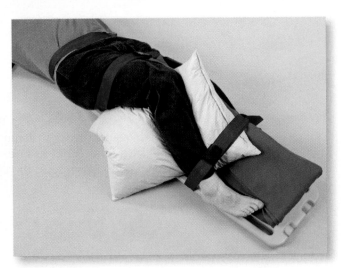

FIGURE 23-27 ▲ Immobilization of a hip injury.

In many cases, a patient with a hip injury will not be able to move the affected leg into a straight position. In these situations, support the affected leg with pillows and rolled blankets between and under the legs. Secure the patient's hips and legs to a long backboard with straps, triangular bandages, or roller gauze to limit movement (Figure 23-27). An injury to the pelvis can also be immobilized with a PASG or pelvic sling. These devices may be used *only* if medical direction allows you to do so. Check with your instructor or medical director.

Injuries to the Upper Thigh (Femur)

Because the femur (thighbone) is protected by large muscles, a great deal of force is required to break it. Most femur fractures involve the middle or upper end of the bone. A broken femur can occur in activities such as skiing, cycling, falls from a great height, and MVCs. It can also occur as a result of child abuse. The injured leg will often appear shorter than the other leg. In addition, the injured leg is often rotated. A broken femur is a true emergency because a patient can easily lose more than a liter of blood internally. Call for ALS personnel immediately. Bone fragments can cause damage to blood vessels, nerves, and soft tissues. Life-threatening bleeding may be present if both femurs are broken.

A fracture of the upper third of the femur is treated as a hip fracture. A closed fracture of the middle third of the femur is best immobilized with a traction splint (Skill Drills 23-2 and 23-3). Applying traction helps stabilize the bone ends and reduces pain. It also reduces the likelihood of a closed fracture becoming an open one and reduces further soft-tissue damage.

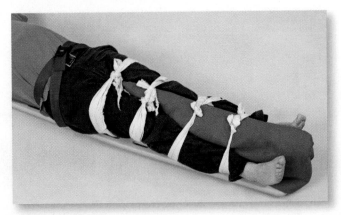

FIGURE 23-26 ▲ Immobilization of an injury to the pelvis or hips.

Applying a Unipolar Traction Splint

STEP 1 ▷ • Expose the fracture site and make sure the injury is a closed, nonangulated midshaft femur fracture.
• Remove the patient's shoe and assess distal pulses, movement, and sensation in the injured leg.

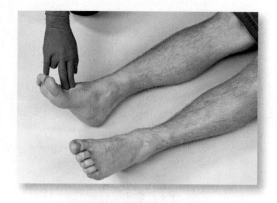

STEP 2 ▷ Place the splint next to the patient's injured leg and adjust the length so that the wheel is even with the patient's heel.

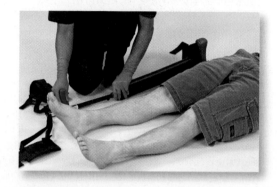

STEP 3 ▷ Place the splint along the inside of the patient's injured leg. Slide the thigh strap up under the thigh. Secure the strap snugly across the thigh.

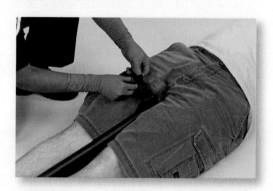

STEP 4 ▷ Apply the ankle hitch to the patient's ankle.

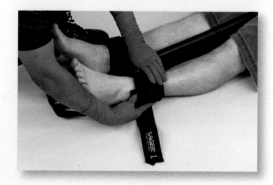

STEP 5 ▶ Apply traction by lengthening the splint. Traction should be applied that is approximately 10% of the patient's body weight, not to exceed 15 pounds of traction.

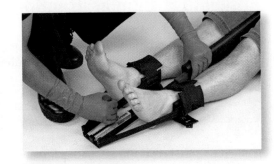

STEP 6 ▶ Fasten the leg straps to secure the leg to the splint. Position the longest strap as high as possible on the thigh. Position the other straps around the knees and lower leg.

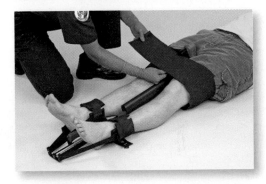

STEP 7 ▶ Reassess distal pulses, movement, and sensation.

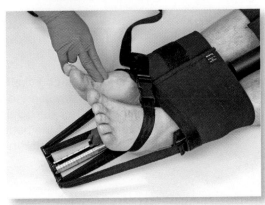

STEP 8 ▶ Place the patient on a long backboard and secure the patient to the board.

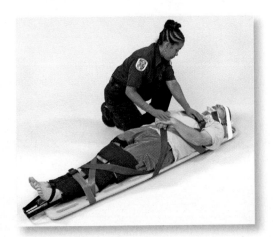

Applying a Bipolar Traction Splint

STEP 1 ▷
- Adjust the traction splint to the proper length. Position the splint next to the patient's uninjured leg, using the bony prominence of the buttock as a landmark. Extend the splint 6-12 inches beyond the patient's uninjured heel. Lock the splint in position.
- Position the support straps at the midthigh, above the knee, below the knee, and above the ankle. Open the straps and fasten them under the splint.

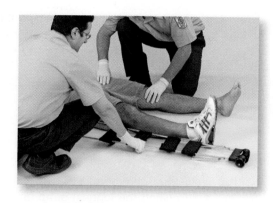

STEP 2 ▷
- Stabilize the injured leg so that it does not move while an assistant fastens the ankle hitch around the patient's foot and ankle.
- Support the leg under the injured area while your assistant applies gentle in-line traction to the injured leg by using the ankle hitch and foot.

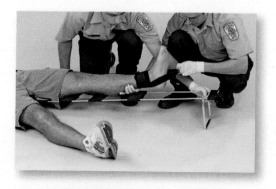

STEP 3 ▷
- While your assistant continues to apply gentle manual traction, position the splint under the injured leg. The ischial pad should rest against the bony prominence of the buttocks.
- Raise the heel stand after the splint is in position.

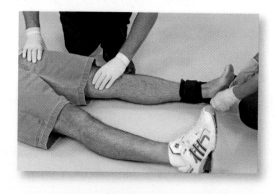

STEP 4 ▷
- Pad the groin area.
- Attach the ischial strap. Secure the strap over the groin and thigh.

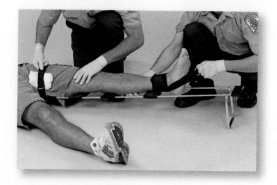

STEP 5 ▷ While your assistant continues to apply gentle manual traction, attach the S hook of the splint to the D ring of the ankle hitch.

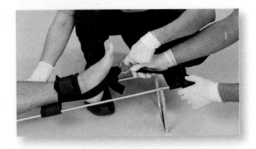

STEP 6 ▷ • While manual traction continues, begin tightening the ratchet on the splint to apply mechanical traction.
   • Continue tightening until mechanical traction is equal to the manual traction and the patient's pain and muscle spasms are reduced. If the patient is unconscious, continue tightening until the length of the injured leg equals that of the uninjured leg.

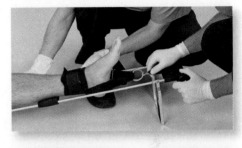

STEP 7 ▷ • Fasten the leg support straps over the injured leg.
   • Recheck the ischial strap and ankle hitch. Make sure both are fastened securely.

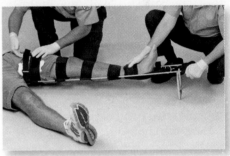

STEP 8 ▷ Reassess distal pulses, movement, and sensation.

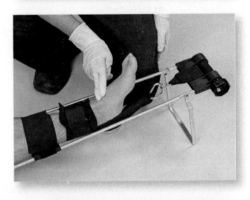

STEP 9 ▷ • Place the patient on a long backboard.
   • Secure the leg and splint in place. Place padding between the splint and the uninjured leg.

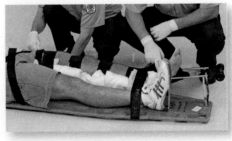

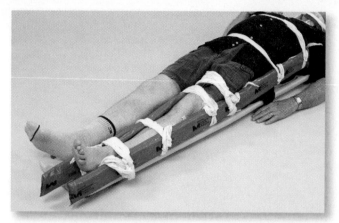

FIGURE 23-28 ▲ Immobilization of a femur fracture.

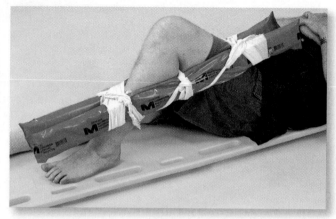

FIGURE 23-29 ▲ Immobilization of the knee in a bent position.

A femur fracture can also be immobilized by using two long boards (Figure 23-28). Use a board on the outside of the leg that extends from the patient's armpit to below the bottom of the foot. Use a board on the inside of the leg that extends from the patient's groin to below the bottom of the foot. Be sure to pad any hollow areas and then secure the boards to the patient with straps, triangular bandages, or roller gauze. Secure the boards under the patient's arms, at the hips, just above the knees, at the calves, and just above the ankles. Be sure the knots are secured on the outside of the boards. Additional straps or triangular bandages must be used when you are securing the patient to a long backboard.

Injuries to the Knee

The knee joint is formed by the lower end of the femur (thighbone), the upper end of the tibia (shinbone), and the patella (kneecap). The kneecap is frequently dislocated from injuries such as a fall. This type of injury usually appears as a lump on the lateral side of the knee. You will often find the patient complaining of pain with his leg in a bent position at the knee. Distal pulses are usually present.

A knee dislocation may result from violent direct force, such as the knee hitting the dashboard during a MVC. This type of injury is serious because the popliteal artery behind the knee can be cut or compressed. The patient is often unable to move his leg. The affected leg is usually grossly deformed around the knee. Extensive swelling is usually present, and distal pulses may be absent. Check distal pulses frequently. Call for ALS personnel immediately.

If you find the patient with his knee in a bent position, support the affected knee with a pillow. To limit movement, place a padded board splint on

each side of the knee from the thigh to the calf (Figure 23-29). Secure the boards in place with triangular bandages or roller gauze above and below the knee.

If the knee is straight, place a long, padded board splint on each side of the knee (Figure 23-30). The board on the outside of the leg should extend from the patient's hip to the ankle. The board on the inside of the leg should extend from the groin to the ankle. Tie triangular bandages or roller gauze above and below the knee, at the uppermost part of the thigh, and just above the ankle. Be sure the ties are positioned on the outside of the splint.

Injuries to the Lower Leg

The tibia and fibula are the bones of the lower leg. A fracture of the tibia is the most common type of long-bone fracture. Fractures of the lower leg usually occur as a result of a direct force injury, such as a fall, an MVC, or a twisting force. A fracture of

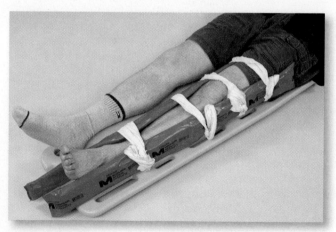

FIGURE 23-30 ▲ Immobilization of the knee in a straight position.

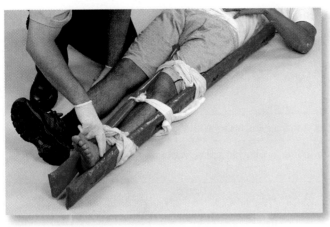
(a)

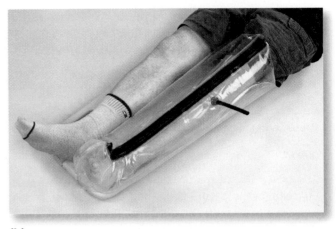
(b)

FIGURE 23-31 ▲ Immobilization of the lower leg. **(a)** Immobilization by means of padded boards. **(b)** Immobilization by means of an air splint.

either the tibia or fibula can occur by itself. However, a tibia fracture is usually associated with a fibula fracture because the force that causes the tibia fracture is transmitted to the fibula. Bruising, swelling, and tenderness are usually present over the fracture site. When the tibia is broken, the patient will complain of pain when he puts weight on it. Because the tibia lies very close to the skin surface, a large number of fractures involving these bones are open fractures.

Immobilize a fracture of the tibia and fibula with a splint that extends from the hip to the foot. Place a padded board splint on each side of the leg (Figure 23-31). The board on the outside of the leg should extend from the patient's hip to the foot. The board on the inside of the leg should extend from the groin to the foot. Make sure to pad behind the knee to keep it in a position of comfort. Use triangular bandages or roller gauze to secure the boards in place. For a closed injury, an air splint that extends above the knee and covers the entire foot may be used instead of padded boards.

Injuries to the Ankle and Foot

The ankle is formed by the lower ends of the tibia and the fibula (the shinbones) and the many smaller bones of the foot. It is difficult to tell when an ankle or foot injury is a fracture or a sprain because both are very painful and swell a great deal. An ankle or foot injury is best immobilized with a preformed lower leg splint, a soft splint such as a pillow or blanket, or an air splint (Figure 23-32).

Splints that can be used for various bone and joint injuries are listed in Table 23-3.

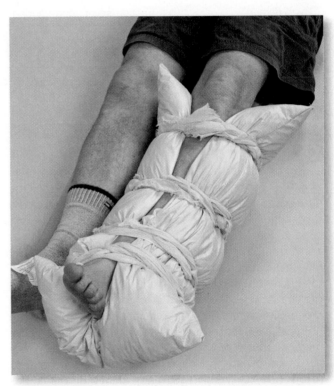

FIGURE 23-32 ▲ Immobilization of an ankle or foot injury.

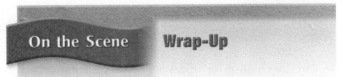
On the Scene   Wrap-Up

You have applied a cervical collar before the Paramedics arrive. The crew chief listens as you give your report. You tell her there are good pulses, movement, and

TABLE 23-3 Possible Splints for Bone and Joint Injuries

Site of Injury	Possible Splints
Shoulder	Sling and swathe
Upper arm (humerus)	Padded board splint, padded wire ladder splint, sling and swathe, SAM Splint
Elbow	Padded board splint, padded wire ladder splint, air splint, vacuum splint, sling and swathe, SAM Splint
Forearm (radius, ulna)	Padded board splint, padded wire ladder splint, air splint, vacuum splint, sling and swathe, SAM Splint
Wrist, hand	Padded board splint, padded wire ladder splint, air splint, vacuum splint, sling and swathe, SAM Splint
Pelvis	Long backboard, scoop stretcher, PASG, pelvic sling
Hip	Long backboard with blanket or pillow between the legs, scoop stretcher, PASG
Thigh (femur)	Traction splint, long padded board splints, other leg used as a splint
Knee	Pillow, padded board splint, SAM Splint, air splint, vacuum splint, other leg used as a splint
Lower leg (tibia, fibula)	Padded board splint, SAM Splint, air splint, vacuum splint, other leg used as a splint
Ankle, foot	Preformed lower leg splint, pillow or blanket, air splint, vacuum splint

sensation distal to each of the patient's injuries. You and your partner apply a traction splint to care for the suspected femur fracture. The Paramedic fashions a rigid splint to support the patient's upper-arm injury. "Pad a formable splint and put it on her right lower arm," the Paramedic instructs you. Your crew carefully reassesses each extremity after the splints are applied to ensure that pulses, movement, and sensation are still present. You apply ice packs to each injured area and move the patient to the ambulance. En route to the hospital, you reassess her vital signs while the Paramedic starts an IV. You call in a report to medical direction, who gives the injured woman some medicine to relieve her pain. As you get ready to step off the ambulance, you notice that your patient's eyes close and her face visibly relaxes. ∎

Sum It Up

▶ The mechanism of injury to bones and joints can be caused by direct forces, indirect forces, and twisting forces:
  • A direct force causes injury at the point of impact.

  • An indirect force causes injury at a site other than the point of impact.
  • A twisting force causes one part of an extremity to remain in place while the rest twists. Twisting injuries commonly affect the joints such as ankles, knees, and wrists. Twisting forces cause ligaments to stretch and tear.
▶ Injuries to bones and joints may be open or closed:
  • In an open injury, the skin surface is broken. An open injury increases the risk of contamination and infection. These injuries can also result in serious blood loss.
  • In closed injuries of bones and joints, the skin surface is not broken. The injury is often painful, swollen, and deformed.
▶ A fracture is a break in a bone. If a bone is broken, chipped, cracked, or splintered, it is said to be fractured.
▶ A dislocation occurs when the ends of bones are forced from their normal positions in a joint.
▶ A subluxation, which is a partial dislocation, means the bone is partially out of the joint. A complete dislocation means it is all the way out. Dislocations and subluxations usually result in temporary

deformity of the joint and may result in sudden and severe pain.

- A sprain is a stretching or tearing of a ligament, the connective tissue that joins the end of one bone with another. Sprains are classified as mild, moderate, and severe.

- A strain is a twisting, pulling, or tearing of a muscle or tendon. A muscle strain usually occurs when a muscle is stretched beyond its limit. A strain often occurs near the point where the muscle joins the tough connective tissue of the tendon.

- Most sprains and strains can be treated with the *RICE* technique:
  - *R*est
  - *I*ce
  - *C*ompression
  - *E*levation

- In assessing extremity injuries, check the pulse, movement, and sensation (PMS) in each extremity.

- A splint is a device used to limit movement of a body part (immobilize) to prevent pain and further injury.
  - In some situations, the patient will have already splinted the injury by holding the injured part close to his body in a comfortable position. Using the body as a splint is called a self-splint or anatomic splint.
  - Before splinting an injured hand or foot, place it in the position of function. The natural position of the hand at rest looks as if you were gently grasping a small object, such as a baseball.

- Rigid splints are made of hard material, such as wood, strong cardboard, or plastic. This type of splint is useful for immobilizing injuries that occur to the middle portion (midshaft) of a bone. Some rigid splints are padded, but others must be padded before they are applied to the patient.

- Semi-rigid (flexible) splints are very useful for immobilizing joint injuries. These splints can be molded to the shape of the extremity. Examples include the SAM Splint and aluminum ladder splints. Semi-rigid splints can be used in combination with other splints, such as a sling and swathe.

- Soft splints are flexible and useful for immobilizing injuries of the lower leg or forearm. Examples of soft splints include a sling and swathe, blanket rolls, pillows, and towels.
  - A sling and swathe is used to immobilize injuries to the shoulder, collarbone, or upper arm bone. A triangular bandage is often used to make a sling. A swathe is a piece of soft material used to secure the injured extremity to the body.

- A traction splint is a device used to immobilize a closed fracture of the thighbone. This type of splint maintains a constant steady pull on the bone. A traction splint keeps broken bone ends in a near-normal position.
  - A unipolar traction splint has one pole that provides external support for the injured leg.
  - A bipolar traction splint uses two external poles, one on each side of the injured leg, to provide external support

- A pneumatic splint requires air to be pumped in or suctioned out of it. An air splint, vacuum splint, and the pneumatic antishock garment (PASG) are examples of pneumatic splints. A pneumatic splint is placed around the injured area and is inflated (air splint or PASG) or deflated (vacuum splint) until it becomes firm.

24 Injuries to the Head and Spine

By the end of this chapter, you should be able to:

Knowledge Objectives ▶

1. State the components of the nervous system.
2. List the functions of the central nervous system.
3. Define the structure of the skeletal system as it relates to the nervous system.
4. Relate mechanism of injury to potential injuries of the head and spine.
5. Describe the implications of not properly caring for potential spine injuries.
6. State the signs and symptoms of a potential spine injury.
7. Describe the method of determining whether a responsive patient may have a spine injury.
8. Relate the airway emergency medical care techniques to the patient with a suspected spine injury.
9. Describe how to stabilize the cervical spine.
10. Discuss indications for sizing and using a cervical spine immobilization device.
11. Establish the relationship between airway management and the patient with head and spine injuries.
12. Describe a method for sizing a cervical spine immobilization device.
13. Describe how to log roll a patient with a suspected spine injury.
14. Describe how to secure a patient to a long spine board.
15. List instances when a short spine board should be used.
16. Describe how to immobilize a patient by using a short spine board.
17. Describe the indications for the use of rapid extrication.
18. List steps in performing rapid extrication.
19. State the circumstances in which a helmet should be left on the patient.
20. Discuss the circumstances in which a helmet should be removed.
21. Identify different types of helmets.
22. Describe the unique characteristics of sports helmets.
23. Explain the preferred methods to remove a helmet.
24. Discuss alternative methods for removal of a helmet.
25. Describe how the patient's head is stabilized to remove the helmet.
26. Differentiate between how the head is stabilized with a helmet and how it is stabilized without a helmet.

Attitude Objectives ▶ **27.** Explain the rationale for immobilization of the entire spine when a cervical spine injury is suspected.

28. Explain the rationale for using immobilization methods apart from the straps on the cots.

29. Explain the rationale for using a short spine immobilization device when moving a patient from the sitting to the supine position.

30. Explain the rationale for using rapid extrication approaches only when they indeed will make the difference between life and death.

31. Defend the reasons for leaving a helmet in place for transport of a patient.

32. Defend the reasons for removal of a helmet before transport of a patient.

Skill Objectives ▶ **33.** Demonstrate opening the airway in a patient with suspected spinal cord injury.

34. Demonstrate evaluating a responsive patient with a suspected spinal cord injury.

35. Demonstrate stabilization of the cervical spine.

36. Demonstrate the 3-person log roll for a patient with a suspected spinal cord injury.

37. Demonstrate securing a patient to a long spine board.

38. Demonstrate using the short board immobilization technique.

39. Demonstrate procedure for rapid extrication.

40. Demonstrate preferred methods for stabilization of a helmet.

41. Demonstrate helmet removal techniques.

42. Demonstrate alternative methods for stabilization of a helmet.

43. Demonstrate completing a prehospital care report for patients with head and spinal injuries.

On the Scene

You and your Emergency Medical Technician partner are dispatched to a construction site for a head injury. Upon arrival, you find a 28-year-old man lying on the floor in the construction site office. Your first impression reveals the patient is awake and aware of your approach. He appears to be breathing normally and his skin color is pink. A coworker is holding a bloodied towel to the side of the patient's head.

The patient states that while he was working, an 8-pound sledgehammer fell from about 8-10 feet above him onto his head. He then walked about 80 feet to his supervisor's office where they laid him down and controlled the bleeding from his head wound. Your partner finds an approximately 1-inch full-thickness laceration to the patient's right temporal area. The patient's initial vital signs are as follows: Pulse 110, strong and regular; respirations 16, unlabored; blood pressure 138/60. The patient denies any loss of consciousness and states that he feels dizzy and nauseated. ∎

THINK ABOUT IT

As you read this chapter, think about the following questions:

- Is the patient's mechanism of injury significant?
- Should the patient receive a rapid trauma assessment or a focused physical examination?
- What emergency care should you provide for this patient?

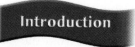

Managing Head and Spine Injuries

Every day in the United States, 30 people experience a spinal cord injury. The most common causes of this injury are motor vehicle crashes (MVCs), sports accidents, falls, penetrating trauma, and industrial mishaps. Sixty percent of these individuals are 30 years of age or younger. If a head or spine injury is missed or improperly treated, permanent disability or death may result. Your initial treatment of a patient with a possible injury to the head or spine can prevent further injury. You must know when to suspect this type of injury and how to provide appropriate care.

Anatomy Review

Nervous System

Central Nervous System

Objectives 1, 2

The nervous system controls the voluntary and involuntary activities of the body. The central nervous system (CNS) is made up of the brain and spinal cord.

The outermost part of the head is called the **scalp.** The scalp contains tissue, hair follicles, sweat glands, oil glands, and a rich supply of blood vessels. The brain occupies the entire space within the cranium. Meninges (literally, membranes) are 3 layers of connective tissue coverings that surround the brain and spinal cord. The **pia mater** (literally, "gentle mother") forms the delicate inner layer that clings gently to the brain and spinal cord. It contains many blood vessels that supply the nervous tissue. The **arachnoid** (literally, "resembling a spider's web") layer is the middle meningeal layer with delicate fibers resembling a spider's web. It contains few blood vessels. The **dura mater** (literally, "hard mother" or "tough mother") is the tough, durable, outermost layer that clings to the inner surface of the cranium.

Cerebrospinal fluid (CSF) surrounds the brain and spinal cord. It acts as a shock-absorber. It also provides a means for exchange of nutrients and wastes between the blood, brain, and spinal cord.

The cerebrum is the largest part of the human brain. It consists of 2 cerebral hemispheres. The corpus callosum joins the 2 hemispheres. Each cerebral hemisphere has 4 lobes:

1. The frontal lobe, which controls motor function
2. The parietal lobe, which receives and interprets nerve impulses from sensory receptors
3. The occipital lobe, which controls eyesight
4. The temporal lobe, which controls hearing and smell

The cerebellum is the second largest part of the human brain. It is responsible for precise control of muscle movements, maintenance of posture, and maintaining balance. The brain stem includes the **midbrain, pons,** and **medulla oblongata.** The midbrain connects the pons and cerebellum with the cerebrum. It acts as a relay for auditory and visual impulses. The pons (literally, "bridge") connects parts of the brain with one another by means of tracts. It influences respiration. The medulla oblongata extends from the pons and is continuous with the upper portion of the spinal cord. It is involved in the regulation of heart rate, blood vessel diameter, respiration, coughing, swallowing, and vomiting.

The spinal cord extends from the medulla of the brain stem to the level of the upper border of the 2nd lumbar vertebra in an adult. An adult's spinal cord is about 16-18 inches in length. The spinal cord is made up of long tracts of nerves that join the brain with all body organs and parts (Figure 24-1). It is the center for many reflex activities of the body. **Motor nerves** carry responses from the brain and spinal cord, stimulating a muscle or organ. **Sensory nerves** send signals to the brain about the activities of the different parts of the body relative to their surroundings. For example, when you want a finger to move, the message, "Attention, finger! Move!" is sent down the spinal cord and through the nerve of the finger, and your finger moves. At about the same time, the finger sends a reply to the brain saying, "Mission complete." If the spinal cord is severely damaged, nerve

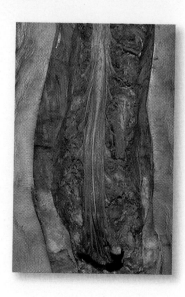

FIGURE 24-1 ▶ A dissected spinal cord and roots of the spinal nerves. © *The McGraw-Hill Companies, Inc./Karl Rubin, photographer.*

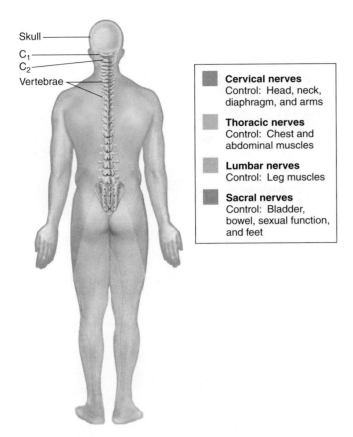

Skull
C₁
C₂
Vertebrae

Cervical nerves
Control: Head, neck, diaphragm, and arms

Thoracic nerves
Control: Chest and abdominal muscles

Lumbar nerves
Control: Leg muscles

Sacral nerves
Control: Bladder, bowel, sexual function, and feet

FIGURE 24-2 ▲ If the patient has a spinal cord injury, his signs and symptoms will depend on the location of the injury.

signals cannot get from the brain to the parts of the body below the injury. The patient's signs and symptoms will depend on the type and location of the injury (Figure 24-2).

Peripheral Nervous System

The peripheral nervous system (PNS) consists of all nervous tissue found outside the brain and spinal cord. There are 12 pairs of cranial nerves. They connect the brain with the neck and structures in the thorax and abdomen. There are 31 pairs of spinal nerves. Sensory nerves transmit messages to the brain and spinal cord *from* the body. Motor nerves transmit messages from the brain and spinal cord *to* the body.

The PNS has two divisions; both divisions contain sensory (afferent) and motor (efferent) nerves. The somatic (voluntary) division has receptors and nerves concerned with the external environment. It influences the activity of the musculoskeletal system. The autonomic (involuntary) division, also called the *autonomic nervous system* (ANS), has receptors and nerves concerned with the internal environment. The ANS controls the involuntary system of glands

and smooth muscle and functions to maintain a steady state in the body. The autonomic division is further divided into the sympathetic division and parasympathetic division. The sympathetic division mobilizes energy, particularly in stressful situations (the "fight-or-flight" response). Its effects are widespread throughout the body. The parasympathetic division conserves and restores energy. Its effects are localized in the body.

The Skeletal System

Objective 3

The skeletal system gives the body shape, support, and form. It protects vital internal organs. The skull protects the brain. The rib cage protects the heart and lungs. The lower ribs protect most of the liver and spleen. The spinal column protects the spinal cord. The skeletal system works with muscles to provide for body movement, stores minerals (such as calcium and phosphorus), and produces red blood cells.

The **skull** is a rigid container that protects the brain from injury. However, damage to the skull can cause damage to the brain. The spinal column consists of 33 bones. The spinal cord is well protected by the spinal column in the back. Injuries associated with a lot of force are usually necessary to cause damage to the spinal cord.

Injuries to the Spine

Mechanism of Injury

Objective 4

Most spinal injuries occur to the cervical spine. The next most commonly injured areas are the thoracic and lumbar spine. The spinal column normally allows a limited amount of movement in a forward, backward, and side-to-side direction. Movement beyond this normal range can result in damage to the spinal column and possibly to the spinal cord. A spinal *column* injury (bony injury) can occur with or without a spinal *cord* injury. A spinal *cord* injury can also occur with or without an injury to the spinal *column*. The spinal cord does not have to be severed in order for a loss of function to occur. In most people with a spinal cord injury, the spinal cord is intact, but the damage to it results in a loss of function. Children and the elderly are most likely to suffer an injury to the spinal cord without damage to the vertebrae.

A compression injury of the spine can drive the weight of the head into the neck, or the pelvis into

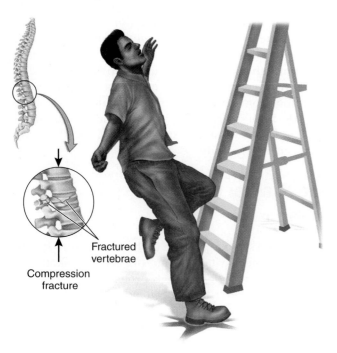

FIGURE 24-3 ▲ A compression injury of the spine can result from a fall from a significant height onto the head or legs. The force of the injury can drive the weight of the head into the neck, or the pelvis into the torso.

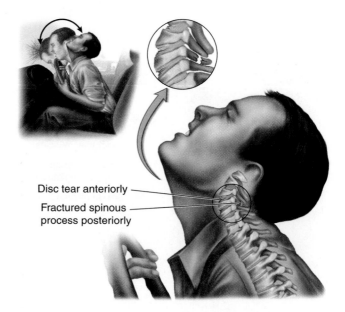

FIGURE 24-4 ▲ Severe backward movement of the head can result if the face hits the windshield in a motor vehicle crash.

Disc tear anteriorly

Fractured spinous process posteriorly

the torso (Figure 24-3). Compression fractures of the spine result in weakened vertebrae. A compression fracture can occur with or without a spinal cord injury. Compression injuries can result from any of the following:

- Contact sports
- MVCs with unrestrained occupants
- Diving into shallow water
- Falls from moving vehicles
- Falls from a significant height onto the head or legs

Severe backward movement (extension) of the head can result from diving into shallow water, banging the face into the windshield in a MVC, or falling and striking the face or chin (usually seen in elderly people) (Figure 24-4). Severe forward movement (flexion) of the head onto the chest can result from diving into shallow water, the sudden slowing of a motor vehicle, or being thrown from a horse or motorcycle (Figure 24-5). Severe rotation of the torso or head and neck can move one side of the spinal column against the other. A rotation injury can result from a motorcycle crash or rollover MVC. Injuries caused by flexion, extension, or rotation can dislocate the disks between the vertebrae, compress the spinal cord, and stretch or tear ligaments in the neck or spine.

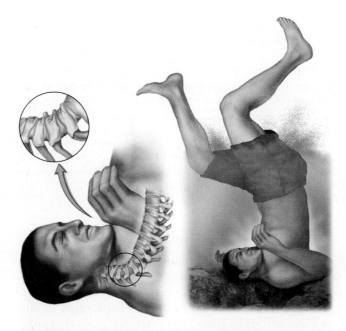

FIGURE 24-5 ▲ Severe forward movement of the head onto the chest can result from diving into shallow water.

Contact sports or "T-bone" MVCs can cause a sudden side impact that moves the torso sideways (lateral bending). The head remains in place until it is moved along by its attachments to the cervical spine. Lateral bending can compress and displace the vertebrae and stretch ligaments (Figure 24-6).

The spine can also be pulled apart (distraction). When the spine is distracted, ligaments and muscles are overstretched or torn and the vertebrae are

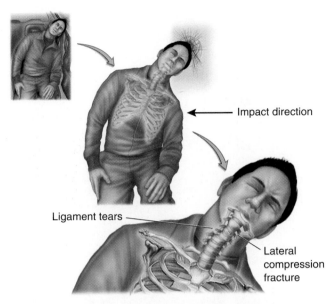

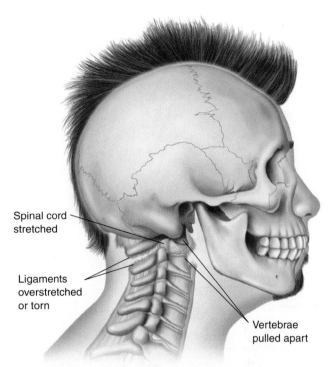

FIGURE 24-6 ▲ T-bone motor vehicle crashes can cause a sudden side impact that moves the torso sideways. The head remains in place until it is moved along by its attachments to the cervical spine.

pulled apart (Figure 24-7). This type of injury occurs in hangings, in schoolyard or playground accidents, or when a snowmobile or motorcycle is ridden under rope or wire. The spine may also be injured as a result of a penetrating wound to the head, neck, or torso.

As is evident from the mechanisms of injury mentioned here, a spinal injury is often seen in a patient with injuries to other areas of the body, such as the head, chest, or abdomen. For this reason, it is important to treat every patient with a significant mechanism of injury as if he has a spinal injury until it is proven otherwise.

You should have a high index of suspicion for a spinal injury in situations involving any of the following mechanisms of injury:

- MVCs
- Blunt trauma (such as an assault)
- Ejection or fall from a transportation device (such as a bicycle, motorcycle, motorized scooter, snowmobile, skateboard, rollerblades)
- Electrical injuries, lightning strike
- Involvement in an explosion
- Unresponsive trauma patients
- Hangings
- Any fall, particularly in an older adult
- Any shallow-water diving incident
- Any injury in which a helmet is broken (including a sports helmet, motorcycle helmet, and industrial hardhat)

FIGURE 24-7 ▲ Ligaments and muscles are overstretched or torn and the vertebrae are pulled apart when the spine is distracted.

- Any injury that penetrates the head, neck, or torso
- Any pedestrian-vehicle crash
- Any high-impact, high-force, or high-speed condition involving the head, spine, or torso

Stop and Think!

The patient's ability to walk, move his extremities, and feel sensation, as well as a lack of pain to the spinal column when you arrive on the scene does *not* rule out the possibility of spinal column or spinal cord damage.

Signs and Symptoms of a Spinal Injury

Objective 5

The most common and devastating spinal injuries occur in the area of the neck (cervical spine). An injury to the spinal cord may be complete or incomplete. A complete injury occurs when the spinal cord is severed. The patient has no voluntary movement or sensation below the level of the injury. Both sides of the body are equally affected. **Paraplegia** is

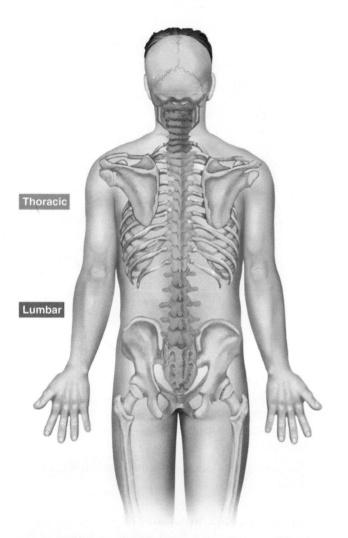

FIGURE 24-8 ▲ Paraplegia results from a spinal cord injury at the level of the thoracic or lumbar vertebrae.

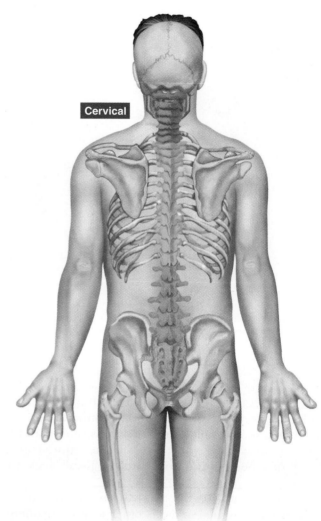

FIGURE 24-9 ▲ Quadriplegia (also called *tetraplegia*) results from a spinal cord injury at the level of the cervical vertebrae.

the loss of movement and sensation of the lower half of the body from the waist down. Paraplegia results from a spinal cord injury at the level of the thoracic or lumbar vertebrae (Figure 24-8). **Quadriplegia** (also called *tetraplegia*) is a loss of movement and sensation in both arms, both legs, and the parts of the body below an area of injury to the spinal cord. Quadriplegia results from a spinal cord injury at the level of the cervical vertebrae (Figure 24-9). In paraplegia and quadriplegia, the spinal cord is damaged so severely that nerve signals cannot be sent to areas below the damaged area or back again. About 3% of patients with a complete spinal cord injury will show some improvement over the first 24 hours after being injured. After 24 hours, improvement is almost never seen.

With an incomplete spinal cord injury, some parts of the spinal cord remain intact. Therefore, the patient has some function below the level of the injury. The patient may be able to move one extremity more than another, may be able to feel parts of the body that cannot be moved, or may have more function on one side of the body than the other. With an incomplete injury, there is potential for recovery because function may be lost only temporarily.

Remember This!

Spinal cord and spinal column injuries are uncommon in children. However, when they do occur, children younger than 8 years of age tend to injure the upper area of the cervical spine (the 1st and 2nd cervical vertebrae). Adults and older children tend to have cervical spine injuries in the lower area of the cervical spine.

The signs and symptoms of a possible spinal injury include the following:

- Tenderness in the injured area
- Pain associated with movement (Do *not* ask the patient to move to see if he has pain. Do *not* move the patient to test for a pain response.)
- Pain independent of movement
- Pain on palpation along the spinal column
- Pain down the lower legs or into the rib cage
- Pain that comes and goes, usually along the spine and/or the lower legs
- Soft-tissue injuries associated with trauma to the head and neck (cuts, bruises)
- Numbness, weakness, or tingling in the extremities
- A loss of sensation or paralysis below the site of injury
- A loss of sensation or paralysis in the upper or lower extremities
- Difficulty breathing
- A loss of bladder or bowel control
- An inability of the patient to walk or move his extremities
- Deformity or muscle spasm along the spinal column

The amount of weakness or loss of sensation your patient has will depend on the extent of the injury. It will also depend on the amount of pressure on the spinal cord or spinal nerves. Be prepared for breathing problems if your patient has an injury to the cervical or thoracic spine. An important nerve that stimulates the diaphragm exits the spinal cord between the 3rd and 5th vertebrae in the neck. "C3, 4, and 5 keep the diaphragm alive." (This saying refers to cervical vertebrae 3, 4, and 5.) If this nerve is severed or compressed, the patient's diaphragm is usually paralyzed. If the diaphragm is paralyzed, you will see shallow abdominal breathing. A spinal cord injury involving the lower neck or upper chest may result in paralysis of the muscles between the ribs. Patients with these injuries will usually need help breathing with a bag-mask (BM) device connected to 100% oxygen.

Assessing the Potential Spine-Injured Patient

Conduct a scene size-up and ensure your safety. Evaluate the mechanism of injury before approaching the patient. Put on appropriate personal protective equipment (PPE).

Making a Difference

Managing a patient with a suspected spinal injury can directly affect the patient's outcome. The early recognition of a spinal injury can help reduce permanent disability and even prevent death. It is *critical* that you have a high index of suspicion for a spinal injury based on the mechanism of injury, even when there are no outward signs of trauma. If the mechanism of injury suggests it, suspect a spinal injury and treat your patient accordingly.

Perform a primary survey and determine the urgency of further assessment and care. If the mechanism of injury suggests the possibility of spinal injury, ask the patient not to move his head while answering questions. Face the patient so he does not have to turn his head to talk with you. Quickly assess the patient's mental status, airway, breathing, and circulation. Identify and treat any life-threatening conditions. If the possibility of a spinal injury exists, ask an assistant to manually stabilize the patient's cervical spine while you assess the patient's airway (Figure 24-10). (Refer to the *Remember This!* box, "Manually Stabilizing the Head and Neck," that follows this section.) Maintain manual stabilization of the patient's cervical spine until the patient has been completely immobilized on a long backboard. Long backboards help stabilize the head, neck and torso, pelvis, and extremities. They are used to immobilize patients found in a lying, standing, or sitting position.

Establish patient priorities. Priority patients are those:

- Who give a poor general impression
- Who have severe pain anywhere
- Who have uncontrolled bleeding
- Who are experiencing difficulty breathing
- Who have signs and symptoms of shock
- Who are unresponsive, with no gag reflex or cough
- Who are responsive and unable to follow commands

In these situations, request Advanced Life Support (ALS) personnel as soon as possible. If ALS personnel are not available, the patient should be transported promptly to the closest appropriate facility.

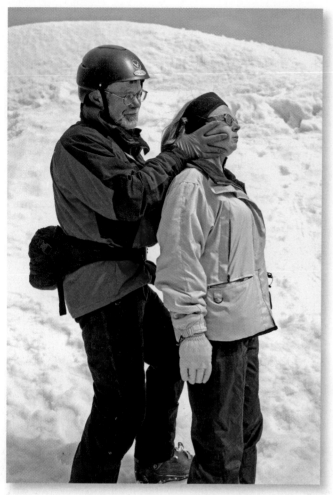

(a)

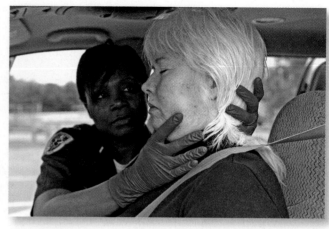

(c)

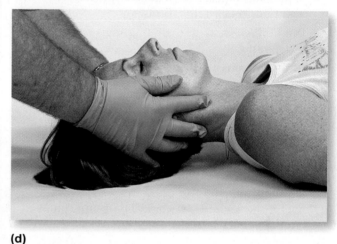

(d)

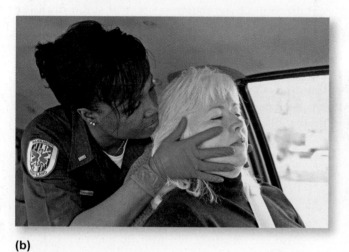

(b)

FIGURE 24-10 ▲ To manually stabilize the patient's head and neck, position yourself so you can place the patient's head between your hands. Place your palms over the patient's ears. Keep his head in a neutral position—eyes facing forward and level—and support the weight of his head. **(a)** Manual stabilization of the head and neck with the patient standing. **(b)** Manual stabilization of the head and neck from behind the patient. **(c)** Manual stabilization of the head and neck from the patient's side. **(d)** Manual stabilization of the head and neck with the patient supine.

Objective 7

Perform a physical examination. If no significant mechanism of injury exists, perform a focused physical examination based on the patient's chief complaint, mechanism of injury, and primary survey findings.

Then assess the patient's baseline vital signs and obtain a SAMPLE history.

If a significant mechanism of injury exists, continue in-line spinal stabilization throughout the examination. Consider the need for ALS personnel and reconsider your transport decision. Perform a rapid trauma assessment to determine life-threatening injuries. In the responsive patient, symptoms should be sought before and during the trauma assessment. If the patient is awake, instruct him not to move during the examination. Look closely at the patient's head, neck, chest, abdomen, pelvis, extremities, and posterior body for cuts (lacerations), scrapes (abrasions), bruises (contusions), deformities, penetrations, and swelling. Feel each area for tenderness, deformity, swelling, and instability. Feel and listen for crepitus, the grating of broken bone ends against each other. Check distal pulses, movement, and sensation (PMS) in each extremity. Compare each extremity to the opposite extremity. To assess sensation, touch the fingers and toes of each extremity and ask the patient to tell you where you are touching. To assess movement, ask the patient if he can:

- Shrug his shoulders
- Spread the fingers of both hands
- Squeeze your fingers and release them
- Wiggle his toes
- Push down with each foot against your hand ("gas pedal") and then pull the foot up

Stop if the patient experiences pain. If the patient is unresponsive, assess movement and sensation by gently pinching each foot and hand. See if the patient responds to pain with facial movements or movement of the pinched extremity.

After assessing the front and back of the patient's neck, apply a rigid cervical collar (also called a *C-collar*). The technique for applying a cervical collar is discussed in the next section. If a cervical collar is applied, the patient will need to be immobilized on a backboard.

Take the patient's vital signs and gather the patient's medical history. Determine the events leading to the present situation by asking the following questions:

- What happened?
- When did the injury occur?
- Where does it hurt?
- Does your neck or back hurt?
- Were you wearing a seat belt?
- Did you pass out before the accident?
- Did you move or did someone move you before we arrived?
- Have your symptoms changed from the time of the injury until the time we arrived?

Emergency Care of a Spinal Injury

To treat a patient with a spinal injury, perform the following steps:

- Establish and maintain an open airway. If the patient is unresponsive, remember that a jaw thrust without head tilt is the preferred method for opening the airway in a patient with a suspected spinal injury. However, according to the American Heart Association, "Because maintaining a patent airway and providing adequate ventilation is a priority in CPR, use a head tilt–chin lift maneuver if the jaw thrust does not open the airway." Insert an oral airway if needed. Suction as necessary. Since an unresponsive patient cannot protect his own airway, it will be important for you to make sure that the patient's airway remains open and free of secretions.

- Remember that injuries to the cervical and thoracic spine may affect the patient's ability to breathe. An injury involving the lower cervical or upper thoracic portion of the spinal cord may result in paralysis of the intercostal muscles. If the patient's breathing is adequate, give oxygen by nonrebreather mask. If it is inadequate, assist his breathing with a BM device connected to 100% oxygen. Whenever possible, positive-pressure ventilation must be performed while the patient's spine is stabilized in an in-line position. Reassess the adequacy of the patient's breathing often while he is in your care.

- Control bleeding, if present. If signs of shock are present or if internal bleeding is suspected, treat for shock.

- Cover open wounds with a sterile dressing.

- Splint any bone or joint injuries. If the mechanism of injury suggests the patient has experienced an injury to the spine, the spine must be immobilized. Spinal stabilization techniques are discussed in the next section.

Stop and Think!

You can use a backboard in specific situations without using a cervical collar. But you must never use a cervical collar without a backboard. For example, a patient in shock from a medical cause may be placed on a backboard. In this situation, a cervical collar is not necessary. However, if you apply a cervical collar because the mechanism of injury warrants it, then the patient's spine needs to be stabilized on a backboard.

- Comfort, calm, and reassure the patient. Keep in mind that injuries to muscles and bones are painful. Your patient may be worried about a permanent loss of function of the injured area or possible disfigurement. Listen to your patient and do your best to comfort him. Perform ongoing assessments every 5 minutes if the patient is in shock and every 15 minutes if the patient is stable.
- Record all patient care information, including the patient's medical history and all emergency care given, on a prehospital care report (PCR).

Remember This!

Manually Stabilizing the Head and Neck

Manual stabilization of the head and neck is also called *in-line stabilization*. Manual stabilization of the head and neck helps prevent further injury to the spine.

- To manually stabilize the patient's head and neck, position yourself so that you can place the patient's head between your hands. You must be able to hold that position comfortably for a significant length of time. Place your palms over the patient's ears. Spread your fingers on each side of the patient's head for added stability. Keep his head in a neutral position and support the weight of his head.
  - When the head and neck are in a neutral ("in-line") position, they are in an anatomically correct position. The eyes are facing forward and level, and the patient's nose is in line with the navel.
- Do *not* excessively move the head forward, backward, or from side to side. Do *not* pull on the patient's head or neck. If the patient is lying on his back, place your forearms on the ground for support. If the patient is sitting or standing, support your forearms by placing them on the patient's back or chest.
- If an attempt to move the patient's head and neck into a neutral position results in any of the following, *stop* any movement and stabilize the head in the position in which it was found:
  - Airway obstruction
  - Difficulty breathing
  - Neck muscle spasm
  - Increased pain

  - An onset or worsening of numbness or tingling, or a loss of movement
  - Resistance that is felt when moving the head to a neutral position

A cervical collar cannot be applied to the patient in these situations. Use rolled towels or blanket rolls secured with tape or triangular bandages to stabilize the head and neck in the position in which it was found.

- Continue manual stabilization of the patient's cervical spine until either a cervical collar has been applied and the patient is fully immobilized on a long backboard or additional Emergency Medical Services (EMS) resources have arrived and have assumed patient care.

Spinal Stabilization Techniques

You may be expected to immobilize or assist with immobilizing a patient with a suspected spinal injury. Equipment used for spinal stabilization includes:

- A cervical collar, large towels, a blanket, or a commercial device to secure the head (such as a head block)
- A long backboard
- Straps, tape, triangular bandages, or 4-inch roller gauze

When stabilizing the patient's spine, remember that the joint above and the joint below the injured area must be immobilized. If an injury to the cervical spine or thoracic spine is suspected, stabilize the patient's spine from the head to the pelvis. If an injury to the lumbar spine is suspected, stabilize the patient's thoracic spine, pelvis, and hips. Since sideways movement of the patient's legs can cause movement of the pelvis, the patient's legs are also secured to the board. In the case of a suspected lumbar spine injury, the patient's head should also be stabilized if a possible cervical spine injury exists. Some of the more common techniques used for spinal stabilization are discussed in the following sections.

Remember This!

Defer to your company policy or consult with medical direction if you are considering not immobilizing the whole patient with a potential cord injury at any point along the vertebral column.

Cervical Collars
Objectives 10, 12

After assessing the front and back of the patient's neck, apply a rigid cervical collar. When used alone, a rigid C-collar does not immobilize the cervical spine. For effective stabilization, a rigid collar must be used with manual stabilization or a spinal stabilization device, such as a backboard. A rigid collar is used to:

- Temporarily splint the head and neck in a neutral position
- Limit movement of the cervical spine
- Support the weight of the patient's head while he is in a sitting position
- Help maintain the cervical spine in a neutral position when the patient is lying on his back
- Remind the patient and other healthcare professionals that the mechanism of injury suggests a possible spinal injury

The technique for applying a cervical collar is shown in (Skill Drill 24-1).

If a cervical collar is not available or does not fit the patient, the patient's head and neck can be stabilized by using a long backboard, rolled towels, or a blanket (Figure 24-11).

You should apply a rigid cervical collar *only* if it fits properly:

- If the collar is too tight, it can apply pressure on the blood vessels in the patient's neck and reduce blood flow.
- If the collar is too loose, it can cover the patient's chin and mouth, causing an airway

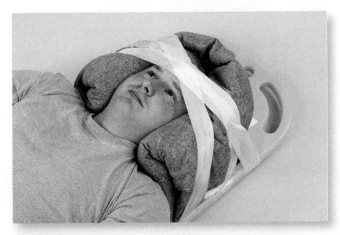

FIGURE 24-11 ▲ If a cervical collar is not available or does not fit the patient, the patient's head and neck can be stabilized by using a long backboard, rolled towels, or a blanket.

obstruction. If it is too loose, it will also not adequately stabilize the head and neck.

- A collar that is too short will not provide adequate stabilization because the patient's head can move forward.

Objective 11

- A collar that is too tall will not provide adequate stabilization because the patient's head will be moved backward by the collar. The collar can also force the jaw closed, limiting access to the airway.

Three-Person Log Roll
Objective 13

You may encounter situations in which you find an unresponsive patient who is lying face down. If the scene suggests that the patient may have experienced some type of trauma such as a fall or a blow to the body, you should assume a spinal injury exists. A log roll is a technique used to move a patient from a face-down or side-lying position to a face-up position while keeping the head and neck in line with the rest of the body. This technique is also used to place a patient with a suspected spinal injury on a backboard. The steps to perform a 3-person log roll are shown in Skill Drill 24-2.

Making a Difference

Remember: Once the patient has been immobilized on the long backboard, he will have limited sight. Explain all movements to him before starting the move so that he will not be frightened.

Immobilization of a Supine Patient on a Long Backboard
Objective 14

After a patient has been log-rolled onto a long backboard, he must be secured to it. To maintain an adult's head and neck in a neutral position, place 1-2 inches of padding on the board under the patient's head (Figure 24-12). Be careful to avoid extra movement. To maintain the head of an infant or a child younger than age 3 in a neutral position, you may need to place padding under the infant's or child's torso. The padding should extend from the shoulders to the pelvis. It should be thick enough for the child's

Applying a Cervical Collar

STEP 1 ▶ • Put on appropriate personal protective equipment. Ask an assistant to maintain manual stabilization of the patient's head and neck in a neutral position.
• Assess distal pulses, movement, and sensation.
• Measure the width of the patient's neck by placing your fingers between the patient's lower jaw and shoulder.

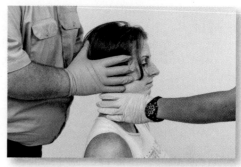

STEP 2 ▶ Select a rigid cervical collar and measure the device. Adjust the size of the collar to fit the patient's measurements as necessary.

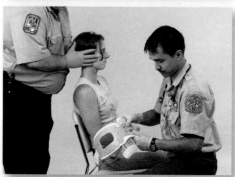

STEP 3 ▶ • Apply the cervical collar to the patient.
• Check to make sure the collar fits according to the manufacturer's instructions.
• Continue manual stabilization of the patient's head and neck until the patient is fully immobilized on a long backboard.
• Remember to check distal pulses, movement, and sensation after applying the collar.

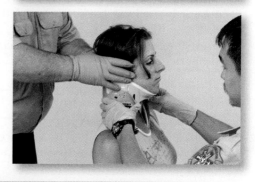

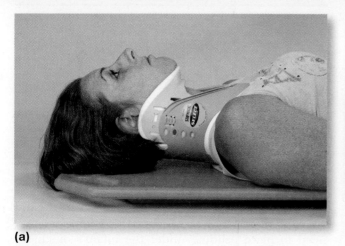

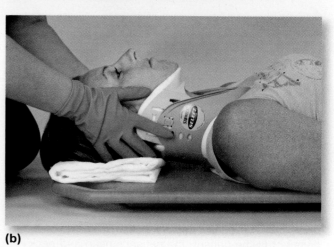

(a) (b)

FIGURE 24-12 ▲ **(a)** Head and neck stabilization of an adult without padding. **(b)** Head and neck stabilization of an adult with 1-2 inches of padding on the board under the patient's head.

Three-Person Log Roll

STEP 1 ▸ • Put on appropriate personal protective equipment.

• Rescuer #1 kneels at the patient's head, maintaining manual in-line immobilization of the patient's head and neck. This rescuer will direct the move.

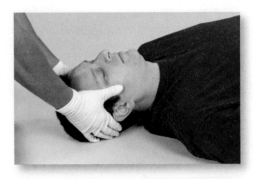

STEP 2 ▸ Rescuer #2 sizes and applies a rigid cervical collar.

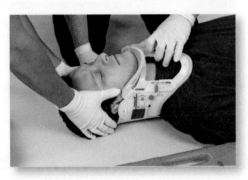

STEP 3 ▸ • Rescuers #2 and #3 position a long backboard at one side of the patient.
• The patient is positioned with his legs and arms straight out at his sides, palms facing in.
• Rescuer #2 is positioned at the patient's mid-chest with his hands placed on the patient's far shoulder and hip.
• Rescuer #3 is positioned at the patient's upper legs with his hands placed on the patient's hip and hand as well as his lower leg.
• If the patient has an injury to his chest or abdomen, he should be rolled onto his uninjured side if possible.

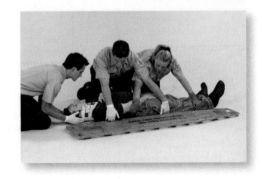

STEP 4 ▸ • When everyone is ready, Rescuer #1 gives the order to roll the patient.
• Rescuer #1 maintains manual stabilization of the patient's head and neck.
• Rescuers #2 and #3 roll the patient on his side toward them. The patient's head, shoulders, and pelvis are kept in line during the roll.

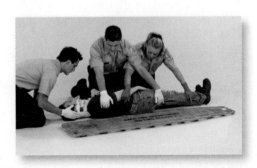

Continued on next page

Three-Person Log Roll (*continued*)

STEP 5 ▶ The patient's back is quickly assessed. A long back-board is positioned under the patient.

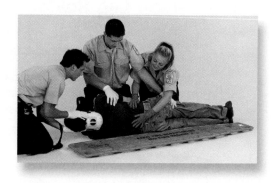

STEP 6 ▶
- When everyone is ready, Rescuer #1 gives the order to roll the patient onto the backboard. If the backboard was angled, the patient and the backboard are lowered to the ground together.
- Manual stabilization of the patient's head and neck is continued until the patient is fully immobilized on the backboard.

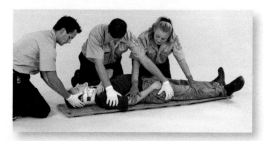

shoulders to be in line with his ear canal (Figure 24-13). An older child may not require padding to obtain a neutral position.

Pad any hollow areas (spaces) between the patient and the board as necessary. These spaces include the small of the back and under the patient's knees. Immobilize the patient's torso to the board. Immobilize the upper torso to the board with one strap over the chest or, preferably, with 2 straps placed in an "X" fashion. Make sure that the straps are tight enough to limit patient movement but not so tight that they restrict breathing. If your patient is a woman, place the chest strap above her breasts and under her arms, not across the breasts.

Immobilize the pelvis to the board with a strap centered over the patient's hips. Secure the patient's

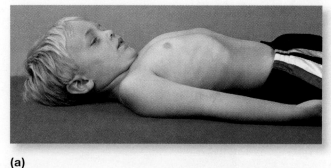

(a)

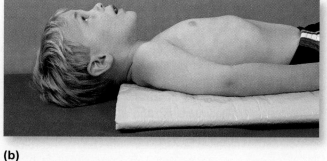

(b)

FIGURE 24-13 ▲ **(a)** Infants and young children have large heads. The size of the head causes it to move forward when placed on a flat surface. **(b)** To maintain the head in a neutral position, you may need to place padding under the child's torso. The padding should extend from the shoulders to the pelvis and be thick enough so that the child's shoulders are in line with the ear canal.

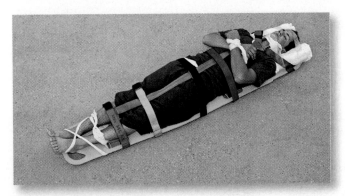

FIGURE 24-14 ▲ A patient fully immobilized on a long backboard.

upper legs to the board with a strap across the legs above the knees. Secure the lower legs with a strap across the legs below the knees. Secure the patient's arms to the board. The head is secured to the board *last*. You must maintain manual stabilization of the head and neck until the head and the rest of the body are secured to the board. Secure the patient's head to the board with a ready-made head immobilizer, rolled towels, or blanket rolls. Place a strap or tape snugly across the patient's lower forehead. Place another strap or tape snugly across the front portion of the cervical collar. Reassess the security of the straps. Reassess pulses, movement, and sensation in all extremities (Figure 24-14).

Stop and Think!

Once a patient has been fully immobilized on a backboard, a healthcare professional must remain with the patient *at all times*. Because immobilization will restrict the patient's ability to keep his airway open, a healthcare professional must assume this responsibility. If the patient vomits, turn the board and patient together as a unit and clear the airway.

Spinal Stabilization of a Seated Patient
Objectives 15, 16

If a patient with a possible spinal injury is found sitting in a chair, stabilize the patient's spine by using a short-backboard immobilization device. However, if the patient must be moved urgently because of his injuries, the need to gain access to others, or dangers at the scene, carefully lower the patient directly onto a long backboard while providing manual spinal stabilization.

There are several types of short-backboard immobilization devices, including vest-type devices and a rigid short backboard. Short backboards help to immobilize a patient's head, neck, and torso. A short backboard is used for the following purposes:

- To immobilize a seated patient who has a suspected spinal injury and stable vital signs
- To immobilize a patient in a confined space
- As a long backboard for a small child

In most areas, vest-type devices are used primarily for extrication. They feature straps to secure the patient's head, chest, and legs. Once the patient has been extricated, he should remain in the device and be secured to a long backboard. The steps used to apply a vest-type device are shown in Skill Drill 24-3.

Spinal Stabilization of a Standing Patient

If the patient with a possible spinal injury is found in a standing position, stabilize the patient's spine by using a long backboard. Skill Drill 24-4 shows the steps for spinal stabilization of a standing patient.

Rapid Extrication
Objectives 17, 18

Rapid extrication is an example of an urgent move (see Chapter 6). Rapid extrication should be performed when there is an immediate threat to life, such as in the following situations:

- Altered mental status
- Inadequate breathing
- Shock (hypoperfusion)

Other indications for rapid extrication include an unsafe scene and situations in which a patient blocks your access to another, more seriously injured, patient.

Rapid extrication must be accomplished quickly, without compromise or injury to the patient's spine. The steps for rapid extrication are shown in Skill Drill 6-2 (Chapter 6, "Lifting and Moving Patients").

You Should Know

Indications for Rapid Extrication

- Unsafe scene
- Altered mental status
- Inadequate breathing
- Shock (hypoperfusion)
- Patient blocking access to another, more seriously injured patient

Spinal Stabilization of a Seated Patient

STEP 1 ▶
- Put on appropriate personal protective equipment. Rescuer #1 manually stabilizes the patient's head and neck.
- Rescuer #2 assesses the patient's pulses, movement, and sensation in all extremities.
- After assessing the front and back of the patient's neck, a rigid cervical collar is applied.

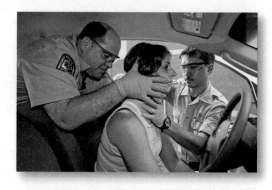

STEP 2 ▶ Rescuer #2 positions the vest-type device behind the patient.

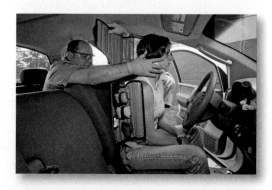

STEP 3 ▶
- Rescuer #2 positions the chest panels snugly into the patient's armpits.
- The device is then secured to the patient's torso. Rescuer #2 fastens all chest straps, making sure that the straps are snug but do not interfere with breathing.

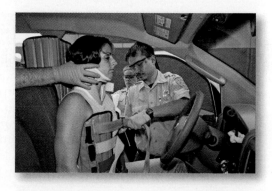

STEP 4 ▶
- Rescuer #2 secures the patient's legs next. The leg straps are loosened and wrapped around the leg on the same side. The straps are then fastened and tightened.
- Rescuer #2 evaluates the position of the device and makes sure all straps are secure.

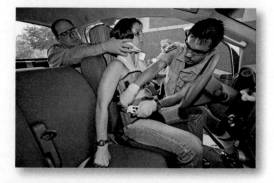

STEP 5 ▷
- To keep the patient's head in a neutral position, Rescuer #2 applies firm padding to any hollow areas between the patient's head and the head-piece of the device.
- Rescuer #2 then positions the head flaps on the side of the patient's head, coordinating with Rescuer #1 to maintain manual stabilization of the head and neck.
- Rescuer #2 then secures the head flaps by using elastic straps or wide tape.

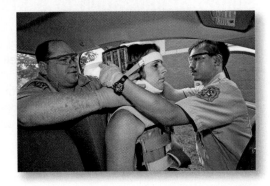

STEP 6 ▷
- After the patient's head is secured to the device, Rescuer #1 releases manual stabilization of the head.
- Rescuer #2 reassesses distal pulses, movement, and sensation in each extremity.

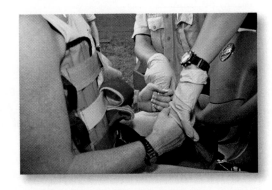

STEP 7 ▷
- The patient is rotated so that his back is to the opening through which he will be removed. A long backboard is positioned through the opening and placed under the patient.
- The patient is lowered onto the long backboard and slid into position on the board.

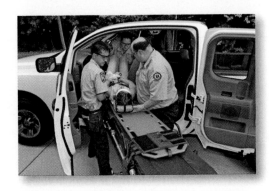

STEP 8 ▷
- The leg straps on the vest-type device are loosened so that the patient can extend his legs out straight. The straps are then retightened.
- The patient is then secured to a long backboard.
- Pulses, movement, and sensation are reassessed in all extremities.

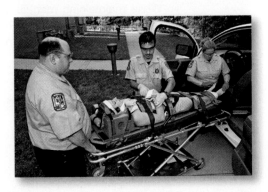

Spinal Stabilization of a Standing Patient

STEP 1 ▶ • Put on appropriate personal protective equipment. Rescuer #1 positions himself behind the patient and manually stabilizes the patient's head and neck. This rescuer will direct the move.
     • Rescuer #2 assesses the patient's pulses, movement, and sensation in all extremities.

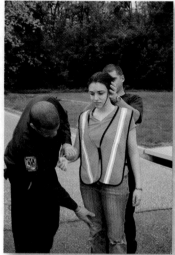

STEP 2 ▶ After assessing the front and back of the patient's neck, a rigid cervical collar is sized and applied. Rescuer #1 continues manual stabilization of the head and neck.

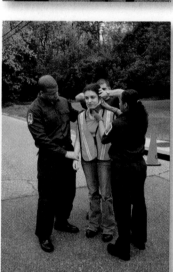

STEP 3 ▶ • Rescuer #2 and Rescuer #3 position a long backboard behind patient, making sure the board is centered behind the patient.
     • While maintaining manual stabilization of the patient's head and neck, Rescuer #1 adjusts the position of his elbows to make room for positioning of the backboard.

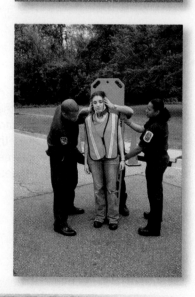

STEP 4 ▶ While Rescuer #1 continues manual stabilization from behind the patient, Rescuer #2 and Rescuer #3 position themselves on either side of the patient. Using the hand that is closest to the patient, Rescuers #2 and #3 reach under the patient's armpits and grasp the board. The board is grasped at the same level as the patient's armpit or higher.

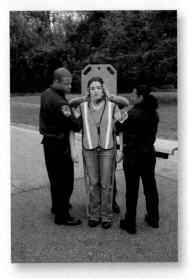

STEP 5 ▶ • While Rescuer #1 continues manual stabilization from behind the patient, he explains to the patient that she must not move as the rescuers begin lowering the patient and board to the ground.
• Rescuer #1 directs the move, walking backward as the patient and board are slowly lowered to the ground. At the same time, Rescuers #2 and #3 begin walking forward.
• At the direction of Rescuer #1, Rescuers #2 and #3 pause as needed to allow Rescuer #1 to adjust his body position.

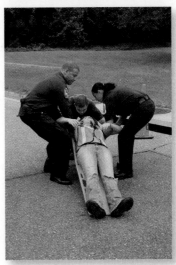

STEP 6 ▶ Once the board is on the ground, Rescuer #1 maintains manual stabilization of the patient's head and neck while the patient is assessed by the other rescuers. The patient is then secured to the board.

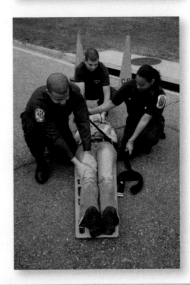

Helmet Removal

Objectives 19, 20, 21, 22, 23, 24, 25, 26

It can be a challenge to properly assess a patient wearing a helmet. There are two main types of helmets: sports helmets and motorcycle helmets. Sports helmets usually open in the front and provide easy access to the patient's airway once the face guard is removed. The face guard can be unclipped, unsnapped, removed with a screwdriver, or cut off with rescue scissors. Some sports helmets, such as those used in football and ice hockey, are custom fitted to the individual. Motorcycle helmets usually have a shield that covers the entire face. The face shield can be unbuckled or snapped off to access the patient's airway.

Do not assume that a helmet must be removed. If your patient has a spinal injury, removing the helmet could worsen the injury. To determine if a helmet should be left in place or removed, you should first ask yourself the following questions:

- Can I access the patient's airway?
- Is the patient's airway clear?
- Is the patient breathing adequately?
- Is there room to apply a face mask if it is necessary to assist the patient's breathing?
- How well does the helmet fit?
- Can the patient's head move within the helmet?
- Can the patient's spine be stabilized in a neutral position if the helmet is left in place?

You should *leave a helmet in place* in the following circumstances:

- There are no impending airway or breathing problems.
- The helmet fits well, with little or no movement of the patient's head within the helmet.
- Helmet removal would cause further injury to the patient.
- Proper spinal stabilization can be performed with the helmet in place.
- The presence of the helmet does not interfere with your ability to assess and reassess airway and breathing.

You should *remove a helmet* in these circumstances:

- You are unable to assess and/or reassess the patient's airway and breathing.
- The helmet limits your ability to adequately manage the patient's airway or breathing.

- The helmet does not fit properly, allowing excessive head movement within the helmet.
- You cannot properly stabilize the patient's spine with the helmet in place.
- The patient is in cardiac arrest.

At least two rescuers are needed to remove a helmet. The method used for helmet removal depends on the type of helmet worn by the patient. Skill Drill 24-5 shows the steps for removing a motorcycle helmet from a patient with a possible spinal injury.

Injuries to the Head

Objectives 4, 11

Head injuries can be caused by a variety of mechanisms that result in pain, swelling, bleeding, and deformity. These mechanisms of injury are similar to those previously described for spinal injuries. Mechanisms of injury such as MVCs and falls often cause the patient to become unresponsive. When a patient loses consciousness, he loses the ability to protect his own airway. Appropriate airway management and breathing support are critical when treating a patient with a head injury.

Injuries to the Scalp

An injury to the scalp may occur because of blunt or penetrating trauma. The scalp contains tissue, hair follicles, sweat glands, oil glands, and a rich supply of blood vessels. Because the brain is protected by a rigid container called the *skull*, a scalp injury may or may not cause an injury to the brain. When injured, these areas may bleed heavily. In children, the amount of blood loss from a scalp wound may be enough to produce shock. In adults, shock is usually not caused by a scalp wound or internal skull injuries. More often, in adults, shock results from an injury elsewhere.

Assess the scalp carefully for cuts because some are not easy to detect. Control bleeding with direct pressure. Do not apply excessive pressure to the open wound if you suspect a skull fracture. Doing so can push bone fragments into the brain.

Injuries to the Skull

Skull injuries may occur from blunt or penetrating trauma. Significant force, such as a severe impact or blow, can result in a skull fracture. The signs of a skull fracture are shown in Figure 24-15.

Helmet Removal

STEP 1 ▶ Rescuer #1 positions himself at the patient's head and removes the face shield from the helmet to assess airway and breathing. If the patient is wearing eyeglasses, they should be removed.

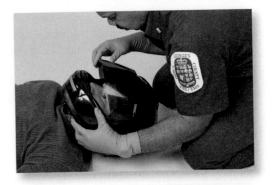

STEP 2 ▶
- Rescuer #1 stabilizes the helmet by placing his hands on each side of the helmet. His fingers should be on the patient's lower jaw to prevent movement.
- Rescuer #2 loosens the helmet strap.

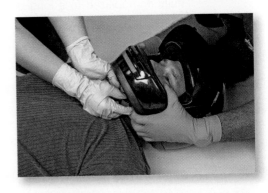

STEP 3 ▶ Rescuer #2 assumes manual stabilization by placing one hand on the patient's lower jaw at the angle of the jaw. The rescuer's other hand goes under the neck and behind the patient's head at the back of the head.

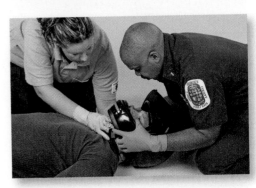

STEP 4 ▶ Rescuer #1 pulls out on the sides of the helmet to clear the patient's ears, gently slips the helmet halfway off the patient's head, and then stops.

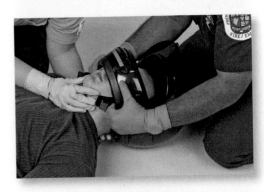

Continued on next page

Helmet Removal (*continued*)

STEP 5 ▶
- Rescuer #2 slides the hand supporting the occiput (the back of the patient's head) toward the top of the patient's head to prevent the head from falling back after complete helmet removal.
- Rescuer #1 tilts the helmet backward to clear the nose and removes the helmet completely.

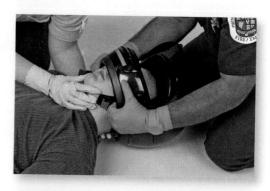

STEP 6 ▶ Manual stabilization is continued until the patient is fully immobilized to a long backboard.

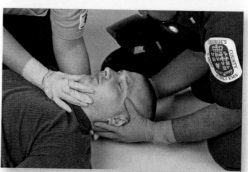

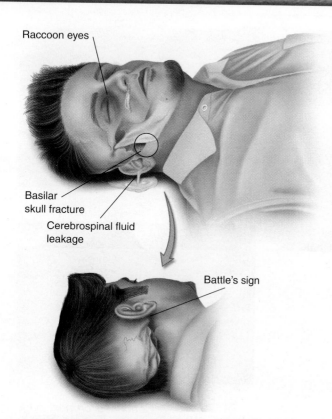

Raccoon eyes

Basilar skull fracture

Cerebrospinal fluid leakage

Battle's sign

FIGURE 24-15 ▲ Signs of a skull fracture.

You Should Know

Signs and Symptoms of a Skull Fracture

- Bruises or cuts to the scalp
- Deformity to the skull
- Discoloration around the eyes (raccoon eyes)
- Discoloration behind the ears (Battle's sign)
- Loss of consciousness
- Confusion
- Convulsions
- Restlessness, irritability
- Drowsiness
- Blood or clear, watery fluid [cerebrospinal fluid (CSF)] leaking from the ears or nose
- Visual disturbances
- Changes in pupils (unequal pupil size or pupils that are not reactive to light)
- Slurred speech
- Difficulties with balance
- Stiff neck
- Vomiting

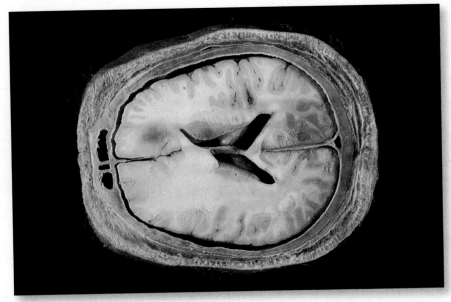

FIGURE 24-16 ▲ The skull is a rigid, closed container. If bleeding occurs within the skull, the pressure within the skull increases as the blood takes up more space within the closed container. © *The McGraw-Hill Companies, Inc./Karl Rubin, photographer.*

A head injury may be open or closed. In a closed head injury, the skull remains intact. However, the brain can still be injured by the forces or objects that struck the skull. The forces that impact the skull cause the brain to move within skull. The brain strikes the inside of the skull, which causes injuries to the brain tissue. The impact and shearing forces that affect the brain can cause direct damage to the brain tissue. These forces can also injure the surrounding blood vessels.

The skull is a rigid, closed container (Figure 24-16). If bleeding occurs within the skull, the pressure within the skull increases as the blood takes up more space within the closed container. If the bleeding continues and the pressure continues to rise, the patient can suffer severe brain damage and even death.

In an open head injury, the scalp is not intact and the risk of infection is increased. Broken bones or foreign objects forced through the skull can cut, tear, or bruise the brain tissue itself. If the skull is cracked, the blood and CSF that normally surrounds the brain and spinal cord can leak through the crack in the skull and into the surrounding tissues. If the forces are strong enough to cause an open head injury, then the brain will most likely sustain an injury as well.

Brain injuries can occur for reasons other than trauma. For example, a nontraumatic injury may result from clots or hemorrhaging. This type of injury occurs when a patient has a stroke. Nontraumatic brain injuries can cause an altered mental status. Their signs and symptoms are similar to those of traumatic brain injuries. The signs and symptoms of a traumatic head injury appear in the following *You Should Know* box.

You Should Know

Signs and Symptoms of a Traumatic Head Injury

- Changes in mental status that range from confusion and repetitive questioning to unresponsiveness
- Deep cuts or tears to the scalp or face
- Exposed brain tissue (a very bad sign)
- Penetrating injuries such as gunshot wounds and impaled objects
- Swelling ("goose eggs"), bruising of the skin
- Edges or fragments of bone seen or felt through the skin
- A deformity of the skull such as "sunken" areas (depressions)
- Swelling or discoloration behind the ears (Battle's sign; may not be seen for hours after the injury)
- Swelling or discoloration around the eyes (raccoon eyes; may not be seen for hours after the injury)
- Pupils that are unequal in size, irregular in shape, or do not react to light equally; dilation of both pupils

- An irregular breathing pattern
- Nausea and/or vomiting
- Seizures
- Blood or clear, watery fluid from the ears or nose
- Weakness or numbness of one side of the body
- A deterioration in vital signs
- A loss of bladder or bowel control

Injuries to the Brain

Concussion

A **concussion** is a traumatic brain injury that results in a temporary loss of function in some or all of the brain. A concussion occurs when the head strikes an object or is struck by an object (Figure 24-17). The injury may or may not cause a loss of consciousness. A headache, loss of appetite, vomiting, and pale skin are common soon after the injury. A patient who experiences a concussion often appears confused and may not remember what happened. The patient may ask the same questions over and over, such as, "What happened? What happened?" This action is called *repetitive questioning.* If memory loss occurs, maximum memory loss usually happens immediately after the injury and returns as time passes. The signs and symptoms of a concussion are an indication of a brain injury. Although the symptoms of a concussion usually disappear within 48 hours, the patient needs to be evaluated by a physician. Worsening symptoms suggest a more serious injury.

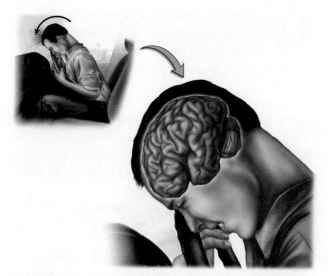

FIGURE 24-17 ▲ A concussion occurs when the head strikes an object or is struck by an object.

Cerebral Contusion

A **cerebral contusion** is a brain injury in which brain tissue is bruised and damaged in a local area. Bruising may occur at both the area of direct impact (coup) and/or on the side opposite (contrecoup) the impact. Bruising of the brain is usually present when the forces involved in the injury were sufficient to cause prolonged unconsciousness. The patient's signs and symptoms depend on the location and size of the bruise. For example, a large bruise in the area of the brain's temporal lobe can cause aggressive or combative behavior.

Remember This!

An altered or decreasing mental status is the best indicator of a brain injury.

Hematomas

Bleeding beneath the dura (subdural) or between the dura and skull (epidural) may be associated with bruising of the brain and other injuries (Figure 24-18). When bleeding occurs in the skull, the pressure within the skull (intracranial pressure) increases as the blood takes up more space within the closed container. As the pressure within the skull increases, blood flow to the brain decreases. When the brain senses a decrease in blood flow, it signals the cardiovascular system to increase blood pressure, thereby increasing blood flow. At the same time, signals are sent to the respiratory system to increase the rate of breathing to increase oxygen. If intracranial pressure continues to rise, the patient's breathing pattern becomes irregular and his heart rate decreases. In a head-injured patient, these 3 findings (increased systolic blood pressure, abnormal breathing pattern, and decreased heart rate) are called **Cushing's triad.** It is very important to recognize these signs. When they are present, you must move quickly and transport rapidly to the closest appropriate facility.

A **subdural hematoma** usually results from tearing of veins located between the dura and the cerebral cortex after an injury to the head. Blood builds up in the space between the dura and the arachnoid layer of the meninges (Figure 24-19). In an acute subdural hematoma, most patients develop signs and symptoms within minutes or hours after the injury because the blood builds up quickly. An example of a situation in which an acute subdural hematoma may occur is a sports-related head injury. In a chronic subdural hematoma, the buildup of blood occurs gradually. This makes signs and symptoms more difficult to recognize.

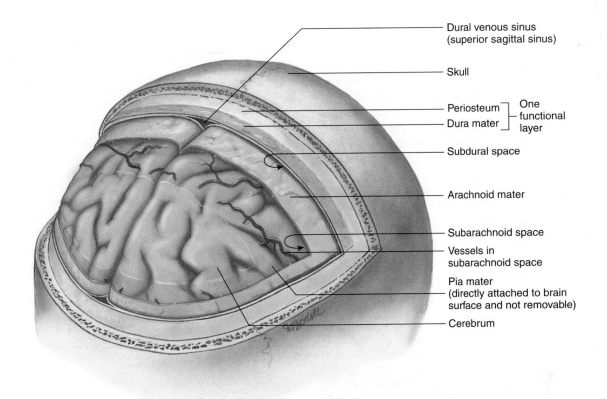

- Dural venous sinus (superior sagittal sinus)
- Skull
- Periosteum ⎱ One
- Dura mater ⎰ functional layer
- Subdural space
- Arachnoid mater
- Subarachnoid space
- Vessels in subarachnoid space
- Pia mater (directly attached to brain surface and not removable)
- Cerebrum

(a)

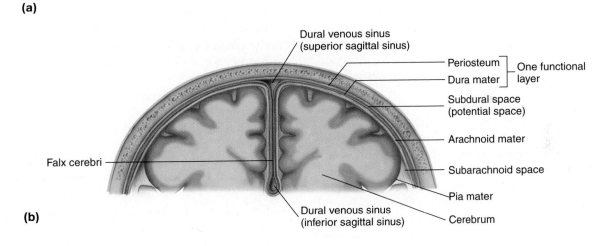

- Dural venous sinus (superior sagittal sinus)
- Periosteum ⎱ One functional
- Dura mater ⎰ layer
- Subdural space (potential space)
- Arachnoid mater
- Subarachnoid space
- Pia mater
- Falx cerebri
- Dural venous sinus (inferior sagittal sinus)
- Cerebrum

(b)

FIGURE 24-18 ▲ **(a)** The meningeal layers that surround the brain and spinal cord. **(b)** A view of the head from the front to show the meninges.

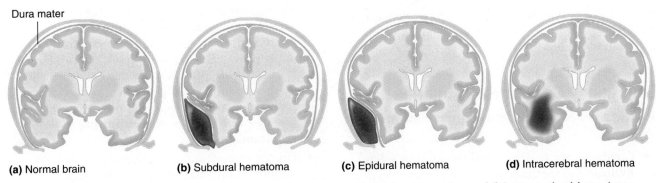

Dura mater

(a) Normal brain   **(b)** Subdural hematoma   **(c)** Epidural hematoma   **(d)** Intracerebral hematoma

FIGURE 24-19 ▲ **(a)** Normal brain. **(b)** Subdural hematoma. **(c)** Epidural hematoma. **(d)** Intracerebral hematoma.

Examples of patients in whom a chronic subdural hematoma may occur include infants who have been subjected to shaken baby syndrome and older adults (because of frequent falls). Signs and symptoms of a subdural hematoma depend on the amount of bleeding within the subdural space and the location of the injury. The patient may appear as if he is having a stroke or is under the influence of drugs or alcohol. Other signs and symptoms can include the following:

- Restlessness
- Headache
- Altered mental status
- Difficulty concentrating
- Slurred speech
- Vomiting
- Seizures

An **epidural hematoma** involves a rapid buildup of blood between the dura and the skull. Most epidural hematomas are associated with an overlying skull fracture. Whereas a subdural hematoma usually involves tearing of veins, an epidural hematoma often involves the tearing of an artery; usually the middle meningeal artery. As blood builds up between the skull and the dura and intracranial pressure increases, most patients will complain of a severe headache. Some patients (less than 30%) experience a loss of consciousness that is followed by a "lucid interval." This means that the patient regains consciousness for a short period (minutes to hours). This is followed by a steady decline in mental status. An early sign of an epidural hematoma is a fixed and dilated pupil on the same side as the injury. A fixed pupil means that the pupil does not react to light. Other signs and symptoms include nausea, vomiting, and seizures. Epidural hematomas occur most often in young adults. This type of brain injury is less common than a subdural hematoma. A patient who has an epidural hematoma must be transported rapidly to the closest appropriate facility with neurosurgical capabilities.

An **intracerebral hematoma** is a collection of blood within the brain. Many intracerebral hematomas are associated with other brain injuries, such as a cerebral contusion. Signs and symptoms depend on the area of the brain involved, the amount of bleeding, and associated injuries.

Emergency Care of Head Injuries

To treat a patient with a head injury, use the following steps:

- Conduct a scene size-up and ensure your safety. Evaluate the mechanism of injury before approaching the patient. Put on appropriate PPE.

Making a Difference

ALS Assist

When caring for a head-injured patient, be alert for changes in the patient's condition that reflect signs of increasing intracranial pressure. These signs include a headache that becomes increasingly severe, confusion, decreasing level of consciousness, vomiting, pupil changes, slow or irregular pulse, irregular breathing, increasing blood pressure, and seizures. If you note any of these signs and symptoms, be sure to relay this information to the ALS personnel who assume responsibility for patient care. This information can help the ALS personnel decide if a tube needs to be placed in the patient's airway, determine the medications that may need to be given, and decide the most appropriate facility to which the patient should be transported.

- Perform a primary survey to identify and treat any life-threatening conditions.
- If the mechanism of injury suggests a head or spinal injury, continue manual stabilization of the patient's head and neck until the patient has been completely immobilized on a long backboard.
- Establish and maintain an open airway. If you must open the patient's airway, use a jaw thrust without head tilt. For an unresponsive patient without a gag reflex, insert an oral airway. Vomiting is common in head-injured patients. Monitor the patient's airway closely while the patient is in your care. Suction as necessary.
- Give oxygen. Inadequate breathing is common in head-injured patients. If the patient's breathing is inadequate, assist his breathing with a BM device connected to 100% oxygen.
- Control bleeding. If bleeding is present from an open head wound, apply firm pressure with a clean cloth to control blood loss over a broad area. If blood soaks through the dressing, apply additional dressings on top and continue to apply pressure. If signs of shock are present or if internal bleeding is suspected, treat for shock. Do not attempt to stop the flow of blood or cerebrospinal fluid from the ears or nose. Cover the area with a loose sterile dressing to absorb the drainage.
- Do not remove a penetrating object. Instead, stabilize it in place with bulky dressings.
- Dress and bandage any open wounds.

- Splint any bone or joint injuries. With any head injury, you must suspect a spinal injury. Stabilize the patient's spine.
- Comfort, calm, and reassure the patient and family members. Remember that the patient may ask the same questions over and over because of his injury. Be prepared for changes in the patient's condition, such as seizures. En route to the receiving facility, perform ongoing assessments as often as indicated. Closely monitor the patient's airway, breathing, pulse, and mental status for deterioration.
- Record all patient care information, including the patient's medical history and all emergency care given on a PCR.

On the Scene   Wrap-Up

Remember that a significant mechanism of injury is one that is likely to produce serious injury. Because this patient experienced a significant mechanism of injury, a rapid trauma assessment should be performed. Provide manual stabilization of the patient's head and neck until the patient has been completely immobilized on a long backboard. Because the patient has experienced a blow to the head and is complaining of nausea, be alert for vomiting and have suction ready. Give 100% oxygen by nonrebreather mask. Dress and bandage the patient's head wound and then prepare the patient for transport to the closest appropriate facility. En route to the receiving facility, perform ongoing assessments every 5 minutes. Closely monitor the patient's airway, breathing, pulse, and mental status for deterioration. ■

Sum It Up

▶ Most spinal injuries occur to the cervical spine. The next most commonly injured areas are the thoracic and lumbar spine. A spinal column injury (bony injury) can occur with or without a spinal cord injury. A spinal cord injury can also occur with or without an injury to the spinal column. The spinal cord does not have to be severed in order for a loss of function to occur.

▶ Compression fractures of the spine result in weakened vertebrae. A compression fracture can occur with or without a spinal cord injury.

▶ Distraction occurs when the spine is pulled apart. When the spine is distracted, ligaments and muscles are overstretched or torn and the vertebrae are pulled apart.

▶ An injury to the spinal cord may be complete or incomplete:
- A complete spinal cord injury occurs when the spinal cord is severed. The patient has no voluntary movement or sensation below the level of the injury. Both sides of the body are equally affected.
  —Paraplegia is the loss of movement and sensation of the lower half of the body from the waist down. Paraplegia results from a spinal cord injury at the level of the thoracic or lumbar vertebrae.
  —Quadriplegia (also called tetraplegia) is a loss of movement and sensation in both arms, both legs, and the parts of the body below the area of injury to the spinal cord. Quadriplegia results from a spinal cord injury at the level of the cervical vertebrae.
- With an incomplete spinal cord injury, some parts of the spinal cord remain intact. The patient has some function below the level of the injury. With this type of injury, there is a potential for recovery because function may be only temporarily lost.

▶ The signs and symptoms of a possible spinal injury include the following:
- Tenderness in the injured area
- Pain associated with movement (Do not ask the patient to move in order to see if he has pain. Do not move the patient to test for a pain response.)
- Pain independent of movement or palpation along the spinal column
- Pain down the lower legs or into the rib cage
- Pain that comes and goes, usually along the spine and/or the lower legs
- Soft-tissue injuries associated with trauma to the head and neck (cuts, bruises)
- Numbness, weakness, or tingling in the extremities
- A loss of sensation or paralysis below the site of injury
- A loss of sensation or paralysis in the upper or lower extremities
- Difficulty breathing
- A loss of bladder or bowel control
- An inability of the patient to walk or move his extremities

▶ Manual stabilization of the head and neck is also called *in-line stabilization*. Manual stabilization of the head and neck helps prevent further injury to the spine.

▶ As an EMT, you may need to apply a rigid cervical collar (also called a *C-collar*) in treating a spinal injury. When used alone, a rigid cervical collar does not immobilize. For effective immobilization, a rigid collar must be used with manual stabilization or a spinal immobilization device, such as a backboard.

▶ A log roll is a technique used to move a patient from a face-down or side-lying position to a face-up position while maintaining the head and neck in line with the rest of the body. This technique is also used to place a patient with a suspected spinal injury on a backboard.

▶ A long backboard helps stabilize the head, neck, torso, pelvis, and extremities. It is used to immobilize patients found in a lying, standing, or sitting position.

▶ A short backboard helps to immobilize a patient's head, neck, and torso. It can also be used as a long backboard for a small child. Examples include vest-type devices and rigid short backboards.

▶ An injury to the scalp may occur because of blunt or penetrating trauma. When injured, the scalp may bleed heavily. In children, the amount of blood loss from a scalp wound may be enough to produce shock.

▶ The skull protects the brain from injury. However, damage to the skull can cause damage to the brain. Skull injuries may occur from blunt or penetrating trauma. Significant force, such as a severe impact or blow, can result in a skull fracture.

▶ A head injury may be open or closed:

• In an open head injury, the scalp is not intact and the risk of infection is increased. Broken bones or foreign objects forced through the skull can cut, tear, or bruise the brain tissue itself.

• In a closed head injury, the skull remains intact. However, the brain can still be injured by the forces or objects that struck the skull. The forces that impact the skull cause the brain to move within skull. The brain strikes the inside of the skull, which causes injuries to the brain tissue.

▶ A concussion is a traumatic brain injury that results in a temporary loss of function in some or all of the brain. A concussion occurs when the head strikes an object or is struck by an object. The injury may or may not cause a loss of consciousness. A headache, loss of appetite, vomiting, and pale skin are common soon after the injury.

▶ A cerebral contusion is a brain injury in which brain tissue is bruised and damaged in a local area. Bruising may occur at both the area of direct impact (coup) and on the side opposite (contrecoup) the impact.

▶ A subdural hematoma usually results from tearing of veins located between the dura and the cerebral cortex after an injury to the head. Blood builds up in the space between the dura and the arachnoid layer of the meninges.

▶ An epidural hematoma involves a rapid buildup of blood between the dura and the skull. An epidural hematoma often involves the tearing of an artery; usually the middle meningeal artery.

▶ An intracerebral hematoma is a collection of blood within the brain. Signs and symptoms depend on the area of the brain involved, the amount of bleeding, and associated injuries.

▶ An altered or decreasing mental status is the best indicator of a brain injury.

▶ To treat a patient with head injury, use the following steps:

• Conduct a scene size-up, ensure safety, and put on appropriate PPE. Evaluate the mechanism of injury.

• Perform a primary survey and ask an assistant to manually stabilize the patient's head and neck while you continue your exam.

• Closely monitor the patient's airway, breathing, pulse, and mental status.

• Perform a physical examination.

• Dress and bandage any open wounds

• Stabilize the patient's spine.

25 Injuries to the Chest, Abdomen, and Genitalia

By the end of this chapter, you should be able to:

Knowledge Objectives ▶

1. List the contents of the chest cavity.
2. List two classifications of chest injuries.
3. State the signs and symptoms and describe the emergency care for:

   a. Rib fractures

   b. Flail chest

   c. Simple pneumothorax

   d. Tension pneumothorax

   e. Hemothorax

   f. Cardiac tamponade

   g. Traumatic asphyxia

   h. Pulmonary contusion

   i. Myocardial contusion

   j. Open pneumothorax

4. State the signs and symptoms of a possible abdominal injury.
5. Describe the emergency care for a patient with a possible abdominal injury.
6. Describe the emergency care for injuries to the external male genitalia.
7. Describe the emergency care for injuries to the external female genitalia.

Attitude Objectives ▶

8. Understand the importance of quickly assessing and treating chest and abdominal injuries.

Skill Objectives ▶

9. Demonstrate assessment of a patient with a suspected chest injury.
10. Demonstrate assessment of a patient with a suspected abdominal injury.
11. Demonstrate assessment of a male patient with a suspected injury to the external genitalia.
12. Demonstrate assessment of a female patient with a suspected injury to the external genitalia.
13. Demonstrate completing a prehospital care report for patients with injuries to the chest, abdomen, or genitalia.

You and your Emergency Medical Technician partner are called to a private residence for a "fall injury." You arrive to find an 81-year-old man lying on the floor in his living room. The patient's wife tells you that she was helping her husband to the bathroom when he suddenly felt weak and fell to the floor, hitting the left side of this chest. The patient is awake, alert, and oriented to person, place, time, and event. You note that his left arm is in a cast. He explains that the cast is the result of a fall 2 days ago. The patient and his wife assure you that he did not hit his head today or lose consciousness. However, the patient did hit his head when he fell 2 days ago.

Using your stethoscope, you hear wheezes on the right side of the chest. Breath sounds are clear on the left side. Palpation of his left rib cage elicits pain, but no instability. The patient says he has had a "terrible headache" all day. He mentions that he had a heart attack 10 years ago, and now takes a "heart pill" daily. His blood pressure is 192/78, pulse 58 (strong and regular). His skin is pink, warm, and dry. His respiratory rate is 36. ∎

THINK ABOUT IT

As you read this chapter, think about the following questions:

- What type of chest injury has this patient sustained?
- After carefully evaluating the patient's vital signs and the historical information he provided, what are possible causes of his headache?
- What additional assessment and care will you need to perform?

Introduction

Managing Injuries to the Chest, Abdomen, and Genitalia

Some injuries to the chest are immediately life threatening and must be identified in the primary survey (Table 25-1). Others are potentially life threatening and need to be identified during the secondary survey. The information in this chapter is enrichment material provided to assist you in learning the types of injuries that may result from trauma to the chest, abdomen, and genitalia. You must know when to suspect these types of injuries and how to provide appropriate care.

TABLE 25-1 Deadly and Potentially Deadly Chest Injuries

Deadly Chest Injuries	Potentially Deadly Chest Injuries
Tension pneumothorax	Pulmonary contusion
Open pneumothorax	Myocardial contusion
Massive hemothorax	
Cardiac tamponade	
Flail chest	

Chest Injuries

Anatomy of the Chest (Thoracic) Cavity

Objective 1

The chest is the upper part of the trunk between the diaphragm and the neck. It contains the mediastinum and pleural cavities. The mediastinum is the area between the lungs that extends from the sternum to the vertebral column. The mediastinum includes all of the contents of the chest cavity (except the lungs), including the esophagus, trachea, heart, and large blood vessels. The right lung is in the right pleural cavity; the left lung is in the left pleural cavity.

The organs of the chest are protected by the rib cage and the upper portion of the spine (Figure 25-1). The rib cage includes the ribs, thoracic vertebrae, and the sternum. The ribs are connected to the vertebrae in back. All but two pairs of ribs are connected by cartilage to the sternum in the front. The rib cage encloses the lungs and heart. Damage to the ribs can result in damage to these organs.

Categories of Chest Injuries

Objective 2

Chest injuries are categorized as closed or open injuries. In closed chest injuries, no break occurs in the skin over the chest wall. These injuries are usually the result of blunt trauma. Underlying structures, such as the heart, lungs, and great vessels, may sustain significant injury. In open chest injuries, a break occurs in the skin over the chest wall. These injuries result from penetrating trauma, such as gunshot wounds, stabbings, or an impaled object.

Closed Chest Injuries

Rib Fractures

Rib fractures are a common injury resulting from blunt trauma to the chest. The presence of a rib fracture suggests significant force caused the injury. Rib fractures may be associated with injury to the underlying lung or the heart.

Although seat belts have reduced the number of deaths and the severity of injuries resulting from motor vehicle crashes (MVCs), they occasionally cause injury. For example, a properly worn 3-point restraint harness can result in rib fractures (Figure 25-2). Lap belts can cause lumbar fractures and abdominal injuries, such as bruising or rupture of the intestines.

The seriousness of a rib fracture increases with age, the number of fractures, and the location of the fracture. Children are less likely to sustain rib fractures than adults are because a child's chest wall is more flexible than that of an adult. Rib fractures most commonly occur in older adults because the ribs of an older adult are more brittle and rigid.

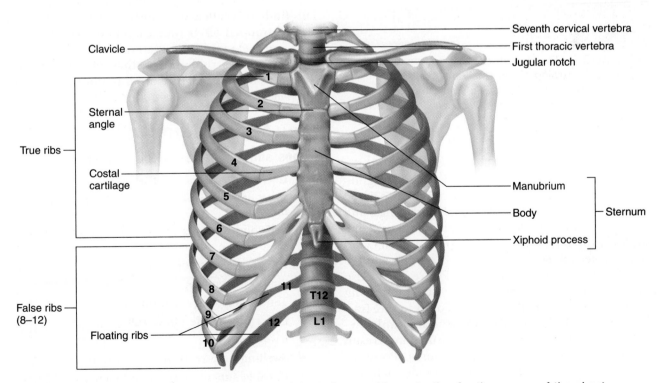

FIGURE 25-1 ▲ The rib cage and upper portion of the spine provide protection for the organs of the chest.

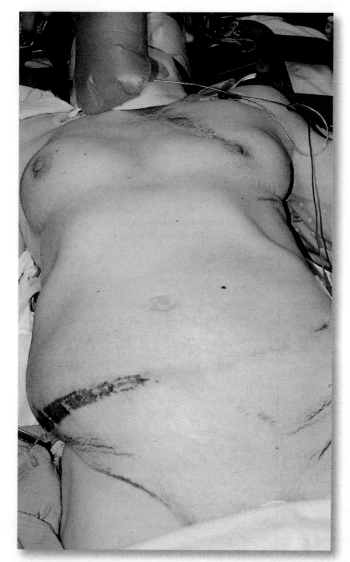

FIGURE 25-2 ▲ This patient experienced multiple rib fractures and bruising of the small intestine from a 3-point seat belt injury. *Courtesy of Stephan Corbett, MD, from Atlas of Emergency Medicine, 2nd edition, McGraw-Hill Company, Inc.*

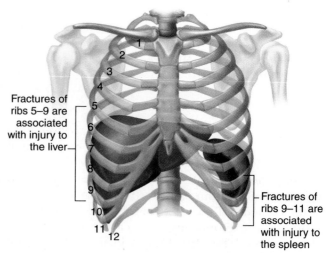

Fractures of ribs 5–9 are associated with injury to the liver

Fractures of ribs 9–11 are associated with injury to the spleen

FIGURE 25-3 ▲ Consider the possibility of injury to underlying structures with lower rib fractures. For example, fractures of ribs 9-11 on the left are associated with rupture of the spleen. Fractures of ribs 5-9 on the right are associated with injury to the liver.

When assessing the chest of a responsive patient who has a rib fracture, you may notice that the patient holds his arm close to his chest. This common finding is the patient's attempt to "splint" the injury because of pain. The patient's pain is usually localized to the injured area and increases when he breathes deeply, coughs, or moves. The patient may breathe shallowly to decrease the pain associated with breathing. You may notice a crackling sensation under your fingers while assessing the patient's chest. This finding is called *subcutaneous emphysema* and represents trapped air between layers of skin. You may hear and feel crepitus, a grating sound produced by bone fragments rubbing together. Other signs and symptoms of a rib fracture are listed in the following *You Should Know* box.

You Should Know

Signs and Symptoms of Rib Fracture

- Localized pain at the fracture site that worsens with deep breathing, coughing, or moving
- Self-splinting of the injury by holding the arm close to the chest
- Pain on inspiration
- Shallow breathing
- Tenderness on palpation
- Deformity of the chest wall
- Crepitus
- Swelling and/or bruising at the fracture site
- Possible subcutaneous emphysema

Ribs 1-3 are protected by the shoulder girdle. Fractures of ribs 1 and 2 are associated with significant trauma. These fractures are often associated with injury to the head, neck, spinal cord, lungs, and the major blood vessels. Ribs 4-9 are the most commonly fractured because these ribs are long, thin, and poorly protected. Fractures of ribs 5-9 on the right are associated with injury to the liver (Figure 25-3). Also consider the possibility of injury to underlying structures with lower rib fractures. For example, fractures of ribs 9-11 on the left are associated with rupture of the spleen. Multiple rib fractures may result in inadequate breathing and pneumonia. Posterior rib fractures are usually the result of deceleration accidents.

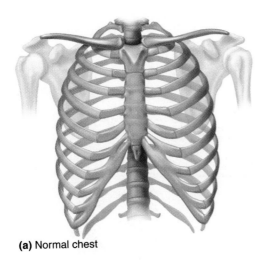

(a) Normal chest

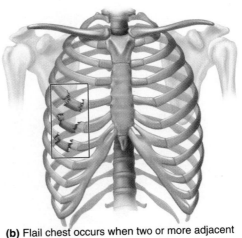

(b) Flail chest occurs when two or more adjacent ribs fracture in two or more places

FIGURE 25-4 ▲ **(a)** Normal chest. **(b)** Flail segment.

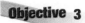

To treat a patient with a rib fracture, perform the following steps:

- Put on appropriate personal protective equipment (PPE).
- If spinal injury is suspected, maintain manual in-line stabilization until the patient is secured to a long backboard. Establish and maintain an open airway.
- Give oxygen. If the patient's breathing is adequate, apply oxygen by nonrebreather mask at 15 L/min if not already done. If the patient's breathing is inadequate, provide positive-pressure ventilation with 100% oxygen. Assess the adequacy of the ventilations delivered.
- Encourage the patient to breathe deeply. Reassess breath sounds often while the patient is in your care.
- Do not apply tape or straps to the ribs or chest wall. Applying tape or straps limits chest wall motion and reduces the effectiveness of ventilation.
- Allow the patient to hold a pillow for comfort, if appropriate. Self-splinting will reduce pain, and a pillow will not provide excessive pressure to reduce ventilatory effectiveness. It also encourages deeper breathing, since the chest wall expands into the soft, padded surface.
- Perform ongoing assessments as often as indicated during transport.
- Record all patient care information, including the patient's medical history and all emergency care given, on a prehospital care report (PCR).

Flail Chest

A flail chest occurs when two or more adjacent ribs are fractured in two or more places or when the sternum is detached (Figure 25-4). The section of the chest wall between the fractured ribs becomes free-floating because it is no longer in continuity with the thorax. This free-floating section of the chest wall is called the *flail segment*. The flail segment does not move with the rest of the rib cage when the patient attempts to breathe (**paradoxical movement**). When the patient inhales, the flail segment is drawn inward instead of moving outward (Figure 25-5). When the patient exhales, the flail segment moves outward instead of moving inward.

A flail chest is a life-threatening injury. Flail chest most commonly occurs in MVCs (especially crushing rollover crashes) but may also occur because of:

- Falls from a height
- Assault
- Industrial accidents
- Neonatal trauma during childbirth

The forces necessary to produce a flail chest cause bruising of the underlying lung (pulmonary contusion). Although instability of the chest wall results in paradoxical movement of the chest wall during breathing, it is the bruising of the underlying lung and pain associated with breathing that contributes to hypoxia. Respiratory failure may occur because of:

- Bruising of the underlying lung and associated hemorrhage of the alveoli, reducing the amount of lung tissue available for gas exchange
- Instability of the chest wall and pain associated with breathing, leading to decreased ventilation and hypoxia
- Interference with the normal "bellows" action of the chest, resulting in inadequate gas exchange

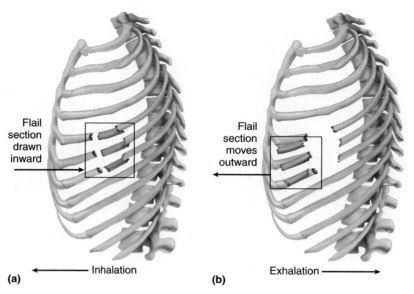

FIGURE 25-5 ▲ Paradoxical movement. **(a)** When the patient inhales, the flail segment is drawn inward instead of moving outward. **(b)** When the patient exhales, the flail segment moves outward instead of moving inward.

Flail chest may be associated with other injuries, including:

- Bruising of the underlying lung (pulmonary contusion)
- Bruising of the heart muscle (myocardial contusion)
- Hemothorax
- Pneumothorax

You Should Know

Signs and Symptoms of Flail Chest

- Crepitus
- Breathing difficulty
- Bruising of the chest wall
- Increased heart rate (tachycardia)
- Pain and self-splinting of the affected side
- Increased respiratory rate (tachypnea)
- Pain in the chest associated with breathing
- Paradoxical chest wall movement

Objective 3

To treat a patient with a flail chest, perform the following steps:

- Put on appropriate PPE. Keep on-scene time to a minimum. Request an early response of Advanced Life Support (ALS) personnel to the scene, or consider an ALS intercept while en route to the receiving facility. Do not delay transport for ALS arrival.

- Suspect associated spinal injuries. Maintain manual in-line stabilization until the patient is secured to a long backboard.
- Establish and maintain an open airway.
- Give oxygen. If the patient's breathing is adequate, apply oxygen by nonrebreather mask at 15 L/min if not already done. If the patient's breathing is inadequate, provide positive-pressure ventilation with 100% oxygen. Assess the adequacy of the ventilations delivered. Monitor closely for development of a tension pneumothorax (discussed later in this chapter).
- If consistent with your local protocol, stabilize the chest wall by applying a bulky dressing to the flail segment.
- Continually monitor and reassess respiratory rate, rhythm, depth, and effort; vital signs (including pulse oximetry); degree of paradoxical chest movement; and skin temperature, color, and condition (moisture).
- Treat for shock if indicated.
- Transport promptly to the closest appropriate facility. Perform ongoing assessments, including vital signs, at least every 5 minutes en route.
- Record all patient care information, including the patient's medical history and all emergency care given, on a PCR.

Simple Pneumothorax

A pneumothorax is a collection of air or gas outside the lung and between the lung and the chest wall. In a **simple pneumothorax,** air enters the chest cavity, causing a loss of negative pressure (vacuum) and a

- Paradoxical movement is probably most readily seen in an unresponsive patient. In patients with thick or muscular chest walls, it may be difficult to observe paradoxical movement. In some conscious patients, spasm and self-splinting of the chest muscles may cause paradoxical motion to go unnoticed.
- Studies show that many patients who have a flail chest injury have long-term problems, including ongoing chest wall pain, deformity, and difficulty breathing with exertion.

partial or total collapse of the lung (Figure 25-6). A simple pneumothorax may occur because of blunt or penetrating chest trauma. For instance, a simple pneumothorax may occur because of a blast injury or diving accident. Air may also enter the chest cavity through a hole in the chest wall (sucking chest wound) or a hole in the lung tissue, bronchus, or the trachea. As air enters and fills the pleural space, lung tissue is compressed. This reduces the amount of lung tissue available for gas exchange.

The patient's signs and symptoms depend on the size of the pneumothorax and the patient's general health. Small tears may self-seal, resolving by themselves. The patient may not experience difficulty breathing or other signs of respiratory distress. Larger tears may progress, resulting in signs and symptoms of respiratory distress. Signs and symptoms of a simple pneumothorax are shown in the following *You Should Know* box.

You Should Know

Signs and Symptoms of Simple Pneumothorax

- Sudden onset of sharp pain in the chest associated with breathing
- Shortness of breath
- Difficulty breathing
- Decreased or absent breath sounds on the affected side
- Increased respiratory rate (tachypnea)
- Increased heart rate (tachycardia)
- Subcutaneous emphysema (may not be present)

A **spontaneous pneumothorax** is a type of pneumothorax that does not involve trauma to the lung. There are 2 types of spontaneous pneumothorax. A **primary spontaneous pneumothorax** occurs in people with no history of lung disease. This condition most

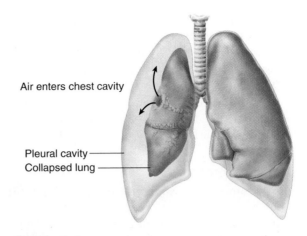

Air enters chest cavity

Pleural cavity
Collapsed lung

FIGURE 25-6 ▲ In a simple pneumothorax, air enters the chest cavity, causing a loss of negative pressure and a partial or total collapse of the lung.

commonly occurs in tall, thin men between the ages of 20 and 40. It rarely occurs in persons older than 40 years. A **secondary spontaneous pneumothorax** most often occurs as a complication of lung disease. Chronic obstructive pulmonary disease (COPD) is the most common underlying disorder. Other lung diseases associated with this condition include asthma, pneumonia, tuberculosis, and lung cancer. A secondary spontaneous pneumothorax usually occurs in older persons. A spontaneous pneumothorax typically occurs while the patient is at rest or during sleep. It is usually caused by the rupture of a **bleb** (a small air- or fluid-filled sac) in the lung. Although they depend on the size of the pneumothorax, common signs and symptoms include a sudden onset of chest pain on the affected side, shortness of breath, an increased respiratory rate, and a cough. The patient's chest pain may be described as dull, sharp, or stabbing.

Objective 3

To treat a patient with a pneumothorax, perform the following steps:

- Put on appropriate PPE.
- If spinal injury is suspected, maintain manual in-line stabilization until the patient is secured to a long backboard. If spinal injury is not suspected, place the patient in a position of comfort. Most patients will be more comfortable sitting up.
- Establish and maintain an open airway.
- Give oxygen. If the patient's breathing is adequate, apply oxygen by nonrebreather mask at 15 L/min if not already done. If the patient's breathing is inadequate, provide positive-pressure ventilation with 100% oxygen. Assess the adequacy of the ventilations delivered.

- Transport promptly to the closest appropriate facility. Perform ongoing assessments as often as indicated. Reassess frequently for signs of a tension pneumothorax (explained in the next section).

- Record all patient care information, including the patient's medical history and all emergency care given, on a PCR.

Tension Pneumothorax

Tension pneumothorax is a life-threatening injury. It can occur because of blunt or penetrating trauma or as a complication of treatment of an open pneumothorax. In an **open pneumothorax,** there is an open wound in the chest wall into the pleural cavity. In a tension pneumothorax, air enters the pleural cavity during inspiration and progressively builds up under pressure. The flap of injured lung acts as a one-way valve, allowing air to enter the pleural space during inspiration but trapping it during expiration. The injured lung collapses completely. Pressure rises, forcing the trachea, heart, and major blood vessels to be pushed toward the opposite side (Figure 25-7). Shifting of the trachea from its normal midline position is called *tracheal deviation* (or *tracheal shift*). In a tension pneumothorax, the trachea shifts to the uninjured lung (the side opposite the injury). To effectively assess tracheal deviation, examine the trachea by feeling for the tubular shape of the trachea between your thumb and index finger just above the sternum in the suprasternal notch. Assessing above this area for tracheal deviation may not reveal a shift of the trachea even if it does exist. Because significant pressure must build up to cause tracheal deviation, it is a late physical examination finding. Shifting of the heart and major blood vessels from their normal position is called **mediastinal shift.** Shifting of the major blood vessels causes them to kink, resulting in a backup of blood into the venous system. The backup of blood into the venous system results in jugular venous distention (JVD), decreased blood return to the heart, and signs of shock. Signs and symptoms of a tension pneumothorax are listed in the following *You Should Know* box.

You Should Know

Signs and Symptoms of Tension Pneumothorax

- Cool, clammy skin
- Increased pulse rate
- Cyanosis (late sign)
- JVD
- Decreased blood pressure
- Severe respiratory distress
- Agitation, restlessness, anxiety
- Bulging of intercostal muscles on the affected side
- Decreased or absent breath sounds on the affected side
- Tracheal deviation toward the unaffected side (late sign)
- Possible subcutaneous emphysema in the face, neck, or chest wall

Objective 3

Follow these steps when providing emergency care for a possible tension pneumothorax:

- Put on appropriate PPE. Keep on-scene time to a minimum. Request an early response of ALS personnel to the scene, or consider an ALS intercept while en route to the receiving facility. Do not delay transport for ALS arrival.

- If spinal injury is suspected, maintain manual in-line stabilization until the patient is secured to a long backboard.

- Establish and maintain an open airway.

- Give oxygen. If the patient's breathing is adequate, apply oxygen by nonrebreather mask at 15 L/min if not already done. If the patient's breathing is inadequate, provide positive-pressure ventilation with 100% oxygen and assess the adequacy of the ventilations delivered.

- Treat for shock if indicated.

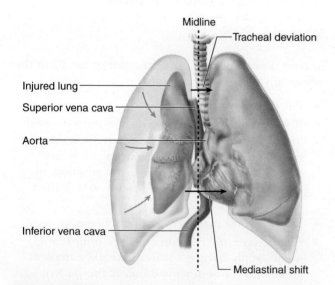

Midline
Tracheal deviation
Injured lung
Superior vena cava
Aorta
Inferior vena cava
Mediastinal shift

FIGURE 25-7 ▲ In a tension pneumothorax, air enters the pleural cavity during inspiration and progressively builds up under pressure.

- If an open chest wound was bandaged with an occlusive dressing, release the dressing. If air is present under tension, air will rush out of the wound. Once the air is released, reseal the wound again with a dressing taped on three sides.
- Transport promptly to the closest appropriate facility, reassessing vital signs at least every 5 minutes en route.
- Record all patient care information, including the patient's medical history and all emergency care given, on a PCR.

Hemothorax

A hemothorax is a collection of blood in the pleural cavity that may result from injury to the chest wall, the major blood vessels, or the lung because of penetrating or blunt trauma (Figure 25-8). Rib fractures are a common cause of a hemothorax. A hemothorax is often seen with a simple or tension pneumothorax.

The chest cavity can hold 2000–3000 mL of blood. The term **massive hemothorax** is used to describe blood loss of more than 1500 mL in the chest cavity. A massive hemothorax is a life-threatening injury. Signs and symptoms of hemothorax are listed in the following *You Should Know* box.

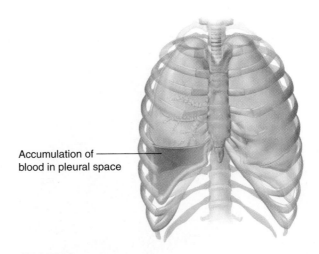

Accumulation of blood in pleural space

FIGURE 25-8 ▲ A hemothorax is a collection of blood in the pleural cavity.

- If spinal injury is suspected, maintain manual in-line stabilization until the patient is secured to a long backboard.
- Establish and maintain an open airway.
- Give oxygen. If the patient's breathing is adequate, apply oxygen by nonrebreather mask at 15 L/min if not already done. If the patient's breathing is inadequate, provide positive-pressure ventilation with 100% oxygen and assess the adequacy of the ventilations delivered.
- Treat for shock if indicated.
- Reassess frequently for development of a tension pneumothorax.
- Transport promptly to the closest appropriate facility, reassessing vital signs at least every 5 minutes en route.
- Record all patient care information, including the patient's medical history and all emergency care given, on a PCR.

You Should Know

Signs and Symptoms of Hemothorax

- Cool, clammy skin
- Weak, thready pulse
- Restlessness, agitation, anxiety
- Coughing up blood (**hemoptysis**) (may not occur)
- Rapid, shallow breathing (tachypnea)
- Flat neck veins (caused by hypovolemia)
- Decreasing blood pressure (hypotension)
- Decreased or absent breath sounds on the affected side

Cardiac (Pericardial) Tamponade

Cardiac tamponade is a life-threatening injury. It most frequently occurs because of penetrating chest trauma, but it can occur because of blunt trauma to the chest. Cardiac tamponade occurs when blood enters the pericardial sac because of:

- Laceration of a coronary blood vessel
- Ruptured coronary artery
- Laceration of a chamber of the heart
- Significant bruising of the heart (myocardial contusion)

The blood in the pericardial sac compresses the heart, decreasing the amount of blood the heart can pump out with each contraction (Figure 25-9). The patient's signs and symptoms depend on how quickly

Objective 3

Follow these steps when providing emergency care to a patient with a possible hemothorax:

- Put on appropriate PPE. Keep on-scene time to a minimum. Request an early response of ALS personnel to the scene, or consider an ALS intercept while en route to the receiving facility. Do not delay transport for ALS arrival.

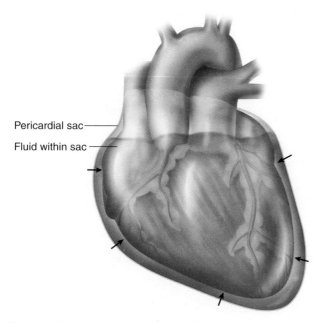

Pericardial sac
Fluid within sac

FIGURE 25-9 ▲ Cardiac tamponade occurs when blood enters the pericardial sac and compresses the heart. This decreases the amount of blood the heart can pump out with each contraction.

blood collects in the pericardial sac. Signs and symptoms of cardiac tamponade are listed in the following *You Should Know* box.

You Should Know

Signs and Symptoms of Cardiac Tamponade

- Cool, clammy skin
- Normal breath sounds
- Narrowing pulse pressure
- Trachea in midline position
- Increased heart rate (tachycardia)
- Cyanosis of head, neck, and upper extremities
- Muffled heart sounds (often difficult to assess in the field)
- Distended neck veins (may not be present in hypovolemia)

Objective 3

Perform the following steps to treat a patient with cardiac tamponade:

- Put on appropriate PPE. Keep on-scene time to a minimum. Request an early response of ALS personnel to the scene, or consider an ALS intercept while en route to the receiving facility. Do not delay transport for ALS arrival.

- If spinal injury is suspected, maintain manual in-line stabilization until the patient is secured to a long backboard.
- Establish and maintain an open airway.
- Give oxygen. If the patient's breathing is adequate, apply oxygen by nonrebreather mask at 15 L/min if not already done. If the patient's breathing is inadequate, provide positive-pressure ventilation with 100% oxygen and assess the adequacy of the ventilations delivered.
- Treat for shock if indicated.
- Transport promptly to the closest appropriate facility, reassessing vital signs at least every 5 minutes en route.
- Record all patient care information, including the patient's medical history and all emergency care given, on a PCR.

Traumatic Asphyxia

Traumatic asphyxia occurs because of a severe compression injury to the chest, such as compression of the chest under a heavy object or between a vehicle's seat and steering wheel. Blood backs up into the veins, venules, and capillaries of the head, neck, extremities, and upper torso, resulting in capillary rupture (Figure 25-10). The skin of the head and neck becomes deep red, purple, or blue. This characteristic finding is called *hooding* or a *purple cape* by Emergency Medical Services (EMS) professionals. Signs and symptoms of traumatic asphyxia are shown in the following *You Should Know* box.

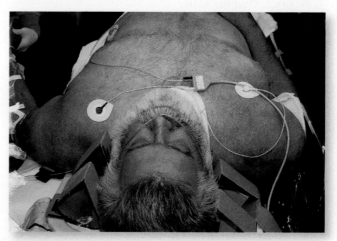

FIGURE 25-10 ▲ Traumatic asphyxia. This 45-year-old man was working under a truck when it fell on his chest. He was pinned under the truck and unable to breathe for 3 to 4 minutes until his coworkers rescued him. Note the discoloration of his upper body. The patient was observed in the hospital overnight and recovered with no complications. *Courtesy of Stephan Corbett, MD, from Atlas of Emergency Medicine, 2nd edition, McGraw-Hill Company, Inc.*

Signs and Symptoms of Traumatic Asphyxia

- JVD
- Swelling of the tongue and lips
- Eyes that appear bloodshot and bulging
- Deep red, purple, or blue discoloration of the head and neck (hooding)
- Low blood pressure once the compression is released
- Normal-looking pink skin below the level of the crush injury (unless other injuries are present)

Objective 3

To treat a patient with traumatic asphyxia, perform the following steps:

- Put on appropriate PPE. Keep on-scene time to a minimum. Request an early response of ALS personnel to the scene, or consider an ALS intercept while en route to the receiving facility. Do not delay transport for ALS arrival.
- Suspect spinal injuries and multiple organ damage. Maintain manual in-line stabilization until the patient is secured to a long backboard.
- Establish and maintain an open airway.
- Give oxygen. If the patient's breathing is adequate, apply oxygen by nonrebreather mask at 15 L/min if not already done. If the patient's breathing is inadequate, provide positive-pressure ventilation with 100% oxygen. Assess the adequacy of the ventilations delivered.
- Control any bleeding, if present. If indicated, treat for shock.

- Transport promptly to the closest appropriate facility, reassessing vital signs at least every 5 minutes en route. Monitor closely for development of a tension pneumothorax and/or cardiac tamponade.
- Record all patient care information, including the patient's medical history and all emergency care given, on a PCR.

Pulmonary Contusion

A pulmonary contusion (bruising of the lung) is a potentially life-threatening injury. A pulmonary contusion occurs in about 75% of patients with flail chest. Most pulmonary contusions occur because of a rapid deceleration injury, such as a fall, high-speed MVC, or other blunt trauma. It can also occur as a result of blunt trauma without rib fracture. A pulmonary contusion is often missed because of the presence of other, associated injuries.

In a pulmonary contusion, the alveoli fill with blood and fluid because of bruising of the lung tissue (Figure 25-11). As a result, the area of the lung available for gas exchange is decreased. The severity of the patient's signs and symptoms depends on the amount of lung tissue injured. Bleeding from a pulmonary contusion may result in a blood loss of 1000–1500 mL. Signs and symptoms of pulmonary contusion are shown in the next *You Should Know* box.

Objective 3

To treat a patient with a pulmonary contusion, perform the following steps:

- Put on appropriate PPE. Keep on-scene time to a minimum. Request an early response of ALS personnel to the scene, or consider an ALS intercept while en route to the receiving facility. Do not delay transport for ALS arrival.

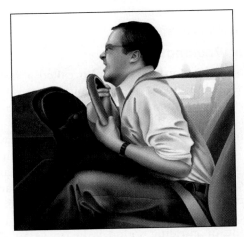 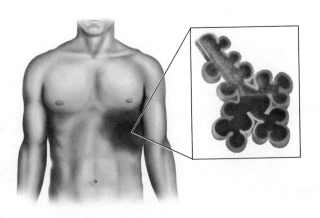

FIGURE 25-11 ▲ In a pulmonary contusion, the alveoli fill with blood and fluid because of bruising of the lung tissue.

- Suspect spinal injuries. Maintain manual in-line stabilization until the patient is secured to a long backboard.
- Establish and maintain an open airway.
- Give oxygen. If the patient's breathing is adequate, apply oxygen by nonrebreather mask at 15 L/min if not already done. If the patient's breathing is inadequate, provide positive-pressure ventilation with 100% oxygen. Assess the adequacy of the ventilations delivered.
- Treat for shock if indicated.
- Transport promptly to the closest appropriate facility, reassessing vital signs at least every 5 minutes en route.
- Record all patient care information, including the patient's medical history and all emergency care given, on a PCR.

Myocardial (Cardiac) Contusion

A **myocardial contusion** is bruising of the heart (Figure 25-12). It occurs because of blunt chest trauma, such as:

- Chest compressions during cardiopulmonary resuscitation (CPR)
- Acceleration/deceleration injuries
- Fractures of the sternum
- Fractures of ribs 1-3

A myocardial contusion is a potentially life-threatening injury. Signs and symptoms of a myocardial contusion include chest pain or discomfort, increased or slowed heart rate, and (possibly) an irregular heart rhythm.

Objective 3

To treat a patient with a myocardial contusion, perform the following steps:

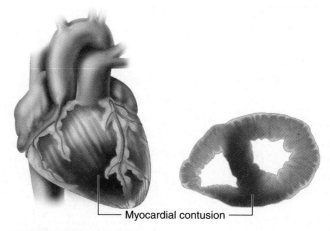

FIGURE 25-12 ▲ A myocardial contusion is a bruise of the heart.

- Put on appropriate PPE. Keep on-scene time to a minimum. Request an early response of ALS personnel to the scene, or consider an ALS intercept while en route to the receiving facility. Do not delay transport for ALS arrival.
- Suspect spinal injuries. Maintain manual in-line stabilization until the patient is secured to a long backboard.
- Establish and maintain an open airway.
- Give oxygen. If the patient's breathing is adequate, apply oxygen by nonrebreather mask at 15 L/min if not already done. If the patient's breathing is inadequate, provide positive-pressure ventilation with 100% oxygen and assess the adequacy of the ventilations delivered.
- Treat for shock if indicated.
- Transport promptly to the closest appropriate facility, reassessing vital signs at least every 5 minutes en route.
- Record all patient care information, including the patient's medical history and all emergency care given, on a PCR.

Open Chest Injuries

Open Pneumothorax

An **open pneumothorax** is also called a *sucking chest wound*. It is a life-threatening injury that is caused by penetrating trauma (see the next *You Should Know* box). Air enters the chest cavity through an open wound in the chest wall into the pleural cavity (Figure 25-13). The severity of an open pneumothorax depends on the size of the wound. If the diameter of the chest wound is more than 2/3 the diameter of the patient's trachea, air will enter the chest wound rather than through the trachea with each breath. A sucking or gurgling sound is heard as air moves in and out of the pleural space through the open chest

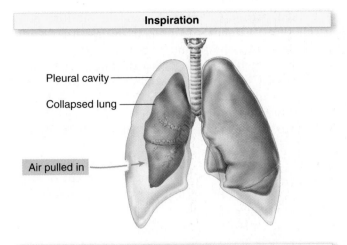

Inspiration

Pleural cavity

Collapsed lung

Air pulled in

Expiration

Air escapes

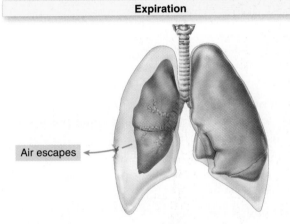

FIGURE 25-13 ▲ An open pneumothorax is a life-threatening injury that is caused by penetrating trauma.

wound. If the flap of chest wall closes during expiration, air will become trapped inside the pleural cavity. As air collects in the pleural cavity, pressure builds with each inspiration. This eventually results in a tension pneumothorax.

You Should Know

Possible Causes of Open Pneumothorax

- Blast injuries
- Knife wounds
- Impaled objects
- Gunshot wounds
- MVCs

Objective 3

To treat a patient with an open pneumothorax, perform the following steps:

- Put on appropriate PPE. Keep on-scene time to a minimum. Request an early response of ALS

You Should Know

Signs and Symptoms of Open Pneumothorax

- Shortness of breath
- Increased heart rate
- Pain at the site of injury
- Increased respiratory rate
- Subcutaneous emphysema
- Sucking sound on inhalation
- Open wound in the chest wall
- Decreased breath sounds on the affected side

personnel to the scene, or consider an ALS intercept while en route to the receiving facility. Do not delay transport for ALS arrival.

- Suspect spinal injuries. Maintain manual in-line stabilization until the patient is secured to a long backboard.
- Establish and maintain an open airway.
- Promptly close the chest wound with an airtight (occlusive) dressing. Plastic wrap and petroleum gauze are examples of dressings that may be used. Make sure that the dressing is large enough so that it is not pulled into the wound during inspiration. Tape the dressing on three sides (1-way valve). The dressing will be sucked over the wound as the patient inhales, preventing air from entering. The open end of the dressing allows air to escape as the patient exhales. If signs and symptoms of a tension pneumothorax develop after an airtight dressing has been applied, release the dressing. Reassess the patient's airway, breathing, circulation, and mental status. If the patient's breathing returns to normal, replace the airtight dressing and again secure it in place over the wound by taping it in place on three sides.
- Give oxygen. If the patient's breathing is adequate, apply oxygen by nonrebreather mask at 15 L/min if not already done. If the patient's breathing is inadequate, provide positive-pressure ventilation with 100% oxygen. Assess the adequacy of the ventilations delivered. Watch closely for development of a tension pneumothorax.
- Control any external bleeding. Treat for shock if indicated.
- Transport promptly to the closest appropriate facility. Perform ongoing assessments every 5 minutes.
- Record all patient care information, including the patient's medical history and all emergency care given, on a PCR.

Abdominal Injuries

In some situations, it will not always be clear if an injury to a patient's torso involves only the chest or the abdomen, or both. For instance, suppose your patient has a stab wound in the area of the 9th rib on the right side of his body. Can you be sure that the damage inflicted by the knife blade is limited to the chest? No, for a couple of reasons. First, remember that the diaphragm divides the chest and abdominal cavities. However, the position of the diaphragm changes with respiration (Figure 25-14). When a person takes a deep breath in, the diaphragm may be well below the lower edge of the rib cage (costal margin). This increases the likelihood of injury to the organs in the chest cavity. With full exhalation, the diaphragm may be at the level of the nipple line. This increases the likelihood of injury to the abdominal organs. Second, the forces involved in producing the injury and the course a penetrating object takes in the body cannot be determined with 100% accuracy by simply looking at the point of impact or penetration. For these reasons, it is best to assume that an injury to the chest or abdomen involves both body cavities. In this way, injuries are less likely to be overlooked.

Types of abdominal injuries include open injuries, in which the skin is broken, and closed injuries, in which the skin is not broken. Closed or open wounds to the abdomen may involve multiple organs and major blood vessels, including the abdominal aorta and inferior vena cava. Deaths from abdominal trauma result mainly from hemorrhage or infection.

Recall from Chapter 4 that the abdomen is divided into 4 quadrants to make things easier when identifying the abdominal organs and the location of pain or injury (Figure 25-15). These quadrants are created by drawing two imaginary lines that intersect with the midline through the navel. Knowing the organs found within each of the 4 quadrants will help you describe the location of a patient's injury (Table 25-2).

The abdomen contains both hollow and solid organs (Table 25-3). If hollow organs are cut or ruptured, their contents spill into the abdominal cavity, causing inflammation. Severe bleeding may result if a solid organ is cut or ruptures.

Objective 4

Signs and symptoms of abdominal injury include the following:

- Patient who lies still, usually on his side, with the legs drawn up to the chest (fetal position)
- Nausea
- Vomiting blood (**hematemesis**)
- Possible blood in the urine (**hematuria**)
- Possible skin wounds and penetrations
- Abdominal pain
- Rigid abdominal muscles
- Distended abdomen
- Rapid, shallow breathing
- Signs of shock
- Protruding organs (evisceration)

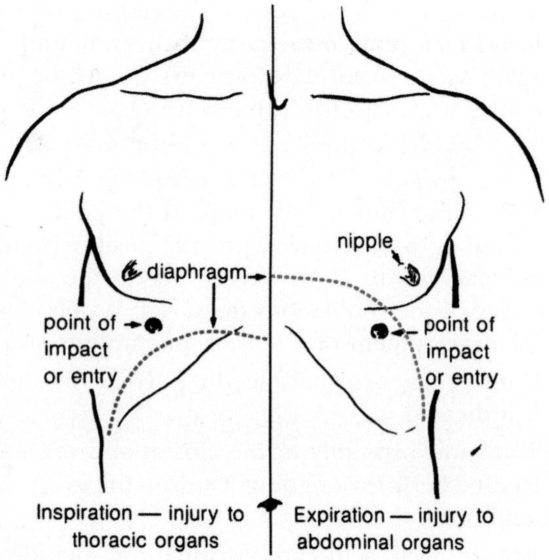

FIGURE 25-14 ▲ The position of the diaphragm changes with respiration.

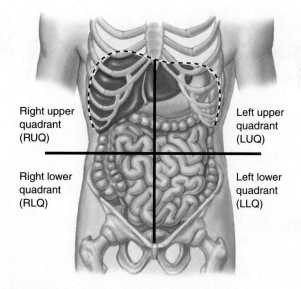

Right upper quadrant (RUQ)

Left upper quadrant (LUQ)

Right lower quadrant (RLQ)

Left lower quadrant (LLQ)

FIGURE 25-15 ▲ The abdominal area is divided into four quadrants.

TABLE 25-2 Abdominal Organs by Quadrant

Abdominal Quadrant	Organs
Right upper quadrant	Liver, gallbladder, portions of the stomach, right kidney, ascending colon, transverse colon, major blood vessels
Right lower quadrant	Appendix, ascending colon, right ovary (female), right fallopian tube (female)
Left upper quadrant	Stomach, spleen, pancreas, transverse colon, descending colon, left kidney
Left lower quadrant	Descending colon, sigmoid colon, left ovary (female), left fallopian tube (female)

TABLE 25-3 Hollow and Solid Abdominal Organs

Hollow Organs	Solid Organs
Stomach	Liver
Intestines	Spleen
Gallbladder	Pancreas
Urinary bladder	Kidneys
Uterus (female)	Adrenal glands
	Ovaries (female)

Objective 5

To treat a patient with an abdominal injury, perform the following steps:

- Put on appropriate PPE. Keep on-scene time to a minimum.
- If spinal injury is suspected, maintain manual in-line stabilization until the patient is secured to a long backboard. If a spinal injury is not suspected, place the patient in a position of comfort.
- Establish and maintain an open airway.
- Give oxygen. If the patient's breathing is adequate, apply oxygen by nonrebreather mask at 15 L/min if not already done. If the patient's breathing is inadequate, provide positive-pressure ventilation with 100% oxygen and assess the adequacy of the ventilations delivered.
- Control any external bleeding. If signs of shock are present or if internal bleeding is suspected, treat for shock.
- Do not remove penetrating objects; rather, stabilize in place with bulky dressings.
- Do not touch protruding organs. Carefully remove clothing from around the wound. Apply a large sterile dressing, moistened with sterile water or saline, over the organs and wound. Secure the dressing in place with a large bandage to retain moisture and prevent heat loss.
- Flex the patient's hips and knees, if they are uninjured and spinal injury is not suspected, to decrease tension on the abdominal muscles.
- Monitor for changes in tenderness or rigidity of the abdomen.
- Transport promptly. Perform ongoing assessments at least every 5 minutes en route.
- Record all patient care information, including the patient's medical history and all emergency care given, on a PCR.

Injuries to the Genitalia

Males

Objective 6

Injuries to the external male genitalia include cuts, bruises, penetrating objects, amputations, and avulsions. If the patient is responsive, explain to him that you will need to view the area and then obtain permission from him to proceed. Be aware that he will most likely be anxious and may be embarrassed. Offer emotional support, maintain the patient's privacy, and protect his modesty. Emergency care for an injury to the male genitalia includes the following:

- Put on appropriate PPE.
- Give oxygen on the basis of the patient's signs, symptoms, and vital signs, including pulse oximetry.
- If spinal injury is suspected, maintain manual in-line stabilization until the patient is secured to a long backboard. If a spinal injury is not suspected, place the patient in a position of comfort.

- Expose the wound site. Control external bleeding by applying direct pressure to the wound with a sterile dressing. If blood soaks through the dressing, apply additional dressings and reapply pressure. Treat for shock, if indicated.
- Do not remove penetrating objects.
- Manage avulsed or amputated parts as other soft tissue injuries.
- Protect the patient's modesty and provide emotional support.
- Perform ongoing assessments as often as indicated en route to the receiving facility.
- Record all patient care information, including the patient's medical history and all emergency care given, on a PCR.

Females

Objective 7

The internal female genitalia are rarely injured except in the pregnant patient or in cases of sexual assault with penetration. Blunt injuries may rupture the uterus, causing loss of life of the fetus and severe hemorrhage. Injuries to the external female genitalia usually result from straddle injuries or sexual assault.

Looking at the external female genitalia is necessary if childbirth is imminent or if the patient complains of bleeding from the vaginal or rectal area. Before visualizing the area, tactfully explain that you will need to view the area and obtain permission from the patient to do so. If possible, it is advisable to have a female EMS professional in attendance during the assessment. Your assessment of the female genitalia is limited to *looking* at the area, while maintaining the patient's privacy and protecting her modesty. You must *never* insert anything into the vagina or attempt to examine the internal female genitalia. These actions are outside the Emergency Medical Technician's scope of practice.

Emergency care for an injury to the female genitalia includes the following:

- Put on appropriate PPE.
- Give oxygen on the basis of the patient's signs, symptoms, and vital signs, including pulse oximetry.
- If spinal injury is suspected, maintain manual in-line stabilization until the patient is secured to a long backboard. If a spinal injury is not suspected, place the patient in a position of comfort.
- To control bleeding from a wound, apply direct pressure to the wound with a sterile dressing. If blood soaks through the dressing, apply additional dressings and reapply pressure. Control

severe vaginal bleeding with external padding. Treat for shock, if indicated.
- Do not remove penetrating objects. Manage avulsed or amputated parts as other soft tissue injuries.
- Nothing should be placed in the vagina.
- Protect the patient's modesty and provide emotional support.
- Perform ongoing assessments as often as indicated en route to the receiving facility.
- Record all patient care information, including the patient's medical history and all emergency care given, on a PCR.

On the Scene   Wrap-Up

A repeat set of vital signs reveals the following: blood pressure 196/70, pulse 56, and respiration 32. You suspect the patient's chest injury is probably a bruised muscle over a rib or rib fracture. However, on the basis of your physical examination findings, the patient's complaint of a severe headache, and his vital signs, you suspect the patient may have a bigger problem—bleeding in his brain. The patient's vital signs are consistent with signs of increasing intracranial pressure. Possible causes include a subdural hematoma (most likely from the fall 2 days ago) or a stroke. Remember that a patient who has a subdural hematoma may appear as if he is having a stroke or is under the influence of drugs or alcohol. Using the Cincinnati Prehospital Stroke Scale, you note that the patient has no facial droop, his speech is clear, and he is able to hold his arms in front of him with no arm drift. You give oxygen, place the patient in a position of comfort, and transport him to the hospital. A few hours later, an Emergency Department nurse calls to compliment you for taking the time to look at the "big picture" and not only the patient's chest trauma. The patient was admitted to the hospital for a subdural hematoma. By recognizing the significance of the patient's abnormal vital signs, you definitely made a difference in his emergency care. ■

Sum It Up

▶ Chest injuries are categorized as closed or open injuries. In closed chest injuries, no break occurs in the skin over the chest wall. These injuries are usually the result of blunt trauma. Underlying structures, such as the heart, lungs, and great vessels, may sustain significant injury. In open chest injuries, a break occurs in the skin over the chest wall. These injuries result from penetrating trauma, such as gunshot wounds, stabbings, or an impaled object.

▶ Rib fractures are a common injury. Fractures of ribs 1 and 2 are associated with significant trauma. Fractures of ribs 9-11 on the left are associated with rupture of the spleen. Fractures of ribs 5-9 on the right are associated with injury to the liver.

▶ Flail chest occurs when two or more adjacent ribs are fractured in two or more places or when the sternum is detached. The section of the chest wall between the fractured ribs becomes free floating because it is no longer in continuity with the thorax. This free-floating section of the chest wall is called a *flail segment*. The flail segment does not move with the rest of the rib cage when the patient attempts to breathe (paradoxical movement).

▶ A pneumothorax is a collection of air or gas outside the lung, between the lung and the chest wall. In a simple pneumothorax, air enters the chest cavity, causing a loss of negative pressure and a partial or total collapse of the lung.

▶ A spontaneous pneumothorax is a type of pneumothorax that does not involve trauma to the lung. It is usually caused by the rupture of a bleb (a small air- or fluid-filled sac) in the lung. A primary spontaneous pneumothorax occurs in people with no history of lung disease. A secondary spontaneous pneumothorax most often occurs as a complication of lung disease, such as COPD, asthma, pneumonia, tuberculosis, or lung cancer.

▶ An open pneumothorax is also called a *sucking chest wound*.

▶ A tension pneumothorax is a life-threatening condition in which air enters the pleural cavity during inspiration and progressively builds up under pressure. The flap of injured lung acts as a one-way valve, allowing air to enter the pleural space during inspiration but trapping it during expiration. The injured lung collapses completely. Pressure rises, forcing the trachea, heart, and major blood vessels to be pushed toward the opposite side. Shifting of the major blood vessels causes them to kink, resulting in a backup of blood into the venous system. The backup of blood into the venous system results in JVD, decreased blood return to the heart, and signs of shock.

▶ A hemothorax is a collection of blood in the pleural cavity that may result from injury to the chest wall, the major blood vessels, or the lung because of penetrating or blunt trauma. A hemothorax is often seen with a simple or tension pneumothorax.

A massive hemothorax is blood loss of more than 1500 mL in the chest cavity.

▶ Cardiac tamponade usually occurs because of penetrating chest trauma, but it can also occur because of blunt trauma to the chest. Cardiac tamponade occurs when blood enters the pericardial sac. The blood in the pericardial sac compresses the heart, decreasing the amount of blood the heart can pump out with each contraction. The patient's signs and symptoms depend on how quickly blood collects in the pericardial sac.

▶ Traumatic asphyxia occurs because of a severe compression injury to the chest, such as compression of the chest under a heavy object or between a vehicle's seat and steering wheel. Blood backs up into the veins, venules, and capillaries of the head, neck, extremities, and upper torso, resulting in capillary rupture.

▶ A pulmonary contusion is bruising of the lung. In a pulmonary contusion, the alveoli fill with blood and fluid because of bruising of the lung tissue. As a result, the area of the lung available for gas exchange is decreased.

▶ A myocardial contusion is bruising of the heart muscle. Signs and symptoms of a myocardial contusion include chest pain or discomfort, increased heart rate, and (possibly) an irregular heart rhythm.

▶ The severity of an open pneumothorax depends on the size of the wound. If the diameter of the chest wound is more than two thirds the diameter of the patient's trachea, air will enter the chest wound rather than through the trachea with each breath. Promptly close the chest wound with an airtight (occlusive) dressing. Plastic wrap and petroleum gauze are examples of dressings that may be used. Make sure that the dressing is large enough so that it is not pulled into the wound during inspiration. Tape the dressing on three sides. If signs and symptoms of a tension pneumothorax develop after an airtight dressing has been applied, release the dressing.

▶ Types of abdominal injuries include open injuries, in which the skin is broken, and closed injuries, in which the skin is not broken. If hollow abdominal organs are cut or rupture, their contents spill into the abdominal cavity, causing inflammation. Severe bleeding may result if a solid organ is cut or ruptures.

▶ Injuries to the external male genitalia include cuts, bruises, penetrating objects, amputations, and avulsions.

▶ The internal female genitalia are rarely injured except in the pregnant patient or in cases of sexual assault with penetration. Injuries to the external female genitalia usually result from straddle injuries or sexual assault.

Division 6

Infants and Children

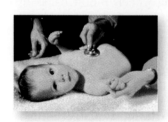

▶ CHAPTER **26**

Infant and Child Emergency Care   591

26 Infant and Child Emergency Care

By the end of this chapter, you should be able to:

Knowledge Objectives ▶

1. Identify the developmental considerations for the following age groups:
   - Infants
   - Toddlers
   - Preschoolers
   - School-age children
   - Adolescents
2. Describe differences in anatomy and physiology of the infant, child, and adult patient.
3. Differentiate the response of the ill or injured infant or child (age specific) from that of an adult.
4. Indicate various causes of respiratory emergencies.
5. Differentiate between respiratory distress and respiratory failure.
6. List the steps in the management of foreign body airway obstruction.
7. Summarize emergency medical care strategies for respiratory distress and respiratory failure.
8. Identify the signs and symptoms of shock (hypoperfusion) in the infant and child patient.
9. Describe the methods of determining end-organ perfusion in the infant and child patient.
10. State the usual cause of cardiac arrest in infants and children versus adults.
11. List the common causes of seizures in the infant and child patient.
12. Describe the management of seizures in the infant and child patient.
13. Differentiate between the injury patterns in adults, infants, and children.
14. Discuss the field management of the infant and child trauma patient.
15. Summarize the indicators of possible child abuse and neglect.
16. Describe the medical-legal responsibilities in suspected child abuse.
17. Recognize need for debriefing after a difficult infant or child transport.

Attitude Objectives ▶

18. Explain the rationale for having knowledge and skills appropriate for dealing with the infant and child patient.
19. Attend to the feelings of the family when dealing with an ill or injured infant or child.

20. Understand the provider's own response (emotional) to caring for infants or children.

Skill Objectives ▶ 21. Demonstrate the techniques of foreign body airway obstruction removal in the infant.
22. Demonstrate the techniques of foreign body airway obstruction removal in the child.
23. Demonstrate the assessment of the infant and child.
24. Demonstrate bag-mask artificial ventilations for the infant.
25. Demonstrate bag-mask artificial ventilations for the child.
26. Demonstrate oxygen delivery for the infant and child.

On the Scene

You are dispatched for a "child with difficulty breathing." As you walk into the room, it is obvious that a 4-year-old girl is struggling to catch her breath. She is pale and leaning forward on the edge of her bed, and her nostrils flare open with each breath. A high-pitched whistle is audible even without use of the stethoscope. "She has asthma," her father tells you, "but it seems worse this time." You count her breathing at 40 breaths/min. Her radial pulse is 146. When you lift her shirt, you can see the skin between her ribs pull in with each breath. ■

THINK ABOUT IT

As you read this chapter, think about the following questions:

• Which signs of respiratory distress have you observed in this child?
• Are her vital signs within normal limits?
• What treatment should you consider for this patient?

Introduction

Caring for Infants and Children

Remember This!

The key to working with children is to "Keep it simple." Children respond very well to basic management skills.

Children are not just small adults. Children have unique physical, mental, emotional, and developmental characteristics that you must consider when assessing and caring for them. You may be anxious when treating a child because of lack of experience in treating children, fear of failure, or identifying the patient with your own child. If you understand the expected physical and developmental characteristics of infants and children of

different ages, you will be able to more accurately assess your patient and provide appropriate care.

You Should Know

Age Classifications of Infants and Children

Life Stage	Age
Newly born infant	Birth to several hours after birth
Neonate	Birth to 1 month
Infant	1 to 12 months of age
	• Young infant: 0 to 6 months of age
	• Older infant: 6 months to 1 year of age
Toddler	1 to 3 years of age
Preschooler	4 to 5 years of age
School-age child	6 to 12 years of age
Adolescent	13 to 18 years of age

Anatomical and Physiological Differences in Children

Objective 2

Head

A child's head is proportionately larger and heavier than an adult's until about 4 years of age. It takes several months for a child to develop neck muscles that are strong enough to support his head. Because the back of a child's head (occiput) sticks out and a child's forehead is large, these areas are susceptible to injury. It isn't unusual for children to have multiple forehead bruises from hitting their heads on tables and floors. Trauma to the head may result in flexion and extension injuries.

The necks of infants and toddlers are flexed when they are lying flat because the back of the skull is large. The chin is then angled toward the chest (Figure 26-1). Appropriate positioning of an infant's or a toddler's head will be one of the most important techniques that you will use when managing children. Proper positioning is an important factor when managing the airway.

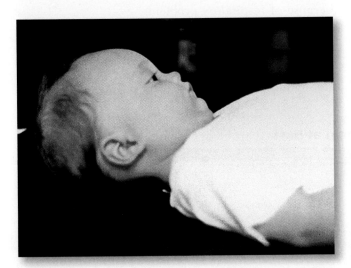

FIGURE 26-1 ▲ Proper positioning of an infant's or a toddler's head is an important consideration during airway management. *EMSC Slide Set (CD-ROM), 1996. Courtesy of the Emergency Medical Services for Children Program, administered by the U.S. Department of Health and Human Service's Health Resources and Services Administration, Maternal and Child Health Bureau.*

The bones of the head of an infant are soft and flexible to allow for growth of the brain. On both the top and back of the head are small diamond-shaped openings called *fontanels* (*soft spots*). These areas will not completely close until about 6 months of age for the rear fontanel and 18 months for the top one. You should assess the fontanels of an infant and toddler for bulging or depression. The soft spots of an infant or toddler are normally nearly level with the skull. Coughing, crying, or lying down may cause the soft spots to bulge temporarily. Bulging in a quiet patient suggests increased pressure within the skull, such as pressure from fluid or pressure on the brain. A depression suggests the patient is dehydrated.

Face

A child's nasal passages are very small, short, and narrow. It is easy for children to develop obstruction of these areas with mucus or foreign objects. Newborns are primarily nose breathers. A newborn will not automatically open his mouth to breathe when his nose becomes obstructed. As a result, any obstruction of the nose will lead to respiratory difficulty. You must make sure the newborn's nose is clear to avoid breathing problems.

Although the opening of the mouth is usually small, a child's tongue is large in proportion to the mouth. The tongue of an infant or child fills the majority of the space in his mouth. The tongue is the most common cause of upper airway obstruction in an unconscious child because the immature muscles of the lower jaw (mandible) allow the tongue to fall to the back of the throat.

Airway

In children, the opening between the vocal cords (glottic opening) is higher in the neck and more toward the front than in an adult. As we grow up, our neck gets longer and the glottic opening drops down. The flap of cartilage that covers this opening, the epiglottis, is larger and floppier in children. Therefore, any injury to or swelling of this area can block the airway.

The windpipe (trachea) is the tube through which air passes from the mouth to the lungs. In children, this area is softer, more flexible, and has a smaller diameter and shorter length than in adults. The trachea has rings of cartilage that keep the airway open. In children, this cartilage is soft and collapses easily, which can then obstruct the airway. Extending or flexing the neck too far can result in crimping of the trachea and a blocked airway. To avoid blocking the airway, place the head of an infant or young child in a neutral or "sniffing" position. This position is covered in more detail later in this chapter.

Breathing

A child's ribs are soft and flexible because they are made up mostly of cartilage. Bone growth occurs with time, filling in the cartilaginous areas from the center out to the ends. Because the rib cage is softer than in an adult, trauma to the chest will be transmitted to the lungs and other internal structures more easily.

The amount of oxygen a child requires is about twice that of an adolescent or adult. The muscles between the ribs (intercostal muscles) help lift the chest wall during breathing. Because these muscles are not fully developed until later in childhood, the diaphragm is the primary muscle of breathing. As a result, the abdominal muscles move during breathing. During normal breathing, the abdominal muscles should move in the same direction as the chest wall. The movement of abdominal muscles opposite each other is called *seesaw breathing* and is abnormal. A child's respiratory rate is faster than an adult's is and decreases with age (Table 26-1). Because the muscles between the ribs are not well developed, a child cannot keep up a rapid rate of breathing (faster than normal for the patient's age) for very long.

The stomach of an infant or child often fills with air during crying. Air can also build up in the stomach if rescue breathing is performed. As the stomach swells with air, it pushes on the lungs and diaphragm. This action limits movement and prevents good ventilation. Infants and young children's breathing is dependent on the diaphragm. Breathing difficulty results if movement of the diaphragm is limited.

Circulation

Children breathe faster than adults, and their hearts beat harder and faster than those of adults. Infants and young children have a relatively smaller blood volume (80 mL/kg). A sudden loss of 1/2 L (500 mL) of the blood volume in a child and 100–200 mL of the blood volume in an infant is considered serious.

A child's heart rate will increase as a result of shock, fever, anxiety, and pain. It will also increase as he loses body fluid (hypovolemia). This condition can occur because of bleeding, vomiting, or diarrhea. Most of an infant's body weight is water, so vomiting and diarrhea can result in dehydration. Blood loss resulting from broken bones and soft-tissue injuries may quickly result in shock. The system of an infant or child tries to make up for a loss of blood or fluid through an increase in heart rate and a constriction of the skin's blood vessels. These actions help to deliver as much blood and oxygen as possible to the brain, heart, and lungs.

A child's rate and effort of breathing will increase when the amount of oxygen in the blood is decreased (as in late shock). This helps to make up for a lack of oxygen. As the child tires and the blood oxygen level becomes very low, the heart muscle begins to pump less effectively. As a result, the child's heart rate slows. If the lack of oxygen is not corrected, the child will stop breathing (respiratory arrest). A child will often survive a respiratory arrest as long as his oxygen level is maintained sufficiently so that the heart does not stop. Normal heart rates for children at rest are shown in Table 26-2.

Remember This!

In children, circulatory problems often develop because of respiratory problems.

If you have the necessary equipment, measure the blood pressure in children older than 3 years of age. The blood pressure of a child is normally lower than

TABLE 26-1 Normal Respiratory Rates in Children at Rest

Life Stage	Age	Breaths per Minute
Newborn	Birth to 1 month	30–50
Infant	1 to 12 months	20–40
Toddler	1 to 3 years	20–30
Preschooler	4 to 5 years	20–30
School-age child	6 to 12 years	16–30
Adolescent	13 to 18 years	12–20

TABLE 26-2 Normal Heart Rates in Children at Rest

Life Stage	Age	Beats per Minute
Newborn	Birth to 1 month	120–160
Infant	1 to 12 months	80–140
Toddler	1 to 3 years	80–130
Preschooler	4 to 5 years	80–120
School-age child	6 to 12 years	70–110
Adolescent	13 to 18 years	60–100

TABLE 26-3 Lower Limit of Normal Systolic Blood Pressure by Age

Life Stage	Age	Lower Limit of Normal Systolic Blood Pressure
Term neonate	0 to 28 days	>60 mm Hg or strong central pulse
Infant	1 to 12 months	>70 mm Hg or strong central pulse
Child /Adolescent	1 to 10 years	>70 + (2 × age in years)
	≥10 years	>90 mm Hg

that of an adult (see Table 26-3). In children 1 to 10 years of age, the following formula may be used to determine the lower limit of a normal systolic blood pressure: 70 + (2 × child's age in years) = systolic blood pressure. The lower limit of normal systolic blood pressure for a child 10 or more years of age is 90 mm Hg. The diastolic blood pressure should be about 2/3 the systolic pressure.

Infants and young children are susceptible to changes in temperature. A child has a large body surface area (BSA) compared with his weight. The larger the BSA that is exposed, the greater the area of heat loss.

An infant's skin is thin with few fat deposits under it. This condition contributes to an infant's sensitivity to extremes of heat and cold. Infants have poorly developed temperature-regulating mechanisms. For example, newborns are unable to shiver in cold temperatures. In addition, their sweating mechanism is immature in warm temperatures. Because infants and children are at risk of hypothermia, it is very important to keep them warm.

The skin of an infant or child will show changes related to the amount of oxygen in the blood. Pale (whitish) skin may be seen in shock, fright, or anxiety. A bluish (cyanotic) tint, often seen first around the mouth, suggests inadequate breathing or poor perfusion. This is a critical sign that requires immediate treatment. The skin may appear blotchy (mottled) in shock, hypothermia, or cardiac arrest. Flushed (red) skin may be caused by fever, heat exposure, or an allergic reaction. Yellowing of the skin (jaundice) and the sclerae of the eyes suggests a liver problem. The tissue in the mouth of a healthy child should be pink and moist, regardless of the child's race. Most children should feel slightly warm to the touch. Their skin should be tight and not dry or flaky.

The Developmental Stages of Children

Infants (Birth to 1 Year of Age)

Objectives 1, 3

Infants are completely dependent on others for their needs (Figure 26-2). They cry for many reasons, including pain, hunger, excessive heat or cold, or a

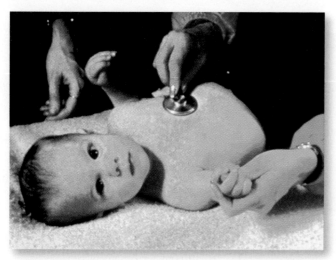

FIGURE 26-2 ▲ Infants are completely dependent on others for their needs. *EMSC Slide Set (CD-ROM), 1996. Courtesy of the Emergency Medical Services for Children Program, administered by the U.S. Department of Health and Human Service's Health Resources and Services Administration, Maternal and Child Health Bureau.*

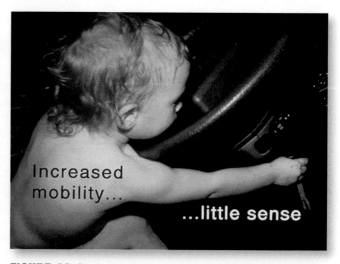

FIGURE 26-3 ▲ Toddlers are always on the move. As a result, they are prone to injury. *EMSC Slide Set (CD-ROM), 1996. Courtesy of the Emergency Medical Services for Children Program, administered by the U.S. Department of Health and Human Service's Health Resources and Services Administration, Maternal and Child Health Bureau.*

dirty diaper. Young infants (birth to 6 months of age) are unafraid of strangers and have no modesty. Older infants (6 months to 1 year of age) do not like to be separated from their caregiver (separation anxiety). They may be threatened by direct eye contact with strangers. They show little modesty.

When providing care for an infant, watch the baby from a distance before making contact. If possible, assess the baby on the caregiver's lap. Avoid loud noises; bright lights; and quick, jerky movements. Smile and use a calm, soothing voice. Allow the baby to suck on a pacifier for comfort, if appropriate. Be sure to handle an infant gently but firmly, always supporting the head and neck if the baby is not on a solid surface.

An infant must be kept warm and covered as much as possible, particularly the head. The head is the largest BSA in infants and young children. Heat loss from this area significantly cools the rest of the body. Make sure your hands and stethoscope are warmed before touching the infant.

You Should Know

Shaken baby syndrome is a severe form of head injury. It occurs when an infant or child is shaken by the arms, legs, or shoulders with enough force to cause the baby's brain to bounce against his skull. This shaking can cause bruising, swelling, and bleeding of the brain. It can lead to severe brain damage or death.

Just 2 to 3 seconds of shaking can cause bleeding in and around the brain. *Never shake or jiggle an infant or child.*

Stop and Think!

An increased risk of a foreign body airway obstruction begins at about 6 months of age, when a child is able to grasp objects. Be careful not to leave small objects within an infant's reach.

Toddlers (1 to 3 Years of Age)

Objectives 1, 3

A toddler is always on the move. A toddler's eye-hand coordination improves, and sitting, standing, and walking begin. As a result, toddlers are prone to injury (Figure 26-3). A toddler responds appropriately to an angry or friendly voice. When separated from their primary caregiver, most toddlers experience strong separation anxiety.

A toddler can answer simple questions and follow simple directions. However, you cannot reason with a toddler. A toddler is likely to be more cooperative if he is given a comfort object like a blanket, stuffed animal, or toy.

Toddlers understand "soon," "bye-bye," "all gone," and "uh-oh." A toddler's favorite words are "no" and "mine," so avoid asking questions that can be answered with a yes or no. If you ask questions that begin with "May I," "Can I," or "Would you like to," a toddler will probably say no. If you then do whatever you asked him anyway, you will immediately lose the toddler's trust and cooperation. You are more likely to have cooperation if you state clearly what you are going to do in simple terms, rather than asking for permission from the child.

Toddlers view illness and injury as punishment. They are distrustful of strangers. Toddlers are likely to resist examination and treatment. When touched, they may scream, cry, or kick. Toddlers do not like having their clothing removed and do not like anything on their faces. They are afraid of being left alone, of monsters, of interruptions in their usual routine, and of getting hurt (such as a fall or cut).

Encourage the child's trust by gaining the cooperation of his caregiver. When he sees you talking with the caregiver first and understands that the adult is not threatened, the child may be more at ease. When possible, allow the child to remain on the caregiver's lap. If this is not possible, try to keep the caregiver within the child's line of vision. Approach the child slowly and address him by name. Talk to him at eye level, using simple words and short phrases. Speak to him in a calm, reassuring tone of voice. Although the child may not understand your words, he will respond to your tone. Try a game such as counting toes or fingers to enlist the child's cooperation.

Assess the child's head last. Start with either his trunk or feet and move upward. Respect the child's modesty by keeping him covered. When it is time to remove an item of clothing, ask the child's caregiver to do so, if possible. Replace clothing promptly after assessing each body area. Be sure to praise the child for cooperative behavior.

Remember This!

Do not tell a child he cannot cry or that he needs to be strong. Instead, reassure the child that it is okay to cry, be angry or frightened, and express emotion. However, you can remind the child that hitting, kicking, or biting is not allowed.

Preschoolers (4 to 5 Years of Age)

Objectives 1, 3

Preschoolers are afraid of the unknown, the dark, being left alone, and adults who look or act mean. They may think their illness or injury is punishment for bad behavior or thoughts (Figure 26-4). Approach the child slowly and talk to him at eye level. Use simple words and phrases and a reassuring tone of voice. Assure the child that he was not bad and is not being punished.

A preschooler may feel vulnerable and out of control when lying down. Assess and treat the child in an upright position when possible. Preschoolers are modest. They do not like being touched or having their clothing removed. When assessing a child, keep in mind that he has probably been told not to let a stranger touch him. Remove clothing, assess the child,

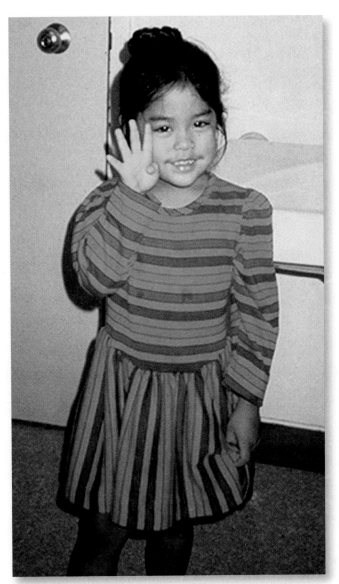

FIGURE 26-4 ▲ Preschoolers are highly imaginative and may think their illness or injury is punishment for bad behavior or thoughts. *EMSC Slide Set (CD-ROM), 1996. Courtesy of the Emergency Medical Services for Children Program, administered by the U.S. Department of Health and Human Service's Health Resources and Services Administration, Maternal and Child Health Bureau.*

and then quickly replace clothing. Allow the caregiver to remain with the child whenever possible.

Preschoolers are curious and like to "help." Encourage the child to participate. Tell the child how things will feel and what is to be done just before doing it. For example, a preschooler may fear being suffocated by an oxygen mask. It may be helpful to use a doll or a stuffed animal to explain the procedure. The child may want to hold or look at the equipment first.

Preschoolers are highly imaginative. When talking with a preschooler, choose your words carefully. Avoid baby talk and frightening or misleading terms. For example, avoid words such as *take, cut, shot, deaden,* or *germs.* Instead of saying, "I'm going to take your pulse," you might say, "I'm going to see how fast your heart is beating." Instead of saying, "I'm going to take your blood pressure," you might say, "I'm going to hug your arm" or "I'm going to see how strong your muscles are." Because they are afraid of blood, dress and bandage wounds right away.

Depending on the child's age, you may find that distracting them is helpful. Remember that children are self-centered—they imagine that the world revolves around them. Paying attention to their world and needs will improve your ability to assess and care for your pediatric patients.

You Should Know

Distractions

- Ask a child about his favorite foods, games, cartoon characters, movies, or computer game.
- Ask the child to visually locate an item in the area.
- Ask the child to sing a song or tell you about school.
- Use a stuffed animal as a distraction or comfort item.

School-Age Children (6 to 12 Years of Age)

Objectives 1, 3

School-age children are less dependent on their caregivers than are younger children. They are usually cooperative (Figure 26-5). They fear pain, permanent injury, and disfigurement. They are also afraid of blood and prolonged separation from their caregivers. A school-age child is very modest and does not like his body exposed to strangers. A child of this age may still view his illness or injury as punishment. Reassure the child that what is happening to him is not related to being punished.

When caring for a school-age child, approach him in a friendly manner and introduce yourself. Talk directly to the child about what happened, even if you also obtain a history from the caregiver. Explain procedures before carrying them out. Because school-age children often view things in concrete terms, choose your words carefully. For example, the phrase "I am going to take your pulse" will concern a school-age child. He will wonder why you are taking it away and when he will get it back. Allow the child to see and touch equipment that may be used in his care.

Honesty is very important when interacting with school-age children. If you are going to do something

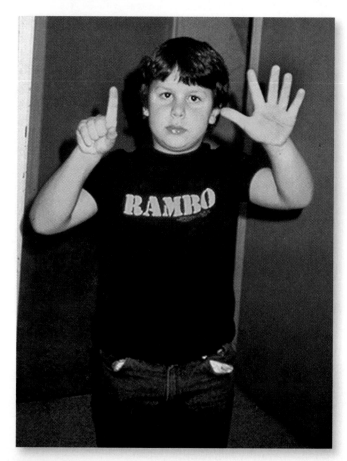

FIGURE 26-5 ▲ School-age children are usually cooperative. *EMSC Slide Set (CD-ROM), 1996. Courtesy of the Emergency Medical Services for Children Program, administered by the U.S. Department of Health and Human Service's Health Resources and Services Administration, Maternal and Child Health Bureau.*

to the child that may cause pain, warn the child just before you do it. Give a simple explanation of what will take place just before the procedure so that he does not have long to think about it. For example, if a child has a possible broken leg and you must move the leg to apply a splint, warn the child just before you move the leg. Do not threaten the child if he is uncooperative.

Adolescents (13 to 18 Years of Age)

Objectives 1, 3

Adolescents often show inconsistent and unpredictable behavior, although they expect to be treated as adults (Figure 26-6). Talk to an adolescent in a respectful, friendly manner, as if speaking to an adult. If possible, obtain a history from the patient instead of a caregiver. Expect an adolescent to have many questions and want detailed explanations about what you are planning to do or what is happening to him. Explain things clearly and honestly. Allow time for questions. Do not bargain with an adolescent in order

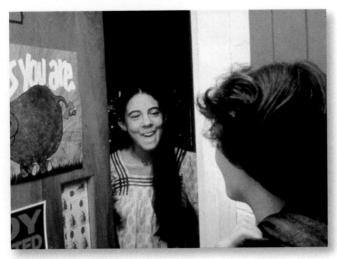

FIGURE 26-6 ▲ Adolescents expect to be treated as adults. *EMSC Slide Set (CD-ROM), 1996. Courtesy of the Emergency Medical Services for Children Program, administered by the U.S. Department of Health and Human Service's Health Resources and Services Administration, Maternal and Child Health Bureau.*

to do what you need to do. Recognize the tendency for adolescents to overreact. Do not become angry with an emotional or hysterical adolescent.

Adolescents fear pain and permanent damage to their bodies that results in a change in appearance, scarring, or death. They may go back and forth between being very modest and openly displaying their bodies. Try to have an adult of the same gender as the child present while you examine the patient. Allow the caregiver to be present during your assessment if the patient wishes. However, some adolescents may prefer to be assessed privately, away from their caregivers.

Peers are a major influence in the life of an adolescent. When you are providing care, an adolescent may prefer to have a peer close by for reassurance. When caring for an adolescent, do not tease or embarrass him—particularly in front of his peers.

Assessment of the Infant and Child

Scene Size-Up

When you are called for an emergency involving a child, quickly determine if the emergency is a result of trauma or a medical condition. If the emergency is a result of trauma, determine the mechanism of injury (Figure 26-7). If the emergency is to the result of a medical condition, determine the nature of the illness. This information can be obtained from the patient, family members, or bystanders, as well as from your observations of the scene.

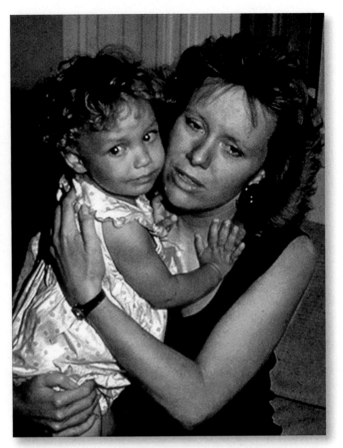

FIGURE 26-7 ▲ Quickly determine if the emergency is to the result of trauma or a medical condition. If the emergency is to the result of trauma, determine the mechanism of injury. *EMSC Slide Set (CD-ROM), 1996. Courtesy of the Emergency Medical Services for Children Program, administered by the U.S. Department of Health and Human Service's Health Resources and Services Administration, Maternal and Child Health Bureau.*

Survey the patient's environment for clues to the cause of the emergency. Note any hazards or potential hazards. For example, open pill bottles or cleaning solutions may indicate a possible toxic ingestion. Look at the child's environment. Does it appear clean and orderly? Do other children appear healthy and well cared for? Determine if you need additional resources, including law enforcement personnel. Remember to wear appropriate personal protective equipment (PPE) before approaching the patient.

Primary Survey

Any incident that involves children will cause some degree of anxiety and stress among every person present. Your emotional response in these situations will play an important part in how effective you can be. Your emotional response may be related to a limited exposure to children as a healthcare professional and/or caregiver. Alternately, caring for an ill or injured child who is the same age as a member of your own family may also affect your response.

In most situations, your approach to an ill or injured infant or child should include the patient's caregiver. Watch the interaction between the caregiver and the child. Does the caregiver appear concerned? Or is he angry or indifferent? Keep in mind that an agitated caregiver results in an agitated child. A calm caregiver results in a calm child. If the child's caregiver is adding to the child's anxiety, give the adult something to do. For example, you might ask the caregiver to locate the child's favorite comfort object. Including the caregiver in the child's care reassures both the child and caregiver. It also allows the adult a chance to take part in the child's recovery. Although a child's caregiver may not have medical training, she is the expert on what is normal or abnormal for her child. She also knows what measures will have a calming effect on the child.

General Impression

Your assessment of an infant or child should begin "across the room." When forming a general impression of an infant or child, look at his appearance, breathing, and circulation. Quickly determine if the child appears sick or not sick.

- *Appearance.* A child should be alert and responsive to his surroundings. Is the child awake and alert? Does the child behave appropriately for his age? Does he recognize his caregiver? Is the child playing or moving around, or does he appear drowsy or unaware of his surroundings? Does the child show interest in what is happening? Does the child appear agitated or irritable? Does he appear confused or combative? If the child appears agitated, restless, or limp or if he appears to be asleep, proceed immediately to the ABCDE assessment.

- *(Work of) Breathing.* With normal breathing, both sides of the chest rise and fall equally. Breathing is quiet and painless and occurs at a regular rate. Is the child sitting up, lying down, or leaning forward? Can you hear abnormal breathing sounds such as stridor (a high-pitched sound), wheezing, or grunting? Stridor suggests an upper airway obstruction. Wheezing suggests narrowing of the lower airways. Do you see retractions (sinking in around the ribs and collarbones), nasal flaring, or shoulder hunching? (Figure 26-8.) Is the child's breathing rate faster or slower than expected? Is his head bobbing up and down toward his chest? If the child appears to be struggling to breathe, has noisy breathing, moves his chest abnormally, or has a rate of breathing that is faster or slower than normal, proceed immediately to the ABCDE assessment.

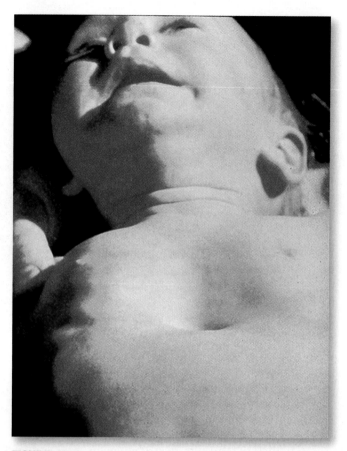

FIGURE 26-8 ▲ Retractions are a sign of an increased work of breathing. *EMSC Slide Set (CD-ROM), 1996. Courtesy of the Emergency Medical Services for Children Program, administered by the U.S. Department of Health and Human Service's Health Resources and Services Administration, Maternal and Child Health Bureau.*

- *Circulation.* Visual signs of circulation relate to skin color, obvious bleeding, and moisture. What color is the child's skin? Is it pink, pale, mottled, flushed, or blue? Do you see any bleeding? If bleeding is present, where is it coming from? How much blood is there? Does the child look sweaty? Or do the child's lips look dry and flaky? If the child's skin looks pale, mottled, flushed, gray, or blue, proceed immediately to the ABCDE assessment.

Remember This!

During your primary survey, find the answers to these 5 questions:

1. Is the child awake and alert?
2. Is the child's airway open?
3. Is the child breathing?
4. Does the child have a pulse?
5. Does the child have severe bleeding?

Once your general impression is complete, perform a hands-on ABCDE assessment. In a responsive infant or child, use a toes-to-head or trunk-to-head approach. This approach should help reduce the infant's or the child's anxiety.

Level of Responsiveness and Cervical Spine Protection

Objective 9

After forming a general impression, assess the patient's level of responsiveness (mental status) and the need for cervical spine protection.

Level of Responsiveness (Mental Status)

Is the child awake and alert? An alert infant or young child (younger than 3 years of age) smiles, orients to sound, follows objects with his eyes, and interacts with those around him. As the infant or young child's mental status decreases, you may see the following changes (in order of decreasing mental status):

- The child may cry but can be comforted.
- The child may show inappropriate, constant crying.
- The child may become irritable and restless.
- The child may be unresponsive.

Assessing the mental status of a child older than 3 years of age is the same as assessing that of an adult. Most children will be agitated or resist your assessment. A child who is limp, allows you to perform any assessment or skill, or does not respond to his caregiver is sick. Unresponsiveness in an infant or child usually indicates a life-threatening condition. If the patient is a child with special healthcare needs, the child's caregiver will probably be your best resource. The caregiver will be able to tell you what "normal" is for the child regarding his mental status, vital signs, and level of activity.

Depending on the child's age, you may ask the child or caregiver, "Why did you call 9-1-1 today?" If the child appears to be asleep, gently rub his shoulder and ask, "Are you okay?" or "Can you hear me?" If the child does not respond, ask the family or bystanders to tell you what happened while you continue your assessment.

Remember This!

An infant or child who does not recognize your presence is sick.

Cervical Spine Protection

If you suspect trauma to the head, neck, or back, or if the child is unresponsive with an unknown nature of illness, take spinal precautions. If the child is awake and you suspect trauma, face him so that he does not have to turn his head to see you. Tell him not to move his head or neck. Use your hands to manually stabilize the child's head and neck in line with his body. Once begun, manual stabilization must be continued until the child has been secured to a backboard with his head stabilized.

Remember This!

If the child complains of pain or if you meet resistance when moving the child's head and neck to a neutral position, stop and maintain the head and neck in the position in which they were found.

A is for Airway

Is the child's airway open? A child who is talking or crying has an open airway. If the child is responsive and the airway is open, assess the child's breathing. If the child is responsive but unable to speak, cry, cough, or make any other sound, his airway is completely obstructed. If the child has noisy breathing, such as snoring or gurgling, he has a partial airway obstruction.

A responsive child may have assumed a position to maintain an open airway. Allow the child to maintain this position as you continue your assessment. For example, in cases of serious upper airway obstruction, the child may instinctively assume a "sniffing" position (Figure 26-9). In this position, the child is seated with his head and chin thrust slightly forward, as if sniffing a flower. In cases of severe respiratory distress, the child may assume a "tripod" position. In this position, the child is seated and leaning forward (Figure 26-10).

If the child is unresponsive and no trauma is suspected, use the head tilt–chin lift maneuver to open the airway. If trauma to the head or neck is suspected, the jaw thrust without head tilt maneuver is the preferred method of opening the airway. Do not hyperextend the neck. Doing so can cause an airway obstruction. To help maintain the proper positioning of the patient's head and neck, you may need to place padding under the torso of an infant or small child. The padding should be firm and evenly shaped and extend from the shoulders to the pelvis. The padding should be thick enough so that the child's shoulders are in alignment with the ear canal (Figure 26-11). Using irregularly shaped or insufficient padding or placing padding only under the shoulders can result in movement or misalignment of the spine.

After opening the airway, look in the mouth of every unresponsive child. To do this, open the child's mouth with your gloved hand. Look for an actual or potential airway obstruction, such as a foreign body,

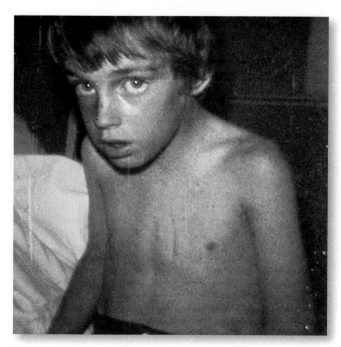

FIGURE 26-9 ▲ In cases of serious upper airway obstruction, the child may instinctively assume a "sniffing" position. In this position, the child is seated with his head and chin thrust forward slightly. *EMSC Slide Set (CD-ROM), 1996. Courtesy of the Emergency Medical Services for Children Program, administered by the U.S. Department of Health and Human Service's Health Resources and Services Administration, Maternal and Child Health Bureau.*

blood, vomitus, teeth, or the child's tongue. If you see a foreign body in the child's mouth, attempt to remove it with your gloved fingers. If there is blood, vomitus, or other fluid in the airway, clear it with suctioning.

Clearing the Airway

Depending on the cause of the obstruction, methods you can use to clear the patient's airway include foreign body airway obstruction maneuvers (see Appendix A), the recovery position, finger sweeps, and suctioning.

If the child is unresponsive, uninjured, and breathing adequately, you can place him on his side. In this position, gravity allows fluid to flow from the child's mouth. Do *not* place a child with a known or suspected spinal injury in the recovery position. You must continue to monitor the child until you transfer care to a qualified healthcare professional.

If you *see* foreign material in an unresponsive child's mouth, remove it by using a finger sweep:

- If the child is uninjured, roll him to his side.
- Wipe any liquids from the airway with your index and middle fingers covered with a 4 × 4-inch gauze pad.
- Remove solid objects with a gloved finger positioned like a hook. Use your little finger when

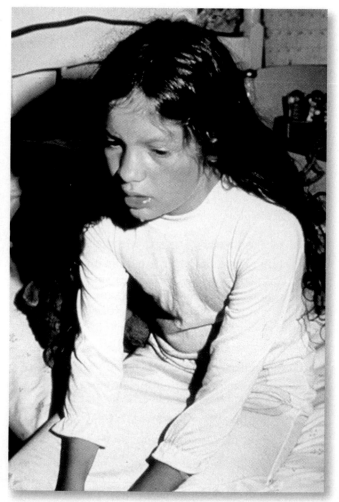

FIGURE 26-10 ▲ In cases of severe respiratory distress, the child may assume a "tripod" position. In this position, the child is seated and leaning forward. *EMSC Slide Set (CD-ROM), 1996. Courtesy of the Emergency Medical Services for Children Program, administered by the U.S. Department of Health and Human Service's Health Resources and Services Administration, Maternal and Child Health Bureau.*

performing a finger sweep in an infant or child. Remember: Blind finger sweeps are *never* performed in an infant or child.

Suctioning may be needed if placing the patient in the recovery position and performing finger sweeps are not effective in clearing the patient's airway. It may also be necessary if trauma is suspected and the patient cannot be placed in the recovery position. Use a rigid suction catheter to remove secretions from the child's mouth. Remember that the catheter should be inserted into the child's mouth no more deeply than the base of his tongue.

A bulb syringe is used to remove secretions from an infant's mouth or nose. To use a bulb syringe, squeeze the bulb before inserting it into the baby's mouth. With the bulb depressed, insert the syringe into the mouth. Release the bulb. Remove the syringe

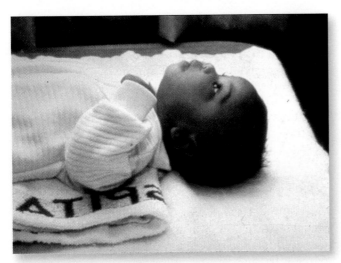

FIGURE 26-11 ▲ To assist in maintaining the proper positioning of the patient's head and neck, it is often necessary to place padding under the torso of an infant or small child. *EMSC Slide Set (CD-ROM), 1996. Courtesy of the Emergency Medical Services for Children Program, administered by the U.S. Department of Health and Human Service's Health Resources and Services Administration, Maternal and Child Health Bureau.*

from the infant's mouth and empty the contents. If both the mouth and nose need to be suctioned, always suction the mouth first and then the nose. Gentle suctioning is usually enough to remove secretions.

Do not suction a newborn for more than 3 to 5 seconds per attempt. When suctioning an infant or child, do not apply suction for more than 10 seconds at a time. The child's heart rate may slow or become irregular because of a lack of oxygen or because the tip of the device stimulates the back of the tongue or throat. If the patient's heart rate slows, stop suctioning and provide ventilation. Give oxygen between each suctioning attempt.

Airway Adjuncts

An oral airway may be used to help keep the airway open in an unresponsive child. Remember that this airway is used only if the patient does not have a gag reflex. If the child gags, coughs, chokes, or spits out the airway, do not use it. A nasal airway may be used to help keep the airway open in an unresponsive or semi-responsive child. Remember to select a device of proper size by aligning the airway on the side of the patient's face and selecting an airway that extends from the tip of the nose to the earlobe.

B is for Breathing

Is the child breathing? After you have made sure that the child's airway is open, assess his breathing. To do this, you must be able to see his chest or abdomen. Watch and listen to the child as he breathes. Look for the rise and fall of the chest. Does the chest rise and fall equally? Count the child's respiratory rate for 30 seconds. Double this number to determine the breaths per minute. If the breathing is irregular, you should count for a full 60 seconds.

Listen for air movement. Determine if breathing is absent, quiet, or noisy. Stridor is a high-pitched sound that is heard when the upper airway passages are partially blocked. Wheezing is heard when the lower airway passages are narrowed. Assess breath sounds. Listen below the collarbones in the midclavicular line and under the armpits along the midaxillary line. Determine if breath sounds are present or absent. Wheezing may be present because of swelling, spasm, secretions, or the presence of a foreign body. If air movement is inadequate, wheezing may not be heard. Listen for a change in the child's voice or cry. Hoarseness may be caused by a foreign body or an inflamed upper airway. Look for signs of increased breathing effort, such as nasal flaring (widening of the nostrils), retractions, head bobbing, seesaw respirations, or the use of accessory muscles. Feel for air movement from the child's nose or mouth against your chin, face, or palm.

If breathing is present, quickly determine if breathing is adequate or inadequate. If the child's breathing is inadequate or absent, you must begin breathing for him immediately. If the chest does not rise, assume the airway is blocked. Depending on the cause of the obstruction, methods you can use to clear the patient's airway include foreign body airway obstruction maneuvers (see Appendix A), the recovery position, finger sweeps, and suctioning. The patient's situation will dictate which technique is most appropriate.

C is for Circulation

Objective 9

Does the child have a pulse? Is severe bleeding present? Note the rate, regularity (rhythm), and quality of the pulse. Pulse regularity normally changes with respirations (increases with inspiration, decreases with expiration). Use the carotid artery to assess the pulse in an unresponsive child older than 1 year of age. Feel for a brachial pulse in an unresponsive infant. Feel for a pulse for about 10 seconds. If there is no pulse, or if a pulse is present but the rate is less than 60 beats/min with signs of shock, you must begin chest compressions.

In infants and children, it is important to compare the pulse of the central blood vessels (such as the femoral artery) with those found in peripheral areas of the body (such as the feet). For example, locate the dorsalis pedis pulse on top of the foot. Then place your other hand in the child's groin area. Compare the strength and rate of the pulses in these areas. They should feel the same. If they do not, a circulatory problem is present. For example, a weak central pulse can be a sign of late shock.

Assess capillary refill in children 6 years of age or younger. To assess capillary refill, firmly press on the child's nail bed until it blanches (turns white) and then release. Observe the time it takes for the tissue to return to its original color. If the temperature of the environment is normal to warm, color should return within 2 seconds. Delayed capillary refill may occur because of shock or hypothermia, among other causes.

Assess blood pressure in children older than 3 years of age. Remember that blood pressure is one of the *least* sensitive indicators of adequate circulation in children. A child may have compromised circulation despite a normal blood pressure. A properly sized cuff must be used to obtain accurate readings. A cuff that is too wide will cause a falsely low reading. A cuff that is too narrow will cause a falsely high reading. The width of the cuff should be about two thirds the length of the long bone used (such as the upper arm or thigh).

If severe bleeding is present, control it by using direct pressure. Assess the child's skin temperature, color, and moisture. Determine if the skin is warm, hot, or cold; moist or dry; and loose or firm. Hot skin suggests fever or heat exposure. Cool skin suggests inadequate circulation or exposure to cold. Cold skin suggests extreme exposure to cold. Clammy (cool and moist) skin suggests shock, among many other conditions. Wet or moist skin may indicate shock, a heat-related illness, or diabetic emergency. Excessively dry skin may indicate dehydration.

Common Problems in Infants and Children

Airway Obstruction

There are many causes of an airway obstruction, including:

- Foreign body
- Mucus plug
- Blood or vomitus
- The tongue
- Trauma to the head or neck
- Infection, such as croup or pneumonia

If a child is unable to speak, cry, cough, or make any other sound, his airway is completely obstructed. If the child has noisy breathing, such as snoring or gurgling, he has a partial airway obstruction. A child with a partial airway obstruction and good air exchange is typically alert and sitting up. You may hear stridor or a crowing sound and see retractions when the child breathes in. The child's skin color is usually normal, and a strong pulse is present. You should allow an older child to assume a position of comfort. Assist a younger child in sitting up. Do not allow him to lie down. He may prefer to sit on his caregiver's lap.

Do not agitate the child. If the child has a foreign body in his airway, agitation could cause the object to move into a position that completely blocks the airway. Encourage the child to cough and allow him to continue his efforts to clear his own airway. Continue to watch the child closely.

Objective 6

You will need to intervene if the child has a complete airway obstruction. You will also need to intervene if the child has a partial airway obstruction that is accompanied by any of the following signs of poor air exchange:

- Ineffective cough
- Increased respiratory difficulty accompanied by stridor
- Loss of responsiveness
- Altered mental status

Clear the child's airway by using the techniques described in the Appendix A for removal of a foreign body airway obstruction. Perform ongoing assessments as often as indicated during transport. Record all patient care information, including the patient's medical history and all emergency care given, on a prehospital care report (PCR).

Respiratory Emergencies

Objective 4

Respiratory emergencies are the most common medical emergencies encountered in children. There are many causes of respiratory emergencies in children. Some conditions affect the upper airway, some affect the lower airway, and some affect both. Upper airway problems usually occur suddenly. Lower airway problems usually take longer to develop. A patient with an upper airway problem is more likely to worsen during the time you are providing care than one with a lower airway problem. You must watch closely for changes in the patient's condition and adjust your treatment as needed.

Objective 5

There are three levels of severity of respiratory problems: (1) respiratory distress, (2) respiratory failure, and (3) respiratory arrest. Most children will present with either respiratory distress or respiratory failure. Respiratory distress is an increased work of breathing (respiratory effort). Respiratory failure is a condition in which there is not enough oxygen in the blood and/or ventilation to meet the demands of body tissues. Respiratory failure is evident when the patient becomes tired and can no longer maintain good oxygenation and ventilation. Respiratory arrest occurs when a patient stops breathing.

Respiratory distress is associated with several signs that you will be able to spot (see the following *You Should Know* box). These signs reflect an increased work of breathing (respiratory effort). The child works harder than usual to breathe in order to make up for the low level of oxygen in his blood.

You Should Know

Signs of Respiratory Distress

- Fear, irritability, anxiousness, restlessness
- Noisy breathing (stridor, grunting, gurgling, wheezing)
- A breathing rate that is faster than normal for the patient's age
- An increased depth of breathing
- Nasal flaring
- A mild increase in heart rate
- Retractions
- Seesaw respirations (abdominal breathing)
- The use of neck muscles to breathe
- Changes in skin color

Remember This!

Give oxygen to *every* infant and child who is experiencing a respiratory problem. There is no medical reason to avoid giving oxygen to an infant or child. Attempts to deliver oxygen should not delay transport.

You will see signs of respiratory failure as the child tires and can no longer maintain good oxygenation and ventilation (see the following *You Should Know* box). A child in respiratory failure looks very sick. The child becomes limp, peripheral pulses become weak, his color worsens, and his heart rate slows down. The breathing rate slows to below 20 breaths/min in an infant and 10 breaths/min in a child. A slow heart rate in a child with respiratory failure is a red flag. Cardiopulmonary arrest will occur soon if the child's oxygenation and ventilation are not corrected quickly.

Making a Difference

When providing care for any patient with a respiratory problem, reassess the patient's condition at least every 5 minutes.

You Should Know

Signs of Respiratory Failure

- Sleepiness or agitation
- Combativeness
- Limpness (the patient may be unable to sit up without help)
- A breathing rate that is initially fast with periods of slowing and then eventual slowing
- An altered mental status
- A shallow chest rise
- Nasal flaring
- Retractions
- Head bobbing
- Pale, mottled, or bluish skin
- Weak peripheral pulses

Objective 7

You can assist a child with respiratory distress by doing the following:

- Help the child into a position of comfort.
- Reposition his airway for better airflow if necessary.
- Give oxygen.

A child with respiratory distress will usually be most comfortable in a sitting position. Do not place a child in a sitting position if trauma is suspected. Do not agitate a child with respiratory distress. For example, do not excite the child by taking a blood pressure. If the child shows signs of respiratory failure or respiratory arrest, prepare for immediate transport to the closest appropriate facility. Keep on-scene time to a minimum. Request an early response of Advanced Life Support (ALS) personnel to the scene, or consider an ALS intercept while en route to the receiving facility. Do not delay transport for ALS arrival.

Assist the child's breathing with a bag-mask (BM) device as needed. BM breathing is also appropriate if you are uncertain about the child's degree of respiratory difficulty. If the child resists your efforts to ventilate him, he is probably not sick enough to need it. On the other hand, if he does not resist your efforts, he most likely does need your help. Deliver each breath over 1 second. Watch for the rise and fall of the patient's chest with each breath. Stop ventilation when you see gentle chest rise. Allow the patient to exhale between breaths. Breathe at a rate of 12 to 20 breaths/min (1 breath every 3 to 5 seconds). If the child does not tolerate a mask, consider using blow-by oxygen (see the following *You Should Know* box). Although not an ideal method of oxygen delivery, blow-by oxygen is better than no oxygen. Be sure to have suction within arm's reach.

You Should Know

Blow-by oxygen refers to blowing oxygen over the face of an infant or child so that the patient breathes oxygen-enriched air. To give blow-by oxygen, connect oxygen tubing to an oxygen source set to at least 5 L/min. Cup your hand around the tubing. Hold the tube close to the patient's nose and mouth. Alternately, insert the oxygen tubing into a paper cup and direct the tubing at the patient's nose and mouth. You can also ask the child's caregiver to hold an oxygen mask near the patient's nose and mouth.

Check the child's pulse every 1 to 2 minutes to see if chest compressions need to be started. Perform ongoing assessments as often as indicated during transport. Record all patient care information, including the patient's medical history and all emergency care given, on a PCR.

Cardiopulmonary Failure

When a person stops breathing, a respiratory arrest occurs. When a person heart stops, a cardiac arrest occurs. When the heart and lungs stop working, a cardiopulmonary arrest results. When respiratory failure occurs together with shock, **cardiopulmonary failure** results. Cardiopulmonary failure is the result of inadequate oxygenation, inadequate ventilation, and poor perfusion (Figure 26-12).

Objective 10

In adults, cardiopulmonary failure and arrest is often the result of underlying heart disease. In children, cardiopulmonary failure and arrest is usually the result of an uncorrected respiratory problem. Some illness and injuries are associated with a high risk of cardiopulmonary failure.

You Should Know

Conditions Associated with a High Risk of Cardiopulmonary Failure

- Massive traumatic injuries
- Burns
- Severe dehydration
- Severe asthma, reactive airway disease
- Drowning
- An upper airway obstruction
- Prolonged seizure
- Coma

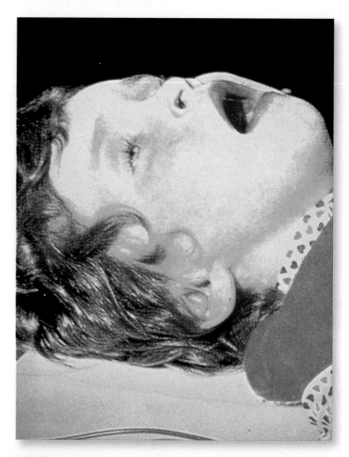

FIGURE 26-12 ▲ Inadequate oxygenation, inadequate ventilation, and poor perfusion can all result in cardiopulmonary failure. *EMSC Slide Set (CD-ROM), 1996. Courtesy of the Emergency Medical Services for Children Program, administered by the U.S. Department of Health and Human Service's Health Resources and Services Administration, Maternal and Child Health Bureau.*

The signs and symptoms of cardiopulmonary failure include:

- Mental status changes
- A weak respiratory effort
- Slow, shallow breathing
- Pale, mottled, or bluish skin
- A slow pulse rate
- Weak central pulses and absent peripheral pulses
- Cool extremities
- A delayed capillary refill

Cardiopulmonary failure will progress to cardiopulmonary arrest unless it is recognized and treated promptly. If your patient is showing signs of cardiopulmonary failure, make sure his airway is open. If trauma is suspected, take spinal precautions as necessary. Assist the child's breathing with a BM or mouth-to-mask device. Perform chest compressions if necessary.

Altered Mental Status

Altered mental status (also called an *altered level of consciousness* [ALOC]) means a change in a patient's level of awareness of his surroundings. For example, a person may be awake and know his name but he may be unable to answer questions about where he is or what happened to him. In order for you to determine if there has been a change in the patient's behavior, you must find out what the patient's normal behavior is. The patient's caregiver is usually the best person to provide this information. In fact, the child's caregiver is often the person who calls 9-1-1 because he has noticed that the child "isn't acting right." A patient with an altered mental status may appear agitated, combative, sleepy, difficult to awaken, or unresponsive.

There are many causes of altered mental status. The most common causes in a pediatric patient are a low level of oxygen in the blood, head trauma, seizures, infection, low blood sugar, and drug or alcohol ingestion.

You Should Know

Causes of Altered Mental Status

- Low blood oxygen level (hypoxia)
- Head trauma
- Seizures
- Brain infection
- Shock
- Low blood sugar
- Drug or alcohol ingestion
- Fever
- Respiratory failure

Any patient with an altered mental status is in danger of an airway obstruction. The patient may lose the ability to keep his own airway open because the soft tissues of the airway and the base of the tongue relax. The tongue falls into the back of the throat, blocking the airway. The patient may also have depressed gag and cough reflexes. A blocked airway can result in low blood oxygen levels, respiratory failure, or respiratory arrest. A pulse oximeter should be routinely used and continuously monitored for any infant or child who has an altered mental status. Many causes of an altered mental status may be associated with vomiting. Be prepared to clear the patient's airway with suctioning. Anticipate the need to place the patient in the recovery position (if no trauma is suspected).

If the equipment is available, check the child's blood glucose level. If the child's glucose level is low, notify medical direction. Give oral glucose if appropriate and if ordered by medical direction. Remember that your patient must be awake, with an intact gag reflex. Remember to comfort, calm, and reassure the patient. Perform ongoing assessments as often as indicated during transport. Record all patient care information, including the patient's medical history and all emergency care given, on a PCR.

Shock

Objective 8

Shock rarely results from a primary cardiac problem in infants and children. Common causes of shock in infants and children include diarrhea and dehydration, trauma, vomiting, blood loss, infection, and abdominal injuries. Less common causes of shock include allergic reactions, poisoning, and cardiac disorders. Signs and symptoms of shock include:

- Rapid respiratory rate
- Pale, cool, clammy skin
- Weak or absent peripheral pulses
- Delayed capillary refill
- Decreased urine output (determined by asking the caregiver about diaper wetting and looking at the child's diaper)
- Mental status changes
- Absence of tears, even when crying

Emergency care for an infant or child in shock includes making sure the patient's airway is open and giving oxygen. Request an early response of ALS personnel to the scene, or consider an ALS intercept while en route to the receiving facility. Do not delay transport for ALS arrival. If the patient's breathing is adequate, give oxygen at 15 L/min by nonrebreather mask. If breathing is inadequate, provide positive-pressure ventilation with 100% oxygen. Assess the adequacy of the ventilations delivered. Because of a child's small blood volume, you must quickly control any bleeding, if present. If the child is experiencing anaphylaxis, contact medical direction and request an order to administer epinephrine, or assist the patient with his own auto-injector.

Keep the patient warm and transport rapidly to the closest appropriate facility. Perform ongoing assessments every 5 minutes during transport. Record all patient care information, including the patient's medical history and all emergency care given, on a PCR.

Fever

Fever is a common reason for infant or child calls. Elevated body temperature may be caused by:

- Infection or inflammation
- Heat exposure

- Certain poisonings, such as aspirin
- Severe dehydration
- Uncontrolled seizures

Seizures are common in children. Seizures, including seizures caused by fever (**febrile seizures**), should be considered potentially life-threatening. Seizures from fever are most common in children under the age of 5. It is the rapid rise of the child's temperature in a short period—not how high the temperature is—that causes the seizure.

Meningitis is an inflammation of the meninges, the membranes covering the brain and spinal cord. It may be caused by a virus (most common type), fungus, or bacteria. In children more than 2 years of age, common signs and symptoms include a high fever, headache, and stiff neck. These findings may develop over several hours (less common) or 1 to 2 days (more common). Fever, headache, and neck stiffness may not be present in newborns and young infants (less than 2 to 3 months). Signs and symptoms in newborns and young infants may include poor feeding, decreased activity, and irritability. A bulging fontanelle or high-pitched cry may also be present. One form of meningitis is potentially life-threatening when the organism that causes it enters the bloodstream. A fever and reddish-purple rash is present in more than half of the patients who develop this form of meningitis (Figure 26-13).

Emergency care for an infant or child with a fever includes the following steps:

- Remember to use appropriate PPE. Position the child so you can maintain an open airway.
- Remove excess clothing.
- Be alert for seizures. Treat for shock if indicated.
- If instructed to begin cooling measures by medical direction, sponge the child with lukewarm water. Do not use cold or ice water or alcohol to

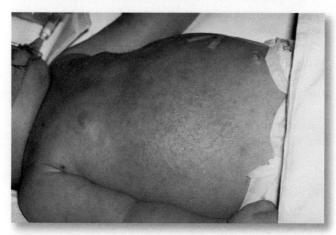

FIGURE 26-13 ▲ A life-threatening form of meningitis is associated with a fever and reddish-purple rash.
© Mediscan.

cool the child. Ice or cold-water baths cause shivering, which is the body's way of generating heat. Alcohol is not used because it can be absorbed through the skin, causing poisoning. Alcohol can also cause very rapid cooling.

- Transport the child for physician evaluation. Perform ongoing assessments as often as indicated en route. Record all patient care information, including the patient's medical history and all emergency care given, on a PCR.

Seizures

Objective 11

A seizure is a temporary change in behavior or consciousness caused by abnormal electrical activity in one or more groups of brain cells. **Status epilepticus** is recurring seizures without an intervening period of consciousness. Status epilepticus is a medical emergency that can cause brain damage or death if it is not treated.

Many conditions can cause seizures, but sometimes the cause is unknown. It is not necessary for you to determine the cause of a seizure in order to manage a patient who is having one.

You Should Know

Known Causes of Seizures

- Low blood oxygen level
- Low blood sugar
- Brain tumor
- Poisoning
- Head injury
- Previous brain damage
- Seizure disorder
- Fever
- Infection
- An abnormal heart rhythm
- Inherited factors

Seizures generally last about 30 to 45 seconds but can continue for minutes to hours. During the seizure, the child may have an altered mental status, changes in behavior, uncontrolled muscle movements, and a loss of bowel or bladder control. Depending on its severity, injuries can occur during a seizure. Injuries may include biting of the tongue or cheek, injury to the head, bruises, and broken bones.

Objective 12

When you arrive on the scene, perform a scene size-up before starting emergency medical care. If the scene is safe, approach the child and perform a primary survey. Complete a physical exam as needed.

Important assessment findings that can help explain the cause of the seizure include a purplish skin rash, signs of a head injury, or hot skin. The child's arms and/or legs may show signs of trauma from muscle movements during the seizure.

It is most likely that once you have arrived, the seizure will be over. Obtaining a good history is very important when treating these patients. Examples of questions to ask the child's caregiver are listed in the following *Making a Difference* box.

Making a Difference

Questions to Ask About a Seizure

Is this the child's first seizure?

If the child has a history of seizures, is he taking a seizure medication? Was this the child's normal seizure pattern? If not, how did it differ?

What did the caregiver do for the child during the seizure?

Could the child have ingested any medications, household products, or any potentially toxic item?

How long did the seizure last?

Does the child have a fever?

Does the child have a history of diabetes (possible low blood sugar)?

If the patient is actively seizing when you arrive, look to see if he has bitten his tongue or hit his head during the seizure. If you witness the seizure, you will need to be able to describe what it looked like when transferring patient care. Important information includes how long the seizure lasted and if the seizure involved full body jerking or movement of only an arm or a leg. Note if the child lost bladder or bowel control. If the seizure has stopped, look for clues to the cause. Check for a medical identification device. Look for evidence of burns or suspicious substances that might indicate poisoning or a toxic exposure. Are there signs of recent trauma? If the equipment is available, check the child's blood glucose level. If the child's glucose level is low, notify medical direction.

Comfort, calm, and reassure the patient while he is in your care. Protect the patient's privacy. Ask bystanders (except the caregiver) to leave the area. During the seizure, protect the child from harm by moving hard or sharp objects out of the way. Never attempt to restrain a child having a seizure. Do not put anything in the patient's mouth. Make sure that suction is available because the child may vomit during or after the seizure.

As soon as the seizure is over, make sure the child's airway is clear. Gently suction the child's mouth if secretions are present. Place the child in the recovery position if there is no possibility of spinal trauma. Loosen tight clothing. Give oxygen by nonrebreather mask. Use blow-by oxygen if necessary. If the child's skin appears blue, assist his breathing with a BM or mouth-to-mask device. If the child's skin is hot and he is bundled in blankets, remove the blankets.

The period after a seizure is called the *postictal phase*. During this recovery period, the child often appears limp, has shallow breathing, and has an altered mental status. This altered mental status may appear as confusion, sleepiness, combativeness, memory loss, unresponsiveness, or difficulty talking. The postictal phase may last minutes to hours.

In most cases, the child should be transported to the hospital without using flashing lights and siren. Flashing lights can cause seizures or agitation in susceptible patients. However, if the patient's condition is critical (such as status epilepticus), use lights and siren as needed. Perform ongoing assessments as often as indicated during transport. Record all patient care information, including the patient's medical history and all emergency care given, on a PCR.

Poisonings

Exposure to toxins can happen by eating and drinking, inhaling, absorption through the skin, injection into the body by needle, or bites and stings. Many calls involving a pediatric poisoning become very emotional. You will need to calm the situation, find out what the exposure was, and contact your local Poison Control Center (PCC) at 1-800-222-1222 (the national PCC number). Ask questions using "Who, What, Where, When, Why, and How" to find out what the child was exposed to (see Chapter 17). Keep in mind that trying to find an antidote for a specific poison is not necessary.

Emergency care for an infant or child toxic exposure includes the following steps:

- Use appropriate protection, or have trained rescuers remove the patient from the poisonous environment. Call for additional resources if needed.

- Follow proper decontamination procedures, if necessary, and prepare the ambulance to receive the patient. Methods used for decontamination will depend on the toxin and type of exposure. Call a poison center for advice, as needed, about decontamination procedures and patient care.

- Establish and maintain an open airway. If a child is found unresponsive or trauma is suspected, remember to consider the possibility of spinal injury and take appropriate precautions as needed. Use gloves to remove pills, tablets, or fragments from the patient's mouth, as needed, without injuring oneself. Be alert for vomiting and have suction within arm's reach.

- Give oxygen. If the child's breathing is adequate, apply oxygen by nonrebreather mask. If the patient's breathing is inadequate, provide positive-pressure ventilation with 100% oxygen. If the child will not tolerate a mask, give blow-by oxygen.

- If the patient has ingested a poison (and is awake), consult medical direction about giving activated charcoal. If the patient is unresponsive or seizing, consult medical direction about checking the child's blood sugar.

- If possible, bring all containers, bottles, labels, and other evidence of suspected poisons to the receiving facility. If the child vomits, save the vomitus in a container (such as a portable suction unit) and transport it to the receiving facility for analysis.

- Anticipate complications, including seizures, vomiting, shock, agitation, and an irregular heart rhythm. Perform ongoing assessments as often as indicated during transport. Record all patient care information, including the patient's medical history and all emergency care given, on a PCR.

Making a Difference

Keep in mind that your line of questioning should not take an accusatory tone. Often, "Why?" questions are misinterpreted as accusations toward the child's caregiver, when most poisonings are quite accidental. The parents or caregivers are already feeling quite guilty, and any untoward comments made by you or other healthcare professionals at the scene will likely cause further grief for the person responsible for the safety of the child.

Drowning

Absence of adult supervision is a factor in most submersion incidents involving infants and children. When you are called to the scene of a possible drowning, first study the scene and determine if approaching the patient is safe. Evaluate the mechanism of injury and determine (if possible) the length of submersion, cleanliness of the water, and temperature of the water. If needed, call for additional help *before* contact with the patient. Perform a primary survey and determine the presence of life-threatening conditions. Stabilize the patient's spine as needed.

Signs and symptoms of drowning will vary depending on the type and length of submersion. Possible signs

and symptoms are shown in the following *You Should Know* box. Assess baseline vital signs. Perform a physical examination, carefully assessing the patient for other injuries. Determine the events leading to the present situation.

- How long was the child submerged?
- What was the water temperature?
- Where did the incident occur (for example: lake, pool, bathtub, toilet, bucket)?
- Was the child breathing when removed from the water?
- Was there a pulse?
- Did the child experience any loss of consciousness?
- Was the incident witnessed? (This information is useful in determining possible head or spinal injury.)
- Does the child have any significant medical problems?
- Are there any signs of abuse or neglect?

You Should Know

Signs and Symptoms of Drowning

- Altered mental status, seizures, unresponsiveness
- Coughing, vomiting, choking, or airway obstruction
- Absent or inadequate breathing
- Difficulty breathing
- Fast, slow, or absent pulse
- Cool, clammy, and pale or cyanotic skin
- Vomiting
- Possible abdominal distention

Emergency care for a drowning victim includes ensuring the safety of all rescue personnel. Remove the patient from the water as quickly and safely as possible. Keep on-scene time to a minimum. Request an early response of ALS personnel to the scene, or consider an ALS intercept while en route to the receiving facility. Do not delay transport for ALS arrival. Protect the patient from environmental temperature extremes. Suction the patient's airway as needed. Give oxygen. If breathing is adequate, administer oxygen at 15 L/min by nonrebreather mask. If breathing is inadequate, provide positive-pressure ventilation with 100% oxygen. Assess the adequacy of the ventilations delivered. Remove wet clothing and dry the patient to prevent heat loss. If trauma is not suspected, place the patient in the recovery position to assist gravity in draining secretions from the patient's airway.

If the patient is unresponsive, is not breathing, and has no pulse or has a pulse rate of less than 60 beats/min with signs of shock, begin CPR once the patient has been removed from the water. If the child has no pulse, attach an automated external defibrillator (AED). Make sure the patient has been dried off before you operate the AED. To avoid electrical injury, take extra precautions to ensure that no one around the patient is in contact with the patient and water or metal during defibrillation.

All drowning victims should be transported to the hospital. Perform ongoing assessments as often as indicated en route. Record all patient care information, including the patient's medical history and all emergency care given, on a PCR.

You Should Know

The American Heart Association's 2005 Resuscitation Guidelines recommend that the following terms related to drowning should no longer be used: near-drowning, dry and wet drowning, active and passive drowning, silent drowning, secondary drowning, and drowned versus near-drowned.

Sudden Infant Death Syndrome

The National Institute of Child Health and Human Development defines **sudden infant death syndrome (SIDS)** as "the sudden and unexpected death of an infant that remains unexplained after a thorough case investigation, including performance of a complete autopsy, examination of the death scene, and review of the clinical history."

About 90% of all SIDS deaths occur during the first 6 months of life. Most deaths occur between the ages of 2 and 4 months. SIDS occurs in apparently healthy infants. Boys are affected more often than girls. Most SIDS deaths occur at home, usually during the night after a period of sleep. The baby is most often discovered in the early morning.

The cause of SIDS is not clearly understood. Research is ongoing. The number of SIDS deaths has decreased significantly since 1992, when caregivers were first told that infants should sleep on their backs and sides rather than on their stomachs. SIDS can be diagnosed only by autopsy.

Although not present in all cases, common SIDS physical exam findings include an unresponsive baby who is not breathing and has no pulse. The skin often appears blue or mottled. You may see frothy sputum or vomitus around the mouth and nose. The underside of the baby's body may look dark and bruised because of pooled blood (dependent lividity). General stiffening of the body (rigor mortis) may be present.

An **apparent life-threatening event (ALTE)**, also called *near-miss SIDS* or *near-SIDS*, is an episode in which an infant was about to die but was found early enough for successful resuscitation. The infant has some combination of apnea (absence of breathing), color change (cyanosis or pallor), marked change in muscle tone (usually extreme limpness), and choking or gagging.

Unless signs of obvious death are present, you should begin resuscitation according to your local protocols. Rigor mortis is an obvious sign of death. Dependent lividity is considered an obvious sign of death only when there are extensive areas of reddish-purple discoloration of the skin on the underside of the body of an unresponsive, breathless, and pulseless patient. In some Emergency Medical Services (EMS) systems, both lividity and rigor mortis must be present to be considered signs of obvious death. Check with your instructor about your local protocols regarding obvious death.

Whether or not resuscitation is performed, you must find out about the events leading up to the call for help. Ask questions as tactfully as possible. Start by asking the caregiver the baby's name. Once the baby's name is given to you, refer to the baby by name. Do not use nonspecific words such as "the baby" or "it." Carefully document what you see at the scene and the caregiver's responses to your questions. Avoid any comments or tone of voice that seems to point blame at the caregiver.

One of the most important skills you can perform on the scene of a SIDS patient is to provide emotional support for the baby's caregiver. The caregiver will usually be very distressed. You may observe crying, screaming, yelling, a stony silence, or physical outbursts. The caregiver's feelings of guilt are often enormous.

If the infant is obviously dead, you will need to tell the caregiver. Speak slowly in a quiet, calm voice. Begin by saying, "This is hard to tell you, but . . ." Explain that the baby is dead. Use the words "dead" or "death." Do not use phrases such as "passed on" or "no longer with us." Explain that there was nothing the caregiver could have done to prevent the baby's death. Pause frequently and ask the caregiver if he understands what you are saying. You may need to repeat information several times.

Before leaving the scene, make sure a friend, relative, member of the clergy, or grief support personnel are available to provide grief support for the family. Remain with the family until law enforcement personnel assume responsibility for the body and grief support personnel are on the scene.

After the call, make sure to assess your own emotional needs. It may be helpful for you and other personnel involved in the call to discuss the feelings that normally follow the death of an infant or child.

Trauma

Injuries are the leading cause of death in infants and children. Blunt trauma is the most common mechanism of serious injury in the pediatric patient. Examples of causes of common blunt trauma injuries are shown in the following *You Should Know* box.

You Should Know

Causes of Common Blunt Trauma Injuries

- Falls
- Bicycle-related injuries
- Motor vehicle–related injuries (restrained and unrestrained passengers)
- Car-pedestrian incidents
- Drowning
- Sports-related injuries
- Abuse and neglect

Objective 13

The injury pattern seen in a child may be different from that seen in an adult. For example, if an adult is about to be struck by an oncoming vehicle, he will typically turn away from the vehicle. This results in injuries to the side or back of the body. In contrast, a child will usually face an oncoming vehicle, resulting in injuries to the front of the body.

In a motor vehicle crash, an unrestrained infant or child will often have head and neck injuries. Restrained passengers often have abdominal and lower spine injuries. Child safety seats are often improperly secured, resulting in head and neck injuries. Contributing factors to pediatric motor vehicle–related injuries include failure to use (or improper use of) passenger restraints, inexperienced adolescent drivers, and alcohol abuse.

Deaths resulting from pedestrian injuries are common among children 5 to 9 years of age. The child is unable to judge the speed of the traffic and typically bolts out into the street. Children are often injured while chasing a toy, friend, or pet into the path of an oncoming vehicle. A child struck by a car is likely to sustain injury to the head, chest or abdomen, and an

extremity (Waddell's Triad). The vehicle first strikes the left side of the child. The bumper contacts the left femur, and the fender strikes the left side of the child's abdomen. The child is thrown against the vehicle's hood or windshield. The child is thrown to the ground, striking his head on the pavement as the vehicle comes to a stop. The child is then often run over by the vehicle.

Bicycle-related injuries often involve head trauma, abdominal injuries (from striking the handlebars) and trauma to the face and extremities. Sports injuries often involve injuries to the head and neck.

Submersion incidents are a significant cause of death and disability in children younger than 4 years of age. Alcohol appears to be a significant risk factor in adolescent drowning.

Most fire-related deaths occur in private residences, usually in homes without working smoke detectors. Smoke inhalation, scalds, and contact and electrical burns are especially likely to affect children younger than 4 years of age.

Injuries caused by a firearm include an entrance wound, exit wound, and an internal wound. Most guns used in unintentional shootings are found in the home and often found loaded in readily accessible places. The presence of a gun in the home has been linked to an increased likelihood of adolescent suicide.

Falls are a common cause of injury in infants and children. Infants and young children have large heads in comparison to their body size, making them more prone to falls. Note the distance of the fall, the surface on which the child landed, and the body area(s) struck. Any fall more than 3 times the child's height should be considered serious. Concrete and asphalt are associated with more severe injuries than other surfaces. Children who land on hard ground or concrete sustain more severe injury than those who hit grass, even when the heights of the falls are similar. If the child fell from a height or was diving into shallow water, suspect injuries to the head and neck.

Head Trauma

Children are prone to head injuries because their heads are large and heavy when compared with their body size. The younger the child, the softer and thinner the skull is. The force of injury is more likely to be transferred to the underlying brain instead of fracturing the skull. The blood vessels of the face and scalp bleed easily. Even a small wound can lead to major blood loss. When the head is struck, it jars the brain. The brain bounces back and forth, causing multiple bruised and injured areas. Signs and symptoms of a head injury vary according to the location and severity of the injury. Possible signs and symptoms are listed in the following *You Should Know* box.

Airway and breathing problems are common with head injuries. The most common cause of a low oxygen level in the unresponsive head injury patient is the tongue obstructing the airway. You must make sure that the child's airway is open and that his breathing is adequate.

Chest, Abdominal, and Pelvic Trauma

Signs of blunt trauma to the chest and abdomen may be hard to see on the body surface. The younger the patient, the softer and more flexible his ribs are. Therefore, rib fractures are less common in children than in adults. However, the force of the injury can be transferred to the internal organs of the chest, resulting in major damage. The presence of a rib fracture in a child suggests that major force caused the injury. Bruising of the lung (pulmonary contusion) is one of the most frequently observed chest injuries in children. This injury is potentially life threatening.

The abdomen is a more common site of injury in children than in adults. The abdomen is often a source of hidden injury. In fact, abdominal trauma is the most common cause of unrecognized fatal injury in children. The abdominal organs of an infant or child are prone to injury because the organs are large and the abdominal wall is thin. As a result, the organs are closer to the surface of the abdomen and less protected. In infants and young children, the liver and spleen extend below the lower ribs. Their location gives them less protection and makes them more susceptible to injury. A swollen, tender abdomen is a cause for concern.

Pelvic fractures are uncommon in children. However, when they do occur, they are often the result of the child's being struck by a moving vehicle. Because the pelvis contains major blood vessels, you must be alert for signs of internal bleeding and shock.

Extremity Trauma

Extremity trauma is common in children. The younger the child, the more flexible his bones are. When a child has multiple injuries, fractures are often missed. Assessing nondisplaced fractures in young children can be difficult because they cannot verbalize well. If a child is not walking on an injured extremity or using an upper extremity during normal activity, suspect a fracture until proven otherwise. Fractures of both thighs can cause a major blood loss, resulting in shock. Extremity injuries in children are managed in the same way as for adults.

Objective 14

When arriving on the scene, complete a scene size-up before beginning emergency medical care. Consider the mechanism of injury and perform a primary survey to determine the presence of life-threatening injuries. Be sure to comfort, calm, and reassure the patient. Keep on-scene time to a minimum. Request an early response of ALS personnel to the scene, or consider an ALS intercept while en route to the receiving facility. Do not delay transport for ALS arrival.

If the child is not alert or the mechanism of injury suggests that the child experienced trauma to the head or neck, stabilize the child's spine. Assume that any patient who has an injury above the collarbones has a spinal injury and immobilize accordingly. An unresponsive infant or child should always be immobilized, especially when the cause is unknown. Remember that you may need to place padding under the child's torso to maintain the cervical spine in a neutral position.

Making sure the child's airway is open and clear of secretions is the most important step in managing a trauma patient. If the patient is unresponsive, use the jaw thrust without head tilt maneuver to open the airway. Vomiting and inadequate breathing are common. Make sure suction is within arm's reach. Suction the mouth as needed with a rigid suction catheter. Insert an oral airway to help keep the airway open. If the child's breathing is inadequate or there is no air movement, assist breathing with BM or mouth-to-mask ventilation. Give oxygen and control obvious bleeding if present. A pulse oximeter should be routinely used and continuously monitored in any head-injured patient.

Check for signs of shock by assessing the child's mental status, heart rate, and skin color. If the child is 6 years of age or younger, assess capillary refill. Remember to keep the child warm. If signs and symptoms of shock are present with a closed head injury, look for signs of other injuries (such as internal bleeding) that may be the cause of the shock. Extremity injuries should be stabilized by immobilizing the joint above and below the fracture site. Remember to assess pulses, motor function, and sensation in the affected extremity before and after immobilization.

Perform ongoing assessments every 5 minutes during transport. Record all patient care information, including the patient's medical history and all emergency care given, on a PCR.

Child Abuse and Neglect

The definitions that appear here are from the National Clearinghouse on Child Abuse and Neglect and the National Child Abuse and Neglect Data System Glossary.

Child maltreatment is an act or failure to act by a parent, caregiver, or other person as defined by state law that results in physical abuse, neglect, medical neglect, sexual abuse, and/or emotional abuse. It is also defined as an act or failure to act that presents an impending risk of serious harm to a child (Figure 26-14). State laws define the specific acts that make up the various forms of abuse. These laws vary from state to state.

Physical abuse refers to physical acts that cause or could cause physical injury to a child. Examples of physical abuse include burning, hitting, punching, shaking, kicking, beating, or otherwise harming a child. **Neglect** is the failure to provide for a child's basic needs (Figure 26-15). Neglect can be medical, physical, educational, or emotional. **Medical neglect** is a type of maltreatment characterized by failure of the caregiver to provide for the appropriate healthcare of the child despite being financially able to do so. The signs of neglect that you may see in the child's environment include:

- Untreated chronic illness (such as a diabetic or asthmatic child with no medication)

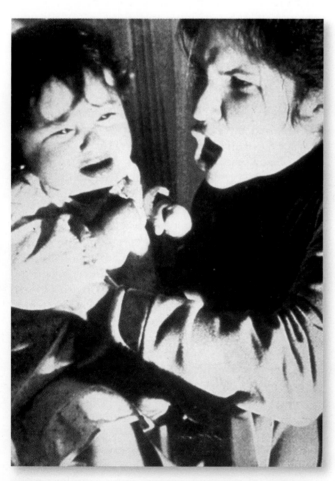

FIGURE 26-14 ▲ *Never* shake or jiggle a baby. *EMSC Slide Set (CD-ROM), 1996. Courtesy of the Emergency Medical Services for Children Program, administered by the U.S. Department of Health and Human Service's Health Resources and Services Administration, Maternal and Child Health Bureau.*

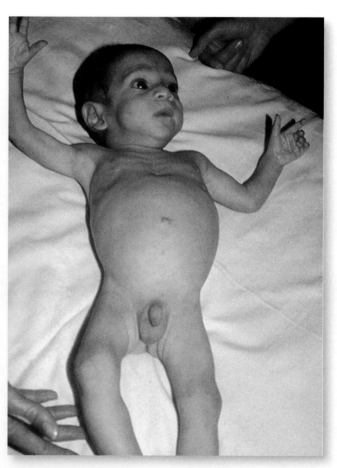

FIGURE 26-15 ▲ Neglect is the failure to provide for a child's basic needs. Neglect can be medical, physical, educational, or emotional. *EMSC Slide Set (CD-ROM), 1996. Courtesy of the Emergency Medical Services for Children Program, administered by the U.S. Department of Health and Human Service's Health Resources and Services Administration, Maternal and Child Health Bureau.*

- Untreated soft-tissue injuries
- A home that is bug or rodent infested
- A lack of adult supervision
- A lack of food or basic necessities
- A child who appears to be malnourished
- Stool or urine present on items in the home
- An unsafe living environment
- The presence of drugs or alcohol paraphernalia

Sexual abuse is inappropriate adolescent or adult sexual behavior with a child. To be considered child abuse, these acts have to be committed by a person responsible for the care of a child (for example, a babysitter, parent, or daycare provider) or related to the child. If a stranger commits these acts, it is considered sexual assault. Any form of sexual abuse is handled by the police and criminal courts. **Psychological maltreatment** is a pattern of caregiver behavior that conveys to children that they are worthless, flawed, unloved, unwanted, endangered, or only of value in meeting another's needs. This type of maltreatment includes verbal abuse, emotional abuse or neglect, psychological abuse, and mental injury.

As a healthcare professional, you must be aware of these conditions and be able to recognize them. Physical abuse and neglect are the two forms of child maltreatment that you are most likely to detect. As an Emergency Medical Technician (EMT), you may be the only trained healthcare professional in the child's environment. You will be able to see things that other healthcare professionals will never see. Your eyes and ears will help them complete the puzzle of suspected abuse.

You Should Know

Physical Signs That May Indicate Abuse

- Multiple bruises in various stages of healing
- Human bite marks
- Inflicted burns—"stocking-like" burns with no associated splash marks; usually present on the buttocks, genitalia, or extremities
- Circular burns from a cigarette or cigar
- Rope burns on the wrists
- Burns in the shape of a household utensil or appliance, such as a spoon or iron
- Fractures
- Head, face, and oral injuries
- Abdominal injuries
- An injury inconsistent with the history or developmental level of the child

Objective 15

According to the National Clearinghouse on Child Abuse and Neglect, you should consider the possibility of physical abuse when the *child:*

- Has unexplained burns, bites, bruises, broken bones, or black eyes
- Has fading bruises or other marks noticeable after an absence from school
- Seems frightened of the caregiver and protests or cries when it is time to go home
- Shrinks at the approach of adults
- Reports injury caused by a parent or another adult caregiver

It is important to recognize that some medical conditions or cultural practices may look like signs of abuse but are not. For example, **impetigo** is a contagious bacterial skin infection that can look like a burn (Figure 26-16). Chickenpox may resemble cigarette burns. **Mongolian spots** are bluish areas usually seen in non-Caucasian infants and young children that may be mistaken for bruises (Figure 26-17). Some cultures, such as those of Southeast Asia, practice **coining.** Coining is a healing remedy in which a coin is heated in hot oil and then rubbed along the patient's spine to heal an illness, such as congestion in the lungs (Figure 26-18). Coining is not considered child abuse.

You should consider the possibility of physical abuse when the *parent or other adult caregiver:*

- Offers conflicting, unconvincing, or no explanation for the child's injury
- Describes the child as "evil," or refers to him in some other very negative way

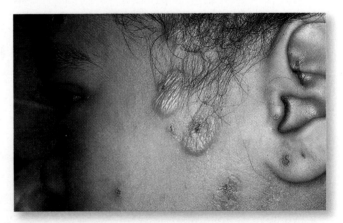

FIGURE 26-16 ▲ Impetigo, a bacterial skin infection, can be mistaken for burns. *Courtesy of Anne W. Lucky, M.D. from Knoop, et al., Atlas of Emergency Medicine, 2nd edition, McGraw-Hill Company, Inc.*

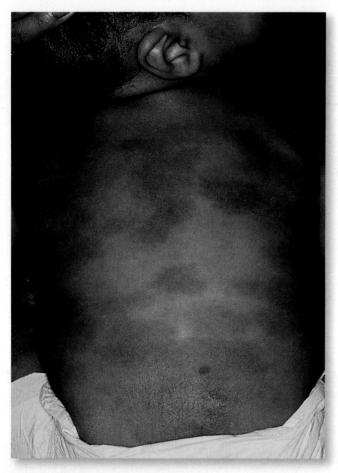

FIGURE 26-17 ▲ Mongolian spots can be mistaken for bruises. *Courtesy of Douglas R. Landry, MD, from Knoop, et al., Atlas of Emergency Medicine, 2nd edition, McGraw-Hill Company, Inc.*

- Uses harsh physical discipline with the child
- Has a history of abuse as a child

You should consider the possibility of neglect when the *child:*

- Is frequently absent from school
- Begs or steals food or money
- Lacks needed medical or dental care, immunizations, or glasses
- Is consistently dirty and has severe body odor
- Lacks sufficient clothing for the weather
- Abuses alcohol or other drugs
- States that there is no one at home to provide care

You should consider the possibility of neglect when the *parent or other adult caregiver:*

- Appears to be indifferent to the child
- Seems apathetic or depressed
- Behaves irrationally or in a bizarre manner
- Is abusing alcohol or other drugs

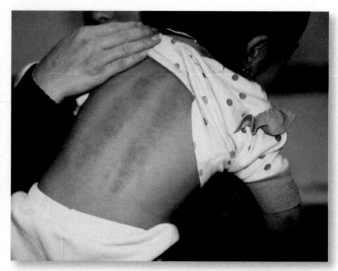

FIGURE 26-18 ▲ Some cultures practice coining, a healing remedy. *Courtesy of Charles Schubert, MD, from Knoop, et al., Atlas of Emergency Medicine, 2nd edition, McGraw-Hill Company, Inc.*

Objective 16

Do not confront or accuse any caregiver of abuse. Accusation and confrontation delay transportation and may endanger the EMT or crew. Keep in mind that the caregiver with the child at the scene may not be the abuser.

Reporting known or suspected child abuse is required by law in most states. Individuals who are typically required to report abuse have frequent contact with children. Some states require all citizens to report suspected abuse or neglect regardless of their profession. It is your responsibility to know what the requirements are in your area.

Carefully document your physical exam findings as well as your observations of the child's environment. Document the caregiver's comments exactly as stated and enclose them in quotation marks. Make sure that your documentation reflects the facts and not your opinion of what may or may not have occurred. Report what you see and hear. Do not comment on what you think. Be objective, and do not document emotions or suspicions. Document only what you see, hear, or witness using your five senses. Report your findings to appropriate personnel when transferring patient care.

Providing care for an infant or child who is ill or injured because of neglect or abuse is stressful for most healthcare professionals. Show a professional and caring attitude as you care for the patient. You must make the interests of an ill or injured infant or child your main concern when making patient care decisions. After the call, assess your own emotional needs. A discussion with other personnel involved in the call may be helpful. If necessary, consult your agency's crisis counseling policies.

Infants and Children with Special Needs

Children with special needs may also be referred to as *technology-assisted children*. These are children experiencing a chronic or terminal illness who are being cared for at home and are dependent on high-technology equipment. Types of children with special needs include:

- Premature babies with lung disease
- Babies and children with heart disease
- Infants and children with neurological disease
- Children with cancer
- Children with chronic disease or altered function from birth

Tracheostomy Tubes

A *tracheostomy* is the creation of a surgical opening into the trachea through the neck, with insertion of a tube to aid passage of air or removal of secretions. The surgical opening created is called a *stoma*. A tracheostomy may be temporary or permanent. A temporary tracheostomy is sewn closed when no longer needed. In a permanent tracheostomy, a tube is inserted to keep the stoma open. Tracheostomy tubes come in a variety of types and sizes. They may be metal or plastic, cuffed or uncuffed. The tube selected depends on the patient's condition and physician preference. Complications that you may encounter include the following:

- Obstruction of the tube by dried secretions, excessive secretions, or airway swelling
- Dislodgment from coughing or patient movement, accidental removal, or inability to reinsert after a routine change
- Bleeding
- Air leak
- Infection

Emergency care includes maintaining an open airway. Request an early response of ALS personnel to the scene, or consider an ALS intercept while en route to the receiving facility. If the tracheostomy tube has become dislodged and the caregiver is unable to replace it, ventilate the patient as needed with a BM device. Seal the BM device over the child's mouth and nose and cover the stoma with a gloved hand. If unsuccessful, cover the stoma with a small mask and attempt to ventilate through the stoma. At the same time, cover the child's mouth and nose with a gloved hand. If needed, suction the tracheostomy tube to clear secretions. Limit suctioning to no more than 5 seconds at a time. If external bleeding is present, apply gentle direct pressure to the bleeding site, being careful not to block the airway or apply pressure to the carotid arteries. Allow the child to maintain a position of comfort. Perform ongoing assessments as often as indicated en route. Record all patient care information, including the patient's medical history and all emergency care given, on a PCR.

Home Mechanical Ventilators

Mechanical ventilators are used to assist breathing in patients who are unable to breathe adequately on their own. Ventilator equipment is usually managed by a supplier that provides 24-hour emergency service. The home ventilator has an internal backup battery in case of power failure. Ventilator malfunction is usually to the result of mechanical failure, power outage, or low oxygen supply.

If the ventilator is malfunctioning and the caregiver cannot quickly determine the cause of the problem, disconnect the child from the ventilator. Request an early response of ALS personnel to the scene, or consider an ALS intercept while en route to the receiving facility. Establish and maintain an open airway. Provide positive-pressure ventilation with a BM device. If the child has a tracheostomy tube in place, the bag-mask device can be connected directly to the tracheostomy tube. Perform ongoing assessments as often as indicated en route. Record all patient care information, including the patient's medical history and all emergency care given, on a PCR.

Central Lines

A **central line** is an intravenous (IV) line placed near the heart for long-term use. Central lines may be used to give medications and nutritional solutions directly into the venous circulation. Central lines may also be referred to by the manufacturers' name, such as Broviac, Hickman, Groshong, or Corcath. Central lines may be placed in the subclavian vein or, often, the femoral vein in children.

A **peripherally-inserted central catheter** is also called a *PICC line*. A PICC line is smaller than those routinely used for central lines. Because of their small size, they are often used for neonates, young children, or those requiring only short-term therapy. Complications include a cracked line, infection, clotting off, and bleeding.

If you are called for a patient who has a problem with a central line, request an early response of ALS personnel to the scene, or consider an ALS intercept while en route to the receiving facility. Establish and maintain an open airway. Give the child oxygen if needed. If the site is bleeding, apply direct pressure to the site with a sterile dressing. Perform ongoing assessments as often as indicated en route. Record all patient care information, including the patient's medical history and all emergency care given, on a PCR.

Gastrostomy Tubes and Gastric Feeding

A **gastrostomy tube** is a special catheter placed directly into the stomach for feeding. It is most often used when passage of a tube through a child's mouth, pharynx, or esophagus is contraindicated or impossible or when the tube must be maintained for a long period. A typical gastrostomy tube sticks out about 12-15 inches from the skin. It is sewn in place. A skin-level "feeding button" may be used in children who require long-term gastrostomy feedings. The "button" is small and sticks out only slightly from the abdomen. The button has a one-way valve that accepts a feeding tube. It allows the child greater mobility and comfort and is easier to care for than a gastrostomy tube.

Emergency care for a child with a gastrostomy tube includes making sure the airway remains open. Request an early response of ALS personnel to the scene, or consider an ALS intercept while en route to the receiving facility. Be prepared to suction if necessary. Be alert for changes in mental status. If the child is a diabetic, he will become hypoglycemic quickly if he cannot be fed. Give oxygen as needed. Check the site for bleeding and control bleeding if present. Transport the child in a sitting (Fowler's) position or lying on the right side, with the head elevated. Perform ongoing assessments as often as indicated en route. Record all patient care information, including the patient's medical history and all emergency care given, on a PCR.

Shunts

Hydrocephalus is a condition in which there is an excess of cerebrospinal fluid (CSF) within the brain. A **ventricular shunt** is a drainage system used to remove the excess CSF. A catheter is surgically implanted in a chamber in the brain. The catheter is connected to a reservoir that collects the fluid. The reservoir can usually be felt through the skin behind the ear. A one-way valve prevents fluid from flowing back into the ventricle. The reservoir is connected to a drainage catheter that empties into the abdominal cavity. The major complications associated with shunts include infection and equipment failure caused by obstruction, kinking, plugging, displacement, or separation of the tubing. If the shunt becomes blocked, excess CSF will collect

in the brain. Because the skull is a rigid vault, pressure within the skull will increase. This will produce signs and symptoms like those of a patient with a head injury. These include changes in mental status, headache, irritability, vomiting, seizures, and respiratory depression.

Request an early response of ALS personnel to the scene, or consider an ALS intercept while en route to the receiving facility. Establish and maintain an open airway. Be prepared to suction if necessary. Give oxygen. If the patient's breathing is adequate, apply oxygen by nonrebreather mask at 15 L/min if not already done. If the patient's breathing is inadequate, provide positive-pressure ventilation with 100% oxygen. Perform ongoing assessments as often as indicated en route. Record all patient care information, including the patient's medical history and all emergency care given, on a PCR.

On the Scene   Wrap-Up

You apply an oxygen mask to your small patient while calmly reassuring her that it will help her. You quickly assess her, contact medical direction, and then begin assisting her with her prescribed metered-dose inhaler. Within a few minutes of starting the drug, her breathing is improving, but her wheezing is still significant. You secure the patient in the ambulance and reassess her every 5 minutes during the 30-mile trip to the hospital. ∎

Sum It Up

▶ The age classification of infants and children is the following:
  • Newly born: Birth to several hours after birth
  • Neonate: Birth to 1 month
  • Infant: 1 to 12 months of age
    —Young infant: 0 to 6 months of age
    —Older infant: 6 months to 1 year of age
  • Toddler: 1 to 3 years of age
  • Preschooler: 4 to 5 years of age
  • School-age child: 6 to 12 years of age
  • Adolescent: 13 to 18 years of age

▶ Perform a primary survey. Begin by forming a general impression of an infant or child from "across the room." Quickly determine if the child appears sick or not sick. Quickly assess:

- *Appearance.* A child should be alert and responsive to his surroundings.
- *(Work of) Breathing.* With normal breathing, both sides of the chest rise and fall equally. Breathing is quiet and painless and occurs at a regular rate.
- *Circulation.* Visual signs of circulation relate to skin color, obvious bleeding, and moisture. If the child's skin looks pale, mottled, flushed, gray, or blue, proceed immediately to the primary survey.

▶ Once your general impression is complete, perform a hands-on ABCDE assessment to determine if life-threatening conditions are present. In a responsive infant or child, use a toes-to-head or trunk-to-head approach. This approach should help reduce the infant or child's anxiety.

▶ During your primary survey, find the answers to these five questions:

1. Is the child awake and alert?
2. Is the child's airway open?
3. Is the child breathing?
4. Does the child have a pulse?
5. Does the child have severe bleeding?

▶ If a child is unable to speak, cry, cough, or make any other sound, his airway is completely obstructed. If the child has noisy breathing, such as snoring or gurgling, he has a partial airway obstruction. You will need to intervene if the child has a complete airway obstruction.

▶ In children, pulse regularity normally changes with respirations (increases with inspiration, decreases with expiration).

▶ Use the carotid artery to assess the pulse in an unresponsive child older than 1 year of age. Feel for a brachial pulse in an unresponsive infant. Feel for a pulse for about 10 seconds. If there is no pulse, or if a pulse is present but the rate is less than 60 beats/min with signs of shock, you must begin chest compressions.

▶ In infants and children, it is important to compare the pulse of the central blood vessels (such as the femoral artery) with those found in peripheral areas of the body (such as the feet). They should feel the same. If they do not, a circulatory problem is present.

▶ Assess capillary refill in children 6 years of age or younger. Delayed capillary refill may occur because of shock or hypothermia, among other causes.

▶ Assess blood pressure in children older than 3 years of age. In children 1 to 10 years older than 1 year of age, the following formula may be used to determine the lower limit of a normal systolic blood pressure: 70 + (2 × child's age in years) = systolic blood pressure. The lower limit of normal systolic blood pressure for a child 10 or more years of age is 90 mm Hg. The diastolic blood pressure should be about two thirds the systolic pressure.

▶ The most common medical emergencies in children are respiratory emergencies. Upper airway problems usually occur suddenly. Lower airway problems usually take longer to develop. Respiratory distress is an increased work of breathing (respiratory effort). Respiratory failure is a condition in which there is not enough oxygen in the blood and/or ventilation to meet the demands of body tissues. Respiratory failure becomes evident when the patient becomes tired and can no longer maintain good oxygenation and ventilation. Respiratory arrest occurs when a patient stops breathing.

▶ Cardiopulmonary arrest results when the heart and lungs stop working. When respiratory failure occurs together with shock, cardiopulmonary failure results. Cardiopulmonary failure will progress to cardiopulmonary arrest unless it is recognized and treated promptly.

▶ A seizure is a temporary change in behavior or consciousness caused by abnormal electrical activity in one or more groups of brain cells. Status epilepticus is recurring seizures without an intervening period of consciousness. Status epilepticus is a medical emergency that can cause brain damage or death if it is not treated.

▶ The most common causes of an altered mental status in a pediatric patient are a low level of oxygen in the blood, head trauma, seizures, infection, low blood sugar, and drug or alcohol ingestion. Any patient with an altered mental status is in danger of an airway obstruction. Be prepared to clear the patient's airway with suctioning.

▶ Sudden infant death syndrome (SIDS) is the sudden and unexpected death of an infant. The cause of SIDS is not clearly understood.

▶ Injuries are the leading cause of death in infants and children. If the child is not alert or the mechanism of injury suggests that the child experienced trauma to the head or neck, stabilize the child's spine. Making sure the child's airway is open and clear of secretions is the most important step in managing a trauma patient. Extremity injuries should be stabilized by immobilizing the joint above and below the fracture site. Remember to assess pulses, motor function, and sensation in the affected extremity before and after immobilization.

- Child maltreatment is an act or failure to act by a parent, caregiver, or other person as defined by state law that results in physical abuse, neglect, medical neglect, sexual abuse, and/or emotional abuse. It is also defined as an act or failure to act that presents an impending risk of serious harm to a child.

- Physical abuse refers to physical acts that cause or could cause physical injury to a child. Examples of physical abuse include burning, hitting, punching, shaking, kicking, beating, or otherwise harming a child.

- Neglect is the failure to provide for a child's basic needs. Neglect can be medical, physical, educational, or emotional. Medical neglect is a type of maltreatment caused by failure of the caregiver to provide for the appropriate healthcare of the child although financially able to do so.

- Sexual abuse is inappropriate adolescent or adult sexual behavior with a child. To be considered child abuse, these acts have to be committed by a person responsible for the care of a child (for example a babysitter, parent, or daycare provider) or related to the child. If a stranger commits these acts, it is considered sexual assault and is handled by the police and criminal courts.

- Psychological maltreatment is a pattern of caregiver behavior that conveys to children that they are worthless, flawed, unloved, unwanted, endangered, or only of value in meeting another's needs. This type of maltreatment includes verbal abuse, emotional abuse or neglect, psychological abuse, and mental injury.

- When providing care for an infant or child who is ill or injured because of neglect or abuse, show a professional and caring attitude for the patient. Report known or suspected child abuse as required by law in your state. Carefully document your physical exam findings as well as your observations of the child's environment. Document the caregiver's comments exactly as stated and enclose them in quotation marks. Your documentation must reflect the facts and not your opinion of what may or may not have occurred. Report your findings to appropriate personnel when transferring patient care. After the call, assess your own emotional needs. A discussion with other personnel involved in the call may be helpful.

- Infants and children with special needs include many different types of children. Examples of these patients include premature babies with lung disease, babies and children with heart disease, infants and children with nervous system disease, and children with chronic disease or altered function from birth.

Division 7

Operations

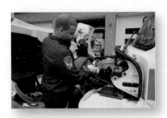
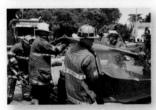
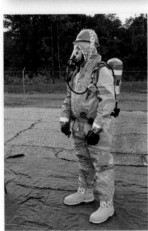

27 Emergency Vehicle Operations

By the end of this chapter, you should be able to:

Knowledge Objectives ▶

1. Discuss the medical and nonmedical equipment needed to respond to a call.
2. List the phases of an ambulance call.
3. Describe the general provisions of state laws relating to the operation of the ambulance and privileges in any or all of the following categories:
   - Speed
   - Warning lights
   - Sirens
   - Right of way
   - Parking
   - Turning
4. List contributing factors to unsafe driving conditions.
5. Describe the considerations that should be given to:
   - Request for escorts
   - Following an escort vehicle
   - Intersections
6. Discuss "due regard for the safety of others" while operating an emergency vehicle.
7. State what information is essential in order to respond to a call.
8. Discuss various situations that may affect response to a call.
9. Differentiate among the various methods of moving a patient to the unit on the basis of injury or illness.
10. Apply the components of the essential patient information in a written report.
11. Summarize the importance of preparing the unit for the next response.
12. Identify what is essential for completion of a call.
13. Distinguish among the terms *cleaning, disinfection, high-level disinfection,* and *sterilization.*
14. Describe how to clean or disinfect items following patient care.

Attitude Objectives ▶

15. Explain the rationale for appropriate report of patient information.
16. Explain the rationale for having the unit prepared to respond.

Skill Objectives ▶ There are no skill objectives for this lesson.

You are looking forward to your first day as an Emergency Medical Technician (EMT). You have arrived early for your shift. You have combed your hair, pressed your uniform, verified that all of your certification cards are current, and studied your local protocols to make sure you are up to date with appropriate treatments. Your partner for the day is a 15-year veteran who is known for her extensive knowledge of prehospital care. She introduces you to the off-going shift and then asks you to sit while she explains how she likes to have things done on "her shift." At exactly 0800, you ask if you should begin checking the equipment for the day. Your partner explains that they have an "arrangement" at this station. No one checks the equipment unless the off-going shift reports that they have not had time to replace anything used on a late call. As the off-going crew has not mentioned anything, she says, "The equipment is fine." For the next hour your partner talks to you about her years of experience as an EMT. You are amazed at the amount of information that she has stored inside her head.

You hear your first alarm, dispatching your unit to a possible cardiac arrest at a local shopping mall. You and your partner respond quickly and efficiently to the proper address. While en route, you review the list of equipment that may be needed at the scene and wonder where it might be located. Your unit is the first to arrive. Your partner states that she will get the stretcher as you get the rest of the equipment. It takes you several minutes to find the needed equipment, as you have never looked inside this vehicle before. In fact, you are unable to find an automated external defibrillator (AED) or an airway kit. You decide to assist your partner with the stretcher and hope that the next unit will have additional equipment. You find the patient lying on the ground next to his vehicle in the mall parking lot. The patient is in cardiac arrest. Your partner begins positive-pressure ventilation with a bag-mask device while you start chest compressions. ■

THINK ABOUT IT

As you read this chapter, think about the following questions:

- Could a lack of proper equipment have an unfavorable effect on the care your patient receives?
- If you could turn back the clock, what would you have done differently when you arrived on the job today?

An Overview of Emergency Vehicle Operations

An Emergency Medical Technician (EMT) must be familiar with emergency vehicle operations, the medical and nonmedical equipment used in patient care, the phases of an emergency call, and appropriate use of air transport services. To minimize the risk of exposure to and transmission of infectious diseases, an EMT must understand the primary methods of decontamination. Although an overview of emergency vehicle operations is presented in this chapter, you should consider completing a standardized Emergency Vehicle Operator's course.

Your patient needs and deserves your best effort at all times, including daily vehicle checks and the cleaning and restocking of your apparatus. Be diligent in all duties, and represent your profession with pride and integrity. Remember your life, your partner's life, and the lives of your patients will literally be in your hands.

Phases of an Emergency Medical Services Call

Preparation Phase

Personnel and Basic Supplies

Objective 1

Preparation for an Emergency Medical Services (EMS) call requires ensuring that appropriately trained personnel are available to respond. Minimum staffing requirements for an ambulance include at least one EMT in the patient compartment. Two EMTs are preferred. In some states, two licensed personnel are required.

To be "certified" as ambulances, emergency transport vehicles are required to carry specific types and quantities of medical equipment. You must check with your local and state regulatory agencies for the specific equipment requirements. Supplies in addition to those in the following *You Should Know* box may be needed to address the specific needs of your agency or the type of calls that are most common in your area.

In addition to basic medical supplies, nonmedical supplies include personal safety equipment as required by local, state, and federal standards and preplanned routes or comprehensive street maps. A ground ambulance must also be equipped to provide, and be capable of providing, voice communication between:

- The ambulance attendant and the dispatch center
- The ambulance attendant and the ground ambulance service's assigned medical direction authority
- The ambulance attendant in the patient compartment and the ground ambulance service's assigned medical direction authority

You Should Know

Ground Ambulance: Basic Medical Equipment and Supplies

- Suction equipment (portable and a fixed apparatus)
- Oxygen cylinders (fixed and portable), each with a variable flow regulator
- Oxygen administration equipment, including tubing, nasal cannula (adult and pediatric), and nonrebreather mask (adult and pediatric)

- Hand-operated, disposable, self-expanding bag-mask (BM) devices (adult and pediatric)
- Adult, child, and infant oral airways
- Nasal airways
- Cervical stabilization devices
- Upper- and lower-extremity splints
- Traction splint
- Full-length spine boards
- Supplies to secure a patient to a spine board
- Cervical-thoracic spinal stabilization device for extrication
- Sterile burn sheets
- Triangular bandages
- Multi-trauma dressings, 10 × 30 inches or larger
- Abdominal bandages, 5 × 7 inches or larger
- Nonsterile 4 × 4-inch gauze sponges
- Nonsterile soft roller bandages, 4 inches or larger
- Nonsterile elastic roller bandages, 4 inches or larger
- Sterile occlusive dressings, 3 × 8 inches or larger
- Adhesive tape rolls, 2 or 3 inches in width
- Sterile obstetrical kit containing towels, 4 × 4-inch dressing, scissors, bulb suction, and clamps or tape for the umbilical cord
- Blood pressure cuffs (child size, adult size, and large adult size)
- Specific emergency medications as determined by protocols
- Automated external defibrillator (AED)
- Stethoscope
- Heavy duty scissors capable of cutting clothing, belts, or boots
- Blankets, sheets
- Infection control materials, including protective gloves, gowns, masks, shoe coverings, filtration masks, protective eye wear, and non-latex gloves

Remember This!

Avoid the temptation to overstock your emergency vehicle. If you believe that there is a need for additional supplies, contact the appropriate individual or committee to change the normal quantity.

Patient Transfer Equipment

Objective 9

In most instances, your agency will have already determined the type of patient transfer equipment that will be available for you to use on each call. You must learn the proper method(s) of using this equipment. The proper use of this equipment and the appropriate techniques for lifting will help ensure your patient's safety and will also reduce your risk of injury during a lifting procedure.

Generally, each patient transport vehicle will have the following basic patient transfer equipment: a wheeled stretcher, a collapsible stretcher, and a long backboard or "Stokes" basket. Some EMS agencies will also have a bariatric stretcher available for use (see Chapter 6).

Wheeled stretchers are used more often than any other patient transfer device (see Chapter 6). A collapsible stretcher is designed to be folded. It is generally used when a standard stretcher is too large to be used on scene. Care should be taken to ensure that your patient is properly secured to the stretcher before moving. Kinds of collapsible stretchers include the stair chair and the roll-up stretcher. When using a collapsible stretcher, remember to plan the move before lifting the patient. Someone must be "in charge" to ensure a coordinated and safe move to the stretcher. In most instances, you will need additional personnel to ensure a safe lift. Never try to move these types of stretchers without a clear path to the main stretcher. A "stair chair" will force your patient into a sitting position. This may cause additional pain or even injury if used improperly. If the patient has experienced trauma or has the potential for any spinal injury, consider the use of a long backboard or the Stokes-style stretcher.

If needed, request additional resources and personnel before moving a patient. Then secure your patient to the device. Explain your plan to the patient before the first move. An unsuspecting patient who is frightened by suddenly being lifted into the air will reach out for support and grab the closest object, which may be you!

Stop and Think!

Think before you lift. Is there a better path? Have you removed any obstacles that may trip you and cause you to drop the patient? Have all personnel on the scene heard the plan, and do they understand their part in the move?

In some instances, you will need to use alternative devices to move a patient during the extrication phase of a rescue. Only trained personnel using proper safety and personal protective equipment (PPE) should attempt these specialty rescues. If you are part of this kind of rescue, take precautions to securely strap your patient onto the rescue board or into the basket. This style of rescue may place your patient at an extreme angle during the extrication. You must prevent movement or slipping in all planes of travel.

Daily Inspections

The importance of careful completion of the preparation phase cannot be overemphasized. Preparing your vehicle for daily operation is important.

Your first preparations for duty start before you arrive at the workplace. The knowledge and skills that you acquired during your initial training must be constantly refreshed and practiced. Careful review of your knowledge base and practice with infrequently used equipment will prepare you to give the most efficient and skilled patient care possible.

Planning for duty includes getting a reasonable amount of rest before your shift. You will be required to move your patients to the stretcher and lift them into the transport vehicle. Staying in shape and exercising will protect your back and ensure the safety of your patients during a lift.

Vehicle Inspection

One of your primary responsibilities will be to check the safe condition of your vehicle and determine if it is ready for operation. Your vehicle inspection begins with a careful consideration of the types of calls that you will respond to and the type of vehicle needed for these responses. The normal operation of an emergency vehicle has the potential to cause wear and damage to the vehicle. You may be held legally responsible if your apparatus is unable to respond or breaks down during an emergency response and the determination is made that the mechanical failure was preventable. At the very least, your patient's life may be endangered. In addition, you may incur legal responsibility if the failure leads to an accident or injury.

Exterior Begin your vehicle inspection with a conversation with the crew that used the apparatus during the previous shift. They should be able to inform you about any needs or deficits in the apparatus. Next, visually inspect your vehicle for any obvious damage or deficits (Figure 27-1). Note any breakage or damage on the appropriate "check-off sheet." Decide if the vehicle needs immediate repair or is safe for operation.

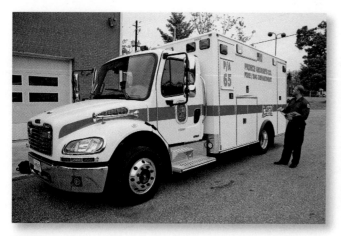

FIGURE 27-1 ▲ Inspect the exterior of the emergency vehicle for any obvious damage. Note any breakage or damage on the appropriate "check-off sheet."

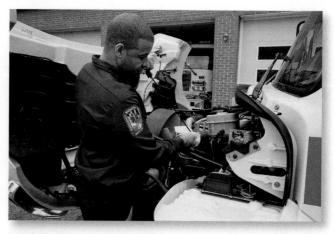

FIGURE 27-3 ▲ Check the vehicle's engine compartment. Inspect the condition of the radiator, hoses and belts, and all fluid levels.

All glass should be inspected and free of breakage, and the windshield wipers should function properly. Tires should have no visible damage to the rims or sidewalls. The tread depth should be no less than the state's accepted minimum. The nationally recognized minimum is about 1/8 inch, and tire pressure should be appropriate to manufacturer's guidelines. In addition, all tire lugs should be inspected for tightness and to ensure that none are missing.

All doors and compartments should open and close with ease. The latching mechanisms should be intact and in working order. External mirrors should be intact and moved to the proper position for vehicle operation. All external lights should function properly and have no damage to the external housing. This inspection must include the activation of all lighting devices (Figure 27-2).

When inspecting the engine, make sure the motor is off. You should wear gloves to protect your hands

from any damage or contamination. Start with a visual inspection of the entire engine compartment, looking for any obviously loose or damaged components. All hoses should be intact and not have any visible cracks or abrasions.

Inspect the radiator for leaks or damage and verify that the fluid reservoir is at the appropriate level. If fluid must be added, contact the maintenance division or consult your local policies to determine the proper type and amount of fluid to add. All belts should be inspected for cracks or unusual wear. The appropriate personnel should immediately replace any damaged belt. Inspect the battery and cables to confirm that they are intact and that the cables are tightly connected to the battery. Pay particular attention to any visible corrosion as this may interfere with the proper connection of the cables to the battery.

Check all fluid levels as detailed by the operator's guide (Figure 27-3). Oil levels should be appropriate to the manufacturer's specifications and generally must be clear or tan in color. Black engine oil is an indication of the need for an oil change or may be indicative of a potential failure. Transmission fluid levels are generally checked after the vehicle has been "warmed up." The vehicle operator's guide should be consulted for the proper method of inspection. Windshield washer fluid should be checked as a standard part of all vehicle inspections. This fluid may be of critical importance during winter driving conditions.

Patient Area Begin inspection of the patient compartment by looking at the general cleanliness of the area. Next, confirm that all safety equipment and seat belts are in good repair and function properly. All patient care equipment must be checked to ensure that there are appropriate stock levels and that each

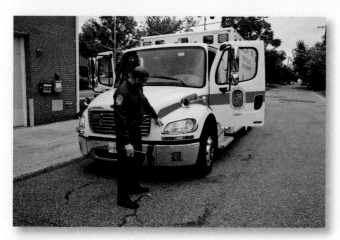

FIGURE 27-2 ▲ Vehicle inspection must include the activation of all lighting devices.

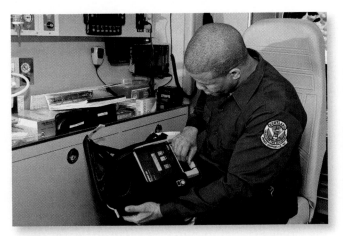

FIGURE 27-4 ▲ Check all patient care equipment to ensure that there are appropriate stock levels and that each item functions as required.

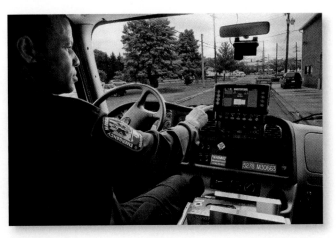

FIGURE 27-5 ▲ In the operator's area, inspect all warning and fluid gauges on the instrument panel to confirm that they are functioning and indicating safe operational levels.

item functions as required (Figure 27-4). This includes cardiac monitors, suction devices, sharps containers, and your response bag or box. The inspection of any battery-powered device must include verification of proper battery levels and the availability of additional batteries for extended responses. The equipment must then be properly stowed and secured in preparation for a response.

Continued inspection of the patient area should confirm the proper functioning of the heating, cooling, and exhaust systems. All oxygen storage devices should be checked to confirm that they contain appropriate levels of oxygen and that the regulators function properly.

In general, most transport vehicles have communications equipment available in the patient area. This equipment must also be checked to confirm that it functions as required.

Operator Area The operator's area requires not only inspection but also the adjustment of some equipment to your specifications. The first piece of equipment to be checked is the operator's seat. It should be placed at a safe and comfortable distance from the steering wheel and operator's floor pedals. Most new apparatus will allow the operator to change the angle and distance of the steering wheel in relation to the operator's console. Many of the inspections required in the operator's area require the vehicle to be started and kept running. This check of equipment while the vehicle is running must be performed outside of any structure or in an area where appropriate exhaust-handling systems are in place. Failure to follow this guideline can lead to the potential exposure to carbon monoxide.

Inspect all warning and fluid gauges on the instrument panel to confirm that all are functioning and indicating safe operational levels (Figure 27-5). Activate and then verify that the turn signals function properly. Note any deficiencies for immediate follow-up and repair before using the vehicle on a call. Although it is important to verify the proper functioning of the horn and siren, in many instances this is prohibited by the placement of the station and the apparatus. Remember to warn all personnel in the area before activating the horn or sirens. Inappropriate use of the horn or siren during vehicle inspection has the potential to cause hearing damage in any nearby personnel who are not wearing the proper protective devices. Always wear hearing protection before and during this testing.

Adjust all mirrors as needed. Adjust safety belts and restraint devices as needed. Confirm that all interior lights function appropriately. Parking brakes should be checked for proper operation. Communications equipment will also need to be checked. Follow local protocol for the safe and proper method to verify the operation of this equipment.

Remember This!

Safe operation of an emergency vehicle affects the safety of the crew, the patient, and the general public. You should not leave the station with a vehicle that is not safe for the road.

Dispatch Phase
Objectives 2, 7

In the dispatch phase of an EMS response, the patient or a witness reports the emergency by calling 9-1-1 or another emergency number. The call to 9-1-1 goes to a

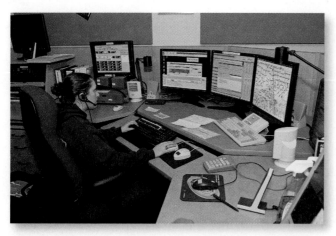

FIGURE 27-6 ▲ An Emergency Medical Dispatcher receives an emergency call, gathers information from the caller, and activates an appropriate EMS response based on the information received.

central communications system that is available 24 hours a day. This system links police, fire, and EMS resources. An Emergency Medical Dispatcher (EMD) receives the call and gathers information from the caller (Figure 27-6). The dispatcher then activates (dispatches) an appropriate EMS response based on the information received. The EMD will attempt to gather important information from the caller, including:

- The nature of the call
- The name, location, and callback number of the caller
- The location of the patient
- The number of patients and the severity of their illness or injury
- Other special problems that can be identified by the caller

The EMD is also responsible for coordinating logistics. An EMD is knowledgeable about the geography of the area, the EMS's capabilities, and the activities of other public service agencies. In most EMS systems, the EMD is trained to relay instructions to the caller for life-saving procedures that can be performed, if necessary, while waiting for trained medical personnel to arrive. A good EMD can make a big difference on a call. He can shave minutes off your response time by getting precise information about the location of your patient. He can keep you safe by asking about hazards on the scene. He can send you appropriate resources in a timely manner.

En Route, or Response, Phase

As you respond to the reported emergency, begin to anticipate the knowledge, equipment, and skills you may need to provide appropriate patient care. Notify the dispatcher that you are responding to the call. Write down the essential information from the dispatcher, including the nature and location of the call.

Determine the responsibilities of the crewmembers before arriving on the scene. For example, while you and your partner are en route to the scene decide who will assess the patient and who will document the call. In most agencies, these responsibilities are determined at the start of a shift instead of on the way to a call.

Most states and many companies encourage or even require all emergency vehicle operators to attend and successfully complete an approved driver-training course. The characteristics of good emergency vehicle operators include the following:

- Being physically and mentally fit
- Being able to perform under stress
- Having a positive attitude about their skills
- Being tolerant of other drivers.

Safe driving is important in the emergency medical care of the ill or injured patient. Your safe arrival (and that of your crew) at the scene will be one of the most important things that happens during your response. Your late arrival at the scene because of an accident while en route will delay the life-saving care that your patient needs. Bluntly stated, you may be the best EMT in the world, but you cannot render care if you don't get there!

As you begin your response to the reported emergency, use preplanned routes and street maps. Select the best route on the basis of weather, traffic patterns, and road conditions. You may need to consider many different factors. For instance, you may need to use a different route depending on the time of day, day of the week, detours, road closings, bridges, railroad crossings, tunnels, schools, heavy traffic areas, weather, or local construction. Plan an alternate route if unforeseen conditions are encountered. Consider the need for additional resources if the call is a large incident with multiple patients. Other factors to consider may include checking the wind direction as you approach the scene to confirm that you are upwind from a possible hazardous materials exposure.

Safety guidelines, such as the use of seat belts, should be exercised during each response. The list of actions shown in the following *Remember This!* box may be used as a guide for your safe response to an incident or emergency.

Remember This!

Response Action List

- Verify the location and type of call.
- Select the most appropriate route.
- Observe weather and road conditions and modify response if needed.
- Apply safety restraint devices.
- Notify the dispatch agency of your response.
- Modify your emergency response on the basis of your knowledge of the characteristics of your response vehicle. Factors such as length, width, and weight will alter the way your vehicle handles.
- Understand appropriate use of lights and siren.
- Obtain additional information from dispatch.
- Drive with due regard for the safety of others.
- Maintain a safe following distance.
- Approach the scene from uphill and upwind as needed.

Emergency Response

Objective 3

The general definition of an **emergency response** is the operation of an emergency vehicle while responding to a medical emergency. Laws pertaining to the proper methods of responding to an emergency vary from state to state. These laws also govern the use of emergency signaling devices, such as lights and sirens. In general, most states require emergency vehicle operators to obey all traffic regulations unless a specific exemption has been made and documented in statute. Most states allow for these exemptions unless their use endangers life or property. In addition, these exemptions are typically granted only when a true emergency exists. The definition of a "true emergency" can be rather vague. A possible definition of a **true emergency** is a situation in which there is a high possibility of death or serious injury and the rapid response of an emergency vehicle may lessen the risk of death or injury.

Objective 6

When driving in emergency mode, the operator of an emergency vehicle must drive with due regard for the safety of others on the roadway. Due regard means that, in similar circumstances, a reasonable and responsible person would act in a way that is safe and considerate of others. The reasonableness of your emergency response will be judged on the basis of some of the following guidelines:

- Emergency vehicles should never operate at a speed greater than is warranted by the nature of the call or the condition of the patient that you are transporting. This speed must also not be greater than traffic, road, and weather conditions allow.
- All emergency vehicle warning systems should be used as intended by the manufacturer and must be in operation during an emergency response.
- All emergency vehicle warning systems must be functioning in the prescribed manner before entering any intersection.

The following guidelines are intended to give an overview of motor vehicle laws and are not intended to supersede any local authority. Contact your local or state regulatory agency for the specifics of an emergency response in your area.

Speed and Speed Limits

The posted speed limit on any road or highway is determined by many factors, such as the type of road surface and the normal driving conditions. Most states allow for the increase of your emergency response speed to a maximum of 10 miles an hour over the posted speed limit. This increase is also based on weather and road conditions. Most emergency response training courses discourage any increase in your response speed over the posted limit. In general, an increase in speed also increases the risk to the responding crews and the general public on the roadways.

Warning Lights and Sirens

Emergency signaling devices such as warning lights and sirens are intended to alert other drivers that an emergency response vehicle is approaching and to request that they yield the right of way to that response vehicle. Transportation engineers and emergency response experts calculate that the use of emergency lights and sirens will decrease your overall response time only by seconds. This overall reduction in your response time comes with the added risk of accident and injury.

There are several factors that must be taken into consideration during your emergency response. Do the drivers around your vehicle know that there is an emergency vehicle approaching them? Do they have enough time to make a choice about what to do? Do they have time and space to respond or carry out their choice in an appropriate manner? It is impossible to determine if the drivers around you will notice your approach and react appropriately. You must be prepared for them to make the worst possible decision about how to respond to your approach.

Right of Way

Your use of lights and sirens does not automatically grant you the right-of-way. Your use of lights and siren is a *request*, not a *demand*, for the right-of-way. The standard rules of the road apply, even if you are in the emergency response mode. Other drivers may not see or hear your vehicle's warning devices because of conversation in their vehicles or the use of air-conditioning or stereo equipment, among other reasons. Before taking the right-of-way, make sure other drivers see your emergency vehicle.

You Should Know

- Headlights are the most visible warning devices on an emergency vehicle because they are mounted at the eye level of other drivers. Use caution during any response that uses lights and siren because of the "excitement factor."
- Most drivers will yield the right-of-way if they notice your approach with lights and siren. However, in many instances they won't know that you are there and may over-correct their vehicle when they see you. This may potentially put your vehicle in jeopardy. You must be extremely alert when driving in emergency response mode. You must be prepared for these situations.

General Considerations

In general, most jurisdictions allow emergency response vehicle drivers to alter standard rules in many of the following situations:

- *Parking or standing.* You may be allowed to park or have the vehicle remain stationary even in posted "No Parking" areas.
- *Red lights, stop signs, intersections.* You must stop at all red lights, stop signs, and

intersections even if you are responding to an emergency. However, once you have assured that the intersection is clear and no traffic is preparing to enter the intersection, you may proceed through the red light at a slow rate of speed.

- *Speed limit.* Maintain your speed at the speed limit or below as weather conditions permit. In general, the vehicle may travel up to 10 miles per hour over the posted speed limit if conditions and traffic allow.
- *Directions of flow and specified turns.* You may use all lanes of travel and even turn against no turn signs to reach the emergency scene. However, you are responsible for any collision and injury, regardless of your response mode.
- *Emergency or disaster routes.* You may be allowed to use any emergency route or access, but do so with extreme caution.
- *School buses.* Do not proceed past a school bus that has stopped to load or unload unless it has specifically yielded to your lights and siren. Approach the school bus that is stopped to pick up passengers with extreme caution. You should make eye contact with the driver to verify that it is safe to proceed before passing this vehicle.

Contributing Factors to Unsafe Driving Conditions

Objective 4

Some of the factors that contribute to unsafe driving conditions include heavy traffic, traffic jams, wind, rain, snow and ice, dust, fog, debris, animals, running or standing water, night driving, and fatigue.

Wind has the potential to influence the handling characteristics of your emergency response vehicle. Most emergency response vehicles have a higher center of gravity than other vehicles. A strong crosswind can cause your vehicle to sway or even overturn. As you encounter other vehicles or changes in terrain, the winds may be blocked or even funneled into stronger gusts. Be prepared for these changes and reduce your speed appropriately. Use extreme caution in high winds, especially around curves or corners and when the roadway is wet or icy.

Rain can reduce tire traction and block your vision during an emergency response. Always verify that the emergency vehicle's windshield wipers are functioning and that there are no cracks or dry spots in the blades. Tire tread depth and design can be a factor when water is on the roadway. Hydroplaning is possible any time there is rain or standing water on the roadway. Reduce speed and be prepared for hydroplaning or tire pull caused by rain.

Snow and ice can be extremely hazardous and tend to reduce tire traction even in small amounts. Be aware of local weather conditions. Be prepared for ice to form, particularly on bridges or shaded portions of the roadway. Tire tread design and depth is a factor that must be considered before your response. Add traction devices or change to traction-type tires when you have advance knowledge of the possibility for adverse weather. The best advice is to *slow down*. Snow and ice can be especially hazardous during braking, turning, and acceleration. Each of these maneuvers may cause sliding. In addition, blowing snow can rapidly reduce visibility. You must reduce speed to avoid collisions during this type of weather. Snow and ice may also build up rapidly on the windshield. You will need good wiper blades and the proper windshield washer fluid to remove it.

Dust and dust storms are a significant hazard in some areas and can reduce driving visibility to zero in just seconds. You must be aware of the potential for these storms. Never knowingly enter a dust storm. If you are already on the roadway when one occurs, reduce your speed and safely exit the roadway as far as you reasonably can. Next, turn off your headlights, emergency lights, and remove your foot from the brake pedal. Traffic on the roadway may mistakenly believe that your taillights are from a moving vehicle on the roadway and may strike you.

Some areas of the country experience fog at almost any time of year. Visibility may be reduced significantly, and your driving will be impaired. Always reduce your speed to match road conditions. Turn on any fog lights with which your vehicle is equipped. Generally, the low-beam setting on your headlights will be more beneficial than the high beams. The increased amount of light produced by the high beams tends to be reflected back by the fog, further reducing visibility. If your vehicle has an Opticom or a strobe that activates traffic signal lights, consider turning it off. Driving for any extended period with this system functioning has the potential to "mesmerize" you or to capture your attention to the reflection and away from the road.

Response to some rural areas can bring you into conflict with everything from livestock to large wild animals. Hitting an elk, moose, or cow even at low speeds can be deadly. Slow down anytime there is the possibility of this type of collision.

Be alert to the possibility of debris in the roadway and reduce your speed to limit the need for extreme maneuvers to dodge this material. Any extreme maneuver such as braking or steering around an object has the potential to cause harm to the personnel and patient in the transport vehicle. It may also contribute to the loss of control of the vehicle.

Standing water has the potential to either cause hydroplaning or even stall out a vehicle, depending on the depth of the water, and should be approached cautiously and at a safe speed. Running water *must not* be entered in any circumstance. Moving water can sweep your vehicle downstream, placing all aboard in jeopardy. In addition, most states that have the possibility of flash flooding have laws that prohibit anyone from entering running water.

Nighttime can cause unsafe driving conditions because of decreased visibility. In addition, the number of sleep-deprived or otherwise impaired drivers increases dramatically at night. Use your headlights to your best advantage. Use your high beams if oncoming traffic will allow. Avoid the tendency to "overdrive" your headlights. Keep your eyes moving between an outside focus and an inside focal point. This will help to reduce eyestrain. As you approach an oncoming vehicle, scan the right shoulder instead of the centerline. This will help to keep your night vision intact.

Fatigue is another factor that must be considered. Fatigue will impair your judgment, vision, and driving skills. It may even impair your patient care skills. When the opportunity for rest arises, take a nap. Know your limits. Do not drive impaired.

Escorts and Multiple-Vehicle Responses
Objective 5

Escorts and multiple-vehicle responses are extremely dangerous. They should be used only when emergency responders are unfamiliar with the location of the patient or receiving facility or when multiple units from the same location are being called to a multiple-casualty incident. Provide a safe following distance (generally a minimum of 500 feet). Stop, and then use the standard right-of-way guidelines to proceed through any intersection. Check your agency's policy regarding the use of siren and/or lights in these situations. Some agencies do not want them used because they may confuse other drivers. Other agencies specify that a different siren time and/or tone must be used to help other motorists distinguish multiple emergency vehicles.

Multiple-vehicle responses pose an even greater-than-normal hazard at intersections. For example, a motorist may see the first emergency vehicle pass and begin to proceed, assuming it was the only emergency vehicle. An accident may occur with the motorist and the second emergency vehicle. Each vehicle must "clear" the intersection by using the guidelines in the following section.

Intersection Crashes

Intersection crashes are the most common collision involving emergency vehicles. Intersection crashes can occur in the following ways:

- The motorist arrives at an intersection as the light changes and does not stop.
- Multiple emergency vehicles are following closely, and a waiting motorist does not expect more than one vehicle.
- Vision is obstructed by vehicles waiting at an intersection, blocking the view of a pedestrian.

All intersections should be approached and cleared by using the following guidelines:

- Your siren should be in "wail" mode at least 300 feet before the intersection. Change your siren to the "yelp" mode 150 feet before the intersection (Figure 27-7).
- Begin deceleration and make sure that your vehicle can be at a complete stop at the cross-walk line. Give two short blasts on the vehicle's air horn. Look to your left first, then straight ahead, then to the right, and then again to your left before entering the intersection.
- Verify that all left lanes are stopped and will remain stopped as you proceed into the intersection. The best method to verify that the driver of a stopped vehicle is aware of your presence in the intersection is to make eye contact with each driver.
- Proceed carefully through the intersection at no more than 10 miles per hour. Use extreme caution when crossing the path of a vacant lane to your left or right. Drivers in these lanes may be unaware of your presence in the intersection.
- Right turns at an intersection where all traffic has stopped can be very hazardous. Verify that all drivers are stopped and are aware of your need to make a right turn in front of them. Proceed with extreme caution.

You must also be aware of the potential for other emergency vehicles responding through the same intersection at the same time as your vehicle. Confirm that they have completely stopped before proceeding with your response.

You Should Know

Contributing Factors to Unsafe Driving Conditions

- Escorts
- Road surface
- Excessive speed
- Reckless driving
- Weather conditions
- Multiple-vehicle response
- Inadequate dispatch information and unfamiliarity with the location
- Failing to heed traffic warning signals
- Disregarding traffic rules and regulations
- Failing to anticipate the actions of other motorists
- Failing to obey traffic signals or posted speed limits

Arrival Phase/Scene Size-Up

Although your approach to an emergency at a residence may not be influenced by topography and weather, your response to a motor vehicle crash (MVC) may require your consideration of these factors. If you receive additional information while en route, consider the need for additional resources, and make the appropriate assignments based on this information.

To ensure the safety of all personnel responding to a scene, you will need to be cautious and look for dangers while approaching the scene. You should also be aware of the presence of or the need for other emergency vehicles. Positioning of your emergency vehicle requires careful consideration of the following potential dangers:

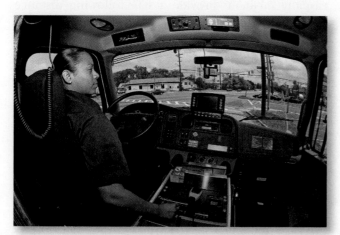

FIGURE 27-7 ▲ When approaching an intersection, your siren should be in "wail" mode at least 300 feet before the intersection. Change your siren to the "yelp" mode 150 feet before the intersection.

- *Hazardous materials.* Indications of hazardous materials dangers may include spills, fumes, and noxious gases. Be alert for the presence of hazardous materials when responding to tractor-trailer accidents, train derailments, industrial incidents, and certain farm incidents.

- *Fires.* Approach the scene of a fire with caution. Avoid driving into a wet area, as the liquid may be flammable. Never drive over hoses unless specifically ordered by fire suppression personnel. Be cautious of smoke clouds as they may be toxic. Coordinate your response and the positioning of your vehicle with the firefighters on scene.

- *Downed power lines.* Power lines that are down or hanging are extremely dangerous. Only trained personnel should try to remove them. Do not touch or try to move any downed power line. Remember that any water or other object that is in contact with a power line may be energized. Set up a **safe zone** (an area safe from exposure or the threat of exposure), also called the *cold zone* or *support zone,* and restrict entry to properly trained personnel only. Stay in the safe zone until cleared by trained personnel.

- *Heavy traffic flow.* Transport vehicles should be parked away from the flow of traffic to ensure the protection of the crew, the patient, and the vehicle itself. Unfortunately, many motorists are very interested in observing the scene of an emergency and may not pay close attention to their driving. This can and will place all emergency responders at risk of an additional accident. In addition, if your vehicle is struck or damaged, your ability to transport the patient may be compromised.

- *Large crowds.* Use extreme caution when approaching a scene where a crowd has gathered. Crowds can become hostile to EMS personnel or may "rush" your vehicle, placing themselves in danger.

- *Violent or terrorist acts.* The potential exists for an emergency call to be a violent situation or even a terrorist event. Allow law enforcement personnel to deal with violent or hostile persons. Position your vehicle out of range of gunfire or other violence. Do not approach the scene without clearance from law enforcement personnel.

Vehicle Placement

The tendency to park your vehicle in the first available clear area and rush to assist with patient care may place you and your apparatus at risk. This can lead to more problems and delays because access to your vehicle and equipment may become dangerous or even impossible.

There are four things to consider when placing an emergency vehicle at the emergency scene. They include scene safety, traffic volume and flow, egress from the scene, and distance from the patient(s) or scene.

Scene Safety

Personal safety, as well as the safety of the crew when accessing the vehicle and the equipment carried in the vehicle, is an important consideration for vehicle placement. If the sides of the vehicle are along the flow of traffic, it will be dangerous for crewmembers to get to the equipment needed for patient care. Park where access to all compartments is out of dangerous traffic flow. Be conscious of obstacles such as guardrails, trees, additional emergency vehicles, and other hazards, which may restrict access to parts of the vehicle if you park too close to them.

Remember This!

When parking, consider access to the patient and the effects of traffic flow, the roadway, known hazards, the public, and other agencies.

In general, the transport vehicle should not be used for scene protection. The primary function of this vehicle is for patient transport. Most jurisdictions have standard operating procedures for these types of situations and use other emergency vehicles, such as fire apparatus, to protect the scene. Fire apparatus is typically parked downward from the scene and in such a way that a traveling vehicle would be more likely to strike the apparatus and not crew members (see Chapter 28). Call for additional resources if necessary. If there are no additional resources available, then you may have to consider the use of your vehicle as a shield for the scene.

Always attempt to park the transport vehicle far enough away from the scene to protect the crew and the patient. In the case of a vehicle wreck, park at least 100 feet beyond the wreckage. This will generally protect the transport vehicle from broken glass and debris from the wreckage and allow access for fire suppression equipment. In addition, you must be aware of any fuel leaking from wrecked vehicles and park uphill or upwind. Park at least 2,000 feet from a hazardous substance. In situations involving a trench rescue, emergency vehicles are parked 300 feet from the excavation site to minimize vibration. Working apparatus at these scenes are positioned at least 100 feet from the excavation site.

Avoid placing the transport vehicle where it will block the access of other emergency personnel and vehicles. Use extreme care if you must park on a hill or any other unstable or uneven surface. Be sure to set the vehicle's parking brake. In addition, position the front wheels so that if the vehicle starts to roll, the wheels will hit the curb.

Traffic Volume and Flow

The transport vehicle should be positioned so that it does not block traffic. In general, placing the transport vehicle in the path of traffic will limit access to the compartments and needed equipment.

Egress from the Scene

Position the emergency vehicle in preparation for an easy and rapid departure. In general, you should always position the transport vehicle pointed in the direction of the appropriate medical facility. Attempt to avoid having to back into traffic or steer around obstacles once the patient has been loaded.

In most situations, you should not use the driveway of a private residence if you are responding to an emergency in a residential area. It may be better to park in the street, especially if the house is near the street or if the driveway is steep or narrow. Parking on the street will prevent your having to back into or out of a driveway. This can be difficult and dangerous on residential streets because of the presence of children, pets, and obstacles like bushes and parked cars.

Distance from the Patient or Scene

Your need for equipment to care for your patient and the necessity for ease of departure may require you to position your vehicle closer than you believe is safe. Use common sense and extreme caution in these instances.

On-Scene Care

When you arrive on the scene, notify the EMD of your arrival. Before initiating patient care, put on appropriate PPE. Make certain that your actions at the scene are efficient and organized, keeping in mind the goals of safe and efficient patient care and transport. Determine the mechanism of injury or nature of the patient's illness. Ask for additional resources before making patient contact and initiate the Incident Command System if needed (see Chapter 29). When it is safe to do so, gain access to the patient. Perform a primary survey and provide essential emergency care.

Transferring the Patient to the Ambulance

If patient transport is needed, prepare the patient. Make sure that dressings and splints, if used, are secure. When you are ready, ask for assistance with lifting and moving the patient to the ambulance, using

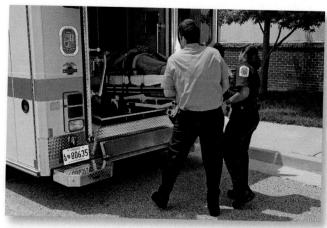

FIGURE 27-8 ▲ Secure the patient to the stretcher and lock the stretcher in place.

the techniques discussed in Chapter 6. The lifting and moving method and the device used will depend on the patient's illness or injury. They will also be determined by the safety of the scene, such as an emergency move at an unsafe scene versus moving a stable medical patient. Secure the patient to the stretcher and lock the stretcher in place (Figure 27-8). Before leaving the scene, the driver should ensure that all outside compartment doors are closed and secure.

Transport Phase

Objective 2

During transport, remember that your safety must be your priority. Wearing a seatbelt is one way to ensure your safety. Although some people may consider it cumbersome to wear a seatbelt during transport, your risk of injury increases if you are not restrained. Notify the dispatcher when you are leaving the scene. Let the dispatcher know your destination. For example:

Medic 51: "Medic 51 (five, one) to Dispatch."

Dispatch Center: "Dispatch. Medic 51 (five, one), go ahead."

Medic 51: "Dispatch, Medic 51 (five, one) is transporting one patient to Anytown Medical Center, emergent."

Dispatch Center: "Received, Medic 51 (five, one). Transporting one patient to Anytown Medical Center, emergent. Time: 1532 (fifteen, three, two)."

Medic 51: "Dispatch, Medic 51 (five, one), received, clear."

Follow your local protocol regarding the communication of additional patient information.

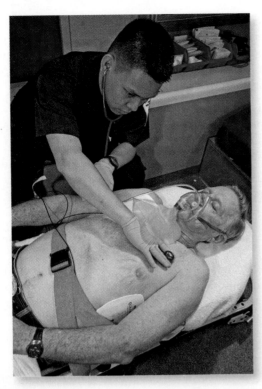

FIGURE 27-9 ▲ Care begun on the scene should be continued throughout patient transport.

Care begun on the scene should be continued throughout patient transport (Figure 27-9). The frequency of performing ongoing patient assessments during transport will be based on the patient's condition. The patient's condition may improve, remain the same, or worsen during transport. A good rule to follow is that if the patient is unstable, he should be reassessed at least every 5 minutes. If the patient is stable, he should be reassessed at least every 15 minutes. Reassure the patient throughout the transport.

Complete your prehospital care report (PCR). Contact the receiving facility, if possible, and use a standardized medical reporting format (Figure 27-10). In most EMS systems, the information that is relayed to the receiving facility includes:

- Your unit's name and level of service (Basic Life Support or Advanced Life Support)
- The estimated time of arrival
- The patient's age and gender
- The patient's chief complaint
- A brief, pertinent history of the present illness
- Major past illnesses
- The patient's mental status and baseline vital signs
- Pertinent physical exam findings
- The emergency medical care given (and by whom)
- The patient's response to emergency medical care

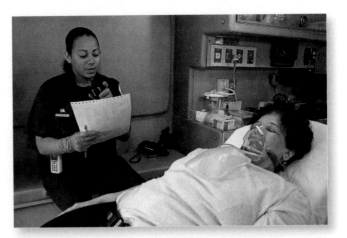

FIGURE 27-10 ▲ When possible, contact the receiving facility while you are en route. Use a standardized medical reporting format to provide patient information.

The following is a sample radio report simulating communication with a receiving facility:

Medic 51: "Anytown Medical Center, Medic 51 (five, one)" Anytown Medical Center: "Anytown Medical Center. Go ahead, Medic 51 (five, one)."

Medic 51: "Anytown Medical Center, EMT Bruck on Medic 51 (five, one). We are en route to your facility. Expected arrival time: 4 minutes. The patient is a 67-year-old man found unresponsive by his wife on the bedroom floor. On arrival, the patient was unresponsive, not breathing, and had no pulse. The patient's wife states he was last seen about 5 minutes before her call to 9-1-1. CPR was performed and the AED applied. One shock delivered while on scene. After resuming CPR, rhythm analysis by the AED indicated no shock advised. Strong carotid pulse present. Patient now responds to verbal stimuli. Vital signs follow: respirations 14; pulse 98, strong and regular; blood pressure 104/62. Exam reveals clear breath sounds bilaterally. There is a healed surgical scar in the center of the patient's chest. The patient's wife says the patient had a 3-vessel coronary bypass 7 months ago. She has provided a typed list of medications. The patient is on oxygen by nonrebreather mask at 15 liters per minute. Any questions or orders?"

Anytown Medical Center: "Medic 51 (five, one), Anytown Medical Center report received (your report may be repeated to ensure accuracy). No orders or questions. Contact us if there is any change in patient condition before arrival. Anytown Medical Center clear."

Medic 51: "Medic 51 (five, one) clear."

Making a Difference

Place yourself in this situation. You have just been involved in an MVC. The local emergency responders have just finished cutting you out of your mangled vehicle. You are strapped onto a hard piece of plastic and placed on a stretcher. You cannot see where you are going, and you feel every bump and corner that the emergency transport vehicle hits or travels around. The EMT in the back of the ambulance is busy writing on a clipboard or talking on a radio and doesn't seem to have time for your questions.

Would you feel comforted during this trip? Is this the type of care that you would like to have rendered to you or a family member?

At some point in our careers, we make a statement that sounds something like this, "I got into this business to help people and make a difference." Now is your chance to prove that you meant what you said. On each call, you have an opportunity to make a difference in someone's life. Yes, you need to complete your report. Yes, you will need to talk to the receiving facility. These tasks pale in importance compared with the need to give comfort and care to your patient. In some instances, this may be as simple as listening to your patient's fears. You are charged with the responsibility to use your knowledge and skills to help people in their time of need. Treat the patient as needed, assess his vital signs, and do all of the things you were trained to do; just don't forget to listen.

Transfer to Definitive Care
Objective 2

Notify the dispatcher as soon as you arrive at the receiving facility.

> **Medic 51:** "Dispatch, Medic 51 (five, one). Arrival at Anytown Medical Center."
>
> **Dispatch Center:** "Received, Medic 51 (five, one). Arrival at Anytown Medical Center at 1535 (fifteen, three, five)."

Once at the hospital, you must give a verbal report to the hospital staff. As the healthcare professional that provided patient care, you become the only link the hospital staff has to the patient's history and what happened at the scene. Information about how you found the patient, how the scene looked, and the care given to him by family members or bystanders before you arrived will be available to the hospital staff only through your report.

You should give a verbal report to the appropriate hospital staff member at the patient's bedside. Introduce the patient by name (if known). Summarize the information already provided by radio or telephone to the receiving facility, including:

- The patient's chief complaint
- Pertinent patient history that was not previously given
- Emergency medical care given en route and the patient's response to the treatment given
- Vital signs taken en route

Provide any additional information collected en route but not transmitted by telephone or radio. Be sure to let hospital staff know if there was any delay in reaching the patient or if there were any unusual circumstances at the scene. Make sure the hospital staff member who listens to your report signs your PCR when you transfer patient care.

Objective 10

Leave a copy of your completed PCR with the hospital staff person. Your report will be included in the patient's hospital medical record. Remember that good documentation accurately and completely tells a story about what happened while the patient was in your care. This includes the patient's condition on arrival at the scene, your assessment findings, the emergency care performed, and the patient's response to the care given. Your documentation should contain facts that are supported by what you see, hear, feel, and smell. It should not contain jargon, slang, bias, opinions, or impressions. Subjective information that can be documented includes what the patient says that pertains to his current illness or complaint.

En Route to the Station
Objective 2

Notify the dispatcher when you are en route to your station and again when you arrive.

> **Medic 51:** "Dispatch, Medic 51 (five, one). En route to the station."
>
> **Dispatch Center:** "Received, Medic 51 (five, one). En route at 1551."
>
> **Medic 51:** "Dispatch, Medic 51 (five, one). Arrival at the station."
>
> **Dispatch Center:** "Received, Medic 51 (five, one). Arrival at your station at 1602 (sixteen, zero, two)."

Most transport vehicles carry enough supplies to run multiple calls. Your vehicle should be cleaned and readied for the next call. In most instances, most of the cleaning will take place at the receiving facility. Your transport vehicle should carry enough cleaning supplies to perform a simple decontamination. Most EMS systems have a limited number of vehicles available at any one given time. Your rapid preparation for the next call can be very beneficial to the entire EMS system. It will be your responsibility to clean and disinfect the ambulance and equipment as needed. You will need to restock any disposable equipment that you may have used and return equipment to its storage area. It is very important that you understand your company's policies and arrangements made with receiving hospitals regarding restocking of supplies.

After the Run

Objectives 2, 12, 13, 14

Refuel your vehicle as needed and remember to file all written reports. Notify the dispatcher as soon as you are available for the next call. Mentally and physically prepare yourself for the next call. Have lunch or dinner, stay hydrated, and try to relax for a few moments. Inspect the vehicle, checking tires, lights, and anything unusual noticed during the run. Replace empty oxygen cylinders. Replace discharged batteries or reconnect them to vehicle chargers. Replace supplies used during the run. Change soiled uniforms.

Complete cleaning and disinfecting the vehicle and/or equipment. **Decontamination** is the use of physical or chemical means to remove, inactivate, or destroy bloodborne pathogens on a surface or item to the point at which it is no longer capable of transmitting infectious particles and the surface or item is considered safe for handling, use, or disposal. Primary methods of decontamination include low-level disinfection, intermediate-level disinfection, high-level disinfection, and sterilization. **Low-level disinfection** destroys most bacteria, some viruses and fungi, but not tuberculosis bacteria or bacterial spores. It is used for routine cleaning of surfaces, such as floors, countertops, and ambulance seats, when no body fluids are visible. Use a household bleach and water solution or a hospital disinfectant registered with the Environmental Protection Agency (EPA).

Intermediate-level disinfection destroys tuberculosis bacteria, vegetative bacteria, and most viruses and fungi, but not bacterial spores. It is used for surfaces that contact intact skin and have been visibly contaminated with body fluids, such as blood pressure cuffs, stethoscopes, backboards, and splints. Use a household bleach and water solution or an EPA-registered hospital disinfectant that claims it is tuberculocidal.

High-level disinfection destroys all microorganisms except large numbers of bacterial spores. It is used for reusable equipment that has been in contact with mucous membranes, such as laryngoscope blades. Use either hot-water pasteurization by placing articles in water 176 to 212°F (80 to 100°C) for 30 minutes or immerse in an EPA-registered chemical sterilizing agent for 10 to 45 minutes according to manufacturer's instructions. Items requiring high-level disinfection should first be cleaned with soap and water to remove debris.

Sterilization destroys all microorganisms, including highly resistant bacterial spores. It is used for instruments that penetrate the skin or contact normally sterile areas of the body during invasive procedures. Methods used include autoclave (steam under pressure) and immersion in an EPA-registered chemical sterilizing agent for 6 to 10 hours. Sterilization is usually performed at the hospital. Items requiring sterilization should first be cleaned with soap and water to remove debris.

Remember This!

Medical equipment should never be disinfected in areas such as the kitchen, bathrooms, or living areas of the station or receiving facility.

Infection Control Procedures

Remove any contaminated clothing. If blood or other potentially infectious material contaminates your clothing, remove it as soon as possible. Bag the clothing for decontamination and place it in an appropriately designated area or container. Thoroughly wash your hands, contaminated skin areas, and areas of skin that were not covered by clothing or PPE. Remember that your hands should be washed after every patient encounter. Also, remember to wash your hands after cleaning and disinfecting procedures are completed. Wear protective gloves, such as cleaning gloves, when cleaning up potentially infectious materials. If splashing is likely, wear face and eye protection.

Contaminated sharps must be discarded immediately in an acceptable sharps container. If leakage is possible, or if the outside of the container has become contaminated, the sharps container must be placed in a secondary container that is closable, labeled or color-coded, and leak resistant. If the sharps container is 1/2 to 3/4 full, close and lock the lid. Follow agency procedures for disposal of the container.

Decontaminate the vehicle and large equipment. Clean up blood and body fluid spills with disposable towels. Dispose of the towels in a biohazard-labeled bag. Decontaminate surfaces with soap and water. Wipe or spray with a disinfectant solution as needed and allow disinfected areas to air dry. Place disposable PPE worn during decontamination procedures in a properly labeled, sealed waste container. Restock the vehicle. Make note of any items needing repair or replacement.

Protective gloves and other appropriate PPE must be worn when handling contaminated laundry. Laundry contaminated with blood or other potentially infectious materials should be handled as little as possible. It must be placed in appropriately marked bags at the location where it was used. Contaminated laundry should be washed according to the uniform or linen manufacturer's recommendations. Contaminated items should always be laundered separately from other laundry to prevent cross-contamination.

Notify dispatch when your tasks are complete and you are ready for another call.

> **Medic 51:** "Dispatch, Medic 51 (five, one). In service and available for traffic."

> **Dispatch Center:** "Received, Medic 51 (five, one). Available for traffic at 1615 (sixteen, one, five)."

Air Medical Transport Considerations

When air medical transport is necessary, the scene is often complex. In most cases, air transportation is used because the condition of one or more patients is critical (Figures 27-11 and 27-12). In these types of scenes, emotions run high, and safety considerations can be overlooked. Remember that the goal in any EMS operation is to ensure the safety of every person at the scene.

It is important to identify the need for air transport as early as possible. The mechanisms of injury that may require helicopter transport include:

- A vehicle rollover with unrestrained passengers
- An incident in which a vehicle strikes a pedestrian at a speed greater than 10 miles per hour
- Falls from a height greater than 15 feet
- An incident in which a motorcyclist is thrown from the motorcycle at a speed of more than 20 miles per hour
- Multiple victims

Time and distance must also be considered before transporting by helicopter. Helicopter transport should be considered in the following circumstances:

- The transport time to a trauma center is more than 15 minutes by ground ambulance.
- The transport time to a local hospital by ground ambulance is more than the transport time to a trauma center by helicopter.
- The patient is entrapped and extrication will take longer than 15 minutes.
- Using local ground ambulance leaves the local community without ground ambulance coverage.
- The patient needs rapid transport to a specialty center (for example, a burn center or pediatric center).

You will need to notify the appropriate agency for help in securing a landing zone (LZ). In most cases,

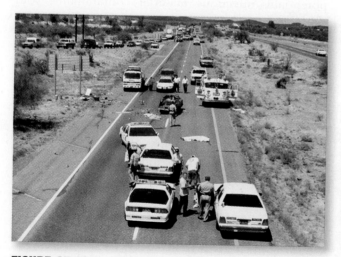

FIGURE 27-11 ▲ When the condition of one or more patients is critical, air medical transportation is often used. © *The McGraw-Hill Companies, Inc./Carin Marter, photographer.*

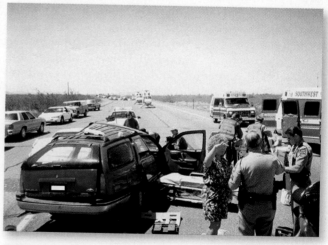

FIGURE 27-12 ▲ Multiple helicopters may be necessary at a multipatient scene. © *Courtesy of AirEvac Services.*

the local fire department will be the agency contacted. However, in some cases, police departments assume this role. When more than one agency is on the scene, each agency should have the ability to communicate on a common radio channel. All healthcare professionals that provide care need to be aware of the location of the LZ and the helicopter's estimated time of arrival (ETA).

If your unit is designated to land the helicopter, you will need to locate a secure LZ. This means that you must locate an area that is easily controlled for traffic and pedestrians. Check with your local helicopter service for LZ requirements. A good rule to follow is to allow *at least* 100 feet by 100 feet for any helicopter. The area should be free of overhead obstacles such as wires, trees, and light poles. The area should be free of debris and relatively level. The ground should be clear of rocks and grooves and must be firm enough to support the aircraft. Mark the corners of the landing area with light sticks or cones. Alternately, you can use emergency vehicles with headlights directed toward the landing area (but not at the approaching aircraft). If the landing area is dirt, lightly moisten the area with water if possible. Under no circumstances should anyone be allowed to enter the LZ after it has been secured.

Constant communication must be maintained throughout the helicopter operation. If you are the ground contact, you may be responsible for relaying important information to the responding flight crew about the patient's condition. All aspects of the LZ, including hazards such as light poles, trees, and power lines, must be relayed to the pilot. The pilot should also be told the approximate ground wind conditions.

As the helicopter approaches, it is important to maintain eye contact with the helicopter and pay attention to any visible hazards on the ground at the same time. At any moment it may be necessary to abort the landing. Your assessment of ground conditions could be the key factor in this decision. As the helicopter is landing (or taking off), lower the face shield on your helmet or turn your head momentarily to avoid getting debris in your eyes from the rotor wash.

Once the helicopter is on the ground, it is very important to pay attention to traffic. The arrival of a helicopter often draws a large crowd with many bystanders. Pay particular attention to bicycles and motorized vehicles because they can approach the scene quickly and without warning. As the patient is moved toward the helicopter, the flight crew will be focused on loading the patient. They may not see all of the hazards on the ground. Your constant attention to the scene is critical to the safety of the

flight crew and all persons on the scene. The rear of a helicopter can be especially dangerous. The tail rotor is often low and invisible when turning. Use extreme caution and follow the instructions of the crew when you are close to the aircraft. Important safety tips to keep in mind around helicopters are shown in the following *Stop and Think!* box.

Stop and Think!

Working Safely Around Helicopters

- Never move toward a helicopter until signaled by the flight crew.
- Always approach the helicopter from the front so that the pilot can see you.
- Wear ear and eye protection when approaching the helicopter.
- Never raise your arms or equipment above your head.
- Remove loose items, such as hats, that can be blown around or sucked into the rotors or engines.
- If the aircraft is parked on a slope, always approach and exit from the downhill side.
- When moving from one side of the helicopter to the other, always cross in front of the helicopter.
- Do not open or pull on any part of the aircraft.
- Do not allow vehicles or non-aircraft personnel within 60 feet of the aircraft.

After the patient is loaded into the helicopter, the pilot will radio you when he is ready for liftoff. A brief response from you that the scene is still clear will assure the pilot that you have been vigilant about surveying the scene for hazards. As the helicopter leaves the scene, advise your coworkers to keep the LZ intact for several minutes. This step is done in case the helicopter must return for an emergency landing.

Make sure your dispatcher is aware of all times associated with helicopter operations. For example, you should notify the EMD when the helicopter has arrived on the scene. You should also notify the dispatcher when the helicopter has left the scene, and you should report its destination. In your PCR, make sure to document the time patient care was transferred to the flight crew, the patient's condition at the time care was transferred, and the patient's destination.

Fortunately, your partner knows where the airway kit and the AED are located on your unit. She quickly grabs the needed equipment. The call runs smoothly. After performing CPR, and shocking when prompted by the AED, the patient begins moaning. You can feel a strong pulse. Using proper body mechanics, you and your partner move the patient from the ground to the stretcher and then into the back of the ambulance. En route to the hospital, you make promises to yourself that you will *always* know where the appropriate equipment is located on an emergency vehicle and that you will perform a complete check of the vehicle and equipment at the start of each shift. ∎

Sum It Up

▶ Preparations for an emergency call include having the appropriate personnel and equipment and an emergency response vehicle that is ready for use. Minimum staffing requirements for an ambulance include at least one EMT in the patient compartment. Two EMTs are preferred. In some states, two licensed personnel are required. Emergency transport vehicles are required to carry specific types and quantities of medical equipment to be "certified" as an ambulance. In addition to basic medical supplies, nonmedical supplies include personal safety equipment as required by local, state, and federal standards, and preplanned routes or comprehensive street maps. Daily inspections of the emergency response vehicle and its equipment are necessary to ensure it is in proper working order.

▶ In the dispatch phase of an EMS response, the patient or a witness reports the emergency by calling 9-1-1 or another emergency number. The EMD receives the call and gathers information from the caller. The dispatcher then activates (dispatches) an appropriate EMS response based on the information received.

▶ En route to the reported emergency, begin to anticipate the knowledge, equipment, and skills you may need to provide appropriate patient care. Notify the dispatcher that you are responding to the call. Determine the responsibilities of the crewmembers before arriving on the scene.

▶ Laws pertaining to the proper methods of responding to an emergency vary from state to state. In general, most states require emergency vehicle operators to obey all traffic regulations unless a specific exemption has been made and documented in statute. Most states allow for such an exemption, as long as it does not endanger life or property. In addition, these exemptions are typically only granted when a true emergency exists. A true emergency is a situation in which there is a high possibility of death or serious injury and the rapid response of an emergency vehicle may lessen the risk of death or injury

▶ When driving in emergency mode, the operator of an emergency vehicle must drive with due regard for the safety of others on the roadway. Due regard means that, in similar circumstances, a reasonable and responsible person would act in a way that is safe and considerate of others. Emergency vehicles should never operate at a speed greater than is warranted by the nature of the call or the condition of the patient that you are transporting. This speed must also not be greater than traffic, road, and weather conditions allow. All emergency vehicle warning systems should be used as intended by the manufacturer and must be in operation during an emergency response. All emergency vehicle warning systems must be functioning in the prescribed manner before entering any intersection.

▶ Escorts and multiple-vehicle responses are extremely dangerous. They should be used only if emergency responders are unfamiliar with the location of the patient or receiving facility. Provide a safe following distance (generally a minimum of 500 feet). Stop and then proceed through any intersection as directed by the standard right-of-way guidelines.

▶ While approaching the scene, be cautious, and look for dangers. Position the emergency vehicle with careful consideration of potential dangers such as fire, hazardous materials, downed power lines, crowds, heavy traffic flow, and potential violence. When you arrive on the scene, notify the EMD of your arrival. Before initiating patient care, put on appropriate PPE. Determine the mechanism of injury or nature of the patient's illness. Ask for additional resources before making patient contact and institute the Incident Command System if needed. When it is safe to do so, gain access to the patient. Perform a primary survey and provide essential emergency care.

▶ If patient transport is needed, prepare the patient. Ask for assistance with lifting and moving the patient to the ambulance. Secure the patient to the stretcher, and lock the stretcher in place. Ensure outside compartment doors are closed and secure.

- During transport, remember that your safety must be your priority. Wearing a seatbelt is one way to ensure your safety. Notify the dispatcher when you are leaving the scene. Perform ongoing patient assessments during transport. Complete your PCR and contact the receiving facility, if possible, using a standardized medical reporting format.

- Notify the dispatcher as soon as you arrive at the receiving facility. Give a verbal report to the hospital staff. Notify the dispatcher when you are en route to your station and again when you arrive. Clean and disinfect the vehicle and equipment as needed in preparation for the next call. Replace supplies used during the run. Notify the dispatcher when your tasks are complete and you are ready for another call.

- Air medical transport may be necessary when the condition of one or more patients is critical. If your unit is designated to land the helicopter, you will need to locate a secure landing zone. You must locate an area that is easily controlled for traffic and pedestrians. You should allow at least 100 feet by 100 feet to land any helicopter. The area should be free of overhead obstacles such as wires, trees, and light poles. It should also be free of debris and should be relatively level. The ground should be clear of rocks and grooves and must be firm enough to support the aircraft.

By the end of this chapter, you should be able to:

Knowledge Objectives ▷ **1.** Describe the purpose of extrication.

2. Discuss the role of the Emergency Medical Technician (EMT) in extrication.

3. Identify what equipment for personal safety is required for the EMT.

4. Define the fundamental components of extrication.

5. State the steps that should be taken to protect the patient during extrication.

6. Evaluate various methods of gaining access to the patient.

7. Distinguish between simple and complex access.

Attitude Objectives ▷ There are no attitude objectives identified for this lesson.

Skill Objectives ▷ There are no skills objectives identified for this lesson.

On the Scene

While driving back to the station, your unit is dispatched to a motor vehicle crash at the intersection of Central Ave and Main Street. While en route, the mobile data computer in the unit advises that this will be a 2-vehicle crash with injuries. Upon arrival, you find a 4-door sedan that has been struck in the passenger side by a full-size pickup truck. There is a patient in the front seat on the passenger side of the 4-door sedan who cannot get out of the vehicle. The vehicle's other occupants are standing outside. ■

THINK ABOUT IT

As you read this chapter, think about the following questions:

- How will you gain access to the interior of the vehicle to treat the patient?
- What types of protection are required for both the patient and yourself while performing extrication?
- How will you determine the route by which to remove the patient from the vehicle?
- What can you determine about the patient's condition from observing the interior and exterior of the vehicle?

Each year thousands of people are involved in motor vehicle collisions on U.S. roadways. Vehicle crashes can range in severity from a minor auto accident involving only damage to the bumpers of the vehicles to a motor vehicle crash (MVC) involving heavy entrapment of the patient.

Objective 1

Extrication is the process of removing machinery from around a patient to facilitate patient care and transport. Situations in which a patient cannot get out of the vehicle by himself or should not because of his injuries will require extrication. It is important to remember that this involves removing the machinery from around the patient, not removing the patient from the machinery. This chapter will prepare you for dealing with patients entrapped in vehicles after a vehicle collision has occurred.

Role of the Emergency Medical Technician on an Extrication Scene

Objective 2

As an Emergency Medical Technician (EMT) on an extrication scene, you may be called to perform a variety of tasks to assist in the extrication process. Your main duty will involve patient care by providing cervical spine stabilization, treating any injuries sustained by the patient(s), and assisting Paramedics on the scene with any special needs. Patient care precedes extrication unless delayed movement would endanger the life of the patient or rescuers. Patient care should include attention to life-threatening emergencies. All patients should be packaged and moved carefully to minimize the danger of further injury or aggravation of existing injuries.

In some areas, the EMTs are also the rescue providers. If this is the case, you must be trained in the use of extrication tools and proper extrication techniques. A chain of command should be established to assure patient care priorities. Give necessary care to the patient before extrication and ensure that the patient is removed in a way that minimizes further injury.

Equipment

Objective 3

Remember that your personal safety is your priority on every call. Protective clothing that is appropriate for the situation must be worn during extrication. This includes protective boots, pants, a coat, eye protection, a helmet, and gloves. Respiratory protection may also be needed if there is a possibility of inhaling particulates from the extrication process. Particulates can come from many sources, such as a deployed airbag or the windshield being cut by a reciprocating saw, just to name a few. Several standards regulate the use of personal protective equipment (PPE) and should be followed when selecting the type of clothing to wear. Hearing protection may also be necessary depending on the amount of noise on the scene. If there is any possibility of a fire, structural firefighting gear should be worn. Fire-resistant jumpsuits are also available and can be worn if your agency permits. A helmet, gloves, boots, and eye protection should be used in conjunction with the jumpsuit. Bloodborne pathogens are another concern and should be addressed with appropriate PPE that is rated against bloodborne pathogens. Structural firefighting gear is rated against bloodborne pathogens, but additional protection may be required, including medical gloves and respiratory protection for airborne pathogens. Always wear the PPE that will give you the most protection from the hazards present at the extrication scene (Figure 28-1).

Stages of Extrication

Objective 4

Preparation

Preparing for the possibility of extrication is the first step in providing good patient care. It begins by doing exactly what you're doing right now: learning. Many textbooks have been written on vehicle extrication that provide valuable information about extrication techniques and procedures for removing patients from motor vehicles. Additionally, several hands-on classes are available that allow for practicing learned techniques in a controlled setting before performing them on an extrication scene.

Once you are working in the field and adequately trained, preparation also includes inspecting any extrication equipment at the beginning of your shift to ensure it is in good condition; has the proper

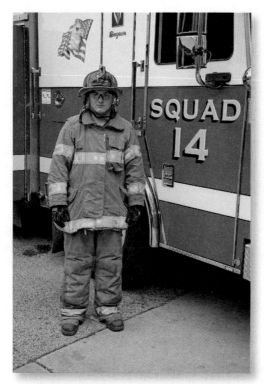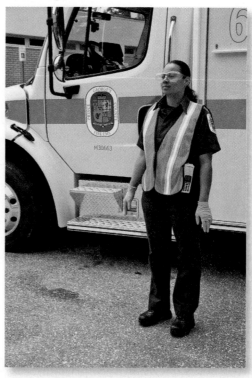

FIGURE 28-1 ▲ Protective clothing that is appropriate for the situation must be worn during extrication.

amount of fuel, if applicable; and is working properly. Post-call reviews from previous calls are also a great way of learning the extrication techniques that proved useful during the call and those that did not. Remember: Continuous training is the key for preparing to handle MVCs that require extrication.

Scene Size-Up

The scene size-up is an important step in the extrication process because it determines the direction the call is going to take. If done properly, the scene size-up will reveal any hazards present and provide information to determine the need for additional resources. It should also give a good indication of the number of persons injured, the types of injury, and which patient or patients require medical attention first.

Scene size-up begins as you respond to the crash scene. En route to the scene, the dispatcher should advise you of any pertinent information regarding conditions on the scene. Once on the scene, park in a **fend-off position.** The fend-off position involves parking your unit downward from the scene and in such a way that allows traveling vehicles to strike your unit and not crew members (Figure 28-2). This provides protection to crew members while they are working on the scene.

Before exiting your unit, make sure that it is safe to do so. Check for passing traffic and any hazards

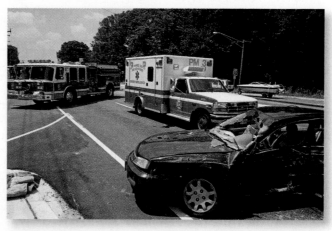

FIGURE 28-2 ▲ Once on the scene, park in a fend-off position. The fend-off position involves parking your unit downward from the scene and in such a way that allows traveling vehicles to strike your unit and not crew members.

that would prevent you from exiting the vehicle (see the following *Stop and Think!* box). Either your partner or you will need to establish command, with the most experienced person being the incident commander. A 360-degree rotation (looking at the scene from all angles) should be made around the entire scene to look for any hazards around and underneath the vehicles. If extrication is required, call for the additional resources that will be necessary.

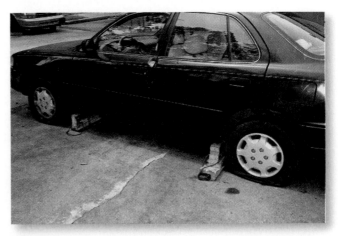

FIGURE 28-3 ▲ If a vehicle is in an upright position, stabilize it by taking four step chocks and placing two behind the front tires and two in front of the rear tires. Make sure that the frame will rest on the step that is closest to the height of the frame.

Vehicle Stabilization

When vehicles collide, they can wind up in a wide array of configurations that may place the vehicles in unstable positions. **Stabilization** is the process of rendering a vehicle motionless in the position in which it is found. The purpose of stabilization is to eliminate potential movement of a vehicle (or structure) that may cause further harm to entrapped patients or rescuers.

Equipment for stabilization may include a come-along (hand winch), cribbing and wedges, airbags, step chocks, hydraulic rams, jacks, and/or chains. Cribbing is usually used to provide a platform for the vehicle to rest on for stabilization. Cribbing is comprised of 4 × 4-inch wooden posts that can range from 18–36 inches long depending upon your needs. Step chocks are another form of cribbing. They provide a stair-like platform for the vehicle's frame to rest on. The bottom stair of the step chock is 24 inches long. As the stairs move up, the length of the stair shortens. This allows the step chock to be used for multiple vehicles of different heights.

If the vehicle is in an upright position, stabilization of the vehicle is straightforward. Begin by taking four step chocks and placing two behind the front tires and two in front of the rear tires. Make sure that the frame will rest on the step that is closest to the height of the frame. This will allow the vehicle to come down the least amount possible (Figure 28-3). If step chocks are not available, use 4 × 4-inch cribbing as a substitute. Next, use a pair of pliers and remove the valve stems from all 4 tires. As the vehicle begins to lower, the frame will rest on the step chocks isolating the frame from the vehicle's springs and tires. Stabilizing the vehicle is the first step in providing spinal stabilization for the patient. If the vehicle is motionless, then the patient will be motionless as well, which protects the patient's spine. With the step chocks in place and the tires deflated, the vehicle is now stable, and the extrication process can begin.

Other tools are available for special situations, including car-on-car situations, vehicles on their sides or roofs, and larger vehicles. These tools include jacks, ratchet straps, and struts, among others. The use of this equipment is covered in advanced extrication courses.

Gaining Access

Objective 6

Gaining access to the patient inside of an entangled vehicle should be accomplished as soon as safely possible after arriving on the scene. Use the path of least resistance. Try opening each door, roll down windows, or have the patient unlock doors. In many cases, the easiest way to gain access to the interior of a vehicle is through the unaffected side of the vehicle. When collision damage extends to the interior of a vehicle, the main hazards are the airbags inside the vehicle. The 5-10-20 rule is the standard rule regarding strike zones from undeployed airbags. This means that you should be at least 5 inches away from the side airbags, 10 inches away from the driver's side airbag, and 20 inches from the passenger side airbag. Placing yourself in the center of the backseat of the vehicle will put you outside of all strike zones from undeployed airbags.

Remember This!

The route used to reach the patient is not necessarily the route through which the patient will be removed.

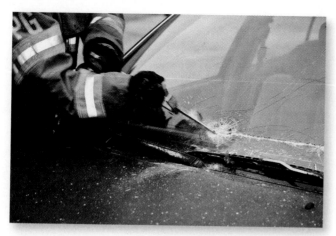

FIGURE 28-4 ▲ The front windshield of most vehicles is made of laminated glass. Remove it by taking an axe and working around the edges of the glass. Continue around the edge until you come back to the starting point, then remove the glass.

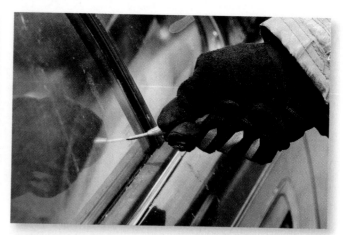

FIGURE 28-5 ▲ A window punch can be used to remove tempered glass from side windows and the rear window.

If the vehicle is not upright or there is heavy damage to the vehicle, you may need to enter through the vehicle's glass. There are two types of glass commonly found in vehicles today. Laminated glass is found in the front windshield of most vehicles. It is composed of two panes of glass with a laminated sheet between them. The laminated sheet allows the glass to remain intact should it be struck by an object. It is best removed by working around the edges of the glass. Start by taking an axe and working around the edges of the glass, using the axe like a can opener. Continue around the edge until you come back to the starting point. The glass can now be removed from the vehicle (Figure 28-4). The other type of glass is tempered, which breaks into small pieces but does not shatter and leave jagged, sharp edges, as most glass does. It is found in side windows and the rear window. A window punch is the best tool for this type of glass. Simply place the tip of the punch against the upper corner of the window and push in. The glass will break into very small pieces but should remain relatively intact until you remove it by hand (Figure 28-5).

You Should Know

When using a window punch, use contact paper or duct tape to help keep the glass together during the breakage and removal. Without this, there is occasionally a problem with the glass shattering and going in different directions, and possibly getting onto the patient. Shield the patient before using a window punch.

Objective 5

After you have gained access to the interior of the vehicle, the next step should be to provide protection for the patient. A heavy tarp or other type of cover specially designed for rescue purposes should be used to protect the patient, and respiratory protection should be used if there is a concern about particulates entering the patient's respiratory tract (Figure 28-6). It is important to remember that the patient does not understand the extrication process and can become frightened by the sounds and procedures occurring around him. It is often desirable for a rescuer working in the interior of the vehicle to provide psychological support from underneath the tarp during the extrication. This will also give you the opportunity to assess the patient continuously throughout the extrication process.

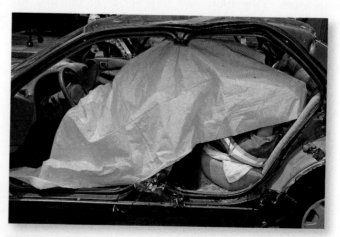

FIGURE 28-6 ▲ A heavy tarp or other type of cover specially designed for rescue purposes should be used to protect the patient during extrication.

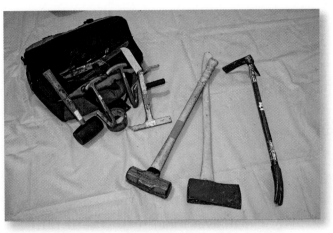

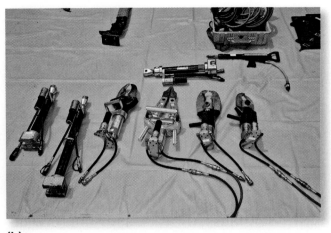

(a)

(b)

FIGURE 28-7 ▲ **(a)** Simple extrication is the use of hand tools in order to gain access to and extricate the patient from the vehicle. **(b)** Complex extrication involves the use of powered hydraulic rescue tools, such as cutters, spreaders, and rams.

Extrication Process

Objective 7

Extrication can be divided into two categories: simple and complex. **Simple extrication** is the use of hand tools in order to gain access and extricate the patient from the vehicle. Simple hand tools include tools such as hammers, hacksaws, battery-operated saws, and pry bars (Figure 28-7a). **Complex extrication** involves the use of powered hydraulic rescue tools such as cutters, spreaders, and rams (Figure 28-7b). The patient's level of entrapment will determine whether the extrication will fall into a simple or complex category.

Degrees of Entrapment

Four levels of entrapment are possible during an MVC (see the following *You Should Know* box). The first level is no entrapment. This means no one is entrapped in the vehicle and occupants were able to get out of the vehicle on their own. Light entrapment means that a door or some other object will need to be opened or moved to get the patient out (Figure 28-8a). Moderate entrapment is more involved, requiring removal of doors or the roof (Figure 28-8b). A patient in a moderate entrapment situation is confined by the wreckage, but a rescuer can access the entire patient. Heavy entrapment is the highest level of entrapment and involves any situation that is above and beyond moderate entrapment. A person who is heavily entrapped in a vehicle is actually pinned by some part of the vehicle that must be moved away from the patient before the patient can be removed from the vehicle (Figure 28-8c).

Light entrapment situations fall into the category of simple extrication. In most cases, only hand tools are needed to gain access to the patient. Moderate entrapment falls into the complex category. It usually involves hydraulic, gas, or electric tools to remove the doors from the vehicle. The same tools can remove the roof and any additional pieces of the vehicle that need to be removed in order to gain patient access and provide egress. Heavy entrapment requires rescuers to actually move a structural component of the vehicle to free the patient for removal from the vehicle.

Removing the Patient

Disentanglement is the moving or removing of material that is trapping a victim. As disentanglement progresses, the patient can be prepared for removal. You should remove the patient from the vehicle in the manner that provides the greatest amount of spinal protection for the patient. Manual cervical spinal stabilization should be performed upon patient contact. Then a cervical collar should be applied for additional protection. The rest of the patient's spine should also be stabilized. This is best accomplished with the use of a short spine immobilizer. One example of a short spine immobilizer is the Kendrick Extrication Device

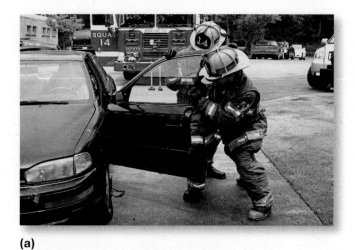

(a)

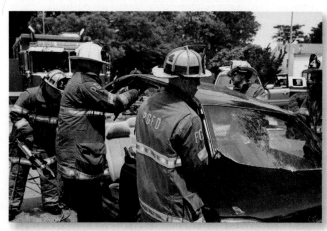

(b)

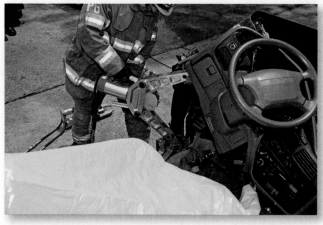

(c)

FIGURE 28-8 ▲ **(a)** Light entrapment requires opening or moving a door or some other object to get the patient out. **(b)** Moderate entrapment requires removal of doors or the roof. **(c)** A person who is heavily entrapped in a vehicle requires that some part of the vehicle must be moved away from the patient before the patient can be moved from the vehicle.

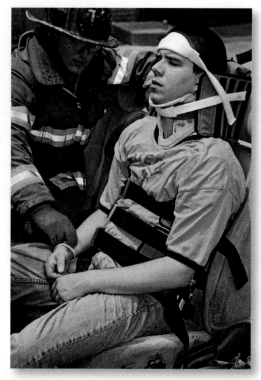

FIGURE 28-9 ▲ A short spine immobilizer, such as the KED, allows the patient's spine to be immobilized from his head to his lower lumbar vertebrae.

(KED). The KED allows the patient's spine to be stabilized from his head to his lower lumbar vertebrae (Figure 28-9). If the patient is a child, use a device of appropriate size, such as a Pedi-Immobilizer, that allows for whole-body stabilization (Figure 28-10). Dress and bandage open wounds and splint or stabilize fractures as time and conditions permit.

In most cases, if an immobilized patient is being removed from the vehicle through a doorway, then he should be taken out feet first onto a backboard (Figure 28-11). Vehicles are designed for occupants to get out feet first so the logical choice for removal is to do the same when placing your patient on a backboard. Several rescuers will be needed to remove a patient from a vehicle. Always call for additional help if needed, and use proper body mechanics to prevent injury while moving any patient.

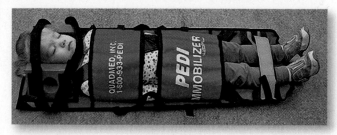

FIGURE 28-10 ▲ A device such as a Pedi-Immobilizer allows for whole-body stabilization.

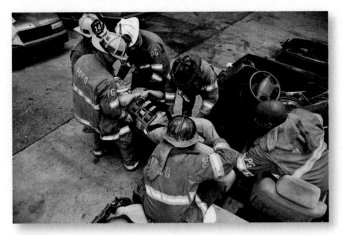

FIGURE 28-11 ▲ In most cases, an immobilized patient who is being removed from the vehicle through a doorway should be taken out feet first onto a backboard.

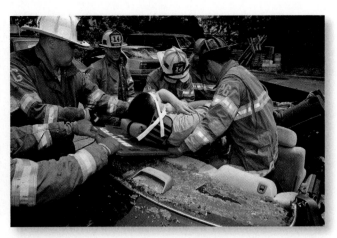

FIGURE 28-12 ▲ Removing a patient over the trunk of a vehicle.

Another method of removal from a vehicle is to place a backboard behind the patient while he is still in his seat. This method requires that the roof be totally removed from the vehicle. First, recline the seat into a position that will allow you to place the backboard behind the victim, positioning the backboard between the patient and the seat. Several rescuers will be needed to accomplish this. One rescuer should be at the patient's head and will be in control of patient movement. When the head rescuer calls for the patient to be moved, every rescuer involved in the process moves at once and brings the patient farther up the backboard until the patient is completely on. With the patient on the backboard, the head should be stabilized last by using materials designed for this purpose (such as soft foam blocks and tape). The straps on the backboard should be joined together. The patient is now ready to be taken away from the vehicle. The rescuers can now lift the patient on either side and take the backboard out over the trunk of the vehicle (Figure 28-12). Continue to protect the patient from hazards.

Transport

The patient is now ready for transport to the hospital. Several factors should be considered when determining whether to go by ground transportation or air, such as time of day, traffic considerations, and weather.

Remember This!

The extrication of patients requires special consideration. For instance, if a patient is pinned by the dash, compartment syndrome can result. The patient can severely decompensate once the dash is removed (blood can rushed into the pinned extremity, which can result in severe circulatory problems from toxins, as well as significant hypotension). If the patient is trapped, try to find out how long the patient has been trapped. If the patient has been trapped for an hour or more, you should suspect crush syndrome. Contact dispatch and request Advanced Life Support (ALS) personnel to the scene. In these situations, it will be important for ALS personnel to begin patient treatment before extrication.

Additional Scene Hazards

With the extrication process over and the patient removed, the next step is to secure any hazards created on the scene. These include any pieces of the vehicle that were removed, fuel leaks, or even vehicles still in the roadway that need to be removed. Address the removed pieces of the vehicle by placing them back into the vehicle that was cut. Fuel leaks should be handled by placing an absorbent material on the spill and then collecting the material for disposal. Any additional vehicles on the scene that can be removed from the roadway should be placed outside of the traffic area.

Making a Difference

After every extrication, a post-call review should be performed to determine which actions proved to be beneficial and which did not. This is not a blame session. It is a tool to facilitate learning for the next extrication you perform. Each experience will help you to become a better EMT.

Any extrication is a complex event that requires great skill and a working knowledge of vehicle design and extrication operations. On the basis of the patient's condition, you decide that this patient needs to be extricated from the vehicle. You perform a 360-degree rotation around the vehicle to check for any hazards; none is found. With your PPE on, you approach the vehicle. Stabilization of the vehicle is accomplished by using cribbing. You then enter the vehicle through the back door on the driver's side. As you enter the vehicle, you notice that there is a significant amount of intrusion of the passenger side of the vehicle. This gives you an indication of the types and severity of the patient's injuries. The extrication team removes the roof of the vehicle, lifts the patient onto a long backboard, and takes the patient out of the vehicle over the trunk. The patient is placed into the back of your ambulance for transport, and you accompany the patient to the hospital. ∎

Sum It Up

▶ Extrication is the process of removing machinery from around a patient to facilitate patient care and transport. The EMT on the extrication scene has an important role both as a care provider for the patient and a support member for the extrication team. Base the extrication on the patient's condition to ensure that the techniques used will provide the fastest access and best egress for the patient from the vehicle.

▶ Protective clothing that is appropriate for the situation must be worn during extrication. This includes protective boots, pants, a coat, eye protection, a helmet, and gloves. Respiratory protection may also be needed.

▶ Scene size-up is an important step in the extrication process. A proper scene size-up will reveal any hazards present and also give a good indication of the number of persons injured, the types of injury, and which patient or patients require medical attention first.

▶ Once on the scene, fire apparatus should be parked in the fend-off position, which involves parking your unit downward from the scene and in such a way that allows traveling vehicles to strike your unit and not crew members.

▶ Stabilization is the process of rendering a vehicle motionless in the position in which it is found. The purpose of stabilization is to eliminate potential movement of a vehicle (or structure) that may cause further harm to entrapped patients or rescuers.

▶ Simple extrication is the use of hand tools in order to gain access and extricate the patient from the vehicle. Complex extrication involves the use of powered hydraulic rescue tools, such as cutters, spreaders, and rams. The patient's level of entrapment will determine whether the extrication will fall into a simple or complex category.

▶ Four levels of entrapment are possible during a motor vehicle crash. The first level is no entrapment. Light entrapment means that a door or some other object will need to be opened or moved to get the patient out. Moderate entrapment is more involved, requiring removal of doors or the roof. Heavy entrapment is the highest level of entrapment and involves any situation that is above and beyond moderate entrapment.

▶ Disentanglement is the moving or removing of material that is trapping a victim.

▶ Continue your education beyond the information contained in this chapter in order to provide the best care for your patient and maintain and improve your skills as you gain more experience in Emergency Medical Services.

By the end of this chapter, you should be able to:

Knowledge Objectives ▶

1. Explain the Emergency Medical Technician's (EMT's) role during a call involving hazardous materials.
2. Describe what the EMT should do if there is reason to believe that there is a hazard at the scene.
3. Describe the actions that an EMT should take to ensure bystander safety.
4. State the role the EMT should perform until appropriately trained personnel arrive at the scene of a hazardous materials situation.
5. Break down the steps to approaching a hazardous situation.
6. Discuss the various environmental hazards that affect Emergency Medical Services (EMS).
7. Describe the criteria for a multiple casualty situation.
8. Evaluate the role of the EMT in the multiple casualty situation.
9. Summarize the components of basic triage.
10. Define the role of the EMT in a disaster operation.
11. Describe basic concepts of incident management.
12. Explain the methods for preventing contamination of self, equipment, and facilities.
13. Review the local mass casualty incident plan.

Attitude Objectives ▶ There are no attitude objectives identified for this lesson.

Skill Objectives ▶ 14. Given a scenario of a mass casualty incident, perform triage.

You drive with caution through the thick, milky fog to the vehicle collision, thankful you are on the ambulance with a seasoned veteran tonight. As you approach the scene, you can see that this is no ordinary car crash. A car has collided with a train. The car lies crushed in the ditch about 10 feet off the road. Bystanders are pointing you to several patients who are scattered in the area.

You and your partner quickly size up the situation. There were six teens in the car—four were ejected and two remain trapped in the mangled wreckage. You open the airway of a young girl. She is not breathing, so you reopen her airway and look, listen, and feel again; there is still no breathing. You know what you have to do, but it's not easy—you tag her black and move on. The others are breathing, but three are unconscious and the remaining two have signs of shock. Your partner radios for more ambulances and equipment, and you begin the overwhelming task of trying to provide some care for your seriously injured patients. ■

THINK ABOUT IT

As you read this chapter, think about the following questions:

- How will you categorize the remaining patients?
- How should incoming units protect the scene from another collision while you move your patients across the road to the ambulance?
- Who will remove the trapped patients?
- What types of additional resources are needed to safely treat all of the patients?

Introduction

You may respond to situations involving hazardous materials or multiple patients. To prevent further illness or injury, you must be able to recognize when a hazardous materials situation exists. You must also understand the basic concepts of incident management and be able to effectively triage patients in multiple-casualty situations.

Hazardous Materials

Objective 6

The National Fire Protection Association (NFPA) defines a hazardous material as "a substance (solid, liquid, or gas) that, when released, is capable of creating harm to people, the environment, and property." Hazardous materials may be found in incidents involving vehicle crashes, railroads, pipelines, storage containers and buildings, chemical plants, and acts of terrorism. Hazardous materials can also be found in the home.

The Role of the Emergency Medical Technician

Objective 1

Management of a hazardous materials incident requires preplanning, specialized emergency care by trained personnel, identifying the substance or material, treatment protocols specific for the material involved, and Emergency Department care by personnel trained to handle this type of medical emergency.

During the early stages of a hazardous materials event, local Emergency Medical Services (EMS) providers will be on their own for the initial phase of the response until specialty teams arrive. You must ensure the safety of yourself and your crew, the patient, and bystanders. To do this effectively, standard operating procedures and protocols must be used. In some cases, you will be able to recognize a hazardous material from the information given by the dispatcher. Alternately, you may be the one who activates the hazardous materials team because you discovered the incident.

Scene Safety and Reporting

Objectives 2, 3, 4, 5

The first phase of dealing with a hazardous materials incident is recognizing that one exists and recognizing the limitations of yourself and your crew. Remember that hazardous materials may pose a threat to the community. As always, your personal safety is your priority in any emergency scene. Dealing with hazardous materials requires extensive training and proper equipment. Without the proper equipment, any intervention could put you and your crew at risk. Access to any patient must not occur without the proper protective equipment. Standard body substance isolation equipment may not be sufficient or appropriate for this type of response.

Protective Equipment

Objective 12

Many chemicals can cause harm to unprotected skin. Corrosives and strong oxidizers can cause contact dermatitis or chemical burns. Many pesticides and poisons can seep into the skin, resulting in toxic effects. Liquefied or cryogenic gases can cause thermal injuries, such as frostbite. Some liquefied gases may present more than one hazard. For example, chlorine stored as a liquefied gas is corrosive, especially to the eyes and moist skin. It is also a thermal hazard because of the frostbite potential as it rapidly evaporates.

Chemical protective clothing (CPC) is designed to protect the skin from exposure to chemicals by either physical or chemical means. Examples of CPC classes include gas-tight encapsulating suits, liquid splash–protective suits, permeable protective suits, nonhazardous chemical–protective clothing, and other protective apparel, such as chemically resistant hoods, gloves, and boots. A variety of materials are used to make the fabric from which CPC is manufactured. Each material provides protection against specific chemicals or mixtures of chemicals but may afford little or no protection against certain others. No material provides satisfactory protection from all chemicals. Protective clothing material needs to be compatible with the chemical substances involved and its use consistent with manufacturers' instructions. When used alone, CPC provides no fire or heat protection.

CPC is commonly categorized as either *limited use* or *heavy use*. Heavy-use CPC is designed to be more highly resistant to abrasions and punctures. Limited-use CPC is generally of lighter-weight construction. It is designed to be used once and then disposed of.

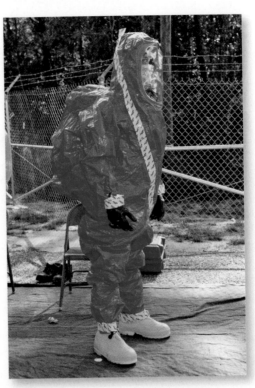

FIGURE 29-1 ▲ Level A protective equipment.

The Environmental Protection Agency has defined four levels of personal protective equipment (PPE). Level A protection is a vapor-protective suit that is encapsulated. This type of suit provides the highest available level of respiratory, skin, and eye protection from solid, liquid, and gaseous chemicals. Level A PPE includes a pressure-demand, full-face mask; self-contained breathing apparatus (SCBA); inner chemical-resistant gloves; and chemical-resistant safety boots (Figure 29-1). Optional equipment includes a cooling system, outer gloves, hard hat, and 2-way radio communications system. Level A protection is intended for situations in which a chemical or chemicals have been identified and pose high levels of hazards to the respiratory system, skin, and eyes. Level A protection is typically used by members of the Hazmat (hazardous material) team for entry into the contaminated area (hot zone).

Level B protection is a liquid splash–protective suit. It includes a pressure-demand, full-face mask; SCBA; inner chemical-resistant gloves; chemical-resistant safety boots; and a hard hat (Figure 29-2). Level B PPE offers the same level of respiratory protection as Level A but less skin protection. It offers no protection against chemical vapors or gases. Level B protection is worn when the chemical or chemicals have been identified but do not require a high level of skin protection. For example, Level B protection is used when evaluation of the scene identifies that hazards of the chemical involved are associated with liquid but not vapor contact.

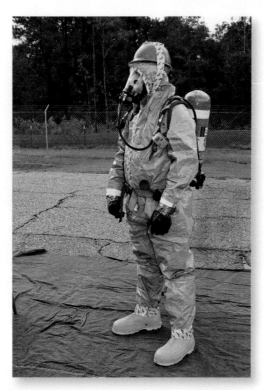

FIGURE 29-2 ▲ Level B protective equipment.

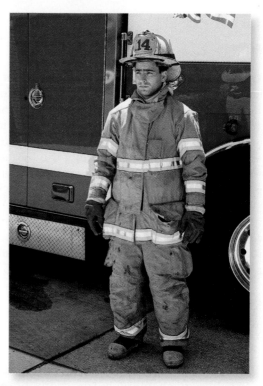

FIGURE 29-4 ▲ Level D protective equipment.

Level C PPE is a support-function protective garment. It includes a full-face mask, chemical-resistant gloves and safety boots, and a canister-equipped respirator that filters chemicals from the air (Figure 29-3).

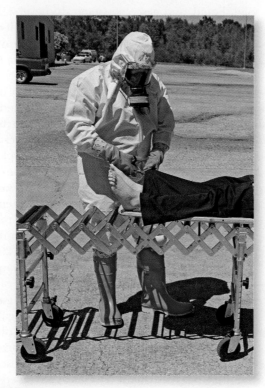

FIGURE 29-3 ▲ Level C protective equipment.

It does not include an SCBA. Level C protective equipment provides the same level of skin protection as Level B but a lower level of respiratory protection. It provides liquid splash protection but no protection against chemical vapors or gases. Level C protection is used when the type of airborne substance is known and contact with the chemical or chemicals will not affect the skin. Level C protective equipment is not acceptable for use in a chemical emergency response.

Level D PPE includes a work uniform, such as firefighter turnout clothing (Figure 29-4). It provides no respiratory protection and minimal skin protection. This level of protective equipment is used when the atmosphere of the involved area contains no known chemical hazards. Level D protective equipment is not acceptable for use in a chemical emergency response. (See Table 29-1 for an overview of the levels of protective equipment.)

Scene Size-Up

To maximize safety, approach and park uphill and upwind of a hazardous materials scene. In this position, you are less likely to become exposed if the hazardous material becomes airborne or a large spill occurs. Examples of incidents that may involve hazardous materials include vehicle crashes (commercial vehicles, pest control vehicles, tankers, cars with alternative fuels, or tractor-trailers), transportation (railroads or pipelines), storage (tanks or storage

TABLE 29-1 Levels of Personal Protective Equipment

Level	When Used	Notes
A	Intended for situations in which the chemical or chemicals have been identified and pose high levels of hazards to the respiratory system, skin, and eyes	• Vapor-protective suit that is encapsulated • Highest available level of respiratory, skin, and eye protection from solid, liquid, and gaseous chemicals
B	Worn when the chemical or chemicals have been identified but do not require a high level of skin protection	• Liquid splash–protective suit • Same level of respiratory protection as Level A but less skin protection • No protection against chemical vapors or gases • Usually worn by decontamination team
C	Used when the type of airborne substance is known and contact with the chemical or chemicals will not affect the skin	• Support-function protective garment • Same level of skin protection as Level B but a lower level of respiratory protection • Liquid splash protection but no protection against chemical vapors or gases • Not acceptable for use in a chemical emergency response
D	Used when the atmosphere of the involved area contains no known chemical hazards	• No respiratory protection and minimal skin protection • Should not be worn in the hot zone • Not acceptable for use in a chemical emergency response

You Should Know

No single combination of protective equipment and clothing can protect you from all hazards. Combining PPE ensembles with other types of protective clothing may be appropriate as additional measures for preventing exposure. For example, although CPC alone provides no fire or heat protection, aluminized radiant heat protection worn over CPC will provide limited protection in potential flash fire situations.

A specific PPE ensemble may protect well against some hazards but poorly, or not at all, against others. In many instances, PPE will not provide continuous protection from a particular hazard. In such cases, exposure times should be reduced as necessary and closely monitored. Technical data provided by the PPE manufacturer must be used when determining the most appropriate PPE for the hazards present.

vessels, warehouses, hardware or agricultural stores), manufacturing operations (such as chemical plants), and acts of terrorism.

On arrival at the scene, obtain scene control and establish a perimeter. If the call was not initially reported as a hazardous materials incident and you are the first on the scene and suspect hazardous materials involvement, an Emergency Medical Dispatcher (EMD) should be notified so that appropriate measures can be taken. Give dispatch the exact location of the incident or perimeter.

If hazardous substances or conditions are suspected, the scene must be secured by qualified personnel wearing appropriate equipment. If you are not qualified and do not have the appropriate equipment, you may need to wait for additional help to arrive before you can attempt entry into the scene. Stage (wait for instructions) a minimum of 2000 feet from a suspected hazardous materials incident.

If you have been trained to do so (and are properly equipped), identify and establish safety zones. Initiate the National Incident Management System (NIMS) plan (discussed later in this chapter). Designate the Incident Commander, and announce the location of the command post. The command post location may be determined by standard operating procedures or other resources. Generally, the command post should not be less than 300 feet away from the scene. In most cases, apparatus should point away from the scene. If possible, attempt to identify the material by sighting placards or identification numbers through binoculars while remaining at a safe distance from the area.

Remember This!

Scene size-up is a continuous process. It allows the Incident Commander to periodically review strategy and tactics in order to effectively position more resources where necessary.

Identifying Hazardous Substances

The substance involved in an incident can be identified by using a number of resources:

- U.S. Department of Transportation (DOT) *Emergency Response Guidebook*
- United Nations (UN) classification numbers
- NFPA 704 placard system
- UN/DOT placards
- Shipping papers
- Material safety data sheets

Department of Transportation Regulations

The DOT regulates all aspects of transporting hazardous materials in the United States. These regulations include the design of the container, the type of container used, and the means by which hazardous materials are transported. If dangerous materials are being transported, the DOT requires that a placard be displayed on shipping containers and transport vessels (railroad cars, trucks, and ships). The color of the placard tells the class of the hazardous material. The presence of a 4-digit number allows more specific identification. This 4-digit number is keyed to the DOT's *Emergency Response Guidebook*. This book is a quick reference guide for hazardous materials incidents. Chemicals are listed in the book alphabetically and by their 4-digit DOT number. Each chemical is given a reference number that corresponds to a set of instructions and precautions, listed in the back of the book, for dealing with that class of chemical.

National Fire Protection Association's Standard 704

The NFPA's Standard 704 designates a hazardous material's classification. The NFPA hazard classification system uses diamond-shaped placards divided into quadrants. Different background colors and

Remember This!

EMTs should attend a 24-hour Hazardous Materials First Responder course. If you have not received specific Hazardous Materials training, use the following rule of thumb. Assume that any material that has a "colored" placard or 4-digit number on it is dangerous to your health and safety and that you must set up a safe zone until trained personnel properly identify the material.

numbers ranging from 0 to 4 (4 representing an extremely high hazard) are used to indicate the dangers presented by the hazardous material:

- Blue quadrant—health hazard
- Red quadrant—flammability hazard
- Yellow quadrant—reactivity hazard
- White quadrant—specific hazard (such as radioactivity, water reactivity, or biological hazard)

Material Safety Data Sheets

Material safety data sheets (MSDSs) provide detailed information about the material. This information includes the name and physical properties of the substance, fire and explosion hazard information, and first aid treatment. The Occupational Safety and Health Administration (OSHA) requires MSDSs to be kept on site anywhere chemicals are used. MSDSs may be used to identify materials or products if they can be obtained safely.

You Should Know

Hazardous Materials Information Resources

Resources for information about hazardous materials include the following:

- Your local hazardous materials (Hazmat) response team
- The Chemical Transportation Emergency Center (CHEMTREC)
  —This organization provides a 24-hour hotline: (800) 424-9300. It can provide product and emergency action information.
- The *Emergency Response Guidebook*, published by the U.S. DOT
- Your regional Poison Control Center (PCC)
  —Your local center can provided detailed information, including decontamination methods and treatment.
- Material safety data sheets (MSDSs)

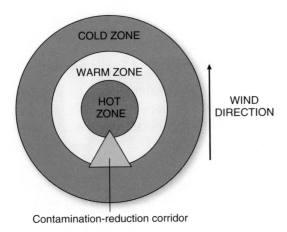

Contamination-reduction corridor

FIGURE 29-5 ▲ Safety zones.

Establishing Safety Zones
Objective 12

Hazardous materials scenes are divided into zones according to safety. If you have been trained to do so (and are properly equipped), identify and establish safety zones (Figure 29-5). The **hot zone** is the area of the incident that contains the hazardous material (contaminant). The hot zone is also known as the *exclusion zone.* This is a dangerous area. The size of the hot zone depends on many factors, including the characteristics of the chemical, the amount released (or spilled or escaped), local weather conditions, the local terrain, and other chemicals in the area. Areas around the contaminant that may be exposed to gases, vapors, mist, dust, or runoff are also part of the hot zone. Only personnel with high-level PPE enter this area. The hot zone is considered contaminated and dangerous until cleared by trained personnel.

The **warm zone** (also called the *contamination reduction zone*) is a controlled area for entry into the hot zone. The warm zone is where most operations will take place as a support area for the hot zone. It also serves as the decontamination area after exiting the hot zone. All personnel in the warm zone must wear appropriate protective equipment. If you have not been trained and do not have the appropriate protective gear, you *must* stay out of the hot and warm zones.

The safe zone (also called the *cold zone* or *support zone*) is an area safe from exposure or the threat of exposure. The cold zone serves as the staging area for personnel and equipment. If there is no risk to you, remove patients to a safe zone. You should not move from this zone or allow anyone else access the scene from this zone unless they have specialized training and PPE. The Incident Command Post is located in the cold zone.

Approaching the Patient

Determine if the scene has been secured to allow for your safe approach to the patient. Do not approach unless you are trained and equipped with appropriate PPE for the situation or the scene has been deemed safe by the proper authorities. Much of the information you will need to properly treat the patient may be gathered initially from a distance with the use of binoculars or spotting scopes.

Remember to stay uphill and upwind as you approach any patient. Patient care must be performed only by trained personnel wearing the appropriate level of PPE, or the patient must have already been decontaminated.

Patients who are unable to walk must be removed from the hot zone by trained personnel. This is usually done by fire department and/or hazardous materials personnel. Even if you have been trained and are properly equipped, emergency care in the hot zone must be limited to spinal stabilization, gross airway management (such as opening the airway, suctioning), and hemorrhage control. Emergency care in the hot zone is limited because of the risk of patient or rescuer exposure to hazardous substances or conditions.

Address life-threatening problems and carry out gross decontamination before giving emergency care. Gross decontamination means removing all suspected contaminated clothing. Brush off any obvious contaminants. Remove the patient's jewelry and watch, if present. Cover wounds with a waterproof dressing after decontamination. If spinal stabilization appears necessary, begin it as soon as feasible. Perform a primary survey at the same time as decontamination. Request Advanced Life Support (ALS) personnel if you suspect hazardous material contamination. Complete a more detailed assessment as conditions allow.

When treating patients, consider the chemical-specific information received from your PCC and other information resources. In multiple-patient situations, begin proper triage procedures according to your local emergency response plan. Triage is discussed later in this chapter.

Decontamination

At every incident involving hazardous materials, there is a possibility that personnel, their equipment, and members of the public will become contaminated. The contaminant poses a threat to the persons contaminated, as well as to other personnel who may subsequently be exposed to contaminated personnel and equipment. Decontamination (decon) is done to reduce and prevent the spread of contamination from persons and equipment used at a hazardous materials incident by physical and/or chemical processes. The process should be directed toward confinement of the contaminant to maintain the safety and health of response personnel, the public, and the environment. Decon should be performed only by trained personnel wearing the appropriate level of PPE. Decon is usually performed in the warm zone. Decon procedures should be continued until it is determined or judged no longer necessary.

Mass Casualty Incidents

Objectives 7, 8

A **mass casualty incident (MCI),** also be called a *multiple casualty incident* or *multiple casualty situation* (MCS), is any event that places a great demand on resources—equipment, personnel, or both. An MCI could be four patients for some communities and a much larger number for others. There is no set number of patients that defines an MCI.

In most EMS situations, emergency care is provided first to the most seriously injured patient(s). In an MCI, the goal is to do the most good for the most people. Priority is given to the most salvageable patients with the most urgent problems. *Triage* is a French word that means "to sort." Triage is sorting multiple victims into priorities for emergency medical care or transportation to definitive care. By quickly sorting the injured patients and identifying the needs of those patients, you are better able to grasp what resources will be needed to care for them.

START Triage System

Objective 9

Many EMS systems use the **START triage system.** START is an acronym for *S*imple *T*riage *A*nd *R*apid *T*reatment. START was developed by the Newport Beach (California) Fire and Marine Department in cooperation with staff at Hoag Hospital in Newport Beach. When you are using the START system, your initial patient assessment and treatment should take less than 30 seconds for each patient. Four areas are evaluated during your initial assessment: (1) the ability to walk (ambulation), (2) respirations, (3) perfusion, and (4) mental status. On the basis of your assessment findings, you then place the patient into one of four categories:

- Red—immediate treatment
- Yellow—delayed treatment
- Green—minor (ambulatory patients; "walking wounded")
- Black—dead or dying

Color-coded triage tags that correspond with these categories are placed on the patient and used to identify the level of injury sustained.

When you begin triaging patients, first identify patients who are able to walk. Patients who are able to walk are called the *walking wounded.* Clear them from the area so that you can triage the more seriously injured patients. For example, instruct patients who can walk to go to a predetermined evaluation and treatment area. These patients should be tagged as "green" or "minor." Next, determine the patients who are injured but have adequate respirations, perfusion, and mental status. For example, you might ask, "If you can hear me, please raise an arm or leg so we can help you!" These patients should be tagged as "yellow" or "delayed." Proceed to the remaining patients. These patients will be tagged as "red" (immediate) or "black" (dead or dying), depending on your assessment. Start with the patient closest to you.

Remember This!

Triaging patients during an MCI goes against your instincts to help everyone you encounter. Practice using the START triage system so it will be easy to use if you are ever faced with an MCI.

To assess the patient by using the START method, assess the patient's respirations. If the patient is not breathing, open his airway. If he is still not breathing, triage the patient as dead. If opening the patient's airway results in breathing, check his respiratory rate. If he is breathing more than 30 times per minute, triage the patient as immediate (red tag). If the patient is breathing less than 30 times per minute, check perfusion. To assess perfusion, check the patient's radial pulse. If a radial pulse is absent, triage the patient as immediate. If a radial pulse is present, check the patient's mental status. If the patient cannot follow simple commands (he is unresponsive or has an altered mental status), triage the patient as immediate. If the patient can follow simple commands, triage the patient as delayed. If the patient is triaged as immediate, repositioning the airway and controlling severe bleeding are the only initial treatment efforts that are performed before moving on to next patient. Continue triaging patients until all patients have been assigned a category. However, do not triage the patients once and think you are done. Triage is an ongoing process. In most MCIs, reassessing the patient is done in the treatment area and again when he is moved to the transportation area. The patient's triage category is updated as needed.

Making a Difference

A rule of triage is to do the greatest good for the greatest number. To make sure you are ready in the event of an MCI, a MCI drill should be a part of regular training for you and your agency.

JumpSTART Triage System

The START system works very well for adults. However, Dr. Lou Romig, a well-known pediatric emergency and EMS physician, identified some weaknesses in the START system when applied to children. As a result, in 1995 she developed a modified START system for use with children. This system is called *JumpSTART Triage*.

In the JumpSTART system, all children who are able to walk are triaged in the minor (green) category. Begin assessing children who are not able to walk as you come to them. First, assess the child's breathing. If he is breathing, assess his respiratory rate. If the child is not breathing or has very irregular breathing, open his airway by using the jaw thrust without head tilt. If the child begins breathing, triage him as immediate (red) and move on to the next patient. If the child does not begin breathing, check for a pulse. If there is no pulse, triage the patient as dead (black) and move on. If the child does have a pulse, give 15 seconds of mouth-to-mask breathing (about 5 breaths). If the child begins breathing, triage him as immediate (red) and move on. If he does not begin breathing, triage the patient as dead (black) and move on.

If a child is breathing on his own when you find him, quickly check his respiratory rate. If the child is breathing faster than 45 times per minute or less than 15 times per minute, or if his breathing is irregular, triage him as immediate. If the child is breathing 15–45 times per minute, assess perfusion. If a pulse is present, assess mental status. If no pulse is present in the least injured limb, triage the child as immediate and move on.

Assess mental status by using the AVPU scale. If the child is alert, responds to a verbal stimulus, or responds appropriately to pain, triage the child as delayed (yellow) and move on. If the child responds inappropriately to pain or is unresponsive, triage him as immediate (red) and move on. As with adults, children will need to be reassessed in the treatment and transportation areas.

Incident Command System

Objectives 10, 11

In 2003, President George W. Bush directed the Secretary of Homeland Security to develop and administer a National Incident Management System (NIMS). The purpose of NIMS is to provide a consistent nationwide template that allows all governmental, private-sector, and nongovernmental agencies to work together during domestic incidents. Examples of domestic incidents include acts of terrorism, wildland and urban fires, floods, hazardous materials spills, nuclear accidents, aircraft accidents, earthquakes, tornadoes, hurricanes, typhoons, and war-related disasters.

The Incident Command System (ICS) (also called the *Incident Management System* [IMS]) is an important part of this comprehensive system. ICS is a standardized system developed to assist with the control, direction, and coordination of emergency response resources. The ICS can be used at an incident of any type and size, from an everyday call to the large and complex incident.

An **Incident Commander (IC)** is the person who is responsible for managing all operations at the incident site. There is only one IC per incident. The Incident Commander has three priorities:

- Life safety (ensuring the safety of the lives and the physical well-being of emergency personnel and the public)
- Incident stability (minimizing the effect the incident may have on the surrounding area while using resources efficiently)
- Property conservation (minimizing damage to property)

Persons on the scene who are familiar with ICS will also be familiar with the following risk-benefit model:

"We will risk our lives a lot within a calculated plan for lives that are savable.

We will risk our lives a little within a calculated plan for property that is savable.

We will not risk our lives at all for lives or property that is already lost."

Objective 8

At the beginning of an incident, the IC is typically the most senior EMS professional who arrives at the scene. As more resources arrive, command is transferred to another person on the basis of who has the primary authority for overall control of the incident. When command is transferred, the outgoing IC must give the incoming IC a full report and notify all staff of the change in command.

The ICS organizational structure can expand or contract in a modular fashion as needed for each incident. For instance, depending on the size of the incident, the IC may assign to others the authority to perform certain activities. Scene operations may be broken down into groups. For example, the treatment group is assigned patient treatment while an extrication group is responsible for extrication.

If you arrive on the scene of an MCI where the ICS has been established, report to the command post. Find out who the IC is. Identify yourself and your level of training. Follow the directions given by the IC about your assignment. In most instances, you will be assigned to the staging area. You will be required to remain available until you are instructed to move to another area. Do not "self-assign." This only creates confusion and may hinder the responses of others working to resolve the incident.

On the Scene Wrap-Up

The fire captain on the first engine that arrives positions his truck to block the road behind the ambulance and assumes command of the scene. He tells the rescue squad to extricate the trapped patients. He establishes a staging area for incoming ambulances. He also asks the police to direct traffic and place flares to alert oncoming cars. As each ambulance crew arrives, you assign them a patient. Within 30 minutes, the last teen is en route to the local hospital. In the debriefing later, you discuss how the weather prevented the use of helicopter transport. Overall, everyone felt that all crews performed well and hoped that they are never again faced with such a scene. ∎

Sum It Up

▶ As defined by the NFPA, a hazardous material is any substance that causes or may cause adverse effects on the health or safety of employees, the general public, or the environment.

▶ A hazardous substance can be identified by using a number of resources:
  • U.S. DOT *Emergency Response Guidebook*
  • UN classification numbers

  • NFPA 704 placard system
  • UN/DOT placards
  • Shipping papers
  • MSDSs

▶ The first phase of dealing with a hazardous materials incident is recognizing that one exists. As always, your personal safety is your priority in any emergency scene. If there is no risk to you (and you are properly trained and equipped to do so), remove patients to a safe zone. The safe zone (also called the *cold zone*) is an area safe from exposure or the threat of exposure. The warm zone is a controlled area for entry into the hot zone. It also serves as the decontamination area after exiting the hot zone. All personnel in the warm zone must wear appropriate protective equipment. The hot zone is the danger zone.

▶ A mass casualty incident (MCI) may also be called a *multiple-casualty incident* or *multiple-casualty situation* (MCS). An MCI is any event that places a great demand on resources—equipment, personnel, or both.

▶ The START triage system is used by many systems in dealing with MCIs. START stands for *Simple Triage And Rapid Treatment*. On the basis of your assessment findings, you categorize each patient according to one of four categories. Color-coded triage tags that correspond with these categories are placed on the patient and used to identify the level of injury sustained.

▶ The JumpSTART triage system was developed for use with children. It specifies how the four color-coded tags are applied to pediatric patients.

▶ The National Incident Management System (NIMS) was created to provide a consistent nationwide template that allows all governmental, private-sector, and nongovernmental agencies to work together during domestic incidents. The Incident Command System (ICS) is an important part of NIMS. ICS is a standardized system developed to assist with the control, direction, and coordination of emergency response resources. The ICS can be used at an incident of any type and size.

▶ An Incident Commander (IC) is the person who is responsible for managing all operations at the incident site. Depending on the size of the incident, the Incident Commander may assign to others the authority to perform certain activities. Scene operations may be broken down into groups, such as treatment and extrication.

▶ If you arrive on the scene of an MCI where the ICS has been established, report to the command post. Find out who the IC is. Identify yourself and your level of training. Follow the directions given by the IC about your assignment.

Division 8

Advanced Airway (Elective)

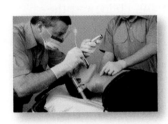

30 Advanced Airway Techniques

By the end of this chapter, you should be able to:

Knowledge Objectives ▶
1. Identify and describe the airway anatomy of the infant, child, and the adult.
2. Differentiate between the airway anatomy of the infant, child, and the adult.
3. Explain the pathophysiology of airway compromise.
4. Describe the proper use of airway adjuncts.
5. Review the use of oxygen therapy in airway management.
6. Describe the indications, contraindications, and technique for insertion of nasogastric tubes.
7. Describe how to perform the Sellick maneuver (cricoid pressure).
8. Describe the indications for advanced airway management.
9. List the equipment required for endotracheal intubation.
10. Describe the proper use of the curved blade for endotracheal intubation.
11. Describe the proper use of the straight blade for endotracheal intubation.
12. State the reasons for and proper use of the stylet in endotracheal intubation.
13. Describe the methods of choosing the appropriate size endotracheal tube for an adult patient.
14. State the formula for sizing an infant or child endotracheal tube.
15. List complications associated with advanced airway management.
16. Define the various alternative methods for sizing the infant and child endotracheal tube.
17. Describe the skill of endotracheal intubation in the adult patient.
18. Describe the skill of endotracheal intubation in the infant and child patient.
19. Describe the skill of confirming endotracheal tube placement in the adult, infant, and child patient.
20. State the consequence of and the need to recognize unintentional esophageal intubation.
21. Describe the skill of securing the endotracheal tube in the adult, infant, and child patient.

Attitude Objectives ▶
22. Recognize and respect the feelings of the patient and family during advanced airway procedures.
23. Explain the value of performing advanced airway procedures.

24. Defend the need for the Emergency Medical Technician (EMT) to perform advanced airway procedures.

25. Explain the rationale for the use of a stylet.

26. Explain the rationale for having a suction unit immediately available during intubation attempts.

27. Explain the rationale for confirming breath sounds.

28. Explain the rationale for securing the endotracheal tube.

Skill Objectives ▶ 29. Demonstrate how to perform the Sellick maneuver (cricoid pressure).

30. Demonstrate the skill of endotracheal intubation of the adult patient.

31. Demonstrate the skill of endotracheal intubation of the infant and child patient.

32. Demonstrate the skill of confirming endotracheal tube placement in the adult patient.

33. Demonstrate the skill of confirming endotracheal tube placement in the infant and child patient.

34. Demonstrate the skill of securing the endotracheal tube in the adult patient.

35. Demonstrate the skill of securing the endotracheal tube in the infant and child patient.

On the Scene

A 67-year-old man collapsed in his living room. You find that he is unresponsive, is not breathing, and has no pulse. Your partner is performing chest compressions. You are 15 minutes from the closest hospital. An Advanced Life Support unit is not available to assist you. While ventilating the patient with a bag-mask (BM) device, you make the decision to insert an advanced airway. ■

THINK ABOUT IT

As you read this chapter, think about the following questions:

- Can you name two advanced airways that may be inserted by an EMT if approved by the EMT's state Emergency Medical Services office?
- Which advanced airway technique requires visualization of the vocal cords?
- Should an advanced airway be inserted before ventilating the patient with a BM device?
- Because your transport time is short, will this factor affect your decision to insert an advanced airway?

Introduction

Advanced airway management by an Emergency Medical Technician (EMT) is an elective module that may be included in an EMT course if approved by the state Emergency Medical Services (EMS) office. Advanced airways include the **esophageal-tracheal Combitube (ETC or Combitube)** and the **endotracheal tube (ET tube)**. An ET tube is a plastic tube that is open at both ends and designed for insertion into a patient's trachea. Endotracheal intubation is the placement of an ET tube into a patient's trachea to keep the airway open. Insertion of an ET tube requires visualization of the structures of the upper airway. Insertion of a Combitube does not. In some states, advanced airways may be inserted by EMTs who have been properly instructed in their use and who receive ongoing education to ensure skill competency.

Airway Anatomy Review

Respiratory System

Objective 1

The respiratory system was discussed in detail in Chapters 4 and 7. In this chapter, our discussion of respiratory system anatomy is limited to the areas pertinent to insertion of advanced airways.

The upper airway includes the nose, the pharynx, and the larynx. The lower airway consists of the trachea and the lungs. The floor of the nasal cavity is bony and is called the *hard palate*. The soft palate is fleshy and extends behind the hard palate. It marks the boundary between the nasopharynx and the rest of the pharynx. The pharynx is a muscular tube that serves as a passageway for food, liquids, and air. The pharynx is made up of three parts.

- *Nasopharynx.* The nasopharynx is located directly behind the nasal cavity. It serves as a passageway for air only. The tissues of the nasopharynx are extremely delicate and bleed easily.

- *Oropharynx.* The oropharynx is the middle part of the throat. It opens into the mouth and serves as a passageway for both food and air. It is separated from the nasopharynx by the soft palate.

- *Laryngopharynx.* The laryngopharynx is the lowermost part of the throat. It surrounds the openings of the esophagus and larynx. It opens in the front into the larynx and in the back into the esophagus. It serves as a passageway for both food and air.

The larynx connects the pharynx with the trachea. The vocal cords stretch across the inside of the larynx. The space between the vocal cords is called the *glottis*. This area is the narrowest part of the adult larynx. The larynx is made up of 9 cartilages connected to each other by muscles and ligaments. The thyroid cartilage (Adam's apple) is the largest cartilage of the larynx. The epiglottis is a special flap of cartilage that covers the trachea during swallowing so that food or liquids do not enter the lungs. When endotracheal intubation is performed by using a straight blade, the tip of the blade is positioned under the epiglottis. When the epiglottis is lifted up with the blade, the opening between the vocal cords (**glottic opening**) is exposed. This allows the ET tube to be passed through the cords and into the trachea. The **vallecula** is the area between the base of the tongue and the epiglottis. When endotracheal intubation is performed by using a curved blade, the tip of the blade is inserted into this important landmark.

The cricoid cartilage is the lowermost cartilage of the larynx. It is the only complete ring of cartilage in the larynx. The cricoid cartilage forms the base of the larynx on which the other cartilages rest. When pressure is applied to the cricoid cartilage of an unresponsive patient, the trachea is pushed backward and the esophagus is compressed (closed) against the cervical vertebrae. This compression helps decrease the amount of air entering the stomach during positive-pressure ventilation.

The trachea is located in the front of the neck. It is kept permanently open by C-shaped cartilages. The esophagus is part of the digestive system. It serves as a passageway for food. The open part of each C-shaped cartilage faces the esophagus. This allows the esophagus to expand slightly into the trachea during swallowing. If the opening between the vocal cords is not clearly visible when an ET tube is being inserted, the tube may enter the esophagus. If this occurs, ventilating the patient will result in air entering the stomach instead of the lungs. If this situation is not recognized, the patient will be deprived of oxygen with devastating results.

The trachea branches into the right and left mainstem bronchi. An ET tube that is inserted too far has a tendency to go down the right mainstem bronchus because it is shorter, wider, and straighter than the left. The point at which the trachea divides into two primary bronchi forms an internal ridge called the *carina*. The mainstem bronchi subdivide into smaller air passages, ending at the alveoli.

Infant and Child Anatomy Considerations

Objectives 2, 3

In general, the structures of the mouth and nose of an infant and child are smaller and more easily obstructed than adults. The tongue of an infant and child is large relative to the mouth. When a patient becomes unresponsive, the tongue falls back into the posterior oropharynx (back of the mouth). This can cause a complete airway obstruction.

The epiglottis of an infant and toddler is large, long, and U-shaped. The trachea of an infant or child is shorter and narrower than an adult's trachea. It is more easily obstructed by swelling. Because the trachea is softer and more flexible in infants and children, head positioning when opening the airway is important. Moving the head too far forward or backward can cause an airway obstruction. Because the trachea is short, an ET tube that has been placed in the trachea can easily become displaced if the patient's head is moved. Once an ET tube is in the proper position, it is very important to secure it in place to prevent displacement.

The larynx of infants and young children looks like a funnel. Their larynx is located higher in the neck than an adult's. For example, in an adult, the larynx is located opposite the 4th to 7th cervical vertebrae (C4-C7). A newborn's larynx is about the same level as C1-C4. The larynx of a 7-year-old is about the same level as C3-C5.

Like other cartilage in young children, the cricoid cartilage is less developed and less rigid than in an adult. The narrowest area of a young child's upper airway is at the level of the cricoid cartilage. In an older child, the narrowest part of the upper airway is at the level of the vocal cords, as it is in an adult.

The chest wall of an infant or child is softer than an adult's. If respiratory distress or respiratory failure is present, retractions may be seen above the clavicles, between the ribs, and below the rib cage. Infants and children tend to depend more heavily on the diaphragm for breathing. If positive-pressure ventilation is performed too aggressively, air can enter the stomach and cause it to swell (gastric distention). This can impair movement of the diaphragm, hindering effective ventilation.

Adequate and Inadequate Breathing

Objective 3

A patient who is breathing adequately:

- Does not appear to be in distress
- Speaks in full sentences without pausing to catch his breath
- Breathes at a regular rate and within normal limits for his age
- Has an equal rise and fall of the chest with each breath
- Has an adequate depth of breathing (tidal volume)
- Has normal skin color

The signs of inadequate breathing include the following:

- Anxious appearance, concentration on breathing
- Confusion, restlessness
- A breathing rate that is too fast or slow for the patient's age
- An irregular breathing pattern
- A depth of breathing that is unusually deep or shallow
- Noisy breathing (stridor, snoring, gurgling, wheezing)
- Sitting upright and leaning forward to breathe
- Being unable to speak in complete sentences

- Pain with breathing
- Skin that looks flushed, pale, gray, or blue; skin that feels cold or sweaty

Objectives 4, 5, 7

Inadequate breathing must be treated aggressively before it becomes absent breathing. Because the use of airway adjuncts, oxygen therapy, suctioning, and cricoid pressure are essential components of airway management, please review this information in Chapter 7. Having suction equipment within arm's reach is critical when managing a patient's airway. Always check your suction unit often. Hoses can get misplaced or displaced. A unit may appear to work and even sound as if it works, yet there is no suction. To ensure your suction is working, place your finger over the end of the connecting tubing and make sure it is functioning. Advanced airway techniques are challenging. They should not be attempted without first ensuring that all necessary equipment is available and in working order.

Remember This!

If your state regulations (and medical direction) permit you to insert an advanced airway, you must remember that the key to successful *advanced* airway techniques is having strong *basic* airway management skills. For example, an advanced airway should not be inserted before attempting to ventilate the patient by another means (such as with a bag-mask [BM] device). If debris is present in the patient's airway, it must be removed with suctioning before (and sometimes during) insertion of an advanced airway. If you are unsuccessful inserting an advanced airway, you can always rely on your basic airway management skills and support your patient's needs. Remember: "BLS before ALS"—Basic Life Support before Advanced Life Support.

Endotracheal Intubation

The most stressful prehospital medical call usually involves a difficult airway. If you are unable to ventilate your patient, he will not likely survive the event. The most definitive method of airway control is endotracheal intubation. All other means of airway control are compared with this standard. Unless an airway obstruction is present, endotracheal intubation gives the healthcare professional an unobstructed path for ventilation. Endotracheal intubation reduces the risk of aspiration, allows for better oxygen delivery, and allows for deeper airway suctioning.

Indications

Objective 8

Endotracheal intubation is an effective means of controlling a patient's airway. Indications for this procedure include the following:

- Prolonged artificial ventilation is required.
- Adequate artificial ventilation cannot be achieved by other methods.
- The patient is unresponsive and has no cough or gag reflex.
- The patient is unable to protect his own airway (cardiac arrest, unresponsive).

Another indication for endotracheal intubation is the presence of respiratory failure or an impending airway obstruction. For example, a patient who has an inhalation injury is at risk of an airway obstruction. A patient who has severe pulmonary edema is at risk of a respiratory arrest as his respiratory muscles tire because of the work of breathing. These situations typically involve patients who are awake and alert or patients who have an altered mental status. ALS personnel will need to manage the patient's airway in situations like these. In many EMS systems, the ALS providers are authorized to give the patient medications to sedate him before inserting an ET tube.

Equipment

Objective 9

Endotracheal intubation requires special equipment and supplies (see the following *You Should Know* box).

Endotracheal Tubes

An ET tube is open at both ends (Figure 30-1). The proximal end of the tube has a 15-mm adapter (connector) plugged into it. This adapter is used to connect to a BM device. (Because the mask of a BM device is not used when ventilating through an ET tube, the device is more correctly called a *bag-valve device*.) The distal tip of an ET tube is beveled to

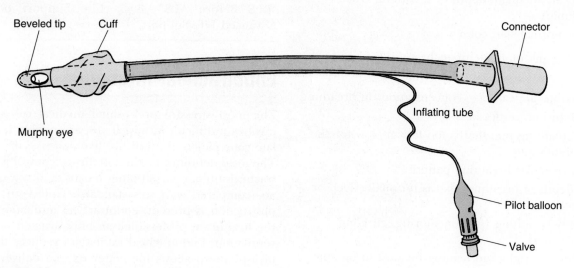

FIGURE 30-1 ▲ Components of an ET tube.

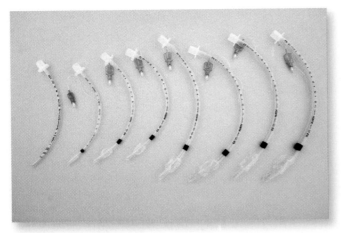

FIGURE 30-2 ▲ ET tubes come in a variety of sizes.

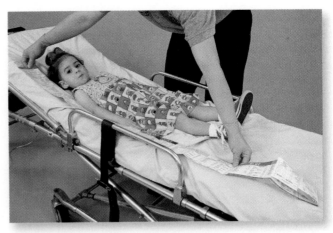

FIGURE 30-3 ▲ Use a length-based tape to determine proper ET tube for an infant or child.

ease passage of the tube between the vocal cords. There is an opening on the side of the ET tube opposite the beveled tip. This opening is called the *Murphy eye*. It helps prevent complete obstruction of the tube if the tip of the ET tube should become blocked.

Some ET tubes have an inflatable cuff near the distal end of the tube. When the cuff is inflated, it forms a seal in the trachea. By sealing off the trachea from the rest of the pharynx, the patient's risk of aspiration is reduced (but not eliminated). If the ET tube has a cuff, a pilot balloon is present on the upper 1/3 of the tube. The pilot balloon is used to detect the status of the cuff. The pilot balloon has an inflation valve in it. If the cuff is inflated, the pilot balloon will be inflated. When checking your equipment before intubation, inflate the cuff to check for leaks and then deflate it. This helps to ensure that the cuff will inflate adequately after the tube is inserted into the patient. After the patient is intubated, you will inflate the pilot balloon with air, using a 10-mL syringe. This in turn inflates the cuff and seals the trachea. After inflating the cuff, you must remember to unhook the syringe or the air will escape out of the cuff and go back into the syringe.

ET tubes come in a variety of sizes (Figure 30-2). The internal diameter (i.d.) of an ET tube is indicated as millimeters (mm) i.d. Internal tube diameters range from 2.5-mm to 4.5-mm (uncuffed) and 5-mm to 10-mm (cuffed). The size you should use depends on your patient. The average-size ET tube for an adult man is 8.0–8.5 mm i.d. For an adult woman, the average size is 7–8 mm i.d. The "emergency rule" is that a 7.5 mm i.d. ET tube will fit most adults in an emergency.

Remember that the narrowest part of an infant or young child's airway is the cricoid cartilage. This is where the distal tip of the ET tube is placed. In general, uncuffed ET tubes are used in patients younger than 8 years of age. The circular narrowing at the level of the cricoid cartilage serves as a functional cuff. Cuffed tubes are usually used for children older than 8 years of age.

When selecting the proper size ET tube for the pediatric patient, you should use a length-based tape (Figure 30-3). The tape provides all recommended ET tube sizes, blade sizes, vital signs, and other information for children who weigh up to about 35 kg. If a length-based tape is not available, you can use the following formulas to estimate the correct ET tube size for children 1 to 10 years of age:

- (age in years + 16)/4 or (age in years/4) + 4 = *uncuffed* ET tube size (mm i.d.)
- (age in years/4) + 3 = *cuffed* ET tube size (mm i.d.)

A good habit to develop is to have an ET tube 0.5 mm larger and a tube 0.5 mm smaller than the size that you calculated that you needed.

Objectives 13, 14, 16

When an ET tube is placed properly, the distal tip of the tube should rest between the patient's vocal cords and carina. An ET tube has markings on it to measure the distance from the distal tip in centimeters. After proper position of the tube has been confirmed, the centimeter marking on the tube at the patient's front teeth should be documented and the tube secured in place. (Some EMS systems use the cm marking at the patient's lip.) In an adult man, the average ET tube depth is 23 cm at the lips and 22 cm at the teeth. In an adult woman, the average ET tube depth is 22 cm at the lips and 21 cm at the teeth. For an estimation of proper ET tube depth in a child older than 2 years of age, the child's age in years + 10 equals the centimeter mark at the lip. For example,

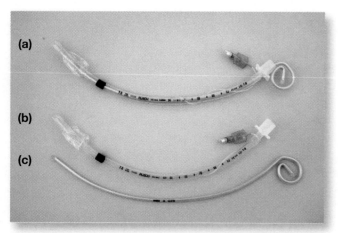

FIGURE 30-4 ▲ **(a)** ET with stylet inserted, **(b)** ET tube, **(c)** Stylet.

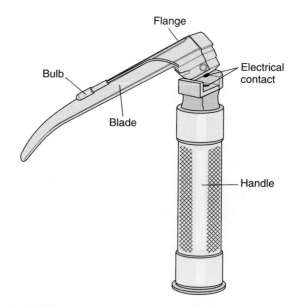

FIGURE 30-5 ▲ A laryngoscope blade has a bulb on its distal tip. A notch on the blade fits onto a locking bar on the laryngoscope handle. Lifting the blade to a right angle locks it into place and turns on the light.

for a 4-year-old child, 4 years + 10 = 14 cm. On arrival at the hospital, an x-ray is usually taken to verify ET tube position and depth. The ET tube has a radiopaque material that runs the length of the tube so that it shows up on an x-ray.

Stylet

Objective 12

A **stylet** is a flexible plastic-coated wire that is inserted into the ET tube to provide stiffness and shape to the ET tube (Figure 30-4). This is especially beneficial in hot environments because the hotter the ET tube gets, the softer it becomes. If allowed to get hot enough, the ET tube could feel like a wet noodle and be difficult to pass through the vocal cords. Once inserted into the ET tube, the stylet should not be inserted beyond the Murphy eye! This will decrease the chance of soft-tissue trauma to the patient's airway.

Laryngoscope Handle and Blades

A **laryngoscope** is an instrument that is used to visualize the glottic opening (the space between the vocal cords). A laryngoscope consists of a handle and blade that are made of plastic or stainless steel. The handle holds batteries. A laryngoscope blade has a bulb on its distal tip or a fiberoptic light source that runs the length of the blade. A notch on the blade fits onto a locking bar on the laryngoscope handle. Lifting the blade to a right angle locks it into place and turns on the light (Figure 30-5). The light should be "bright, white, and tight." When checking your equipment before intubation, it is important to have spare batteries on hand for the laryngoscope handle as well as spare bulbs in assorted sizes for the blades.

Objectives 10, 11

There are two types of laryngoscope blades—straight and curved. Straight blades are available in sizes ranging from 0 to 4 (Figure 30-6). Sizes 0 to 2 are used for infants and children. Sizes 3 and 4 are used for adults. A straight blade is used to lift the epiglottis in order to see the glottic opening and vocal cords. A straight blade is preferred in children and infants. Curved blades are available in sizes ranging from 0 to 4 (Figure 30-7). The tip of a curved blade is inserted into the vallecula. This indirectly lifts the epiglottis in order to see the glottic opening and vocal cords. To select a laryngoscope blade of the proper size, hold the blade next to the patient's face. A blade of proper size should reach between the patient's lips and larynx.

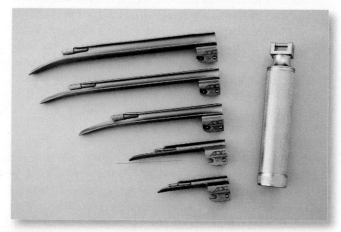

FIGURE 30-6 ▲ Straight laryngoscope blades.

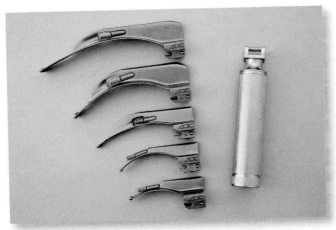

FIGURE 30-7 ▲ Curved laryngoscope blades.

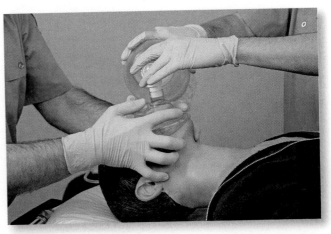

FIGURE 30-8 ▲ Put on appropriate personal protective equipment. Ask your assistants to ventilate the patient with 100% oxygen as you prepare the intubation equipment.

Remember This!

The benefits of endotracheal intubation must outweigh the risks associated with the procedure. If you are using BLS skills and the patient's oxygenation and ventilation are adequate, you must ask yourself, "Is it worth the risks to perform this procedure?"

Studies have shown that there is a high incidence of misplaced and displaced tracheal tubes in the prehospital setting. Current resuscitation guidelines recommend that if your transport time is short, oxygenation and ventilation of a patient by using a BM device is recommended over endotracheal intubation.

Procedure

Objectives 17, 18

Before intubating a patient, put on appropriate personal protective equipment (PPE) (Figure 30-8). This should include gloves, protective eyewear, and a mask. At least two EMS professionals should be assigned to manage the patient's airway. One person will open the patient's airway, hold the mask of a BM device in place, and maintain the patient's head in proper position. A second person is needed to squeeze the bag. Listen to the patient's breath sounds to establish a baseline. Attach the pulse oximeter to the patient (if not already done).

Assemble and test all intubation equipment (Figure 30-9). This includes testing the suction unit, laryngoscope batteries, and the bulb on the laryngoscope blade. If the ET tube you will be using has a cuff, test the cuff for leaks. If there are no leaks, completely deflate the cuff. Leave the syringe filled with air attached to the inflation valve. If you will be using a stylet, insert it into the ET tube. Check to be sure that the end of the stylet is recessed at least

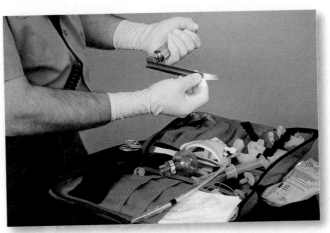

FIGURE 30-9 ▲ Assemble and test all equipment.

1/2 inch from the tip of the ET tube. To keep the stylet in proper position, bend the proximal end of the stylet over the ET tube. Lubricate the distal end of the ET tube with water-soluble lubricant. Prepare the tape or securing device.

Remember This!

Items such as suction, batteries, and the bulb in the laryngoscope blade should be checked at the beginning of your shift. The time that it is needed should not be the first time that it is checked.

Place the patient in a position that enables total control of the airway. If needed, move the patient away from structures or objects that are in your way. If trauma is not suspected, place the patient's head in the "sniffing position" to make visualization of the vocal cords

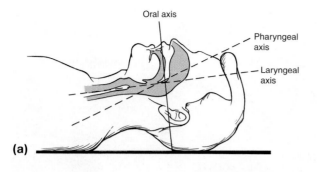

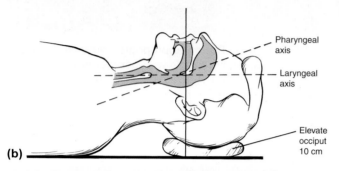

FIGURE 30-10 ▲ **(a)** The axes of the mouth, pharynx, and trachea. **(b)** If trauma is not suspected, placing the patient's head in the sniffing position creates a straight line between the teeth and the vocal cords.

and glottic opening easier (Figure 30-10). To achieve the sniffing position, it may be necessary to place a small amount of padding under the patient. In many cases, placing padding under the base of the skull or under the shoulders (depending on the patient's age) will help you achieve better head positioning. If trauma is suspected, do not place the patient in a sniffing position. Instead, you must have an assistant manually stabilize the patient's head and neck in a neutral position and intubate the patient while he is in this position.

As you prepare to open the patient's mouth, it will be necessary for your assistant to temporarily stop positive-pressure ventilation. Once ventilation stops, you have 30 seconds to complete the intubation and resume ventilating the patient.

Open the patient's mouth. Suction blood, secretions, vomitus, and debris from the patient's mouth, if present. If dentures are present, remove them. Ask an assistant to apply cricoid pressure. Cricoid pressure should be continued until the ET tube is secured in place. If the patient begins vomiting, discontinue cricoid pressure until the vomiting stops and the airway has been cleared with suctioning.

Holding the laryngoscope in your left hand, gently insert the laryngoscope blade into the right corner of the patient's mouth (Figure 30-11). When intubating an infant or child, the patient's large tongue makes intubation a challenge. Using a sweeping motion, move the tongue to the left so that it is out of the way.

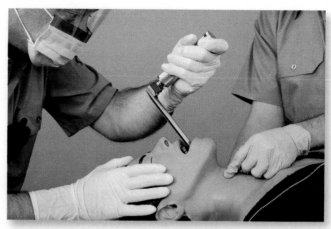

FIGURE 30-11 ▲ Holding the laryngoscope in your left hand, gently insert the laryngoscope blade into the right corner of the patient's mouth. Using a sweeping motion, move the tongue to the left so that it is out of the way.

Advance the laryngoscope blade until the distal end reaches the base of the tongue. If you are using a straight blade, place the blade under the epiglottis (Figure 30-12). If you are using a curved blade, place the blade tip into the vallecula (Figure 30-13). When intubating the pediatric patient, it is recommended that you use a straight blade with the curved blade technique. This means that instead of inserting the straight blade under the epiglottis, you should insert the straight blade into the vallecula. This technique is recommended because the epiglottis in the pediatric patient is longer and harder to control.

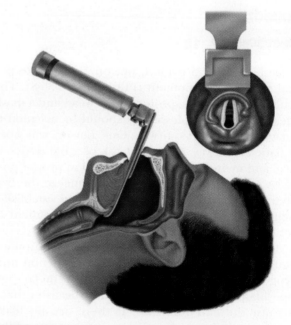

FIGURE 30-12 ▲ Advance the laryngoscope blade until the distal end reaches the base of the tongue. If you are using a straight blade, place the blade under the epiglottis.

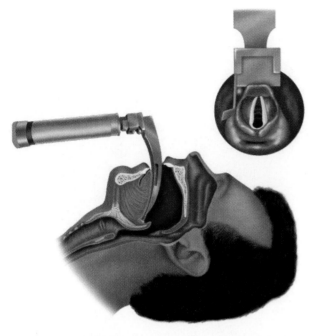

FIGURE 30-13 ▲ The tip of a curved blade is inserted into the vallecula.

Gently lift the laryngoscope up and away from the patient (Figure 30-14). (Think of the laryngoscope blade as a large tongue depressor.) Do not allow the blade to touch the patient's teeth. To increase your ability to see the vocal cords and decrease your chances of causing trauma to the patient, be sure to keep your wrists straight, and don't use the patient's teeth or gums as a fulcrum.

Objective 21

Once you see the vocal cords and glottic opening, you will use your right hand to introduce the ET tube

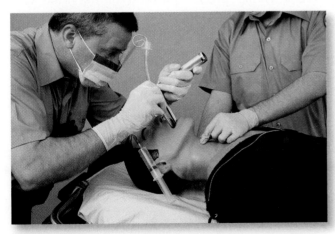

FIGURE 30-14 ▲ Gently lift the laryngoscope up and away from the patient. Do not allow the blade to touch the patient's teeth. Using your right hand, insert the ET tube from the right side of the patient's mouth.

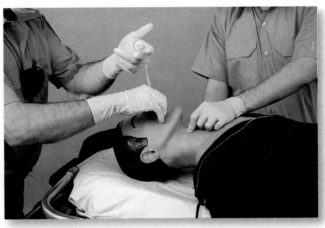

FIGURE 30-15 ▲ Using your right hand, insert the ET tube from the right side of the patient's mouth. Gently advance the ET tube between the vocal cords. Position the cuff just past the vocal cords and then stop. Make a note of the centimeter marking at the lip and have someone document this number. Gently remove the laryngoscope blade. Immediately fold the blade to extinguish the light. While holding onto the ET tube with one hand, gently remove the stylet if used.

into the glottic opening. From the right side of the patient's mouth, gently advance the ET tube between the vocal cords (Figure 30-15). Position the cuff just past the vocal cords (about 1/2–1 inch beyond the cords) and then stop. Make a note of the centimeter marking at the lip and have someone document this number. Gently remove the laryngoscope blade. Make it a habit to immediately fold the blade to extinguish the light. This helps conserve your batteries for the next intubation. Use caution during the removal of the blade so that you don't accidentally remove or displace the tube. While holding onto the ET tube with one hand, gently remove the stylet from the tube (if one was used). Inflate the ET tube cuff via the pilot balloon (Figure 30-16). After inflation,

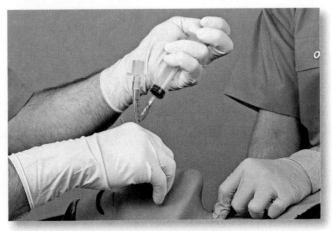

FIGURE 30-16 ▲ Inflate the ET tube cuff. After inflation, disconnect the syringe from the inflation valve.

remember to disconnect the syringe from the inflation valve as soon as possible. After confirming proper position of the tube (discussed later in this chapter), secure it in place with a commercially available tube holder or tape.

Remember This!

Because of the small size of their airway, infants and children are at increased risk of accidental ET tube displacement. Movement of the head or movement of the ET tube less than 2 cm can displace the ET tube. Pediatric patients have a high incidence of respiratory infections. This can cause them to produce a large amount of secretions. It is easy for a pediatric ET tube to become blocked because of its small diameter.

Confirming Tube Placement

Objectives 19, 20

In the field, there is a significant risk of the ET tube of an intubated patient becoming displaced. This is because of the amount of times a patient is moved. Because a misplaced or dislodged tube can be fatal, confirmation of ET tube placement is an ongoing assessment. It must be done frequently while the patient is in your care. ET tube placement should be checked immediately after insertion, after securing the tube, during transport, and whenever the patient is moved.

When initially confirming placement of the tube (and while using 1 hand to make sure the ET tube does not move), place your stethoscope over the upper portion of the patient's stomach (epigastrium) (Figure 30-17). With the stethoscope on the epigastrium, have an assistant attach the bag-valve device to the ET tube and begin positive-pressure ventilation. You should not hear gurgling or air entry over the epigastrium. If gurgling or air entry is heard over this area, you most likely have intubated the esophagus instead of the trachea. Remove the ET tube *immediately*, attach a mask to the bag-valve device, and provide BM ventilation.

If you do not hear air entry or gurgling over the epigastrium, the tube is most likely not in the epigastrium. Next, look at your patient, starting with the chest. Is chest rise and fall symmetrical and adequate? Look at the patient's general appearance. If the ET tube is in proper position, the patient's color should be improving. Connecting an exhaled carbon dioxide (CO_2) detector to the ET tube is useful

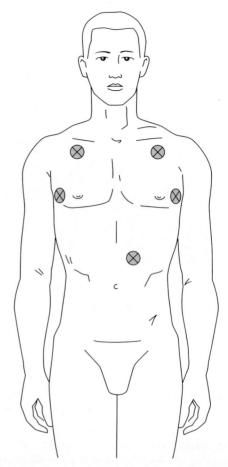

FIGURE 30-17 ▲ Begin confirming the position of the ET tube by listening for sounds over the epigastrium. If the ET tube is properly placed in the trachea, you should not hear gurgling or air entry over the epigastrium. If no sounds are heard over the epigastrium, listen to breath sounds on both sides of the chest.

in confirming proper position of the tube (see below). Do not let go of the tube until its placement is confirmed and it has been secured to the patient.

Listen to breath sounds. Listen to the apex (top) of the left lung. Compare this with the air entry in the right apex. Breath sounds should be equal bilaterally. Then, listen over the left side of the chest, just below the armpit laterally. Listen and compare to the same area on the right. Finally, compare the base of the left lung with the base of the right lung. All breath sounds should be equal bilaterally.

If baseline breath sounds were present on the left side before intubation and are now diminished or absent on that side, you most likely have a right mainstem intubation. Deflate the ET tube cuff, place your stethoscope on the left chest, and slowly pull the ET tube back, 1 cm at a time until you have equal, bilateral breath sounds. Take care not to

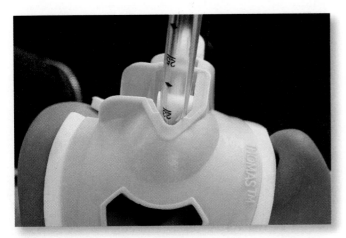

FIGURE 30-18 ▲ After confirming an ET tube is in proper position, secure it in place. Document the centimeter mark on the tube at the lip.

remove the tube from the patient by pulling the ET tube back too far. Once the tube is in the proper place, secure it and make note of the centimeter mark on the tube at the lip (Figure 30-18).

If an ET tube becomes displaced, remove the tube. Insert an oral airway and ventilate the patient by using a BM device with 100% oxygen. When able, try again to intubate the patient. If an ET tube becomes displaced and you do not detect it, the patient can die from a lack of oxygen. The use of a CO_2 detector can help decrease the chance of an esophageal intubation. This has become a standard in the prehospital environment.

After the patient has been successfully intubated, it is your responsibility to maintain an open airway. This requires frequent ongoing assessments with endotracheal suctioning as needed. Signs that your patient requires suctioning include the following:

- Decreased compliance (stiff lungs are harder to ventilate with a bag-valve device)
- Agitation
- Coughing
- Wheezing
- Wet breath sounds
- Decreased oxygen saturation values
- Mucus in the ET tube
- Increased or decreased heart rate

When suctioning an ET tube, use a flexible suction catheter that is equal to 1/2 the diameter of the ET tube. Remember this helpful hint: If you double the ET tube size, that number will equal the largest size flexible catheter that you can use. For example, if you initially use a size 7 ET tube, $7 \times 2 = 14$. The largest size flexible catheter than you can use is a 14.

Remember This!

Remember that an adult in cardiac arrest is ventilated at a rate of 10 to 12 breaths/min (one ventilation every 5 to 6 seconds). Once an advanced airway is in place and its position confirmed, the rate of ventilation is decreased to 8 to 10 breaths/min. When an advanced airway is in place, chest compressions can be performed continuously. There is no need to pause compressions to deliver ventilations.

Exhaled Carbon Dioxide Detectors

The measurement of exhaled CO_2 levels is called **capnometry.** In patients who have adequate perfusion, the use of an exhaled CO_2 detector (also called an *end-tidal CO_2 detector*) is considered the most reliable method for verifying tube placement. In a patient who has poor perfusion, an exhaled CO_2 detector may not be reliable. This is because the CO_2 produced by the patient may not be enough to register on the CO_2 detector.

Exhaled CO_2 detectors are available as electronic monitors or disposable colorimetric devices. When using an exhaled CO_2 detector, place the device between the ET tube and the bag-valve device (Figure 30-19). Before using the device to confirm ET tube placement, ventilate the patient at least 6 times. This is done to quickly wash out any CO_2 that may have entered the patient's esophagus and stomach with BVM ventilation. A pediatric CO_2 detector should be used for patients weighing 4.4 pounds to 33 pounds (2 to 15 kg). Use an adult CO_2 detector if the patient weighs more than 33 pounds.

Electronic CO_2 detectors indicate the presence of CO_2 by means of a number or a waveform. The wave-

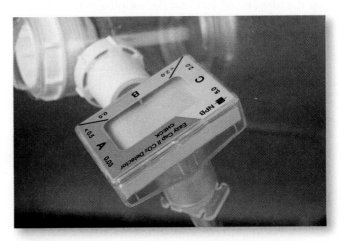

FIGURE 30-19 ▲ When an exhaled-CO_2 detector is used, the device is placed between the ET tube and the bag-valve device.

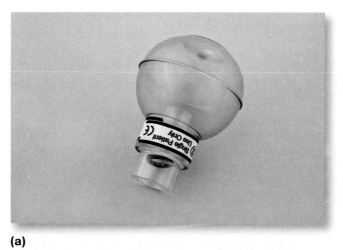
(a)

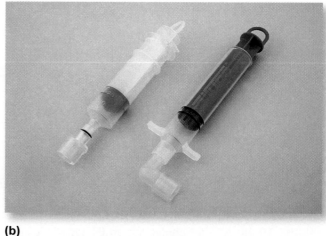
(b)

FIGURE 30-20 ▲ Esophageal detector devices. **(a)** Self-inflating bulb. **(b)** Syringe-type device.

form correlates with the patient's respiratory cycle. Electronic CO_2 detectors can detect much lower levels of CO_2 than colorimetric devices.

A disposable colorimetric device contains special paper that changes color according to the amount of CO_2 detected. In a patient who has adequate perfusion, a lack of color change during exhalation suggests that the ET tube is in the esophagus.

Esophageal Detector Device

An **esophageal detector device (EDD)** is an inexpensive, easy-to-use tool that may be used as an aid in confirming the position of an ET tube. An EDD may be used in children 5 years of age or older or those who weigh more than 20-kg.

There are two types of EDDs, a self-inflating bulb and a syringe-type device (Figure 30-20). Unlike an exhaled CO_2 detector, the accuracy of an EDD does not depend on adequate perfusion. Instead, an EDD relies on the anatomical fact that the esophagus is a soft, collapsible tube and the walls of the trachea are rigid.

If the syringe-type EDD is used and an ET tube is in the trachea, the rigid tracheal walls allow airflow and there is no resistance when drawing back on the plunger of the syringe. If the ET tube is in the esophagus, the soft walls of the esophagus will collapse when drawing back on the plunger. As a result, resistance is felt and air cannot be aspirated easily.

The self-inflating-bulb EDD is compressed before it is connected to the ET tube. As the pressure on the bulb is released, a vacuum is created. Refilling of the bulb in less than 5 seconds is generally considered an indicator of placement of the tube in the trachea. The bulb will remain collapsed if the ET tube is in the esophagus.

When using an EDD, attach the device to the ET tube adapter after intubation but *before* ventilating the

patient. If the patient is ventilated before an EDD is used, an EDD may rapidly reinflate regardless of the tube's location. Studies have shown that results may be misleading in patients who are morbidly obese or who have severe asthma, patients in late pregnancy, and patients who have a significant amount of secretions in the trachea.

Remember This!

No one method is 100% reliable in confirming placement of an ET tube. Use at least two methods to confirm placement. Methods used should include a combination of assessment methods (such as breath sounds, chest rise and fall) and mechanical methods (such as the use of an exhaled CO_2 detector and/or esophageal detection device). Ongoing assessments are essential to ensure proper position of the tube.

Complications

Objective 15

There are many possible complications associated with endotracheal intubation. Most of them are preventable if proper technique is used before, during, and after the procedure. Complications include:

- Slowing of the heart rate. The structures of the upper airway are sensitive to stimulation. Stimulation can cause a slow heart rate, especially in children.
- Soft-tissue trauma to the lips, teeth, tongue, gums, and airway structures
- Inadequate oxygenation resulting from prolonged or unsuccessful intubation attempts

- Intubation of the right mainstem bronchus
- Intubation of the esophagus
- Removal of the tube by the patient (self-extubation)
- Vomiting and aspiration
- Vocal cord damage
- Obstruction of the tube by secretions
- Swelling of the larynx or trachea

Remember This!

Patient movement is a primary cause of displaced tubes. Be sure to reassess chest wall motion, breath sounds, and use a CO_2 detector after every major move—from the scene to the ambulance and from the ambulance to the receiving facility.

The Esophageal-Tracheal Combitube

In some states, an EMT is authorized to insert an esophageal-tracheal Combitube (commonly called the *Combitube*). The Combitube is also called a *dual-lumen airway* because it consists of two (esophageal and tracheal) tubes. This permits ventilation if the tube is inserted into the esophagus (most common) or into the trachea. The Combitube also has two balloon cuffs (Figure 30-21). One balloon is large. It is located near the halfway point of the tube and is called the *pharyngeal balloon*. The second balloon cuff is located near the end of the tube. When the pharyngeal balloon is inflated with air, the balloon fills the space between the base of the tongue and the soft palate. This anchors the Combitube in position and helps prevent the escape of air through the

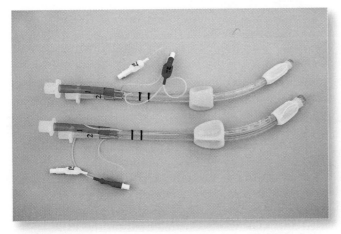

FIGURE 30-21 ▲ The components of the Combitube.

nose or mouth. Unlike endotracheal intubation, insertion of a Combitube does not require visualization of the vocal cords to ventilate the trachea. After the Combitube is inserted, the cuffs are inflated with air and the patient is ventilated through the tube with a BM device.

Indications
- Respiratory arrest
- Cardiac arrest

Contraindications
- Intact gag reflex
- Height less than 4 feet
- Known esophageal disease
- Recent ingestion of a caustic substance
- Known or suspected foreign body obstruction of the larynx or trachea.

Equipment
- PPE
- Oxygen source
- BM device
- Suction device
- Combitube Small Adult (SA) or Combitube
- Syringes—140 mL, 20 mL
- Water-soluble lubricant
- Adhesive tape
- Stethoscope
- Exhaled CO_2 detector

Insertion Procedure

Put on appropriate PPE. While you assemble and test the equipment needed to insert the Combitube, ask two EMS professionals to manage the patient's airway. Have one person open the patient's airway, hold the mask of a BM device in place, and maintain the patient's head in proper position. Ask a second person to squeeze the bag. Listen to the patient's breath sounds to establish a baseline.

Assemble and test all equipment. Select the correct size Combitube on the basis of the patient's height. Use the Combitube SA for patients 4 to 5.5 feet tall (Figure 30-22). Use the Combitube for patients over 5 feet tall. Test the balloons and cuffs for leaks. If you are using the Combitube SA, inflate the pharyngeal balloon with 85 mL of air. Inflate the distal cuff with 12 mL of air. If you are using the Combitube,

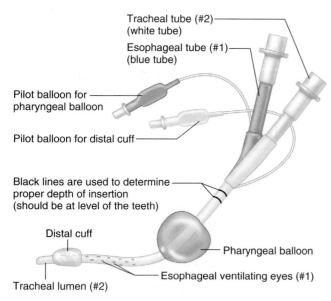

Tracheal tube (#2)
(white tube)

Esophageal tube (#1)
(blue tube)

Pilot balloon for
pharyngeal balloon

Pilot balloon for distal cuff

Black lines are used to determine
proper depth of insertion
(should be at level of the teeth)

Distal cuff

Pharyngeal balloon

Tracheal lumen (#2)

Esophageal ventilating eyes (#1)

FIGURE 30-22 ▲ A Combitube is available in two sizes. The Combitube Small Adult is used for patients 4 to 5.5 feet tall. The Combitube is used for patients over 5 feet tall.

inflate the pharyngeal balloon with 100 mL of air (Figure 30-23). Inflate the distal cuff with 15 mL of air. If there are no leaks, deflate the pharyngeal balloon and distal cuff. Lubricate the distal end of the tube with water-soluble lubricant.

Ask your assistant to temporarily stop positive-pressure ventilation. Once BM ventilation stops, you have 30 seconds to complete the Combitube insertion procedure and resume ventilating the patient. Using a gloved hand, grasp the patient's tongue and lower jaw between your thumb and index finger and lift upward. With your other hand, insert the Combitube following the natural curvature of the pharynx.

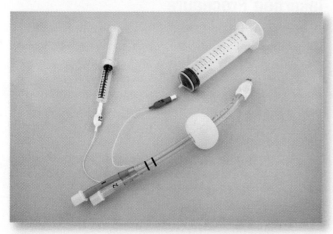

FIGURE 30-23 ▲ The pharyngeal balloon inflated with air.

Maintaining a midline position, gently advance the Combitube along the base of the tongue and into the airway until the heavy black lines on the tube are positioned at the level of the patient's teeth (or gums, if the patient lacks teeth). As you insert the device, make sure the patient's teeth do not snag and tear the cuffs on the tube.

Next, inflate the pharyngeal balloon. To do this, inflate the blue pilot balloon, using 100 mL of air for the Combitube and 85 mL of air for the Combitube SA. As you inflate the pharyngeal cuff, you may see the Combitube move slightly from the patient's mouth. Inflate the distal cuff via the white pilot balloon, using 15 mL of air for the Combitube and 12 mL of air for the Combitube SA. Remember to remove the syringe from the pilot balloon after inflating the balloon/cuff.

Using a bag-mask device, begin ventilation through the blue (esophageal) tube (Figure 30-24). Ventilation begins with the esophageal tube because the Combitube usually enters the esophagus after it is inserted. Watch for chest rise. Using a stethoscope, listen for sounds over the epigastrium. Then listen over each lung. The Combitube is in the esophagus if the chest rises, breath sounds are present on both sides of the chest, and no sounds are heard over the epigastrium. Continue to ventilate through the blue tube. Once placement of the Combitube in the esophagus is confirmed, you can decompress the stomach by inserting a gastric suction catheter (provided in the airway kit) into the clear tube (tube #2). Secure the tube and reassess the patient's vital signs at least every 5 minutes. When available, an exhaled CO_2 detector and pulse oximeter should be used and their values documented on the prehospital care report (PCR). Remember that an exhaled CO_2 detector may be unreliable if the patient has poor perfusion, such as in cardiac arrest. Reassess the position of the Combitube whenever the patient is moved.

If the chest does not rise or sounds are heard over the epigastrium, attach the bag-valve device to the ET tube and immediately begin ventilating (Figure 30-25). Confirm placement of the Combitube in the trachea by listening again over the epigastrium and for breath sounds over each lung. If the Combitube is in the trachea, the chest should rise during ventilation through the clear tube. In addition, breath sounds should be present on both sides of the chest, and no sounds should be heard over the epigastrium. If the Combitube is in the trachea, continue ventilation through the clear tube. Secure the tube and reassess the patient's vital signs at least every 5 minutes. When available, an exhaled CO_2 detector and pulse oximeter should be used and their values documented on the PCR.

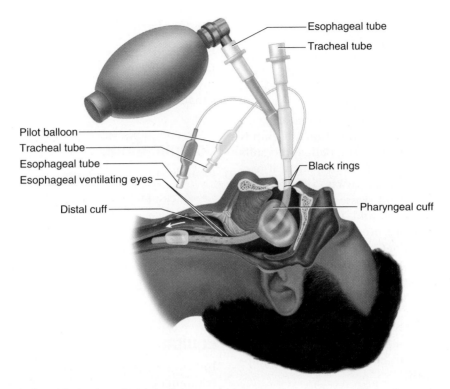

FIGURE 30-24 ▲ The Combitube inserted into the esophagus.

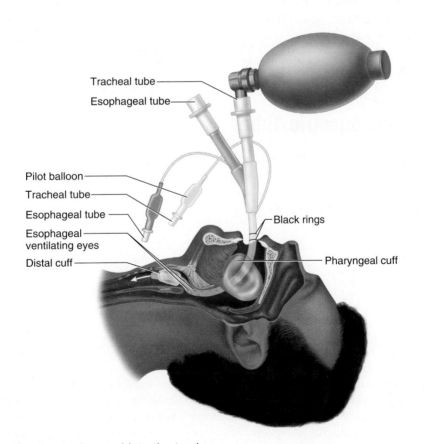

FIGURE 30-25 ▲ The Combitube inserted into the trachea.

If breath sounds are absent and no sounds are heard over the epigastrium, the Combitube may have been advanced too far. Deflate the tube cuffs, starting with the blue tube. Slowly withdraw the tube 2 to 3 cm out of the patient's mouth. Then reinflate the cuffs (blue first). Ventilate and reassess placement. If breath sounds are now present and no sounds are heard over the epigastrium, continue ventilation. If breath sounds and epigastric sounds are still absent, deflate the cuffs and remove the tube. Then suction the patient if necessary, insert an oral or nasal airway, ventilate the patient with a BM device, and reassess.

Ongoing assessments should include assessing the patient for spontaneous breathing and the presence of a pulse. Remove the Combitube if the patient develops a gag reflex or becomes conscious or ventilation is inadequate because of placement of the Combitube. If any of these situations occur, ventilate the patient by using basic airway techniques. When a Combitube is removed, be prepared for vomiting. Turn the patient on his side (if there are no contraindications) and be sure to have your suction equipment within arm's reach.

Complications

Complications of Combitubes include the following:

- Improper placement
- Trauma to the esophagus or trachea because of poor insertion technique or use of wrong size Combitube

Nasogastric and Orogastric Tubes

A **nasogastric (NG) tube** is a long, flexible tube that is passed through the nose, into the posterior nasopharynx, down the esophagus, and into the stomach. An **orogastric (OG) tube** is passed through the mouth and into the stomach.

Indications

Objective 6

In the prehospital setting, indications for insertion of an NG/OG tube include an unresponsive patient and the inability to artificially ventilate a patient because of gastric distention. After insertion, you are able to empty the stomach of unwanted air and undigested food. This increases lung compliance by allowing the diaphragm to flatten during positive pressure ventilation, making it easier to ventilate the lungs. It also decreases the chance of vomiting, which in turn decreases the risk of aspiration.

Contraindications

Contraindications include the presence of major facial, head, or spinal trauma. Insertion of an OG tube instead of an NG tube is preferred in these situations.

Complications

Complications of NG tubes include the following:

- Accidental entry of the NG/OG tube into the trachea
- Nasal or oral trauma
- Vomiting
- Passage of the NG/OG tube into the cranium in cases of basilar skull fractures

Equipment

Insertion of an OG or NG tube requires the following equipment:

- NG/OG tubes in assorted sizes. Use a length-based tape to determine the appropriate size for an infant or child. If a length-based tape is not available, the following sizes may be used as a general guideline:
  —Newborn/infant: 8 French
  —Toddler/preschooler: 10 French
  —School-age children: 12 French
  —Adolescent: 14-16 French
- 60-mL syringe
- Water-soluble lubricant
- Emesis basin
- Tape to secure the tube (a Veniguard works well for this)
- Stethoscope
- Suction unit and suction catheters

Insertion Procedure

- Put on appropriate PPE.
- Prepare and assemble all equipment.
- Determine the correct distance to insert the tube by measuring from the tip of the nose to the earlobe. Then, add the distance from the earlobe to a point midway between xiphoid process and umbilicus (Figure 30-26). Mark the measured distance with a piece of tape on the tube. (The method of measurement for an OG tube is the same as that for an NG tube).

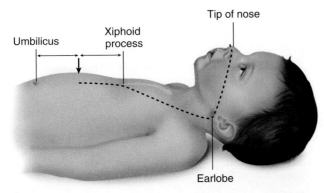

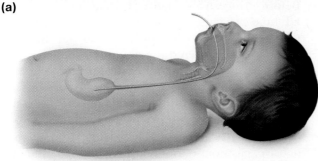

(a)

(b)

FIGURE 30-26 ▲ **(a)** Determine the correct distance to insert the tube by measuring from the tip of the nose to the earlobe. Then, add the distance from the earlobe to a point midway between xiphoid process and umbilicus. **(b)** An orogastric tube in proper position.

- If the tube will be inserted into the nose, lubricate the distal end of the tube with water-soluble lubricant.
- If trauma is not suspected, place the patient in a semi-Fowler's position with the head slightly tilted forward.
- If the tube is being inserted into the nose, pass the tube through one nostril along the floor of the nose. When the tube reaches the back of the nose, direct the tube downward through the nasopharynx. If the tube does not slide easily into the nostril, try inserting it into the other nostril. Never force the tube into the nostril. Encourage the patient to swallow, as this will help passage of the NG tube.
- If the tube is being inserted into the mouth, pass the tube to the back of the tongue and then direct the tube downward through the oropharynx. Encouraging the patient to swallow will help in the process.
- Advance the tube until the tape mark is at the nostril or the lip. If you meet resistance, the patient's breathing changes, his color changes, or if the tube coils in the patient's mouth, remove the tube.

- Check placement of the NG/OG tube by:
  - —Aspirating stomach contents with a syringe
  - —Listening with a stethoscope over the stomach while injecting 10-20 mL of air into the tube
- Aspirate stomach contents to decompress the stomach.
- Secure the tube in place with tape (or use a Veniguard).

On the Scene Wrap-Up

Advanced airways include the Combitube and the ET tube. Not all states permit EMTs to insert these devices. Be sure to check with your instructor about your state's regulations pertaining to EMTs and advanced airways. Insertion of an ET tube requires visualization of the structures of the upper airway; insertion of a Combitube does not. An advanced airway should not be inserted before attempting to ventilate the patient by another means, such as with a BM device. Remember: "BLS before ALS." Current resuscitation guidelines recommend that if your transport time is short, oxygenation and ventilation of a patient with a BM device is recommended over endotracheal intubation. In this scenario, your transport time to the closest appropriate facility was about 15 minutes. Keeping current resuscitation guidelines in mind, a reasonable course of action in this situation would be to continue CPR, transport quickly, and maintain the patient's airway with BLS maneuvers during your short transport time (unless specified otherwise by your local protocols or medical direction). ■

Sum It Up

▶ In some states, advanced airways may be inserted by EMTs who have been properly instructed in their use and who receive ongoing education to ensure skill competency. Advanced airways include the esophageal-tracheal Combitube (ETC or Combitube) and the endotracheal (ET) tube. Insertion of an ET tube requires visualization of the structures of the upper airway; insertion of a Combitube does not.

▶ An ET tube is a plastic tube that is open at both ends and designed for insertion into a patient's trachea. Endotracheal intubation is the placement of an ET tube into a patient's trachea to keep the airway open.

▶ Indications for endotracheal intubation include the following:

- Prolonged artificial ventilation is required.
- Adequate artificial ventilation cannot be achieved by other methods.
- The patient is unresponsive and has no cough or gag reflex.
- The patient is unable to protect his own airway (cardiac arrest, unresponsive).

▶ The average size ET tube for an adult man is 8.0-8.5 mm i.d. For an adult woman, the average size is 7-8 mm i.d. The "emergency rule" is that a 7.5 mm i.d. ET tube will fit most adults in an emergency. When selecting the proper size ET tube for the pediatric patient, you should use a length-based tape.

▶ There is a high incidence of misplaced and displaced tracheal tubes in the prehospital setting. Current resuscitation guidelines recommend that if your transport time is short, oxygenation and ventilation of a patient with a BM device is recommended over endotracheal intubation.

▶ A straight laryngoscope blade is placed under the epiglottis. The tip of a curved blade is placed into the vallecula.

▶ Infants and children are at increased risk of accidental ET tube displacement. Movement of the head or movement of the ET tube less than 2 cm can displace the ET tube.

▶ The measurement of exhaled CO_2 levels is called capnometry. In patients who have adequate perfusion, the use of an exhaled CO_2 detector is considered the most reliable method for verifying tube placement. In a patient who has poor perfusion, an exhaled CO_2 detector may not be reliable.

▶ Use at least two methods to confirm ET tube placement. Methods used should include a combination of assessment methods (such as breath sounds, chest rise and fall) and mechanical methods (such as the use of an exhaled CO_2 detector and/or esophageal detection device). Ongoing assessments are essential to ensure proper position of the tube.

▶ Before using an exhaled CO_2 detector to confirm ET tube placement, ventilate the patient at least 6 times. This is done to quickly wash out any CO_2 that may have entered the patient's esophagus and stomach with BM ventilation. Patient movement is a primary cause of displaced tubes. Be sure to reassess chest wall motion and breath sounds, and use a CO_2 detector after every major move.

▶ An esophageal detector device (EDD) is an inexpensive, easy-to-use tool that may be used as an aid in confirming the position of an ET tube.

▶ The Combitube is called a *dual-lumen airway* because it consists of two (esophageal and tracheal) tubes. This permits ventilation if the tube is inserted into the esophagus (most common) or into the trachea. After the Combitube is inserted, the cuffs on the device are inflated with air and the patient is ventilated through the tube with a bag-mask device.

▶ In the prehospital setting, indications for insertion of an NG/OG tube include an unresponsive patient and the inability to artificially ventilate a patient because of gastric distention.

A Cardiopulmonary Resuscitation

One-Rescuer Adult Cardiopulmonary Resuscitation

STEP 1 ▷
- Make sure the scene is safe for providing emergency care. If the scene is safe, quickly check the patient's level of responsiveness. Gently squeeze the patient's shoulders and shout, "Are you all right?"
- If the patient does not respond, shout for help. If you are alone and there is no response to your shout for help, contact your dispatcher and request additional resources, including an AED (if you do not have an AED with you).

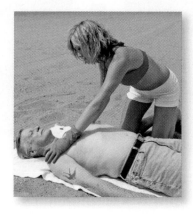

STEP 2 ▷
- If the patient is unresponsive and you do not suspect trauma, open his airway by using the head tilt–chin lift maneuver.

  —If trauma is suspected, open the airway by using the jaw thrust without head tilt maneuver.
  —If trauma is suspected but you are unable to maintain an open the airway by using the jaw thrust maneuver, open the airway by using the head tilt–chin lift maneuver.

- Suction any blood, vomit, or other fluid that may be present from the patient's airway.

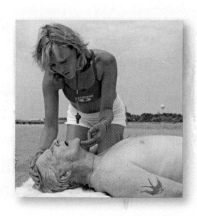

STEP 3 ▷ Place your face near the patient and look, listen, and feel for adequate breathing. Check for at least 5 seconds but not for more than 10 seconds.

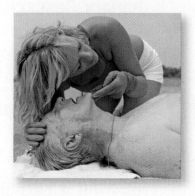

STEP 4 ▷ If the patient's breathing is not adequate, begin rescue breathing by using a pocket mask, mouth-to-barrier device, or BM device. Give 2 breaths (each breath over 1 second), with just enough pressure to make the chest rise with each breath.

—If the first rescue breath does not result in chest rise, reposition the patient's head and try again to ventilate.
—If there is still no chest rise, move on to the next step.

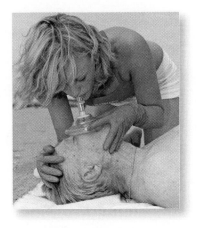

STEP 5 ▷ • Assess the carotid pulse on the side of the patient's neck nearest you. Feel for a pulse for 5 to 10 seconds.
• If you definitely feel a pulse, give 1 breath every 5 to 6 seconds. Reassess the patient's pulse every 2 minutes.
• If you do not definitely feel a pulse within 10 seconds, or if you are uncertain, begin chest compressions.

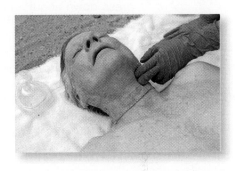

STEP 6 ▷ • If there is no pulse, begin cycles of 30 compressions and 2 breaths. Kneel beside the patient's chest.
• Place the heel of one hand in the center of the patient's chest, between the nipples. Place your other hand on top of the first hand. Interlock the fingers of both hands to keep your fingers off the patient's ribs.

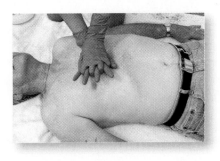

continued on next page

One-Rescuer Adult Cardiopulmonary Resuscitation *(continued)*

STEP 7 ▶ Position yourself directly above the patient's chest so that your shoulders are directly over your hands.

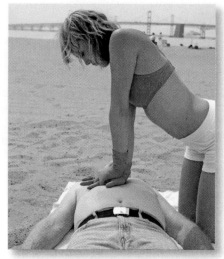

STEP 8 ▶
- With your arms straight and your elbows locked, press down about $1\frac{1}{2}$–2 inches on the patient's breastbone with the heels of your hands. Compress at a rate of 100 per minute.
- Release pressure (let up) after each compression to allow the patient's chest to recoil.

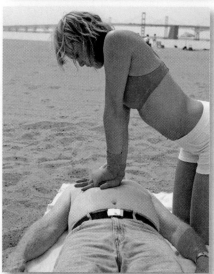

STEP 9 ▶ After 30 compressions, open the patient's airway and deliver 2 breaths.

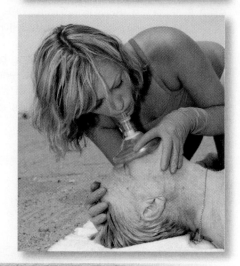

Two-Rescuer Adult Cardiopulmonary Resuscitation

STEP 1 ▷
- Make sure the scene is safe for providing emergency care. If the scene is safe, quickly check the patient's level of responsiveness. Gently squeeze the patient's shoulders and shout, "Are you all right?"
- If the patient does not respond, one rescuer should call for help.

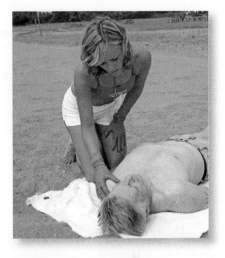

STEP 2 ▷
- If the patient is unresponsive and you do not suspect trauma, open his airway by using the head tilt–chin lift maneuver.

  —If trauma is suspected, open the airway by using the jaw thrust without head tilt maneuver.

  —If trauma is suspected but you are unable to maintain an open the airway by using the jaw thrust maneuver, open the airway by using the head tilt–chin lift maneuver.

- Suction any blood, vomit, or other fluid that may be present from the patient's airway.

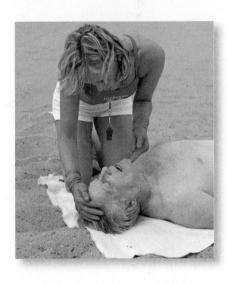

STEP 3 ▷ Place your face near the patient and look, listen, and feel for adequate breathing. Check for at least 5 seconds but not for more than 10 seconds.

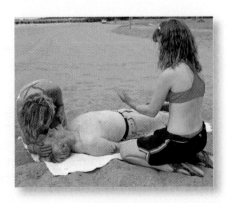

continued on next page

Two-Rescuer Adult Cardiopulmonary Resuscitation *(continued)*

STEP 4 ▷   If the patient's breathing is not adequate, the first rescuer should begin rescue breathing by using a pocket mask, mouth-to-barrier device, or BM device. Give 2 breaths (each breath over 1 second), with just enough pressure to make the chest rise with each breath.

—If the first rescue breath does not result in chest rise, reposition the patient's head and try again to ventilate.
—If there is still no chest rise, move on to the next step.

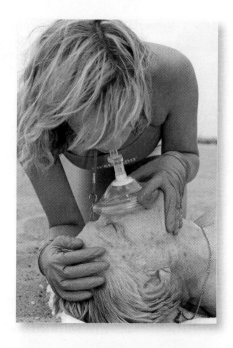

STEP 5 ▷   • The first rescuer should assess the carotid pulse on the side of the patient's neck nearest the rescuer. Feel for a pulse for 5 to 10 seconds.
     • If you definitely feel a pulse, give 1 breath every 5 to 6 seconds. Reassess the patient's pulse every 2 minutes. If you do not definitely feel a pulse within 10 seconds, or if you are uncertain, begin chest compressions.

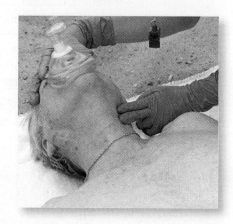

STEP 6 ▷   • If there is no pulse, begin cycles of 30 compressions and 2 breaths.
     • The second rescuer should kneel beside the patient's chest and then place the heel of one hand in the center of the patient's chest, between the nipples.
     • The rescuer should then place her other hand on top of the first, interlocking the fingers of both hands to keep her fingers off the patient's ribs.

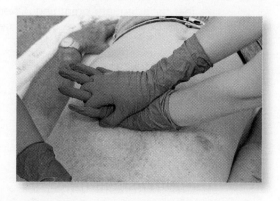

STEP 7 ▶ Position yourself directly above the patient's chest so that your shoulders are directly over your hands.

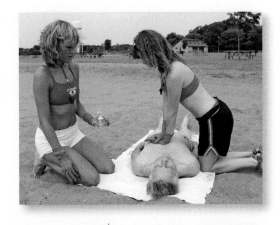

STEP 8 ▶ • With your arms straight and your elbows locked, press down about $1\frac{1}{2}$–2 inches on the patient's breastbone with the heels of your hands. Compress at a rate of 100 per minute.
• Release pressure (let up) after each compression to allow the patient's chest to recoil.

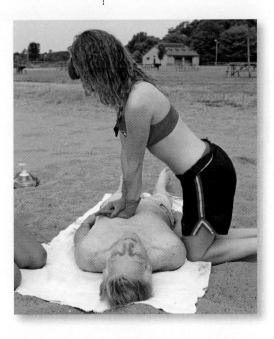

STEP 9 ▶ After 30 compressions, the first rescuer should open the patient's airway and deliver 2 breaths.

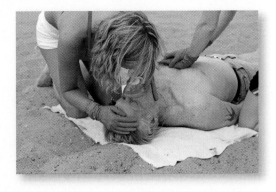

continued on next page

Two-Rescuer Adult Cardiopulmonary Resuscitation *(continued)*

STEP 10 ▶   Because performing chest compressions is tiring, rescuers should switch roles about every 2 minutes or 5 cycles of CPR. The "switch" should ideally take place in 5 seconds or less.

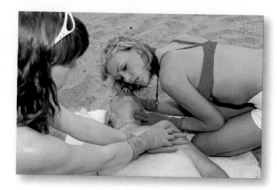

One-Rescuer Child Cardiopulmonary Resuscitation

STEP 1 ▶
- Make sure the scene is safe for providing emergency care. If the scene is safe, quickly check the patient's level of responsiveness. Gently squeeze the patient's shoulders and shout, "Are you all right?"
- If the patient does not respond, you are alone, and you saw the child collapse, phone for help and get an AED, and then begin CPR.
- If the child does not respond, you are alone, and you did not witness the child's collapse, begin CPR. After about 2 minutes of CPR, phone for help and get an AED.

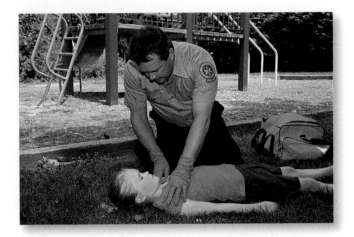

STEP 2 ▶
- If the patient is unresponsive and you do not suspect trauma, open the airway by using the head tilt–chin lift maneuver. Push down on the child's forehead with one hand. Place the fingers of your other hand on the bony part of the chin. Gently lift the chin.

  —If trauma is suspected, open the airway by using the jaw thrust without head tilt maneuver.

  —If trauma is suspected but you are unable to maintain an open the airway by using the jaw thrust maneuver, open the airway by using the head tilt–chin lift maneuver.

- Look for an actual or a potential airway obstruction, such as a foreign body, blood, vomit, teeth, or the patient's tongue. Suction the airway if necessary.

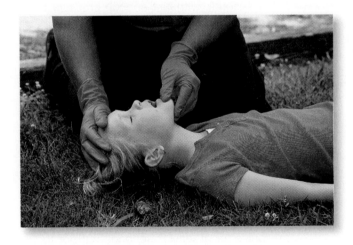

continued on next page

One-Rescuer Child Cardiopulmonary Resuscitation *(continued)*

STEP 3 ▶ Hold the airway open and look, listen, and feel for breathing for at least 5 seconds but not for more than 10 seconds.

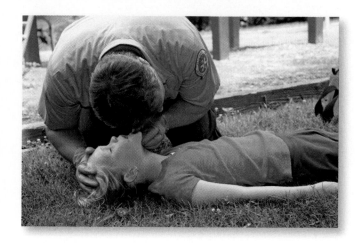

STEP 4 ▶ If the patient's breathing is not adequate, begin rescue breathing by using a pocket mask, mouth-to-barrier device, or BM device. Give 2 breaths (each breath over 1 second), with just enough pressure to make the chest gently rise with each breath.

—If the first rescue breath does not result in chest rise, reposition the patient's head and try again to ventilate.

—If there is still no chest rise, move on to the next step.

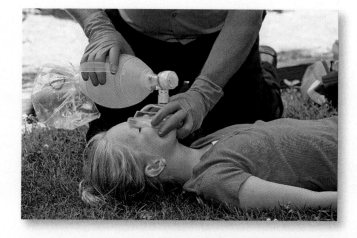

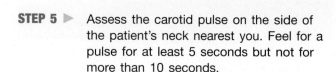

STEP 5 ▶ Assess the carotid pulse on the side of the patient's neck nearest you. Feel for a pulse for at least 5 seconds but not for more than 10 seconds.

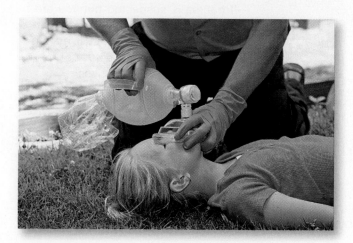

STEP 6 ▶ • If you definitely feel a pulse, give 1 breath every 3 to 5 seconds. Reassess the patient's pulse every 2 minutes. If you do not definitely feel a pulse within 10 seconds, if you are uncertain, or if a pulse is present but the heart rate is less than 60 beats/ min with signs of poor perfusion (pale, cool, mottled skin), begin chest compressions.

• Begin cycles of 30 compressions and 2 breaths. Kneel beside the patient's chest. Place the heel of one hand in the center of the patient's chest, between the nipples. Use one or two hands as needed to compress the child's chest 1/3 to 1/2 the depth of the chest. Give compressions at a rate of about 100 per minute.

• Release pressure (let up) after each compression to allow the patient's chest to recoil.

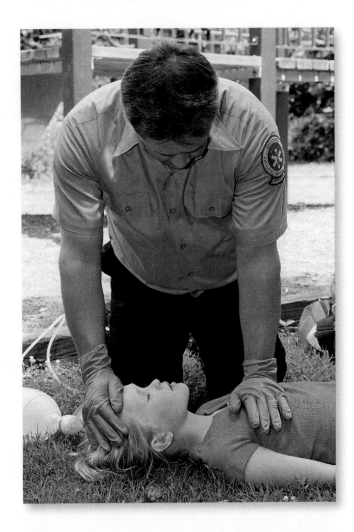

STEP 7 ▶ After 30 compressions, open the airway and deliver 2 breaths.

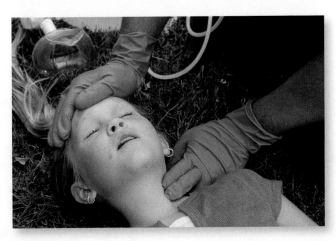

One-Rescuer Infant Cardiopulmonary Resuscitation

STEP 1 ▶
- Make sure the scene is safe for providing emergency care. If the scene is safe, quickly check the infant's level of responsiveness (if the infant is not obviously awake) by gently tapping the infant's feet.
- If the patient does not respond, you are alone, and you saw the infant collapse, phone for help and then begin CPR.
- If the infant does not respond, you are alone, and you did not witness the infant's collapse, begin CPR. After about 2 minutes of CPR, phone for help, then resume CPR.

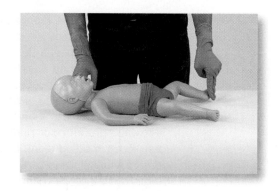

STEP 2 ▶ If the infant is unresponsive and you do not suspect trauma, open his airway by using the head tilt–chin lift maneuver.

 —If trauma is suspected, open the airway by using the jaw thrust without head tilt maneuver.
 —If trauma is suspected but you are unable to maintain an open the airway by using the jaw thrust maneuver, open the airway by using the head tilt–chin lift maneuver.

- Suction any blood, vomit, or other fluid that may be present from the infant's airway.

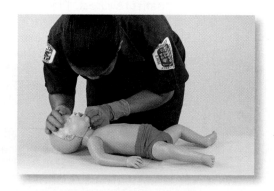

STEP 3 ▶ Hold the airway open and look, listen, and feel for breathing for at least 5 second but not for more than 10 seconds.

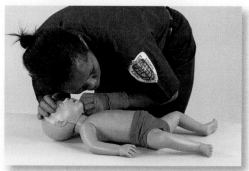

STEP 4 ▶ If the patient's breathing is not adequate, begin rescue breathing by using a pocket mask, mouth-to-barrier device, or BM device. Give 2 breaths (each breath over 1 second), with just enough pressure to make the chest gently rise with each breath.

 —If the first rescue breath does not result in chest rise, reposition the patient's head and try again to ventilate.
 —If there is still no chest rise, move on to the next step.

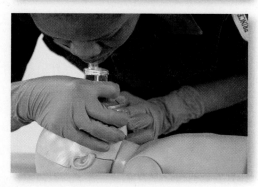

STEP 5 ▶ • Assess the brachial pulse on the inside of the upper arm. Feel for a pulse for at least 5 seconds but not for more than 10 seconds.

• If you definitely feel a pulse, give 1 breath every 3 to 5 seconds. Reassess the patient's pulse every 2 minutes. If you do not definitely feel a pulse within 10 seconds, if you are uncertain, or if a pulse is present but the heart rate is less than 60 beats/min with signs of poor perfusion (pale, cool, mottled skin), begin chest compressions.

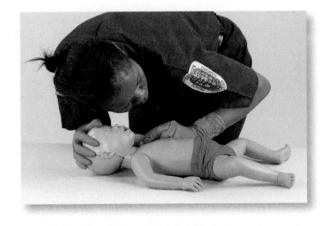

STEP 6 ▶ • Begin cycles of 30 compressions and 2 breaths. Imagine a line between the nipples. Place the flat part of your middle and ring fingers about one finger's width below this imaginary line. Use your other hand to hold the infant's head in a position that keeps the airway open.

• Give compressions at a rate of about 100 per minute. Depress the breastbone 1/3 to 1/2 the depth of the chest.

• Release pressure (let up) after each compression to allow the infant's chest to recoil.

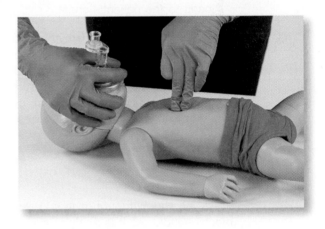

STEP 7 ▶ After 30 compressions, open the airway and deliver 2 breaths.

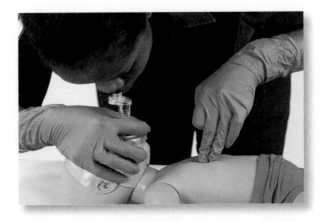

Adult Automated External Defibrillator Sequence

STEP 1 ▶
- If you arrive on the scene and see an adult collapse (you witness a cardiac arrest), assess the patient's airway, breathing, and circulation, and then quickly apply an AED. Perform CPR until the AED is ready. Your medical director may recommend that if you arrive at the scene of an adult cardiac arrest, did not witness the patient's collapse, and your response time is more than 4 to 5 minutes, provide 5 cycles of CPR (about 2 minutes) and then analyze the patient's rhythm with an AED.
- Be sure the patient is lying face up on a firm, flat surface. Place the AED near the rescuer who will be operating it. Turn on the power of the AED. If more than one rescuer is present, one rescuer should continue CPR while the other readies the AED for use. One rescuer should apply the AED pads to the patient's chest.

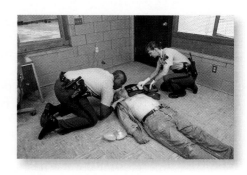

STEP 2 ▶ Analyze the patient's heart rhythm. Do not touch the patient while the AED is analyzing the rhythm. If the AED advises that a shock is indicated, check the patient from head to toe to make sure no one is touching the patient (including you) before pressing the shock control. Shout, "Stand clear!"

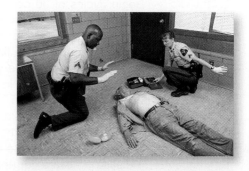

STEP 3 ▶ Press the shock control once it is illuminated and the machine indicates it is ready to deliver the shock.

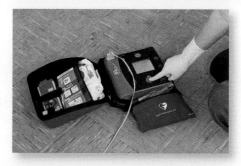

STEP 4 ▶ After delivery of the shock, quickly resume CPR, beginning with chest compressions. After about 2 minutes of CPR, reanalyze the rhythm.

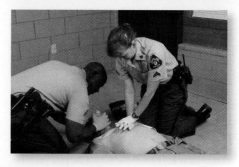

Clearing a Foreign Body Airway Obstruction in a Conscious Adult

STEP 1 ▶
- Find out if the patient can speak or cough. Ask, "Are you choking?"
- If the patient can cough or speak, encourage him to cough out the obstruction. Watch him closely to make sure the object is expelled.

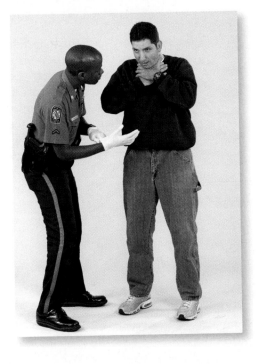

STEP 2 ▶
- If the patient cannot cough or speak, perform abdominal thrusts (the Heimlich maneuver).
- Stand behind the patient and wrap your arms around his waist.
- Make a fist with one hand. Place your fist, thumb side in, just above the patient's navel.

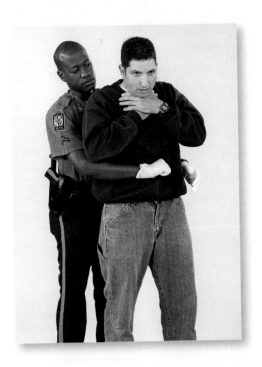

continued on next page

Clearing a Foreign Body Airway Obstruction in a Conscious Adult *(continued)*

STEP 3 ▶
- Grab your fist tightly with your other hand. Pull your fist quickly inward and upward.
- Continue performing abdominal thrusts until the foreign body is expelled or the patient becomes unresponsive. Perform each abdominal thrust with the intent of relieving the obstruction. If abdominal thrusts are not effective, consider the use of chest thrusts to relieve the obstruction.

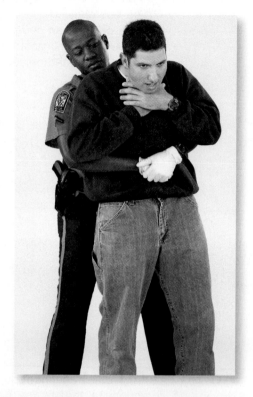

STEP 4 ▶ If your patient is obese or in the later stages of pregnancy, perform chest thrusts instead of abdominal thrusts:

—Place your arms around the patient's chest, directly under the armpits. Press your hands backward, giving quick thrusts into the middle of the breastbone. Do not place your hands on the patient's ribs or on the bottom of the breastbone (xiphoid process). The xiphoid process can easily be broken off the breastbone and can cut underlying organs, such as the liver.

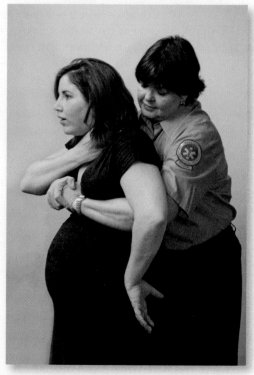

Clearing a Foreign Body Airway Obstruction in an Unconscious Adult

STEP 1 ▷
- Make sure the scene is safe for providing emergency care. If the scene is safe, quickly check the patient's level of responsiveness. Gently squeeze the patient's shoulders and shout, "Are you all right?" If the patient does not respond, shout for help.
- If the patient is unresponsive and you do not suspect trauma, open his airway by using the head tilt–chin lift maneuver. If trauma is suspected, open the airway by using the jaw thrust without head tilt maneuver. If trauma is suspected but you are unable to maintain an open airway by using the jaw thrust maneuver, open the airway by using the head tilt–chin lift maneuver.
- Check the nose and mouth for secretions, vomit, a foreign body, or other obstruction. Suction fluids from the airway as needed. If you *see* a solid object in the patient's upper airway, remove it. Do not blindly sweep the mouth in search of a foreign object.

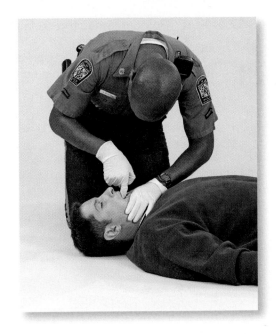

STEP 2 ▷
- Place your face near the patient and look, listen, and feel for adequate breathing. Check for at least 5 seconds but not for more than 10 seconds.
- If the patient's breathing is not adequate, begin rescue breathing by using a pocket mask, mouth-to-barrier device, or BM device. Give 2 breaths (each breath over 1 second), with just enough pressure to make the chest rise with each breath.

  —If the first rescue breath does not result in chest rise, reposition the patient's head and try again to ventilate.

  —If there is still no chest rise, begin CPR. Check the patient's mouth for the foreign body each time you open the airway to give rescue breaths. If you see a solid object in the patient's upper airway, remove it. If no foreign body is seen, continue CPR.

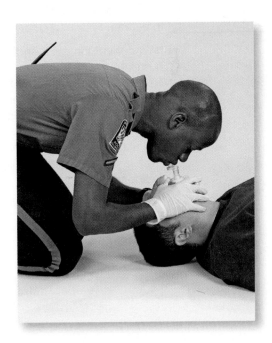

Clearing a Foreign Body Airway Obstruction in a Conscious Child

STEP 1 ▶
- Find out if the child can speak or cough. Ask, "Are you choking?"
- If the patient can cough or speak, encourage her to cough out the obstruction. Watch her closely to make sure the object is expelled.

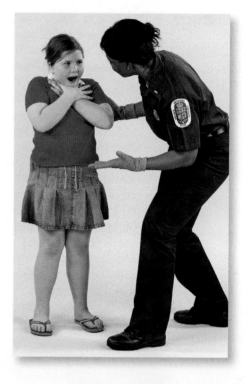

STEP 2 ▶ If the child cannot cough or speak, perform abdominal thrusts (the Heimlich maneuver).

—Stand behind the child and wrap your arms around her waist.
—Make a fist with one hand. Place your fist, thumb side in, just above the patient's navel. Grab your fist tightly with your other hand. Pull your fist quickly inward and upward.
—Continue performing abdominal thrusts until the object is expelled or the child becomes unresponsive.

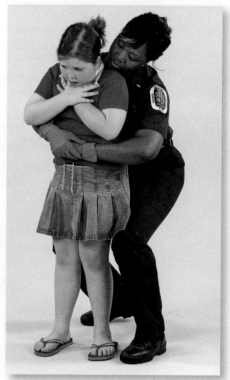

Clearing a Foreign Body Airway Obstruction in an Unconscious Child

STEP 1 ▶
- Make sure the scene is safe for providing emergency care. If the scene is safe, quickly assess the child's level of responsiveness. Gently squeeze the patient's shoulders and shout, "Are you all right?" If the patient does not respond, shout for help.
- If the child is unresponsive and you do not suspect trauma, open her airway by using the head tilt–chin lift maneuver. If trauma is suspected, open the airway by using the jaw thrust without head tilt maneuver. If trauma is suspected but you are unable to maintain an open the airway by using the jaw thrust maneuver, open the airway by using the head tilt–chin lift maneuver.
- Check the nose and mouth for secretions, vomit, a foreign body, or other obstruction. Suction fluids from the airway as needed. If you see a solid object in the patient's upper airway, remove it. Do not blindly sweep the mouth in search of a foreign object.

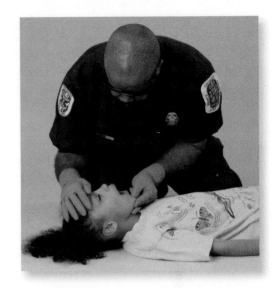

STEP 2 ▶
- Place your face near the patient and look, listen, and feel for adequate breathing. Check for at least 5 seconds but not for more than 10 seconds.
- If the patient's breathing is not adequate, begin rescue breathing by using a pocket mask, mouth-to-barrier device, or BM device. Give 2 breaths (each breath over 1 second), with just enough pressure to make the chest rise with each breath.

  —If the first rescue breath does not result in chest rise, reposition the patient's head and try again to ventilate.

  —If there is still no chest rise, begin CPR. Check the patient's mouth for the foreign body each time you open the airway to give rescue breaths. If you see a solid object in the patient's upper airway, remove it. If no foreign body is seen, continue CPR.

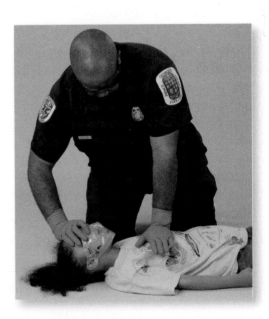

Clearing a Foreign Body Airway Obstruction in a Conscious Infant

STEP 1 ▶ While supporting the infant's head, place the infant facedown over your forearm. You may find it helpful to rest your forearm on your thigh to support the weight of the infant. Keep the infant's head slightly lower than the rest of the body.

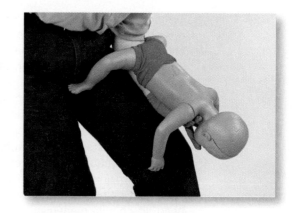

STEP 2 ▶ Using the heel of one hand, forcefully deliver up to 5 back blows (slaps) between the infant's shoulder blades.

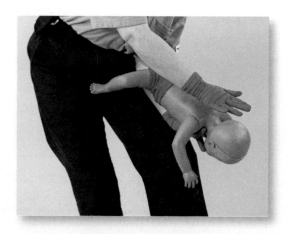

STEP 3 ▶ • If the foreign body is not expelled, deliver chest thrusts. Place your free hand on the infant's back. Turn the infant over onto his back while supporting the back of the head with the palm of your hand. Imagine a line between the infant's nipples. Place the flat part of one finger about one finger width below this imaginary line. Place a second finger next to the first on the infant's sternum. Deliver up to 5 downward chest thrusts at a rate of about 1 per second.
• Check the infant's mouth. If you see the foreign body, remove it.
• Continue alternating up to 5 back slaps and up to 5 chest thrusts and attempting to visualize the object until the object is expelled or the infant becomes unconscious.

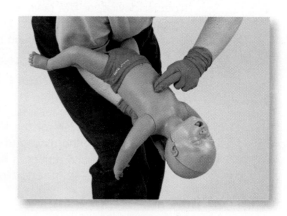

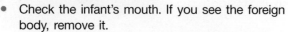

Clearing a Foreign Body Airway Obstruction in an Unconscious Infant

STEP 1 ▶
- Make sure the scene is safe for providing emergency care. If the scene is safe, quickly assess the infant's level of responsiveness. After confirming that the infant is unresponsive, place the infant on his back on a flat surface or on your forearm. Support the infant's head.
- If the infant is unresponsive and you do not suspect trauma, open his airway by using the head tilt–chin lift maneuver. If trauma is suspected, open the airway by using the jaw thrust without head tilt maneuver. If trauma is suspected but you are unable to maintain an open the airway by using the jaw thrust maneuver, open the airway by using the head tilt–chin lift maneuver.
- Check the nose and mouth for secretions, vomit, a foreign body, or other obstruction. Suction fluids from the airway as needed. If you see a solid object in the infant's upper airway, remove it. Do not blindly sweep the mouth in search of a foreign object.

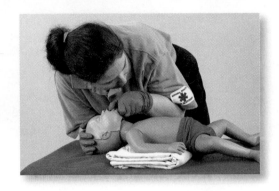

STEP 2 ▶
- Place your face near the infant and look, listen, and feel for adequate breathing. Check for at least 5 seconds but not for more than 10 seconds.
- If the infant's breathing is not adequate, begin rescue breathing by using a pocket mask, mouth-to-barrier device, or BM device. Give 2 breaths (each breath over 1 second), with just enough pressure to make the chest rise with each breath.

  —If the first rescue breath does not result in chest rise, reposition the patient's head and try again to ventilate.
  —If there is still no chest rise, begin CPR. Check the infant's mouth for the foreign body each time you open the airway to give rescue breaths. If you see a solid object in the infant's upper airway, remove it. If no foreign body is seen, continue CPR.

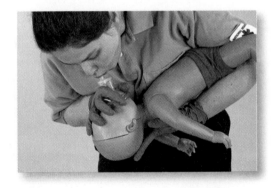

B Older Adults

Introduction

In 2003, the number of persons in the United States age 65 years or older was estimated at 35.9 million. That number is projected to grow to almost 71.5 million by 2030. The term *elderly* refers to persons 65 years of age and older. Elderly people are rapidly becoming the largest group of patients that are encountered in the prehospital setting (Figure AB-1).

Because of the advances in medical technology and treatment, patients are living longer with diseases that were once terminal or required prolonged hospitalization. This has resulted in prehospital professionals dealing with patients who have increased medical needs.

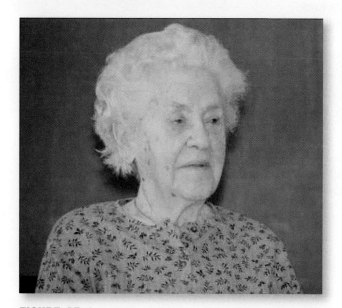

FIGURE AB-1 ▲ Elderly patients are rapidly becoming the largest group of patients that emergency personnel encounter in the prehospital setting. © *Administration on Aging.*

Many older adults have at least one chronic medical condition. Some have multiple medical conditions, such as high blood pressure, heart disease, and arthritis. Many of them are on multiple medications. Some may be technology dependent. Technology-dependent patients have special healthcare needs. These patients depend on medical devices for their survival. Although some elderly people have multiple medical conditions, do not assume that every elderly patient will have age-related health problems. Many elderly patients are healthy and active even into their later years.

You Should Know

Patients over the age of 65 are the largest population transported to the hospital by ambulance.

Communication During the Interview Process

Many physical changes take place as we age, including changes associated with hearing, vision, taste, smell, and touch. In addition, reaction times are slowed as a result of changes in the central nervous system. Most muscle and organ systems also undergo changes. Because of these changes, your patient may be unable to communicate with you at the speed you would like. *Be patient!* Allow the patient time to process your questions (Figure AB-2). Do not be too hasty in assuming that he has a hearing impairment or does not understand.

When communicating with your patients, be respectful and willing to listen. You can build trust by letting the patient know that you are interested in what he has to say. Do not use phrases such as "hon" or "dear" when speaking to an older adult. Phrases such as these are disrespectful and unprofessional. Address your patient as "Mr." or "Mrs." unless the patient instructs you to do otherwise.

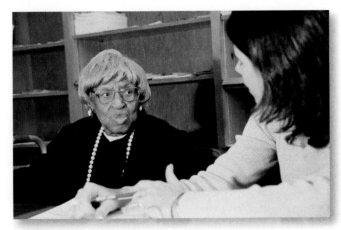

FIGURE AB-2 ▲ Be patient when speaking with an elderly person. Allow your patient time to process your questions. © *Administration on Aging.*

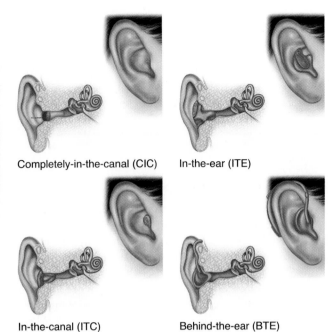

Completely-in-the-canal (CIC)   In-the-ear (ITE)

In-the-canal (ITC)   Behind-the-ear (BTE)

FIGURE AB-3 ▲ Examples of hearing aids.

Making a Difference

Your patients are individuals of varying ages with a wide range of life experiences, knowledge, reasoning abilities, skills, and medical needs. Remember this when providing care.

Hearing Impairments

Some patients will experience a loss of hearing that can lead to an inability to communicate. Because a patient has a hearing impairment does not mean that he lacks intelligence. Many deaf patients do not consider a lack of hearing a disability. In fact, they often resent being treated as if they have a disability.

A common mistaken belief of some emergency care professionals is that speaking more slowly and loudly than usual helps the patient understand. Not only does this not work, but it may actually confuse the patient. When you speak more slowly than normal, you have a tendency to overemphasize the way you move your mouth when you speak. This can lead to a greater misunderstanding if the patient is trying to read your lips. Try not to drastically change the way you speak. Use your normal tone of voice and speak at your normal speed—as if you were carrying on a conversation with any other patient.

If the patient has a sound amplification device or hearing aid, you may need to help him put it in place (Figure AB-3). Family members are a good resource because they have experience communicating with the patient regularly. Keep in mind that a hearing aid may not restore hearing to normal.

You may have to get your patient's attention with a gentle touch on the shoulder. Face your patient directly so that he can see your face and mouth.

Make sure that there is adequate lighting so the patient can see your face and mouth clearly. When speaking, do not move your head around. Doing so makes it difficult for the patient to follow what you are saying. If the patient has some limited ability to hear, try to reduce any unnecessary background noise. For example, shut off televisions, radios, dishwashers, or other noisy appliances while talking with the patient. You may even resort to the use of paper and pen to communicate.

When questioning your patient about his condition, think about the questions you want to ask. Then ask him short, direct questions that require a very specific answer. Make sure to actually speak or say every word in your question. Ask one question at a time and follow up on the answer before starting another line of questioning. Doing so will allow you and the patient to focus on one problem at a time. It can even lead to a better interview. It is unlikely that the patient or a family member will understand confusing medical terms. Use common terms when asking questions and explaining the care you will provide. Avoid the use of sign language unless you are very skilled.

Your treatment of a hearing-impaired patient should be based on his medical condition. The care you provide will generally not require extraordinary changes in your usual treatment plan. Remember to explain any procedure before providing care. When transferring patient care, be sure to inform the receiving healthcare professional of the patient's hearing impairment.

- Not all hearing-impaired people hear the same sounds in the same way.
- Keep in mind that family members have a tendency to reword your questions and the patient's answers.

Speech Impairments

Many patients can experience speech difficulties as a result of a brain injury or a lack of oxygen to the brain. For example, a stroke patient may be unable to speak but may be able to understand your questions. You may be able to establish some other means of communication, such as a hand squeeze or even eye blinks. If your patient appears to understand your questions but is unable to answer, stop asking the questions but continue to talk to the patient. Let him know that you understand he is unable to talk. It may be comforting to the patient to know that you are aware of his situation.

Children and adults may have language problems that stem from a hearing impairment, a congenital learning disorder, a speech delay, or cerebral palsy. Other speech problems may occur when a patient has difficulty with his speech pattern, such as stuttering. A patient who has cancer of the larynx may have a hoarseness or harshness in his voice. Such patients may have only a limited ability to respond to your questions. Try to keep your questions short and to the point. In some situations, it may be helpful to ask questions that can be answered with a yes or no. Allow the patient time to respond in his own way. Rushing the patient to answer may only increase his anxiety and frustration. Pay attention and listen carefully to what the patient has to say. He may even use hand gestures or a notepad to communicate his needs.

Your treatment of a patient with speech impairment should be based on his medical condition. The care you provide will generally not require unusual changes in your treatment plan.

You Should Know

Sometimes a person's inability to say certain sounds or words is only temporary. For example, a person who has ingested too much alcohol or taken too many narcotics may slur his words, use words incorrectly, or be unable to recall some words.

Making a Difference

Never assume that a person who cannot speak clearly lacks intelligence. A severe speech deficit can be completely unrelated to intelligence.

Vision Impairments

The term *visual impairment* applies to a variety of vision disturbances. Visual impairments range from blindness and lack of usable sight to low vision. **Low vision** is a visual impairment that interferes with a person's ability to perform everyday activities. It cannot be corrected to normal vision with standard eyeglasses, contact lenses, medicine, or surgery. Low vision can result from a variety of diseases, disorders, and injuries that affect the eye.

A patient may have a visual impairment as a result of a medical emergency, a traumatic injury, or a preexisting condition. As a general rule, a patient who has a sudden change in vision needs immediate transport to the closest appropriate medical facility. A vision change may be due to a lack of oxygen to the brain. It may also result from physical damage to the eyes, the optic nerve, or even the brain. If the vision disturbance is due to a preexisting condition, continue with your assessment and treatment.

When communicating with a blind patient, begin by identifying yourself in a normal voice. Most blind persons are not hearing impaired, so there is no need to raise your voice or shout when talking to them. If family members or others are present, address the patient by name so that it is clear to whom you are talking. Clearly explain any care you are going to provide before doing so. In this way, you do not surprise or startle the patient. Be sure to talk directly to the patient, not through a family member.

If the patient requires evaluation at the hospital, guide your patient carefully to the stretcher if he is able to walk. Offer the patient your arm and let him hold on just above your elbow. Guide the patient by leading him. It can be very helpful to "verbalize" the location of your equipment. When giving directions, indicate left and right according to the way the patient is facing.

A very strong bond can form between a visually impaired patient and his guide dog. Make every attempt to keep them together if at all possible. Do not pet or otherwise distract a guide dog. A blind person's safety depends on the animal's full attention. If the animal has been injured, contact your dispatcher for the appropriate care as soon as possible.

Altered Mental Status

You may be called to assess an elderly patient with an altered mental status. One of your first goals must be to determine the patient's normal level of consciousness. It may be difficult for you to find out whether the patient's symptoms are due to a medical emergency or an ongoing (chronic) medical problem, or are a part of normal aging. To help find out what the patient's normal mental status is, ask someone who knows the patient to give you this information. For example, ask a family member or neighbor how the patient appears to him today. Ask the family, "What is different today? Is he confused? Behaving inappropriately? Having hallucinations? Does his speech sound normal to you?" Then ask the person providing information to compare how your patient appears today with how he was 2 or 3 days ago.

Medications

Some older adults are on several medications because they have multiple medical problems. If your elderly patient's chief complaint is unclear or does not seem to fall within the "normal" signs and symptoms of a particular disease, it may be due to his not taking his medication as prescribed. The patient may not take his pills at all, may take them every now and then, or may accidentally overdose from taking too much medication.

A patient who is not taking his medication as prescribed may be doing so because he simply cannot afford it. Some prescribed medications are expensive. Many older adults are on fixed incomes and may have to choose between taking their medicine or paying for food and utilities. Some older adults see several doctors. If they fail to tell each doctor about the drugs another physician has prescribed, they may be prescribed drugs that can cause serious health problems when taken with the other medicines. Be respectful but firm when questioning the patient about his medical history, including any prescribed medicines and their proper dosages.

Some of the medicines that older adults take can "hide" the signs and symptoms of other illness. For example, some patients take heart or blood pressure medicines that keep the heart rate low. If they have a blood loss, the drug will prevent the heart rate from increasing to compensate for the shock. When you assess them, you may think that they are stable because the heart rate remains normal despite shock.

Pain Perception

If your older adult patient is complaining of pain or discomfort, ask carefully worded questions about the discomfort he is having. Because pain sensation can be lessened or absent in older adults, the patient can easily misjudge how serious his condition is. Older adults may live with chronic pain and "underreport" the discomfort associated with their current medical problem. Asking an older adult to rate his discomfort on a scale from 0 to 10 may not give a true picture of the pain he is experiencing. Look for visual cues that your patient is in pain. For example, grimacing, wincing, or stiff muscles may be indicators that the patient is experiencing pain.

The elderly patient may not tell you about important symptoms because he is afraid of being hospitalized. He may be afraid that once he is at the hospital, he will never come home or he may not be able to make decisions about his care. Try to reassure the patient that he will receive the best of care from the hospital. It is extremely important to acknowledge these fears, as they are often justified concerns. You have a greater chance of successfully transporting your patient for appropriate care if you simply listen with empathy to his concerns and carefully explain what you will be doing and what the patient can anticipate at the hospital. Often, encouraging a loved one to meet you at the hospital will help diffuse fears of loss of control.

Physical Examination Considerations

Physical examination of the elderly patient can be a real challenge. Conduct your physical examination in the same general order as with patients in other age groups. Make sure to explain any procedure or exam that you are going to perform before actually performing it or touching the patient. This explanation is especially important when examining an older adult with a vision problem. Remember to be sensitive to the patient's modesty.

Older adults often wear multiple layers of clothing, which can get in the way of your exam. Keep in mind that an elderly patient's temperature-regulating system becomes depressed. An elderly patient's temperature may generally be lower than normal because of a slower metabolic rate and decreased activity. In

You Should Know

Elder abuse is on the rise. If you survey the scene and find evidence of violence or neglect, it should be reported as soon as possible so that police can treat the scene as a possible crime scene and the violence can stop.

addition, the skin loses subcutaneous fat and becomes less effective at responding to changes in heat or cold. Some medications change the body's ability to control temperature. As a result of these factors, the elderly are more likely to be affected by environmental temperature extremes. They may also tire easily and have difficulty tolerating the exam.

Remember This!

An older adult who has fallen and has lain on the floor for many hours may have a low body temperature.

It can be hard to tell the difference between signs of a medical emergency and those of an ongoing medical condition. For example, the patient's breathing may be very quiet because older adults often do not breathe as fast or as deeply or move as much air as a younger person. An older adult's cough reflex is diminished, decreasing his ability to clear secretions. The patient may have an underlying respiratory problem that causes him to have noisy respirations. On the other hand, these findings can also be signs of a respiratory emergency. Swelling of the legs may be due to poor circulation and inactivity, or it may be due to a heart problem.

Making a Difference

As many as 20% of older adults who seek emergency care are malnourished. The physical signs of malnutrition are not always easy to spot. While you are in a patient's home, take a moment to look around you. Does the patient have adequate food in the house? Is he able to prepare food for himself? Also look for hazards in the home that can contribute to falls, such as extension cords, loose rugs, slick or wet floors, inadequate lighting, a lack of stair or bath rails, and uneven flooring. Be sure to let appropriate personnel within your organization and/or at the receiving facility know your findings.

Use care when taking an older adult's blood pressure. An elderly patient's skin is often dry, thin, transparent, and wrinkled. Capillaries are fragile, and the skin bruises easily. Your patient may also be on medications, such as steroids, that can cause the skin to become thin and tear easily.

The physical changes associated with aging must be considered when immobilizing an older adult or moving the patient from his home to an ambulance. As we age, bones become brittle. In addition, muscle fibers decrease in number and become weaker. The curves of the cervical and thoracic spine become more pronounced. Cartilage in the joints breaks down, resulting in stiffness and a loss of flexibility. Rough handling may cause tissue damage or even fractures. Padding a backboard may be necessary to allow for changes in the shape of the patient's spine. Use gentle care when moving your patient.

C Intravenous Monitoring

Introduction

Intravenous (IV) monitoring by an Emergency Medical Technician (EMT) is most likely to occur in Emergency Medical Services (EMS) systems with limited Advanced Life Support (ALS) personnel. If permitted to do so by state law, your ability to assist with this procedure will be a significant benefit to your ALS partner and to your patient's well-being.

Purpose of Intravenous Therapy

The word **intravenous** means "within a vein." **Intravenous (IV) cannulation** is the placement of a catheter (also called a *cannula*) into a vein to gain access to the body's venous circulation. Although starting an IV is considered an ALS skill, you may be required to monitor an IV after it has been started by an ALS provider. Proper protective equipment must be worn while monitoring any IV or handling any IV equipment.

The technique of piercing a patient's vein with a needle is called **venipuncture.** Venipuncture is performed to withdraw a blood sample from a patient and to give IV fluids or medications. **Intravenous therapy** is the giving of a liquid substance, such as IV fluids or medications, directly into the venous circulation.

Types of Intravenous Access

A patient's venous circulation is usually accessed by using peripheral veins. The veins of the arm, hand, and sometimes the neck, are most commonly used. If an infant is ill or injured and an arm or hand vein is not readily accessible, an ALS provider may choose to use the veins on the infant's scalp as an alternate IV site. An IV catheter inserted into a peripheral vein is referred to as a *peripheral line* or *peripheral IV.* A peripheral IV provides an effective route for giving fluids and medications. If an ALS provider is unsuccessful at starting a peripheral IV, direct pressure can be easily applied to the site to control bleeding. You may be asked to apply direct pressure to the site while an ALS provider attempts an IV start in a different peripheral vein.

Inserting an IV catheter into one of the body's major veins is called **central venous access.** The subclavian and internal jugular veins are examples of central veins that ALS providers typically access. An IV catheter that is inserted into a central vein is commonly referred to as a *central line.* A central line provides a more direct route to the venous circulation than a peripheral IV line. Central venous access requires more skill than insertion of a peripheral IV line. It is also associated with a higher rate of complications.

A patient who has a long-term illness may have a special type of central line in place. Common central IV catheters inserted for long-term use include the Hickman catheter and Broviac catheter. By having such a catheter in place, the patient is exposed to fewer needle sticks and IV starts.

Types and Sizes of Intravenous Catheters

Types of Intravenous Catheters

There are several types of IV catheters. A hollow needle IV catheter is made of steel and has flexible plastic wings (Figure AC-1). A hollow needle is also called a *butterfly catheter, scalp vein needle,* or *winged infusion set.* When this type of IV catheter is used, the ALS provider holds onto the wings of the device and then pierces the patient's skin with the metal needle.

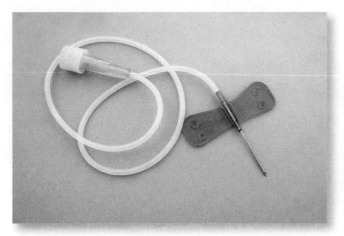

FIGURE AC-1 ▲ A hollow needle IV catheter is also called a *butterfly catheter.*

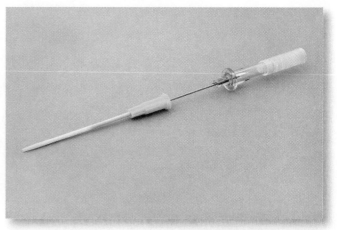

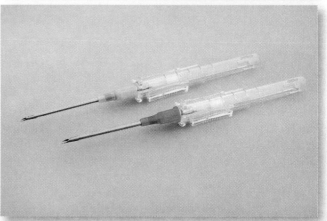

Once the vein has been entered, the needle remains in place and is secured with tape.

The most common type of IV catheter used is an over-the-needle catheter. There are many manufacturers of this type of IV catheter, such as Angiocath, Jelco, and Insyte, to name a few. As its name implies, an over-the-needle catheter consists of a hollow IV needle that is surrounded by a soft catheter made of plastic or plastic-like material (Figure AC-2). The length of the catheter is limited by the length of the needle. The plastic hub of the catheter is rigid and remains outside the skin. It varies in color depending on the size of the catheter. When an over-the-needle catheter is used, the ALS provider pierces the patient's skin and vein with the needle. Once the vein has been entered, the catheter is slid into the vein and the needle is withdrawn. The catheter is then secured in place. The hub of the IV catheter is then connected to IV tubing, which is connected to a bag containing IV solution. Medications and fluids can then be given through the IV tubing to the patient.

Needle Size

A needle's gauge refers to its outside diameter. Gauge is expressed as a number. The smaller the number, the larger the diameter. For example, a 10-gauge needle has a very large diameter. A 26-gauge needle has a very small diameter. The length of an IV catheter varies from 1/2 inch to 3 inches, depending on the catheter's gauge.

IV needles that have a gauge of 16 or less are considered "large-bore" IV catheters. An ALS provider will use a 12-, 14-, or 16-gauge IV needle when a large volume of fluid must be given over a short period or when he anticipates the patient's condition may quickly worsen (Figure AC-3). He will use an 18- or 20-gauge IV needle for an older child, adolescent, or adult patient who has stable vital signs. A 22-gauge IV needle is often used for

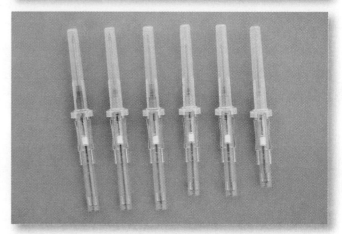

FIGURE AC-2 ▲ Over-the-needle catheters.

young children. A 24- or 26-gauge IV needle is usually used for newborns, infants, children, and adults who have fragile veins (Figure AC-4).

Saline Lock

A saline lock is used in some EMS systems. A **saline lock** is an IV catheter that has a medication port on its end (Figure AC-5). It is used when a patient needs (or is likely to need) IV medications but does not need IV fluid.

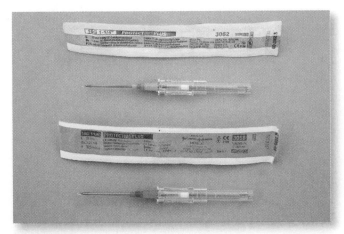

FIGURE AC-3 ▲ Examples of "large-bore" IV needles.

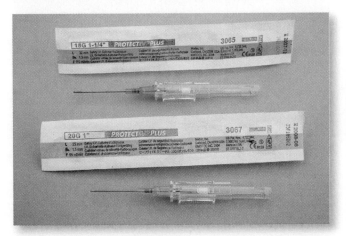

(a)

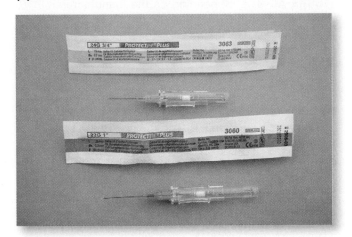

(b)

FIGURE AC-4 ▲ **(a)** Examples of 18- and 20-gauge IV needles. **(b)** Examples of 22- and 24-gauge IV needles.

Intravenous Administration Tubing

Although IV drugs can be given directly into a vein with a needle and syringe, this method of drug administration is uncommon. Drugs are more com-

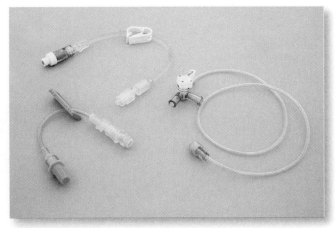

FIGURE AC-5 ▲ A saline lock is an IV catheter that has a medication port on its end.

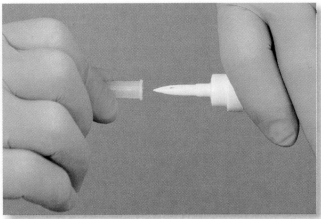

FIGURE AC-6 ▲ Be careful not to contaminate the spike on an IV administration set when removing its protective sheath.

monly given intermittently or by continuous infusion. IV drugs may be given rapidly (bolus) or slowly (infusion) directly into the bloodstream. An **intravenous drip** (also called an *IV infusion*) is the continuous administration of a drug or fluids by means of an IV line.

Once an IV catheter has been inserted into a vein, it is connected to IV tubing. Other names for IV tubing include a *primary IV set* and an *IV administration set*. An IV administration set consists of clear tubing that is usually 60 inches in length or longer. The tubing is packaged in a sterile container. One end of the IV tubing has a pointed end that is sharp. This is called the *spike*. When the IV tubing is removed from its sterile packaging, the spike has a protective covering to keep it sterile. The protective sheath must be removed before the spike is inserted into a port on the bag of IV solution (Figure AC-6). *Do not use your teeth* to remove the sheath. Nonvented spikes are used for collapsible IV bags, such as those used in the field.

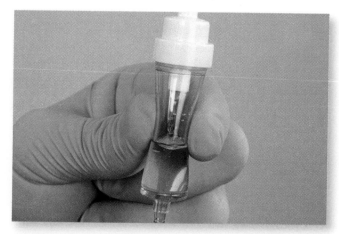

FIGURE AC-7 ▲ When filling IV tubing with solution from an IV bag for the first time, squeeze the drip chamber until it is about 1/3 to 1/2 full.

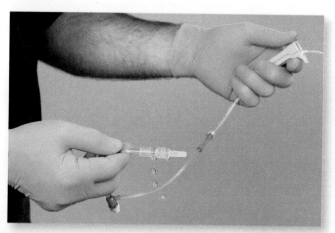

FIGURE AC-8 ▲ Close the clamp on the IV tubing when IV fluid drips from its end.

Vented spikes are used for noncollapsible IV bottles. Inserting the spike tip into the IV bag is called *spiking the bag*. It is very important not to contaminate the spike when inserting its tip into the IV bag.

Remember This!

When spiking an IV bag, hold the bag and connected IV tubing at about a 45-degree angle, with the bag above the tubing. Squeeze the drip chamber once or twice to move fluid into the end of the chamber. Holding the bag and tubing at an angle will decrease the number of air bubbles that you must clear from the tubing.

A clear drip chamber attached to the IV tubing enables you to see fluid flowing from the bag through the tubing, one drop at a time. When the IV tubing is filled with solution from the IV bag for the first time,

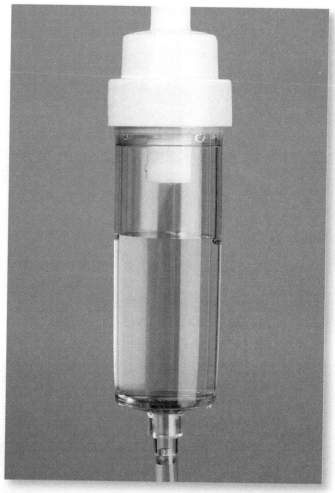

FIGURE AC-9 ▲ Depending on the manufacturer, macrodrip IV tubing can deliver 10, 15, or 20 drops per milliliter of IV fluid.

the drip chamber is squeezed until it is about 1/3 to 1/2 full (Figure AC-7). A clamp (also called a *flow regulator*) attached to the tubing allows you to set and monitor how quickly or slowly the fluid flows through the tubing. When the IV tubing is initially filled with solution, the clamp is slowly opened and the cap at the end of the tubing is loosened but not removed. This is called *priming the tubing* and allows air to be flushed from the tubing. If air bubbles are present, the tubing is flicked with a finger to remove them. The clamp is then closed when IV fluid drips from the end of the tubing (Figure AC-8). If the cap at the end of the tubing is removed and the exposed tubing contacts the ground, floor, bed, or other contaminated surface, it must be replaced with a clean administration set.

The drops visible in the drip chamber of the IV tubing vary in size depending on the type of IV administration set used. A **macrodrip IV administration set** forms large drops of IV fluid. Depending on the manufacturer, macrodrip IV tubing can deliver 10, 15, or 20 drops per milliliter of IV fluid (Figure AC-9). A

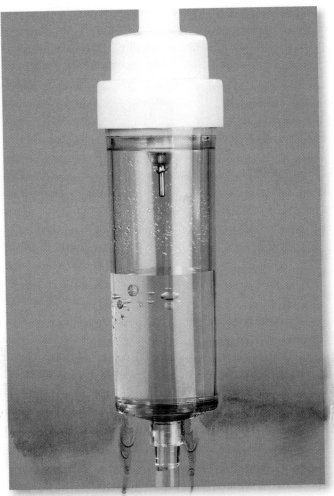

FIGURE AC-10 ▲ A microdrip administration delivers 60 drops per milliliter of IV fluid.

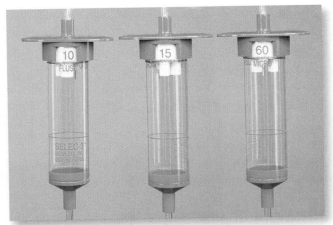

FIGURE AC-11 ▲ Some products function as a multipurpose IV set, allowing delivery of 10, 15, or 60 drops per milliliter of IV fluid.

microdrip IV administration set (also called a *minidrip*) forms very small drops, delivering 60 drops per milliliter of IV fluid (Figure AC-10). Some products function as a multipurpose IV set, allowing for the delivery of 10, 15, or 60 drops per milliliter (Figure AC-11).

The type of IV administration set used will depend on the reason the IV was started. For example, macrodrip IV tubing is used when it is known or anticipated that the patient will need a large amount of fluid. A microdrip IV administration set is used in situations where a patient needs an IV line for possible medication administration but does not need a large volume of IV fluid. For instance, an ALS provider may start an IV in a patient with congestive heart failure (CHF) to give him drugs that will help him eliminate excess fluid from his body. Because a patient in CHF does not need additional IV fluid, a microdrip IV administration set (or saline lock) is used.

When the bag of IV solution and administration set has been assembled, the patient is readied for the venipuncture. If the venipuncture is successful, the clamp on the IV tubing is opened and then the flow rate is regulated. If the IV bag is placed above the level of the patient, the fluid from the bag will flow into the patient by gravity. Some EMS systems use IV infusion pumps, which allow better control over the flow rate and amount of fluid delivered.

Making a Difference

ALS Assist

There may be instances when you are asked to assist an ALS provider in preparing an IV administration set. While this practice may be commonplace in some areas, you should be aware of the responsibility and liability that you incur when assisting in this way. Always confirm that you are not exceeding your scope of practice. Know your state rules and regulations concerning this practice.

Calculating Intravenous Flow Rates

When monitoring an IV, you will be expected to calculate the infusion rate of the IV solution. In order to calculate an IV infusion rate, there are three things you must know:

1. The amount (volume) of IV solution to be infused
2. The time over which the fluid is to be infused
3. The number of drops per milliliter (also called the *drop factor*) that the IV administration set delivers

Once this information is known, you can calculate the IV infusion rate (in drops per minute) by using the following formula:

$$\frac{\text{Volume to be infused} \times \text{drop factor (drops/mL) of IV set}}{\text{Total time of infusion in minutes}} = \text{Drops/min}$$

Example #1. Your patient is to receive 250 mL of IV solution over 20 minutes. The IV administration set delivers 10 drops (gtt) per milliliter. How many drops per minute (gtt/min) should this patient receive?

$$\frac{\text{Volume} \times \text{drop factor}}{\text{Time in minutes}} = \frac{250 \text{ mL} \times 10 \text{ gtt/mL}}{20 \text{ min}}$$

$$= \frac{2500 \text{ gtt}}{20 \text{ min}}$$

$$= 125 \text{ gtt/min}$$

Example #2. Your patient is to receive 500 mL of IV solution over 12 hours. The IV administration set delivers 60 gtt/mL. How many drops per minute should this patient receive?

$$\frac{\text{Volume} \times \text{drop factor}}{\text{Time in minutes}} = \frac{500 \text{ mL} \times 60 \text{ gtt/mL}}{720 \text{ min}}$$

$$= \frac{30000 \text{ gtt}}{720 \text{ min}}$$

$$= 83 \text{ gtt/min}$$

Types of Intravenous Fluids

There are many types of IV solutions. Solutions that are commonly used in the prehospital setting include 0.9% saline (normal saline) and Lactated Ringer's solution. These solutions are isotonic. In a person who has normal fluid balance, an **isotonic solution** does not cause body cells to gain or lose water. A solution of 5% dextrose in water (D5W) is less often used.

After the ALS provider has selected the IV solution to be used, the protective covering must be removed from the IV bag. The IV bag itself must then be closely inspected. Check the expiration date on the bag to

Stop and Think!

Most states do not allow an EMT to transport any patient with an IV infusion other than normal saline or patient-administered pain medications. Contact your local or state health department for specific guidelines and protocols.

be sure that it is not outdated. Make sure there are no leaks in the IV bag. Look at the clarity of the IV solution. It should not be cloudy. Gently agitate the bag and look for particulate matter ("floaties"). Discard the bag if it is outdated, leaking, or cloudy or if particulates are present.

Complications of Intravenous Therapy

General Complications

A common complication encountered with IV drug or fluid administration is an interruption in fluid flow. This is usually due to some type of blockage or restriction with the IV tubing. To prevent this common problem, make sure that you can see all parts of the IV tubing at all times. Some of the most common causes of fluid flow restriction include a closed flow regulator, a closed clamp, tubing that may be caught under the patient or backboard, or a tourniquet left around the patient's arm by the ALS provider. This restriction may also be due to blood clots developing in the IV catheter itself, especially if the fluid flow is too slow. The typical flow rate needed to keep a vein free of clots is at least 1 drop through the drip chamber about every 2 to 4 seconds.

Fluid flow may also be restricted if the tubing has been kinked. Verify that all IV lines are straight and not compressed by patient restraints or clothing. It may be necessary to reposition the patient's arm and/or equipment. You may need to apply a splint to the patient's arm to keep it straight.

Occasionally the patient's movements may cause the IV tubing to become disconnected. If this occurs, immediately occlude the catheter by placing your gloved hand on the IV site to occlude the distal end of the catheter. There is a significant risk of infection if the end of the tubing has been exposed to any material, including the patient's skin. The IV line should be reconnected only by an ALS provider. In almost every case, the IV line will need to be discontinued and a new line started.

Local Complications

Local complications of IV therapy occur at or near the IV insertion site. Examples of local complications include infiltration, hematoma (bruise), **thrombosis** (the presence of a clot within a blood vessel), and phlebitis.

Infiltration occurs when an IV medication or solution leaks out of the vein and into the tissues surrounding the IV insertion site. This complication can occur when an IV catheter shifts from its normal position inside the vein. The tissue surrounding the area may be injured, depending on the IV solution being infused. Signs of infiltration usually include swelling or coolness of the tissue at the IV insertion site. The patient may or may not complain of pain or discomfort at the IV site. Other signs of infiltration can include the following:

- An IV that won't flow, or flows sluggishly
- An IV that continues to flow even when pressure is applied to the vein above the tip of the IV catheter
- An IV that results in no backflow of blood into the IV tubing when the regulator clamp is opened and the IV bag is lowered below the IV site

If you suspect that infiltration is occurring, you should immediately notify ALS personnel. Depending on your state regulations, you may be allowed only to monitor this line. In some states, you may be permitted to discontinue the IV. If you are permitted to discontinue the IV, first close the clamp on the IV tubing to shut down the flow. After carefully removing the tape or other device securing the IV catheter in place, remove the needle or catheter while holding pressure on the skin at the IV site. Carefully inspect the needle or catheter to be sure that it appears intact. Then place the needle or catheter in the appropriate sharps container. Next, apply an adhesive strip to the IV insertion site and a pressure dressing to the infiltration site. Continue to monitor the site for any bleeding or additional swelling. Document all signs, symptoms, and the actions taken to alleviate this problem. Make sure to notify the receiving facility staff about this problem on your arrival.

A hematoma may develop near the IV insertion site, or a clot (thrombus) may form at the tip of the IV catheter. This can cause the IV infusion to slow or stop. If the clot causes irritation, the vein may become inflamed (**phlebitis**). Phlebitis may occur simply because a foreign body (the IV catheter) is present. The patient's skin may be warm and red around the IV site. The patient's extremity may be swollen, and the patient may complain of throbbing pain in the limb. If any of these complications occur, immediately notify ALS personnel. Follow the steps outlined previously if you are instructed (and permitted) to discontinue the IV line.

Systemic Complications

Systemic problems that may be encountered as a complication of intravenous therapy include air embolism, sepsis, and fluid overload.

An embolism can occur when air, blood, or any other foreign material enters the bloodstream through the IV site. While it is considered uncommon, an air embolism may be fatal to an ill person at volumes of less than 30 mL of air. The general signs and symptoms of an embolus may include low blood pressure; cyanosis; a weak, rapid pulse; complaint of shortness of breath; and possible loss of consciousness. If your protocols allow, immediately close the IV tubing and notify the ALS provider. Give high-flow oxygen and contact medical control.

Sepsis will generally not be noted during the prehospital phase of an emergency. However, you may note it during an interfacility transport. Signs of sepsis may include fever, low blood pressure, and a loss of consciousness. Immediately notify the ALS provider. Give high-flow oxygen and contact medical control. Do not discontinue the flow through the IV unless specifically instructed to do so by medical control.

Fluid overload can occur when an IV has been allowed to flow too fast or at an uncontrolled rate. This can result in high blood pressure, which burdens the patient's circulatory system, and even heart failure. Complications can occur very rapidly in infant, children, and older adults. Immediately notify the ALS provider if this problem occurs.

D Weapons of Mass Destruction

Note: This appendix is not intended to replace the need for a Hazardous Materials, First Responder Course.

Introduction

Our world has changed dramatically in just a few short years. Events involving weapons of mass destruction or hazardous material once would have been unthinkable outside the movie theater but now must be considered possible (in the real world). **Weapons of mass destruction (WMD)** are materials used by terrorists that have the potential to cause great harm over a large area.

Terrorists use fear to bring about political change. They want to cause panic and disrupt normal activities. Their goal is to injure (incapacitate), not necessarily kill, large numbers of people. By injuring as many victims as possible, terrorists cause mass confusion and panic. This could affect an already overloaded Emergency Medical Services (EMS) system, bringing it to a standstill. Additionally, healthcare professionals and emergency responders are prime targets. Incapacitating them ensures other victims do not recover. Military experts agree that "incapacitating" a victim creates the need for a minimum of two healthcare professionals to begin any type of care.

There are six main categories of WMD. B-NICCE is a simple way to remember these categories:

- *B*iological
- *N*uclear/radiological
- *I*ncendiary
- *C*hemical
- *C*yber/technological
- *E*xplosive

Any material that has a harmful effect on the body can be used as a weapon of mass destruction or as a weapon of mass confusion. The sad reality is that there is an amazing amount of "terrorist" information about such materials available on the Internet. Fortunately, it is hard to "weaponize" most of these materials. For instance, some biological agents must come into contact with the victim's lung tissue to have a harmful effect and thus must be dispersed into the air. Other types of materials, such as nerve agents, need only to come in contact with the victim's skin to have a harmful effect.

Remember This!

We must prepare for the "unthinkable" at all levels of training.

Types of Weapons of Mass Destruction

Biological Weapons

Biological weapons involve the use of bacteria, viruses, rickettsia, or toxins to cause disease or death (Figure AD-1). Diseases can be spread by:

- Inhalation of substances dispersed by spray devices (aerosols)
- Ingestion of contaminated food or water supplies
- Absorption through direct skin contact with the substance
- Injection into the skin

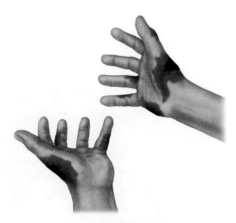

Bacteria: anthrax, tularemia (rabbit fever)

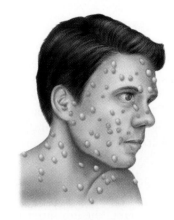

Virus: smallpox, Ebola virus

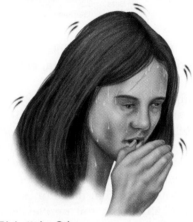

Rickettsia: Q fever

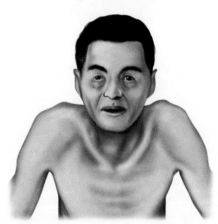

Toxin: ricin, botulism, enterotoxin B

FIGURE AD-1 ▲ Biological weapons involve the use of bacteria, viruses, rickettsia, or toxins to cause disease or death.

Bacteria are germs that can cause disease in humans, plants, or animals. Bacteria can live outside the human body and do not depend on other organisms to live and grow. Examples of diseases caused by bacteria that may be used as biological weapons include anthrax and tularemia (rabbit fever).

A **virus** is a type of infectious agent that depends on other organisms to live and grow. Viruses that could serve as biological weapons include the smallpox virus and those that cause viral hemorrhagic fevers, such as the Ebola virus. Infection with a hemorrhagic virus causes bleeding from many body tissues. The person may die from shock or from lack of oxygen caused by severe bleeding.

Rickettsia are very small bacteria that require a living host to survive. Rickettsias are transmitted by bloodsucking parasites such as fleas, lice, and ticks. An example of a disease caused by rickettsia is Q fever.

Toxins are substances produced by an animal, plant, or microorganism. Toxins are not the same as chemical agents. Toxins are natural substances and are generally more deadly than chemical agents, which are manmade. Toxins that could serve as biological weap-

ons include ricin (made from the waste left over from processing castor beans), botulism (found in improperly canned food and in contaminated water supplies, such as rivers and lakes), and enterotoxin B.

Indicators of possible biological weapon use are shown in the following *You Should Know* box.

You Should Know

Indicators of Possible Biological Weapon Use

- Dead or dying animals, fish, or birds
- Unusual casualties
- Unusual widespread illness not typical for that region

Creating a biological weapon is not complicated. It can be done by using materials purchased at a local hardware store and techniques learned in a high school chemistry course. Large quantities of biological weapons can often be produced in a few days to a few weeks.

The Centers for Disease Control and Prevention (CDC) categorize biological weapons according to their risk to national security. "Category A" diseases and agents are most likely to be used in an attack and include germs that are rarely seen in the United States. Category A diseases and agents include organisms that pose a risk to national security because they:

- Can be easily spread from person to person
- Result in high death rates and have the potential for major public health impact
- Might cause public panic
- Require special action for public health preparedness

Examples of Category A diseases and agents include anthrax, botulism, plague, smallpox, tularemia, and viral hemorrhagic fevers.

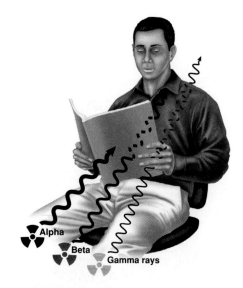

FIGURE AD-2 ▲ Nuclear radiation gives off three main types of radiation: alpha, beta, and gamma.

"Category B" diseases and agents are the second highest priority to the CDC because they are fairly easy to spread but cause moderate amounts of disease and low death rates. These weapons require specific public-health action, such as improved diagnostic and detection systems. These agents include Q fever, brucellosis, glanders, ricin, enterotoxin B, viral encephalitis, food safety threats, water safety threats, and typhus fever.

"Category C" diseases and agents include germs that could be engineered for mass distribution in the future because they are fairly easy to obtain, produce, and spread. They can produce high rates of disease and death. Examples of Category C diseases and agents include Nipah virus and hantavirus.

Nuclear Weapons

Nuclear weapons may be used in the form of ballistic missiles or bombs. Nuclear power plants, nuclear medicine machines in hospitals, research facilities, industrial construction sites, and vehicles used to transport nuclear waste may be possible targets for terrorist groups.

Nuclear radiation gives off three main types of radiation: alpha, beta, and gamma (Figure AD-2). It is the charge that makes radiation an immediate problem and disruptive to cell function and structure.

Alpha particles are large, heavy, charged, and cannot penetrate very far into matter. Because clothing or a sheet of paper is of sufficient thickness to stop them, external exposure to alpha particles usually has no effect on people. This is because the outermost dead layer of skin (epidermis) stops the particles from entering a person's body. However, if a person eats, drinks, or breathes in material that is contaminated

with alpha-emitting particles, the alpha radiation can cause significant damage inside his body with exposure of live tissues.

Beta particles are much smaller, travel more quickly, have less charge, and can penetrate more deeply than alpha particles. Beta particles can be stopped by layers of clothing or thin metal or plastic, such as several sheets of aluminum foil or Plexiglas. Generally, skin burns (called *beta burns*) can occur if the skin is exposed to large amounts of beta radiation. Internal damage can occur if a person eats, drinks, or breathes in material that is contaminated with beta-emitting particles.

Gamma rays are waves of very high energy, similar to light. These waves of energy penetrate very deeply and can easily go right through a person. To reduce exposure from gamma rays, thick material such as lead must be used. Because gamma rays can penetrate tissues and organs, nausea, vomiting, high fever, hair loss, and skin burns may result if a person is exposed to a large amount of gamma radiation in a short period.

According to the CDC, a dirty bomb is a mix of explosives, such as dynamite, with radioactive powder or pellets. A dirty bomb is also known as a *radiological weapon*. When the dynamite or other explosives are set off, the blast carries radioactive material into the surrounding area. The impact of a dirty bomb depends on factors such as the size of the explosive, the amount and type of radioactive material used, and weather conditions. Any terrorist explosion or WMD incident has the potential of being a dirty bomb.

Remember This!

You cannot see, smell, feel, or taste radiation. The longer you are exposed to it, the worse the effect.

Incendiary Weapons

Incendiary materials are substances that burn with a hot flame for a specific period. An incendiary system consists of the materials needed to start a fire, such as the initiator (the source that provides the first fire, such as a match), a delay mechanism (if needed), an igniter or fuse, and incendiary material or filler.

Most terrorist attacks involve the use of explosives, improvised explosive devices, and incendiary materials. Incendiaries are mainly used to set fire to wooden structures and other burnable targets. Firebombs are examples of incendiaries. They may range from a Molotov cocktail (bottle, gasoline, rag, and match) to much larger and sophisticated bombs. Firebombs may contain napalm or other flammable fluid. They are usually ignited with a fuse. Some incendiaries are used to melt, cut, or weld metal.

Chemical Weapons

Chemical agents are poisonous substances that injure or kill people when inhaled, ingested, or absorbed through the skin or eyes. There are five broad categories of chemical weapons: nerve agents, blister agents, blood agents, choking agents, and irritants (Table AD-1). Indicators of possible chemical weapon use are shown in the next *You Should Know* box. The general symptoms of exposure will vary by individual and depend on many factors such as:

- The substance involved
- The concentration of the substance
- The duration of exposure
- The number of exposures
- The route of entry (inhalation, ingestion, injection, or absorption)

Other factors that influence how an individual is affected include the person's age, gender, general health, allergies, smoking habits, alcohol consumption, and medications.

You Should Know

Indicators of Possible Chemical Weapon Use

- Dead or dying animals, fish, or birds
- Lack of insects
- Unexplained casualties
- Multiple victims
- Serious illnesses
- Unusual liquid, spray, vapor, or droplets
- Unexplained odors
- Low clouds or fog unrelated to the weather
- Suspicious devices or packages, including metal debris, abandoned spray devices, unexplained weapons

Irritants are often used for personal protection and by police in riot control. Examples include Mace,

TABLE AD-1 Chemical Agents

Chemical Agent	Effects	Examples
Nerve agents	Interrupt nerve signals, causing a loss of consciousness within seconds and death within minutes of exposure	Tabun, Sarin, Soman, VX
Blister agents	Produce effects like those of a corrosive chemical, such as lye or a strong acid; result in severe burns to the eyes, skin, and tissues of the respiratory tract	Distilled mustard, forms of nitrogen mustard
Blood agents	Cause rapid respiratory arrest and death by blocking the absorption of oxygen to the cells and organs through the bloodstream	Cyanide, arsine, hydrogen chloride
Choking (pulmonary) agents	Inhaled chlorine mixes with the moisture in the lungs and becomes hydrochloric acid, which causes fluid to build up in the lungs (pulmonary edema), interferes with the body's ability to exchange oxygen, and results in asphyxiation that resembles drowning	Chlorine
Irritants	Results in immediate tearing of the eyes, coughing, difficulty breathing, nausea, and vomiting	Mace, pepper spray, tear gas

pepper spray, and tear gas. These substances cause burning and intense pain to exposed skin areas. Exposure results in immediate tearing of the eyes, coughing, difficulty breathing, nausea, and vomiting.

Medical attention is needed for any of the following:

- Unconsciousness
- Confusion
- Lightheadedness
- Anxiety
- Dizziness
- Changes in skin color
- Shortness of breath
- Burning of the upper airway
- Coughing or painful breathing
- Drooling
- Chest tightness
- Loss of coordination
- Seizures
- Nausea, vomiting
- Abdominal cramping
- Diarrhea
- Loss of bowel or bladder control
- Dim, blurred, or double vision
- Tingling or numbness of the extremities

All of these signs and symptoms can be indicative of some type of chemical exposure. They should be considered as the first warning signs that the call may be a WMD event. The reality of these types of situations is that responders may have already treated a large number of patients before recognizing that this is a WMD situation. Treating a large number of patients with the same signs and symptoms at the same scene should trigger the thought of a WMD event. Can you imagine the difficulty with recognizing the problem when the patients have been transported to multiple hospitals over a period of several days? You must be conscientious in recognizing and reporting these types of scenes.

A growing number of EMS operational systems are or will be carrying auto-injected medications called *Mark One Kits*. In the event of a mass exposure to a nerve agent, these kits are designed for self-treatment and treatment of other members of the initial emergency response team, as well as the general public.

Cyber and Technological Weapons

Cyber and technological terrorism involves the use of computers to steal, alter, or destroy information. Cyber weapons include computer viruses and unauthorized access into computer systems. These weapons can cause computer systems to fail or malfunction. Computer hackers can alter computer system access and destroy or change important information stored in a computer.

Explosives

Most terrorist attacks involve the use of explosives. Explosives are associated with a very rapid release of gas and heat. Examples of explosives include:

- Grenades
- Rockets
- Missiles
- Mines
- Pipe bombs
- Vehicle bombs
- Package or letter bombs
- Bombs carried in devices, such as a knapsack

Weapons of Mass Destruction Incident Response

A scene involving WMD is a crime scene. At a possible WMD incident, your primary responsibilities will be to:

- Isolate the scene
- Preserve evidence and deny entry
- Ask for additional help (see the following *Remember This!* box) and coordinate efforts with other responding fire, EMS, and law enforcement personnel
- Recognize signs of a potential WMD incident and alert the proper authorities
- Recognize potential of a secondary explosion or attack on emergency responders
- Make sure you, as well as additional responders, are safe

Depending on the type of WMD incident, additional resources that may be needed include:

- Law enforcement personnel
- Fire, hazardous materials, and other special rescue teams
- Gas, electric, water companies
- Hospitals
- Environmental Protection Agency (EPA)
- CDC
- State health department
- Military
- Public transportation
- Disaster services (Red Cross, Salvation Army)

To work effectively, you must use standard operating procedures (SOP) and protocols according to your local emergency response plan (LERP). Try to assess the potential for an exposure by using the guidelines in the following sections.

Because a terrorist event is a crime scene, it is important that you disturb the scene as little as possible.

Pre-Arrival Response

From the dispatch information you are given, listen for specific clues that may indicate a possible terrorist incident, such as:

- Type of incident
- Incident location
- Number of reported casualties

Prearrival information may be your only opportunity to recognize a WMD incident before you become part of the situation. Your knowledge of the terrain, local events, and local weather may be very important in recognizing a possible WMD event. For instance, knowing that a large open-air event is going on in your response area should trigger the thought of the potential for a mass casualty incident in the event of an exposure.

Arrival Response

As you approach the scene, consider the safest approach, such as uphill, upwind, or even upstream. Be aware of the terrain and try to avoid "bottlenecks"

or traps. Don't become a victim yourself by rushing in haphazardly.

Be alert for indicators of possible terrorist activity or WMD. Be prepared for a possible rush of contaminated patients. Use the dispatch information provided, your senses, and any other information available. As you approach, you may smell odors indicating a gas leak, chemical spill, or fire. Look for:

- An unusually large number of people with burns or "blast" injuries
- Large numbers of people running from the scene or on the ground
- Danger of fire, explosion, electrical hazards, or structural collapse
- Weapons, explosive devices
- Signs of corrosion
- Evidence of use of chemical agents

Listen for:

- Screaming
- Explosion
- Breaking glass
- Hissing sounds indicating pressure releases
- Information from victims or bystanders

Remember that responders to the scene may be the target! This means *you*. Terrorists may use a secondary explosive device (equipped with a timer or trigger mechanism) designed to detonate after responders have arrived at a location. The intention is clear: to injure or kill responders.

The location of an incident may also be a clue to the type of problem. For example, targeted locations may include an abortion clinic, religious function, or political event. Approach any large or special event with caution. Examples of high-risk targets include:

- Landmarks: the White House, the Hoover Dam, the Statue of Liberty
- Transportation sites: highways, railways, airports, bridges, tunnels
- Energy sources: nuclear power plants, oil or gas pipelines
- Financial institutions: the Federal Reserve, the Stock Exchange
- Government or public safety buildings: military, EMS, police, fire

- High-attendance sites: amusement parks, concerts, sporting events, graduations
- Communications centers

The anniversary of an event can be significant. For instance, the 1995 bombing of the Alfred P. Murrah Federal Building in Oklahoma City, Oklahoma, took place on the second anniversary of a 1993 standoff between Branch Davidians and the Federal Bureau of Investigation (FBI) near Waco, Texas. Unfortunately, the significance of a date may not be realized until after the incident has occurred.

Other factors to consider at a possible WMD incident include:

- Time of day
- Temperature
- Wind intensity and direction
- Humidity
- Cloud cover
- Precipitation

These factors can be very important. For example, time of day can be an indicator of the increased possibility of the use of a biological agent. In most cases, wind speed is slower at night, and biological agents will not disperse or thin out as rapidly.

On arrival at the scene, obtain scene control and establish a perimeter. Give dispatch the exact location of the incident or perimeter. Alert responders to potential hazards or danger. Always err on the side of caution.

A WMD is a hazardous material. The presence of hazardous materials is not always easy to detect. In a WMD incident, the presence of identifying placards may not be accurate because the placards may have been deliberately altered by terrorists. If hazardous substances or conditions are suspected, the scene must be secured by qualified personnel wearing appropriate equipment. If you are not qualified and do not have the appropriate equipment, you may need to wait for additional help to arrive before you can attempt entry into the scene (see Chapter 29). Try to quickly identify the type of incident (e.g., biological, nuclear, chemical). Relay the information to dispatch as soon as possible. Knowing the type of incident is important so that you can take appropriate precautions when providing emergency care.

Approaching the Patient

Access to any patient must not occur without the proper personal protective equipment. Standard body substance isolation equipment may not be sufficient or appropriate for this type of response.

In most respects, a contaminated patient is like any other patient except that emergency responders must protect themselves and others from dangers resulting from secondary contamination. The goals for emergency responders at a scene involving WMD include

- Terminating the patient's exposure to the contaminant
- Maintaining rescuer safety
- Removing the patient from danger
- Providing emergency patient care

Determine if the scene has been secured to allow for your safe approach to the patient. In many instances, there will be no clear signals that this is a potential WMD event. Approach with caution.

Assuming that you are properly trained and equipped to do so, emergency care in the hot zone must be limited to spinal stabilization, gross airway management (such as opening the airway and suctioning), and hemorrhage control. Remember that the patient will be further exposed to any airborne contaminants when you open his airway. Address life-threatening problems and gross decontamination before giving emergency care. If spinal stabilization appears necessary, begin it as soon as feasible.

Stop and Think!

Do not go into the hot zone unless you are properly trained and equipped.

Begin your primary survey at the same time as decontamination. Look for clues that suggest the presence of some type of exposure. Is he having a seizure? This may alert you to the presence of some type of nerve agent. Assess the patient's level of responsiveness by shouting a question to him from a distance away. If the patient responds to your voice or is moving, you can safely make some assumptions about the amount of blood flow to his brain. Look at the patient closely. Is he breathing? Can you see the rise and fall of his chest? Is his breathing regular, or is he gasping for breath? As you get closer to the patient, look at his body and limb position. Do you see any obvious signs of trauma, such as limbs in an abnormal position? This may be a sign that there has been some force applied to the patient's body. Is his clothing intact or has it been torn or shredded? Is there evidence of any foreign material on his clothing or skin? This may be indicative of some type of explosive device. Request ALS personnel if you suspect WMD contamination.

Complete a more detailed assessment as conditions allow. When treating patients, consider the chemical-specific information received from your Poison Control Center (PCC) and other information resources. In multiple patient situations, begin proper triage procedures according to your local emergency response plan.

Key Safety Points

Always consider the possibility of multiple hazards. Only those emergency personnel wearing appropriate protective gear and actively involved in performing emergency operations should work inside the contaminated area.

Stop and Think!

Rushing into a possible WMD event only increases confusion and the potential for harm to yourself and other emergency responders. Stay alert and remain suspicious of unusual events or circumstances.

Identify the materials involved in the incident *only* from a safe distance. Do not approach anyone coming from a contaminated area. They may be the perpetrator, or they may be contaminated.

E Rural and Frontier EMS

Emergency Response in Rural and Frontier Areas

Emergency Medical Services (EMS) is an important part of rural and frontier healthcare. Rural and frontier areas have been defined as the wilderness of woods, hills, mountains, plains, islands, and desert outside of urban and suburban centers. In most areas of the United States, when people place a 9-1-1 call for a medical emergency, they expect an immediate dispatch of an ambulance and/or fire equipment. In many areas of the United States, including many rural areas, EMS consistently meets this expectation. However, this expectation is not being met in some rural and frontier areas for a variety of reasons.

The Challenges of Rural and Frontier Emergency Medical Services

Healthcare Resources

The number of hospital and medical practice closures in rural and frontier areas has increased. This increase has resulted in shrinking healthcare resources in these communities. Because of the heavy demands of rural healthcare (such as long hours and no backup), it is hard for many rural areas to recruit and retain doctors, nurses, and other healthcare personnel. Doctors and nurses who choose to work in rural and frontier areas often have limited contact with EMS personnel. They are often unfamiliar with the different levels of EMS professionals and their capabilities.

You Should Know

In 2004, the National Rural Health Association (NRHA), the National Organization of State Offices of Rural Health (NOSORH), and the National Association of State EMS Directors (NAS-EMSD) released the final draft of the *Rural/Frontier EMS Agenda for the Future.* This document offers recommendations to support and improve emergency services in rural and frontier communities by focusing on restructuring, reimbursement, and recruitment issues.

As the residents of rural and frontier areas age, their need for medical care increases. Residents must often travel great distances to see specialists. As their local healthcare resources disappear, residents of these areas call upon EMS professionals for assistance. Requests for help may include an unofficial assessment, advice, or emergency care.

Some rural and frontier communities are using EMS professionals in doctor's offices, healthcare clinics, hospice, and home health settings. In some settings, EMS professionals are used between EMS calls to supplement the hospital staff. In others, they are used for regular shift coverage. Using EMS professionals in this way helps to fill the gap in the community's healthcare resources.

Response Times

In urban areas, fire departments and ambulance services try hard to arrive at the patient's side within 4 to 8 minutes of the patient's call for help. This goal is unrealistic in rural and frontier areas. Rural and frontier EMS professionals cover large, sparsely populated areas, using minimal resources to respond to the scene. Response times in rural and frontier settings may be long because of the following:

- A delay in volunteers' response from home or work
- A failure to respond
- The physical distance that must be covered
- The type of transportation that must be used (land, air, water)
- The type and condition of the roadway, airway, or waterway
- Bad weather, difficult access, unmarked roads, and houses not visible from the street (addresses unmarked and fewer landmarks to help guide response vehicles)

Limited access to communications may delay the detection and reporting of a need for emergency care. When traveling on land, remote locations and unpredictable road conditions (including unmarked roads) can delay the arrival of EMS professionals on the scene.

Emergency Medical Services Workforce

Many rural and frontier EMS professionals often work a full-time job outside of their EMS roles. They frequently volunteer their time to provide emergency medical care and transportation to members of their community. When a volunteer receives a request to respond to an EMS call, he often leaves a full-time job to respond in his private vehicle. In areas where an emergency response vehicle is available, the volunteer must travel to the station, pick up the emergency vehicle, and then respond to the emergency. When an EMS call is over, the volunteer returns home, returns to his regular job, or goes back to the station to return the emergency vehicle. Rural and frontier EMS professionals

- Often know their patient
- Often know about the patient's condition
- Understand the environment in which the patient lives and works
- Know what the patient needs

Rural and frontier EMS systems rely heavily on volunteers. However, the increasing expectations of rural and frontier residents about the level and type of prehospital care may result in a demand for services that cannot easily be provided by volunteers. In rural and frontier settings, the level of Emergency Medical Responder and Emergency Medical Technician (EMT) prehospital care is more likely to be available than is advanced-level care. This situation is partly the result of

the costs, time, and travel needed to obtain advanced-level training. States have been pressured to use EMT as the national minimum level of care for personnel who provide patient care on ambulances. Some EMS leaders are concerned that increased training, testing, and certification requirements will jeopardize the interest and availability of their volunteers. At the same time, the number of interested EMS volunteers may be decreasing because of the following factors:

- The increase in two-wage-earner households
- Limited EMS pay or a lack of pay
- Increasing exposure to the risks of providing EMS care
- The belief that there is increased personal liability when providing EMS care
- A lack of EMS leadership in the community
- Limited funding or a lack of funding for training, equipment, and supplies
- An increased number of nursing home and routine transfer calls instead of emergency calls

Individuals who do become Advanced EMTs and Paramedics often do not remain in the rural or frontier area after their training is finished. Low call volumes in some areas make it difficult for some advanced care professionals to keep up their skills. Continuing education opportunities may be limited, and training resources (including qualified instructors) are often scarce.

As in the urban setting, EMS professionals in rural and frontier communities should seek out opportunities for continuing education. Some colleges are recognizing the unique needs of busy professionals and are providing Internet refresher and continuing education courses for rural and long-distance students so that they do not have to leave their communities to obtain education.

Illness and Injury

Many rural and frontier residents are employed in some of the most hazardous occupations in our country—logging, mining, farming, fishing, and hunting. Work-related deaths occur more frequently among these groups of workers than among workers as a whole.

A number of factors may contribute to the severity of injuries and the greater number of injury-related deaths seen in rural and frontier areas:

- There may be long delays between the time of the injury and its discovery by a passerby.
- It may take a considerable amount of time to get a patient from the scene of an accident to a hospital because of distances between the scene, the ambulance service, and the hospital.
- Prehospital care in many rural areas may be performed by volunteers who are unable to provide advanced airway management or fluid resuscitation.
- Emergency Departments in small rural hospitals may be staffed by physicians who do not have the knowledge or skills needed to manage critical trauma patients.
- There may be relatively few trauma cases at the rural hospital, making it difficult for physicians and nurses to maintain their skills.
- Rural hospitals may not have 24-hour physician coverage. In addition, laboratory and x-ray services may not be available 24 hours a day.
- In situations involving multiple victims, delays may occur in the initial stabilization of patients because there are too few emergency responders, physicians, or nurses available.
- Injuries from all-terrain vehicles, snowmobile collisions, and other recreational activities are common in rural settings.
- Injuries may occur as a result of farming activities. Adults and children may be injured while operating heavy machinery, operating dangerous tools, caring for large livestock, or handling dangerous pesticides or other chemicals (Figure AE-1). Responses to situations that involve large livestock can be unsafe to rescuers. Farm rescues may include hazards such as poisonous gases or low-oxygen atmospheres found in silos, confined-space situations, and unique extrication situations involving farm machinery.
- Industries located in rural and frontier areas may pose potential hazards (Figure AE-2).
- Rural emergencies may also include wilderness-related medical situations. These situations

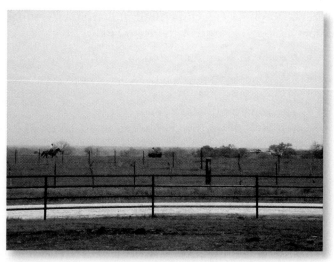

FIGURE AE-1 ▲ Adults and children may be injured as a result of farm activities. In this picture, a horse and an all-terrain vehicle are being used to herd cattle.

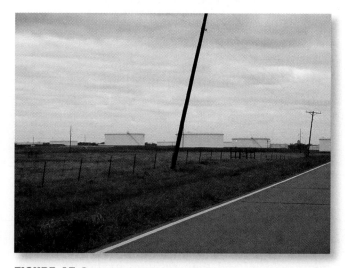

FIGURE AE-2 ▲ Industries located in rural and frontier areas may pose potential hazards.

include envenomation from poisonous snakes; heat-, cold-, and water-related emergencies; and poisoning from plants.

Factors that may contribute to higher rates of motor-vehicle-related injury and death in rural and frontier areas include:

- Poor road conditions
- The absence of safety features (guard rails, appropriately placed shoulder reflectors)
- A greater likelihood of high-speed travel (65 mph or more)
- A greater use of utility vehicles and pickup trucks
- A lack of effective safety measures (seatbelts)
- Greater distances between emergency facilities

A motor vehicle crash occurring along an infrequently traveled rural road may not be detected for hours. When the crash is detected, access to the EMS system may be further delayed because phones or other forms of communication may not be readily available. The patient may sustain injuries that require the use of specialized services such as a Trauma Center. Trauma Centers are usually not immediately available in rural and frontier areas. It is often necessary to contact an air medical service for patient transport. The air transport team may be located some distance away from the accident site, which delays transporting the patient from the crash site to the hospital.

Making a Difference

In a rural or frontier EMS system, long distances, minimal resources, and road conditions that are less than optimal usually allow for a significant length of time for interaction between you and the patient. This prolonged patient contact time will give you an opportunity to talk with your patient, reassess his condition, perform additional skills, and provide frequent reassurance.

If a cardiac arrest occurs, cardiopulmonary resuscitation (CPR) must be started as quickly as possible. Some rural and frontier communities have improved emergency cardiac care in their areas by providing citizen CPR programs. In addition, they have trained Basic Life Support personnel to use automated external defibrillators (AEDs). AEDs are particularly well suited to the needs of rural and frontier areas because they are easy to use. They are also more affordable now than ever before. Many states have grants and financial assistance programs available. These programs enable agencies to purchase AEDs for use in their community.

Making a Difference

If you will be working in a rural or frontier area, find out from your instructor how you can become a CPR instructor. Teaching CPR regularly and placing AEDs in public areas could save the life of a cardiac arrest patient in your community.

You Should Know

The Unique Training Needs of Rural and Frontier EMS Professionals

In some areas, organizations are working to develop and deliver training programs that meet the unique needs of rural and frontier EMS professionals. Examples of innovative programs include the following:

- The Southern Coastal Agromedicine Center (SCAC), in collaboration with the North Carolina Forestry Association, has developed a Timber Medic program to improve logging-injury outcomes.

- Cornell University offers a First on the Scene program that teaches farm family members, farm employees, and the general community how to make important decisions at the scene of a farm emergency. The program is intended for all farm groups, such as farm managers, employees, spouses, and 4-H and Future Farmers of America groups. Some of the available topics include tractor overturns, machinery entanglements, grain bin emergencies, and silo emergencies.

- The Farmedic Training Program, now housed at Cornell University, provides rural fire and rescue responders with a systematic approach to farm rescue procedures that addresses the safety of both patients and responders (Figure AE-3). This program has trained more than 22,000 students since it began in 1981. For more information, visit the following website: http://www.farmedic.com/training/.

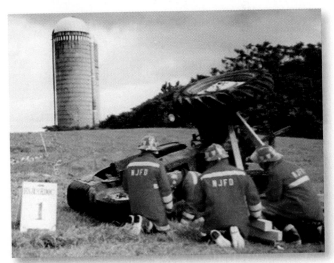

FIGURE AE-3 ▲ Farmedic Provider course in North Java, New York. The student team is stabilizing an overturned tractor to rescue the patient that is pinned under the tractor cowling. © www.farmedic.com. Cornell Farmedic Training Program. Cornell Agricultural Health and Safety Program. Cornell University, Ithaca, NY 14850.

- Airway Oxygen and Ventilation Skills—Upper Airway Adjuncts and Suction
- Bag Mask—Apneic Patient
- Bleeding Control/Shock Management
- Cardiac Arrest Management/AED with Bystander CPR in Progress
- Immobilization Skills—Joint Injury
- Immobilization Skills—Long Bone Injury
- Immobilization Skills—Traction Splinting
- Mouth to Mask with Supplemental Oxygen

- Oxygen Administration
- Patient Assessment/Management—Medical
- Patient Assessment/Management—Trauma
- Spinal Immobilization—Seated Patient
- Spinal Immobilization—Supine Patient
- Ventilatory Management—Dual Lumen Device Insertion Following an Unsuccessful Endotracheal Intubation Attempt
- Ventilatory Management—Endotracheal Intubation

AIRWAY, OXYGEN AND VENTILATION SKILLS
UPPER AIRWAY ADJUNCTS AND SUCTION

Start Time: _____

Stop Time: _____ Date: _____

Candidate's Name: _____

Evaluator's Name: _____

OROPHARYNGEAL AIRWAY	Points Possible	Points Awarded
Takes, or verbalizes, body substance isolation precautions	1	
Selects appropriately sized airway	1	
Measures airway	1	
Inserts airway without pushing the tongue posteriorly	1	
Note: The examiner must advise the candidate that the patient is gagging and becoming conscious		
Removes the oropharyngeal airway	1	

SUCTION

	Points Possible	Points Awarded
Note: The examiner must advise the candidate to suction the patient's airway		
Turns on/prepares suction device	1	
Assures presence of mechanical suction	1	
Inserts the suction tip without suction	1	
Applies suction to the oropharynx/nasopharynx	1	

NASOPHARYNGEAL AIRWAY

	Points Possible	Points Awarded
Note: The examiner must advise the candidate to insert a nasopharyngeal airway		
Selects appropriately sized airway	1	
Measures airway	1	
Verbalizes lubrication of the nasal airway	1	
Fully inserts the airway with the bevel facing toward the septum	1	
Total:	13	

Critical Criteria

_____ Did not take, or verbalize, body substance isolation precautions

_____ Did not obtain a patent airway with the oropharyngeal airway

_____ Did not obtain a patent airway with the nasopharyngeal airway

_____ Did not demonstrate an acceptable suction technique

_____ Inserted any adjunct in a manner dangerous to the patient

BAG-VALVE-MASK
APNEIC PATIENT

Start Time: _____

Stop Time: _____ Date: _____

Candidate's Name: _____

Evaluator's Name: _____

	Points Possible	Points Awarded
Takes, or verbalizes, body substance isolation precautions	1	
Voices opening the airway	1	
Voices inserting an airway adjunct	1	
Selects appropriately sized mask	1	
Creates a proper mask-to-face seal	1	
Ventilates patient at proper rate and adequate volume **(The examiner must witness for at least 30 seconds)**	1	
Connects reservoir and oxygen	1	
Adjusts liter flow to 15 liters/minute or greater	1	
The examiner indicates arrival of a second EMT. The second EMT is instructed to ventilate the patient while the candidate controls the mask and the airway		
Voices re-opening the airway	1	
Creates a proper mask-to-face seal	1	
Instructs assistant to resume ventilation at proper rate and adequate volume **(The examiner must witness for at least 30 seconds)**	1	
Total:	11	

Critical Criteria

_____ Did not take, or verbalize, body substance isolation precautions

_____ Did not immediately ventilate the patient

_____ Interrupted ventilations for more than 20 seconds

_____ Did not provide high concentration of oxygen

_____ Did not provide, or direct assistant to provide proper volume/breath or rate
(more than 2 ventilation errors per minute)

_____ Did not allow adequate exhalation

BLEEDING CONTROL/SHOCK MANAGEMENT

Start Time: _____

Stop Time: _____ Date: _____

Candidate's Name: _____

Evaluator's Name: _____	Points Possible	Points Awarded
Takes, or verbalizes, body substance isolation precautions	1	
Applies direct pressure to the wound	1	
Elevates the extremity	1	
Note: The examiner must now inform the candidate that the wound continues to bleed.		
Applies an additional dressing to the wound	1	
Note: The examiner must now inform the candidate that the wound still continues to bleed. The second dressing does not control the bleeding.		
Locates and applies pressure to appropriate arterial pressure point	1	
Note: The examiner must now inform the candidate that the bleeding is controlled		
Bandages the wound	1	
Note: The examiner must now inform the candidate the patient is now showing signs and symptoms indicative of hypoperfusion		
Properly position the patient	1	
Applies high concentration oxygen	1	
Initiates steps to prevent heat loss from the patient	1	
Indicates the need for immediate transportation	1	
Total:	10	

Critical Criteria

_____ Did not take, or verbalize, body substance isolation precautions

_____ Did not apply high concentration oxygen

_____ Applied a tourniquet before attempting other methods of bleeding control

_____ Did not control hemorrhage in a timely manner

_____ Did not indicate a need for immediate transportation

CARDIAC ARREST MANAGEMENT/AED
WITH BYSTANDER CPR IN PROGRESS

Start Time: _____

Stop Time: _____ Date: _____

Candidate's Name: _____

Evaluator's Name: _____

	Points Possible	Points Awarded
ASSESSMENT		
Takes, or verbalizes, body substance isolation precautions	1	
Briefly questions the rescuer about arrest events	1	
Turns on AED power	1	
Attaches AED to the patient	1	
Directs rescuer to stop CPR and ensures all individuals are clear of the patient	1	
Initiates analysis of the rhythm	1	
Delivers shock	1	
Directs resumption of CPR	1	
TRANSITION		
Gathers additional information about the arrest event	1	
Confirms effectiveness of CPR (ventilation and compressions)	1	
INTEGRATION		
Verbalizes or directs insertion of a simple airway adjunct (oral/nasal airway)	1	
Ventilates, or directs ventilation of the patient	1	
Assures high concentration of oxygen is delivered to the patient	1	
Assures adequate CPR continues without unnecessary/prolonged interruption	1	
Continues CPR for 2 minutes	1	
Directs rescuer to stop CPR and ensures all individuals are clear of the patient	1	
Initiates analysis of the rhythm	1	
Delivers shock	1	
Directs resumption of CPR	1	
TRANSPORTATION		
Verbalizes transportation of the patient	1	
Total:	20	

Critical Criteria

_____ Did not take, or verbalize, body substance isolation precautions

_____ Did not evaluate the need for immediate use of the AED

_____ Did not immediately direct initiation/resumption of CPR at appropriate times

_____ Did not assure all individuals were clear of patient before delivering a shock

_____ Did not operate the AED properly or safely (inability to deliver shock)

_____ Prevented the defibrillator from delivering any shock

IMMOBILIZATION SKILLS
JOINT INJURY

Start Time: _____

Stop Time: _____ Date: _____

Candidate's Name: _____

Evaluator's Name: _____	Points Possible	Points Awarded
Takes, or verbalizes, body substance isolation precautions	1	
Directs application of manual stabilization of the shoulder injury	1	
Assesses motor, sensory and circulatory function in the injured extremity	1	
Note: The examiner acknowledges "motor, sensory and circulatory function are present and normal."		
Selects the proper splinting material	1	
Immobilizes the site of the injury	1	
Immobilizes the bone above the injured joint	1	
Immobilizes the bone below the injured joint	1	
Reassesses motor, sensory and circulatory function in the injured extremity	1	
Note: The examiner acknowledges "motor, sensory and circulatory function are present and normal."		
Total:	8	

Critical Criteria

_____ Did not support the joint so that the joint did not bear distal weight

_____ Did not immobilize the bone above and below the injured site

_____ Did not reassess motor, sensory and circulatory function in the injured extremity before and after splinting

IMMOBILIZATION SKILLS
LONG BONE INJURY

Start Time: _____

Stop Time: _____ Date: _____

Candidate's Name: _____

Evaluator's Name: _____	Points Possible	Points Awarded
Takes, or verbalizes, body substance isolation precautions	1	
Directs application of manual stabilization of the injury	1	
Assesses motor, sensory and circulatory function in the injured extremity	1	
Note: The examiner acknowledges "motor, sensory and circulatory function are present and normal"		
Measures the splint	1	
Applies the splint	1	
Immobilizes the joint above the injury site	1	
Immobilizes the joint below the injury site	1	
Secures the entire injured extremity	1	
Immobilizes the hand/foot in the position of function	1	
Reassesses motor, sensory and circulatory function in the injured extremity	1	
Note: The examiner acknowledges "motor, sensory and circulatory function are present and normal"		
Total	10	

Critical Criteria

_____ Grossly moves the injured extremity

_____ Did not immobilize the joint above and the joint below the injury site

_____ Did not reassess motor, sensory and circulatory function in the injured extremity before and after splinting

IMMOBILIZATION SKILLS
TRACTION SPLINTING

Start Time: _____

Stop Time: _____ Date: _____

Candidate's Name: _____

Evaluator's Name: _____

	Points Possible	Points Awarded
Takes, or verbalizes, body substance isolation precautions	1	
Directs application of manual stabilization of the injured leg	1	
Directs the application of manual traction	1	
Assesses motor, sensory and circulatory function in the injured extremity	1	
Note: The examiner acknowledges "motor, sensory and circulatory function are present and normal"		
Prepares/adjusts splint to the proper length	1	
Positions the splint next to the injured leg	1	
Applies the proximal securing device (e.g..ischial strap)	1	
Applies the distal securing device (e.g..ankle hitch)	1	
Applies mechanical traction	1	
Positions/secures the support straps	1	
Re-evaluates the proximal/distal securing devices	1	
Reassesses motor, sensory and circulatory function in the injured extremity	1	
Note: The examiner acknowledges "motor, sensory and circulatory function are present and normal"		
Note: The examiner must ask the candidate how he/she would prepare the patient for transportation		
Verbalizes securing the torso to the long board to immobilize the hip	1	
Verbalizes securing the splint to the long board to prevent movement of the splint	1	
Total:	14	

Critical Criteria

_____ Loss of traction at any point after it was applied

_____ Did not reassess motor, sensory and circulatory function in the injured extremity before and after splinting

_____ The foot was excessively rotated or extended after splint was applied

_____ Did not secure the ischial strap before taking traction

_____ Final immobilization failed to support the femur or prevent rotation of the injured leg

_____ Secured the leg to the splint before applying mechanical traction

Note: If the Sagar splint or the Kendricks Traction Device is used without elevating the patient's leg, application of manual traction is not necessary. The candidate should be awarded one (1) point as if manual traction were applied.

Note: If the leg is elevated at all, manual traction must be applied before elevating the leg. The ankle hitch may be applied before elevating the leg and used to provide manual traction.

MOUTH TO MASK WITH SUPPLEMENTAL OXYGEN

Start Time: _____

Stop Time: _____ Date: _____

Candidate's Name: _____

Evaluator's Name: _____	Points Possible	Points Awarded
Takes, or verbalizes, body substance isolation precautions	1	
Connects one-way valve to mask	1	
Opens patient's airway or confirms patient's airway is open (manually or with adjunct)	1	
Establishes and maintains a proper mask to face seal	1	
Ventilates the patient at the proper volume and rate	1	
Connects the mask to high concentration or oxygen	1	
Adjusts flow rate to at least 15 liters per minute	1	
Continues ventilation of the patient at the proper volume and rate	1	
Note: The examiner must witness ventilations for at least 30 seconds		
Total:	8	

Critical Criteria

_____ Did not take, or verbalize, body substance isolation precautions

_____ Did not adjust liter flow to at least 15 liters per minute

_____ Did not provide proper volume per breath
(more than 2 ventiliation errors per minute)

_____ Did not ventilate the patient at a rate of 10-12 breaths per minute

_____ Did not allow for complete exhalation

OXYGEN ADMINISTRATION

Start Time: _____

Stop Time: _____ Date: _____

Candidate's Name: _____

Evaluator's Name: _____

	Points Possible	Points Awarded
Takes, or verbalizes, body substance isolation precautions	1	
Assembles the regulator to the tank	1	
Opens the tank	1	
Checks for leaks	1	
Checks tank pressure	1	
Attaches non-rebreather mask to oxygen	1	
Prefills reservoir	1	
Adjusts liter flow to 12 liters per minute or greater	1	
Applies and adjusts the mask to the patient's face	1	
Note: The examiner must advise the candidate that the patient is not tolerating the non-rebreather mask. The medical director has ordered you to apply a nasal cannula to the patient.		
Attaches nasal cannula to oxygen	1	
Adjusts liter flow to 6 liters per minute or less	1	
Applies nasal cannula to the patient	1	
Note: The examiner must advise the candidate to discontinue oxygen therapy		
Removes the nasal cannula from the patient	1	
Shuts off the regulator	1	
Relieves the pressure within the regulator	1	
Total:	15	

Critical Criteria

_____ Did not take, or verbalize, body substance isolation precautions

_____ Did not assemble the tank and regulator without leaks

_____ Did not prefill the reservoir bag

_____ Did not adjust the device to the correct liter flow for the non-rebreather mask
(12 liters per minute or greater)

_____ Did not adjust the device to the correct liter flow for the nasal cannula
(6 liters per minute or less)

Patient Assessment/Management - Medical

Start Time: _____

Stop Time: _____ Date: _____

Candidate's Name: _____

Evaluator's Name: _____

		Points Possible	Points Awarded
Takes, or verbalizes, body substance isolation precautions		1	
SCENE SIZE-UP			
Determines the scene is safe		1	
Determines the mechanism of injury/nature of illness		1	
Determines the number of patients		1	
Requests additional help if necessary		1	
Considers stabilization of spine		1	
INITIAL ASSESSMENT			
Verbalizes general impression of the patient		1	
Determines responsiveness/level of consciousness		1	
Determines chief complaint/apparent life threats		1	
Assesses airway and breathing	Assessment	1	
	Indicates appropriate oxygen therapy	1	
	Assures adequate ventilation	1	
Assesses circulation	Assesses/controls major bleeding	1	
	Assesses pulse	1	
	Assesses skin (color, temperature and condition)	1	
Identifies priority patients/makes transport decisions		1	
FOCUSED HISTORY AND PHYSICAL EXAMINATION/RAPID ASSESSMENT			
Signs and symptoms (Assess history of present illness)		1	

Respiratory	Cardiac	Altered Mental Status	Allergic Reaction	Poisoning/ Overdose	Environmental Emergency	Obstetrics	Behavioral
*Onset?	*Onset?	*Description of the episode.	*History of allergies?	*Substance? When did you ingest/become exposed?	*Source? *Environment? *Duration? *Loss of consciousness? *Effects- general or local?	*Are you pregnant? *How long have you been pregnant? *Pain or contractions? *Bleeding or discharge? *Do you feel the need to push? *Last menstrual period?	*How do you feel? *Determine suicidal tendencies. *Is the patient a threat to self or others? Is there a medical problem? Interventions?
*Provokes?	*Provokes?	*Onset?	*What were you exposed to?				
*Quality?	*Quality?	*Duration?		*How much did you ingest?			
*Radiates?	*Radiates?	*Associated Symptoms?	*How were you exposed?	*Over what time period?			
*Severity?	*Severity?	*Evidence of Trauma?	*Effects?	*Interventions?			
*Time?	*Time?	*Interventions?	*Progression?	*Estimated weight?			
*Interventions?	*Interventions?	*Seizures?	*Interventions?				
		*Fever?					

	Points Possible	Points Awarded
Allergies	1	
Medications	1	
Past pertinent history	1	
Last oral intake	1	
Event leading to present illness (rule out trauma)	1	
Performs focused physical examination (assesses affected body part/system or, if indicated, completes rapid assessment)	1	
Vitals (obtains baseline vital signs)	1	
Interventions (obtains medical direction or verbalizes standing order for medication interventions and verbalizes proper additional intervention/treatment)	1	
Transport (re-evaluates the transport decision)	1	
Verbalizes the consideration for completing a detailed physical examination	1	
ONGOING ASSESSMENT (verbalized)		
Repeats initial assessment	1	
Repeats vital signs	1	
Repeats focused assessment regarding patient complaint or injuries	1	
Critical Criteria Total:	30	

Critical Criteria

_____ Did not take, or verbalize, body substance isolation precautions when necessary

_____ Did not determine scene safety

_____ Did not obtain medical direction or verbalize standing orders for medical interventions

_____ Did not provide high concentration of oxygen

_____ Did not find or manage problems associated with airway, breathing, hemorrhage or shock (hypoperfusion)

_____ Did not differentiate patient's need for transportation versus continued assessment at the scene

_____ Did detailed or focused history/physical examination before assessing the airway, breathing and circulation

_____ Did not ask questions about the present illness

_____ Administered a dangerous or inappropriate intervention

Patient Assessment/Management - Trauma

Start Time: _____

Stop Time: _____ Date: _____

Candidate's Name: _____

Evaluator's Name: _____

		Points Possible	Points Awarded
Takes, or verbalizes, body substance isolation precautions		1	
SCENE SIZE-UP			
Determines the scene is safe		1	
Determines the mechanism of injury		1	
Determines the number of patients		1	
Requests additional help if necessary		1	
Considers stabilization of spine		1	
INITIAL ASSESSMENT			
Verbalizes general impression of the patient		1	
Determines responsiveness/level of consciousness		1	
Determines chief complaint/apparent life threats		1	
Assesses airway and breathing	Assessment	1	
	Initiates appropriate oxygen therapy	1	
	Assures adequate ventilation	1	
	Injury management	1	
Assesses circulation	Assesses/controls major bleeding	1	
	Assesses pulse	1	
	Assesses skin (color, temperature and conditions)	1	
Identifies priority patients/makes transport decision		1	
FOCUSED HISTORY AND PHYSICAL EXAMINATION/RAPID TRAUMA ASSESSMENT			
Selects appropriate assessment (**focused or rapid assessment**)		1	
Obtains, or directs assistance to obtain, baseline vital signs		1	
Obtains S.A.M.P.L.E. history		1	
DETAILED PHYSICAL EXAMINATION			
Assesses the head	Inspects and palpates the scalp and ears	1	
	Assesses the eyes	1	
	Assesses the facial areas including oral and nasal areas	1	
Assesses the neck	Inspects and palpates the neck	1	
	Assesses for JVD	1	
	Assesses for tracheal deviation	1	
Assesses the chest	Inspects	1	
	Palpates	1	
	Auscultates	1	
Assesses the abdomen/pelvis	Assesses the abdomen	1	
	Assesses the pelvis	1	
	Verbalizes assessment of genitalia/perineum as needed	1	
Assesses the extremities	1 point for each extremity includes inspection, palpation, and assessment of motor, sensory and circulatory function	4	
Assesses the posterior	Assesses thorax	1	
	Assesses lumbar	1	
Manages secondary injuries and wounds appropriately **1 point for appropriate management of the secondary injury/wound**		1	
Verbalizes re-assessment of the vital signs		1	
	Total:	40	

Critical Criteria

_____ Did not take, or verbalize, body substance isolation precautions

_____ Did not determine scene safety

_____ Did not assess for spinal protection

_____ Did not provide for spinal protection when indicated

_____ Did not provide high concentration of oxygen

_____ Did not find, or manage, problems associated with airway, breathing, hemorrhage or shock (hypoperfusion)

_____ Did not differentiate patient's need for transportation versus continued assessment at the scene

_____ Did other detailed physical examination before assessing the airway, breathing and circulation

_____ Did not transport patient within (10) minute time limit

SPINAL IMMOBILIZATION
SEATED PATIENT

Start Time: _____

Stop Time: _____ Date: _____

Candidate's Name: _____

Evaluator's Name: _____

	Points Possible	Points Awarded
Takes, or verbalizes, body substance isolation precautions	1	
Directs assistant to place/maintain head in the neutral in-line position	1	
Directs assistant to maintain manual immobilization of the head	1	
Reassesses motor, sensory and circulatory function in each extremity	1	
Applies appropriately sized extrication collar	1	
Positions the immobilization device behind the patient	1	
Secures the device to the patient's torso	1	
Evaluates torso fixation and adjusts as necessary	1	
Evaluates and pads behind the patient's head as necessary	1	
Secure the patient's head to the device	1	
Verbalizes moving the patient to a long board	1	
Reassesses motor, sensory and circulatory function in each extremity	1	
Total:	12	

Critical Criteria

_____ Did not immediately direct, or take, manual immobilization of the head

_____ Released, or ordered release of, manual immobilization before it was maintained mechanically

_____ Patient manipulated, or moved excessively, causing potential spinal compromise

_____ Device moved excessively up, down, left or right on the patient's torso

_____ Head immobilization allows for excessive movement

_____ Torso fixation inhibits chest rise, resulting in respiratory compromise

_____ Upon completion of immobilization, head is not in the neutral position

_____ Did not assess motor, sensory and circulatory function in each extremity after voicing immobilization to the long board

_____ Immobilized head to the board before securing the torso

SPINAL IMMOBILIZATION
SUPINE PATIENT

Start Time: _____

Stop Time: _____ Date: _____

Candidate's Name: _____

Evaluator's Name: _____	Points Possible	Points Awarded
Takes, or verbalizes, body substance isolation precautions	1	
Directs assistant to place/maintain head in the neutral in-line position	1	
Directs assistant to maintain manual immobilization of the head	1	
Reassesses motor, sensory and circulatory function in each extremity	1	
Applies appropriately sized extrication collar	1	
Positions the immobilization device appropriately	1	
Directs movement of the patient onto the device without compromising the integrity of the spine	1	
Applies padding to voids between the torso and the board as necessary	1	
Immobilizes the patient's torso to the device	1	
Evaluates and pads behind the patient's head as necessary	1	
Immobilizes the patient's head to the device	1	
Secures the patient's legs to the device	1	
Secures the patient's arms to the device	1	
Reassesses motor, sensory and circulatory function in each extremity	1	
Total:	14	

Critical Criteria

_____ Did not immediately direct, or take, manual immobilization of the head

_____ Released, or ordered release of, manual immobilization before it was maintained mechanically

_____ Patient manipulated, or moved excessively, causing potential spinal compromise

_____ Patient moves excessively up, down, left or right on the device

_____ Head immobilization allows for excessive movement

_____ Upon completion of immobilization, head is not in the neutral position

_____ Did not assess motor, sensory and circulatory function in each extremity after immobilization to the device

_____ Immobilized head to the board before securing the torso

VENTILATORY MANAGEMENT
DUAL LUMEN DEVICE INSERTION FOLLOWING
AN UNSUCCESSFUL ENDOTRACHEAL INTUBATION ATTEMPT

Start Time: _____

Stop Time: _____ Date: _____

Candidate's Name: _____

Evaluator's Name: _____

	Points Possible	Points Awarded
Continues body substance isolation precautions	1	
Confirms the patient is being properly ventilated with high percentage oxygen	1	
Directs the assistant to pre-oxygenate the patient	1	
Checks/prepares the airway device	1	
Lubricates the distal tip of the device (may be verbalized)	1	
Note: The examiner should remove the OPA and move out of the way when the candidate is prepared to insert the device		
Positions the patient's head properly	1	
Performs a tongue-jaw lift	1	

USES COMBITUBE	USES THE PTL	Points Possible	Points Awarded
Inserts device in the mid-line and to the depth so that the printed ring is at the level of the teeth	Inserts the device in the mid-line until the bite block flange is at the level of the teeth	1	
Inflates the pharyngeal cuff with the proper volume and removes the syringe	Secures the strap	1	
Inflates the distal cuff with the proper volume and removes the syringe	Blows into tube #1 to adequately inflate both cuffs	1	
Attaches/directs attachment of BVM to the first (esophageal placement) lumen and ventilates		1	
Confirms placement and ventilation through the correct lumen by observing chest rise, auscultation over the epigastrium and bilaterally over each lung		1	
Note: The examiner states, "You do not see rise and fall of the chest and hear sounds only over epigastrium"			
Attaches/directs attachment of BVM to the second (endotracheal placement) lumen and ventilates		1	
Confirms placement and ventilation through the correct lumen by observing chest rise, auscultation over the epigastrium and bilaterally over each lung		1	
Note: The examiner states, "You see rise and fall off the chest, there are no sounds over the epigastrium and breath sounds are equal over each lung"			
Secures device or confirms that the device remains properly secured		1	
		Total: 15	

Critical Criteria

_____ Did not take or verbalize body substance isolation precautions

_____ Did not initiate ventilations within 30 seconds

_____ Interrupted ventilations for more than 30 seconds at any time

_____ Did not pre-oxygenate the patient prior to placement of the dual lumen airway device

_____ Did not provide adequate volume per breath (maximum 2 errors/minute permissable)

_____ Did not ventilate the patient at a rate of 10-12 breaths per minute

_____ Did not insert the dual lumen airway device at a proper depth or at the proper place within 3 attempts

_____ Did not inflate both cuffs properly

_____ **Combitube** - Did not remove the syringe immediately following inflation of each cuff

_____ **PTL** - Did not secure the strap prior to cuff inflation

_____ Did not confirm, by observing chest rise and auscultation over the epigastrium and bilaterally over each lung that the proper lumen of the device was being used to ventilate the patient

_____ Inserted any adjunct in a manner that was dangerous to the patient

VENTILATORY MANAGEMENT
ENDOTRACHEAL INTUBATION

Start Time: _____

Stop Time: _____ Date: _____

Candidate's Name: _____

Evaluator's Name: _____

Note: If a candidate elects to initially ventilate the patient with a BVM attached to a reservoir and oxygen, full credit must be awarded for steps denoted by "**" provided first ventilation is delivered within the initial 30 seconds

	Points Possible	Points Awarded
Takes, or verbalizes, body substance isolation precautions	1	
Opens the airway manually	1	
Elevates the patient's tongue and inserts a simple airway adjunct (oropharyngeal/nasopharyngeal airway)	1	
Note: The examiner must now inform the candidate, "No gag reflex is present and the patient accepts the airway adjunct."		
**Ventilates the patient immediately using a BVM device unattached to oxygen	1	
**Ventilates the patient with room air	1	
Note: The examiner must now inform the candidate that ventilation is being properly performed without difficulty		
Attaches the oxygen reservoir to the BVM	1	
Attaches the BVM to high flow oxygen (15 liter per minute)	1	
Ventilates the patient at the proper volume and rate of 10-12 breaths per minute	1	
Note: After 30 seconds, the examiner must auscultate the patient's chest and inform the candidate that breath sounds are present and equal bilaterally and medical direction has ordered endotracheal intubation. The examiner must now take over ventilation of the patient.		
Directs assistant to pre-oxygenate the patient	1	
Identifies/selects the proper equipment for endotracheal intubation	1	
Checks equipment · Checks for cuff leaks	1	
Checks equipment · Checks laryngoscope operation and bulb tightness	1	
Note: The examiner must remove the OPA and move out of the way when the candidate is prepared to intubate the patient.		
Positions the patient's head properly	1	
Inserts the laryngoscope blade into the patient's mouth while displacing the patient's tongue laterally	1	
Elevates the patient's mandible with the laryngoscope	1	
Introduces the endotracheal tube and advances the tube to the proper depth	1	
Inflates the cuff to the proper pressure	1	
Disconnects the syringe from the cuff inlet port	1	
Directs assistant to ventilate the patient	1	
Confirms proper placement of the endotracheal tube by auscultation bilaterally and over the epigastrium	1	
Note: The examiner must ask, "If you had proper placement, what would you expect to hear?"		
Secures the endotracheal tube (may be verbalized)	1	
Total:	21	

Critical Criteria

_____ Did not take or verbalize body substance isolation precautions when necessary

_____ Did not initiate ventilation within 30 seconds after applying gloves or interrupts ventilations for greater than 30 seconds at a time

_____ Did not voice or provide high oxygen concentrations (15 liter/minute or greater)

_____ Did not ventilate the patient at a rate of 10-12 breaths per minute

_____ Did not provide adequate volume per breath (maximum of 2 errors per minute permissible)

_____ Did not pre-oxygenate the patient prior to intubation

_____ Did not successfully intubate the patient within 3 attempts

_____ Used the patient's teeth as a fulcrum

_____ Did not assure proper tube placement by auscultation bilaterally over each lung **and** over the epigastrium

_____ The stylette (if used) extended beyond the end of the endotracheal tube

_____ Inserted any adjunct in a manner that was dangerous to the patient

_____ Did not immediately disconnect the syringe from the inlet port after inflating the cuff

Glossary

A

Abandonment   Terminating patient care without making sure that care will continue at the same level or higher.

Abdomen   The part of the body trunk below the ribs and above the pelvis.

Abdominal Cavity   The body cavity located below the diaphragm and above the pelvis. It contains the stomach, intestines, liver, gallbladder, pancreas, and spleen.

Abnormal Behavior   A way of acting or conducting oneself that is not consistent with society's norms and expectations, that interferes with the individual's well-being and ability to function, and that may be harmful to the individual or others.

Abortion   The termination of pregnancy before the fetus is able to live on its own outside the uterus.

Abrasion   Damage to the outermost layer of skin (epidermis) by shearing forces (such as rubbing or scraping).

Abruptio Placentae   A condition that occurs when a normally implanted placenta separates prematurely from the wall of the uterus during the last trimester of pregnancy.

Absence (Petit Mal) Seizure   A type of generalized seizure in which the patient experiences a brief loss of consciousness (for 5 to 10 seconds) without a loss of muscle tone.

Absorption   The process of moving nutrients, water, and electrolytes into the circulatory system so they can be used by body cells.

Accessory Muscles for Breathing   Muscles between the ribs, above the collarbones, and in the abdomen used for breathing during periods of respiratory distress.

Accessory Organs of Digestion   The teeth and tongue, salivary glands, liver, gallbladder, and pancreas.

Acetabulum   A socket of the hip bone.

Acidosis   A buildup of acid in the blood and tissues.

Acrocyanosis   Blueness of the hands and feet.

Active Rewarming   The act of adding heat directly to the surface of the patient's body.

Acute Coronary Syndromes (ACSs)   Conditions caused by temporary or permanent blockage of a coronary artery as a result of coronary artery disease.

Acute Myocardial Infarction (Acute MI; "Heart Attack")   The death of heart tissue that occurs when a coronary artery becomes severely narrowed or is completely blocked, usually by a blood clot (thrombus).

Addiction   A psychological and physical dependence on a substance that has gone beyond voluntary control.

Adrenal Glands   Endocrine glands located on top of each kidney that release epinephrine in response to stress.

Advance Directive   A legal document that details a person's healthcare wishes when he or she becomes unable to make decisions for him or herself.

Agonal Breathing   Slow and shallow breathing that is sometimes seen just before the onset of respiratory failure.

Air Embolism   The entry of air into the circulation through a blood vessel that is torn and exposed to the air.

Airborne Diseases   Infections that are spread by droplets produced by coughing or sneezing.

Airway Adjuncts   Devices used to help keep a patient's airway open.

Alcohol Withdrawal Syndrome   A series of signs and symptoms that occur 6 to 48 hours after a chronic alcoholic reduces his intake or stops consuming alcohol.

Allergen   An antigen that causes signs and symptoms of an allergic reaction.

Allergic Asthma   Asthma that is triggered by an allergic reaction.

Allergic Reaction   An exaggerated response by the body's immune system to a substance.

Altered Mental Status   A change in a patient's level of awareness; also called an *altered level of consciousness* (ALOC).

Alveoli   Grapelike sacs at the end of bronchioles where oxygen and carbon dioxide are exchanged between the air and blood.

Amniotic Sac   The sac of fluid that surrounds the fetus inside the uterus; also called *bag of waters.*

Amputation   The separation of a body part from the rest of the body.

Anal Canal   The end of the large intestine, about 1-2 inches long, that remains closed except during defecation.

Anaphylactic Shock   Shock caused by a severe allergic reaction.

Anaphylaxis   A severe allergic reaction; a life-threatening emergency.

Anatomic Splint   Use of the body as a splint; also called self-splint.

Anatomical Position   A position in which a person stands with arms to the sides and with the palms turned forward, feet close together, the head pointed forward, and the eyes open.

Anatomy   The study of the structure of an organism (such as the human body).

Anesthesia   Without sensation; a loss of feeling.

Aneurysm   An abnormal bulging of a blood vessel.

Angina Pectoris   A symptom of coronary artery disease that occurs when the heart's need for oxygen exceeds its supply; literally, "choking in the chest."

Angioplasty   A procedure in which a balloon–tipped catheter is inserted into a partially blocked coronary artery. When the balloon is inflated, plaque is pressed against the walls of the artery, improving blood flow to the heart muscle.

Anisocoria   Unequal pupil size that is normal in about 2-4% of the population.

Ankle Drag   Emergency move in which the rescuer grasps the patient's ankles or pant cuffs and drags the patient to safety.

Anterior   The front portion of the body or body part.

Antibody   A substance produced by white blood cells to defend the body against bacteria, viruses, or other antigens.

Antidote   A substance that neutralizes a poison.

Antigen   Any substance that is foreign to an individual and causes antibody production.

Anxiety   A state of worry and agitation that is usually triggered by a real or imagined situation.

Anxiety Disorder   Condition that involves excessive anxiety ranging from uneasiness to terror.

Aorta   The largest artery in the body.

Aortic Valve   A semilunar valve located at the junction of the left ventricle and aorta.

Apparent Life-Threatening Event (ALTE)   An episode in which an infant was about to die but was found early enough for successful resuscitation; also called *near-miss SIDS* or *near-SIDS*.

Appendicular Skeleton   The upper and lower extremities (arms and legs), the shoulder girdle, and the pelvic girdle.

Arachnoid   Literally, "resembling a spider's web." The middle meningeal layer with delicate fibers that resemble a spider's web. It contains few blood vessels.

Arteries   Large blood vessels that carry blood away from the heart to the rest of the body.

Arterioles   The smallest branches of arteries leading to the capillaries.

Arteriosclerosis   Hardening (*-sclerosis*) of the walls of the arteries (*arterio-*).

Arthropods   Animals that have a segmented body, jointed legs, a digestive tract and, in most cases, a hard outer shell, but no backbone.

Ascending Colon   The part of the large intestine that passes upward from the cecum to the lower edge of the liver where it turns to become the transverse colon.

Aspiration   The entry of secretions or foreign material into the trachea and lungs.

Assault   Threatening, attempting, or causing a fear of offensive physical contact with a patient or another person.

Asymmetrical   Unevenness.

Atherosclerosis   Narrowing and thickening of the inner lining (endothelium) of the walls of large and medium-size arteries because of a buildup of plaque.

Atria   The two upper chambers of the heart, which receive blood from the body and lungs (singular = *atrium*).

Atrioventricular (AV) Valves   Heart valves that lie between an atrium and ventricle.

Aura   A peculiar sensation that comes before a seizure.

Automated External Defibrillator (AED)   A machine that analyzes a patient's heart rhythm and, if indicated, delivers an electrical shock.

Automatic Vehicle Locator (AVL)   A device that uses the Global Positioning System (GPS) to track a vehicle's location.

Automaticity   The ability of specialized electrical (pacemaker) cells in the heart to produce an electrical impulse without being stimulated by another source, such as a nerve.

Automatisms   Purposeless repetitive behavior, such as lip smacking, eye blinking, chewing or swallowing movements, fumbling of the hands, or shuffling of the feet.

Autonomic Division   The division of the peripheral nervous system that has receptors and nerves concerned with the internal environment. It controls the involuntary system of glands and smooth muscle and functions to maintain a steady state in the body.

AVPU Scale   A memory aid used to identify a patient's mental status. Each letter of the scale refers to a level of awareness. A = alert, V = responds to verbal stimuli, P = responds to painful stimuli, U = unresponsive. A patient who is oriented to person, place, time, and event is said to be "alert and oriented $\times$ ('times') 4" or "A and O $\times$ 4."

Avulsion   A soft-tissue injury in which a flap of skin or tissue is torn loose or pulled completely off.

Axial Skeleton   The part of the skeleton that includes the skull, spinal column, sternum, and ribs.

Axilla   Armpit.

B

Bacteria   Germs that can cause disease in humans, plants, or animals.

Bag-Mask (BM) Device   A self-inflating bag used to force air into a patient's lungs; also called a bag-valve-mask device.

Bandage   Material used to secure a dressing in place.

Barotrauma   Injury to tissue caused by excess pressure.

Barrier Device   A thin film of plastic or silicone that is placed on the patient's face to prevent direct contact with the patient's mouth during positive-pressure ventilation.

Base Station   A transmitter/receiver at a stationary site such as a hospital, mountaintop, or public safety agency.

Baseline Vital Signs   An initial set of vital sign measurements.

Basket Stretcher   A patient transfer device that is usually made of plastic and shaped like a long basket and can accommodate a scoop stretcher or a long backboard. It is used for moving patients over rough terrain and is often used in water rescues or high-angle rescues; also called a *Stokes basket* or *basket litter*.

Battery   The unlawful touching of another person without consent.

Battle's Sign   A bluish discoloration behind the ear that is a sign of a possible skull fracture.

Behavior   The way in which a person acts or performs.

Behavioral Emergency   A situation in which a patient displays abnormal behavior that is unacceptable to the patient, family members, or community.

Bilateral   Pertaining to both sides.

Binaurals The metal pieces of the stethoscope that connect the earpieces to the plastic or rubber tubing.

Biological Weapons The use of bacteria, viruses, rickettsia, or toxins to cause disease or death.

Bipolar Disorder A brain disorder that causes alternating episodes of mood elevation (mania) and depression; also known as *manic-depressive illness.*

Birth Canal A muscular tube that serves as a passageway between the uterus and the outside; also called the *vagina.*

Blanket Drag Emergency move in which the rescuer places the patient on a blanket and drags the blanket.

Blastocyst A cluster of cells that forms a few days after the joining of a sperm and egg. In human development, a blastocyst is preceded by a zygote (fertilized egg), and succeeded by an embryo.

Bleb A small air- or fluid-filled sac.

Blood Glucose Meter (Glucometer) A device used to measure the amount of glucose in a blood sample.

Blood Pressure (BP) The force exerted by the blood on the inner walls of the heart and the walls of the arteries.

Bloodborne Diseases Infections that are spread by contact with the blood or body fluids of an infected person.

Bloody Show Mucus and blood that may come out of the vagina as labor begins.

Blow-by Oxygen A method of oxygen delivery in which the device used to deliver the oxygen does not make actual contact with the patient.

Blunt Trauma Trauma in which a forceful impact occurs to the body but there is no break in the skin.

Body The main part of skeletal muscle; also, the middle portion of the sternum.

Body Cavity A hollow space in the body that contains internal organs.

Body Mechanics The coordinated effort of the musculoskeletal and nervous systems to maintain proper balance, posture, and body alignment during lifting, bending, moving, and other activities of daily living.

Body Substance Isolation (BSI) Precautions Self-protection against all body fluids and substances; also referred to as *Standard Precautions* and *Universal Precautions.*

Body Temperature The balance between the heat produced by the body and the heat lost from the body.

Bradypnea A slower-than-normal respiratory rate for a patient's age.

Brainstem The portion of the brain that consists of the midbrain, pons, and medulla oblongata.

Breach of Duty Violating the standard of care that applies in a given situation.

Breathing The mechanical process of moving air into and out of the lungs; also called *pulmonary ventilation.*

Breech Delivery A delivery in which the presenting part of the infant is the buttocks or feet instead of the head.

Bronchioles Small, thin-walled branches of a bronchus.

Bronchus Large passageway for air to and from the alveoli.

Bruise A collection of blood under the skin caused by bleeding capillaries.

Buccal Pertaining to the cheek.

C

Capillaries The very thin blood vessels that connect arteries and veins.

Capillary Refill An assessment tool used in infants and children. It is performed by pressing on the patient's skin or nailbeds and determining the time for return to initial color. Normal capillary refill in infants and children is less than two seconds; delayed (greater than two seconds) capillary refill suggests circulatory compromise.

Caplet An oval-shaped tablet that has a film-coated covering.

Capnometry The measurement of exhaled carbon dioxide levels.

Capsule A small gelatin container that contains a medication dose in powder or granule form.

Cardiac Arrest A condition that occurs when the contraction of the heart stops. It is confirmed by unresponsiveness, absent breathing, and absent pulses.

Cardiac Muscle Involuntary muscle found only in the heart.

Cardiac Tamponade A condition that occurs when blood enters the pericardial sac because of laceration of a coronary blood vessel, a ruptured coronary artery, laceration of a chamber of the heart, or a significant cardiac contusion. The blood in the pericardial sac compresses the heart, decreasing the amount of blood the heart can pump out with each contraction.

Cardiogenic Shock Shock that occurs when the heart muscle does not have enough force to pump blood effectively to all parts of the body.

Cardiopulmonary Failure Respiratory failure that occurs together with shock.

Cardiopulmonary Resuscitation (CPR) The combination of rescue breathing and external chest compressions.

Cardiovascular Disease Disease of the heart and blood vessels.

Cardiovascular System The heart, blood vessels, and blood.

Carina The internal ridge formed at the point at which the trachea divides into two primary bronchi.

Carpals Wrist bones.

Cecum A blind pouch or cul-de-sac that forms the first part of the large intestine.

Cells The basic building blocks of the body.

Centers for Disease Control (CDC) A federal agency of the U.S. government that promotes health and quality of life by preventing and controlling disease, injury, and disability.

Central Line An intravenous line placed near the heart for long-term use.

Central Nervous System (CNS) The brain and spinal cord.

Central Pulse A pulse found close to the trunk of the body.

Central Venous Access Inserting an intravenous catheter into one of the body's major veins, such as the subclavian or internal jugular vein.

Cephalic Delivery A delivery in which an infant emerges head first from the birth canal.

Cerebellum The second largest part of the human brain. It is responsible for the precise control of muscle movements and the maintenance of posture and equilibrium.

Cerebral Contusion A brain injury in which brain tissue is bruised and damaged in a local area.

Cerebrospinal Fluid (CSF)   A clear liquid that acts as a shock absorber for the brain and spinal cord and provides a means for the exchange of nutrients and wastes among the blood, brain, and spinal cord.

Cerebrum   The largest part of the brain, made up of two hemispheres.

Certification   A designation that ensures a person has met predetermined requirements to perform a particular activity.

Cervix   The narrow opening at the lower end of the uterus that connects the uterus to the vagina.

Chain of Survival   The ideal series of events that should take place immediately after recognizing an injury or the onset of sudden illness.

Chemical Agents   Poisonous substances that injure or kill people by absorption through the skin or eyes, or through inhalation or ingestion.

Chemical Name   A description of a drug's composition and molecular structure.

Chemical Protective Clothing (CPC)   Materials designed to protect the skin from exposure to chemicals by either physical or chemical means.

Chief Complaint   The reason EMS has been called, usually in the patient's own words.

Childbirth   The emergence of an infant from its mother's uterus.

Child Maltreatment   An act or failure to act by a parent, caregiver, or other person as defined by state law that results in physical abuse, neglect, medical neglect, sexual abuse, and/or emotional abuse; an act or failure to act that presents an impending risk of serious harm to a child.

Chronic Bronchitis   Sputum production for three months of a year for at least two consecutive years.

Chyme   Partially digested food that is moved through the digestive tract by peristalsis.

Circumferential Burn   Swelling from a burn that encircles an extremity.

Cleaning   The process of washing a contaminated object with soap and water.

Clenched-Fist Injury   An injury in which the fist of an individual strikes the teeth of another; also called a *fight bite*. The skin on the hand may or may not be broken.

Closed Soft-Tissue Injury   A soft-tissue injury that results when the body is struck by a blunt object. There is no break in the skin, but the tissues and vessels beneath the skin surface are crushed or ruptured.

Closed Wound   An injury that occurs when the soft tissues under the skin are damaged but the surface of the skin is not broken.

Clothes Drag   Emergency move in which a rescuer pulls on the patient's clothing in the neck and shoulder area; also called the *clothing pull* or *shirt drag*.

Coining   A healing remedy practiced by some cultures in which a coin is heated in hot oil and then rubbed along the patient's spine to heal an illness, such as congestion in the lungs.

Comfort Care   Measures used to ease the symptoms of an illness or injury; also called *palliative care* or *supportive care*.

Communicable Disease   A contagious infection that can be spread from one person to another.

Communication   The process of sending and receiving information.

Compartment Syndrome   A compression injury that develops when the pressure within a compartment causes compression and abnormal function of nerves and blood vessels.

Competence   A patient's ability to understand the questions you ask of him or her and understand the implications of the decisions he or she makes concerning his or her care.

Completed Suicide   Death by a self-inflicted, consciously intended action.

Complex Extrication   The use of powered hydraulic rescue tools, such as cutters, spreaders, and rams, to gain access to and extricate the patient from the vehicle.

Complex Partial Seizure   A type of partial seizure in which the patient's consciousness, responsiveness, or memory is impaired; also called a *temporal lobe seizure* or *psychomotor seizure*.

Compliance   The ability of a patient's lung tissue to distend (inflate) with ventilation.

Compulsions   Recurring behaviors or rituals performed with the hope of preventing obsessive thoughts or making them go away.

Computer-Aided Dispatch (CAD)   A computer system that aids dispatch personnel in handling and prioritizing emergency calls.

Concussion   A traumatic brain injury that results in a temporary loss of function in some or all of the brain.

Conduction   The transfer of heat between objects that are in direct contact.

Congestive Heart Failure (CHF)   A condition in which one or both sides of the heart fail to pump efficiently.

Conjunctiva   A paper-thin mucous membrane that covers the sclera (the white of the eye).

Consent   Permission.

Contraindications   Condition(s) for which a drug should not be used because it may cause harm to the patient or offer no improvement of the patient's condition or illness.

Contralateral   Opposite side.

Contributing Risk Factors   Risk factors that can be part of the cause of a person's risk of heart disease.

Contusion   Bruise.

Convection   The transfer of heat by the movement of air current.

Convulsions   The jerking movements during the clonic phase of a tonic-clonic seizure.

Coronary Artery Bypass Graft (CABG)   A surgical procedure in which a graft is created from a healthy blood vessel from another part of the patient's body to reroute blood flow around a diseased coronary artery; pronounced "cabbage".

Coronary Artery Disease (CAD)   A term used for diseases that slow or stop blood flow through the arteries that supply the heart muscle with blood.

Coronary Heart Disease (CHD)   Disease of the coronary arteries and the complications that result, such as angina pectoris or a heart attack.

Corpus Callosum   A collection of nerve fibers in the brain that connect the left and right cerebral hemispheres.

Crackles Abnormal breath sounds that sound like hair rolled between the thumb and forefinger close to one's ear, indicating the presence of fluid in the alveoli or larger airways; also called *rales.*

Cradle Carry A move in which the rescuer kneels next to the patient, places one hand under the patient's shoulders and the other under the patient's knees, and then stands up, carrying the patient to safety; also called the *one-person arm carry.*

Cranial Cavity The body cavity located in the head that contains the brain.

Cranial Nerves Twelve pairs of nerves that connect the brain with the neck and structures in the chest and abdomen.

Cranium The portion of the skull that encloses the brain.

Crepitation (Crepitus) A crackling sensation heard and felt beneath the skin caused by bone ends grating against each other or air trapped between layers of tissue.

Cricoid Cartilage The most inferior of the cartilages of the larynx.

Cricoid Pressure The application of pressure to the cricoid cartilage. This pressure pushes the trachea backward and compresses the esophagus against the cervical vertebrae, decreasing the amount of air entering the stomach during positive-pressure ventilation; also called the *Sellick maneuver.*

Critical Incident A situation that causes a healthcare provider to experience unusually strong emotions.

Critical Incident Stress Debriefing (CISD) A formal group meeting led by a mental health professional and peer counselors.

Critical Incident Stress Management (CISM) A program developed to assist emergency workers in coping with stressful situations.

Croup An infection that affects the larynx and the area just below it.

Crowing A long, high-pitched sound heard on inhalation.

Crowning The stage of birth when the presenting part of the infant is visible at the vaginal opening.

Crush Injury Trauma caused by a compressing force applied to the body; also called a *compression injury.*

Crush Syndrome A compression injury that can occur when a large amount of skeletal muscle is compressed for a long period (usually four to six hours, although it may be as little as one hour) and compromises local blood flow.

Cumulative Stress Tension that results from repeated exposure to smaller stressors that build up over time.

Cushing's Triad Three findings (increased systolic blood pressure, abnormal breathing pattern, and decreased heart rate) that indicate increasing intracranial pressure in a patient with a head injury.

Cyanosis Blue-gray color of the skin or mucous membranes that suggests inadequate oxygenation or poor perfusion.

D

DCAP-BTLS Memory aid used for patient assessment: *deformities, contusions, abrasions, punctures or penetrations, burns, tenderness, lacerations, and swelling.*

Decompression Sickness A diving-related injury that results from dissolved nitrogen in the blood and tissues; also called *the bends.*

Decontamination The use of physical or chemical means to remove, inactivate, or destroy bloodborne pathogens on a surface or item to the point at which it is no longer capable of transmitting infectious particles and the surface or item is considered safe for handling, use, or disposal.

Defecation The elimination of undigested waste from the body.

Defibrillation The delivery of an electrical shock to a patient's heart to end an abnormal heart rhythm.

Defibrillator A machine that delivers electrical shocks to the heart.

Defusing A short, informal meeting, usually led by peer counselors, that is held for rescuers immediately or within a few hours after a critical incident.

Delayed Drowning A type of drowning that occurs when a victim appears to have survived an immersion or submersion episode but later dies from respiratory failure or an infection; also called *secondary drowning.*

Delirium Tremens (DTs) Signs and symptoms associated with alcohol withdrawal that have progressed beyond the usual symptoms of withdrawal and are potentially fatal.

Delivery The actual birth of the baby at the end of the second stage of labor.

Delusions False beliefs that the patient believes are true, despite facts to the contrary.

Denial A defense mechanism used to create a buffer against the shock of dying or dealing with an illness or injury.

Dependent Lividity The settling of blood in dependent areas of the body (those areas on which the body has been resting).

Depression A normal response to the loss of a significant other or the loss of some bodily function; a state of mind characterized by feelings of sadness, worthlessness, and discouragement.

Dermis The thick layer of skin below the epidermis that contains hair follicles, sweat and oil glands, small nerve endings, and blood vessels.

Descending Colon The part of the large intestine descending from the left colic (splenic) flexure to the brim of the pelvis.

Diabetic Ketoacidosis (DKA) Severe, uncontrolled hyperglycemia (usually over 300 mg/dL); also called *diabetic coma.*

Diaphragm The dome-shaped muscle below the lungs that is the primary muscle of respiration.

Diastolic Blood Pressure The pressure in the arteries when the heart is at rest.

Diencephalon The part of the brain between the cerebrum and the brainstem. It contains the thalamus and hypothalamus.

Diffusion The movement of gases or particles from an area of higher concentration to an area of lower concentration.

Digestion The chemical process of breaking down food into small parts so absorption can occur.

Direct Ground Lift A non-urgent move used to lift and carry a patient with no suspected spine injury from the ground to a bed or stretcher.

Direct Pressure Firm pressure applied to a bleeding site with gloved hands or bandages to control bleeding.

Direct Questions Questions that require a yes or no answer.

Disentanglement The moving or removing of material that is trapping a victim.

Disinfecting Cleaning with chemical solutions such as alcohol or chlorine.

Dislocation Forceful movement of the ends of bones from their normal positions in a joint.

Distal Farther away from the midline, or center area, of the body.

Distention Bulging or swelling.

Do Not Resuscitate (DNR) Order Instructions written by a physician that notify medical professionals not to provide medical care to a patient who has experienced a cardiac arrest.

Dose The amount of a drug that should be given to the patient.

Draw Sheet A narrow sheet placed crosswise on a bed under the patient; used to assist in moving a patient or in changing soiled bedsheets.

Dressing Absorbent material placed directly over a wound.

Drowning A process that results in harm to the respiratory system from submersion or immersion in a liquid.

Dry Drowning Drowning in which the larynx closes to prevent the passage of water into the lungs.

Duodenum The portion of the small intestine that connects the stomach and jejunum.

Duplex System A mode of radio transmission that uses two frequencies to transmit and receive messages, allowing simultaneous two-way communication.

Dura Mater Literally, "hard" or "tough mother." The tough, durable, outermost layer of the meninges that adheres to the inner surface of the cranium.

Duty to Act A formal contractual or an implied legal obligation to provide care to a patient requesting services.

Dyspnea A sensation of shortness of breath or difficulty breathing.

E

Ecchymosis Bluish discoloration caused by leakage of blood into the skin or mucous membrane.

Eclampsia A condition of pregnancy characterized by high blood pressure, swelling, protein in the urine, and seizures.

Ectopic Pregnancy A condition that occurs when a fertilized egg implants outside the uterus. An ectopic pregnancy that occurs in a fallopian tube is called a tubal pregnancy.

Edema Swelling.

Elective Abortion An abortion performed at the request of the mother.

Elixirs Clear liquids made with alcohol, water, flavors, or sweeteners.

Embolus A clot that travels through the circulatory system.

Embryo In human development, the 3rd to the 8th week of gestation. At the end of the 8th week, the essentials of the organ systems are present.

Emergency An unexpected illness or injury that requires immediate action to avoid risking the life or health of the person being treated.

Emergency Medical Radio Service (EMRS) A group of frequencies designated by the FCC exclusively for use by EMS providers.

Emergency Medical Responder (EMR) A person who has the basic knowledge and skills necessary to provide lifesaving emergency care while waiting for the arrival of additional EMS help; formerly called *First Responder*.

Emergency Medical Services (EMS) System A network of resources that provides emergency care and transportation to victims of sudden illness or injury.

Emergency Medical Technician (EMT) A member of the Emergency Medical Services team who responds to emergency calls, provides efficient emergency to ill or injured patients, and transports the patient to a medical facility.

Emergency Move A method used to move, lift, or carry a patient when there is an immediate danger to the rescuer or the patient.

Emergency Response Operation of an emergency vehicle while responding to a medical emergency.

Emergency Transportation The process of moving a patient from the scene of an emergency to an appropriate healthcare facility.

Empathy To understand, be aware of, and be sensitive to the feelings, thoughts, and experience of another.

Emphysema An irreversible disease that leads to destruction of the walls of the alveoli, distention of the alveolar sacs, and loss of lung elasticity.

Emulsions Mixtures of two liquids, one distributed throughout the other in small globules.

Endocrine System A system of ductless glands that secrete chemicals, such as insulin and adrenalin, which regulate and influence body activities and functions.

Endometriosis A condition in which uterine tissue is located outside the uterus, causing pain and bleeding.

Endotracheal (ET) Tube A plastic tube that is open at both ends and designed for insertion into a patient's trachea.

Endotracheal Intubation The placement of a plastic tube into a patient's trachea to keep the airway open.

End-Tidal Carbon Dioxide Detector A device that measures a person's exhaled carbon dioxide.

Enhanced 9-1-1 (E9-1-1) A system that routes an emergency call to the 9-1-1 center closest to the caller and automatically displays the caller's phone number and address.

Enteric-Coated Tablets Tablets that have a special coating so that they break down in the intestines instead of the stomach.

Epidermis The outer layer of the skin.

Epidural Hematoma A buildup of blood between the dura and the skull that often involves the tearing of an artery; usually the middle meningeal artery.

Epiglottis Leaf-shaped cartilage that covers the opening to the larynx during swallowing, preventing food and liquids from entering the airway.

Epiglottitis A bacterial infection of the epiglottis.

Epilepsy A condition of recurring seizures in which the cause is usually irreversible.

Erect Standing upright.

Erythrocytes Red blood cells; formed elements of blood.

Esophageal Detector Device (EDD) An inexpensive, easy-to-use tool used as an aid in confirming the position of an endotracheal tube.

Esophageal-Tracheal Combitube (ETC or Combitube) A dual-lumen airway that consists of two tubes (esophageal and tracheal) and that permits ventilation if the tube is inserted into the esophagus (most common) or into the trachea; commonly called the *Combitube.*

Esophagus A muscular tube about 9 inches long (in adults) that is a passageway for food.

Ethics Principles of right and wrong, good and bad, that affect our actions and lead to consequences.

Evaporation A loss of heat by vaporization of moisture on the body surface.

Evisceration The protrusion of an organ through an open wound.

Exhalation The process of breathing out and moving air out of the lungs.

Expiration (Exhalation) The process of breathing out and moving air out of the lungs.

Exposure Direct or indirect contact with infected blood, body fluids, tissues, or airborne droplets.

Expressed Consent A type of consent in which a patient gives specific permission verbally, in writing, or nonverbally for care and transport to be provided.

External Bleeding Bleeding that can be seen.

External Nares Nostrils.

Extrication To free from entrapment.

F

Fainting A sudden, temporary loss of consciousness that occurs when one or both sides of the heart do not pump out a sufficient amount of blood, resulting in inadequate blood flow to the brain.

Fallopian Tubes (Oviducts) In the female, tubes that receive and transport the ovum to the uterus after ovulation.

False Ribs Rib pairs 8 through 10. These ribs attach to the cartilage of the seventh ribs.

Fascia A tough sheet of fibrous tissue that covers the skeletal muscles of the body.

Fasciotomy A surgical procedure in which a physician cuts the tough sheet of fibrous tissue covering a muscle to relieve pressure.

Febrile Seizures Seizures caused by fever.

Federal Communications Commission (FCC) The U.S. government agency responsible for regulation of interstate and international communications by radio, television, wire, satellite, and cable.

Femur The thigh bone. It extends from the hip to the knee.

Fend-Off Position The parking of an emergency vehicle downward from the scene and in such a way that allows traveling vehicles to strike the vehicle and not crew members.

Fetus In human development, the 8th week of gestation through the time of birth.

Fibula The bone that lies next to the tibia along the outer side of the lower leg.

Field Impression The conclusion an EMT reaches about what is wrong with the patient.

Firefighter's Carry A move involving a series of maneuvers in which the patient is positioned lengthwise across the rescuer's shoulders and carried to safety.

Firefighter's Drag Emergency move in which the patient is placed on his back with his wrists crossed and secured. While the rescuer straddles the patient, the patient's arms are lifted over the rescuer's head so that his or her wrists are behind the rescuer's neck. The rescuer then crawls forward, dragging the patient to safety.

Flail Chest A condition in which two or more adjacent ribs are fractured in two or more places or when the sternum is detached. The section of the chest wall between the fractured ribs becomes free floating because it is no longer in continuity with the chest. This free-floating section of the chest wall is called the *flail segment.*

Flexible Stretcher A patient transfer device made of canvas or synthetic flexible material with carrying handles. A flexible stretcher is useful when space is limited to access the patient, such as in narrow hallways, stairs, or cramped corners; examples include the Reeves stretcher, SKED, and Navy stretcher.

Floating Ribs Rib pairs 11 and 12. These ribs have no attachment to the sternum (rib pairs 11 and 12).

Flow Meter A valve that controls the liters of oxygen delivered per minute.

Flow-Restricted, Oxygen-Powered Ventilation Device (FROPVD) A manually triggered ventilation (MTV) device used to give positive-pressure ventilation with 100% oxygen.

Focused Physical Examination An assessment of specific body areas that relate to a patient's illness or injury.

Focused Trauma Assessment A focused physical exam performed on an injured patient.

Foodborne Diseases Infections that are spread by the improper handling of food or by poor personal hygiene.

Foramen Magnum The large opening in the base of the skull through which the spinal cord passes.

Forearm Drag Emergency move in which the rescuer's hands are positioned under the patient's armpits, the patient's forearms are grasped, and the patient dragged to safety; also called the *bent-arm drag.*

Fowler's Position Lying on the back with the upper body elevated at a 45- to 60-degree angle.

Fracture A break in a bone.

Full-Thickness Burn A burn in which the epidermis and dermis are destroyed; also called a *third-degree burn.* The burn may also involve subcutaneous tissue, muscle, and bone.

G

Gallbladder A pear-shaped sac on the undersurface of the liver that stores bile until it is needed by the small intestine.

Gastrostomy Tube A special catheter placed directly into the stomach for feeding.

Gelcap A small gelatin container that contains a liquid medication dose.

Gels Clear or translucent semisolid substances that liquefy when applied to the skin or a mucous membrane.

General Impression An "across-the-room" assessment of a patient that is completed in 60 seconds or less to decide if the patient looks "sick" or "not sick"; also called a *first impression.*

Generalized Seizure A type of seizure that begins suddenly and involves a period of altered mental status.

Generic Name The name given to a drug by the company that first manufactures it; also called the *nonproprietary name.*

Gestational Diabetes   Diabetes that begins during pregnancy.

Global Position System (GPS)   Technology that uses a system of satellites and receiving devices to compute the receiver's geographic position on the Earth.

Glottic Opening   The space between the vocal cords.

Glottis   The space between the vocal cords.

Glucagon   A hormone released from alpha cells in the pancreas that stimulates cells in the liver to break down stores of glycogen into glucose to increase the blood glucose level.

Golden Hour   The first sixty minutes after the occurrence of major trauma; the period from the time of the injury to the time the patient should receive definitive care in an operating room.

Great Vessels   The body's major blood vessels: pulmonary arteries and veins, the aorta, and the superior and inferior vena cavae.

Greater Trochanter   The large, bony prominence on the lateral shaft of the femur to which the buttock muscles are attached.

Greenstick Fractures   A break in a bone that occurs in a child where the bone breaks on one side but not the other, like bending a green tree branch.

Grief   A normal response that helps a person cope with the loss of someone or something that had great meaning to them.

Growth Plate   An area of growing tissue near the end of a long bone in children and adolescents.

Gurgling   A wet sound that suggests that fluid is collecting in the patient's upper airway.

Gynecology   The study of the female reproductive system.

H

Hallucinations   False sensory perceptions that are seen, heard, or felt by a person but not by others.

Hard Palate   The bony floor of the nasal cavity.

Hazardous Material   A substance (solid, liquid, or gas) that, when released, is capable of creating harm to people, the environment, and property.

Head Bobbing   An indicator of increased work of breathing in infants. When the baby breathes out, the head falls forward; the baby's head comes up when the baby breathes in and its chest expands.

Head Tilt–Chin Lift Maneuver   An effective method for opening the airway in a patient with no known or suspected trauma to the head or neck.

Health Insurance Portability and Accountability Act (HIPAA)   A law passed by Congress in 1996 to ensure the confidentiality of a person's health information.

Healthcare System   A network of people, facilities, and equipment designed to provide for the general medical needs of the population.

Heart   The primary organ of the cardiovascular system. It lies in the thoracic cavity (mediastinum) behind the sternum and between the lungs.

Hematemesis   The vomiting of blood.

Hematoma   A localized collection of blood beneath the skin caused by a tear in a blood vessel.

Hematuria   Possible blood in the urine.

Hemophilia   A disorder in which the blood does not clot normally.

Hemoptysis   The coughing up of blood.

Hemorrhage   An extreme loss of blood from a blood vessel; also called *major bleeding*.

Hemorrhagic Shock   Shock caused by severe bleeding.

Hemorrhagic Stroke   A stroke caused by bleeding into the brain.

Hemothorax   Blood in the pleural space.

High-Fowler's Position   A position in which a patient sits upright at a 90-degree angle.

High-Level Disinfection   A method of decontamination that destroys all microorganisms except large numbers of bacterial spores. It is used for reusable equipment that has been in contact with mucous membranes, such as laryngoscope blades.

History of the Present Illness   A chronological record of the reason a patient is seeking medical assistance that includes the patient's chief complaint and the patient's answers to questions about the circumstances that led up to his request for medical help.

Homeostasis   The property of an organism allowing it to regulate its internal processes to maintain a constant internal environment; also called *steady state*.

Hot Zone   An identified safety zone at a hazardous materials incident that contains the hazardous material (contaminant); also known as the *exclusion zone*.

Human Crutch Move   A move in which a rescuer places the patient's arm across the rescuer's shoulders, holds the patient's wrist with one hand, and places the rescuer's other hand around the patient's waist to help him to safety; also called the *rescuer assist* or *walking assist*.

Humerus   The upper arm bone.

Hydrocephalus   A condition in which there is an excess of cerebrospinal fluid within the brain.

Hyperglycemia   A higher-than-normal blood sugar level.

Hyperthermia   A high core body temperature.

Hyphema   Blood in the anterior chamber of the eye.

Hypoglycemia   A lower-than-normal blood sugar level. In adults, hypoglycemia is a blood glucose level less than 70 mg/dL.

Hypothalamus   A part of the brain that plays an important role in the control of thirst, hunger, and body temperature. It also serves as a link between the nervous and endocrine systems.

Hypothermia   A core body temperature of less than 95°F (35°C).

Hypovolemic Shock   Shock caused by a loss of blood, plasma, or other body fluid.

Hypoxia   A lack of oxygen, which may be generalized in the body or limited to a particular area of the body (tissue hypoxia).

Hypoxic Drive   The stimulation of breathing by low levels of oxygen in the blood instead of an increase in carbon dioxide levels.

I

Ileum   The last portion of the small intestine that connects with the cecum, which is the first part of the large intestine.

Immersion Covering of the face and airway in water or other fluid.

Impaled Object An object that remains embedded in an open wound.

Impetigo A contagious bacterial skin infection that can look like a burn.

Implantable Cardioverter-Defibrillator (ICD) A surgically implanted device placed in a person who has had, or is at high risk of having, heart rhythm problems. The device is programmed to recognize heart rhythms that are too fast or life threatening and deliver a shock to reset the rhythm.

Implied Consent Consent assumed from a patient requiring emergency care who is mentally, physically, or emotionally unable to provide expressed consent.

Incendiary Materials Substances that burn with a hot flame for a specific period.

Incident Commander (IC) The person who is responsible for managing all operations during domestic incidents.

Incident Command System (ICS) A standardized system developed to assist with the control, direction, and coordination of emergency response resources at an incident of any type and size; also called the *Incident Management System* (IMS).

Incompetent A patient who does not have the ability to understand the questions asked of him or her or does not understand the implications of the decisions he or she makes regarding his or her care.

Incomplete Abortion An abortion in which part of the products of conception have been passed, but some remain in the uterus.

Index of Suspicion Anticipating potential injuries based on the patient's chief complaint, mechanism of injury, and assessment findings. In the case of a medical patient, anticipating potential complications of an illness on the basis of the patient's chief complaint, SAMPLE history, and assessment findings.

Indications The condition(s) for which a drug has documented usefulness.

Infection An illness that results when the body is invaded by germs capable of producing disease.

Inferior In a position lower than another.

Infiltration A complication of intravenous (IV) therapy that occurs when an IV medication or solution leaks out of the vein and into the tissues surrounding the IV insertion site.

Informed Consent A type of consent in which the patient understands the risks and benefits of the EMT's care.

Ingestion Taking in nutrients, water, and electrolytes into the body's digestive system.

Inhalants Household and commercial products that can be abused by intentionally breathing the product's gas or vapors for its mind-altering effects.

Inhalation The process of breathing in and moving air into the lungs.

In-Line Stabilization A technique used to minimize movement of the head and neck.

Insertion The movable attachment to a bone.

Inspiration (Inhalation) The process of breathing in and moving air into the lungs.

Insulin A hormone released from beta cells in the pancreas that helps glucose enter the body's cells to be used for energy.

Insulin Resistance A condition in which the cells of the body fail to respond to the presence of insulin, thus not allowing glucose to enter the cells.

Integumentary System The body system made up of the skin, hair, nails, sweat glands, and oil (sebaceous) glands.

Interagency Radio Advisory Committee (IRAC) The federal agency responsible for coordinating radio use by agencies of the federal government.

Intercostal Muscles Muscles located between the ribs.

Intercostal Retractions Indentations of the skin between the ribs.

Intermediate-Level Disinfection A method of decontamination that destroys tuberculosis bacteria, vegetative bacteria, and most viruses and fungi, but not bacterial spores. It is used for surfaces that contact intact skin and have been visibly contaminated with body fluids, such as blood pressure cuffs, stethoscopes, backboards, and splints.

Internal Bleeding Bleeding that occurs inside body tissues and cavities.

Intracerebral Hematoma A collection of blood within the brain.

Intracerebral Hemorrhage Bleeding within the brain caused by a ruptured blood vessel within the brain itself.

Intramuscular Route Injection of a liquid form of medication directly into a skeletal muscle.

Intravenous Within a vein.

Intravenous (IV) Cannulation Placement of a catheter (also called a *cannula*) into a vein to gain access to the body's venous circulation.

Intravenous Drip The continuous administration of a drug or fluids by means of an IV line; also called an IV infusion.

Intravenous Therapy The giving of a liquid substance, such as fluids or medications, directly into the venous circulation.

Ipsilateral Same side.

Ischemia Decreased blood flow to an organ or tissue.

Ischemic Stroke A stroke caused by a blood clot (thrombus) or embolus.

Islets of Langerhans Structures located in the pancreas, which is a part of the endocrine system. Alpha cells secrete glucagon, which increases blood glucose concentration; beta cells secrete insulin, which decreases blood glucose concentration.

Isotonic Solution A solution that does not cause body cells to gain or lose water.

J

Jaw Thrust Without Head Tilt Maneuver A preferred method of opening the airway of an unresponsive patient when trauma to the head or neck is suspected; also called the *jaw thrust without head extension maneuver.*

Jejunum The middle portion of the small intestine that connects the duodenum and ileum.

Joint A place where two bones come together.

Jugular Venous Distention (JVD) Bulging of the neck veins when the patient is placed in a sitting position at a 45-degree angle.

K

Kidney One of two organs located at the back of the abdominal cavity on each side of the spinal column that produces urine, maintains water balance, aids in the regulation of blood pressure, and regulates levels of many chemicals in the blood.

Kinematics The science of analyzing the mechanism of injury and predicting injury patterns.

Kinetic Energy The energy of motion.

Kussmaul Respirations A breathing pattern in which the patient breathes deeply and rapidly in an attempt to get rid of excess acid by "blowing off" carbon dioxide.

L

Labor The process in which the uterus repeatedly contracts to push the fetus and placenta out of the mother's body. It begins with the first uterine muscle contraction and ends with delivery of the placenta.

Laceration A break in the skin of varying depth that may be linear (regular) or stellate (irregular); caused by forceful impact with a sharp object (such as a knife, razor blade, or glass).

Lancet A device used to prick a patient's skin to obtain a blood sample.

Large Intestine (Colon) The portion of the digestive system that extends from the ileum of the small intestine to the anus. It is subdivided into the following sections (listed in the order in which food passes through them): cecum, ascending colon, transverse colon, descending colon, sigmoid colon, rectum, and anal canal.

Laryngeal Stoma Surgical opening in the neck.

Laryngectomy The surgical removal of the larynx.

Laryngopharynx The lowermost part of the throat. It serves as a passageway for both food and air.

Laryngoscope An instrument that consists of a handle and blade that are made of plastic or stainless steel and used to visualize the glottic opening (the space between the vocal cords).

Laryngospasm Contraction of the sensitive tissue near the vocal cords.

Larynx The voice box.

Lateral Toward the side of the body.

Lateral Recumbent Position Lying on the side. Left side = left lateral recumbent position, right side = right lateral recumbent position.

Leukocytes White blood cells; formed elements of blood.

Licensure The granting of a written authorization by an official or legal authority.

Limb Presentation A delivery in which the presenting part of the infant is an arm or a leg instead of the head.

Liver The largest organ of the body and one that is responsible for many functions, including the production of bile, the storage of minerals and fat-soluble vitamins, and the storage of blood.

Local Cold Injury Tissue damage to a specific area of the body that occurs when a body part, such as the nose, ears, cheeks, chin, hands, or feet, is exposed to prolonged or intense cold; also called *frostbite*.

Local Effect An effect of a drug that usually occurs at the site of drug application.

Log Roll A technique used to move a patient from a face-down to a face-up position while maintaining the head and neck in line with the rest of the body.

Long Backboard A device that is 6-7 feet long and commonly made of wood, metal, or plastic with holes spaced along the head and foot ends and sides of the board for handholds and the insertion of straps.

Lotion A preparation applied to protect the skin or treat a skin disorder.

Low-Level Disinfection A method of decontamination that destroys most bacteria, and some viruses and fungi, but not tuberculosis bacteria or bacterial spores. It is used for the routine cleaning of surfaces, such as floors, countertops, and ambulance seats, when no body fluids are visible.

Low Vision Visual impairment, not correctable by standard glasses, contact lenses, medicine, or surgery, that interferes with a person's ability to perform everyday activities.

Lungs Spongy, air-filled organs that bring air into contact with the blood so that oxygen and carbon dioxide can be exchanged in the alveoli.

Lymphatic System Lymph, lymph nodes, lymph vessels, tonsils, spleen, and thymus gland.

M

Macrodrip IV Administration Set Intravenous (IV) tubing that forms large drops of IV fluid. Depending on the manufacturer, macrodrip IV tubing can deliver 10, 15, or 20 drops per milliliter of IV fluid.

Major Bleeding An extreme loss of blood from a blood vessel; also called *hemorrhage*.

Mammalian Diving Reflex A reflex triggered by cold water stimulation of the temperature receptors in the skin that causes shunting of blood to the brain and heart from the skin, gastrointestinal tract, and extremities, resulting in slowing of the victim's heart rate in response to the increased volume of blood in the body's core.

Mammary Glands (Breasts) Glands in the female that function in milk production after delivery of an infant.

Mandible Lower jawbone.

Manual Defibrillator A machine that requires the rescuer to analyze and interpret the patient's cardiac rhythm.

Manubrium The uppermost portion of the breastbone. It connects with the clavicle and the first rib.

Mass Casualty Incident (MCI) Any event that places a great demand on resources—equipment, personnel, or both; also called a *multiple casualty incident* or *multiple casualty situation* (MCS).

Massive Hemothorax A life-threatening injury that involves blood loss of more than 1500 mL in the chest cavity.

Material Safety Data Sheets (MSDSs) Papers required by the Occupational Safety and Health Administration to be kept on site anywhere chemicals are used. These sheets include the name of the substance, the physical properties of the substance, fire and explosion hazard information, and guidelines for emergency first-aid treatment.

Maxilla   Upper jawbone.

Mechanism of Action   How a drug exerts its effect on body cells and tissues.

Mechanism of Injury (MOI)   The way in which an injury occurs as well as the forces involved in producing the injury.

Meconium   Thick, sticky material that collects in the intestines of a fetus and forms the first stools of a newborn. It is usually greenish to black in color.

Medial   Toward the midline of the body.

Mediastinal Shift   Shifting of the heart and major blood vessels from their normal position.

Mediastinum   The part of the thoracic cavity between the lungs that contains the heart, major vessels, esophagus, trachea, and nerves.

Medical Director   A physician who provides medical oversight and is responsible for ensuring that actions taken on behalf of ill or injured people are medically appropriate.

Medical Neglect   A type of maltreatment characterized by failure of the caregiver to provide for the appropriate healthcare of the child despite being financially able to do so.

Medical Oversight   The process by which a physician directs the emergency care provided by Emergency Medical Services personnel to an ill or injured patient; also referred to as *medical control* or *medical direction*.

Medical Patient   An individual whose condition is caused by an illness.

Medical Practice Act   A state law that grants authority to provide medical care to patients and determines the scope of practice for healthcare professionals.

Medulla Oblongata   A part of the brainstem that extends from the pons and is continuous with the upper portion of the spinal cord. It is involved in the regulation of heart rate, blood vessel diameter, respiration, coughing, swallowing, and vomiting.

Melatonin   A naturally occurring hormone that has a role in regulating daily rhythms, such as sleep.

Meninges   Literally, membranes; three layers of connective tissue coverings that surround the brain and spinal cord.

Meningitis   An inflammation of the membranes covering the brain and spinal cord.

Menstruation   The periodic discharge of blood and tissue from the uterus; also called a *period*.

Metacarpals   The bones that form the support for the palm of the hand.

Metatarsals   The bones that form the part of the foot to which the toes attach.

Microdrip IV Administration Set   Intravenous (IV) tubing that forms very small drops, delivering 60 drops per milliliter of IV fluid; also called a *minidrip administration set*.

Midaxillary Line   An imaginary vertical line drawn from the middle of the armpits (axillae); parallel to the midline of the body.

Midbrain   A part of the brainstem that acts as a relay for auditory and visual impulses.

Midclavicular Line   An imaginary vertical line drawn through the middle portion of the collarbone (clavicle) and nipple; parallel to the midline of the body.

Midline   An imaginary line down the center of the body that divides the body into right and left sides.

Minimum Data Set   The recommended minimum information that should be included in a prehospital care report.

Minute Volume   The amount of air moved in and out of the lungs in one minute; the tidal volume multiplied by the respiratory rate.

Mitral (Bicuspid) Valve   An atrioventricular valve located between the left atrium and left ventricle.

Mobile Data Computer (MDC)   A computer mounted in an emergency vehicle that displays information pertaining to the calls for which EMS personnel are dispatched.

Mobile Two-Way Radio   A vehicular-mounted communication device that usually transmits at a lower power than base stations.

Modifiable Risk Factors   Risk factors that can be changed.

Mongolian Spots   Bluish areas usually seen in non-Caucasian infants and young children that may be mistaken for bruises.

Motor Nerves   Nerves that carry responses *from* the brain and spinal cord, stimulating a muscle or organ.

Mottling   An irregular or patchy skin discoloration that is usually a mixture of blue and white; usually seen in patients in shock, with hypothermia, or in cardiac arrest.

Mouth-to-Mouth Ventilation   The delivery of a rescuer's exhaled air to a patient while making mouth-to-mouth contact.

Multiplex System   A mode of radio transmission that permits simultaneous transmission of voice and other data using one frequency.

Muscle Tone   The constant tension produced by muscles of the body over long periods.

Myocardial Contusion   Bruising of the heart.

N

Nasal Airway   A soft, rubbery tube with a hole in it that is placed in a patient's nose to keep the tongue from blocking the upper airway.

Nasal Cannula   An oxygen delivery device that consists of plastic tubing with two soft prongs that are inserted into the patient's nostrils and through which oxygen is delivered to the patient.

Nasal Flaring   Widening of the nostrils when a patient breathes in; a sign of increased breathing effort.

Nasogastric (NG) Tube   A long, flexible tube that is passed through the nose, into the posterior nasopharynx, down the esophagus, and into the stomach.

Nasopharynx   The portion of the throat located directly behind the nasal cavity. It serves as a passageway for air only.

National EMS Education Standards   A document that specifies the competencies, clinical behaviors, and judgments that each level of EMS professional must meet when completing their education.

National EMS Scope of Practice Model   A document that defines four levels of EMS professionals and what each level of EMS professional legally can and cannot do.

National Incident Management System (NIMS) A system used to control, direct, and coordinate the activities of multiple agencies.

Nature of the Illness (NOI) The medical condition that resulted in the patient's call to 9-1-1.

Near Syncope (Presyncope) Warning symptoms of an impending loss of consciousness.

Neglect Failure to provide for a child's basic needs.

Negligence A deviation from the accepted standard of care resulting in further injury to the patient.

Neurons Cells of the nervous system.

Non-Allergic Asthma Asthma that is triggered by factors not related to allergies.

Non-Modifiable Risk Factors Risk factors that cannot be changed.

Nonrebreather (NRB) Mask An oxygen delivery device with a reservoir that is designed to deliver high concentration oxygen.

Non-Urgent Move A method used to move, lift, or carry patients with no known or suspected injury to the head, neck, spine, or extremities.

O

Objective Findings A medical or trauma condition of the patient that can be seen, heard, smelled, measured, or felt; also called *signs* or *clinical findings*.

Obsessions Recurring thoughts, impulses, or images that cause the person anxiety.

Obsessive-Compulsive Disorder (OCD) A type of anxiety disorder in which recurring thoughts, impulses, or images cause a person anxiety, which causes the individual to perform recurring behaviors or rituals with the hope of preventing the obsessive thoughts or making them go away.

Obstetric Emergency An emergency related to pregnancy or childbirth.

Occlusive Airtight.

Occupational Safety and Health Administration (OSHA) A branch of the federal government responsible for safety in the workplace.

Off-Line Medical Direction The medical supervision of EMS personnel through the use of policies, protocols, standing orders, education, and quality management review; also called *indirect, retrospective,* or *prospective* medical direction.

Olecranon The elbow.

Onboard Oxygen Large oxygen cylinders carried on an ambulance.

Ongoing Assessment Reassessment of the patient to ensure the delivery of appropriate patient care.

On-Line Medical Direction Direct communication with a physician (or his or her designee) by radio or telephone, or face-to-face communication at the scene, before a skill is performed or care is given.

Open (Compound) Fracture A broken bone that penetrates the skin.

Open-Ended Questions Questions that require a patient to answer with more than a "yes" or "no," such as "What is troubling you today?" or "How can I help you?"

Open Pneumothorax The entry of air through an open wound in the chest wall into the pleural cavity; also called *sucking chest wound.*

Open Soft-Tissue Injury A soft-tissue injury in which a break occurs in the skin.

Open Wound An injury in which the skin surface is broken.

Oral Airway A curved device made of rigid plastic that is inserted into a patient's mouth and used to keep the tongue away from the back of the throat.

Organ At least two different types of tissue that work together to perform a particular function. Examples include the brain, stomach, and liver.

Organ System Tissues and organs that work together to provide a common function; also called body system. Examples of organ systems include the respiratory system and nervous system.

Origin The stationary attachment of a skeletal muscle to a bone.

Orogastric (OG) Tube A long, flexible tube that is passed through the mouth, down the esophagus, and into the stomach.

Oropharynx The middle portion of the throat that opens into the mouth and serves as a passageway for both food and air.

Orthopnea Breathlessness when lying flat that is relieved or lessened when the patient sits or stands.

Osteoporosis A condition that develops when the rate of old bone removal occurs too quickly or when old bone replacement occurs too slowly, resulting in bones that are brittle and tend to break easily.

Ovaries Paired, almond-shaped organs in a woman's body that produce eggs. They are located on either side of the uterus in the pelvic cavity.

Ovary One of two glands in the female that produce the female reproductive cell (the ovum) and the hormones estrogen and progesterone.

Overdose An intentional or unintentional overmedication or ingestion of a toxic substance.

Ovulation Release of an egg from an ovary.

P

Pack-Strap Carry A move in which the rescuer kneels in front of a seated patient with the rescuer's back to patient. The patient's arms are placed over the rescuer's shoulders and crossed over the rescuer's chest. The rescuer grasps the patient's wrists, leans forward, rises up on his or her knees, and pulls the patient up onto the rescuer's back.

Palpitations An abnormal awareness of one's heart beat.

Pancreas A gland that secretes juices that contain enzymes for protein, carbohydrate, and fat digestion into the small intestine.

Panic Attack An intense fear that occurs for no apparent reason.

Paradoxical Uneven, inconsistent.

Paradoxical Movement When a segment of the chest wall moves in an opposite direction from the rest of the chest during respiration.

Paranoia A mental disorder characterized by excessive suspiciousness or delusions.

Paraplegia A loss of movement and sensation of the lower half of the body from the waist down.

Parasympathetic Nervous System The division of the autonomic nervous system that conserves and restores energy. It provides the "rest and digest" response.

Parathyroid Glands Glands located behind the thyroid gland that secrete a hormone that maintains the calcium level in the blood.

Paresthesias Abnormal sensations such as tingling, burning, numbness, or a "pins-and-needles" feeling.

Parietal Pleura The outer pleural lining that lines the wall of the thoracic cavity.

Paroxysmal Nocturnal Dyspnea A sudden onset of difficulty breathing that occurs at night because of a buildup of fluid in the alveoli or pooling of secretions during sleep.

Partial Seizure A category of seizures in which nerve cells fire abnormally in one hemisphere of the brain. This category of seizures includes simple partial seizures and complex partial seizures.

Partial-Thickness Burn A burn that involves the epidermis and dermis; also called a *second-degree burn*.

Passive Rewarming Warming of a patient with minimal or no use of heat sources other than the patient's own heat production. Methods include placing the patient in a warm environment, applying clothing and blankets, and preventing drafts.

Patella The flat, triangular, movable bone that forms the anterior part of the knee; the kneecap.

Patent Open.

Pathogens Germs capable of producing disease, such as bacteria and viruses.

Patient assessment The process of evaluating a person for signs of illness or injury.

Patient History The part of a patient assessment that provides pertinent facts about the patient's current medical problem and medical history.

Pelvic Cavity The body cavity below the abdominal cavity. It contains the urinary bladder, part of the large intestine, and the reproductive organs.

Pelvic Girdle The bones that enclose and protect the organs of the pelvic cavity. It provides a point of attachment for the lower extremities and major muscles of the trunk and supports the weight of the upper body.

Pelvis The bony ring formed by three separate bones that fuse to become one in an adult.

Penetrating Chest Injury A break in the skin over the chest wall.

Penetrating Trauma Any mechanism of injury that causes a cut or piercing of the skin.

Penis The male external organ that serves as the outlet for sperm and urine.

Perfusion The flow of blood through an organ or a part of the body.

Pericardial Cavity The body cavity containing the heart.

Perineum The area between the vaginal opening and the anus.

Peripheral Artery Disease Atherosclerosis that affects the arteries that supply the arms, legs, and feet.

Peripheral Nervous System (PNS) All nervous tissue found outside the brain and spinal cord.

Peripherally-Inserted Central Catheter An intravenous (IV) line often used for neonates, young children, or patients requiring only short-term IV therapy for the delivery of medications and nutritional solutions directly into the venous circulation; also called a *PICC line*.

Peristalsis The involuntary wavelike contraction of smooth muscle that moves material through the digestive tract.

Peritonitis Inflammation of the abdominal lining.

Personal Space The invisible area immediately around each of us that we declare as our own.

Pertinent Negative A finding expected to accompany the patient's chief complaint but not found during the patient assessment. For instance, clear lung sounds in a patient complaining of difficulty breathing is a pertinent negative.

Phalanges The bones of the fingers and toes.

Pharmacology The study of drugs or medications and their effect on living systems.

Pharynx The throat.

Phlebitis Inflammation of a vein.

Phobia An irrational and constant fear of a specific activity, object, or situation (other than a social situation).

Physical Abuse Acts that cause or could cause physical injury to a child.

Physical Examination A head-to-toe assessment of the patient's entire body.

Physiology The study of the normal functions of an organism (such as the human body).

Pia Mater Literally, "gentle mother." The delicate inner layer of the meninges that clings gently to the brain and spinal cord. It contains many blood vessels that supply the nervous tissue.

Piggyback Carry A move in which the rescuer kneels in front of a seated patient with the rescuer's back to patient. The patient's arms are placed over the rescuer's shoulders and crossed over the rescuer's chest. The rescuer grasps the patient's wrists, leans forward, rises up on his knees, and pulls the patient up onto the rescuer's back. The rescuer's forearms are positioned under the patient's knees and his wrists grasped while the patient is carried to safety.

Pineal Gland A small gland located near the center of the brain that is responsible for producing produces the hormone melatonin.

Pituitary Gland A small gland located just beneath the hypothalamus in the brain that regulates growth and controls other endocrine glands; the "master gland" of the body.

Placenta A specialized organ through which the fetus exchanges nourishment and waste products during pregnancy; also called *afterbirth*.

Placenta Previa A condition that occurs when part or all of the placenta implants in the lower part of the uterus, covering the opening of the cervix.

Plasma The liquid portion of the blood.

Platelets Thrombocytes, which are essential for the formation of blood clots. They function to stop bleeding and repair ruptured blood vessels.

Pleurae Serous (oily), double-walled membranes that enclose each lung.

Pleural Cavities The body cavities containing the lungs. The right lung is located in the right pleural cavity and the left lung is located in the left pleural cavity.

Pleural Space   A space between the visceral and parietal pleura, filled with a small amount of oily fluid, that allows the lungs to glide easily against each other.

Pneumonia   A respiratory infection that may involve the lower airways and alveoli, part of a lobe, or an entire lobe of the lung.

Pneumothorax   A buildup of air between the outer lining of the lung and the chest wall causing a complete or partial collapse of the lung.

Pocket Mask   A piece of equipment used for mouth-to-mask ventilation that provides a physical barrier between the rescuer and the patient's nose, mouth, and secretions; also called a *pocket face mask, ventilation face mask,* or *resuscitation mask.*

Poison   Any substance taken into the body that interferes with normal body function.

Poison Control Center (PCC)   A medical facility that provides free telephone advice to the public and medical professionals in case of exposure to poisonous substances.

Poisoning   Exposure to a substance that is harmful in any dosage.

Pons.   Literally, "bridge." A part of the brainstem that connects parts of the brain with one another by means of tracts and influences respiration.

Portable Radio   A handheld communication device used for radio communication away from the emergency vehicle.

Position of Function   The natural position of the hand or foot at rest.

Positive-Pressure Ventilation   Forcing air into a patient's lungs.

Posterior   The back side of the body or body part.

Postictal Phase   The period of recovery that follows a seizure.

Powder   Drugs ground into fine particles.

Power Grip (Underhand Grip)   A method of placing ones hands on an object that is designed to take full advantage of the strength of the rescuer's hands and forearms.

Power Lift   A technique used to lift a heavy object.

Preeclampsia   A condition of high blood pressure and swelling that occurs in some women during the third trimester of pregnancy; also called *pregnancy-induced hypertension* or *toxemia of pregnancy.*

Premature Infant   An infant born before the 37th week of gestation or weighing less than 5.5 pounds (2.5 kilograms); also called a *preemie.*

Premature Labor   Labor before a woman's 37th week of pregnancy; also called *preterm labor.*

Presenting Part   The part of an infant that emerges first during delivery.

Pressure Bandage   Material, such as roller gauze, that is applied snugly to create pressure on a wound and hold a dressing in place over it.

Pressure Regulator   A device used to reduce pressure in an oxygen cylinder to a safe range, allowing the release of oxygen from the cylinder in a controlled manner.

Primary Spontaneous Pneumothorax   A collection of air or gas outside the lung and between the lung and the chest wall that most commonly occurs in tall, thin men between the ages of 20 and 40.

Primary Survey   A rapid assessment of the patient to find and care for immediate life-threatening conditions.

Prone   Facedown.

Prospective Medical Direction   Activities performed by a physician medical director before an emergency call.

Prostate Gland   In the male, a gland that secretes fluid that enhances sperm motility and neutralizes the acidity of the vagina during intercourse.

Protected Health Information (PHI)   Information that relates to a person's physical or mental health, treatment, or payment; that identifies the person or gives a reason to believe that the individual can be identified; and that is transmitted or maintained in any form.

Protocols   Written instructions to provide emergency care for specific health-related conditions.

Proximal   Closer to the midline or center area of the body.

Proximate Cause   Actions or inactions of the healthcare professional that caused the injury or damages.

Pruritus   Itching.

Psychological Maltreatment   A pattern of caregiver behavior that conveys to children that they are worthless, flawed, unloved, unwanted, endangered, or only of value in meeting another's needs.

Public Service Answering Point (PSAP)   A facility equipped and staffed to receive and control 9-1-1 access calls.

Pulmonary Contusion   Bruising of the lung.

Pulmonary Edema   A buildup of fluid in the alveoli, most commonly caused by failure of the left ventricle of the heart.

Pulmonary Embolus   A clot that travels through the circulatory system, eventually becoming trapped in the smaller branches of the pulmonary arteries, causing a partial or complete blood flow obstruction.

Pulmonic Valve   A semilunar valve located at the junction of the right ventricle and pulmonary artery.

Pulse   The rhythmic contraction and expansion of the arteries with each beat of the heart.

Pulse Oximetry   A method of measuring the amount of oxygen saturated in the blood.

Puncture Wound   Piercing of the skin with a pointed object such as a nail, pencil, ice pick, splinter, piece of glass, bullet, or a knife that results in little or no external bleeding (although internal bleeding may be severe); also called a *penetration wound.*

Putrefaction   The decomposition of organic matter, such as body tissues.

Q

Quadriplegia   A loss of movement and sensation in both arms, both legs, and the parts of the body below an area of injury to the spinal cord; also called *tetraplegia.*

Quality Management   A system of internal and external reviews and audits of all aspects of an EMS system.

R

Raccoon Eyes   Bilateral bluish discoloration (ecchymosis) around the eyes that suggests a possible skull fracture.

Radiation The transfer of heat, as infrared heat rays, from the surface of one object to the surface of another without contact between the two objects.

Radius The bone on the thumb (lateral) side of the forearm.

Rapid Medical Assessment A quick head-to-toe assessment of a medical patient who is unresponsive or has an altered mental status.

Rapid Trauma Assessment A quick head-to-toe assessment of a trauma patient with a significant mechanism of injury.

Reasonable Force The amount of force necessary to keep a patient from injuring you, himself, or others.

Recovery Position Placing an unresponsive patient who is breathing and in no need of CPR (and in whom trauma is not suspected) on the patient's side to help keep his or her airway open.

Rectum The lower part of the large intestine, about 5 inches long, between the sigmoid colon and the anal canal.

Regression A return to an earlier or former developmental state.

Repeater A device that receives a transmission from a low-power portable or mobile radio on one frequency and then retransmits it at a higher power on another frequency so that it can be received at a distant location.

Reproductive System Organs that make cells (sperm, eggs) that allow continuation of the human species.

Respiration The act of breathing air into the lungs (inhalation) and out of the lungs (exhalation); the exchange of gases between a living organism and its environment.

Respiratory Arrest An absence of breathing.

Respiratory Distress Increased work of breathing (respiratory effort).

Respiratory Failure Inadequate blood oxygenation and/or ventilation to meet the demands of body tissues.

Retractions "Sinking in" of the soft tissues between and around the ribs or above the collarbones.

Retrospective medical direction Activities performed by a physician after an emergency call.

Rhonchi Abnormal breath sounds produced when air flows through passages narrowed by mucus or fluid.

Rickettsia Very small bacteria that require a living host to survive.

Rigor Mortis The stiffening of body muscles that occurs after death.

Risk Factors Conditions that may increase a person's chance of developing a disease.

Route of Administration The route and form in which a drug should be given to a patient.

Rule of Nines A guide used to estimate the affected body surface area of a burn.

S

Safe Zone An identified safety zone at a hazardous materials incident that is an area safe from the exposure or the threat of exposure and that serves as the staging area for personnel and equipment; also called the *cold zone* or *support zone*.

Saline Lock An intravenous (IV) catheter that has a medication port on its end. It is used when a patient needs (or is likely to need) IV medications but does not need IV fluid.

SAMPLE A memory aid that serves to remind healthcare professionals of the information that should be gathered when obtaining a patient history. SAMPLE stands for *s*igns and symptoms, *a*llergies, *m*edications, *p*ertinent past medical history, *l*ast oral intake, and *e*vents leading to the injury or illness.

Saturation of Peripheral Oxygen (SpO$_2$) A pulse oximeter's calculation of the amount of hemoglobin saturated with oxygen.

Scalp The outermost part of the head that contains tissue, hair follicles, sweat glands, oil glands, and a rich supply of blood vessels.

Scene Safety An assessment of the entire scene and surroundings to ensure your well-being and that of other rescuers, the patient(s), and bystanders.

Scene Size-Up The first phase of patient assessment that includes body substance isolation precautions, evaluation of scene safety, determining the mechanism of injury or the nature of the patient's illness, determining the total number of patients, and determining the need for additional resources.

Schizophrenia A group of mental disorders characterized by hallucinations, delusions, disordered thinking, and bizarre or disorganized behavior.

Scoop (Orthopedic) Stretcher A patient transfer device made of metal and consisting of four sections: Two sections support the upper body and two sections support the lower body. In the absence of spinal injury, the scoop stretcher may be used to carry a supine patient up or down stairs or in other confined spaces; also called a *split litter*.

Scope of Practice State laws that detail the medical procedures and functions that can be legally performed by a licensed or certified healthcare professional.

Scrotum A loose sac of skin that houses the male testes.

Secondary Spontaneous Pneumothorax A collection of air or gas outside the lung and between the lung and the chest wall that most often occurs as a complication of lung disease.

Secondary Survey A full body assessment performed to discover medical conditions and/or injuries that are not immediately life threatening but may become so if left untreated. In addition to a head-to-toe (or focused) assessment, it includes obtaining vital signs; reassessing changes in the patient's condition; and determining the patient's chief complaint, history of present illness, and significant past medical history.

Seesaw Breathing Abnormal breathing in which the abdominal muscles move in a direction opposite the chest wall.

Seizure A temporary change in behavior or consciousness caused by abnormal electrical activity within one or more groups of brain cells.

Semi-Fowler's Position A position in which a patient sits up with his or head at a 45-degree angle and his or her legs out straight.

Semilunar Valves Heart valves shaped like half-moons.

Seminal Vesicles Accessory glands in the male that secrete fluid that nourishes and protects sperm.

Semi-Synthetic Drugs Naturally occurring substances that have been chemically altered, such as antibiotics.

Sensitization The production of antibodies in response to the body's first exposure to an antigen.

Sensory Nerves Nerves that send signals *to* the brain about the activities of the different parts of the body relative to their surroundings.

Septic Shock Shock caused by a severe infection.

Septum A wall between two cavities.

Sexual Abuse Inappropriate adolescent or adult sexual behavior with a child.

Sexually Transmitted Diseases Infections that are spread by either blood or sexual contact.

Shaken Baby Syndrome A severe form of head injury that occurs when an infant or child is shaken by the arms, legs, or shoulders with enough force to cause the baby's brain to bounce against his skull.

Shock (Hypoperfusion) The inadequate flow of blood through an organ or a part of the body.

Shock Position A position in which the patient lays on his or her back with his or her feet elevated approximately 8-12 inches; this position is no longer recommended.

Short Backboard A device made of wood, aluminum, or plastic that is 3-4 feet long and serves as an intermediate device for stabilizing the spine of a stable patient found in a seated position. It must be used in conjunction with a long backboard for full spinal stabilization; also called a *half board.*

Shoulder Drag Emergency move in which the rescuer's hands are positioned under the patient's armpits and the patient dragged to safety.

Shoulder Girdle The bony arch formed by the collarbones (clavicles) and shoulder blades (scapulae).

Side Effects Expected (and usually unavoidable) effects of a drug.

Sigmoid Colon The lower part of the descending colon between the iliac crest and the rectum, shaped like the letter S.

Sign A medical or trauma condition of the patient that can be seen, heard, smelled, measured, or felt; also called *objective findings* or *clinical findings.*

Simple Extrication The use of hand tools in order to gain access and extricate the patient from the vehicle.

Simple Partial Seizure A type of partial seizure that involves motor or sensory symptoms with no change in mental status; also called a *focal seizure* or *focal motor seizure.*

Simple Pneumothorax A condition in which air enters the chest cavity, causing a loss of negative pressure (vacuum) and a partial or total collapse of the lung.

Simplex System A mode of radio transmission that uses a single frequency to transmit and receive messages.

Sinuses Spaces or cavities inside some cranial bones.

Skeletal Muscles Voluntary muscles. Most skeletal muscles are attached to bones.

Skull The bony skeleton of the head that protects the brain from injury and gives the head its shape.

Small Intestine The portion of the digestive system between the stomach and beginning of the large intestine that consists of three parts: the duodenum, the jejunum, and the ileum. It receives food from the stomach and secretions from the pancreas and liver, and completes the digestion of food that began in the mouth and stomach.

Smooth Muscle An involuntary muscle found in many internal organs (except the heart).

Snoring A loud breathing sound that suggests the upper airway is partially blocked by the tongue.

Social Phobia An extreme anxiety response in situations in which the individual may be seen by others, caused by the individual's fear that he will act in an embarrassing or shameful manner.

Soft Palate The fleshy portion of the nasal cavity that extends behind the hard palate. It marks the boundary between the nasopharynx and the rest of the pharynx.

Soft Tissues Layers of the skin and the fat and muscle beneath them.

Solutions Liquid preparations of one or more chemical substances, usually dissolved in water.

Somatic Division The voluntary division of the peripheral nervous system that has receptors and nerves concerned with the external environment.

Somatostatin A hormone released by delta cells in the pancreas that inhibits the release of insulin and glucagon.

Sphygmomanometer A device used to take a blood pressure.

Spinal Cavity The body cavity that extends from the bottom of the skull to the lower back and contains the spinal cord.

Spinal Cord Nervous tissue that extends from the base of the skull down the back and responsible for relaying electrical signals to and from the brain and peripheral nerves.

Spinal Nerves –Any of 31 pairs of nerves that branch from the spinal cord.

Spinal Precautions Precautions made to stabilize the head, neck, and back in a neutral position to prevent movement that could cause injury to the spinal cord.

Spirits Volatile substances dissolved in alcohol.

Splint A device used to limit the movement of an injured arm or leg and reduce bleeding and discomfort.

Spontaneous Abortion The loss of a fetus as a result of natural causes before the 20th week of pregnancy; also called *miscarriage.*

Spontaneous Pneumothorax A type of pneumothorax that does not involve trauma to the lung.

Sprain The stretching or tearing of a ligament.

Stabilization The process of rendering a vehicle motionless in the position in which it is found.

Stable Angina Pectoris Angina pectoris that is relatively constant and predictable in terms of severity, signs and symptoms, precipitating events, and the patient's response to therapy.

Stair Chair A commercially made patient transfer device designed for patients who can assume a sitting position while being carried to an ambulance. The stair chair is useful for moving patients up or down stairs, through narrow corridors and doorways, into small elevators, and in narrow aisles in aircraft or buses.

Standard of Care The minimum level of care expected of similarly trained healthcare professionals; based on education, experience, laws, and protocols.

Standing Orders Written instructions that authorize EMS personnel to perform certain medical interventions before establishing direct communication with a physician.

START Triage System A nationally recognized method of sorting patients by the severity of their illness or injury.

START is an acronym for *Simple Triage And Rapid Treatment*.

Status Epilepticus Recurring seizures without an intervening period of consciousness.

Statutes Laws established by Congress and state legislatures.

Stent A small plastic or metal tube that is inserted into a vessel or duct to help keep it open and maintain fluid flow through it.

Sterilization A method of decontamination that destroys all microorganisms, including highly resistant bacterial spores. It is used for instruments that penetrate the skin or contact normally sterile areas of the body during invasive procedures.

Sterilizing A process that uses boiling water, radiation, gas, chemicals, or superheated steam to destroy all of the germs on an object.

Sternum The breastbone; the flat bone that joins the clavicles (collarbones) and the first seven pairs of ribs.

Stethoscope An instrument used to hear sounds within the body, such as respirations.

Stoma An artificial opening.

Strain The twisting, pulling, or tearing of a muscle.

Stress A chemical, physical, or emotional factor that causes bodily or mental tension.

Stressor Any event or condition that has the potential to cause bodily or mental tension.

Stridor A harsh, high-pitched sound (like the bark of a seal) that is associated with severe upper airway obstruction and is most often heard during inhalation.

Stroke An interruption of the blood supply in the brain caused by blockage or rupture of an artery; also called a *cerebrovascular accident* or *brain attack*.

Stylet A flexible plastic-coated wire that is inserted into an endotracheal tube to provide stiffness and shape to the tube.

Subarachnoid Hemorrhage Bleeding in the brain caused by a ruptured blood vessel in the subarachnoid space in the brain.

Subcostal Retractions Indentations of the skin below the rib cage.

Subcutaneous Emphysema Air trapped beneath the skin; a crackling sensation under the fingers that suggests laceration of a lung and the leakage of air into the pleural space.

Subcutaneous Layer The thick skin layer that lies below the dermis and is loosely attached to the muscles and bones of the musculoskeletal system.

Subcutaneous (SubQ) Route Injection of a liquid form of medication underneath the skin into the subcutaneous tissue.

Subdural Hematoma A buildup of blood in the space between the dura and the arachnoid layer of the meninges that usually results from the tearing of veins located between the dura and the cerebral cortex after an injury to the head.

Subjective Findings A patient's interpretation and description of his or her complaint; also called *symptoms*.

Sublingual Medication given under the tongue.

Subluxation A partial dislocation.

Submersion An incident in which the victim's entire body, including his airway, is under the water or other fluid

Substance Abuse The deliberate, persistent, and excessive self-administration of a substance in a way that is not medically or socially approved.

Substance Misuse The self-administration of a substance for unintended purposes, or for appropriate purposes but in improper amounts or doses, or without a prescription for the person receiving the medication.

Sucking Chest Wound A chest injury in which air moves into the pleural cavity through an open chest wound, creating a sucking or gurgling sound when air escapes from the wound when the patient breathes in.

Suctioning A procedure used to vacuum vomitus, saliva, blood, food particles, and other material from a patient's airway.

Sudden Cardiac Death (SCD) The unexpected death from cardiac causes early after symptom onset (immediately or within one hour) or without the onset of symptoms.

Sudden Infant Death Syndrome (SIDS) The sudden and unexpected death of an infant that remains unexplained after a thorough case investigation, including performance of a complete autopsy, examination of the death scene, and review of the clinical history.

Sudden Sniffing Death Syndrome A condition that can occur when a person sniffs highly concentrated amounts of the chemicals in solvents or aerosol sprays.

Suicide Attempt Self-destructive behavior for the purpose of ending one's life that, for unanticipated reasons, fails.

Suicide Gesture Self-destructive behavior that is unlikely to have any possibility of being fatal.

Superficial Burn A burn that affects only the epidermis; also called a *first-degree burn*.

Superior Above or in a higher position than another portion of the body.

Supine Lying face up.

Suppository Drugs mixed in a firm base such as cocoa butter that, when placed into a body opening, melt at body temperature.

Supraclavicular Retractions Indentations of the skin above the collarbones (clavicles).

Surfactant A thin substance that coats each alveolus and prevents the alveoli from collapsing.

Suspensions Drug particles that are mixed with, but not dissolved in, a liquid.

Swathe A piece of soft material used to secure an injured extremity to the body.

Symmetry Evenness.

Sympathetic Nervous System The division of the autonomic nervous system that mobilizes energy, particularly in stressful situations; the "fight-or-flight" response.

Symptom A condition described by the patient, such as shortness of breath; also called *subjective findings*.

Syncope (Fainting) A brief loss of responsiveness caused by a temporary decrease in blood flow to the brain; sometimes called a *blackout*.

Synthetic Drugs Drugs that are made in a laboratory.

Syrups Drugs suspended in sugar and water.

Systemic Effect An effect of a drug on the whole body rather than just a single area or part of the body.

Systolic Blood Pressure   The pressure in an artery when the heart is pumping blood.

T

Tablet   Powdered drug, molded or compressed into a small form.

Tachypnea   A faster-than-normal respiratory rate for an individual's age.

Tarsals   The bones of the heel and back part of the foot.

Tendons   Strong cords of connective tissue that stretch across joints. When muscles contract, they create a pull between bones.

Tension Pneumothorax   A life-threatening condition in which air enters the pleural cavity during inspiration and progressively builds up under pressure.

Terminal Illness   A disease that cannot be cured and is expected to lead to death.

Testis   One of two male reproductive glands located in the scrotum that produce reproductive cells and secrete testosterone.

Thalamus   An area of the brain that functions as a relay station for impulses going to and from the cerebrum.

Therapeutic Abortion   An abortion performed for medical reasons, often because the pregnancy posed a threat to the mother's health.

Thoracic (Chest) Cavity   The body cavity located below the neck and above the diaphragm. It contains the heart, major blood vessels, and lungs.

Threatened Abortion   A condition in which a woman is less than 20 weeks pregnant and experiences vaginal spotting or bleeding and possible mild uterine cramping. The cervix remains closed and the fetus remains in the uterus.

Thrombosis   The formation or presence of a clot (thrombus) inside a blood vessel.

Thrombus   A blood clot.

Thymus Gland   A ductless organ that produces lymphocytes, which play a role in the body's immune system.

Thyroid Cartilage   The Adam's apple; the largest cartilage of the larynx.

Thyroid Gland   The endocrine gland that lies in the neck, just below the larynx. It regulates the metabolic rate.

Tibia   The shinbone; the larger of the two bones of the lower leg.

Tidal Volume   The amount of air moved into or out of the lungs during a normal breath.

Tinctures   Alcohol solutions prepared from an animal or vegetable drug or chemical substance.

Tissues   A group of similar cells that cluster together to perform a specialized function.

Tolerance   Requiring progressively larger doses of a drug to achieve the desired effect.

Tonic-Clonic Seizure   A seizure that involves stiffening and jerking of the patient's body; also called a *generalized motor seizure*; formerly called a *grand mal seizure.*

Tourniquet   A tight bandage that surrounds an arm or leg and is used to stop the flow of blood in the extremity.

Toxidrome   Signs, symptoms, and characteristics that often occur together in toxic exposures.

Toxin   A poisonous substance.

Trachea   The windpipe; the tube through which air passes to and from the lungs. It extends down the front of the neck from the larynx and divides in two to form the mainstem bronchi.

Tracheal Deviation   Shifting of the trachea from a midline position.

Tracheal Stoma   A permanent opening at the front of the neck that extends from the skin surface into the trachea opening the trachea to the atmosphere.

Tracheostomy   The surgical formation of an opening into the trachea.

Traction Splint   A device used to maintain a constant, steady pull (traction) on a closed fracture of the femur.

Trade Name   A drug's brand name; also called the *proprietary name.*

Transient Ischemic Attack (TIA)   A temporary interruption of the blood supply to the brain; sometimes called a *mini-stroke.*

Transmitter   A device that sends out data on a given radio frequency.

Transverse Colon   The portion of the large intestine that extends across the abdomen.

Trauma Patient   An individual who has experienced an injury from an external force.

Traumatic Asphyxia   A condition that occurs because of a severe compression injury to the chest, resulting in a backup of blood into the veins, venules, and capillaries of the head, neck, extremities, and upper torso, and subsequent capillary rupture.

Treatment Protocol   A list of steps to be followed during provision of emergency care to an ill or injured patient.

Trendelenburg Position   Lying on the back, with the head of the bed lowered and the feet raised in a straight incline.

Triage   Sorting multiple victims into priorities for emergency medical care or transportation to definitive care.

Tricuspid Valve   An atrioventricular valve located between the right atrium and the right ventricle.

Tripod Position   Sitting up and leaning forward with the weight of the upper body supported by the hands on the thighs or knees. This position allows a patient to draw in more air and better expand his lungs than if he were lying on his back or leaning back in a sitting position.

True Emergency   A situation in which there is a high possibility of death or serious injury and the rapid response of an emergency vehicle may lessen the risk of death or injury.

True Ribs   Rib pairs 1–7. These ribs are attached anteriorly to the sternum by cartilage

Turbinates   Several shelf-like projections that protrude into the nasal cavity that help protect structures of the lower airway from foreign body contamination.

Two-Person Carry   A move in which rescuers place one arm under the patient's thighs and the other across the patient's back. Each rescuer grasps the arms of the other, locking them in position at the elbows, forming a "seat." Both rescuers rise to a standing position and carry the patient to safety; also called the *two-person seat carry.*

Type 1 Diabetes Mellitus   A disease in which little or no insulin is produced by beta cells in the pancreas, resulting in a buildup of glucose in the blood. It usually begins during childhood or young adulthood.

Type 2 Diabetes Mellitus   A disease caused by a combination of insulin resistance and relative insulin shortage that usually affects people older than 40 years of age, especially those who are overweight.

U

UHF   Ultra-high frequency radio band (a band is a group of radio frequencies close together).

Ulna   The bone on the medial side of the forearm.

Umbilical Cord   An extension of the placenta through which the fetus receives nourishment while in the uterus.

Unified Command   An application of the Incident Command System that is used when multiple organizations involved in the incident coordinate an effective incident response while carrying out their own jurisdictional responsibilities at the same time.

Unstable Angina Pectoris   Angina pectoris that progressively worsens, occurs at rest, or is brought on by minimal physical exertion.

Ureter   One of two tubes that carry urine from the kidneys to the urinary bladder.

Urethra   A canal that passes urine from the urinary bladder to the outside of the body.

Urgent Move   A method used to move a patient when there is an immediate threat to life.

Urinary Bladder   A temporary storage site for urine.

Urticaria   Hives.

Uterus   A hollow, muscular organ in a female in which a fertilized ovum implants and receives nourishment until birth.

Uterus   A hollow, muscular organ of the female reproductive system where a fertilized egg implants and develops into a fetus; also called the *womb*.

Uvula   The small piece of tissue that looks like a punching bag and that hangs down in the back of the throat.

V

Vagina (Birth Canal)   In the female, a muscular tube that serves as a passageway between the uterus and the outside. It receives the penis during intercourse and serves as a passageway for menstrual flow and the delivery of an infant.

Vallecula   The area between the base of the tongue and the epiglottis. When endotracheal intubation is performed by using a curved blade, the tip of the blade is inserted into this landmark.

Veins   Blood vessels that return blood to the heart.

Venipuncture   The technique of piercing a patient's vein with a needle to withdraw a blood sample from a patient and to give intravenous fluids or medications.

Ventricles   The two lower chambers of the heart; the right ventricle pumps blood to the lungs and the left ventricle pumps blood to the body.

Ventricular Fibrillation (VF or Vfib)   An abnormal heart rhythm in which the heart's electrical impulses are completely disorganized and the heart cannot pump blood effectively.

Ventricular Shunt   A drainage system used to remove excess cerebrospinal fluid in a patient who has hydrocephalus.

Venules   The smallest branches of veins leading to the capillaries.

VHF   A very high frequency radio band (a band is a group of radio frequencies close together).

Visceral Pleura   The inner pleural layer that covers the surface of the lungs.

Virus   A type of infectious agent that depends on other organisms to live and grow.

Vital Organs   The organs essential for life, such as the brain, heart, and lungs.

Vital Signs   Measurements of breathing, pulse, temperature, pupils, and blood pressure.

Voice over Internet Protocol (VoIP)   Technology that allows users to make telephone calls by means of a broadband Internet connection instead of using a regular telephone line; also known as *Internet Voice*.

W

Warm Zone   An identified safety zone at a hazardous materials incident that serves as a controlled area for entry into the hot zone and where most operations take place. It also serves as the decontamination area after exiting the hot zone; also called the *contamination reduction zone*.

Weapons of Mass Destruction (WMD)   Materials used by terrorists that have the potential to cause great harm over a large area.

Wet Drowning   The entry of water into the trachea and lungs.

Wheezes   Musical whistling sounds caused by the movement of air through narrowed airways.

Wheezing   A high- or low-pitched whistling sound that is usually heard on exhalation. Wheezing suggests that the lower airways are partially blocked with fluid or mucus.

Withdrawal   The condition produced when an individual stops using or abusing a drug to which he or she is physically or psychologically addicted.

Wound   An injury to the soft tissues of the body.

X

Xiphoid Process   A piece of cartilage that makes up the inferior portion of the breastbone.

Z

Zygote   Fertilized egg.

Text and Line Art Credits

Table 1.6: From Therapeutic Communications for Health Professionals 2nd edition by TAMPARO/LINDH. 2000. Reprinted with permissions of Delmar Learning, a division of Thomson Learning: www.thomsonrights.com. Fax: 800 730-2215.

Figure 4.2: From Shier, et al., Human Anatomy & Physiology, 9e, Fig. 1.7, p. 13, © 2002. Reprinted with permission of the McGraw-Hill Publishing Companies, Inc.

Figure 4.3: From Saladin, *Anatomy and Physiology, 3e,* Fig. 8.1, p. 245 © 2004. Reprinted with permission of the McGraw-Hill Publishing Companies, Inc.

Figure 4.4: From Saladin, *Anatomy and Physiology, 3e,* Fig. 8.3, p. 248 © 2004. Reprinted with permission of the McGraw-Hill Publishing Companies, Inc.

Figure 4.4(b): From Shier, et al., Human Anatomy & Physiology, 9e, Fig. 1.22 p. 24, © 2002. Reprinted with permission of the McGraw-Hill Publishing Companies, Inc.

Figure 4.5: From Saladin, *Anatomy and Physiology, 3e,* Fig. 8.18, p. 262 © 2004. Reprinted with permission of the McGraw-Hill Publishing Companies, Inc.

Figure 4.6: From Seeley, *Anatomy & Physiology, 6e,* Fig. 7.26, p. 223, © 2003. Reprinted with permission of the McGraw-Hill Publishing Companies, Inc.

Figure 4.6(b): From Lewis, *Life, 4e,* Fig. 34.6, p. 678, © 2002. Reprinted with permission of the McGraw-Hill Publishing Companies, Inc.

Figure 4.7: From Shier, et al., Human Anatomy & Physiology, 9e, Fig. 19.1 p. 780, © 2002. Reprinted with permission of the McGraw-Hill Publishing Companies, Inc.

Figure 4.7(b) From Seeley, *Anatomy & Physiology, 6e,* Fig. 6.2, p. 168, © 2003. Reprinted with permission of the McGraw-Hill Publishing Companies, Inc.

Figure 4.9: From Mader, *Human Biology, 7e,* Fig. 7.13, p. 135, © 2002. Reprinted with permission of the McGraw-Hill Publishing Companies, Inc.

Figure 4.13: From Shier, et al., Human Anatomy & Physiology, 9e, Fig. 1.7, p. 13, © 2002. Reprinted with permission of the McGraw-Hill Publishing Companies, Inc.

Figure 4.13: From Saladin, *Anatomy and Physiology, 3e,* Fig. 8.1, p. 245 © 2004. Reprinted with permission of the McGraw-Hill Publishing Companies, Inc.

Figure 4.13(b): From Seeley, *Anatomy & Physiology, 6e,* Fig. 7.34, p. 225, © 2003. Reprinted with permission of the McGraw-Hill Publishing Companies, Inc.

Figure 4.14: From Saladin, *Anatomy and Physiology, 3e,* Fig. 8.3, p. 248 © 2004. Reprinted with permission of the McGraw-Hill Publishing Companies, Inc.

Figure 4.14(b): From Seeley, *Anatomy & Physiology, 6e,* Fig. 7.34, p. 225, © 2003. Reprinted with permission of the McGraw-Hill Publishing Companies, Inc.

Figure 4.15: From Saladin, *Anatomy and Physiology, 3e,* Fig. 7.34, p. 230, © 2004. Reprinted with permission of the McGraw-Hill Publishing Companies, Inc.

Figure 4.15(b): From Shier, et al., *Human Anatomy & Physiology, 9e,* Fig. 7.14, p. 208, © 2002. Reprinted with permission of the McGraw-Hill Publishing Companies, Inc.

Figure 4.16: From Seeley, *Anatomy & Physiology, 6e,* Fig. 7.26, p. 223, © 2003. Reprinted with permission of the McGraw-Hill Publishing Companies, Inc.

Figure 4.16(b): From Seeley, *Anatomy & Physiology, 6e,* Fig. 23.1, p. 814, © 2003. Reprinted with permission of the McGraw-Hill Publishing Companies, Inc.

Figure 4.17: From Shier, et al., *Human Anatomy & Physiology, 9e,* Fig. 19.1 p. 780, © 2002. Reprinted with permission of the McGraw-Hill Publishing Companies, Inc.

Figure 4.18: From Mader, Human Biology, 7e, Fig. 5.3, p. 84, © 2002. Reprinted with permission of the McGraw-Hill Publishing Companies, Inc.

Figure 4.19: From Mader, *Human Biology, 7e,* Fig. 7.13, p. 135, © 2002. Reprinted with permission of the McGraw-Hill Publishing Companies, Inc.

Figure 4.19(b): From Shier, et al., *Human Anatomy & Physiology, 9e,* Fig. 19.12 p. 787, © 2002. Reprinted with permission of the McGraw-Hill Publishing Companies, Inc.

Figure 4.20: From Seeley, *Anatomy & Physiology, 6e,* Fig. 23.7, p. 822, © 2003. Reprinted with permission of the McGraw-Hill Publishing Companies, Inc.

Figure 4.22: From Shier, et al., *Human Anatomy & Physiology, 9e,* Fig. 19.20 p. 792, © 2002. Reprinted with permission of the McGraw-Hill Publishing Companies, Inc.

Figure 4.23: From Seeley, *Anatomy & Physiology, 6e,* Fig. 23.10, p. 825, © 2003. Reprinted with permission of the McGraw-Hill Publishing Companies, Inc.

Figure 4.25: From Anspaugh, et al., *Wellness, 5e,* fig. 45.15, p. 962, © 1999. Reprinted with permission of the McGraw-Hill Publishing Companies, Inc.

Figure 4.26: From Guttman, *Biology,* Fig. 45.15, p. 962, © 1999. Reprinted with permission of the McGraw-Hill Publishing Companies, Inc.

Figure 4.30: From Seeley, *Anatomy & Physiology, 6e,* Fig. 11.1, p. 364, © 2003. Reprinted with permission of the McGraw-Hill Publishing Companies, Inc.

Figure 4.32: From Lewis, *Life, 4e,* Fig. 30.8, p. 602, © 2002. Reprinted with permission of the McGraw-Hill Publishing Companies, Inc.

Figure 4.33: From Lewis, *Life, 4e,* Fig. 37.6, p. 738, © 2002. Reprinted with permission of the McGraw-Hill Publishing Companies, Inc.

Figure 4.34: From Mader, *Human Biology, 7e,* Fig. 15.2, p. 294, © 2002. Reprinted with permission of the McGraw-Hill Publishing Companies, Inc.

Figure 4.35: From Lewis, *Life, 4e,* Fig. 40.6, p. 795, © 2002. Reprinted with permission of the McGraw-Hill Publishing Companies, Inc.

Figure 4.36: From Lewis, *Life, 4e,* Fig. 40.7, p. 798, © 2002. Reprinted with permission of the McGraw-Hill Publishing Companies, Inc.

Figure 4.37: From Mader, *Human Biology, 7e,* Fig. 10.2, p. 188, © 2002. Reprinted with permission of the McGraw-Hill Publishing Companies, Inc.

Index

Page numbers with *f* indicate figures; page numbers with *t* indicate tables.

Brown recluse spiders, 421*f*, 422*f*
    signs and symptoms of bites of, 422
Bruising, 479, 489, 489*f*, 524
    cerebral, 568
    pulmonary, 223, 583–584, 583*f*
Buccal drugs, 282, 282*f*
Buddy taping, 534
Bulb syringe in clearing airway in infants and
    children, 602–603
Burn centers, 15*f*
    treatment of burns in, 504–505
Burns, 501–508, 502*f*, 503*f*, 504*f*, 507*f*
    alkali, 499
    chemical, 499, 506
    circumferential, 505
    depth of, 501–502, 502*f*, 503*f*
    determining severity of, 501
    electrical, 507–508, 507*f*
    extent of, 502–503, 503*ft*
    friction, 492
    full-thickness, 502, 503*f*
    in infants and children, 504
    location of, 504
    nonchemical, 499
    in older adults, 504
    partial-thickness, 501–502, 502*f*, 504
    rug, 492
    stocking-like, 504, 504*f*
    superficial, 501, 502*f*
    thermal, 450, 505–506
    treatment of, in burn center, 504–505
Butterfly catheter, 707
Bystanders
    assistance from, in emergencies, 121
    communicating with, 250–251
    responses of, to injury or illness, 34
    safety of, 188

C

Calcium, 516
Call
    in communications network, 244
    en route to, 246
Canal, 94
Capillaries, 88, 322
Capillary bleeding, 473–474, 473*f*, 474
Capillary/cellular exchange, 151
Capillary refill, 107–108, 107*f*
    assessing, in children and infants, 604
    in primary survey, 210
Capnometry, 673
Carbon dioxide, 149, 151, 293
Cardiac arrest, 333, 335–343
    cause of, 86
    during transport, 343
Cardiac muscle, 80, 81*f*
Cardiac (pericardial) tamponade, 581–582, 582*f*
Cardiogenic shock, 413, 481
Cardiopulmonary failure in infants and children,
    606, 606*f*
Cardiopulmonary resuscitation (CPR), 34,
    77, 333
    automated external defibrillator
        maintenance, 345
    fundamentals of early, 335–336, 335*f*
    guidelines for, 339*t*
    interruption of, 343
    one-rescuer adult, 682–684*f*
    one-rescuer child, 689–691*f*
    one-rescuer infant, 692–693
    stopping, 345
    training and sources of information, 345
    two-rescuer adult, 685–688*f*
Cardiovascular disease, 323
    acute coronary syndromes, 323–331
Cardiovascular emergencies, 315–345
    automated external defibrillator
        maintenance, 345
    cardiac arrest, 333, 335–343
        during transport, 343
    circulatory system, 317
    disease, 323
        acute coronary syndromes, 323–331
        congestive heart failure, 326

patient assessment and emergency care,
    336–343
    assessing responsiveness, 336–341
physiology of circulation, 322–323, 323*f*
postresuscitation care, 343
stopping cardiopulmonary resuscitation, 345
support of family, 343
system, 317–323
    blood, 322
    blood vessels, 320–322
    heart, 317–318, 317*f*, 318*f*, 319
training and sources of information, 345
Cardiovascular system, 317–323, 400
    blood, 322
    blood vessels, 320–322
    heart, 317–318, 317*f*, 318*f*, 319
    signs and symptoms of allergic reaction
        by, 375*t*
Carina, 83
Carotid arteries, 89, 102, 321, 364
Carotid pulse, 89, 102, 209*f*, 321*f*
Carpals, 77, 519
Carries, 125, 128–131
    cradle, 129, 130*f*
    firefighter's, 128–129, 129*f*
    pack-strap, 129–130, 130*f*
    piggyback, 130–131, 130*f*
    procedure on stairs, 125
    two-person, 131, 131*f*
Cartilage, 519
Cat bites, 425–426
    emergency care for, 426
Cecum, 94
Cells, 70
Cellular telephones, 243
Centers for Disease Control and Prevention
    (CDC), 43
Central lines, 617–618
Central nervous system, 73, 91–93, 91*f*,
    546–547
Central pulses, 91, 102–103, 103*t*, 322
Central venous access, 707
Cephalic (head) delivery, 453
Cerebellum, 92
Cerebral contusion, 568
Cerebral hemorrhages, 364
Cerebrospinal fluid (CSF), 92, 546
Cerebrovascular accident, 363
Cerebrum, 92, 92*f*, 546
Certification, 25
Cervical collars, 553, 554, 555, 555*f*, 556*f*
Cervical spine
    injuries to, 547
    protection of
        in infants and children, 601
        in primary survey, 207, 207*f*
Cervical vertebrae, 77, 518
Cervix, 442
Chain of Survival, 335
Charcoal, activated, for ingested poisons, 282*f*,
    284, 285*t*, 392–395, 393*f*
CHART, 268
Chemical burns, 499, 506
    emergency care of, 506
Chemical names, 280, 280*t*
Chemical protective clothing (CPC), 653
Chemical weapons, 717–718, 717*t*
Chest (thorax), 77, 78*f*, 518
    in head-to-toe examination, 223
    managing injuries to, 574
    trauma to, in infants and children, 613
Chest compressions
    adult, 337
    child, 338
    infant, 338, 338*f*
Chest injuries
    anatomy of, 575, 575*f*
    categories of, 575
    closed, 575–584
    deadly and potentially deadly, 574*t*
    open, 575, 584–585, 585*f*
    penetrating, 496, 496*f*
    sucking wound, 496
Chickenpox (Varicella), 47, 47*t*
Chief complaint, 204–205, 214
    focused medical assessment by, 220*f*

Child abuse
    burns and, 504, 504*f*
    neglect and, 614–617, 614*f*, 615*f*, 616*f*
Child anatomy, infant airway and, 151
Child cardiopulmonary resuscitation,
    one-rescuer, 689–691, 691*f*
Children
    age classification of, 592
    anatomical and physiological differences in
        airway, 593
        breathing, 594, 594*t*
        circulation, 594–595, 595*t*
        face, 593
        head, 593, 593*f*
    assessment of
        primary survey, 599–604, 600*f*, 602*f*, 603*f*
        scene size-up, 599, 599*f*
    burns in, 504, 504*f*
    caring for, 592
    clearing foreign body airway obstruction
        in conscious, 698*f*
        in unconscious, 699*f*
    common problems in
        airway obstruction in, 604
        altered mental status, 607
        cardiopulmonary failure, 606, 606*f*
        chest, abdominal, and pelvic trauma, 613
        drowning, 610–611
        fever, 607–608
        poisonings, 609–610
        respiratory emergencies, 604–606
        seizures, 608–609
        shock, 607
        sudden infant death syndrome, 611–612
        trauma, 612–614
    communication with, 248, 248*f*
    developmental stages of
        adolescents (13 to 18 years of age),
            598–599, 599*f*
        infants (birth to 1 year of age), 595–596, 596*f*
        preschoolers (4 to 5 years of age),
            597–598, 597*f*
        school-age (6 to 12 years of age), 598, 598*f*
        toddlers (1 to 3 years of age),
            596–597, 596*f*
    fractures in, 521–522
    level of responsiveness in, 206–207, 207*f*
    maltreatment of, 614
    musculoskeletal system in, 80–81
    respiratory system in, 86, 297, 663–664
    shock in, 483, 483*f*
    with special needs
        central lines, 617–618
        gastrostomy tubes and gastric feeding, 618
        home mechanical ventilators, 617
        shunts, 618
        tracheostomy tubes, 617
    ventilating, 174
China white, 389
Choking, 149, 294
Cholinergic, 386*t*
Chronic bronchitis, 307, 308*f*
    emergency care of, 307
    signs and symptoms of, 307
Chronic obstructive pulmonary disease
    (COPD), 296
Chronic respiratory diseases, 297
Chyme, 94
Cincinnati Prehospital Stroke Scale, 365
Circulation, 594–595, 595*t*
    assessment of, 235, 337
    in infants and children, 603–604
    physiology of, 91, 322–323, 323*f*
    in primary assessment of infants and children,
        600–601
    in primary survey, 209–210
Circulatory system, 87–91, 98*t*, 317
Circumferential burn, 505
Clammy (cool and moist) skin, 107, 107*f*, 108*f*
Clavicles, 75, 77, 517
Cleaning, 48
Clenched-fist injury, 426
Closed chest injuries, 575–584
    cardiac (pericardial) tamponade, 581–582, 582*f*
    flail chest, 577–578, 577*f*, 578*f*
    hemothorax, 581, 581*f*

Great vessels, 87
Greenstick fracture, 522
Grief, 29, 30*f*
    changes in circumstances that contribute, 30
    stages of, 29–31, 30*f*
Ground ambulance, 12
    basic medical equipment and supplies for, 624
Growth plate, 522, 522*f*
Grunting, 299
Gunshot wounds, 493, 523
    pregnancy and, 449–450
Gurgling, 106, 162, 299
Gynecological emergencies, 466–468
Gynecology. *See* Obstetrics and gynecology

H

Hallucinations, 434
    auditory, 434
    tactile, 434
    visual, 434
Hallucinogens, 389
Hand, injuries to, 533–534, 534*f*
Hand-off report, 252
Handwashing, 43–44, 43*f*
Hard palate, 81, 664
Hard suction catheter, 155, 156*f*
Hazardous materials, 49–50, 49*f*, 652–658
    approaching patient, 657
    decontamination, 658
    establishing safety zones, 657
    protective equipment with, 653–654,
        653*f*, 654*f*
    role of emergency medical technician, 652
    scene safety and reporting with, 653
    scene size-up, 654–656
Hazardous substances, identifying, 656
Head
    in children, 593, 593*f*
    in head-to-toe examination, 221–222, 221*f*
    manual stabilization of, 554
    severe backward movement of, 548, 548*f*
    severe forward movement of, 548, 548*f*
    trauma to, 593
Head bobbing, 297
Head injuries, 564, 566
    anatomy and, 546–547, 546*f*, 547*f*
    closed, 567
    emergency care of, 570–571
    managing, 546
    open, 567
    signs and symptoms of traumatic, 567–568
Head or ear bandage, 511*f*
Head tilt-chin lift maneuver, 152–153, 153*f*,
    205, 601
Head-to-toe examination
    abdomen in, 220–231
    chest in, 223
    ears in, 222
    extremities in, 231–232
    eyes in, 222
    face in, 221–222, 221*f*
    head in, 221–222, 221*f*
    neck in, 223
    pelvis in, 231
    posterior body in, 232
    reassessment of mental status, 221
Head trauma, 612–613
    in infants and children, 612–613
Health and Human Services, U.S. Department
    of (HHS), 6
    Division of Trauma and EMS (DTEMS), 6
Healthcare resources in emergency response in
    rural and frontier areas, 722
Healthcare system, 9–10
Health Insurance Portability and Accountability
    Act (1966) (HIPAA), 64–65, 253
Health Resources and Services Administration
    (HRSA), 12
Hearing impairments. *See also* Ears
    communications and, 249–250, 249*f*
    in older adults, 703, 703*f*
Heart, 80, 87, 87*f*, 88*f*, 317–318, 317*f*, 318*f*,
    319, 327
    valves of, 318, 319*f*
Heart attack, atypical signs and symptoms of, 327*t*

Heart/cardiovascular centers, 15*f*
Heart disease risk factors, 324*t*
Heart rate
    in newborn, 459–460
    possible causes of rapid, 104
    possible causes of slow, 104
Heat, exposure to, 408–410
    predisposing factors, 408
Heat exhaustion, 408
    signs and symptoms of, 409
Heat loss, 401–402, 401*f*
Heat production, 400–401
Heat-related emergencies
    emergency care of patients with,
        409–410
    types of, 408–409
Heat strokes, 408–409
Helicopters
    transport by, 638–639, 638*f*
    working safely around, 639
Helmet removal, 564, 565–566*f*
Hematemesis, 586
Hematomas, 489, 568, 569*f*, 570
    epidural, 570
    intracerebral, 570
    subdural, 568, 569*f*, 570
Hematuria, 586
Hemoglobin, 88, 113, 322
Hemophilia, 473
Hemorrhage, 472. *See also* Bleeding
    intracerebral, 364
    subarachnoid, 364
Hemorrhagic shock, 480
Hemorrhagic strokes, 364
Hemothorax, 230, 581, 581*f*
    massive, 581
Hepatitis B, 46–47
High-Efficiency Particulate Air (HEPA) filter,
    163, 164*f*
High-Efficiency Particulate Air (HEPA) mask,
    45, 46*f*
High-Fowler's position, 140, 140*f*
High-level disinfection, 637
Highway Safety Act (1966), 5
Hinge joint, 519
Hip, 519
    injuries to, 534–535, 535*f*
History of present illness (HPI), 214
Homeland Security Act (2002), 7
Home mechanical ventilators, 617
Homeostasis, 70
Hooding, 582
Hospital care, 14
Hot skin, 210
Hot zone, 657
Human bites, 426
    emergency care for, 426
Human crutch move, 131, 131*f*
Human resources and education, 11–12
Humerus, 77, 518, 519
    injuries to, 532, 532*f*
Humidifiers, 175, 176*f*
Hydrocephalus, 618
Hymen, 97
Hymenoptera stings, 423–424, 424*f*
    emergency care for, 424
Hyoid bone, 76, 82
Hyperbaric centers, 15*f*
Hyperglycemia, 353–354, 353*t*
Hyphema, 222
Hypoglycemia, 352–353, 353*t*
Hypoperfusion, 472, 480
Hypothalamus, 92, 400
Hypothermia, 402–403
    emergency care of patients with, 405–406
    factors that contribute to, 403
    signs and symptoms of, 404*t*
Hypovolemia, 594
Hypovolemic shock, 480, 481*f*, 491
Hypoxia, 114, 298, 577
Hypoxic drive, 85

I

Ice for emergency vehicles, 631
Ileum, 94

Illnesses
    in emergency response in rural and frontier
        areas, 724–725
    events leading to, 117
    nature of, 195, 196*f*
    patient's response to, 31–32, 32*f*
    responses of family, friends, or bystanders to, 34
    stress-induced, 37
Immersion, 410
Immobilization of supine patient on long
    backboard, 555, 558–560, 558*f*, 559*f*, 560*f*
Immunizations, 46–47
Impaled objects, 493, 494*f*, 497
Impetigo, 615, 615*f*
Implantable cardioverter-defibrillator, 338
Implied consent, 59
Implied duty, 63
Inadequate breathing, 665
Incendiary weapons, 717
Incident Command System (ICS), 10, 659–660
Incident response to weapons of mass
    destruction (WMD), 718–721
Incompetence, 57
    mental, 59
Incomplete abortion, 445
Index of suspicion, 216
Indirect force injury, 521, 521*f*
Infants (birth to 1 year of age), 595–596, 596*f*
    age classification of, 592
    assessment of
        primary survey, 599–604, 600*f*, 602*f*, 603*f*
        scene size-up, 599, 599*f*
    burns in, 504
    caring for, 592
    child anatomy and airway of, 151
    clearing foreign body airway obstruction
        in conscious, 700*f*
        in unconscious, 701*f*
    common problems in
        airway obstruction in, 604
        altered mental status, 607
        cardiopulmonary failure, 606, 606*f*
        chest, abdominal, and pelvic trauma, 613
        drowning, 610–611
        fever, 607–608
        poisonings, 609–610
        respiratory emergencies, 604–606
        seizures, 608–609
        shock, 607
        sudden infant death syndrome, 611–612
        trauma, 612–614
    level of responsiveness in, 206–207, 207*f*
    musculoskeletal system in, 80–81
    one-rescuer cardiopulmonary resuscitation for,
        692–693
    respiratory system in, 86, 297, 663–664
    shock in, 483, 483*f*
    with special needs
        central lines, 617–618
        gastrostomy tubes and gastric feeding, 618
        home mechanical ventilators, 617
        shunts, 618
        tracheostomy tubes, 617
    ventilating, 174
Infection, 42
    factors that increase susceptibility, 42
Infection control, 43
    procedures in emergency medical services
        call, 637–638
Inferior, 71
Inferior vena cava, 322
Infiltration, 712–713
Influenza, 47
Information. *See also* Documentation
    falsification of, on prehospital care reports, 266
    protected health, 57, 65
    sources of
        on cardiovascular emergencies, 345
        on drugs, 280
Informed consent, 58–59
Ingested poisons, 392–395
    activated charcoal for, 282*f*, 284, 285*t*,
        392–395, 393*f*
    emergency care for, 392–395
    patient assessment in, 392
Ingestion, 94, 385*f*
Inhalants, 395

Inhalation, 104–105, 295, 385*f*
  signs and symptoms of possible injury, 505
Inhalation drug route, 282, 283*f*
Inhaled poisons, 395–396
  emergency care for, 396
  patient assessment in, 396
Inhaled steroids, 310
Injected poisons, 396–397
  emergency care for, 396–397
  patient assessment for, 396
Injection, 385*f*
Injuries
  in emergency response in rural and frontier
    areas, 724–725
  events leading to, 117
  intentional, 189*t*
  mechanism of, 189–195, 189*t*, 190*f*, 191*f*,
    192*ft*, 193*t*, 194*t*
  patient's response to, 31–32, 32*f*
  prevention programs for, 16
  responses of family, friends, or bystanders
    to, 34
  unintentional, 189*t*
Injury Control Act (1990), 6
Injury Prevention Act (1986), 6
In-line stabilization, 207, 207*f*
Insertion of skeletal muscle, 519, 520*f*
Inspiration, 85, 86
Insulin, 96, 350
Insulin shock, 353
Integumentary system, 93, 94*f*, 98*t*
  signs and symptoms of allergic reaction
    by, 375*t*
Intentional abuse, 386–387
Intentional injuries, 189*t*
Interagency liaison, 224
Interagency Radio Advisory Committee
    (IRAC), 241
Intercostal muscles, 85
Intercostal retractions, 299
Intermediate-level disinfection, 637
Internal bleeding, 478–480, 479*f*, 494
  emergency care of, 479–480, 479*f*
Internet Voice, 11, 244
Intersection crashes in emergency medical
    services call, 632, 632*f*
Intracerebral hematoma, 570
Intracerebral hemorrhage, 364
Intramuscular route, 283, 283*f*
Intravenous (IV) therapy
  calculating flow rates, 711–712
  cannulations, 707
  catheters in
    needle size, 708, 708*f*, 709*f*
    saline lock, 708, 709*f*
    types of, 707–708, 708*f*
  complications of, 712–713
  drip in, 709
  infusion in, 709
  monitoring, 707
    purpose of, 707
    types of access, 707
  tubing in administration of, 709–711,
    709*f*, 710*f*
  types of access, 707
  types of fluids in, 712
Ipsilateral, 71
Irreversible shock, 482
Ischemia, 324
Ischemic strokes, 363, 364*f*
Islets of Langerhans, 96

J

Jaundiced skin, 106*f*, 107, 210
Jaw fracture, 500
Jaw thrust
  without head extension maneuver, 153
  without head tilt, 153–154, 154*f*, 205, 205*f*
Jejunum, 94
Joints, 519, 519*f*
  ball-and-socket, 519
  hinge, 519
  splinting, 533
Jugular venous distention (JVD), 223, 580
JumpSTART triage system, 659

K

Kendrick Extrication Device, 647–648, 648*f*
Kidneys, 97
Kimberly-Clark Self-Adherent Wrap, 510
Kinematics, 189
Kinetic energy, 189
Kling, 510
Knee, 519
  injuries to, 540, 540*f*
Knee bandage, 511*f*
Knee-chest position, 464, 464*f*
Knocked-out (avulsed) tooth, 500
Knowledge. *See also* Information
  maintaining, 25
Knuckle bandage, 510
Kübler-Ross, Elizabeth, 30
Kussmaul respirations, 354

L

Labia majora, 97
Labia minora, 97
Labor, 442
  false, 453, 454*f*
  normal, 452–453
  premature, 445
  stages of, 452–453, 453*f*
Labored breathing, 105
Laceration, 492–493, 492*f*
Lancet, 356
"Landmark Paper," 5
Large intestine, 94
Larrey, Baron Dominique Jean, 4
Laryngeal stoma, 223
Laryngectomy, 171
Laryngopharynx, 82, 664
Laryngoscope, 668
  handle and blades, 668, 668*f*, 669*f*
Laryngospasm, 412
Larynx, 81, 82, 149*f*, 150, 664
Lateral, 71
Lateral recumbent position, 72
Latex allergy, 371
  foods causing allergic reactions in people
    with, 373*t*
  products causing, 373*t*
Left lower quadrant (LLQ), 73, 73*f*
Left upper quadrant (LUQ), 73
Legal and ethical care
  abandonment, 63
  advance directives, 60–61, 62*f*
  assault and battery, 62–63
  communications and, 253
  confidentiality, Health Insurance Portability
    and Accountability Act (HIPAA) and,
    64–65
  consent, 58–59
    expressed, 58–59
    implied, 59
    refusals, 59–60
    special situations, 59
  documentation, 67
  do-not-resuscitate (DNR) orders, 60–61, 62*f*
  duties in, 56
  importance of, 55
  negligence, 63
    breach of duty, 64
    damages, 64
    duty to act, 63
    proximate cause, 64
  prehospital care reports in, 258
  scope of practice
    competence, 57–58
    ethical responsibilities, 57
    legal duties, 56
    responsibilities, 57
  special situations, 66
    crime scenes, 66
    medical identification devices, 66
    organ donation, 66
    reporting requirements, 66
Legal competence, 57
Legislation and regulation, 10
Leukocytes, 88

Level A personal protective equipment (PPE),
  653, 653*f*, 655*t*
Level B personal protective equipment (PPE),
  653, 654*f*, 655*t*
Level C personal protective equipment (PPE),
  654, 654*f*, 655*t*
Level D personal protective equipment (PPE),
  654, 654*f*, 655*t*
Level of responsiveness (mental status), in
  primary survey, 205, 206*f*, 207
Licensure, 25
Life-threatening conditions, examples of, 151
Lift
  direct ground, 134, 135*f*
  extremity, 134, 136*f*
Ligaments, 519
Lily of the valley, 390
Limb presentation, 464, 464*f*
Line-of-sight radio coverage problems, 241
Liquid drugs, 281, 281*t*
Listening, with empathy, 33
Liver, 95
Local cold injury, 406–407, 407*f*
  emergency care of patients with, 406–407
Local effect of drugs, 281
Log roll, 125
Long backboard, 143–144, 625
Long bone, splinting, 532
Love Drug, 389
Lower airway, 294, 664
Lower extremities, 79
  injuries to, 534–535, 535*f*, 536–539*f*, 540, 540*f*,
    541–542, 541*f*, 542*t*
Lower leg, injuries to, 540–541, 541*f*
Low-level disinfection, 637
Low vision, 250, 704
Lumbar spine, injuries to, 547
Lumbar vertebrae, 77, 518
Lungs, 83–84, 84, 149*f*, 150, 294, 295
Lymphatic system, 87
Lysergic acid diethylamine (LSD), 389

M

Macrodrip intravenous (IV) administration
  set, 710
Males, injuries to genitalia in, 587–588
Mammalian diving reflex, 411
Mammary glands, 96
Mandible, 76, 518
Manual defibrillator, 338
Manually triggered ventilation (MTV)
  device, 171
Manual stabilization, 207, 207*f*
Manubrium, 77, 518
Marine life stings, 424–425
Masks, 45, 48
Mass casualty incidents, 658–659
  documentation of, 269, 269*f*
  JumpSTART triage system, 659
  START triage system, 658–659
Massive hemothorax, 581
Material Safety Data Sheet (MSDS), in
  identifying hazardous substances, 656
Maxilla, 76, 518
MDMA (3,4-Methylenedioxymethamphetamine)
  ("ecstasy"), 389
Measles, signs and symptoms, 47*t*
Measles-mumps-rubella (MMR) vaccine, 47
Mechanism of action, 284
Mechanism of injury, 189–195, 189*t*, 190*f*, 191*f*,
    192*ft*, 193*t*, 194*t*
  predictable injuries based on common,
    192–193*t*
  sources of energy and, 189*t*
  in trauma patient, 215–218, 217*f*
Meconium, 458–459
Medial, 71
Mediastinal shift, 580
Mediastinum, 84
Medical abbreviations, common, 269–272
Medical direction
  communicating with, 251, 251*f*
  off-line, 13
  on-line, 13, 13*f*
  prospective, 14

quality management and, 341–342
    retrospective, 14
Medical director, 13
Medical history
    patient's, 214–215
    pertinent past, 116–117
Medical identification devices, 66
Medical neglect, 614
Medical oversight, 13–14, 13*f*, 56
Medical patient, 189, 219, 219*f*
    assessment of, 219*f*
    responsive, 220–221
    unresponsive, 219–220
Medical practice acts, 13
Medical/situational competence, 58
Medical uses of prehospital care reports,
    257–258
Medications, 116. *See also* Drugs
    administration of emergency medical services
        unit, 284, 286*t*
    assisting with prescribed, 285, 287
    in older adults, 705
Medulla, 92
Medulla oblongata, 546
Melatonin, 95
Meninges, 92, 546
Meningitis, 92, 608
Menstruation, 442
Mental competence, 57–58
Mental incompetence, 59
Mental status
    in infants and children, 601
    reassessment of, in head-to-toe
        examination, 221
Mescaline (street names), 389
Metacarpals, 77, 519
Metatarsal bones, 79
Metered-dose inhaler (MDI), 282, 283*f*,
    310–313, 311*f*
    assisting patient with, 312–313
        contraindications, 313
        procedure, 313
    indications, 310
    medication actions, 310, 311*t*
Mexican brown, 389
Mexican milk snake, 418*f*
Microdrop intravenous (IV) administration
    set, 711
Midaxillary line, 71, 72*f*
Midbrain, 546
Midclavicular line, 72, 72*f*
Midline, 71
Mini-stroke, 364
Minors, 59
    emancipated, 59
Minute volume, 151, 299
Miscarriage, 445
Mitral (bicuspid) valve, 318
Mobile Army Surgical Hospital (MASH), 5
Mobile data computer (MDC), 243
Mobile data terminal (MDT), 243
Mobile two-way radio, 242–243, 242*f*
Modifiable risk factors, 324
MONA, 329
Mongolian spots, 615, 616*f*
Morning sickness, 444
Mother, caring for, in childbirth, 460–462, 462*f*
Motor nerves, 546, 547
Motor vehicle crashes (MVCs), 190–192, 191*f*, 192*f*
    potential hazards at scene, 50
    pregnancy and, 449
    rescue scenes and, 50–51
    statistics of, 195
Motor vehicle-pedestrian crashes, 194–195
Mottling, 106*f*, 107, 210
Mounted suction devices, 155, 155*f*
Mouth, 149, 149*f*, 294
    injuries to, 500, 500*f*
    opening, 152, 152*f*
Mouth-to-barrier device ventilation, 166, 166*f*
Mouth-to-mask ventilation, 163–164, 165*f*
Mouth-to-mouth ventilation, 5, 166–167
Multiple births, 465
Multiple-vehicle responses for emergency
    vehicles, 631
Multiplex system, 244
Mumps, signs and symptoms of, 47*t*

Murphy eye, 667
Muscles, 74, 519
    cardiac, 80, 81*f*
    skeletal, 79–80, 81*f*, 519, 520*f*
    smooth, 80, 81*f*
Muscle tone, 80
Muscular system, 79–81, 98*t*, 519, 520*f*
Musculoskeletal care, 515–543
    managing injuries in, 516
    system, 516–520
Musculoskeletal injuries
    care of specific, 530, 531*f*, 532–535, 533*f*,
        534*f*, 535*f*, 536–539*f*, 540–542, 540*f*,
        541*f*, 542*t*
    emergency care of, 525–526, 526*f*
    mechanisms of, 521, 521*f*
    signs and symptoms of, 524
    splinting, 526–530, 528*f*, 529*f*, 530*f*
    types of, 521–524, 522*f*, 523*f*, 524*f*
Musculoskeletal system, 74–81, 74*f*
Myocardial contusion, 584, 584*f*

N

Narcotics (opiates), 387, 388
    examples of, 388
Narrative, 268–269
Nasal airway, 157, 160, 160*f*
    sizing and inserting, 161*f*
Nasal bones, 76
Nasal cannula, 180, 180*f*
Nasal cavity, 149, 149*f*, 293, 294*f*
Nasal flaring, 222
Nasogastric tubes
    complications, 678
    contraindications, 678
    equipment, 678
    indications, 678
    insertion procedure, 678–679, 679*f*
Nasopharyngeal airway, 157
Nasopharynx, 82, 664
National Academy of Sciences-National Research
    Council (NAS/NRC), 5
National Association of Emergency Medical
    Technicians (NAEMT), 6
National Association of State EMS Directors, 259
National Center for Injury Prevention and
    Control, 6
National Emergency Medical Services
    Information System (NEMSIS), 259
National Emergency Number Association
    (NENA), 10
National EMS
    Core Content document, 7
    Education Standards, 11, 25
    Scope of Practice Model, 7, 11–12, 56
National Fire Protection Association (NFPA), 49
    defining of hazardous materials by, 652
    Standard 704 in identifying hazardous
        substances, 656
National Highway Traffic Safety Administration
    (NHTSA), 259
    First There, First Care program, 12
    Technical Assessment Program, components
        of, 6
National Incident Management System (NIMS),
    7, 10
    plan under, 655–656
National Registry of Emergency Medical
    Technicians (NREMT), 5
National Research Council, 6
National Safety Council, 4
Nature of illness, 195, 196*f*
Near-miss sudden infant death syndrome
    (SIDS), 611
Near-sudden infant death syndrome (SIDS), 611
Near syncope, 366
    questions to ask about patient with, 367
    signs and symptoms of, 367
Neck
    in head-to-toe examination, 223
    injuries to, 497–498, 498*f*
    manual stabilization of, 554
Neglect, 614, 614*f*
    medical, 614
Negligence, 63

breach of duty, 64
    damages, 64
    duty to act, 63
    proximate cause, 64
Nerves
    motor, 546, 547
    sensory, 546, 547
    spinal, 77, 547
Nervous system, 91–93, 91*f*, 98*t*
    central, 91–93, 91*f*, 546–547
    peripheral, 547
    signs and symptoms of allergic reaction by, 375*t*
Neurons, 91
Newborn, caring for, 458–460, 459*f*, 460*f*,
    461*ft*, 462*f*
Nicotine, risk of local cold injury and, 406
9-1-1 service, 10, 244
Nitroglycerin (NTG), 282, 283*f*, 288*t*, 326
    assisting patient with prescribed, 330–331,
        332–333*f*, 333*t*
    assisting patient with prescribed spray,
        334–335*f*
Nonadherent pads, 509, 509*f*
Non-allergic asthma, 305, 306
Nonbreather mask, 179–180, 179*f*
Nonbreathing patient, flow-restricted, oxygen-
    powered ventilation for, 172*f*
Nonchemical burn, 499
Non-English-speaking patients, communicating
    with, 249
Noninvasive blood pressure (NIBP) monitor, 110
Non-modifiable risk factors, 324
Nonpurposeful movement, 221
Nonurgent moves, 121, 134
Norepinephrine, 95
Normal labor, 452–453
Nose, 149, 149*f*, 293, 294*f*, 664
Nosebleeds, 500–501, 501*f*
Nuclear weapons, 716, 716*f*

O

Objective findings, 102
Obsessions, 432
Obsessive-compulsive disorder (OCD), 432
Obstetrics and gynecology, 440–469
    anatomy and physiology of female
        reproductive system, 441–444, 442*f*, 443*f*
    assessing pregnant patient, 450–452
    caring for mother and baby, 441
    caring for mother in childbirth, 460–462, 462*f*
    complications of delivery, 462–465, 463*f*,
        464*f*, 465*f*
    complications of pregnancy, 445–446
    emergencies in, 451
    emergency care of newborn and mother,
        458–462, 459*f*, 460*f*, 461*ft*, 462*f*
    gynecological emergencies, 466–468
    normal delivery, 454–458
    normal labor, 452–453
    normal pregnancy, 444–445
    structures of pregnancy, 443–444, 443*f*
    trauma and pregnancy, 449–450, 450*f*
Occipital bone, 75
Occipital lobes, 92, 546
Occlusive, 223
Occlusive dressings, 509, 509*f*
Occupational Safety and Health Administration
    (OSHA), 43
Off-line medical direction, 13
Older adults, 702–706, 702*f*
    altered mental status in, 705
    burns in, 504
    communication during interview process,
        702–705
    communication with, 248
    hearing impairments in, 703, 703*f*
    medications in, 705
    pain perception in, 705
    physical examination considerations in,
        705–706
    speech impairments in, 704
    vision impairments in, 704
Oleander, 390
Olecranon, 77
Onboard oxygen, 174, 174*t*

One rescuer
  adult cardiopulmonary resuscitation, 682–684f
  child cardiopulmonary resuscitation, 689–691f
  infant cardiopulmonary resuscitation, 692–693
Ongoing assessment, 232, 234f
  components of, 232–233, 235
  purpose of, 232
On-line medical direction, 13, 13f
On-scene care in emergency medical services call, 634
Open chest injuries, 575, 584–585, 585f
Open-ended questions, 214
Open fracture, 477, 522–523
Open head injury, 567
Open pneumothorax, 580, 584–585, 585f
  signs and symptoms of, 585
Open wounds, 472, 492–495, 492f, 493f, 494f, 495f
  emergency care of, 495
Operator area in emergency vehicle, 627, 627f
Opiates, 387, 388
  examples of, 388
OPQRST, 117, 214–215, 215t
Oral airway, 156–157m157f
  sizing and inserting, 158–159, 159f
Oral cavity, 149, 149f, 294
Oral glucose, 286t, 356, 358, 358t
  giving, 359f
Oral route of drug administration, 281, 281f
Orbits, 76
Organs, 70
  donation of, 66
  vital, 70
Organ systems, 70, 98
Origin of skeletal muscle, 519, 520f
Orogastric tubes
  complications, 678
  contraindications, 678
  equipment, 678
  indications, 678
  insertion procedure, 678–679, 679f
Oropharyngeal airway, 156–157, 157f
Oropharynx, 82, 664
Osteoporosis, 517
Ovaries, 96, 441
Overdose, 387
  general care for, 389–391
Ovulation, 441
Oxygen, 286t, 293
  cylinders of, 174, 174ft
  delivery devices
    blow-by-oxygen, 180–181, 180f, 181f
    nasal cannula, 180, 180f
    nonrebreather mask, 179–180, 179f
  delivery system
    discontinuing, 178f
    setting up, 176–177f
  supplemental, 174
  using safely, 175

P

Pack-strap carry, 129–130, 130f
Padded sprint, 532
Pain
  assessment of, 115, 117–118, 117f
  perception of, in older adults, 705
Palate
  hard, 81, 664
  soft, 81, 664
Pale skin, 210
Palpitations, 326
  measuring blood pressure by, 112
Pancreas, 95, 350
Pancreatic cell function, 351t
Panic attacks, 432
  signs and symptoms common to, 432
Paradoxical movement, 223, 577, 578f, 579
Paramedics, 11
Paranoia, 433–434
Paraplegia, 549–550, 550f
Parasympathetic division, 93, 547
Parasympathetic simulation, effects of, 93t
Parathyroid glands, 95
Paresthesias, 490
Parietal bones, 75

Parietal lobes, 92, 546
Parietal pleura, 84
Paroxysmal nocturnal dyspnea, 298
Partial seizures, 361
Partial-thickness burns, 501–502, 502f, 504
Passive rewarming, 405
Patella, 79, 519
Patent (open) airway, 205
Pathogens, 42
Patient area in emergency vehicle, 626–627, 627f
Patient assessment, 18, 19f, 20–21, 199–236
  in absorbed poisons, 397
  importance of, 201
  in ingested poisons, 392
  in inhaled poisons, 396
  for injected poisons, 396
  overview of, 201–202, 202f
  performing primary survey, 202–212, 203t
    airway, 205, 205f
    breathing, 208–209, 208f
    capillary refill, 210
    cervical spine protection, 207, 207f
    circulation, 209–210
    disability, 211, 212t
    exposure of patient, 211–212
    general impression, 203–204, 204f
    identifying priority patients, 212
    level of responsiveness (mental status), 205–206, 206f
    obvious bleeding, 209
    pulses in, 209–210, 209f, 210f
    skin color, 210
    skin condition, 210
    skin temperature, 210
Patient history, 115–116
Patient package inserts, 280
Patient positioning, 134, 140–141
Patients
  advocacy for, 22–23
  altered, 58
  approaching, in hazardous materials scenes, 657
  calming, in behavioral emergencies, 436
  complaints and possible significant injury, 194t
  dealing with ill and injured, 32–34
  documentation of refusals by, 264, 265f, 266f
  gaining access to, 20
  helping dying, 35–36
  helping family of dying, 36–37, 36f
  lifting and moving safely, 21
  medical, 189
  medical history of, 214–215
  number of, in scene size-ups, 196
  principles of moving, 121
  recognizing need for control of, 33
  removing, in entrapment, 647–649
  response to illness and injury of, 31–32, 32f
  restraining, with behavioral emergencies, 436–438
  safety of, 188, 188f
  spinal stabilization
    of seated, 559, 561f
    of standing, 559, 562–563f
  transfer
    to ambulance, 634, 634f
    to definitive care, 636
    equipment in, 625
  trauma, 188
  treating, with respect, 32, 32f
PCP (angel dust), 389
Pedal pulse, 89, 322
Pediatric centers, 15f
Pedi-Immobilizer, 648–649
Pedis pulses, 322
Pelvic bone, 519
Pelvic cavity, 73
Pelvic fractures, 613
Pelvic girdle, 75, 517–518
Pelvis, 77, 79, 519
  in head-to-toe examination, 231
  injuries to, 534–535, 535f
  trauma to, in infants and children
Penetrating chest injuries, 496, 496f
Penetrating trauma, 190, 190f
Penetration, 493, 493f
Penis, 96

Penlight, 102
Pentobarbital (Nembutal), 388
Perfusion, 91, 322, 472
Pericardial cavity, 73
Pericardial tamponade, 581–582, 582f
Perinatal centers, 15f
Perineum, 97, 443
Peripheral artery disease (PAD), 324
Peripheral Intravenous (IV), 707
Peripheral line, 707
Peripherally inserted central catheter (PICC line), 617
Peripheral nervous system, 93, 547
Peripheral pulses, 91, 103, 103t
Peripheral (surface) temperature, 400
Peristalsis, 94
Peritonitis, 231
Persian white, 389
Personal health, 23
Personal protective equipment (PPE), 20, 44–45, 44f, 45f
  exposure to bleeding and, 474
  in extrication, 643
  guidelines for using, 46t
  levels of, 653–654, 655t
Personal safety, 23, 187–188, 187f, 188f
Personal space, 23
  common zones of, 24t
Pertinent past medical history, 116–117
Phalanges, 77, 79, 519
Pharmacology, 276–291
  defined, 277
  drug administration
    assisting with prescribed medications, 285, 287
    carried in emergency medical services unit, 284, 286t
    general guidelines, 284
  drug administration procedure, 289–291
  drug forms, 280–281, 281t
  drug legislation in United States, 277, 278–279t
  drug names, 280, 280t
  drug sources, 277
  federal regulatory agencies and services, 277
  routes of drug administration, 281–283
  sources of drug information, 280
Pharyngeal balloon, 675
Pharynx, 81, 82, 664
Phenobarbital (Luminal), 388
Phlebitis, 713
Phobias, 432
  common, 433t
  social, 432
Physical abuse, 614
Physical examination, 213
  considerations in older adults, 705–706
Physician's Desk Reference (PDR), 280
Physiology, 70
  of circulation, 322–323, 323f
Pia mater, 92, 546
Piggyback carry, 130–131, 130f
Pineal gland, 95
Pink puffer, 307
Pituitary glands, 95
Pit vipers, 417
  signs and symptoms of bites of, 418f
Placenta, 443–444, 443f, 444
  delivery of, 461–462
Placental abruption, 448
Placenta previa, 447–448, 447f
Plaque, 323–324
Plasma, 88, 322
Platelets, 74, 88
Pleura, 84
  parietal, 84
  visceral, 84
Pleural cavity, 73
Pleural space, 84
Pneumatic antishock garments (PASG), 477, 477f
Pneumatic splints, 529–530, 530f
Pneumonia
  bacterial, 309
  emergency care of, 309
  signs and symptoms of, 309
  viral, 309

Pneumothorax, 223
  primary spontaneous, 579
Pneumothorax (*cont.*)
  secondary spontaneous, 579
  simple, 578–579, 579*f*
  spontaneous, 579
  tension, 580–581, 580*f*
Pocket face mask, 163, 164*f*
Poison(s)
  absorbed, 397–398
    emergency care in, 397–398
    patient assessment in, 397
  common, 385*t*
  defined, 384
  ingested, 392–395
    activated charcoal for, 282*f*, 284, 285*t*,
      392–395, 393*f*
    emergency care for, 392–395
    patient assessment in, 392
  inhaled, 395–396
    emergency care for, 396
    patient assessment in, 396
  injected, 396–397
    emergency care for, 396–397
    patient assessment for, 396
Poison centers, 15*f*
Poison Control Center (PCC), 384
Poisonings, 384
  examples of accidental, 384
  general care for, 389–391
  in infants and children, 609–610
  primary survey in, 389–390
  scene size-ups in, 389
  secondary survey in, 390–391
  snake, 416*t*
Pons, 92, 546
Popliteal arteries, 89
Portable radio, 243, 243*f*
Portable stretcher, 142, 142*f*
Position of function, 527, 528*f*
Positive-pressure ventilation, 163, 209
  rates for, 166*t*
Posterior, 71
Posterior body in head-to-toe examination, 232
Posterior nosebleed, 500–501
Posterior tibial pulse, 89, 103, 103*t*
Postictal phase, 609
  of tonic-clonic seizures, 361
Postresuscitation care, 343
Power grip, 123, 124*f*
Power lift, 123
  two-person, 124, 124*f*
Power lines, 51
Predictable injuries, based on common
  mechanisms of injury, 192–193*t*
Preeclampsia, 446–447
Preexisting medical conditions, burns and, 504
Pregnancy
  abruptio placentae and, 448, 448*f*, 449
  ectopic, 445–446, 446*f*
  emergency care of complications of,
    451–452
  gestational diabetes in, 352
  normal, 444–445
  structure of, 443–444, 443*f*
  trauma and, 449–450, 450*f*
  vaginal bleeding in late, 447–448, 449*f*
Prehospital care report (PCR), 22, 256
  electronic, 257
  elements of, 259–263
  quality management and, 259
  uses of, 67
    administrative uses, 258
    educational and research uses, 258–259
    legal uses, 258
    medical uses, 257–258
Prehospital education, levels of, 11–12, 11*t*
Premature birth, 465
Premature labor, 445
Preparation for possibility of extrication,
  643–644
Preparation phase in emergency medical services
  call, personnel and basic supplies, 624
Preschoolers (4 to 5 years of age), 597–598, 597*f*
  communicating with, 248–249
Prescribed metered-dose inhaler, 287*t*

Presenting part, 453
Pressure bandage, 475, 475*f*
Pressure immobilization technique for coral
  snake bite, 420*f*
Pressure points in controlling external bleeding,
  476–477, 476*f*
Pressure regulators, 175, 175*f*
Pressure splints in controlling external bleeding,
  477, 477*f*
Presyncope, 366
Preterm labor, 445
Primary spontaneous pneumothorax, 579
Primary survey
  in assessing patient with breathing difficulties,
    298–300
  for infant and child, 599–604, 600*f*, 602*f*, 603*f*
    general impression, 600–601
    levels of responsiveness and cervical spine
      protection, 601–604
  performing, 202–212, 203*t*
    airway, 205, 205*f*
    breathing, 208–209, 208*f*
    capillary refill, 210
    cervical spine protection, 207, 207*f*
    circulation, 209–210
    disability, 211, 212*t*
    exposure of patient, 211–212
    general impression, 203–204, 204*f*
    identifying priority patients, 212
    level of responsiveness (mental status),
      205–206, 206*f*
    obvious bleeding, 209
    pulses in, 209–210, 209*f*, 210*f*
    skin color, 210
    skin condition, 210
    skin temperature, 210
  in poisoning, 389–390
  repeating, in ongoing assessment, 233
Priority patients
  factors to consider when identifying, 194*t*
  identifying, 212
  transport of, 218
Professional help, 40
Prolapsed cord, 462–463, 463*f*
Prone position, 72
Proprietary name, 280
Prospective medical direction, 14
Prostate gland, 96
Protected health information (PHI), 57, 65
Protective equipment with hazardous materials,
  653–654, 653*f*, 654*f*
Protocols, 56
Proximal, 71
Proximate cause, 64
Pruritus, 374
PSAP, 11
Psychological crises in behavioral changes and,
  431–435
Psychological maltreatment, 615
Psychomotor seizure, 361
Public access and communications, 10–11
Public education and prevention, 16, 16*t*
Public Safety Answering Point (PSAP), 10, 244
Pulling, guidelines for safe, 125–126
Pulmonary arteries, 320, 321
Pulmonary contusion, 223, 583–584, 583*f*
Pulmonary edema, 326
Pulmonary embolism, 309
  emergency care of, 309
  signs and symptoms of, 309
Pulmonary ventilation, 85
Pulmonic valve, 318
Pulse ox, 113
Pulse oximetry, 113–115, 114*f*
Pulses, 91, 102–104, 322
  brachial, 103, 103*t*, 210*f*, 321, 321*f*
  carotid, 89, 102, 209*f*, 321
  central, 91, 102–103, 322
  dorsalis pedis, 103, 103*t*
  femoral, 102–103, 321*f*, 322
  normal rates at rest, 104*t*
  pedal, 322
  pedis, 322
  peripheral, 91, 103, 103*t*
  posterior tibial, 103, 103*t*
  in primary survey, 209–210, 209*f*, 210*f*

quality of, 104
radial, 103, 103*t*, 213, 321
strong, 104
thready, 104
Puncture wound, 493, 493*f*
Pupils, 108
  abnormal findings, 109*t*
  dilated, 108
  nonreactive, 108
  unequal, 108
Purple cape, 582
Purposeful movement, 221
Pushing, guidelines for safe, 125–126
Putrefaction, 35

Q

Quadriplegia, 550, 550*f*
Quality management, 16
  medical direction and, 341–342
  prehospital care reports and, 259
  role in, 16
Questions
  to ask concerning difficulty in breathing, 301
  direct, 214
  open-ended, 214

R

Raccoon eyes, 222
Radial arteries, 89, 321
Radial pulse, 89, 103, 103*t*, 213, 321
Radiation, 401, 401*f*
Radio
  frequencies and ranges in communications,
    241–242
  mobile two-way, 242–243, 242*f*
  portable, 243, 243*f*
Radius, 77, 519
Rain, effect of, on emergency vehicle, 630–631
Rainbows, 388
Rales, 230
Rapid extrication, 131–133, 132–133*f*, 559
Rapid medical assessment, 213, 219
Rapid trauma assessment, 213
Rash, road, 492
Rattlesnakes, 417, 417*f*, 418*f*
Reaching, guidelines for safe, 125
Reactivity, 108
Reasonable force, 437
Receiving facility
  arrival at, 252, 253*f*
  en route to, 251–252
Record keeping/data collection, 22
Recovery position, 134, 134*f*, 154, 154*f*
Rectum, 94
Red blood cells, 74, 88, 322
Reds, 388
Refresher courses, 25
Refusals, 59–60
  examples of high-risk, 60
Regressions, 31
Rehabilitation services, 15–16
Relaxation techniques, practicing, 39
Remote, hands-free, or hands-off
  defibrillation, 341
Repeater, 241, 243
Reperfusion injury, 491
Reproductive ducts, 96
Reproductive system, 96–97, 96*f*, 97*f*, 98*t*
Rescue breathing, 170
Rescuer assist, 131
Rescuer safety, 187–188, 187*f*, 188*f*
Research uses of prehospital care reports,
  258–259
Resources, additional, in scene size-ups, 196
Respect, treating patient with, 32, 32*f*
Respirations, 85, 104–106
  control of, 297
  counting, 105
Respiratory arrest, 162, 304, 605
  signs and symptoms of, 162
Respiratory depression, 388
Respiratory disorders, 303
  acute pulmonary edema, 309–310